Contemporary Medical Imaging

Series Editor

U. Joseph Schoepf
Department of Radiology and Radiological Science
Medical University of South Carolina
Charleston, SC, USA

The *Contemporary Medical Imaging* series focuses on the most recent developments in imaging technology and their applications in areas such as cardiology, pulmonology, endocrinology, and neurology. Individual volumes present the core principles in diagnosing and treating disorders via modalities such as radiofrequency ablation, angiography, computed tomography, magnetic resonance imaging, positron emission tomography, and hybrid techniques such as PET/CT. Each title is developed by authoritative radiologists who cover the most important topics in this rapidly advancing field.

More information about this series at https://link.springer.com/bookseries/7687

Carlo N. De Cecco • Marly van Assen
Tim Leiner
Editors

Artificial Intelligence in Cardiothoracic Imaging

Humana Press

Editors
Carlo N. De Cecco
Division of Cardiothoracic Imaging
Department of Radiology and Imaging Sciences
Emory University
Atlanta, GA, USA

Marly van Assen
Division of Cardiothoracic Imaging
Department of Radiology and Imaging Sciences
Emory University
Atlanta, GA, USA

Tim Leiner
Department of Radiology
Mayo Clinic
Rochester, MN, USA

ISSN 2626-6431 ISSN 2626-6423 (electronic)
Contemporary Medical Imaging
ISBN 978-3-030-92086-9 ISBN 978-3-030-92087-6 (eBook)
https://doi.org/10.1007/978-3-030-92087-6

This Humana imprint is published by the registered company Springer Nature Switzerland AG
The registered company address is: Gewerbestrasse 11, 6330 Cham, Switzerland

"To Costanza and Matilde Romana, my strength and serenity."
Carlo N. De Cecco

"To Esther, Willemijn, Jasper, Mycroft, and Pieter for all the joy you bring to my life."
Tim Leiner

"To my parents, who taught me how to dream and to always follow them."
Marly van Assen

Preface

What is now proved was once only imagined.

William Blake

Artificial intelligence (AI) is everywhere these days. AI has quietly entered our lives, and we are often using AI algorithms without even noticing it. However, the medical field is quite different from everyday life. AI is entering at a slower pace with more stringent regulations, and more extensive validation and testing is necessary. *Ça va sans dire*, the application of AI to medicine is one of the most exciting areas for those interested in pushing the boundaries to revolutionize healthcare and medical practice.

From opposite sides of the Atlantic Ocean, Tim, Marly, and I have experienced the marvel and frustrations of AI development for medical imaging, and in particular the opportunities, limitations, and concerns when it comes to its clinical implementation. This book was born from our endless discussions about the use of AI technology in cardiothoracic imaging, whether at conferences or in private. Our last in-person discussion was in January 2020 during a conference in Curaçao, in a world before the pandemic. On that occasion, we agreed on the need for a comprehensive manual that introduces the development of AI and its applications to cardiothoracic imaging to the medical community and all the professionals involved in this exciting endeavor.

Shortly after our last meeting, Prof. U. Joseph Schoepf reached out to invite us to be the editors of a volume on AI in cardiothoracic imaging. We seized the opportunity to combine the experience of the best international groups involved in AI development and cardiothoracic imaging in a book that provides a comprehensive picture of this complex and exciting new world that is unfolding right before our eyes. AI technology is rapidly evolving and reaching maturity in many fields, so this is the perfect time to discuss the status of AI in the field of cardiothoracic imaging.

Modern-day medicine has become more advanced and technically complex than ever. This is especially true for the field of cardiothoracic radiology. The field has been propelled forward by hardware improvements made to CT scanners, the development of high-end MRI sequences, and a variety of novel quantitative analysis approaches for all modalities used, which vastly increases the amount of data available for interpretation. The impact of AI can be conceptualized as an additional "layer" of technological development that can be used to optimize the entire imaging pipeline from patient selection, image acquisition, image reconstruction, and image analysis to reporting and derivation of prognostic information. AI applications can be used to help physicians handle this influx of data in their daily clinical routine, in turn improving preventive actions and interventions. However, for these technical advancements to reach their optimal potential, multidisciplinary collaboration is indispensable. AI is here to improve healthcare forever. However, seizing this opportunity and implementing it in clinical practice is a daunting challenge. Even with the development of a perfect clinical AI algorithm, there are social, ethical, and legal considerations that come into play when bringing AI into the clinical arena. Thus, to make AI in cardiothoracic imaging a reality instead of just an opportunity, it will require a strong, multidisciplinary collaboration between physicians, statisticians, mathematicians, data scientists, computer scientists, and ethicists to work together and have a basic understanding of each other's fields. Physicians need to understand not only the possibilities that AI offers but also its limitations and how these would affect their daily practice. Scientists need to understand the unique challenges that AI faces in the medical field, and how the algorithms can be seamlessly implemented in the clinical practice without disrupting the workflow or placing any risk for the patient.

This book is written for everyone interested in AI for cardiothoracic imaging, either from a clinical or technical background, to understand both the opportunities and challenges that lie ahead on the path to clinical implementation. The book is divided into five parts, each discussing different aspects of the use of AI for cardiothoracic imaging. The first part discusses the basic technological consideration and fundamentals of AI. The entire workflow of AI development is discussed including AI algorithm development and optimization, data preparation, performance metrics, and algorithm validation and testing. Part II discusses both the general approaches to AI and its applications covering the entire clinical workflow. General applications in the field of medical imaging is discussed such as standardized reporting, image reconstruction, and contrast medium and radiation dose optimization. In Part III, the chapters focus on cardiac applications for data analysis including coronary calcium scoring, coronary plaque evaluation, CAD-RADS, CT-FFR, and other cardiac flow measurements. Applications for different imaging modalities are outlined. Part IV does the same for thoracic applications such as COPD, COVID-19, and lung cancer, among others. Finally, Part V gives the readers a view on important considerations regarding the use of AI in the medical field and discusses legislation, patenting, ethical concerns, economics, and cybersecurity.

This book has been made possible by the work of many. An astounding number of international experts from both the medical and technical field came together to present the readers with the most up-to-date data. As editors, we are thankful to all the contributors; their commitment in the preparation of the chapters while facing a pandemic is something remarkable and speaks volumes about their dedication. Finally, our gratitude goes to Prof. U. Joseph Schoepf for offering us this opportunity, and to the Springer team, in particular Margaret Moore and Prakash Jagannathan, for the outstanding support during the preparation of the book.

We hope that the material in this book will be of use to all those interested in developing and applying artificial intelligence to cardiothoracic imaging, inspiring them to embrace this opportunity to improve healthcare and benefit our patients.

Atlanta, GA, USA — Carlo N. De Cecco
Rochester, MN, USA — Tim Leiner
Atlanta, GA, USA — Marly van Assen

Contents

Editors and Contributors

About the Editors

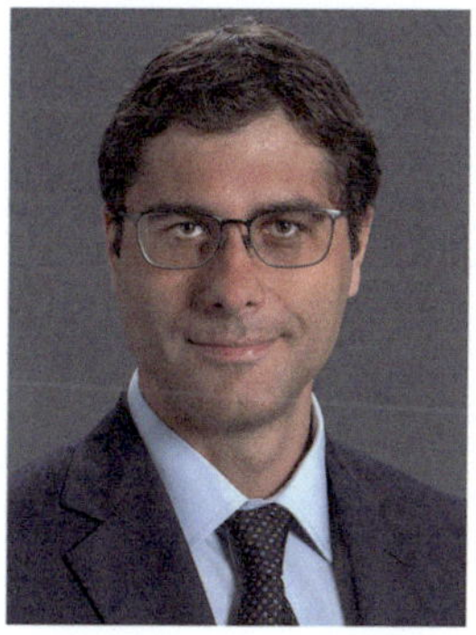

Carlo N. De Cecco MD, PhD, is Associate Professor of Radiology and Biomedical Informatics, and director of the Translational Laboratory for Cardiothoracic Imaging and Artificial Intelligence in the Department of Radiology and Imaging Sciences at Emory University in Atlanta, USA. He is editor of the Springer books *MDCT and MRI of the Heart* (2014) and *Dual Energy CT in Oncology* (2015).

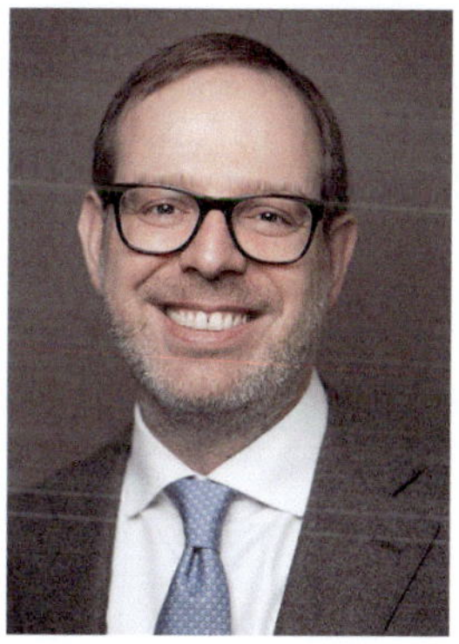

Tim Leiner MD, PhD, is Professor of Radiology at Mayo Clinic, Rochester, USA, MN, and at Utrecht University Medical Center in the Netherlands with a strong interest in development and clinical implementation of AI.

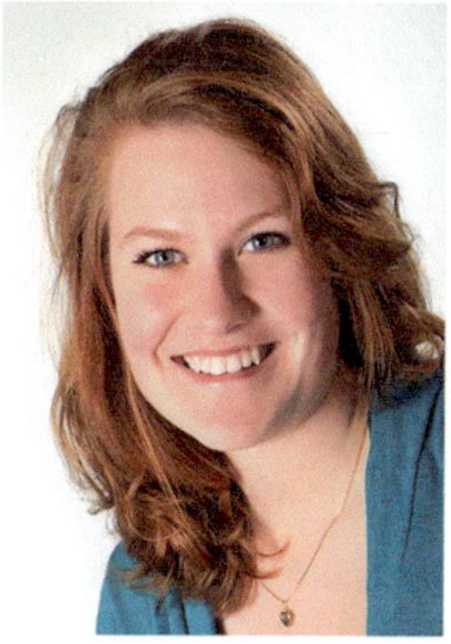

Marly van Assen MSc, PhD, is a postdoctoral fellow and vice-director of the Translational Laboratory for Cardiothoracic Imaging and Artificial Intelligence in the Department of Radiology and Imaging Sciences at Emory University.

Contributors

Musa Abdulkareem, MSc PhD National Institute for Health Research (NIHR) Barts Biomedical Research Centre, William Harvey Research Institute, Queen Mary University of London, London, UK

Barts Heart Centre, St Bartholomew's Hospital, Barts Health National Health Service (NHS) Trust, London, UK

Mehmet Akçakaya, PhD Department of Electrical and Computer Engineering, University of Minnesota, Minneapolis, MN, USA

Center for Magnetic Resonance Research, University of Minnesota, Minneapolis, MN, USA

Subhi J. Al'Aref, MD Division of Cardiology, Department of Medicine, University of Arkansas for Medical Sciences (UAMS), Little Rock, AR, USA

Hatem Alkadhi, MD, MPH Institute of Diagnostic and Interventional Radiology, University Hospital Zurich, Zurich, Switzerland

Mouaz H. Al-Mallah, MD Department of Cardiology, Houston Methodist DeBakey Heart & Vascular Center, Houston, TX, USA

Zaid Almarzooq, MBBCh Brigham and Women's Hospital Heart and Vascular Center, Boston, MA, USA

Nay Aung, PhD National Institute for Health Research (NIHR) Barts Biomedical Research Centre, William Harvey Research Institute, Queen Mary University of London, London, UK

Barts Heart Centre, St Bartholomew's Hospital, Barts Health National Health Service (NHS) Trust, London, UK

Bettina Baessler, MD Institute of Diagnostic and Interventional Radiology, University Hospital Zurich, Zurich, Switzerland

Institute of Diagnostic and Interventional Radiology, University Hospital Würzburg, Würzburg, Germany

Andrea Baggiano, MD Centro Cardiologico Monzino, IRCCS, Milan, Italy

Imon Banerjee, PhD Department of Computer Science, University of Arizona, Tucson, AZ, USA

Department of Biomedical Informatics & Department of Radiology & Imaging Sciences, Emory School of Medicine, Atlanta, GA, USA

Department of Radiology, Mayo Clinic, Phoenix, Arizona, USA

Department of Computer Engineering, SCAI, Arizona State University, Tempe, USA

Dhiraj Baruah, MD Division of Cardiovascular Imaging, Department of Radiology and Radiological Science, Medical University of South Carolina, Charleston, SC, USA

Division of Thoracic Imaging, Department of Radiology and Radiological Science, Medical University of South Carolina, Charleston, SC, USA

Kathrin Bäumler, PhD Department of Radiology, School of Medicine, Stanford University, Stanford, CA, USA

Anton S. Becker, MD, PhD Memorial Sloan Kettering Cancer Center, New York, NY, USA

Yun Bian, MD Department of Radiology, Changhai hospital, Naval medical University, Shanghai, China

Nikolaos Bonaros, MD Department of Cardiac Surgery, Innsbruck Medical University, Innsbruck, Austria

Verena Brandt, MD Division of Cardiovascular Imaging, Department of Radiology and Radiological Science, Medical University of South Carolina, Charleston, SC, USA

Department of Cardiology, Robert-Bosch-Krankenhaus, Stuttgart, Germany

Nynke Breimer, LLM, MBA Global Product Manager Radiology AI & Amplifier Marketplace, Sectra, Linköping, Sweden/Almere, the Netherlands

Jeremy R. Burt, MD Division of Cardiovascular Imaging, Department of Radiology and Radiological Science, Medical University of South Carolina, Charleston, SC, USA

Division of Thoracic Imaging, Department of Radiology and Radiological Science, Medical University of South Carolina, Charleston, SC, USA

Davide Capra, MD Department of Biomedical Sciences for Health, Università degli Studi di Milano, Milan, Italy

Damiano Caruso, MD, PhD Department of Medical Surgical Sciences and Translational Medicine, Sapienza University of Rome - Sant' Andrea University Hospital, Rome, Italy

Federica Catapano, MD Department of Radiological, Oncological and Pathological Sciences, Sapienza University of Rome, Rome, Italy

Claudio Cau, MD Department of Radiology, Azienda Ospedaliero Universitaria (A.O.U.), di Cagliari - Polo di Monserrato, Cagliari, Italy

Riccardo Cau, MD Department of Radiology, Azienda Ospedaliero Universitaria di Cagliari, Cagliari, Italy

Leo Anthony Celi, MD, MS Institute for Medical Engineering and Science, Massachusetts Institute of Technology, Cambridge, MA, USA

Division of Pulmonary, Critical Care and Sleep Medicine, Beth Israel Deaconess Medical Center, Boston, MA, USA

Department of Biostatistics, Harvard T.H. Chan School of Public Health, Boston, MA, USA

Mattia Chiesa, PhD Centro Cardiologico Monzino, IRCCS, Milan, Italy

Teodora Chitiboi, PhD Siemens Healthineers, Princeton, NJ, USA

Marina Codari, MSc, PhD Department of Radiology, School of Medicine, Stanford University, Stanford, CA, USA

Ramon Correa, PhD Student Department of Biomedical Informatics, Emory School of Medicine, Atlanta, GA, USA

Giulia Cundari, MD Department of Radiological, Oncological and Pathological Sciences, Sapienza University of Rome, Rome, Italy

Erfan Darzi, MSc Department of Radiation Oncology and Data Science Center in Health, University Medical Center Groningen, Groningen, The Netherlands

Melissa Davis, MD Department of Radiology & Imaging Sciences, Emory University, Atlanta, GA, USA

Aline L. de Araujo, MD, PhD Segmed, Inc, Menlo Park, CA, USA

Department of Ophthalmology and Visual Sciences, Universidade Federal de São Paulo, São Paulo, Brazil

Jaap de Bruin, MSc Utrecht Health Seed Fund, Utrecht, the Netherlands

Utrecht Holdings, Utrecht University, Utrecht, the Netherlands

Carlo N. De Cecco, MD, PhD Division of Cardiothoracic Imaging, Department of Radiology and Imaging Sciences, Emory University, Atlanta, GA, USA

Josua A. Decker, MD Division of Cardiovascular Imaging, Department of Radiology and Radiological Science, Medical University of South Carolina, Charleston, SC, USA

Department of Diagnostic and Interventional Radiology, University Hospital Augsburg, Augsburg, Germany

Andre Dekker, MSc, PhD Department of Radiation Oncology (MAASTRO), GROW School for Oncology and Developmental Biology, Maastricht University Medical Centre+, Maastricht, The Netherlands

Domenico De Santis, MD Department of Medical Surgical Sciences and Translational Medicine, Sapienza University of Rome - Sant' Andrea University Hospital, Rome, Italy

Bob D. de Vos, PhD Department of Biomedical Engineering and Physics, Amsterdam University Medical Centers – location AMC, University of Amsterdam, Amsterdam, the Netherlands

Amsterdam Cardiovascular Sciences, Amsterdam University Medical Centers, Amsterdam, the Netherlands

Damini Dey, PhD Biomedical Imaging Research Institute, Cedars-Sinai Medical Center, Los Angeles, CA, USA

Matthias Eberhard, MD Institute of Diagnostic and Interventional Radiology, University Hospital Zurich, Zurich, Switzerland

Tilman Emrich, MD Division of Cardiovascular Imaging, Department of Radiology and Radiological Science, Medical University of South Carolina, Charleston, SC, USA

Department of Diagnostic and Interventional Radiology, University Medical Center of the Johannes Gutenberg University Mainz, Mainz, Germany

German Centre for Cardiovascular Research (DZHK), Partner Site Rhine-Main, Mainz, Germany

Antonio Esposito, MD Experimental Imaging Center, IRCCS San Raffaele Scientific Institute, Milan, Italy

School of Medicine, Vita-Salute San Raffaele University, Milan, Italy

Li Fan, MD Department of Radiology, Changzheng Hospital, Naval Medical University, Shanghai, China

Gudrun M. Feuchtner, MD, MBA Department of Radiology, Innsbruck Medical University, Innsbruck, Austria

Peter D. Filev, MD Department of Radiology and Imaging Sciences, Emory University School of Medicine, Atlanta, GA, USA

Dominik Fleischmann, MD Department of Radiology, School of Medicine, Stanford University, Stanford, CA, USA

Cardiovascular Institute, Stanford University, Stanford, CA, USA

Thomas Flohr, PhD Siemens Healthcare GmbH, Computed Tomography, Forchheim, Germany

Marco Francone, MD, PhD, EBCR Department of Biomedical Sciences, Humanitas University, Via Rita Levi Montalcini, Pieve Emanuele (MI), Italy

IRCCS Humanitas Research Hospital, via Manzoni, Rozzano (MI), Italy

Laura Fusini, MD Centro Cardiologico Monzino, IRCCS, Milan, Italy

Alexander Fyrdahl, PhD Department of Radiology, University of Michigan, Ann Arbor, MI, USA

Ernest V. Garcia, PhD Department of Radiology and Imaging Sciences, Emory University School of Medicine, Atlanta, GA, USA

Pablo Garcia-Polo, MSc General Electric Healthcare, Madrid, Spain

Judy Wawira Gichoya, MD, MS Department of Radiology, Emory University, Atlanta, GA, USA

Department of Biomedical Informatics, Emory University, Atlanta, GA, USA

Vicky Goh, MA, MBBChir, MD, MRCP, FRCR Department of Cancer Imaging, School of Biomedical Engineering and Imaging Sciences, King's College London, London, UK

Department of Radiology, Guy's and St Thomas' NHS Foundation Trust, London, UK

Hunter N. Gray, BS Division of Cardiovascular Imaging, Department of Radiology and Radiological Science, Medical University of South Carolina, Charleston, SC, USA

Stefan Großkopf, PhD Siemens Healthcare GmbH, Computed Tomography, Forchheim, Germany

Yu Guan, MM Department of Radiology, Changzheng Hospital, Naval Medical University, Shanghai, China

Andrea I. Guaricci, MD Institute of Cardiovascular Disease, Department of Emergency and Organ Transplantation, University Hospital "Policlinico Consorziale" of Bari, Bari, Italy

Marco Guglielmo, MD Centro Cardiologico Monzino, IRCCS, Milan, Italy

Ralf Gutjahr, PhD Siemens Healthcare GmbH, Computed Tomography, Forchheim, Germany

Lewis Hahn, MD Division of Cardiothoracic Imaging, Department of Radiology, UC San Diego School of Medicine, La Jolla, CA, USA

Jesse I. Hamilton, PhD Department of Radiology, University of Michigan, Ann Arbor, MI, USA

Department of Biomedical Engineering, University of Michigan, Ann Arbor, MI, USA

Kerstin Hammernik, PhD AI in Healthcare and Medicine, Technical University of Munich, Munich, Germany

Department of Computing, Imperial College London, London, UK

Nils Hampe, PhD Department of Biomedical Engineering and Physics, Amsterdam University Medical Centers – location AMC, University of Amsterdam, Amsterdam, the Netherlands

Amsterdam Cardiovascular Sciences, Amsterdam University Medical Centers, Amsterdam, the Netherlands

Cailin Hardell, MS Segmed, Inc, Menlo Park, CA, USA

Kyle Hasenstab, PhD Department of Mathematics and Statistics, San Diego State University, San Diego, CA, USA

Giselle Heleg, LLB Laboratory on Innovation and Artificial Intelligence (IALAB), Faculty of Law, University of Buenos Aires, Buenos Aires, Argentina

Babs M. F. Hendriks, MD Department of Radiology and Nuclear Medicine, Maastricht University Medical Center, Maastricht, The Netherlands

CARIM School for Cardiovascular Diseases, Maastricht University, Maastricht, The Netherlands

Virginia Hinostroza, MSc Department of Radiology, School of Medicine, Stanford University, Stanford, CA, USA

Thomas Wesley Holmes, PhD Department of Radiology and Imaging Sciences and Winship Cancer Institute, Emory University, Atlanta, GA, USA

Carolyn Horst, AB, MA, MBBS, PhD Department of Cancer Imaging, School of Biomedical Engineering and Imaging Sciences, King's College London, London, UK

Department of Radiology, Guy's and St Thomas' NHS Foundation Trust, London, UK

Praveen Indraratna, MBBS Department of Radiology, St. Paul's Hospital, Vancouver, Canada

University of British Columbia, Vancouver, Canada

Ivana Išgum, PhD Department of Biomedical Engineering and Physics, Amsterdam University Medical Centers – location AMC, University of Amsterdam, Amsterdam, the Netherlands

Amsterdam Cardiovascular Sciences, Amsterdam University Medical Centers, Amsterdam, the Netherlands

Department of Radiology and Nuclear Medicine, Amsterdam University Medical Centers – location AMC, University of Amsterdam, Amsterdam, the Netherlands

Martin A. Janich, PhD General Electric Healthcare, Munich, Germany

Muralikrishnan R. Kartha, MHM, MSc, PhD King's Technology Evaluation Centre, School of Biomedical Engineering and Imaging Sciences, King's College London, London, UK

King's Health Economics, Kings College London, London, UK

Jane Ko, MD Department of Radiology, New York University Grossman School of Medicine, New York, NY, USA

Márton Kolossváry, MD, PhD Cardiovascular Imaging Research Center, Massachusetts General Hospital, Boston, MA, USA

Wojciech A. Koszek, MS Segmed, Inc, Menlo Park, CA, USA

Sebastian Kozerke, PhD Institute for Biomedical Engineering, ETH Zurich and University Zurich, Zurich, Switzerland

Andrea Laghi, MD Department of Medical Surgical Sciences and Translational Medicine, Sapienza University of Rome - Sant' Andrea University Hospital, Rome, Italy

Roberta Eufrasia Ledda, MD Scienze Radiologiche, Department of Medicine and Surgery (DiMeC), University of Parma, Parma, Italy

Enzo Maria Le Fevre, PhD Laboratory on Innovation and Artificial Intelligence (IALAB), Faculty of Law, University of Buenos Aires, Buenos Aires, Argentina

Tim Leiner, MD, PhD Department of Radiology, Mayo Clinic, Rochester, MN, USA

Jonathon Leipsic, MD Department of Radiology, St. Paul's Hospital, Vancouver, Canada

University of British Columbia, Vancouver, Canada

Andrew Lin, MBBS, PhD Biomedical Imaging Research Institute, Cedars-Sinai Medical Center, Los Angeles, CA, USA

Shiyuan Liu, MD Department of Radiology, Changzheng Hospital, Naval Medical University, Shanghai, China

Bin Lu, MD Department of Radiology, Fuwai Hospital, State Key Laboratory of Cardiovascular Disease, National Centre for Cardiovascular Diseases, Chinese Academy of Medical Sciences and Peking Union Medical College, Beijing, China

Michele Maddalo, MSc Servizio di Fisica Sanitaria, Azienda Ospedaliera-Universitaria di Parma, Parma, Italy

Abdallah Malkawi, MD Division of Cardiology, Department of Medicine, University of Arkansas for Medical Sciences (UAMS), Little Rock, AR, USA

Livia Marchitelli, MD Department of Radiological, Oncological and Pathological Sciences, Sapienza University of Rome, Rome, Italy

Bibi Martens, MD Department of Radiology and Nuclear Medicine, Maastricht University Medical Center, Maastricht, The Netherlands

CARIM School for Cardiovascular Diseases, Maastricht University, Maastricht, The Netherlands

Domenico Mastrodicasa, MD Department of Radiology, Stanford University School of Medicine, Center for Academic Medicine, Palo Alto, CA, USA

Evan Masutani, CPhil Department of Bioengineering, UC San Diego, La Jolla, CA, USA

Pál Maurovich-Horvat, MD, PhD, MPH MTA-SE Cardiovascular Imaging Research Group, Heart and Vascular Center, Semmelweis University, Budapest, Hungary

Carolyn Meltzer, MD Department of Radiology & Imaging Sciences, Emory University, Atlanta, GA, USA

Casper Mihl, MD, PhD Department of Radiology and Nuclear Medicine, Maastricht University Medical Center, Maastricht, The Netherlands

CARIM School for Cardiovascular Diseases, Maastricht University, Maastricht, The Netherlands

Gianluca Milanese, MD, PhD Scienze Radiologiche, Department of Medicine and Surgery (DiMeC), University of Parma, Parma, Italy

Caterina B. Monti, MD, PhD Department of Biomedical Sciences for Health, Università degli Studi di Milano, Milan, Italy

William Moore, MD Department of Radiology, New York University Grossman School of Medicine, New York, NY, USA

Anirban Mukhopadhyay, PhD Department of Informatics, Technische Universität Darmstadt, Darmstadt, Germany

Emanuele Muscogiuri, MD Division of Cardiothoracic Imaging, Department of Radiology and Imaging Sciences, Emory University, Atlanta, GA, USA

Department of Radiology, Sapienza University of Rome, Rome, Italy

Giuseppe Muscogiuri, MD, PhD Centro Cardiologico Monzino, IRCCS, Milan, Italy

Vivek Muthurangu, MD UCL Centre for Cardiovascular Imaging, University College London, London, UK

Janice Newsome, MD Department of Radiology & Imaging Sciences, Emory University, Atlanta, GA, USA

Robert O'Shea, MB BCh, BAO, MSc Department of Cancer Imaging, School of Biomedical Engineering and Imaging Sciences, King's College London, London, UK

John N. Oshinski, PhD Wallace Coulter Department of Biomedical Engineering, Georgia Institute of Technology and Emory University, Emory University School of Medicine, Atlanta, GA, USA

Department of Radiology and Imaging Sciences, Emory University School of Medicine, Atlanta, GA, USA

Matthijs Oudkerk, MD, PhD, FNASCI, EBCR Faculty of Medical Sciences, University of Groningen, Groningen, The Netherlands

Institute for Diagnostic Accuracy, Groningen, The Netherlands

Anna Palmisano, MD, PhD Experimental Imaging Center, IRCCS San Raffaele Scientific Institute, Milan, Italy

School of Medicine, Vita-Salute San Raffaele University, Milan, Italy

Tiziano Passerini, PhD Siemens Healthineers, Princeton, NJ, USA

Eva S. Peper, PhD Institute for Biomedical Engineering, ETH Zurich and University Zurich, Zurich, Switzerland

Steffen E. Petersen, Msc, MPH, MD, DPhil Barts Heart Centre, St Bartholomew's Hospital, Barts Health National Health Service (NHS) Trust, London, UK

National Institute for Health Research (NIHR) Barts Biomedical Research Centre, William Harvey Research Institute, Queen Mary University of London, London, UK

The Alan Turing Institute, London, UK

Marina Piccinelli, PhD Department of Radiology and Imaging Sciences, Emory University School of Medicine, Atlanta, GA, USA

Fabian Plank, MD, PhD Department of Internal Medicine III and Cardiology, Innsbruck Medical University, Innsbruck, Austria

Tiziano Polidori, MD Department of Medical Surgical Sciences and Translational Medicine, Sapienza University of Rome - Sant' Andrea University Hospital, Rome, Italy

Gianluca Pontone, MD, PhD Centro Cardiologico Monzino, IRCCS, Milan, Italy

Michele Porcu, MD Department of Radiology, Azienda Ospedaliero Universitaria di Cagliari, Cagliari, Italy

Amir Pourmorteza, PhD Department of Radiology and Imaging Sciences and Winship Cancer Institute, Emory University, Atlanta, GA, USA

Department of Biomedical Engineering, Georgia Institute of Technology, Atlanta, GA, USA

Chen Qin, B.Eng, MSc, PhD Institute for Digital Communications, School of Engineering, University of Edinburgh, Edinburgh, UK

Mark G. Rabbat, MD Loyola University of Chicago, Chicago, IL, USA

Edward Hines Jr. VA Hospital, Hines, IL, USA

Jacques Remy, MD Department of Thoracic Imaging, Hospital Calmette, University Lille, CHU Lille, Lille, France

Martine Remy-Jardin, MD, PhD Department of Thoracic Imaging, Hospital Calmette, University Lille, CHU Lille, Lille, France

Yael Rodriguez-Guadarrama, BEng, MSc Wellcome EPSRC Centre for Medical Engineering, School of Biomedical Engineering and Imaging Sciences, King's College London, London, UK

King's Technology Evaluation Centre, School of Biomedical Engineering and Imaging Sciences, King's College London, London, UK

Department of Primary Care and Population Health, Faculty of Population Health Sciences, University College London, London, UK

Tiago Rua, MSc, PhD Covid-19 Vaccination Programme, Guy's and St Thomas' NHS Foundation Trust, London, UK

King's Health Economics, Kings College London, London, UK

Daniel Rueckert, PhD Department of Computing, Imperial College London, London, UK

Klinikum rechts der Isar, Technical University of Munich, Munich, Germany

Luca Saba, MD Department of Radiology, Azienda Ospedaliero Universitaria di Cagliari, Cagliari, Italy

Nabile Safdar, MD Department of Radiology, Emory University, Atlanta, GA, USA

Thiago Santos, MS Department of Computer Science, Emory University, Atlanta, GA, USA

Francesco Sardanelli, MD Department of Biomedical Sciences for Health, Università degli Studi di Milano, Milan, Italy

Unit of Radiology, IRCCS Policlinico San Donato, San Donato Milanese, Milan, Italy

Max Schöbinger, PhD Siemens Healthcare GmbH, Computed Tomography, Forchheim, Germany

U. Joseph Schoepf, MD Division of Cardiovascular Imaging, Department of Radiology and Radiological Science, Medical University of South Carolina, Charleston, SC, USA

Chris Schwemmer, MS Siemens Healthcare GmbH, Computed Tomography, Forchheim, Germany

Francesco Secchi, MD, PhD Department of Biomedical Sciences for Health, Università degli Studi di Milano, Milan, Italy

Unit of Radiology, IRCCS Policlinico San Donato, San Donato Milanese, Milan, Italy

Aurelio Secinaro, MD Advanced Cardiovascular Imaging Unit, Department of Imaging, Bambino Gesù Children's Hospital, IRCCS, Rome, Italy

Karthik Seetharam, MD West Virginia University Medicine Heart & Vascular Institute, Morgantown, WV, USA

Nicole Seiberlich, PhD Department of Radiology, University of Michigan, Ann Arbor, MI, USA

Department of Biomedical Engineering, University of Michigan, Ann Arbor, MI, USA

Partho P. Sengupta, MD, DM West Virginia University Medicine Heart & Vascular Institute, Morgantown, WV, USA

Rutgers Robert Wood Johnson Medical School, Rutgers University, New Jersey, NJ, USA

Jun Shi, PhD School of Communication and Information Engineering, Shanghai University, Shanghai, China

Nannan Shi, MM Department of Radiology, Shanghai Public Health Clinical Center, Fudan University, Shanghai, China

Yuxin Shi, MD Department of Radiology, Shanghai Public Health Clinical Center, Fudan University, Shanghai, China

Mario Silva, MD, PhD Scienze Radiologiche, Department of Medicine and Surgery (DiMeC), University of Parma, Parma, Italy

Piotr J. Slomka, PhD Artificial Intelligence in Medicine Program, Cedars-Sinai Medical Center, Los Angeles, CA, USA

Nikos Sourlos, MSc Department of Radiology, University of Medical Center Groningen/ University of Groningen, Groningen, Netherlands

Jennifer A. Steeden, PhD UCL Centre for Cardiovascular Imaging, University College London, London, UK

Arthur E. Stillman, MD, PhD Department of Radiology and Imaging Sciences, Emory University School of Medicine, Atlanta, GA, USA

Michael Sühling, PhD Siemens Healthcare GmbH, Computed Tomography, Forchheim, Germany

Jasjit S. Suri, PhD, MBA, FIEEE, FAIMBE, FAIUM Stroke Monitoring and Diagnostic Division, AtheroPoint™, Roseville, CA, USA

Nicola Sverzellati, MD, PhD Scienze Radiologiche, Department of Medicine and Surgery (DiMeC), University of Parma, Parma, Italy

Yasasvi Tadavarthi, MD Department of Radiology, Washington University in St. Louis, St. Louis, MO, USA

Qian Tao, PhD Department of Imaging Physics, Delft University of Technology, Delft, The Netherlands

Department of Radiology, Leiden University Medical Center, Leiden, The Netherlands

Amara Tariq, PhD Department of Radiology, Mayo Clinic, Phoenix, Arizona, USA

Christian Tesche, MD Division of Cardiovascular Imaging, Department of Radiology and Radiological Science, Medical University of South Carolina, Charleston, SC, USA

Department of Cardiology, Robert-Bosch-Krankenhaus, Stuttgart, Germany

Department of Cardiology, Munich University Clinic, Ludwig-Maximilians-University, Munich, Germany

Department of Internal Medicine, St. Johannes-Hospital, Dortmund, Germany

Giovanni Tessarin, MD Division of Cardiothoracic Imaging, Department of Radiology and Imaging Sciences, Emory University, Atlanta, GA, USA

Department of Radiology, University of Padua, Padua, Italy

Hari Trivedi, MD Department of Radiology, Emory University, Atlanta, GA, USA

Department of Biomedical Informatics, Emory University, Atlanta, GA, USA

Valery L. Turner, MD Department of Radiology, School of Medicine, Stanford University, Stanford, CA, USA

Wenting Tu, MM Department of Radiology, Changzheng Hospital, Naval Medical University, Shanghai, China

Ijeoma Uchegbu, MPharmS, MSc National Institute for Health Research (NIHR) Barts Biomedical Research Centre, William Harvey Research Institute, Queen Mary University of London, London, UK

Barts Heart Centre, St Bartholomew's Hospital, Barts Health National Health Service (NHS) Trust, London, UK

Leonardus B. van den Oever, MSc Department of Radiation Oncology and Data Science Center in Health, University Medical Center Groningen, Groningen, The Netherlands

Rob J. van der Geest, PhD Department of Radiology, Leiden University Medical Center, Leiden, The Netherlands

Marly van Assen, MSc, PhD Division of Cardiothoracic Imaging, Department of Radiology and Imaging Sciences, Emory University, Atlanta, GA, USA

Peter M. A. van Ooijen, MSc, Phd, CPHIMS Department of Radiation Oncology and Data Science Center in Health, University Medical Center Groningen, Groningen, The Netherlands

Pim van Ooij, PhD Department of Radiology & Nuclear Medicine, Amsterdam University Medical Centers, Location AMC, Amsterdam, The Netherlands

Department of Pediatric Cardiology, Wilhelmina Children's Hospital, University Medical Center Utrecht, Utrecht, The Netherlands

Sanne G. M. van Velzen, PhD Department of Biomedical Engineering and Physics, Amsterdam University Medical Centers – location AMC, University of Amsterdam, Amsterdam, the Netherlands

Amsterdam Cardiovascular Sciences, Amsterdam University Medical Centers, Amsterdam, the Netherlands

Akos Varga-Szemes, MD, PhD Division of Cardiovascular Imaging, Department of Radiology and Radiological Science, Medical University of South Carolina, Charleston, SC, USA

Holger Veenhuis, Dipl.-Phys., Dr. rer. nat. Eisenführ Speiser, Bremen, Germany

Bremen University, Bremen, Germany

Davide Vignale, MD Experimental Imaging Center, IRCCS San Raffaele Scientific Institute, Milan, Italy

School of Medicine, Vita-Salute San Raffaele University, Milan, Italy

Rozemarijn Vliegenthart, MD, PhD Department of Radiology, University of Medical Center Groningen/University of Groningen, Groningen, Netherlands

Lance A. Waller, BS, PhD Department of Biostatistics and Bioinformatics, Rollins School of Public Health, Emory University, Atlanta, GA, USA

Thomas Weikert, PhD Department of Radiology, University Hospital Basel, University of Basel, Basel, Switzerland

Jack Wessell, BS College of Arts and Sciences, Emory University, Atlanta, GA, USA

Joachim E. Wildberger, MD, PhD Department of Radiology and Nuclear Medicine, Maastricht University Medical Center, Maastricht, The Netherlands

CARIM School for Cardiovascular Diseases, Maastricht University, Maastricht, The Netherlands

Martin J. Willemink, MD, PhD Segmed, Inc, Menlo Park, CA, USA

Department of Radiology, Stanford University School of Medicine, Stanford, CA, USA

Andreas Wimmer, PhD Siemens Healthcare GmbH, Computed Tomography, Forchheim, Germany

Jelmer M. Wolterink, PhD Department of Applied Mathematics, Technical Medical Centre, University of Twente, Enschede, Netherlands

Jie Wu, PhD Segmed, Inc, Menlo Park, CA, USA

Yitong Yang, BS Wallace Coulter Department of Biomedical Engineering, Georgia Institute of Technology and Emory University, Emory University School of Medicine, Atlanta, GA, USA

Marta Zerunian, MD Department of Medical Surgical Sciences and Translational Medicine, Sapienza University of Rome - Sant' Andrea University Hospital, Rome, Italy

Jie Zhang, PhD Department of Radiology, Fuwai Hospital, State Key Laboratory of Cardiovascular Disease, National Centre for Cardiovascular Diseases, Chinese Academy of Medical Sciences and Peking Union Medical College, Beijing, China

Sunyi Zheng, MSc Department of Radiation Oncology, University Medical Center Groningen/ University of Groningen, Groningen, The Netherlands

Xiuxiu Zhou, MM Department of Radiology, Changzheng Hospital, Naval Medical University, Shanghai, China

Vitalijs Zujs, MD Department of Cardiac Surgery, Innsbruck Medical University, Innsbruck, Austria

Part I

Artificial Intelligence: Technical Considerations and Fundamentals

Artificial Intelligence: A Century-Old Story

1

Marly van Assen, Emanuele Muscogiuri, Giovanni Tessarin, and Carlo N. De Cecco

Introduction

Artificial intelligence (AI) is one of the fastest expanding fields of informatics. However, AI is not a new invention by any means with a history dating back almost 100 years ago. Over the past three quarters of a century, the field of AI went through several highs and lows. This chapter describes a brief history of the main accomplishments that led AI to the technology, as we know it today. Figure 1.1 shows a schematic timeline of the events discussed in this chapter.

First Half of the Twentieth Century: The Birth of AI

During the first half of the twentieth century, the concept of a machine capable of learning in similar ways as humans started to be considered, as a result of the replacement of mechanics with electronics [1, 2].

The father of artificial intelligence (AI), as considered by many, is Alan M. Turing, a British mathematician, born in London in 1912, known also for his work in deciphering the Enigma code, used by Germans during World War II to encrypt their military communications [3]. In 1936, Turing introduced the concept of the Turing Machine, an abstract computing device, capable of computing any effectively calculable function [4, 5].

In 1948, Turing wrote a report titled "Intelligent Machinery," which is now considered as the first AI manifesto. This manifest also introduced the "imitation game," later discussed in more detail in his most famous paper "Computing machinery and intelligence," published in October 1950. This "imitation game" formed the basis of what is now known as the Turing test [6]. In this theory, Turing raised the question whether machines are capable of playing the aforementioned imitation game, which is to imitate a human in a way that an interrogator cannot detect the difference between a human and a machine. He suggested that in order to make a machine pass for a human, it would be important to make it learn in a similar way as the brain of children; see Fig. 1.2. In addition, he also stated that only true artificial intelligence would be able to pass the "Turing test," and from then on, the Turing test became a yardstick to measure the intelligence of AI algorithms [7, 8]. It was used to test the earliest chatbots, for example, ELIZA and PARRY, in the late 1960s and early 1970s. However, it would take almost 60 years for the first machine to pass the test. In 2014, a chatbot named Eugene Goostman, posing as a 13-year-old Ukrainian boy, earned the title of the first machine to pass the Turing test by convincing a third of the judges he spoke to that he was human.

Another algorithm that was claimed to have passed the Turing test was Google Duplex, presented in 2016, that was able to fool a hairdresser during a call. However, one could ask whether these algorithms used deception as a strategy to fool the interrogator to hide the lack of real intelligence [9, 10]. In addition, questions were raised whether the Turing test is able to test true AI or if it is to focus on mimicking human behavior. With the increased variety of applications for which AI is used, the Turing test's practicality came into question, since not all AI systems use natural language processing (NLP).

M. van Assen, MSc, PhD · C. N. De Cecco, MD, PhD (✉)
Division of Cardiothoracic Imaging, Department of Radiology and Imaging Sciences, Emory University, Atlanta, GA, USA
e-mail: carlo.dececco@emory.edu

E. Muscogiuri, MD
Division of Cardiothoracic Imaging, Department of Radiology and Imaging Sciences, Emory University, Atlanta, GA, USA

Department of Radiology, Sapienza University of Rome, Rome, Italy

G. Tessarin, MD
Division of Cardiothoracic Imaging, Department of Radiology and Imaging Sciences, Emory University, Atlanta, GA, USA

Department of Radiology, University of Padua, Padua, Italy

C. N. De Cecco et al. (eds.), *Artificial Intelligence in Cardiothoracic Imaging*, Contemporary Medical Imaging,
https://doi.org/10.1007/978-3-030-92087-6_1

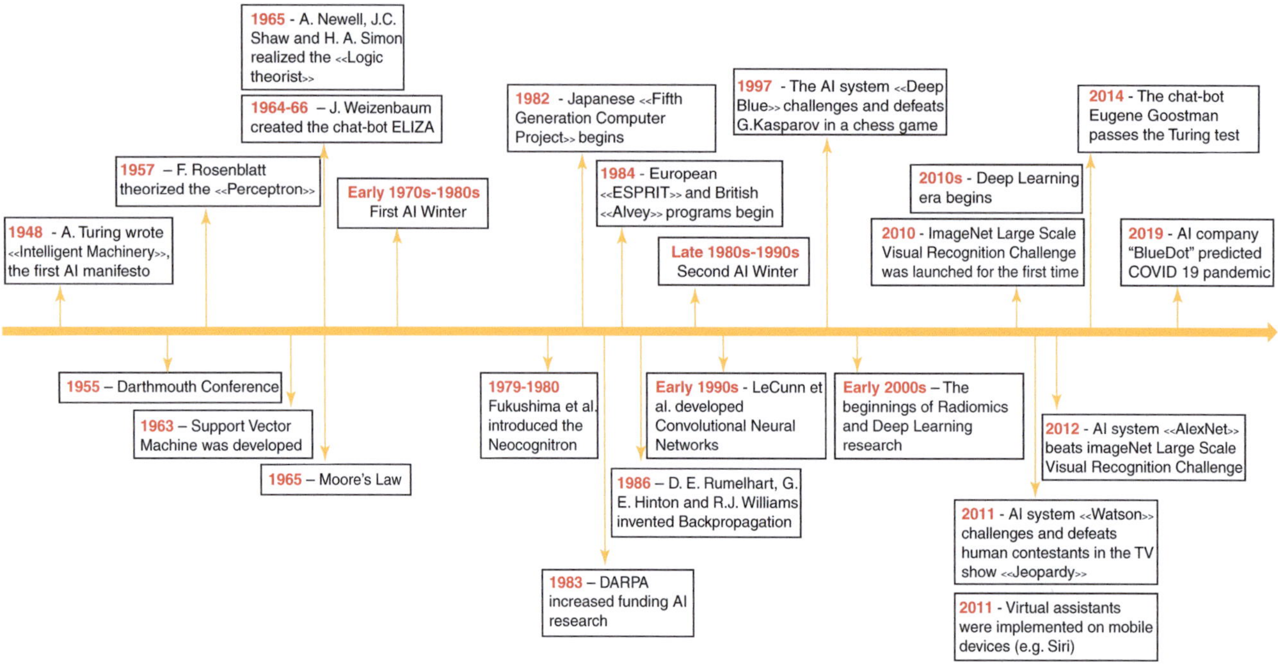

Fig. 1.1 Timeline of main events propelling AI forward to reach the current status

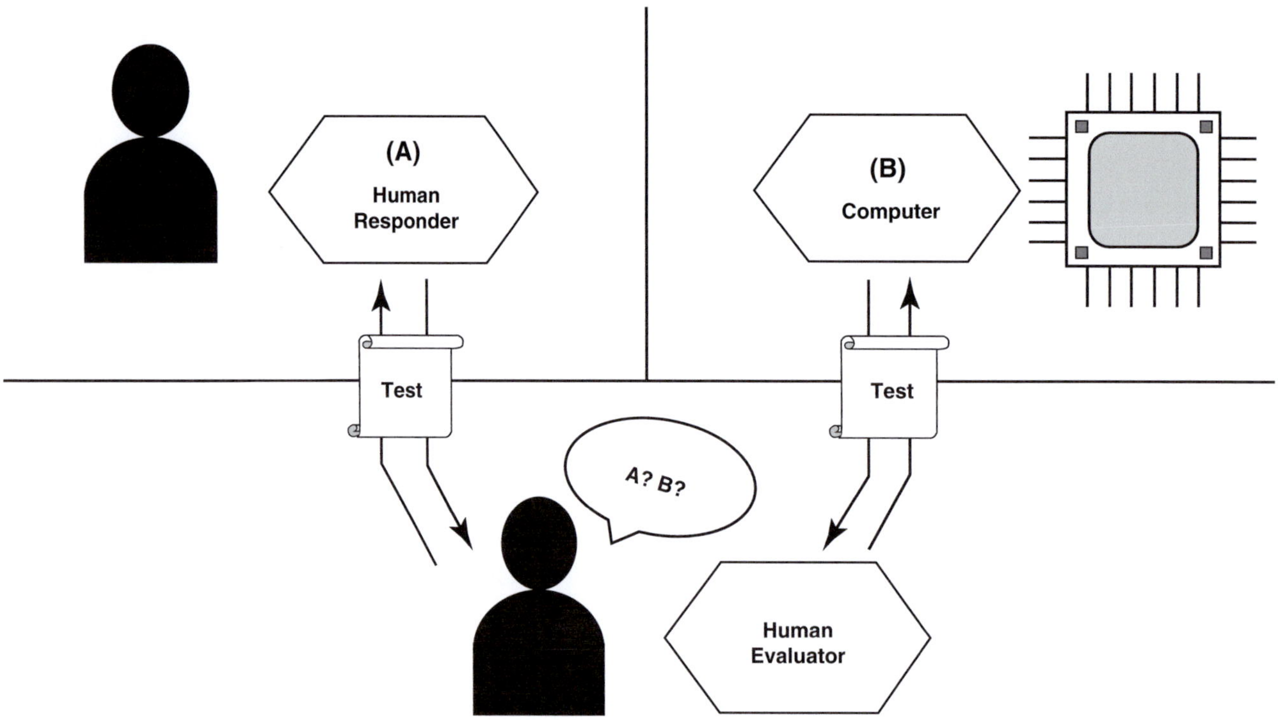

Fig. 1.2 Stylized representation of the Turing test. This test setting is composed by three terminals, each of which is physically separated by the other. One terminal is operated by a computer, while the remaining two are operated by humans. A human evaluator provides test questions to the human responder (A) and the computer (B). If the evaluator is not able to discern between A and B, based upon the answers received from both the contestants, the computer showed reasoning abilities similar to those of humans and it has passed the test. (Image of Alan Turing, considered the father of AI)

Another important milestone that deserves mention is that of McCulloch and Pitts in 1943. Based on the concepts of Turing's first works, their paper titled "A logical calculus of the ideas immanent in nervous activity" proposed a model (MCP from McCulloch and Pitts) to explain the functioning of neural networks in the human brain. It was one of the first attempts to describe biological systems using logical calculus, taking one step toward the goal of finding similarities between animals and logic. This type of model proved to be able to recognize sophisticated patterns; however, it does not explain where information is stored and how the learning process exactly works. McCulloch and Pitts's work is considered to be one of the pillars of both the design of digital computers and neural network(NN) algorithms, currently very popular in the field of AI and radiology [1, 5, 11–14].

The Dartmouth Conference

In 1955, several years after Alan Turing's landmark paper, John McCarthy from Dartmouth, Marvin Minsky from Harvard, Nathaniel Rochester from the IBM Corporation, and Claude E. Shannon from Bell Telephone Laboratories proposed a conference to be held at Dartmouth College in New Hampshire. The goal of this meeting was to gather a select group of scientists to work together for 2 months in order to make significant advances in the field of AI [15]. The so-called Dartmouth Summer Research Project on Artificial Intelligence (DSRPAI), funded by the Rockefeller Foundation, took place in the summer of 1956. This conference was the first time the term "artificial intelligence" made its appearance, proposed by McCarthy himself, to call the science of making intelligent machines [1, 3, 16, 17]. Scientists at the Dartmouth Conference were well aware of the technical limitations of computer memory capacity and speed at the time. However, they believed that with joint efforts, the field of AI could make great progress [15]. After the Dartmouth Conference, specialized centers for AI development such as those at Carnegie Mellon University, the Massachusetts Institute of Technology (MIT), and Stanford University started to grow [18].

The AI Golden Age: The 1960s

In the following years, until the mid-1970s, the field of AI made great advancements, and this is considered a prosperous period. In 1965, A. Newell and J. C. Shaw from the RAND Corporation and H. A. Simon from the Carnegie Institute of Technology realized the Logic Theorist (LT), a program to find proof to theorems, using not just "brute force" but also a heuristic process, in a way similar to the human mind [19, 20]. A more complex program and successor of the LT, the General Problem Solver (GPS), was produced by the same scientists and used means-end analysis as a heuristic system to solve problems difficult for humans [3, 21–23]. The novelty of this approach lay in the fact that until that moment programs were able to prove theorems and solve single tasks such as writing music and playing chess whereas the GPS was the first time a computer program in theory was not limited to a single specific task [21]. This program nevertheless gained some critiques. It was argued that the capabilities of the GPS were limited to the field of riddles and games [24]. In 1967, the limits of the program became clear: the program itself simply occupied too much space in the computer memory, and there was not enough memory left to store data generated during the problem-solving process of elaborate problems. For this reason, the project was discontinued [25, 26].

Where these projects focused specifically on problem-solving, other scientists focused on realizing software capable of interaction with humans. Between 1964 and 1966, Joseph Weizenbaum, a professor of mathematics at MIT, created a computer program called ELIZA that was able to hold a conversation with a human being, often deceiving the user into believing that he was talking to a real person [3]. The first script of this program was called DOCTOR and imitated a psychotherapist [27, 28]. Weizenbaum believed that one of the main goals of AI was deception, the illusion of intelligence, rather than the ability to reach intelligence itself [27, 29].

Most of the progress was made in the field of "symbolic AI" or classic AI, as opposed to another field of AI called "connectionism." The former approach is based on the belief that intelligence could be reached through the use and manipulation of symbols and through explicit rules that explain the relationship between these symbols. Connectionism, on the other hand, aims to replicate the complexity of human mind with the creation of small single processing elements connected to one another, like neurons in the brain, the so-called Artificial Neural Networks (ANN). In this second approach, knowledge resides not in symbols but rather in the strength of the connection between single units [30–32].

In 1957, Frank Rosenblatt, a research psychologist at Cornell Aeronautical Laboratory, contributed to the field of connectionism by proposing the Perceptron, a single-layer model explaining brain function; see Fig. 1.3. Rosenblatt tried to overcome the limits of the MCP model and proposed a neural network capable of information storing and, more importantly, learning and improving. The idea was that

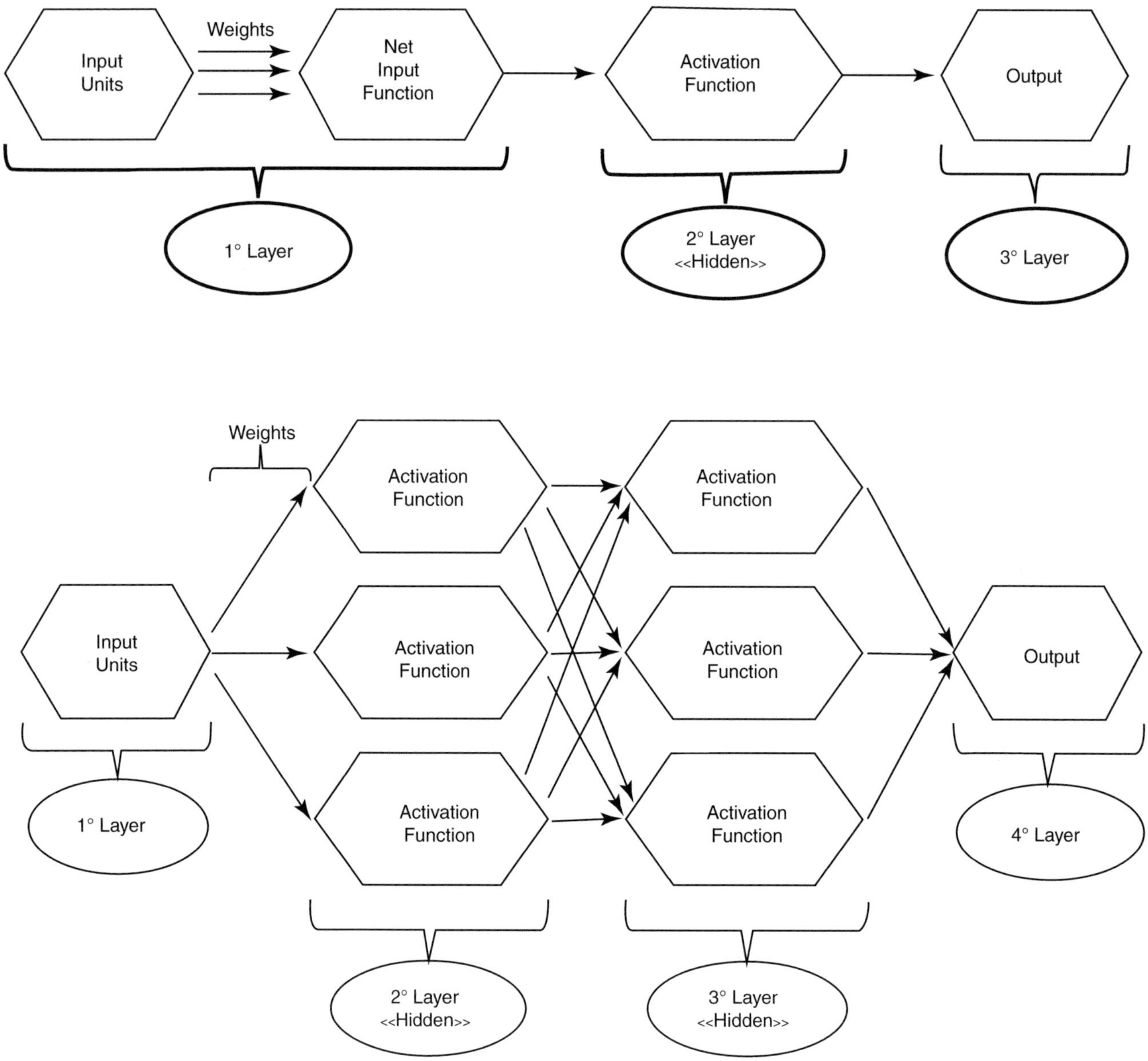

Fig. 1.3 Top image: Schematic diagram representing the Perceptron, the first neural network prototype. Bottom image: Schematic diagram representing the multilayer Perceptron (MLP), the evolution of the Perceptron. As it is possible to notice, this system appears to be more complex than the top figure network, featuring two or more interconnected hidden layers

information was stored as connections between neurons rather than accumulated in a specific location. The goal was to minimize the error made by the algorithm, by simply trying to lower the difference between the obtained and the expected output, using a so-called cost function. Moreover, Rosenblatt's Perceptron was a system that relied on external training; laying the basis for future supervised and unsupervised training approaches. Rosenblatt was also able to turn his theories into a real program for IBM, called Mark I [13, 33–39].

During this period, there was faith in the capabilities and possibilities of AI resulting in many developments and funding opportunities. Marvin Minsky, also from MIT and one of the pioneers of the field, stated in 1970 that within 3–8 years, a machine with capabilities similar to an average human being would be invented [3].

Nevertheless, there were great technological limitations at the time, especially with regard to computational power. Early neural networks were based on analog computers that were inconveniently large, reaching the dimension of a whole laboratory room for the Mark I Perceptron. As stated by Gordon Moore in 1965, the number of components per integrated circuit on a chip, an indication of computational power, will double every year or every other year for at least another decade; this statement is known as "Moore's law." This increase in chip content would be at the basis of many other innovations and advances in technology, such as smartphones, laptops, and GPS. It has also contributed to today's breakthroughs in AI by enabling machine-learning algorithms to assess and use massive amounts of data.

AI's First Winter: The 1970s

The initial limitations of AI started to surface in 1968, when Minsky and Papert published a book titled "Perceptrons: An Introduction to Computational Geometry." In this book, they described the limitations of the Perceptron models proposed by Rosenblatt 10 years earlier. The major limitation was that Perceptrons were single-layer ANNs because at that time, there was no efficient way to train multiple layer ANNs. These single-layer ANNs were not even able to perform simple tasks. The learning process for a single-layer ANN was time-consuming, and computational power was insufficient at the time to carry on the large simulations required [14, 40, 41]. This limitation caused the scientific community to progressively lose interest in the development of ANNs for the next 15 years [40, 42]. The real setback in AI development came in the early 1970s when James Lighthill, a British mathematician, was commissioned by the chair of the British Science Research Council (SRC), Brian Flowers, to file a report on the state of AI in the UK. The request came with the intent to evaluate the expenses of SRC, one of the main contributors of AI development and research in the UK [43]. Lighthill submitted his report in 1972 and divided the field of AI in three categories: the first dealing with automatization (category A), the second one interested in the field of central nervous system-inspired research (category C), and the last one aimed to bridge together the former two, building robots (category B). Lighthill stated that while categories A and B had clear aims and thrived, category B failed to fulfill its expectation. He also highlighted a well-known problem called "combinatory explosion." Extending AI solutions found for toy problems to real-world problems would led to complex operations beyond the possibilities of current hardware [44]. Following the publication of this report in 1973, the British SRC lost faith in the capabilities of AI and started to reduce funding. In the same period, also US Advanced Research Projects Agency (ARPA), later renamed the Defense Advanced Research Projects Agency (DARPA), reduced funding for AI in the USA [45, 46]. The lack of investments started what would become known as the first AI winter [3].

The Way Out: The 1980s

A decade later, several initiatives changed this negative view on AI. In 1982, Japan's Ministry of International Trade and Industry together with eight Japanese electronics manufacturers formed the Institute for New Generation Computer Technology. They started a 10-year project called the Fifth Generation Computer Project with its main aim to make progress in the field of computer architecture and capabilities and subsequently in the field of AI [47]. Following Japan's example and seeing the Fifth Generation Computer Project as a threat to their primate on AI research, the USA, mainly DARPA, progressively increased the annual funding for AI, starting from 1983, reaching $400 million in 1988. Europe and the UK also tried to keep up with the progressively increasing funding. The European ESPRIT and UK Alvey programs began in 1984 with annual AI expenditures of over $200 million [45]. Because of the lost faith in connectionism, the rise of AI was first driven by symbolic AI. These major economical efforts led to the development and diffusion of expert systems. The idea behind expert systems is to transfer specific knowledge into a computer program and, subsequently, to use that program to solve specific issues, such as making a medical diagnosis or predicting structure of chemical compounds [48–52]. The first achievements in this field date back to 1965 with the initial results produced by Feigenbaum and his program DENDRAL, a set of programs developed at Stanford University with an application in the field of chemistry [53]. DENDRAL was followed by MYCIN in the early 1970s, also developed at Stanford University, and used for medical diagnosis [48]. However, it was only in the 1980s that expert systems became widely successful. One of the most successful expert systems built was XCON, designed by Digital Equipment Corporation to help in the configuration of PDP (Programmable Data Processor) and VAX (Virtual Address eXtension) computers. Before the implementation of XCON, configuring a VAX for a costumer was a very complex task, since every component from the software to the cables must be ordered separately and it was not unusual for a costumer to receive the wrong configuration, leading to costumer dissatisfaction. XCON helped the sales department in configuration of the correct VAX set up to costumer's needs. Between 1980 and 1985, this expert system already yielded 15 million dollars in savings [54].

The first Very Large-Scale Integration (VLSI) computer with more computational power and more storage capability was designed in the 1980s. It was made possible by the higher density of transistors per chip. The von Neumann model of computers, based on separation between memory and central processing unit, began to show its limitation, mainly in the speed of computation. This piqued the interest in different types of computers and computing approaches, such as parallel computing, which used multiple processors simultaneously. The increase in computer power and speed sparked a renewed interest in ANN development. With the problem of computing power solved, the limiting factor of the multilayer ANN was that there was still no efficient way to train them. The issue with such complex neural network was that for a neural network to be properly trained, one has to know the derivatives of the errors made by the algorithm in order to adjust the weights of the connections between layers. As long as there are only an input layer and an output layer, the process is simple and the expected results can be compared directly with the obtained result of the output layer. However, adding multiple layers makes this task more complicated, and for years, researchers tried to find an efficient way to adjust the weights within the multiple layers [40].

The first step forward was made by Ackley et al. in 1985, with the creation of the Boltzmann algorithm. Even though this algorithm was not very efficient and was still time-consuming, this method brought researchers one step closer [40, 55]. In 1986, a real game changer for AI came with the invention of backpropagation by D. E. Rumelhart, G. E. Hinton, and R. J. Williams. Backpropagation offers an efficient approach to train and optimize multilayer ANNs. It calculates the derivatives by simply going backward from the output to the hidden layers. The process of minimizing the errors (the cost function) is subsequently completed with the mathematical function called gradient descent [41, 56–59]. Rumelhart, Hinton, and Williams were not the sole inventors of this learning procedure, and it is important to mention other figures that independently came to similar conclusions. Paul Werbos, a Harvard social scientist, developed a technique called dynamic forward in the 1970s. Although similar in principle to that of backpropagation, it was never applied to AI. With the invention of backpropagation, it finally became possible to train and optimize multilayer neural networks in a more time- and computational efficient way.

Back to Reality: The 1990s

As time went by, expert systems showed their limitations. They were limited in their field of applications and were unable to perform complex tasks. In 1984, Mc Carty wrote a paper highlighting some other limitations of expert systems such as the lack in common sense, the inability to learn from their own experience, and the need of continuous updates. With time, it became clear that expert systems were expensive and difficult to maintain [17, 40, 60]. Backpropagation came with some inherent problems too. With the limited computational power available at the time, the learning process was still too time-consuming, especially when the cost function presented deep depressions, called ravines, where small changes in the weights produce big changes in the cost function. Therefore, backpropagation was still limited in its use to simple neural networks in which there were only a few weights to adjust [59, 61–64]. All of these problems together made researchers concentrate on the development of support vector machine (SVM), a simpler algorithm for supervised learning, first invented in 1963 and then refined in 1992. SVMs are one of the most robust types of AI algorithms, being based on statistical learning frameworks. Faith and funding on AI and especially neural networks once again fell, leading to a new AI winter [1, 17, 45].

The Game Changers: Big Data and High Performance Computing

Another important change of paradigm has occurred in the last two decades, mainly due to two major improvements. First, there is much more data to work with in the current era of "big data." For an AI algorithm, in order to be accurate, large quantities of data are needed [46]. Second, computers are finally becoming powerful enough to optimize multilayer neural networks and other AI algorithms used for tasks that are more complex. The increase in computational power and later the implementation of graphics processing units (GPU) were the answer to the need of high performance computing [65–68]. The first signs that something was changing came again from the field of expert systems in 1997 when an artificial intelligence chess playing computer called Deep Blue, developed by IBM, challenged Garry Kasparov, the world champion at that time. At the end of the sixth game, Deep Blue defeated Garry Kasparov for the first time in history. This was a great achievement for the AI community [69–71]. As for ANNs, interest started to rise again in the 1990s with the introduction of a particular type of neural network by LeCun et al. called Convolutional Neural Network (CNN). The specialty of these networks is extracting and recognizing features and pattern in images, thanks to the use of particular filters. This characteristic made CNNs particularly helpful in tasks such as speech recognition, document reading, and, later, face recognition. The use of CNNs grew progressively over time [58, 72, 73]. In 2011, AI reached another important milestone, when Watson, a program invented by IBM based on a DeepQA architecture, was able to defeat two champions in the quiz game called Jeopardy by using natural language processing (NLP) and ML algorithms [74]. Since that time, we have seen AI applications enter everyday life, for example, with the implementation of virtual assistants starting in 2011 with Siri by Apple, followed by Microsoft's Cortana, Amazon's Alexa, and finally Google Assistant [46, 75].

The increased interest in AI combined with the increase in data and computing power availability has led to the advancement of AI into the use of deep learning algorithms. In 2000, this term was first associated with the concept of ANNs by Aizenberg and collegues [76]. Deep learning (DL) is one of the fastest expanding branches of AI. DL distinguishes itself from other AI fields by skipping the manual process of feature extraction and directly uses data or images to evaluate patterns and solve the tasks at hand. This process takes full advantage of multiple layers in ANNs, extracting more complex and abstract features in deeper layers of the network, hence the term deep learning [77, 78]. A milestone of deep learning was reached in 2010, when the ImageNet Large Scale Visual Recognition Challenge was launched. The dataset (ImageNet) and algorithms created for this challenge are still considered the benchmark for object classification and detection. In 2012, AlexNet was developed by Alex Krizhevsky (a former student of Geoffrey Hinton) and colleagues for this challenge. With an error rate of 15.3%, they won the challenge. In 2014, the GoogLeNet algorithm reached an error rate dropped to 6.67%, and in 2015, a Microsoft team based in Beijing reached an even lower error rate of 3.57% with ResNet [79–83]. These algorithms are still frequently used as basis for AI development for image-related tasks.

AI in Medicine

AI is being rapidly integrated into many fields, including medicine. The use of AI in the field of medicine has been steadily growing, especially in research settings. However, many steps are yet to be taken for AI to be widely accepted and implemented in clinical practice. AI offers the opportunity to shift toward a model of medicine that is tailored to the individual (personalized medicine) [17, 84]. Moreover, AI can provide models that can be used for multiple purposes. For example, it can optimize the diagnostic process, assess therapy response and thus prognostic evaluation, or even set up prevention programs [17]. Furthermore, AI has the potential to automate several tasks, commonly performed by medical professionals, therefore increasing efficiency and simultaneously reducing the workload, potentially reducing the costs of healthcare [17].

Early AI Systems: Rule-Based Expert Models

In the early 1970s, research focused on the creation of AI-based computational systems aimed to assist clinical decision-making. The first of these systems mimicked human reasoning by performing a deduction process to diagnose a variety of diseases. One example is MYCIN, a software developed in 1972 that was aimed to assist the physician in the identification of disease-causing microorganisms and simultaneously advise on the optimal antimicrobial therapy [17, 85]. MYCIN was one of the earliest algorithms designed to solve a problem through deduction, to generate new information and to give advice using a knowledge-based and an inference mechanism. Using approximately 500 rules encoded in an "if-then structure," MYCIN was able to provide a potential diagnosis with the appropriate therapy after a series of questions [86]. A domain-independent version of MYCIN was developed in 1980, called EMYCIN, allowing the creation of other similar knowledge-based systems. Some examples of EMYCIN-derived systems are BLUEBOX and HEADMED (psychopharmacology advisers) and ONCOCIN (a program designed to assist the physician regarding the therapeutic management of oncologic patients) [85].

In 1973, together with leading specialists in ophthalmology, a group of researchers developed a causal-associational network (CASNET) model for glaucoma patients. This system is a particular type of knowledge framework that consists of nodes representing the concepts, events, characteristics, and values of interest in a system, as well as branches specifying the relationships between said nodes [85, 87]. The workflow of this software implies the recording of observations that were matched with pathological findings. The latter were causally related forming a network that ultimately leads to disease classification. Treatments were then advised on the basis of both clinical observations and the disease classification [85].

In 1975, different research groups were involved in the creation of the Stanford University Medical Experimental – Artificial Intelligence in Medicine (SUMEX-AIM) laboratory for providing advanced computer capabilities (PDP-10's), connecting and supporting research of all the participating groups. This laboratory allowed several researchers with interest in AI research to perform critical comparisons concerning different systems and the methods to perform tasks such as knowledge representation, inference, and problem-solving [88].

In the 1980s and 1990s, several innovations were introduced regarding the algorithms used for computer-assisted diagnosis. One example was the implementation of a modified Bayesian belief network, which was used in the development of DXplain. This system was developed in 1986 to support physicians in making differential diagnoses. Developers provided DXplain with a huge knowledge database, containing more than 65,000 relationships between clinical manifestations and diseases. This system used a selection rule that took advantage of conditional probabilities and a scoring system similar to a Bayesian computation. Therefore, after giving clinical information as an input, the system was able to provide a list of probable diagnoses, also giving a probability score [89]. This program continued to be developed, and it was also widely used in the clinical practice for over 30 years, constantly expanding its database and implementing new functions [90, 91].

The Rise of Deep Learning

The early 2000s were characterized by a renewed interest regarding the research in AI and its application in medicine, propelled forward by the increase in computer power, storage space, and data variability [17, 84]. In 2007, IBM researchers developed the software "Watson." After its initial success, Watson was applied to the field of medicine, proving useful in many different settings. For example, in 2017, Watson was used to identify novel RNA-binding proteins (RBPs) associated to amyotrophic lateral sclerosis (ALS) by performing literature research and, applying this text-based knowledge on all RBPs in the genome, identifying possible candidates by semantic similarity [92]. The 2010s also saw the development and rise of DL in medicine, with several applications in different fields. DL-based systems can use and explore many different types of healthcare data (images, clinical data, laboratory values), bestowing versatility to this new technology [93].

DL has proven potentially useful to perform many different tasks in a variety of clinical settings. For example, these systems can improve medical imaging analysis by performing segmentation tasks, they can perform advanced analysis of electronic health records, etc. [93–95] As a result, DL also found applications in many different specialized fields of medicine such as genomics, oncology, ophthalmology, and radiology, although mostly in research as the implementation into clinical practice is still lagging [96–101].

Another evolution of AI systems aimed to support physicians is the introduction of chatbots. They are "humanized" platforms that simulate the interaction between two human beings, opening the era of "machine conversation." [102] The most prominent chatbots developed for medical use are MANDY and PHARMABOT. MANDY is a chatbot developed for primary care by L. Ni et al. in a summer research project funded by Precision Driven Health (a public-private research partnership of New Zealand). The system conducts an interview with the patient, proactively gathering useful clinical data and registering the most important symptoms, reliably understanding the patient through its natural language processing module. Subsequently, the program provides a thorough report to the referring physician, reporting both symptoms and differential diagnoses [103]. PHARMABOT is a chatbot developed for physician or pharmacology students with the aim of acting as a consulting pediatric pharmacist. After receiving patient-related data, this system is able to provide the most appropriate and safest drug, including appropriate dosing information [104].

Nowadays, AI is exponentially developing, increasing its influence on the day-to-day medical practice. One example may be the support provided by AI during the still ongoing SARS-CoV-2 pandemic. Indeed, AI proved to be promising in the aggregation of big data useful for epidemiologic studies: one AI company (BlueDot) even predicted the outbreak and warned its customers on December 31, 2019, a week before the first official warning by the Centers for Disease Control and Prevention [105]. Furthermore, AI has also played a pivotal role in drug repurposing, a process that involves the use of a known drug to cure a condition for which it was not originally designed for. AI provided a set of different molecules that represented possible candidates to be an effective therapy against SARS-CoV-2 [106].

AI in Medical Imaging

Concerning digital technology, the field of medical imaging has always been on the forefront. Radiologists have been among the first to use computer science in their clinical practice, and they currently are the most digitally informed healthcare professionals [107]. In this paragraph, we provide an outlook on the history of AI for medical imaging purposes.

The Beginning: Artificial Neural Networks and Computer-Aided Detection Systems

The role of AI in medical imaging is continuously increasing, with many of the basic AI processes, such as pattern recognition, being one of the pillars of the field of radiology. Among the first applications of AI are the computer-aided detection (CAD) systems in the 1980s. These systems applied ML algorithms on medical images aiming to detect abnormalities that were undetectable to the human eye, thus supporting the work of the radiologist. CAD systems were applied to different imaging modalities, such as computed tomography (CT) and magnetic resonance imaging (MRI). Trials have been performed to evaluate the diagnostic performance. However, until the early 2000s, these CAD systems did not show promising results [108]. One famous example is the multicenter trial performed by Fenton et al. The authors compared the diagnostic performance of mammography screening between facilities who adopted a CAD system to those who did not, during a period of 4 years (1998–2002). Surprisingly, the use of the CAD system decreased specificity and positive predictive value of mammography from 90.2% to 87.2% and from 4.1% to 3.2%, respectively [109].

CAD systems were the ultimate results of years of research in AI. Among the different AI algorithms, ANNs have been widely applied in radiology. Multilayer perceptron (MLP) networks (see Fig. 1.3) were later used in medical imaging with different applications. An example is the study of Fujita et al. from 1992, when MLP was used in a

CAD system aimed to improve the diagnostic performance of single-photon emission computed tomography (SPECT) in the detection of coronary artery disease [110].

The sense of sight is a basic human capability; however, it is difficult to emulate with computer modeling. MLP could be used to perform visual tasks; however, their structure does not take advantage of the position of the spatial information encoded in images. In the early 1980s, Fukushima et al. introduced the "Neocognitron," which is considered one of the first complex AI models facilitating imaging-related tasks. The Neocognitron model was further improved by LeCun et al., who proposed the first CNN trained with backpropagation, which was called LeNet. CNNs have been widely applied in medical imaging, starting from the early 1990s. Among the most common applications of CNN are image related like object detection and tissue characterization. We can cite some examples, such as the study performed by Lin et al. [112] regarding a CNN aimed to improve the nodule detection in digital chest radiographs and the study performed by Wu et al. [111] aimed to elaborate a model able to differentiate between benign and malignant microcalcifications in radiographs of pathologic breast specimens [111, 112].

Future Perspectives

In the future, AI is expected to further develop and is likely to have an increasing impact on the field of medical imaging. AI has the ability to affect many parts of the clinical radiology workflow, such as patient selection, acquisition of images, image reconstruction, and analysis and automated generation of reports using the development of different types of AI algorithms throughout the decades. For example, regarding CT, DL algorithms have been developed with the aim to reconstruct low-noise images from low-dose scans, which are considerably noisier, compared to a standard CT acquisition protocol. Concerning MRI, DL algorithms have been developed to improve the image quality while reducing the time of acquisition [113]. With the increasing availability of datasets and the speed of algorithm development, AI will continue to branch out to new areas and solve problems in the field of radiology that are left unsolved so far. Although it is expected that the role of AI in radiology will grow, the field of AI is still in its infancy, and it is unlikely that AI will replace radiologist any time soon, if at all. On the contrary, radiology residency programs should include a dedicated training in AI in order to provide the future radiologist with the necessary knowledge to use these techniques. The ultimate aim of AI throughout the years has been and will be to improve the diagnostic and therapeutic performance of the radiologist, who has to be aware not only of the potential but also of the flaws of these new technologies [114].

Conclusion

The development of AI has greatly increased since its beginnings in the first half of the twentieth century, following an exponential pattern that paralleled that of computer technology. These advances implied a progressive improvement concerning AI's ability of dealing with increasingly complex tasks to the extent that it outperformed human cognitive abilities. Accordingly, AI systems have become more and more prominent in medicine, especially in the field of radiology, which has been traditionally considered the field most dependent on technology. In the future, it will be of the uttermost importance to integrate basic AI notions in medical imaging training, since the main goal of AI is to be integrated in clinical practice and not only be used in research settings.

References

1. Muthukrishnan N, et al. Brief history of artificial intelligence. Neuroimaging Clin N Am. 2020;30:393–9.
2. Jones LV. Beyond babbage. Psychometrika. 1963;28:315–31.
3. Haenlein M, Kaplan A. A brief history of artificial intelligence: on the past, present, and future of artificial intelligence. Calif Manag Rev. 2019;61:5–14.
4. Turing AM. On computable numbers, with an application to the entscheidungsproblem. London: Mathematical Society; 1936.
5. Piccinini G. The first computational theory of mind and brain: a close look at McCulloch and Pitts's 'logical calculus of ideas immanent in nervous activity'. Synthese. 2004;141:175–215.
6. Chandru V. The Turing test. Resonance. 1997;2:2–2.
7. Turing AM. Computing machinery and intelligence. In: Machine intelligence: perspectives on the computational model, vol. LIX 1–28. Hoboken: Taylor and Francis; 2012.
8. Pinar Saygin A, Cicekli I, Akman V. Turing Test: 50 Years Later. Minds and Machines. 2000;10;463–518. https://doi.org/10.1023/A:1011288000451.
9. O'Leary DE. GOOGLE'S duplex: pretending to be human. Intell Syst Account Finance Manag. 2019;26:46–53.
10. Neufeld E, Finnestad S. In defense of the Turing test. AI Soc. 2020;35:819–27.
11. McCulloch WS, Pitts W. A logical calculus of the ideas immanent in nervous activity. Bull Math Biophys. 1943;5:115–33.
12. Abraham TH. (Physio)logical circuits: the intellectual origins of the McCulloch-Pitts neural networks. J Hist Behav Sci. 2002;38:3–25.
13. Krogh A. What are artificial neural networks? Nat Biotechnol. 2008;26:195–7.
14. Sondak NE, Sondak VK. Neural networks and artificial intelligence. In: Proceedings of the twentieth SIGCSE technical symposium on computer science education – SIGCSE'89. Association for Computing Machinery (ACM); 1989. p. 241–5. https://doi.org/10.1145/65293.71221.
15. McCarthy J, Minsky ML, Rochester N, Shannon CE. A proposal for the Dartmouth summer research project on artificial intelligence. AI Mag. 2006;27:12–4.
16. Moor J. Artificial intelligence conference: the next fifty years. AI Mag. 2006;27:87–91.
17. Kaul V, Enslin S, Gross SA. History of artificial intelligence in medicine. Gastrointest Endosc. 2020;92:807–12.
18. Cordeschi R. AI turns fifty: revisiting its origins. Appl Artif Intell. 2007;21:259–79.

19. Newell A, Simon HA. The logic theory machine a complex information processing system. IRE Trans Inf Theory. 1956;2:61–79.
20. Newell A, Shaw JC, Simon HA. Elements of a theory of human problem solving. Psychol Rev. 1958;65:151–66.
21. Newell A, Simon HA. Computer simulation of human thinking. Science (80-). 1961;134:2011–7.
22. Newell A, Shaw JC, Simon H. A general problem solving program for a computer. Comput Autom. 1959;8:10–6.
23. Simon HA, Newell A. Human problem solving: the state of the theory in 1970. Am Psychol. 1971;26:145–59.
24. Garvey CS. The 'general problem solver' does not exist: Mortimer Taube and the art of AI criticism. IEEE Ann Hist Comput. 2021. https://doi.org/10.1109/MAHC.2021.3051686.
25. Dreyfus HL. What computers still can't do: a critique of artificial reason. Cambridge: MIT Press; 1992.
26. Ernst GW, Newell A. Generality and GPS. 1967.
27. Natale S. If software is narrative: Joseph Weizenbaum, artificial intelligence and the biographies of ELIZA. New Media Soc. 2019;21:712–28.
28. Weizenbaum J. ELIZA-A computer program for the study of natural language communication between man and machine. Commun ACM. 1966;9:36–45.
29. Epstein J, Klinkenberg WD. From Eliza to internet: a brief history of computerized assessment. Comput Hum Behav. 2001;17:295–314.
30. Harnad S. The symbol grounding problem. Phys D Nonlinear Phenom. 1990;42:335–46.
31. Smolensky P. Connectionist AI, symbolic AI, and the brain. Artif Intell Rev. 1987;1:95–109.
32. Garnelo M, Shanahan M. Reconciling deep learning with symbolic artificial intelligence: representing objects and relations. Curr Opin Behav Sci. 2019;29:17–23.
33. Block HD. A review of "perceptrons: an introduction to computational geometry". Inf Control. 1970;17:501–22.
34. Rosenblatt F. The perceptron: a probabilistic model for information storage and organization in the brain. Psychol Rev. 1958;65:386–408.
35. Rosenblatt F. Perceptron simulation experiments. Proc IRE. 1960;48:301–9.
36. Nagy G. Neural networks—Then and now. IEEE Trans Neural Netw. 1991;2:316–8.
37. Block HD. The perceptron: a model for brain functioning. I. Rev Mod Phys. 1962;34:123–35.
38. Hay JC, Murray AE, Rosenblatt F, Stieber A, Wolf RA. Mark I perceptron operators' manual. 1960.
39. Eberhart RC, Dobbins RW. Early neural network development history: the age of Camelot. IEEE Eng Med Biol Mag. 1990;9:15–8.
40. Olazaran M. A sociological history of the neural network controversy. Adv Comput. 1993;37:335–425.
41. Wythoff BJ. Backpropagation neural networks. A tutorial. Chemom Intell Lab Syst. 1993;18:115–55.
42. Basheer IA, Hajmeer M. Artificial neural networks: fundamentals, computing, design, and application. J Microbiol Methods. 2000;43:3–31.
43. Agar JON. What is science for? The Lighthill report on artificial intelligence reinterpreted. Br J Hist Sci. 2020;53:289–310. Cambridge University Press.
44. Lighthill J. Part I artificial intelligence a general survey by Sir James Lighthill FRS Lucasian Professor of Applied Mathematics, 1 Introduction 2 The ABC of the subject. 1972. p. 1–22.
45. Grudin J. AI and HCI: two fields divided by a common focus. AI Mag. 2009;30:48–57.
46. van Assen M, Banerjee I, De Cecco CN. Beyond the artificial intelligence hype: what lies behind the algorithms and what we can achieve. J Thorac Imaging. 2020;35. https://doi.org/10.1097/RTI.0000000000000485.
47. Moto-oka T, Stone HS. Fifth-generation computer systems: a Japanese project. Computer (Long Beach Calif). 1984;17:6–13.
48. Duda RO, Shortliffe EH. Expert systems research. Science. 1983;220:261–8.
49. Goel A. The reality and future of expert systems a manager's view of AI research issues. Inf Syst Manag. 1994;11:53–2.
50. Gill TG. Early expert systems: where are they now? MIS Q. 1995;19:51–70.
51. Metaxiotis K, Samouilidis J-E, Psarras J. Expert systems in medicine: academic illusion or real power? J Innov Health Inform. 2000;9:3–8.
52. Liebowitz J. Expert systems: a short introduction. Eng Fract Mech. 1995;50:601–7.
53. Lindsay RK, Buchanan BG, Feigenbaum EA, Lederberg J. DENDRAL: a case study of the first expert system for scientific hypothesis formation. Artif Intell. 1993;61:209–61.
54. Sviokla JJ. An examination of the impact of expert systems on the firm: the case of XCON. MIS Q. 1990;14:127–40.
55. Ackley DH, Hinton GE, Sejnowski TJ. A learning algorithm for Boltzmann machines. Cogn Sci. 1985;9:147–69.
56. Rumelhart DE, Hinton GE, Williams RJ. Learning representations by back-propagating errors. Nature. 1986;323:533–6.
57. Werbos PJ. Backpropagation through time: what it does and how to do it. Proc IEEE. 1990;78:1550–60.
58. Lecun Y, Bengio Y, Hinton G. Deep learning. Nature. 2015;521:436–44.
59. Rumelhart DE, et al. Learning internal representations by error propagation. Ft. Belvoir: Defense Technical Information Center; 1985.
60. McCarthy J. Some expert systems need common sense. Ann N Y Acad Sci. 1984;426:129–37.
61. Silva FM, Almeida LB. Speeding up backpropagation. In: Advanced neural computers. Elsevier; 1990. p. 151–8. https://doi.org/10.1016/b978-0-444-88400-8.50022-4.
62. Sutton R. Two problems with back propagation and other steepest descent learning procedures for networks. In: Proceedings of the eighth annual conference of the Cognitive Science Society; 1986. p. 823–32.
63. Fahlman SE. An empirical study of learning speed in backpropagation networks. Pittsburgh: Carnegie Mellon University; 1988.
64. Gori M, Tesi A. On the problem of local minima in backpropagation. IEEE Trans Pattern Anal Mach Intell. 1992;14:76–86.
65. Ongsulee P. Artificial intelligence, machine learning and deep learning. In: International conference on ICT and knowledge engineering. IEEE Computer Society; 2018. p. 1–6. https://doi.org/10.1109/ICTKE.2017.8259629.
66. Schlegel D. Deep machine learning on GPUs. Semin Talk-Deep Mach Learn Gpus. 2015;1.
67. Baji T. Evolution of the GPU device widely used in AI and massive parallel processing. In: 2018 IEEE Electron Devices Technol. Manuf. Conf. EDTM 2018 – Proc; 2018. p. 7–9. https://doi.org/10.1109/EDTM.2018.8421507.
68. van Assen M, Lee SJ, De Cecco CN. Artificial intelligence from A to Z: from neural network to legal framework. Eur J Radiol. 2020. https://doi.org/10.1016/j.ejrad.2020.109083.
69. Newborn M. Deep Blue's contribution to AI. Ann Math Artif Intell. 2000;28:27–30.
70. Campbell M, Hoane AJ, Hsu FH. Deep blue. Artif Intell. 2002;134:57–83.
71. Schaeffer J, Plaat A. Kasparov versus deep blue: the rematch. J Int Comput Games Assoc. 1997;20:95–101.
72. LeCun Y, et al. Handwritten digit recognition with a back-propagation network. In: Touretzky D, editor. Advances in neural information processing systems, vol. 2. San Mateo: Morgan-Kaufmann; 1990.

73. Albawi S, Mohammed TA, Al-Zawi S. Understanding of a convolutional neural network. In: Proceedings of 2017 international conference on engineering and technology, ICET 2017, vols. 2018-January 1–6. Institute of Electrical and Electronics Engineers Inc.; 2018.
74. Ferrucci DA. Introduction to 'This is Watson'. IBM J Res Dev. 2012;56:1:1–1:15.
75. Hoy M, Alexa B. Siri, Cortana, and More: an introduction to voice assistants. Med Ref Serv Q. 2018;37:81–8.
76. Aizenberg IN, et al. Multiple-valued threshold logic and multi-valued neurons. In: Multi-valued and universal binary neurons. Springer US; 2000. p. 25–80. https://doi.org/10.1007/978-1-4757-3115-6_2.
77. Chen J, et al. Deep learning-based model for detecting 2019 novel coronavirus pneumonia on high-resolution computed tomography: a prospective study. medRxiv 2020.02.25.20021568. 2020. https://doi.org/10.1101/2020.02.25.20021568.
78. Rusk N. Deep learning. Nat Methods. 2015;13:35.
79. Russakovsky O, et al. ImageNet large scale visual recognition challenge. Int J Comput Vis. 2015;115:211–52.
80. Krizhevsky A, Sutskever I, Hinton GE. ImageNet classification with deep convolutional neural networks. Commun ACM. 2017;60:84–90.
81. Szegedy C, et al. Going deeper with convolutions. In: Proceedings of the IEEE computer society conference on computer vision and pattern recognition, vols. 07–12-June 1–9. IEEE Computer Society; 2015.
82. Ballester P, Araujo R. On the performance of GoogLeNet and AlexNet applied to sketches. In: Proceedings of the AAAI conference on artificial intelligence, vol. 30(1). 2016. https://ojs.aaai.org/index.php/AAAI/article/view/10171.
83. He K, Zhang X, Ren S, Sun J. Deep residual learning for image recognition. In: Proceedings of the IEEE computer society conference on computer vision and pattern recognition, vols. 2016-Decem. IEEE Computer Society; 2016. p. 770–78.
84. Xing L, Giger M, Min JK. Artificial intelligence in medicine: technical basis and clinical applications. Asmterdam The Netherlands: Elsevier; 2020.
85. Perry CA. Knowledge bases in medicine: a review. Bull Med Libr Assoc. 1990;78:271–82.
86. Shortliffe EH. Computer-based medical consultations, MYCIN. Asmterdam The Netherlands: Elsevier; 1976.
87. Kulikowski CA. Beginnings of Artificial Intelligence in Medicine (AIM): computational artifice assisting scientific inquiry and clinical art – with reflections on present AIM challenges. Yearb Med Inform. 2019;28:249–56.
88. Kulikowski CA. An opening chapter of the first generation of artificial intelligence in medicine: the first Rutgers AIM workshop, June 1975. Yearb Med Inform. 2015;10:227–33.
89. Barnett GO, Cimino JJ, Hupp JA, Hoffer EP. DXplain. An evolving diagnostic decision-support system. JAMA. 1987;258:67–74.
90. Hoffer EP, Feldman MJ, Kim RJ, Famiglietti KT, Barnett GO. DXplain: patterns of use of a mature expert system. AMIA Annu Symp Proc. 2005;2005:321–5.
91. Martinez-Franco AI, et al. Diagnostic accuracy in family medicine residents using a clinical decision support system (DXplain): a randomized-controlled trial. Diagnosis (Berl). 2018;5:71–6.
92. Bakkar N, et al. Artificial intelligence in neurodegenerative disease research: use of IBM Watson to identify additional RNA-binding proteins altered in amyotrophic lateral sclerosis. Acta Neuropathol. 2018;135:227–47.
93. Esteva A, et al. A guide to deep learning in healthcare. Nat Med. 2019;25:24–9.
94. Litjens G, et al. A survey on deep learning in medical image analysis. Med Image Anal. 2017;42:60–88.
95. Shickel B, Tighe PJ, Bihorac A, Rashidi P. Deep EHR: a survey of recent advances in deep learning techniques for electronic health record (EHR) analysis. IEEE J Biomed Health Inform. 2018;22:1589–604.
96. Leung MK, Xiong HY, Lee LJ, Frey BJ. Deep learning of the tissue-regulated splicing code. Bioinformatics. 2014;30:i121–9.
97. van Grinsven MJ, van Ginneken B, Hoyng CB, Theelen T, Sanchez CI. Fast convolutional neural network training using selective data sampling: application to hemorrhage detection in color fundus images. IEEE Trans Med Imaging. 2016;35:1273–84.
98. Young JD, Cai C, Lu X. Unsupervised deep learning reveals prognostically relevant subtypes of glioblastoma. BMC Bioinformatics. 2017;18:381.
99. Maji D, Santara A, Ghosh S, Sheet D, Mitra P. Deep neural network and random forest hybrid architecture for learning to detect retinal vessels in fundus images. Annu Int Conf IEEE Eng Med Biol Soc. 2015;2015:3029–32.
100. Premaladha J, Ravichandran KS. Novel approaches for diagnosing melanoma skin lesions through supervised and deep learning algorithms. J Med Syst. 2016;40:96.
101. Yasaka K, Abe O. Deep learning and artificial intelligence in radiology: current applications and future directions. PLoS Med. 2018;15:e1002707.
102. Safi Z, Abd-Alrazaq A, Khalifa M, Househ M. Technical aspects of developing chatbots for medical applications: scoping review. J Med Internet Res. 2020;22:e19127.
103. Chen J, Supnithi T, Tang X, Theeramunkong T. Knowledge and systems sciences: 18th International Symposium, KSS 2017, Bangkok, Thailand, November 17–19, 2017, Proceedings. In: Communications in computer and information science, 1 online resource. 2017, XX, p. 267, 84 illustrations. https://doi.org/10.1007/978-981-10-6989-5.
104. Comendador BEV, Francisco BMB, Medenilla JS, Nacion SMT, Serac TBE. Pharmabot: a pediatric generic medicine consultant chatbot. J Autom Control Eng. 2015;3:137–40.
105. Long JB, Ehrenfeld JM. The role of augmented intelligence (AI) in detecting and preventing the spread of novel Coronavirus. J Med Syst. 2020;44:1–2.
106. Zhou Y, Wang F, Tang J, Nussinov R, Cheng F. Artificial intelligence in COVID-19 drug repurposing. Lancet Digit Health. 2020;2:e667–76.
107. Pesapane F, Codari M, Sardanelli F. Artificial intelligence in medical imaging: threat or opportunity? Radiologists again at the forefront of innovation in medicine. Eur Radiol Exp. 2018;2:35.
108. Tang X. The role of artificial intelligence in medical imaging research. BJR Open. 2020;2:20190031.
109. Fenton JJ, et al. Influence of computer-aided detection on performance of screening mammography. N Engl J Med. 2007;356:1399–409.
110. Fujita H, Katafuchi T, Uehara T, Nishimura T. Application of artificial neural network to computer-aided diagnosis of coronary artery disease in myocardial SPECT bull's-eye images. J Nucl Med. 1992;33:272–6.
111. Wu YC, et al. Classification of microcalcifications in radiographs of pathologic specimens for the diagnosis of breast cancer. Acad Radiol. 1995;2:199–204.
112. Lin JS, Ligomenides PA, Freedman MT, Mun SK. Application of artificial neural networks for reduction of false-positive detections in digital chest radiographs. Proc Annu Symp Comput Appl Med Care. 1993:434–8. PMID: 8130511; PMCID: PMC2248546.
113. Lakhani P, et al. Machine learning in radiology: applications beyond image interpretation. J Am Coll Radiol. 2018;15:350–9.
114. Langlotz CP. Will artificial intelligence replace radiologists? Radiol Artif Intell. 2019;1:e190058.

2 Demystifying Artificial Intelligence Technology in Cardiothoracic Imaging: The Essentials

Jelmer M. Wolterink and Anirban Mukhopadhyay

Introduction

Few technologies have impacted radiology research in recent years as artificial intelligence (AI) has. New journals have been launched on the topic of radiology AI, dozens of start-up companies have been founded to bring AI to the clinic, and radiological conferences have seen a steady increase in AI-focused contributions. The number of FDA and CE-marked radiology products using AI is growing [1], and the first reimbursements for AI tools have been announced. AI will undoubtedly have a major impact on radiology in years to come. Yet the technological innovation of AI is often confused with the AI readiness of radiological practice. While the technological maturity of AI is a prerequisite for adoption in the clinic, it is in no way a sufficient condition for the direct adaptation of AI in radiology. One potential roadblock to AI adaptation lies in the difficulties that radiologists may experience in critically appreciating the technology, as AI can be hard to grasp as a concept [2]. Terminology is often used interchangeably, which may make understanding challenging. This lack of clarity could lead to incorrect perceptions, misunderstanding of the potential of this technique, and unmet expectations.

This chapter provides a gentle introduction to modern AI and its most relevant manifestations for radiological applications. This introduction is not intended to provide a complete technical overview of artificial intelligence techniques. For this, the interested reader is referred to works by Bishop et al. [3] and Goodfellow et al. [4]. Nor do we aim to provide a comprehensive review on AI applications in cardiothoracic image analysis. For this, several excellent reviews have recently been published [5, 6]. Instead, we aim to provide an accessible introduction to AI, occasionally drawing examples from cardiothoracic imaging to make concepts clear and tangible.

Disambiguating Terminology

The terms artificial intelligence, machine learning, and deep learning are frequently used interchangeably, yet their scope is quite different. The three terms have nested scopes, where artificial intelligence (AI) is most general and deep learning (DL) most specific (Fig. 2.1). It is good to be aware that deep learning is only a subfield of AI and that what is often presented as AI is only one manifestation – albeit a very successful one – of a much larger endeavor.

Artificial intelligence is a large and diverse, decades-old scientific field in which researchers aim to let computers perform tasks that would otherwise require human intelligence. Classic examples of such tasks are the ability to have conversations that appear to be natural or to play games like chess at a level otherwise reserved only for the best human players. Over the past few years, tremendous strides have been made in tackling such AI problems. For instance, computers can extract patterns from large amounts of texts and reuse these to compose complex new texts and have plausible conversations with humans [7]. As another example, advances in AI have led to computers that can beat even the best human players at games like chess and Go [8]. Nevertheless, AI as a field is still very much in development. The tasks that AI systems are being developed for are narrow, and extrapolation or generalization to slightly different problems is still a significant challenge.

J. M. Wolterink, PhD (✉)
Department of Applied Mathematics, Technical Medical Centre, University of Twente, Enschede, Netherlands
e-mail: j.m.wolterink@utwente.nl

A. Mukhopadhyay, PhD
Department of Informatics, Technische Universität Darmstadt, Darmstadt, Germany
e-mail: anirban.mukhopadhyay@gris.informatik.tu-darmstadt.de

C. N. De Cecco et al. (eds.), *Artificial Intelligence in Cardiothoracic Imaging*, Contemporary Medical Imaging, https://doi.org/10.1007/978-3-030-92087-6_2

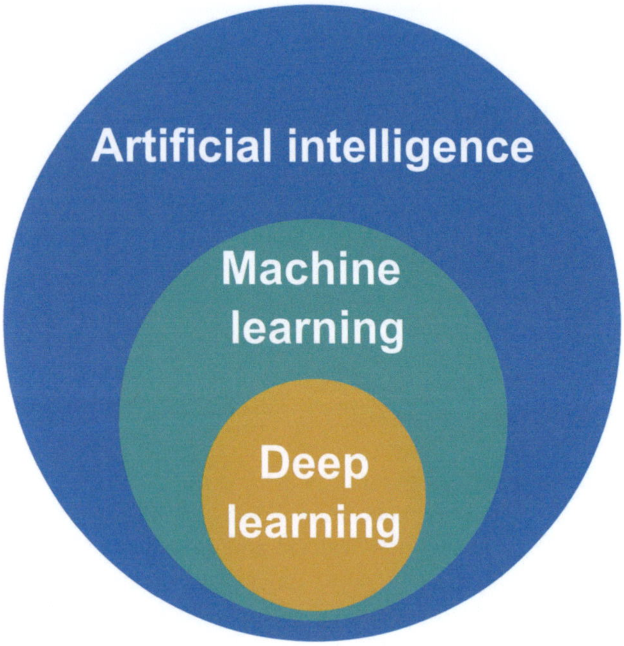

Fig. 2.1 Artificial intelligence, machine learning, and deep learning are related terms with different scope. Artificial intelligence is the scientific field aiming to let machines perform tasks that would otherwise be reserved for humans. Machine learning is the subfield of artificial intelligence focusing on algorithms that can learn without being explicitly programmed. Deep learning is a subfield of machine learning that uses artificial neural networks

There are many different approaches to AI, and the success, popularity, and perception of these different approaches have fluctuated over the years. Success is closely linked to scientific development, but external factors such as the availability of large data sets and computing power also play a role. One family of AI approaches is formed by machine learning techniques. Machine learning (ML) is a large subfield of AI in which the overarching theme is that a model learns about a particular kind of data, such as radiographic images, based on example data or *samples*. This contrasts with approaches that are hardcoded to perform a particular task. A model is typically learned with respect to a particular combination of data and a task. For example, an ML model could be trained to assign an anatomical label to each pixel in an image, i.e., image segmentation. Another example of an ML model could be one that distinguishes between radiographs showing some abnormality and radiographs that do not show this abnormality (Fig. 2.2). Because an ML model does not depend on hardcoded knowledge, it cannot distinguish between categories of images without ever having seen any images. Instead, it must learn to distinguish classes based on example images.

While all machine learning methods share a common purpose, they differ in the way that an internal model is defined. For example, methods that use a model defined by separating hyperplanes, such as support vector machines, have previ-

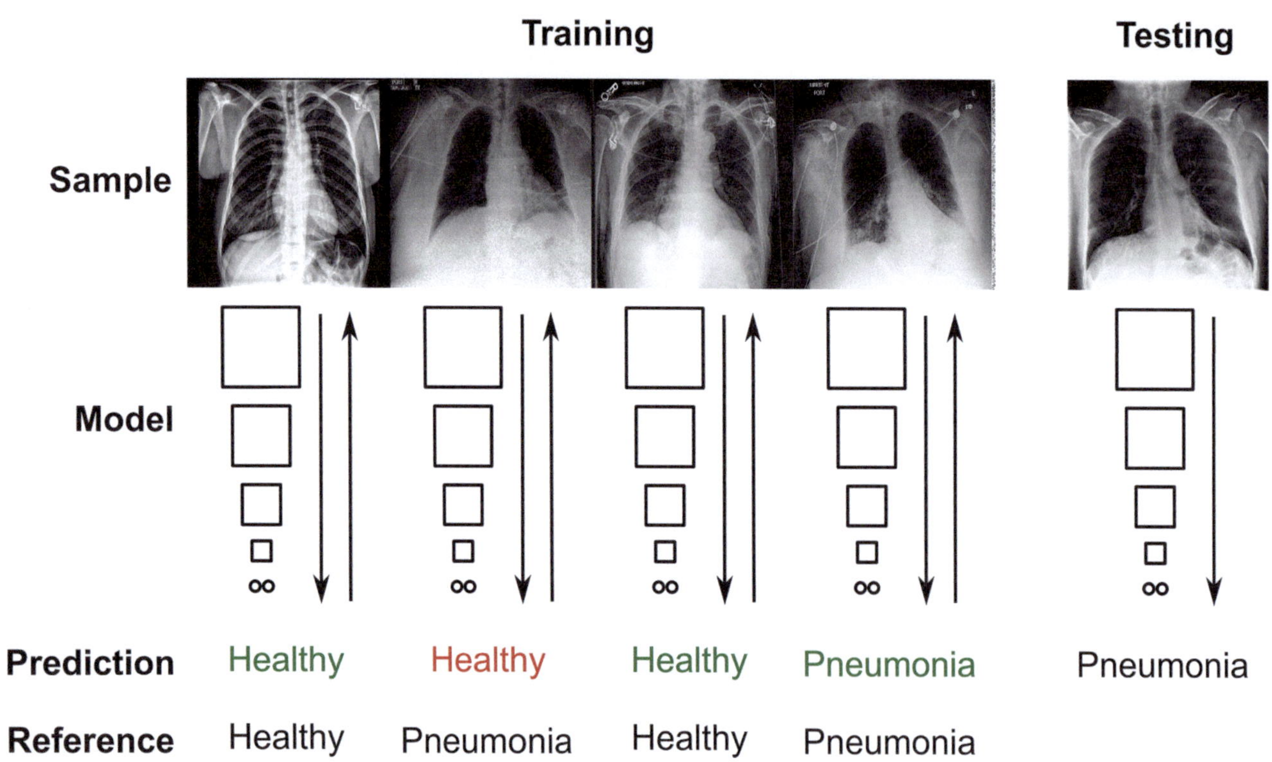

Fig. 2.2 Application of a machine learning model typically consists of a training stage and a testing stage. During training, the parameters of the model are optimized to provide correct predictions for the training data. During testing, new and unseen data is provided and processed by the trained model

ously been successfully applied in cardiothoracic imaging [9]. Alternatively, decision trees use a tree-like model of decisions and their possible consequences and can be encoded algorithmically with only conditional statements. Such models have also been widely used in machine learning and radiological image analysis [10]. Regardless of the type of model, input data needs to be represented in a way that the algorithm can understand. For most machine learning methods, this means that each data sample is represented by a set of features. These are quantitative characteristics that describe the data sample. For example, a medical image could be described by the histogram of its grayscale values or the response of a particular filter on the image. Designing representative features is an art and often requires a large amount of domain knowledge.

Deep learning (DL) is a subfield of ML that stands out from other ML methods for the way in which internal models are defined and for the way in which data features are extracted. DL methods model data using artificial neural networks (ANNs). These ANNs are loosely based on natural neural networks found in the human brain. A neuron or unit in such an ANN is an extreme abstraction of a human neuron, with input and output connections that have varying strengths and connect the unit to other units in the network (akin to synapses). Based on its connections to other units and the activations of those other units, the unit itself achieves a particular activation. Connecting thousands or millions of such artificial neurons through weights in an ANN provides a model that can be trained for a wide range of tasks. The main benefit of ANNs is that they can directly learn descriptive feature representations from input data without the need for hand-crafted features. This alleviated the need for knowledge-based feature design, which may be strongly based on and biased to a human's understanding of the data. Empirical studies have shown that this is highly valuable, in particular for (medical) image analysis. Given the enormous scope of AI, the limited space available in this chapter, and current trends in radiology AI, the remainder of the chapter will focus on deep learning.

Artificial Neural Networks

Artificial neural networks (ANNs) are at the heart of deep learning and have been shown to be extremely effective and versatile for a range of tasks. An ANN consists at least of an input layer to which an input sample is fed and an output layer that provides the desired prediction. An ANN typically also contains hidden layers, which can number in the tens or hundreds. These hidden layers are used to transform input information or features into the desired output (Fig. 2.3). Each layer in an ANN consists of one or multiple units, and each unit is associated with an activation value. The activation of units in the input layer is simply that of the input sample. The activation in subsequent layers depends on input activations and on trainable parameters or weights in the network associated with connections between the units.

Although ANNs can appear to be extremely complex, it is important to realize that everything that goes on inside an ANN is determined by simple mathematical equations that combine activation values, weights, and activation functions. In the ANN illustrated in Fig. 2.3, the activation value a_{out} of a hidden unit depends on the activation values a_0 and a_1 of two input units, the weights w_0 and w_1 between these units and the hidden unit, the weight w_{bias} between a bias node and the unit, and an activation function. Hence, three trainable parameters determine the activation value of the hidden unit: w_0, w_1, and w_{bias}. To compute the activation value, one obtains a weighted sum of incoming activations and passes this sum through a nonlinear activation function $f(x)$. In this case, we use a rectified linear unit (ReLU) activation function (shown in the inset of Fig. 2.3). Neural network units and layers can be combined in infinitely many configurations. We typically refer to these configurations as neural network architectures.

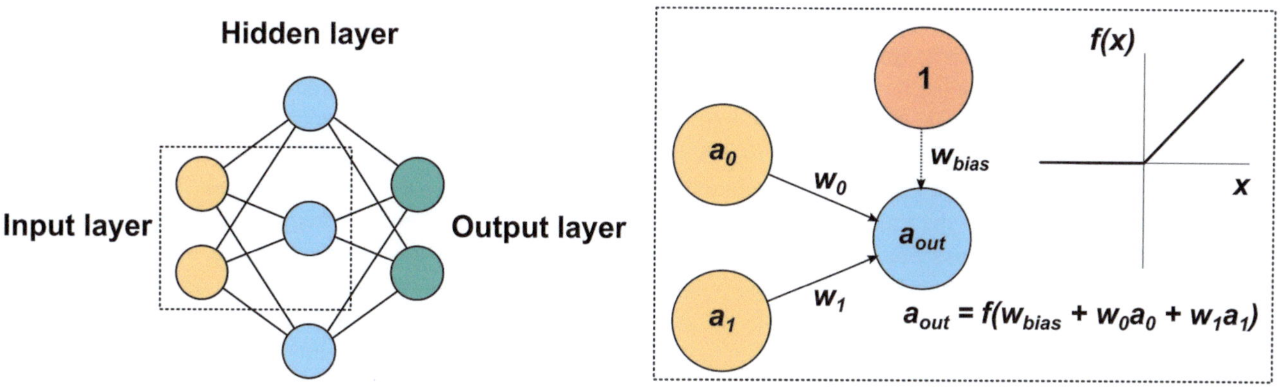

Fig. 2.3 An artificial neural network (ANN) consists of an input layer, one or more hidden layers, and an output layer with units that are connected by weights. (Inset) The output activation a_{out} of each unit depends on the activations of its input units, e.g., a_0 and a_1; the weights between these input units and the unit, w_0 and w_1; and a bias weight w_{bias}. A linear combination of these terms is transformed by a nonlinear activation function f(x), which in this case is a rectified linear unit (ReLU)

Well-known architectures are, for example, the LeNet-5 [11] or ResNet architectures [12].

ANNs are initialized with randomly picked weight values. Hence, they are unlikely to immediately provide the desired predictions on any part of the data set. Therefore, deep learning always requires a *training stage* in which the ANN is optimized based on sampled data, such as images. This is followed by a *testing stage* in which the model is applied to new and unseen data. Depending on how data is used during the training stage, a distinction can be made between supervised learning, unsupervised learning, or semi-supervised machine learning methods.

Learning Paradigms

Supervised Learning

In supervised learning, a model is optimized to provide a prediction for new and unseen data based on what it has learned from fully labeled samples during the training stage. All data samples, such as images, provided during the training stage have a corresponding ground truth label that is assumed to be correct. In the example in Fig. 2.2, samples are chest radiographs of patients presenting with or without pneumonia. Hence, possible labels are *healthy* and *pneumonia*. During training, an objective function is optimized so that for each training sample, the correct label is predicted. For each training sample, the predicted label and ground truth label can be directly compared, and the loss is computed based on their correspondence. The short-term goal of supervised learning is thus to obtain optimal values on the objective function for the training set. In the example in Fig. 2.2, the model predicts an incorrect label in the second sample, and thus, the objective function is not yet optimal. The arrows in Fig. 2.2 indicate how information flows from the sample to the prediction and back from the prediction to the sample, fitting the model to the data.

However, the long-term goal in supervised learning is to train a model that can *generalize* to new and unseen data. In itself, a model that only works for the training data but not for new samples has limited value. Therefore, once training has been finalized, the trained model can be used to process new and unseen samples in a testing stage. Now, information only flows from the sample to the prediction, and no reference label is required. This is the scenario in which radiology AI models will most likely be deployed in the clinic. Supervised learning is by far the most common way to train a deep learning model.

Unsupervised Learning

Unsupervised learning methods do not assume that a ground truth label is available for each training sample and thus put far fewer constraints on the training data. In principle, this makes unsupervised learning ideally suited for medical images, of which large quantities without detailed labels are acquired daily. However, as one can imagine, learning from unlabeled data is much harder than learning from properly labeled data, and thus, unsupervised learning methods are often used for specific tasks. These include clustering or the identification of groups of samples according to their characteristics [13].

Unsupervised learning methods can also be used to generate new data. So-called generative models learn a distribution of data and allow sampling from this distribution to generate new data. This contrasts with discriminative models that can differentiate between classes of samples. Popular generative models include generative adversarial networks (GANs), which have been widely used to synthesize medical images. In GANs, two neural networks play a game, in which the first network tries to synthesize data that the second network cannot distinguish from a set of real samples. This way, the first network learns the real data distribution by using only very *weak* labels of the data samples, i.e., that they are real. Examples in cardiothoracic radiology include works that focus on the synthesis of lung nodules as they would appear in computed tomography (CT) images [14]. The interested reader is referred to [15], in which we provide a primer on GANs for radiologists.

Semi-supervised Learning

In semi-supervised learning, a combination of supervised and unsupervised learning is used. It is assumed that for some samples, ground truth labels are available, while for other samples, no such labels are provided. Labels are available for part of the data set. Given the huge numbers of medical images that are available but do not necessarily contain high-quality labels, such approaches may be valuable.

Although unsupervised and semi-supervised models have the potential to leverage the vast amounts of weakly labeled medical images that are acquired on a daily basis, supervised learning is by far the most commonly used approach for radiologic applications. The remainder of this chapter will assume a supervised learning problem, i.e., one in which each sample has a corresponding ground-truth label.

Optimizing an Artificial Neural Network

Optimization of an ANN for any learning paradigm entails minimizing a loss function. This loss function is highly task specific and different for regression problems and classification problems. For example, in the classification problem in Fig. 2.2, we would want the network to predict the probability that a radiograph x shows pneumonia, and the value of this probability f(x) is between 0 and 1. The loss function then quantifies the difference between the predicted and the reference label for a radiograph. An adequate and often-used loss function for such a binary problem is the binary cross-entropy loss. A radiograph x that does not show pneumonia has a reference label $y = 0$, and the loss should be low if the network also predicts $f(x) = 0$. In mathematical terms, this can be written as $L(y, f(x)) = -\log(1 - f(x))$. On the other hand, a radiograph that does show pneumonia has a reference label $y = 1$, and the loss is low if the network predicts $f(x) = 1$. In mathematical terms, this means that for these samples, $L(y, f(x)) = -\log f(x)$ should be low (Fig. 2.4).

The loss function is used in an iterative process in which each iteration consists of several steps. First, data samples are processed by the ANN. The prediction of the network on these samples is compared to the reference labels, and a loss value is computed using the loss function. The contribution of each of the weights of the network to this loss is computed. Subsequently, an *optimizer* makes a tiny change to each weight so that the loss would be lower if the same data would be passed through the network again. The magnitude of this weight change depends on a learning rate, which needs to be carefully selected. Higher learning rates may lead to faster training but could also make optimization unstable. The process of weight adaptation based on the loss contribution of each individual weight is called backpropagation of errors. This iterative process is repeated with random samples data until the loss value has converged to a sufficiently low value.

Figure 2.5 illustrates this optimization process in an example with only two parameters. The parameter values are initialized at a point (indicated by a dot), and small steps are repeatedly taken based on the local slope of the loss landscape so that the parameter values change and the loss L(y, f(x)) gets lower. The example in Fig. 2.3 shows a network with just three layers, 17 units, and 17 trainable parameters. In practice, an ANN can have millions or billions of parameters, and optimization can require thousands of steps. Different optimizers exist, most of which are based on a process called gradient descent. By locally determining the direction in parameter space that decreases the loss function,

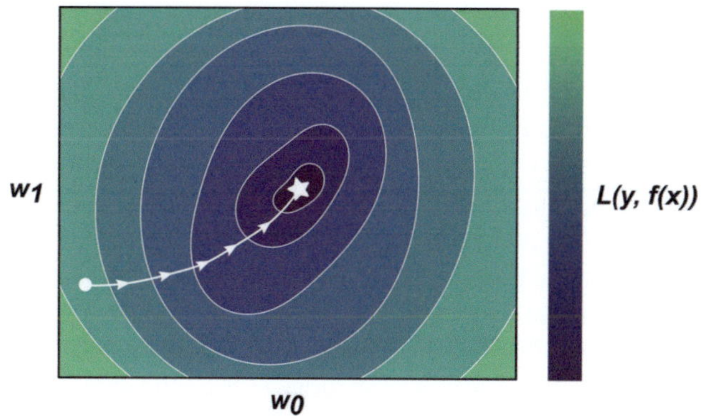

Fig. 2.5 To optimize a neural network, small steps are taken from an initial point (dot) in the parameter space until a set of parameters is found (star) that minimizes a loss function, i.e., a local minimum. In this toy example, there are only two weights, w0 and w1, but in practice, an artificial neural network can have millions or billions of trainable parameters

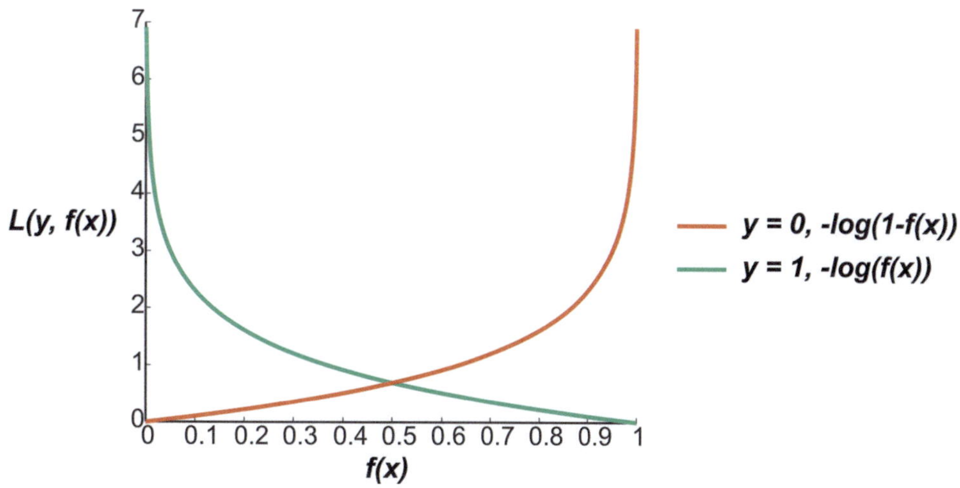

Fig. 2.4 Binary cross-entropy loss as a function of the predicted probability x by an artificial neural network, f(x). For samples with a label $y = 0$, the loss is low if the artificial neural network predicts $f(x) = 0$. For samples with a label $y = 1$, the loss is low if the artificial neural network predicts $f(x) = 0$. For samples with a label $y = 1$, the loss is low if $f(x) = 1$

small steps are taken. Because data sets are often too large to pass through the network and back again in one pass, mini-batches of samples are typically used, leading to a process called *stochastic gradient descent*.

Training, Validation, and Test Sets

To train a supervised machine leaning model, data sets are often divided into three sets. First, a *training set* is used to perform the actual model optimization. The model is directly penalized if it fails to make correct predictions on the training set or, conversely, rewarded if it provides the correct response. The training set is used to find the correct values for the potential thousands or millions of parameters in the machine learning using the aforementioned iterative process.

In addition to the low-level parameters of the model, other parameters determine the model's behavior. For example, the performance of a neural network depends on factors like the depth of the network or the width of its layers. Such freedom is captured in *hyperparameters*, parameters that typically do not change during model optimization but have a potential impact on the performance of the model. A validation set can be used to find the optimal values for these hyperparameters. The model can be trained multiple times with different settings for the hyperparameters, and its performance can be quantified by comparing predictions in the validation set to reference labels in the validation set. Note that these reference labels are not used to optimize all the low-level parameters of the network, and thus, an individual network with set hyperparameters is not optimized to learn the validation set.

Nevertheless, finding and using the optimal set of hyperparameters for the validation set through repeated training may lead to a model that works well on the training as well as the validation data, but not on new and unseen data. Therefore, it is common practice to set aside part of the data in a *test set*, which is not used during method development and only touched once for evaluation at the very end of the machine learning development pipeline. This test set is used as a surrogate for all data that the network has not seen yet, and performance on the test set is typically the only relevant metric that is reported in the literature, as it is least likely to be biased by tuning of either the network's parameters or hyperparameters.

This separation of data into training, validation, and test sets is very common in machine learning but may provide an incomplete assessment of the performance of a method. In practice, only around 30% of data is used for validation and testing, while around 70% of data is used for training. To more efficiently use often scarce data, *N*-fold cross-validation provides an alternative popular experimental set up. In cross-validation, the full data set is split up in *N* nonoverlapping subsets. In each experiment, one of these subsets is used as the validation set, while the other sets are used for training [16].

Convolutional Neural Networks

Many recent advances in AI in radiology are due to the use of ANNs. However, ANNs that consist of only fully connected input, hidden, and output layers have limitations when applied directly to images. The number of trainable parameters in an ANN grows very rapidly with the number of units in the network because layers are fully connected. This makes ANNs less reliable for image analysis applications, where every image pixel would be fed to an input unit (Fig. 2.6). Even for this small 8 × 7-pixel image, the ANN would already contain 56 units in the input layer. For example, with a hidden layer of 50 units, this would lead to more than 2900 trainable parameters. Now imagine such a network for a chest radiograph of 256 × 256 pixels, i.e., a severely downsampled radiograph. A simple one-layer ANN as in Fig. 2.6 with 1000 hidden units would already have over 65 million trainable parameters. Given the limited number of samples in a typical data set, it is likely that these millions of parameters would be tuned well to the training samples but would perform worse on new and unseen data, an effect called overfitting to the training set.

In overfitting, the loss on the training set keeps decreasing during training, while the loss on the validation set at some points starts to diverge (Fig. 2.7). This is undesirable behavior, as it implies that there will be a generalization error between the network's performance on the training set and its performance on new and unseen data. To prevent networks from overfitting, they require *regularization*. This can be achieved in several ways. For example, the objective function can be modified, the values that the network parameters can take on could be constrained, or specific neural network layers such as dropout [17] and batch normalization [18] can be used.

In another strategy to make ANNs for image analysis less susceptible to overfitting, an observation about images comes in hand. Typical images contain a hierarchy of patterns, in which complex patterns can be assembled from smaller and simpler patterns. For example, an image of a car may consist of wheels and rectangles, which in turn may consist of edges and corners. Such patterns can be emphasized using convolution kernels, which are small, typically square filters that are moved over every pixel in an image (Fig. 2.8). ANNs can be adapted to include convolutional layers, which apply such filters to images. Each filter consists of trainable weights, and the number of weights is independent of the size of the image that it is applied to. At each point in the image, the kernel emphasizes the same patterns. The application of one

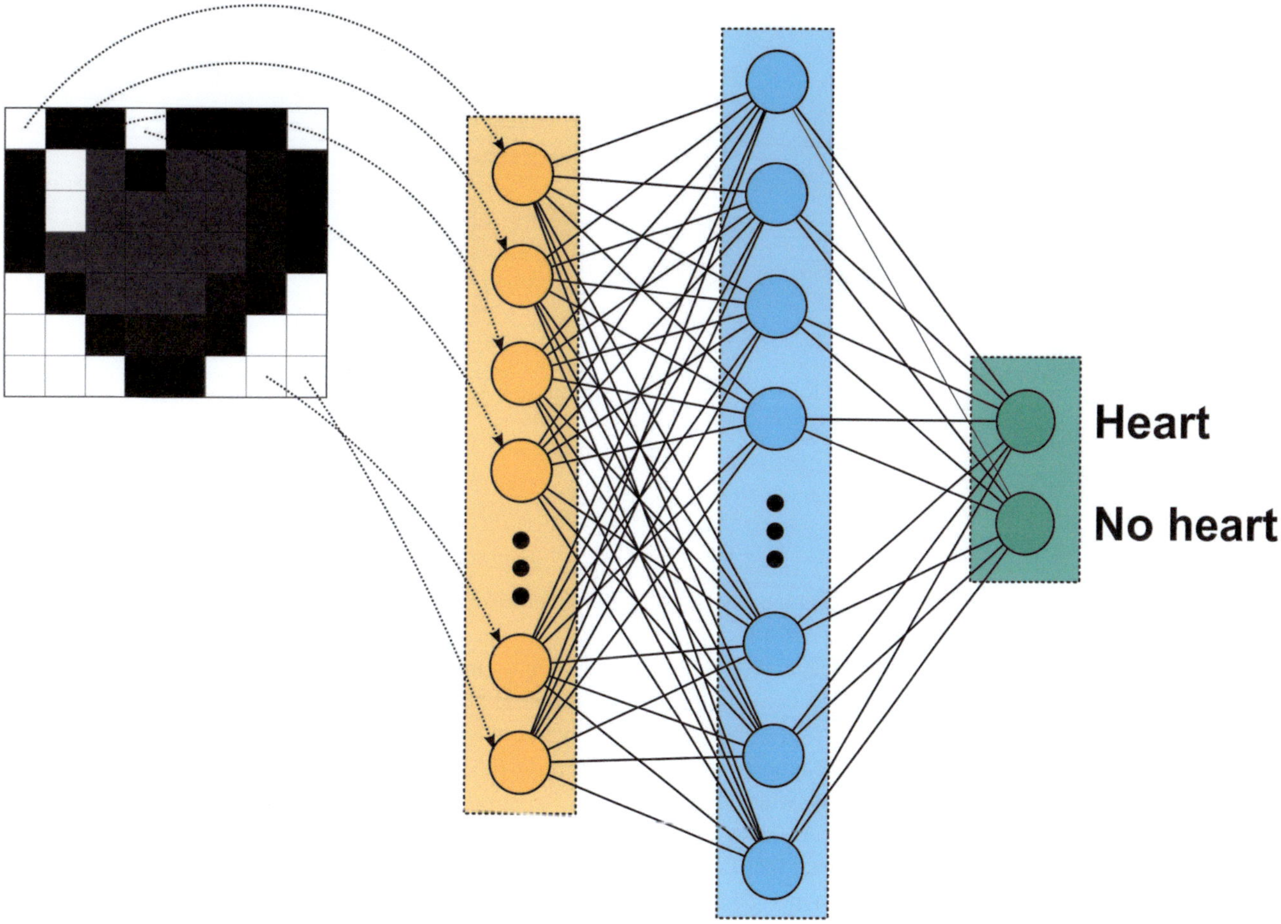

Fig. 2.6 ANNs consisting of only fully connected layers are not ideal for direct application to images. In this example, every input pixel in the input image is fed to an input unit. In a small network with just one hidden layer, the number of parameters increases rapidly with the number of input pixels. Note that most units and weights are not shown for visual clarity

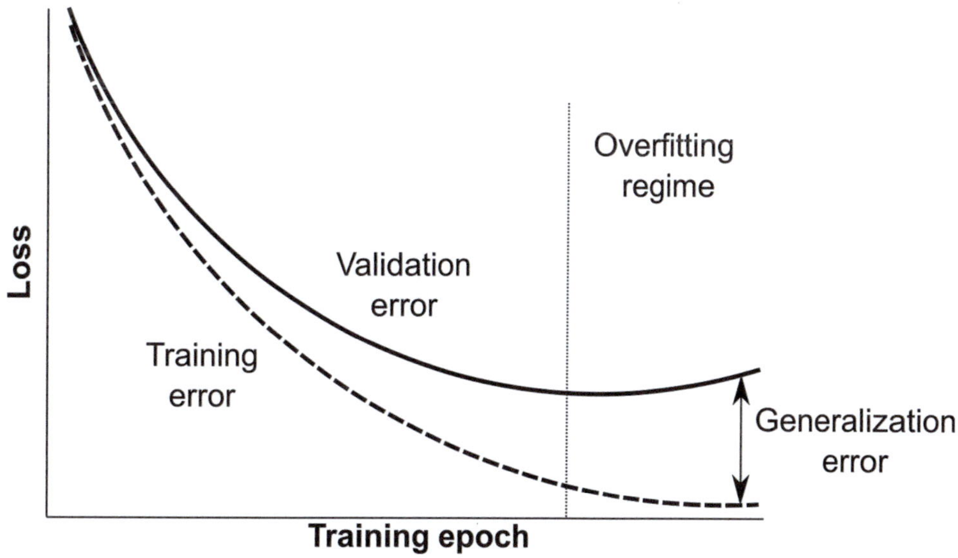

Fig. 2.7 A machine learning model is trained to minimize a predefined loss or error. As training progresses, the training error is reduced, and – ideally – so is the validation error. At some point, the validation error may start to increase again, and the model enters the overfitting regime. The difference between the training and validation error is called the generalization error

kernel emphasizes one pattern, but multiple kernels can emphasize multiple patterns, resulting in multiple filtered images that themselves can again be processed in the next convolutional layer. By applying the same filter at each location in the image, the number of parameters in the network can be drastically reduced, while the network can learn

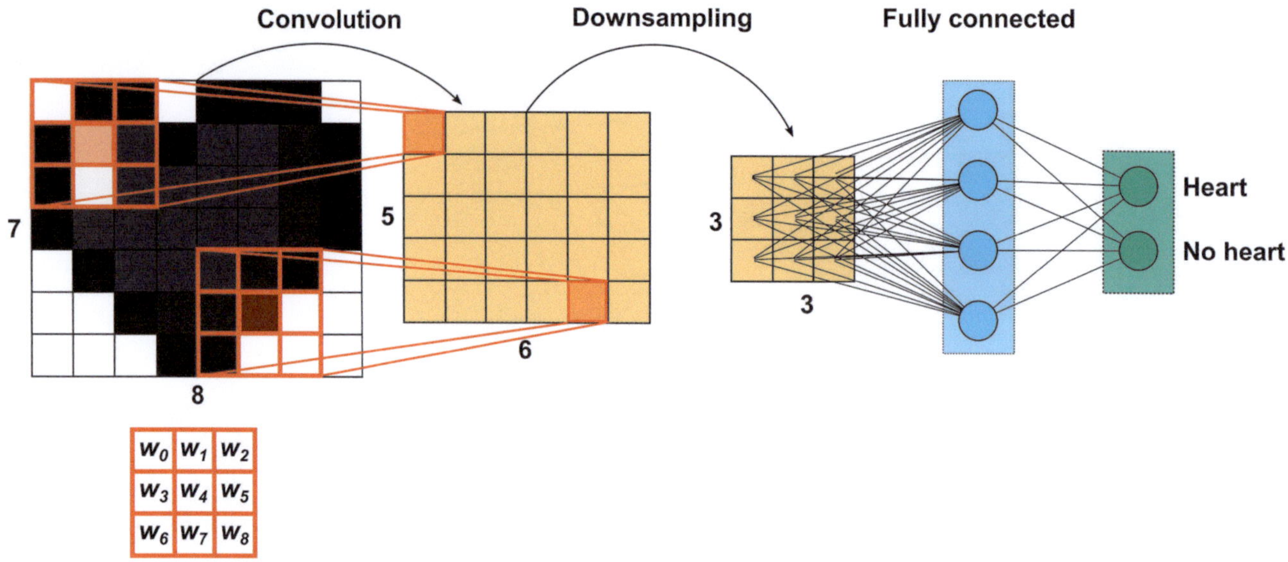

Fig. 2.8 A convolutional neural network typically consists of convolution layers, downsampling layers, and fully connected layers

high-quality representations of the input image. ANNs that include such convolutional layers are called convolutional neural networks (CNNs).

In addition to convolutional layers, convolutional neural networks often contain downsampling layers, which reduce the size of the images or feature maps in hidden layers. This has the benefit of preserving the most relevant features that the network learns and – after several such layers – connecting these features to a fully connected layer. These fully connected layers connect the features to the output layer.

Convolutional neural networks can be trained in the same way as regular ANNs. The weights are now no longer only the connections between units in the network but are in fact the elements of the filters applied to the images in the network. In Fig. 2.8, this means that the elements in the convolution kernel now correspond to weights w_0, w_1, w_2, etc., that are optimized during training. Again, this is done using backpropagation of errors. While LeCun et al. used backpropagation of errors to train CNNs as early as 1989 [11], the effectiveness and widespread popularity of CNNs are due to the AlexNet CNN architecture, which won the ImageNet Large Scale Visual Recognition Challenge in 2012 [19]. Subsequently, CNNs have become immensely valuable in the domain of medical image analysis [20]. Of particular relevance to medical image analysis are fully convolutional networks such as the popular U-Net architecture [21] that efficiently provide one prediction per pixel or voxel, instead of one prediction per image. Such architectures can be used for tasks like image segmentation or cross-modality synthesis. Convolutional neural networks have been widely used in cardiothoracic image analysis for tasks such as image classification and segmentation. In conjunction with new architectures, new task-specific loss functions have been designed, for example, image segmentation [22]. Moreover, convolutional neural networks have opened new avenues for classical image analysis problems, such as the registration of chest CT images [23].

Big Data

In combination with novel ML models and optimization strategies, large data sets are expected to be critical for further developments in AI for radiology. As a rule of thumb, machine learning methods depend on large and diverse data sets to improve their generalization to new and unseen data. While many studies are still based on single-center proprietary data, there is a growing realization that the availability of large and diverse public data sets is crucial to further developments in radiology AI. The need for high-quality, well-annotated, publicly available data sets is becoming more and more evident, and several excellent initiatives to support this exist.

One group of initiatives focuses on the organization of so-called challenges. These are benchmarks on specific medical imaging problems often organized in conjunction with medical imaging conferences such as MICCAI and ISBI. An overview of such challenges is maintained on the Grand Challenge website [24]. These challenges focus on a wide range of tasks and applications in different imaging modalities. Of particular relevance in the cardiothoracic domain are challenges on, for example, automatic coronary artery scoring [25], pulmonary nodule detection [26], and segmentation of organs at risk in chest CT images [27]. Moreover, the Radiological Society of North America (RSNA) has organized challenges on pneumonia detection and pulmonary embolism detection in 2018 and 2020, respectively. Challenges typically have a competitive character, in which a dynamic leaderboard ranks participating methods, and the best performing method is awarded. Although post hoc experiments have shown that such rankings are often not robust [28], they provide an additional incentive for participants to submit their results.

In addition to these challenges, large public databases for medical imaging data are being set up. One example of such a database is The Cancer Imaging Archive [29], which hosts a large number of data sets relating to cancer, such as the National Lung Screening Trial. Alternatively, large-scale national databases are under construction using either centralized data storage or so-called federated learning, in which data stays in place but models move around [30]. Moreover, during the COVID-19 pandemic, multiple large public databases containing X-ray or chest CT images of COVID-19 patients have been set up. While this has facilitated a surge of papers on chest image analysis, clinical use of these models may be limited [31]. One possible reason for this may be the substantial overlap between data sets [32], thus highlighting the need for high-quality, well-curated data sets.

Among all of these initiatives, standardization of data collection and annotation is important. Most supervised machine learning methods are only as good as the data provided to them, and high-quality training data is key. Ideally, data is acquired and reported in a manner that matches the desired clinical workflow but also allows reuse in artificial intelligence applications [33]. Moreover, issues regarding patient privacy should be taken into account.

Discussion and Conclusion

In this chapter, we have provided the reader with an introduction to machine learning and deep learning methods and introduced the reader to some terms that undoubtedly return throughout this book. The number of publications on AI, ML, and DL is still growing at an incredible pace, but hopefully, the interested reader has found some handles in this chapter to follow this ever-increasing body of literature.

While AI is a large scientific field, we have here focused on those manifestations most relevant to current radiological image analysis. Hence, this chapter has a strong focus on deep learning as a subfield of machine intelligence and thus of artificial intelligence. Deep learning is shaped by the use of artificial neural networks, but it is important to realize that not all machine learning methods use artificial neural networks to represent their model. Models like support vector machines and decision trees are still ubiquitous in machine learning, and methods using these have been extremely successful in a range of classification and regression tasks. For data sets in which features have been clearly defined or *hand-crafted*, simple multilayer perceptron artificial neural networks are often outperformed by competing machine learning methods. However, it is in problems in which features are not clearly defined or useful patterns might be hidden in the input data that deep learning methods thrive.

With the advent of deep learning in radiological image analysis, there has been a lot of interest in opening the black box or identifying why it is that a network makes a particular decision. The mechanisms underlying convolutional neural networks allow back projection of the network's decisions to the original image to provide heat maps [34]. An example of this is provided in work by De Vos et al., who performed automatic calcium scoring and provided a heat map of calcification locations determined by back projecting the prediction to the input image [35]. Similarly, interpretable methods can play a large role in the analysis of chest radiographs [36]. Interpretability and explainability of AI methods are likely to be a prerequisite for adoption in the clinic, as are methods to determine the uncertainty in predictions provided by AI methods. The development of such methods is an ongoing endeavor.

In the next few years, we will likely see more extensive big data sets being organized as existing data repositories are merged or new prospective databases are set up at an (inter) national level. This development will undoubtedly further accelerate innovation in AI-based radiological image analysis and enlarge the opportunities and potential of this technique in radiology.

References

1. van Leeuwen KG, Schalekamp S, Rutten MJCM, van Ginneken B, de Rooij M. Artificial intelligence in radiology: 100 commercially available products and their scientific evidence. Eur Radiol [Internet]. 2021 [cited 2021 May 7]:1–8. Available from: https://link.springer.com/10.1007/s00330-021-07892-z.
2. Huisman M, Ranschaert E, Parker W, Mastrodicasa D, Koci M, Pinto de Santos D, Coppola F, Morozov S, Zins M, Bohyn C, Koç U, Wu J, Veean S, Fleischmann D, Leiner T, Willemink MJ. An international survey on AI in radiology in 1,041 radiologists and radiology residents part 1: fear of replacement, knowledge, and attitude. Eur Radiol [Internet]. 2021 [cited 2021 May 6]. Available from: https://pubmed.ncbi.nlm.nih.gov/33744991/.
3. Bishop CM. Pattern recognition and machine learning. New York: Springer; 2006.
4. Goodfellow I, Bengio Y, Courville A. Deep learning. Cambridge: MIT Press; 2016.
5. Litjens G, Ciompi F, Wolterink JM, de Vos BD, Leiner T, Teuwen J, Išgum I. State-of-the-art deep learning in cardiovascular image analysis. JACC Cardiovasc Imaging. Elsevier Inc. 2019;12:1549–65.
6. Dey D, Slomka PJ, Leeson P, Comaniciu D, Shrestha S, Sengupta PP, Marwick TH. Artificial intelligence in cardiovascular imaging: JACC state-of-the-art review [Internet]. J Am Coll Cardiol. Elsevier USA. 2019 [cited 2021 Mar 10];73:1317–35. Available from: https://doi.org/10.1016/j.jacc.2018.12.054.
7. Brown TB, Mann B, Ryder N, Subbiah M, Kaplan J, Dhariwal P, Neelakantan A, Shyam P, Sastry G, Askell A, Agarwal S, Herbert-

Voss A, Krueger G, Henighan T, Child R, Ramesh A, Ziegler DM, Wu J, Winter C, Hesse C, Chen M, Sigler E, Litwin M, Gray S, Chess B, Clark J, Berner C, McCandlish S, Radford A, Sutskever I, Amodei D. Language models are few-shot learners [Internet]. NeurIPS. arXiv. 2020 [cited 2021 Mar 10]. Available from: http://arxiv.org/abs/2005.14165.
8. Silver D, Huang A, Maddison CJ, Guez A, Sifre L, Van Den Driessche G, Schrittwieser J, Antonoglou I, Panneershelvam V, Lanctot M, Dieleman S, Grewe D, Nham J, Kalchbrenner N, Sutskever I, Lillicrap T, Leach M, Kavukcuoglu K, Graepel T, Hassabis D. Mastering the game of go with deep neural networks and tree search. Nature. 2016;529(7587):484–9.
9. Išgum I, Prokop M, Niemeijer M, Viergever MA, Van Ginneken B. Automatic coronary calcium scoring in low-dose chest computed tomography. IEEE Trans Med Imaging [Internet]. 2012 [cited 2021 May 7];31(12):2322–34. Available from: https://pubmed.ncbi.nlm.nih.gov/22961297/.
10. Criminisi A, Shotton J, Konukoglu E. Decision forests: a unified framework for classification, regression, density estimation, manifold learning and semi-supervised learning. Found Trends Comput Graph Vis. 2011;7:81–227.
11. LeCun Y, Bottou L, Bengio Y, Haffner P. Gradient-based learning applied to document recognition. Proc IEEE. 1998;86(11):2278–323.
12. He K, Zhang X, Ren S, Sun J. Deep residual learning for image recognition. Proc IEEE Comput Soc Conf Comput Vis Pattern Recognit [Internet]. IEEE Computer Society. 2016 [cited 2021 May 8]:770–8. Available from: http://image-net.org/challenges/LSVRC/2015/.
13. Zheng Q, Delingette H, Fung K, Petersen SE, Ayache N. Pathological cluster identification by unsupervised analysis in 3,822 UK Biobank Cardiac MRIs. Front Cardiovasc Med [Internet]. 2020 [cited 2021 May 7];7:539788. Available from: /pmc/articles/PMC7701336/.
14. Chuquicusma MJM, Hussein S, Burt J, Bagci U. How to fool radiologists with generative adversarial networks? A visual turing test for lung cancer diagnosis. In: Proceedings – international symposium on biomedical imaging. IEEE Computer Society; 2018. p. 240–4.
15. Wolterink JM, Mukhopadhyay A, Leiner T, Vogl TJ, Bucher AM, Išgum I. Generative adversarial networks: a primer for radiologists. RadioGraphics [Internet]. 2021 [cited 2021 Apr 30]:200151. Available from: http://pubs.rsna.org/doi/10.1148/rg.2021200151.
16. King RD, Orhobor OI, Taylor CC. Cross-validation is safe to use. Nat Mach Intell [Internet]. 2021 [cited 2021 Apr 30];3(4):276. Available from: http://www.nature.com/articles/s42256-021-00332-z.
17. Srivastava N, Hinton G, Krizhevsky A, Salakhutdinov R. Dropout: a simple way to prevent neural networks from overfitting [Internet]. J Mach Learn Res. 2014 [cited 2021 May 8];15. Available from: http://jmlr.org/papers/v15/srivastava14a.html.
18. Ioffe S, Szegedy C. Batch normalization: accelerating deep network training by reducing internal covariate shift [Internet]. PMLR. 2015 [cited 2021 May 8]. Available from: http://proceedings.mlr.press/v37/ioffe15.html.
19. Krizhevsky A, Sutskever I, Hinton GE. ImageNet classification with deep convolutional neural networks. Commun ACM [Internet]. 2017 [cited 2020 Apr 14];60(6):84–90. Available from: http://code.google.com/p/cuda-convnet/.
20. Litjens G, Kooi T, Bejnordi BE, Setio AAA, Ciompi F, Ghafoorian M, van der Laak JAWM, Van Ginneken B, Sánchez CI. A survey on deep learning in medical image analysis. Med Image Anal. 2017;42:60–88.
21. Ronneberger O, Fischer P, Brox T. U-net: convolutional networks for biomedical image segmentation. In: Lecture notes in computer science (including subseries lecture notes in artificial intelligence and lecture notes in bioinformatics) [Internet]. Cham: Springer; 2015 [cited 2019 Jan 15]. p. 234–41. Available from: http://link.springer.com/10.1007/978-3-319-24574-4_28.
22. Milletari F, Navab N, Ahmadi S-A. V-Net: fully convolutional neural networks for volumetric medical image segmentation. In: 2016 fourth international conference on 3D vision (3DV) [Internet]. IEEE; 2016 [cited 2019 Feb 17]. p. 565–71. Available from: http://ieeexplore.ieee.org/document/7785132/.
23. Hering A, van Ginneken B, Heldmann S. mlVIRNET: multilevel variational image registration network. In: Lecture notes in computer science (including subseries lecture notes in artificial intelligence and lecture notes in bioinformatics) [Internet]. Springer; 2019 [cited 2021 Apr 30]. p. 257–65. Available from: https://link.springer.com/chapter/10.1007/978-3-030-32226-7_29.
24. Grand challenge [Internet]. [cited 2021 Apr 30]. Available from: https://grand-challenge.org/.
25. Wolterink JM, Leiner T, de Vos BD, Coatrieux J-L, Kelm BM, Kondo S, Salgado RA, Shahzad R, Shu H, Snoeren M, Takx RAP, van Vliet LJ, van Walsum T, Willems TP, Yang G, Zheng Y, Viergever MA, Išgum I. An evaluation of automatic coronary artery calcium scoring methods with cardiac CT using the orCaScore framework. Med Phys [Internet]. 2016;43(5):2361–73. Available from: http://doi.wiley.com/10.1118/1.4945696.
26. Setio AAA, Traverso A, de Bel T, Berens MSN, Bogaard C van den, Cerello P, Chen H, Dou Q, Fantacci ME, Geurts B, Gugten R van der, Heng PA, Jansen B, de Kaste MMJ, Kotov V, Lin JYH, Manders JTMC, Sóñora-Mengana A, García-Naranjo JC, Papavasileiou E, Prokop M, Saletta M, Schaefer-Prokop CM, Scholten ET, Scholten L, Snoeren MM, Torres EL, Vandemeulebroucke J, Walasek N, Zuidhof GCA, Ginneken B van, Jacobs C. Validation, comparison, and combination of algorithms for automatic detection of pulmonary nodules in computed tomography images: the LUNA16 challenge. Med Image Anal [Internet]. 2017 [cited 2021 May 7];42:1–13. Available from: https://pubmed.ncbi.nlm.nih.gov/28732268/.
27. Lambert Z, Petitjean C, Dubray B, Kuan S. SegTHOR: segmentation of thoracic organs at risk in CT images. In: 2020 10th International conference on image processing theory, tools and applications, IPTA 2020. Institute of Electrical and Electronics Engineers Inc.; 2020.
28. Maier-Hein L, Eisenmann M, Reinke A, Onogur S, Stankovic M, Scholz P, Arbel T, Bogunovic H, Bradley AP, Carass A, Feldmann C, Frangi AF, Full PM, van Ginneken B, Hanbury A, Honauer K, Kozubek M, Landman BA, März K, Maier O, Maier-Hein K, Menze BH, Müller H, Neher PF, Niessen W, Rajpoot N, Sharp GC, Sirinukunwattana K, Speidel S, Stock C, Stoyanov D, Taha AA, van der Sommen F, Wang C-W, Weber M-A, Zheng G, Jannin P, Kopp-Schneider A. Why rankings of biomedical image analysis competitions should be interpreted with care. Nat Commun [Internet]. 2018 [cited 2019 Jul 25];9(1):5217. Available from: http://www.nature.com/articles/s41467-018-07619-7.
29. Clark K, Vendt B, Smith K, Freymann J, Kirby J, Koppel P, Moore S, Phillips S, Maffitt D, Pringle M, Tarbox L, Prior F. The cancer imaging archive (TCIA): maintaining and operating a public information repository. J Digit Imaging [Internet]. 2013 [cited 2021 Apr 30];26(6):1045–57. Available from: https://link.springer.com/article/10.1007/s10278-013-9622-7.
30. Rieke N, Hancox J, Li W, Milletarì F, Roth HR, Albarqouni S, Bakas S, Galtier MN, Landman BA, Maier-Hein K, Ourselin S, Sheller M, Summers RM, Trask A, Xu D, Baust M, Cardoso MJ. The future of digital health with federated learning. npj Digit Med [Internet]. 2020 [cited 2021 May 7];3(1):1–7. Available from: https://doi.org/10.1038/s41746-020-00323-1.
31. Roberts M, Driggs D, Thorpe M, Gilbey J, Yeung M, Ursprung S, Aviles-Rivero AI, Etmann C, McCague C, Beer L, Weir-McCall JR, Teng Z, Gkrania-Klotsas E, Ruggiero A, Korhonen A, Jefferson E, Ako E, Langs G, Gozaliasl G, Yang G, Prosch H, Preller J, Stanczuk J, Tang J, Hofmanninger J, Babar J, Sánchez LE, Thillai

M, Gonzalez PM, Teare P, Zhu X, Patel M, Cafolla C, Azadbakht H, Jacob J, Lowe J, Zhang K, Bradley K, Wassin M, Holzer M, Ji K, Ortet MD, Ai T, Walton N, Lio P, Stranks S, Shadbahr T, Lin W, Zha Y, Niu Z, Rudd JHF, Sala E, Schönlieb CB. Common pitfalls and recommendations for using machine learning to detect and prognosticate for COVID-19 using chest radiographs and CT scans. Nat Mach Intell [Internet]. 2021 [cited 2021 Apr 30];3(3):199–217. Available from: https://doi.org/10.1038/s42256-021-00307-0.

32. Garcia B, Cruz S, Nicolás Bossa M, Sölter J, Husch AD. Public Covid-19 X-ray datasets and their impact on model bias – a systematic review of a significant problem. medRxiv [Internet]. 2021 [cited 2021 Apr 30];2021.02.15.21251775. Available from: https://doi.org/10.1101/2021.02.15.21251775.
33. Willemink MJ, Koszek WA, Hardell C, Wu J, Fleischmann D, Harvey H, Folio LR, Summers RM, Rubin DL, Lungren MP. Preparing medical imaging data for machine learning [Internet]. Radiology. Radiological Society of North America Inc.; 2020 [cited 2021 Apr 30];295:4–15. Available from: https://doi.org/10.1148/radiol.2020192224.
34. Gotkowski K, Gonzalez C, Bucher A, Mukhopadhyay A. M3d-CAM: a PyTorch library to generate 3D data attention maps for medical deep learning. Inform aktuell [Internet]. 2020 [cited 2021 May 6]:217–22. Available from: http://arxiv.org/abs/2007.00453.
35. de Vos BD, Wolterink JM, Leiner T, de Jong PA, Lessmann N, Isgum I. Direct automatic coronary calcium scoring in cardiac and chest CT. IEEE Trans Med Imaging [Internet]. 2019 [cited 2019 Feb 20]:1–1. Available from: https://ieeexplore.ieee.org/document/8643342/.
36. Brunese L, Mercaldo F, Reginelli A, Santone A. Explainable deep learning for pulmonary disease and coronavirus COVID-19 detection from X-rays. Comput Methods Prog Biomed. 2020;196:105608.

Artificial Intelligence Algorithm Development for Biomedical Imaging

3

Peter M. A. van Ooijen and Leonardus B. van den Oever

Introduction

The development of artificial intelligence (AI) in imaging gained momentum with the ability to use deep learning for image classification purposes in the image challenge that was won by Geoff Hinton and his team [1]. From the moment of this feat, medical imaging became one of the prominent areas of research of artificial intelligence and deep learning up to a point where the same Geoff Hinton claimed in a statement in November 2016 at the Machine Learning and Market for Intelligence Conference in Toronto that "we should stop training radiologists now" because they would be replaced by deep learning in a couple of years' time [2]. Since then, a lot of progress has been made, but we are far from replacing medical doctors with AI and the sentiment has changed to the view of AI as an addition to the human expert or augmented intelligence instead of artificial intelligence.

Traditional medical imaging tasks that were supported by conventional image processing software are the segmentation of anatomy or pathology, the detection of pathology, and the classification of pathology. Artificial intelligence started to play its role in these domains but also opened possibilities that were not seen before, such as the generation of synthetic images and the implementation of image data-based predictive algorithms for preventive medicine and treatment planning.

The fast and diverse developments in both the hardware required and the software supporting the development and deployment of AI algorithms create an environment in which the capabilities of AI flourish. However, actual clinical application is still not widespread. Besides ethical and legal reasons, which are enforced because of the weight that medical decisions often carry, this also has technical reasons. The "black-box" nature of deep learning makes it difficult to reproduce and/or explain experimental results and, therefore, renders AI based decision-making incomprehensible for both physicians and patients. This lack of transparency and explainability is also often regarded the main reason that trust in AI among its potential users is still low.

However, it is highly probable that this will change in the coming years when repeated validation of designed AI models will result in more robust and explainable AI implementations, thereby increasing the trust in AI. That hard work is being done to get to that stage as soon as possible can be seen from the sharp increase in the number of papers published on AI, machine learning, and deep learning in cardiology and cardiovascular imaging in the past decade [3]. These papers cover a wide variety of application areas of AI in cardiovascular imaging, ranging from acquisition and reconstruction to prediction and reporting and spanning the full range of data acquisition devices used in cardiovascular imaging from echocardiography [4, 5] to computed tomography (CT) and magnetic resonance imaging (MRI) [6]. With this, it should be noted that all of these currently developed AI systems are so-called narrow AI solutions, or in a more popular term, they are "one-trick ponies." This means that the AI systems developed nowadays are only good in performing one specific task in a very controlled environment and will fail when, for example, unknown new data or data of different quality is presented as input.

Based on the papers published, we can observe reported performance gradually increasing to a level where it is equal to or even better than the human expert. Therefore, it seems that we are on the brink of a more widespread implementation of AI-based tools and many publications have discussed and demonstrated this AI future of cardiovascular imaging [3, 6, 7]. To help get an overview of these rising possibilities and what is technically required to achieve them, this chapter provides insight in the different tasks that can be performed by AI tools based on cardiovascular imaging data and gives an overview of the steps involved in the AI development process.

P. M. A. van Ooijen, MSc, PhD, CPHIMS (✉)
L. B. van den Oever, MSc
Department of Radiation Oncology and Data Science Center in Health, University Medical Center Groningen, Groningen, The Netherlands
e-mail: p.m.a.van.ooijen@umcg.nl; l.b.van.den.oever@umcg.nl

C. N. De Cecco et al. (eds.), *Artificial Intelligence in Cardiothoracic Imaging*, Contemporary Medical Imaging,
https://doi.org/10.1007/978-3-030-92087-6_3

AI in Medical Imaging

AI can have impact on all steps in the medical imaging process from image acquisition to predictive medicine (Fig. 3.1) to provide additional capabilities, automation of tasks, and augmentation of the human operator by providing automated support in a user-guided task.

Image Acquisition

Part of the image acquisition process is the determination of the image quality of the data produced. On the one hand, this is important to the AI algorithms using the data; on the other hand, AI algorithms could also be employed to determine the image quality. This utilization of AI algorithms to assess image quality is especially important in imaging modalities that can have a high variety in image accuracy and quality depending on the equipment used and/or have a high dependency on user experience and skills such as echocardiography. In echocardiography, AI-based image quality assessment could be implemented and used during the actual image acquisition process in real time to guide the user to obtain consistent images of high quality of the correct anatomical positions independent of the experience and skill of the user [4, 8].

Another step in the process of echocardiography acquisition that could benefit from AI is view classification. In clinical practice, the classification of the plane of recorded echocardiography videos is done manually and susceptible to misreporting. Therefore, automatic classification could reduce the workload of the analysts and reduce mistakes. This automation can be achieved using convolutional neural networks (CNN) with cluster analysis to sort input images into five predetermined standard views (e.g., standard cardiac MR views such as short axis, long axis, 2 chamber, 3 chamber, 4 chamber), with a reported accuracy for such classification models of 91–98% [4, 9, 10].

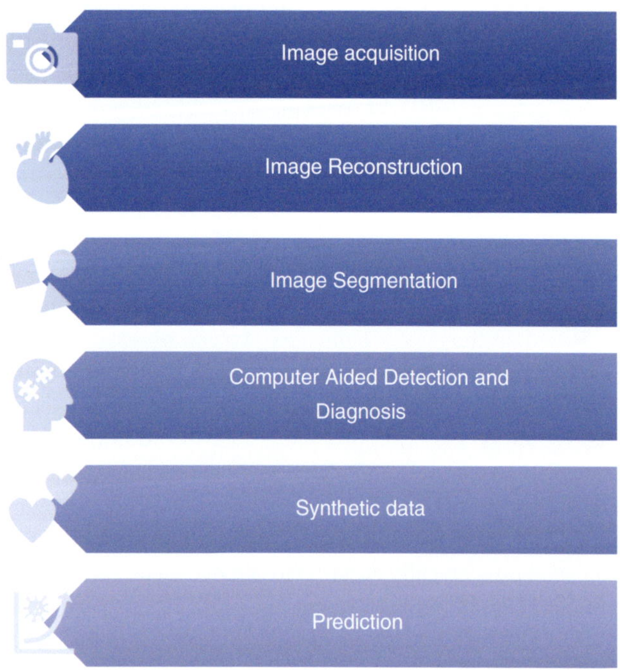

Fig. 3.1 Different possible applications of AI in cardiovascular imaging

In combination, these kinds of models could be applied to guide the user in obtaining the right images for a certain clinical question, thus allowing less experienced operators to acquire high-quality data of the different views.

Another application of AI in image acquisition is the guidance of the technologist in the acquisition of CT or MR examinations to automatically target the right field of view with optimal settings for the individual patient.

Image Reconstruction

Noise reduction is one of the applications of AI during the image reconstruction phase. To achieve noise reduction, a deep learning network is trained – for example – to transform (ultra)low-dose CT data into data that closely resembles the image quality of a full-dose diagnostic CT. This would allow to decrease dose even further and still obtaining diagnostic images. Both convolutional neural networks (CNNs) and generative adversarial networks (GANs) are reported to be able to perform such noise reduction without deterioration of the structure of the image and retaining the diagnostic value of the images [11, 12].

Another benefit of deep learning in the phase of image reconstruction is the ability to decrease the time required to perform cardiac MRI (CMR) examinations by undersampling data collection and using deep learning to estimate the sparse domain based on existing data [13, 14]. Like many AI applications, this method requires large amounts of data to properly train, something that has often been an issue in CMR-related research. Current work, therefore, is restricted to only very specific MR sequences.

Image Segmentation

The most popular application of AI in cardiovascular imaging is undoubtedly the segmentation of cardiac structures in the acquired imaging data, and it is applied to echocardiography, MRI, and cardiac CT in over 100 publications to segment a variety of anatomical and pathological structures [14]. According to the current knowledge base of published work, there is not one specific AI methodology most favorable for the segmentation task. Selected algorithms depend on factors like the imaging modality, protocol used, and cardiac structure to be segmented [15].

One of the possible implementations of automated image segmentation in cardiovascular disease is the segmentation of the cardiac chambers. Several imaging methodologies such as echocardiography, CT, and MRI can employ AI to perform cardiac chamber segmentation, and based on these segmentations, assessment of dynamic parameters such as left ventricular function and size can be automated. High performance is reported on echocardiography using CNNs with an accuracy of 84% [16]. In comparison, left ventricle (LV) segmentation on CT with CNN reported a Dice similarity coefficient of 0.85 with a mean absolute surface distance of 1.1 mm [17]. Most of the work on segmentation of the cardiac chambers using CNN was, however, done in MRI with a variety of techniques. Dice coefficients of 0.94 (Hausdorff distance, 3.5 mm; average symmetric surface distance (ASSD), 0.7 mm) and 0.95 (average perpendicular distance, 1.81 mm) using CNN [18] and CNN with stacked autoencoders [19], respectively, were achieved. Other publications on CNN [20, 21] and deep belief network combining deep learning and level sets [22] also report good performance resembling manual expert segmentation.

Other publications have shown the applicability of AI on segmentation of cardiac valves [23], coronary calcifications [24, 25], and coronary arteries [26, 27].

Computer-Aided Detection and Diagnosis

Classification into multiple categories is a task that can be performed in a supervised or unsupervised manner depending on the task at hand and the available dataset. In a supervised method, both the source data and the corresponding annotations/labels that are the required outcome or endpoint are available. With unsupervised training, only the source data is used to determine clusters of datapoints with similar properties.

Although most of the developed AI applications employ the supervised method, some demonstrations of successful unsupervised methods are available in the literature. For example, Cikes et al. used an unsupervised clustering approach based on a set of parameters to identify patients with heart failure that benefit from cardiac resynchronization therapy [28], and Shah et al. used unsupervised phenomapping to diagnose heart failure with preserved ejection fraction with an AUC of 0.70–0.76 [29].

Supervised AI was employed to determine myocardial disease from a variety of imaging modalities based on quantification. Examples of such applications using echocardiography imaging are the automatic determination of the left ventricular ejection fraction using CNN with high accuracy of 81–95% [4, 16, 30–32], the detection of mitral regurgitation with accuracy >99% using a support vector machine (SVM) [33], and myocardial infarction diagnosis with accuracy ranging from 87% [34] to 99.5% [35]. Wall motion abnormalities could be classified using CNN with a reported AUC of 0.97 [36] and accuracy of 75% [37] and using conventional machine learning classifiers with an accuracy of 96% [38].

Additionally, in cardiac MR, projects on the determination and calculation of cardiac function parameters have reported high accuracy and low mean absolute difference ranging from 3 to 8.5 mL between manual and automatic measurement of the left ventricular end-diastolic volume, end-systolic volume, stroke volume, ejection fraction, and mass [39, 40].

Where MR and echocardiography have their focus on the functional parameters of the heart, CT has mainly been applied to explore the presence and extent of coronary plaque or calcium and the presence and severity of stenotic lesions. For example, for determination of the coronary calcium score, Wolterink et al. described a method where candidates were extracted by intensity-based thresholding and described by location features derived from estimated coronary artery positions, as well as size, shape, and intensity features. Next, a two-class classifier distinguished between coronary calcifications and negatives or a multiclass classifier labeled CAC per coronary artery. Candidates that could not be labeled with high certainty were identified by entropy-based ambiguity detection and presented to an expert for review and possible relabeling with an intra-class correlation coefficient of 0.95 [41].

Both machine learning techniques such as boosted ensemble algorithms [42] and CNNs [43] were used for the quantitative analysis of coronary stenosis and plaque measurement with reported accuracies of >80%. Another application utilizing machine learning is the determination of fractional flow reserve (FFR) based on CT, resulting in an accuracy of up to 83% [44, 45].

Synthetic Data Generation

AI also allows to use available (imaging) data to generate new data, so-called synthetic data. This ability to create synthetic data got a lot of public attention because of demonstrations from Deepfake and sites like http://thispersondoesnotexist.com but so far has not proven to be very popular to apply in medical imaging research. A technique that is commonly used to construct synthetic data is the generative adversarial network (GAN) as proposed by Goodfellow et al. in 2014 [46]. A GAN makes use of two neural networks that compete against each other, a generative and a discriminative network. The generative network generates an image based on a random input, and the discriminative network tries to distinguish between real data and the generated fake. When the discriminative network is unable to make the distinction, the result is a successful fake (or synthetic) image. The error or loss of the discriminative network is, therefore, the reverse loss of the generative network. The higher the loss of the discriminative network, the lower the loss of the generative network, hence the name adversarial network. The generative network can then be used to generate more synthetic data.

For cardiovascular imaging applications, different varieties of synthetic data can be constructed that could prove useful in clinical practice.

First, synthetic data can be generated based on an available database to increase the number of samples that can be used for training a deep learning network. For example, Diller et al. used a dataset of 303 cardiac MRI scans of tetralogy of Fallot patients to generate 100,000 new synthetic images that were then used as a training set to train a U-net segmentation [47]. They found that on visual inspection, all synthetic samples were classified as anatomically plausible by human observers and that the U-net trained on synthetic data performed comparable to the same U-net architecture trained on real patient data. This shows that the use of synthetic data to extend a training set in order to train a deep learning network is a feasible solution when the amount of available data is limited.

A second application of synthetic data generation is the transition from data acquired on one imaging modality to a new synthetic dataset that looks like it was acquired on another imaging modality. Common transitions under investigation in different domains are to synthesize CT data from an acquired MRI or to synthesize CT data from an acquired cone beam CT. Applications that could benefit from synthetic data generation are MR-only radiotherapy planning or synthetic CT based on cone beam CT (CBCT) obtained during radiation therapy in order to enable adaptive treatment planning [48]. Direct applications of this type of data conversions in cardiovascular imaging are not yet found.

Another possibility of using generative networks is synthetic contrast enhancement, where contrast media enhancement is synthetically added to a non-contrast enhanced scan. Although not many papers exist on this particular topic, it shows promise for some clinical applications and could be valuable for patients that are allergic to the contrast agent or to further reduce the amount or concentration of contrast media administered. Santini et al. showed synthetic contrast enhancement in cardiac CT with deep learning to be feasible and achieved a high Dice score of 0.88 ± 0.03 and a low volume percentage error of $9.1 \pm 6.2\%$ for segmentation of the synthetically enhanced left ventricle [49]. However, they only used a small dataset and limited themselves to a 2D representation of the long axis view of the cardiac chambers, thus not providing actual 3D information.

Prediction

Predictive algorithms can be applied to implement early prediction of disease in order to start preventive treatment or to determine future treatment response to allow patient-specific treatment selection.

One concrete example of the prediction possibilities is the prediction of major adverse cardiac events (MACE) based on a combination of clinical, stress-testing, and imaging-derived variables. This kind of prediction relies on the discovery of features in a multi-layered model [6].

Motwani et al. performed prediction of all-cause mortality among patients with suspected coronary artery disease by employing ML techniques (boosted ensemble algorithm) in cardiac CT achieving an AUC of 0.79 [50]. Comparable results with an AUC of 0.771 were achieved by van Rosendael et al. also using a boosted ensemble algorithm (XGBoost) on CT data to predict risk score for all-cause death and non-fatal myocardial infarction during a >3-year follow-up [51]. Based on MRI, Dawes et al. reported an AUC of 0.73 for predictive modeling of survival in patients with pulmonary hypertension using principal component analysis [52]. Also using MRI, Samad et al. performed predictive modeling of deterioration of left ventricular function in patients with a repaired tetralogy of Fallot using a SVM classifier, resulting in an AUC of 0.82 for predicting any deterioration [53].

It is common in ML techniques that use clinical or image-derived variables to first reduce the number of variables used for the targeted prediction. The higher the number of input variables, the more difficult it becomes for an ML technique to train correctly and achieve high accuracy. These dimensionality reduction techniques use one of two basic techniques, feature elimination or feature extraction. The aforementioned XGBoost, a feature elimination method, tests the input variables for their impact on the accuracy of the ML algorithm and discards variables that have little impact on the prediction results, making the ML algorithm more efficient and easier to train. Feature extraction creates new variables by combining the old variables and then dropping all the old variables and the new combined variables that do not add to the prediction accuracy.

AI Development Process

For all of the previously described AI developments, the process is quite similar regardless of whether developing a tool for the technician supporting image acquisition or one for a radiologist or cardiologist to provide outcome prediction (Fig. 3.2). However, differences do exist in certain steps because of the inherent difference in the different methodologies available to the data scientist or AI engineer.

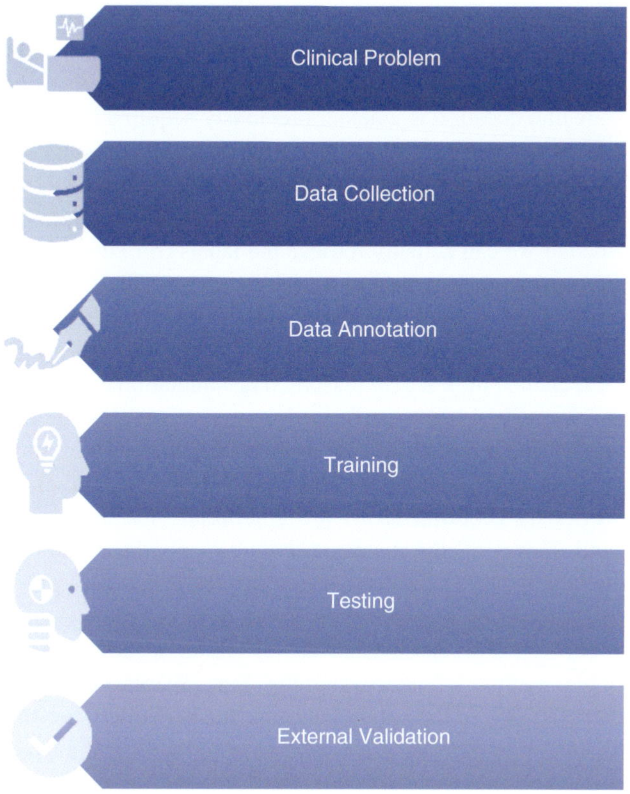
Clinical Problem
Data Collection
Data Annotation
Training
Testing
External Validation

Fig. 3.2 Steps in the AI development process

Machine learning or deep learning methodologies can roughly be divided into three groups, being supervised learning, unsupervised learning, and reinforcement learning.

In *supervised learning*, the system learns by knowing the truth for the training dataset and using the difference between the truth and the prediction (based on the so-called loss function) to iteratively improve the prediction. The known "truth" that is connected to the data can be in the form of annotations or labels to the image. Annotation involves the actual selection of the region of interest on the image itself. This is often used for segmentation tasks. The selection can vary from just identifying the region of interest by placement of a rough bounding box to the full (manual) segmentation of the region of interest by detailed contour drawing. Labeling involves the linking of a textual or numerical label to the image without annotation on the image itself. Such a label could, for example, be a diagnosis (e.g., the existence of a certain disease visible in the image) or a number (e.g., the number of abnormalities shown in the image). Another distinction that can be made in the labeling is a simple binary (yes/no) labeling or a multi-class labeling describing a number of different outcomes. The same holds for annotations where a single region of interest can be available indicating one region with specific properties, or multiple regions can be selected each with their own specific properties. In supervised learning, there are two kinds of learning tasks: classification and regression. Classification models try to predict distinct classes, while regression models predict numerical values.

In *unsupervised learning*, the system tries to discover the hidden structure of data or associations between variables. In that case, training data consists of instances without any corresponding labels or annotations. The associations between variables are defined in the form of clusters. Clusters are informative patterns occurring through clustering, which means the separation of a whole dataset into groups of data, so that instances belonging to the same group are as similar as possible and instances belonging to different groups differ as much as possible.

The term *reinforcement learning* is a general term given to a family of techniques in which the system attempts to learn through direct interaction with the environment so as to maximize some notion of a cumulative reward. It is important to mention here that the system has no prior knowledge about the behavior of the environment and the only way to find out is through trial and error. Reinforcement learning is mainly applied to autonomous systems due to its independence in relation to its environment but can also play a role in medical imaging by providing systems that learn by doing. In such a system, there is no pre-definition of the labels or annotations of the data, but they are provided by the user while the system is learning in the background. After providing sufficient input to the model to obtain a certain level of confidence, the model will start providing the predictions to the user who can then provide input by correcting mistakes to further train and improve the model. One of the major challenges of such systems in clinical practice is that they keep learning and thus change behavior over time, which hampers the legal acceptance and quality assurance of such a model. The learning/training process is dependent on the experience of the user. When a less experienced user is feeding such a system with wrong answers, the system will also learn from this faulty input assuming that it is correct, and eventually the system will adjust itself and start producing answers tailored to the faulty input.

Because of the complex nature, in almost every step of the AI process, the collaboration in a multidisciplinary group of healthcare professionals, data scientists, and deep learning experts is crucial to get to the optimal result.

Clinical Problem

The clinical problem should be the start of every AI project. This problem could be related to the inability of a human observer to retrieve the required information from imaging data, or the time-consuming process of manual processing of images, but also about the inability of the human observer to provide predictions of future events or progression of disease because of the vast amount of data available, which makes it impossible for a human observer to assess it all. All these could lead to the exploration of the support of artificial intelligence to solve the problem. After definition of the clinical problem faced, multiple subsequent steps have to be taken to perform in the AI development process.

Data Collection

The next step to develop an AI algorithm is the collection of a large enough dataset of high quality that represents the target population and holds as little bias as possible. The quality of such a dataset is one of the most important factors of the AI development process and very often the limiting factor. Just as in conventional image processing, the adage "garbage in is garbage out" also holds in the case of artificial intelligence; consistent quality of the data is of utmost importance as is standardization.

When collecting data, it is important to do this based on the clinical question. The data collection should resemble the target population of the eventual tool, contain a large enough portion per subset related to the different endpoints, and have as little bias as possible.

The challenge of bias lies not only in the obvious target population features such as gender, age, and race but also in the data origin. This becomes even more difficult in medical imaging, where the anatomy of patients has a large variation. For training purposes, this means that a dataset needs to include as many samples as possible. In case of limited availability of data, this is often achieved by using either patches from volumes or extracting 2D slices out of volumes, which are often remarkably similar, or by data augmentation during the training phase.

Many of the publications mentioned in this chapter only provide results of an AI system trained, tested, and validated on a single-institution dataset. However, radiological images can vary a lot in their presentation because of the dependency on the imaging equipment used. Because of the bias introduced by training on a database with images of the locally used equipment, acquisition and reconstruction parameters, similar performance is not guaranteed on a database obtained at another institution where these factors differ. For example, Biondetti et al. demonstrated that CNNs can learn to distinguish the scanner manufacturer and that this bias can substantially impact model performance for both classification and segmentation tasks [54].

Data Annotation or Labeling

Besides the data itself, the quality of the annotations or labels connected to the data is also extremely important. The training, test, and validation phase of supervised learning approaches heavily rely on the quality of these data annotations and labeling. Therefore, a number of questions can be asked concerning the annotation and labeling.

A first question is whether previously acquired labels are already available. The previous labels could be obtained from the clinical databases or the reports from a clinical trial or research project. However, this leads to the question whether we can actually retrieve the labels from the clinical or research system used in a usable and readable format. It could therefore also be necessary to specifically (re)label the data because no previous labels exist, or they are not usable for technical or practical reasons. The annotation or labeling is – in many cases – performed by one or multiple human experts and provided as consensus or majority vote of those human experts. This leads to the next question of whether the previously acquired labels are appropriate for the task at hand. This concerns questions about not only the strength of the label but also the consistency of labels that were previously added by multiple people with different methodology or experience. It is important for an ML algorithm to learn a single method of annotating the data. Biases caused by inconsistency of the labels can cause the network to become less accurate. Similarly, for validation and testing, the labels need to be consistent. The ML algorithm will learn to annotate the data in a certain method; if the validation data is then inconsistently labeled, mismatches will negatively influence accuracy. Once we have a labeled or annotated dataset, we also need to consider if there is class balance between the different labels.

In some cases, additional information about the ground truth can be obtained besides the labeling of human observers; if this is possible – for example, pathology results for malignancy prediction – these could be used to strengthen the labels provided.

Training and Testing

The dataset collected will be divided into a train and a test set, often 80% and 20% of the total dataset. This split can be performed in different ways. First, a random split can be performed. However, this will only be sufficient if the dataset is large enough to avoid unwanted bias in either the train or test set. Therefore, a balanced split is also possible where certain factors are balanced over the train and test set, for example, concerning the population (age/gender) or the outcomes (same distribution of the outcomes in both training and test set).

Due to the nature of medical data, most of the times, the classes in a dataset are very imbalanced, usually either toward the healthy prediction or the opposite. This makes the algorithm predictions incline to the majority class, creating poor accuracy on the minority classes that are usually the diseased classes. It should be noted that some quantification methods commonly used will still find high accuracy for these algorithms, since the error will be small if the minority class is also a minority in the test dataset. Oversampling the minority class and undersampling the majority class are techniques commonly employed in the training phase of an ML algorithm to alleviate the class imbalance problem.

The training itself is an iterative process in which a training dataset is provided to the AI model, which will then produce predictions. These predictions are – in case of supervised learning – compared in smaller batches to the true labels, and the difference (or loss) is used to tweak the model to reduce the loss by changing its weights after each batch. After each iteration over the complete training dataset, a separate validation will be done with a part of the dataset that is not used for the training. After *n* iterations (or epochs) over the full dataset, the training will be complete and result in a trained model.

So in this process, the AI model learns by calculating how wrong its predictions are by using the provided correct in- and output.

Many of the deep learning networks are data hungry when training the network and require a lot of data. The number of cases presented to the training phase can be extended by so-called data augmentation. In the case of imaging data, this means that besides the original images, also slightly adjusted images are fed to the deep learning network to expose it to a higher variety of images with different presentations. Possible augmentation adjustments are image mirroring, rotation, zooming, and stretching. This data augmentation is usually performed on the fly during the training process.

External Validation

Sometimes, internal validation is performed by providing a part of the dataset to the model that it never saw before from the own dataset (e.g., by dividing it into 60%/20%/20%). However, a better approach is to obtain a true independent validation by including an external validation set obtained from one or more different institutions. This could be collected, dedicated for this one occasion, but often publicly available datasets are used that are posted on open repositories or were previously released as part of a data science challenge. Using such a set also allows to compare algorithms that report on using the same dataset in their published work.

Multistage Pipelines

Currently, the capabilities of AI software are often not advanced enough for single neural networks to solve the complex problems seen in medical imaging and clinical workflows. Therefore, multistage pipelines of combined neural networks, each for a specific task, are used. One of the examples would be the reduction of variables as discussed in the prediction subchapter. More convoluted problems, such as locating a pneumothorax, will first identify and segment the lungs with a neural network and then train another neural network to classify the segmented image for the presence of a pneumothorax. During development of these kinds of workflows, the pipelines are usually based on clinical workflow. When reading a chest x-ray, intuitively, a reader would identify the lungs and then look for abnormalities. AI does not have intuition, so we have to help it with these steps.

Conclusion

As can be observed from the successful implementations showcased in the growing number of publications, artificial intelligence shows great promise in cardiovascular imaging for different goals [55]. However, most of the studies published are descriptive in nature, and its widespread implementation is still hampered by low availability and reproducibility. Therefore, in the development of AI, careful attention to the different steps in the development process should be taken to avoid suboptimal training of the network. Many challenges still exist in the development of AI tools such as suboptimal training data with bias or incorrect labels, insufficient training and validation, and many more.

However, it can also be observed that AI has made great progress in the past decade and has already made impact in cardiovascular imaging in both acquisition and diagnosis. This shows that AI has the potential to increase the quality of care and reduce the burden on both the healthcare professional and the patient.

References

1. Krizhevsky A, Sutskever I, Hinton GE. ImageNet classification with deep convoluational neural networks. Adv Neural Inf Process Syst. 2012;25:1–9.
2. [Online]. Available: https://www.youtube.com/watch?v=2HMPRXstSvQ.
3. Verjans J, Leiner T. Artificial intelligence for the general cardiologist. Neth Hear J. 2019;27:389–91.
4. Kusunose K. Steps to use artficial intelligence in echocardiography. J Echocardiogr. 2020;Oct 12 (online ahead of print):1–7.
5. Zhang J, Gajjala S, Agrawal P, Tison GH, Hallock LA, Beussink-Nelson L, Lassen MH, Fan E, Aras MA, Jordan C, Fleischmann KE, Melisko M, Qasim A, Shah SJ, Bajcsy R. Fully automated echocardiogram interpretation in clinical practice. Circulation. 2018;138(16):1623–35.
6. Siegersma K, Leiner T, Chew D, Appelman Y, Hofstra L, Verjans J. Artificial intelligence in cardiovascular imaging: state of the art and implications for the imaging cardiologist. Neth Hear J. 2019;27:403–13.

7. Kittanawong C, Zhang H, Wang Z, Aydar M, Kitai T. Artificial intelligenve in precision cardiovascular medicine. J Am Coll Cardiol. 2017;69(21):2657–64.
8. Liao Z, Girgis H, Abdi A, Vaseli H, Hetherington J, Rohling R, Gin K, Tsang T, Abolmaesumi P. On modelling label uncertainty in deep neural networks: automatic estimation of intra-observer variability in 2d echocardiography quality assessment. IEEE Trans Med Imaging. 2020;39(6):1868–83.
9. Madani A, Arnaout R, Mofrad M, Arnaout R. Fast and accurate view classifcation of echocardiograms using deep learning. NPJ Digit Med. 2018;1:6.
10. Kusunose K, Haga A, Inoue M, Fukuda D, Yamada H, Sata M. Clinically feasible and accurate view classifcation of echocardiographic images using deep learning. Biomol Ther. 2020;10(5):665.
11. Wisselink HJ, Pelgrim GJ, Rook M, van den Berge M, Slump K, Nagaraj Y, van Ooijen P, Oudkerk M, Vliegenthart R. Potential for dose reduction in CT emphysema densitometry with post-scan noise reduction: a phantom study. Br J Radiol. 2020;93(1105):20181019.
12. Woltering J, Leiner T, Viergever M, Isgum I. Generative adversarial networks for noise reduction in low-dose CT. IEEE Trans Med Imaging. 2017;36(12):2536–45.
13. Bustin A, Fuin N, Botnar RM, Prieto C. From compressed-sensing to artificial intelligence-based cardiac MRI reconstruction. Front Cardiovasc Med. 2020;7:17.
14. Lekadir K, Leiner T, Young AA, Petersen SE. Editorial: current and future role of artificial intelligence in cardiac imaging. Front Cardiovasc Med. 2020;7:137.
15. Dey D, Slomka PJ, Leeson P, Comaniciu D, Shrestha S, Sengupta PP, Marwick TH. Aritificial intelligence in cardiovascular imaging. J Am Coll Cardiol. 2019;73(11):1317–35.
16. Leclerc S, Smistad E, Pedrosa J, Ostvik A, Cervenansky F, Espinosa F, Espeland T, Berg EAR, Jodoin P-M, Grenier T, Lartizien C, D'hooge J, Lovstakken L, Bernard O. Deep learning for segmentation using an open large-scale dataset in 2D echocardiography. IEEE Trans Med Imaging. 2019;38(9):2198–210.
17. Zreik M, Leiner T, de Vos BD, van Hamersvelt RW, Viergever MA, Isgum I. Automatic segmentation of the left ventricle in cardiac CT angiography using convolutional neural networks. In: 2016 IEEE 13th International Symposium on Biomedical Imaging (ISBI). Prague; 2016.
18. Bratt A, Kim J, Pollie M, Beecy AN, Tehrani NH, Codella N, Perez-Johnston R, Palumbo MC, Alakbarli J, Colizza W, Drexler IR, Azevedo CF, Kim RJ, Devereux RB, Weinsaft J. Machine learning derived segmentation of phase velocity encoded cardiovascular magnetic resonance for fully automated aortic flow quantification. J Cardiovasc Magn Reson. 2019;21(1):1–11.
19. Avendi M, Kheradvar A, Jafarkhani H. A combined deeplearning and deformable-model approach to fully automatic segmentation of the left ventricle in cardiac MRI. Med Image Anal. 2016;30:108–19.
20. Tan LK, Liew YM, Lim E, McLaughlin RA. Convolutional neural network regression for short-axis left ventricle segmentation in cardiac cine MR sequences. Med Image Anal. 2017;39:78–86.
21. Zheng Q, Delingette H, Duchateau N, Ayache N. 3-D consistent and robust segmentation of cardiac images by deep learning with spatial propagation. IEEE Trans Med Imaging. 2018;37(9):2137–48.
22. Ngo TA, Lu Z, Carneiro G. Combining deep learning and levelset for the automated segmentation of the left ventricle of the heart from cardiac cine magnetic resonance. Med Image Anal. 2017;35:159–71.
23. Astudillo P, De Beule M, Dambre J, Mortier P. Towards safe and efficient preoperative planning of transcatheter mitral valve interventions. Morphologie. 2019;103(343):139–47.
24. van Assen M, Martin SS, Varga-Szemes A, Rapaka S, Cimen S, Sharma P, Sahbaee P, De Cecco CN, Vliegenthart R, Leonard TJ, Burt JR, Schoepf UJ. Automatic coronary calcium scoring in chest CT using a deep neural network in direct comparison with non-contrast cardiac CT: a validation study. Eur J Radiol. 2020;21(134):109428.
25. Gharaibeh Y, Prabhu D, Kolluru C, Lee J, Zimin V, Bezerra H, Wilson D. Coronary calcification segmentation in intravascular OCT images using deep learning: application to calcification scoring. J Med Imaging (Bellingham). 2019;6(4):045002.
26. Yang S, Kweon J, Roh J-H, Lee J-H, Kang H, Park L-J, Kim DJ, Yang H, Hur J, Kang D-Y, Lee PH, Ahn J-M, Kang S-J, Park D-W, Lee S-W, Kim Y-H, Lee CW. Deep learning segmentation of major vessels in X-ray coronary angiography. Sci Rep. 2019;9(1):16897.
27. Huang W, Huang L, Lin Z, Huang S, Chi Y, Zhou J, Zhang J, Tan R-S, Zhong L. Coronary artery segmentation by deep learning neural networks on computed tomography coronary angiographic images. Annu Int Conf IEEE Eng Med Biol Soc. 2018;2018:608–11.
28. Cikes M, Sanchez-Martinez S, Claggett B, Duchateau N, Piella G, Butakoff C, Pouleur A, Knappe D, Biering-Sørensen T, Kutyifa V, Moss A, Stein K, Solomon S, Bijnens B. Machine learning-based phenogrouping in heart failure to identify responders to cardiac resynchronization therapy. Eur J Heart Fail. 2018;21:74–85.
29. Shah SJ, Katz DH, Selvaraj S, Burke MA, Yancy CW, Gheorghiade M, Bonow RO, Huang C-C, Deo RC. Phenomapping for novel classification of heart failure with preserved ejection fraction. Circulation. 2015;131:268–79.
30. Tabassian M, Sunderji I, Erdei T, Sanchez-Martinez S, Degiovanni A, Marino P, Fraser AG, D'hooge J. Diagnosis of heart failure with preserved ejection fraction: machine learning of spatiotemporal variations in left ventricular deformation. J Am Soc Echocardiogr. 2018;31(12):1272–84.
31. Asch FM, Poilvert N, Abraham T, Jankowski M, Cleve J, Adams M, Romano N, Hong H, Mor-Avi V, Martin RP, Lang RM. Automated echocardiographic quantifcation of left ventricular ejection fraction without volume measurements using a machine learning algorithm mimicking a human expert. Circ Cardiovasc Imaging. 2020;12(9):e009303.
32. Kusunose K, Haga A, Yamaguchi N, Abe T, Fukuda D, Yamada H, Harada M, Sata M. Deep learning for assessment of left ventricular ejection fraction from echocardiographic images. J Am Soc Echocardiogr. 2020;33(5):632–5.
33. Moghaddasi H, Nourian S. Automatic assessment of mitral regurgitation severity based on extensive textural features on 3D echocardiography videos. Comput Biol Med. 2016;73:47–55.
34. Tabassian M, Alessandrini M, Herbots L, Mirea O, Pagourelias E, Jasaityte R, Engvall J, De Marchi L, Masetti G, D'hooge J. Machine learning of the spatio-temporal characteristics of echocardiographic deformation curves for infarct classification. Int J Cardiovasc Imaging. 2017;33:1159–67.
35. Sudarshan Vidya K, Ng E, Rajendra Acharya U, Meng Chou S, San Tan R, Ghista DN. Computer-aided diagnosis of myocardial infarction using ultrasound images with DWT, GLCM and HOS methods: a comparative study. Comput Biol Med. 2015;62:86–93.
36. Kusunose K, Abe T, Haga A, Fukuda D, Yamada H, Harada M, Sata M. A deep learning approach for assessment of regional wall motion abnormality from echocardiographic images. JACC Cardiovasc Imaging. 2020;13(2 Pt 1):374–81.
37. Omar H, Domingos JS, Patra A, Upton R, Leeson P, Noble JA. Quantifcation of cardiac bull's-eye map based on principal strain analysis for myocardial wall motion assessment in stress echocardiography. In: 2018 IEEE 15th International Symposium on Biomedical Imaging (ISBI 2018). Washington, DC; 2018.
38. Raghavendra U, Fujita H, Gundigar A, Shetty R, Nayak K, Pai U, Samath J, Acharya UR. Automated technique for coronary artery disease characterization and classification using DD-DTDWT in ultrasound images. Biomed Signal Process Control. 2018;40:324–34.
39. Bai W, Sinclair M, Tarroni G, Oktay O, Rajchl M, Vaillant G, Lee AM, Aung N, Lukaschuk E, Sanghvi MM, Zemrak F, Fung K, Paiva

JM, Carapella V, Kim YJ, Suzuki H. Automated cardiovascular magnetic resonance image analysis with fully convolutional networks. J Cardiovasc Magn Reson. 2018;20(65):1–12.

40. Suinesiaputra A, Sanghvi MM, Aung N, Paiva JM, Zemrak F, Fung K, Lukaschuk E, Lee AM, Carapella V, Kim YJ, Francis J, Piechnik SK, Neubauer S, Greiser A, Jolly M-P. Fully-automated left ventricular mass and volume MRI analysis in the UK Biobank population cohort: evaluation of initial results. Int J Cardiovasc Imaging. 2018;34(2):281–91.
41. Wolterink JM, Leiner T, Takx RA, Viergever MA, Isgum I. Automatic coronary calcium scoring in non-contrast-enhanced ECG-triggered cardiac CT with ambiguity detection. IEEE Trans Med Imaging. 2015;34(9):1867–78.
42. Dey D, Gaur S, Ovrehus KA, Slomka PJ, Betancur J, Goeller M, Hell MM, Gransar H, Berman DS, Achenbach S, Botker HE, Jensen JM, Lassen JF, Norgaard BL. Integrated prediction of lesion-specific ischaemia from quantitative coronary CT angiography using machine learning: a multicentre study. Eur Radiol. 2018;28(6):2655–64.
43. Zreik M, van Hamersvelt RW, Wolterink JM, Leiner T, Viergever MA, Isgum I. A recurrent CNN for automatic detection and classification of coronary artery plaque and stenosis in coronary CT angiography. IEEE Trans Med Imaging. 2019;38(7):1588–98.
44. Itu L, Rapaka S, Passerini T, Georgescu B, Schwemmer C, Schoebinger M, Flohr T, Sharma P, Comaniciu D. A machine-learning approach for computation of fractional flow reserve from coronary computed tomography. J Appl Physiol. 2016;121(1):42–52.
45. Coenen A, Kim Y-H, Kruk M, Tesche C, De Geer J, Kurata A, Lubbers ML, Daemen J, Itu L, Rapaka S, Sharma P, Schwemmer C, Persson A, Schoepf UJ, Kepka C, Yang D. Diagnostic accuracy of a machine-learning approach to coronary computed tomographic angiography-based fractional flow reserve result from the MACHINE Consortium. Circ Cardiovasc Imaging. 2018;11(6):e007217.
46. Goodfellow IJ, Pouget-Abadie J, Mirza M, Xu B, Warde-Farley D, Ozair S, Courville A, Bengio Y. Generative adverserial networks. 10 June 2014. [Online]. Available: https://arxiv.org/abs/1406.2661. Accessed 17 Nov 2020.
47. Diller G-P, Vahle J, Radke R, Benesch Vidal ML, Fischer AJ, Bauer UM, Sarikouch S, Berger F, Beerbaum P, Baumgartner H, Orwat S. Utility of deep learning networks for the generation of artificial cardiac magnetic resonance images in congenital heart disease. BMC Med Imaging. 2020;20:113.
48. Chen L, Liang X, Shen C, Jiang S, Wang J. Synthetic CT generation from CBCT images via deep learning. Med Phys. 2019;47(3):1115–25.
49. Santini G, Zumbo LM, Martini N, Valvano G, Leo A, Ripoli A, Avogliero F, Chiappino D, Della Latta D. Synthetic contrast enhancement in cardiac CT with deep learning. 2 July 2019. [Online]. Available: https://arxiv.org/pdf/1807.01779.pdf. Accessed 17 Nov 2020.
50. Motwani M, Dey D, Berman DS, Germano G, Achenbach S, Al-Mallah M, Adreini D, Budoff MK, Cademartiri F, Callister TQ, Chang H-J, Chinnaiyan K, Chow BJ, Cury R, Dey D. Machine learning for prediction of all-causemortality in patients with suspected coronary artery disease: a 5-year multicentre prospective registry analysis. Eur Heart J. 2017;38(7):500–7.
51. van Rosendael AR, Maliakal G, Kolli KK, Beecy A, Al'Aref SJ, Dwivedi A, Singh G, Panday M, Kumar A, Ma X, Achenbach S, Al-Mallah MH, Andreini D, Bax JJ, Berman DS. Maximization of the usage of coronary CTA derived plaque information using a machine learning based algorithm to improve risk stratification; insights from the CONFIRM registry. J Cardiovasc Comput Tomogr. 2018;12(3):204–9.
52. Dawes TJ, de Marvao A, Shi W, Fletcher T, Watson GM, Wharton J, Rhodes CJ, Howard LS, Gibbs JSR, Rueckert D, Cook SA, Wilkins MR, O'Regan DP. Machine learning of three-dimensional right ventricular motion enables outcome prediction in pulmonary hypertension: a cardiac MR imaging study. Radiology. 2017;283(2):381–90.
53. Samad MD, Whener GJ, Arbabshirani MR, Jing L, Powell AJ, Geva T, Haggerty CM, Fornwalt BK. Predicting deterioration of ventricular function in patients with repaired tetralogy of Fallot using machine learning. Eur Heart J Cardiovasc Imaging. 2018;19(7):730–8.
54. Biondetti GP, Gauriau R, Bridge CP, Lu C, Andriole KP. "Name that manufacturer". Relating image acquisition bias with taks complexity when training deep learning models: experiments on head CT. 19 August 2020. [Online]. Available: https://arxiv.org/abs/2008.08525. Accessed 20 Nov 2020.
55. Benjamins J, Hendriks T, Knuuti J, Juarez-Orozco L, van der Harst P. A primer in artificial intelligence in cardiovascular medicine. Neth Heart J. 2019;27:392–402.

Data Preparation for Artificial Intelligence

4

Aline L. de Araujo, Cailin Hardell, Wojciech A. Koszek, Jie Wu, and Martin J. Willemink

Introduction

Artificial intelligence (AI) is broadly defined as the development of computerized systems, which are able to perform tasks that normally need human intelligence. It is well known that AI has tremendous potential in the medical imaging space [1]. Machine learning (ML) and deep learning (DL) models in cardiovascular imaging have been developed for three purposes: (i) to improve workflow in radiology, (ii) to assist the radiologist by automating specific tasks, and (iii) to assist the radiologists and clinicians by quantifying specific imaging features. An example for workflow improvements includes lowering or eliminating gadolinium dose for cardiac magnetic resonance imaging (MRI) [2]. An example for automatic tasks for assisting radiologists includes automatic segmentation of the left cardiac ventricle from cardiac cine MRI exams [3, 4]. An example of automatic image quantification includes coronary artery calcium quantification on non-contrast cardiac computed tomography (CT) [5]. Even though there are many potentially interesting applications of ML/DL models in cardiovascular imaging, the deployment in the clinical setting of these models is limited. A multiple of reasons hinders the implementation of ML/DL models in clinical practice, such as regulatory challenges. The biggest obstacle for model implementation is the lack of available well-curated imaging data for training, validation, and testing of cardiovascular ML/DL models [6].

A. L. de Araujo, MD, PhD
Segmed, Inc, Menlo Park, CA, USA

Department of Ophthalmology and Visual Sciences, Universidade Federal de São Paulo, São Paulo, Brazil
e-mail: aline@segmed.ai

C. Hardell, MS · W. A. Koszek, MS · J. Wu, PhD
Segmed, Inc, Menlo Park, CA, USA
e-mail: cailin@segmed.ai; adam@segmed.ai; jie@segmed.ai

M. J. Willemink, MD, PhD (✉)
Segmed, Inc, Menlo Park, CA, USA

Department of Radiology, Stanford University School of Medicine, Stanford, CA, USA
e-mail: willemink@stanford.edu

Currently, access to medical image data is limited for the majority of academic researchers and industry companies. This is especially true for high-quality well-curated medical imaging datasets. Datasets with smaller sample sizes are oftentimes used, even though these data lack diversity in terms of geography, scanner/machine type, and race/ethnicity, which hinders generalizability and accurate clinical performance of ML/DL models [7]. Datasets with a smaller sample size are oftentimes sufficient for the development of ML/DL models in an academic research setting. However, for the development of commercial and clinically used ML/DL models, larger datasets with heterogeneous data are essential. Large datasets are needed for clinical ML/DL model development [8].

Many medical centers do not have the means to share a large amount of medical imaging data. One of the main issues is that medical data oftentimes is stored in isolated silos and it is difficult to extract the right information. This is suboptimal for the development of medical imaging DL/ML models, as the data is inaccessible to technical developers. Simply allowing these technical developers to gain access to the medical data is not sufficient for adequate ML/DL model development. In addition to getting access, it is essential that data is curated, analyzed, and labeled before it can be used for clinically relevant ML/DL models.

In this chapter, we explain the process of gaining ethical approval, access to the data, querying the right data, de-identification of data, transferring data, controlling the quality, structuring the data, and finally labeling the data. We provide an in-depth overview of multiple strategies to share data in a responsible way, resulting in impactful cardiovascular applications of ML/DL models (Fig. 4.1).

Sources of Data

Before diving into the process of preparing medical imaging data originating at the local hospital or imaging center of the ML/DL developer, it is important to note that there are other

C. N. De Cecco et al. (eds.), *Artificial Intelligence in Cardiothoracic Imaging*, Contemporary Medical Imaging,
https://doi.org/10.1007/978-3-030-92087-6_4

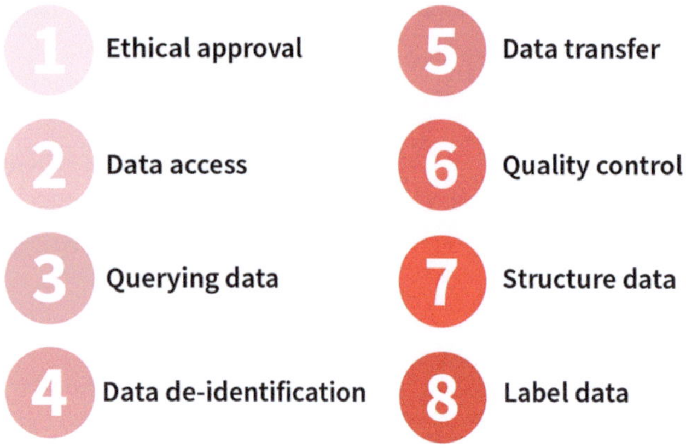

Fig. 4.1 Different steps to be taken to prepare medical imaging data for machine learning and deep learning

sources of data. Some academic institutions have made medical imaging data available to the public. These datasets range from breast imaging [9, 10], neuroradiology [11–16], chest X-rays [17, 18], and musculoskeletal radiology [19]. To the best of our knowledge, there are not many cardiovascular imaging datasets publicly available. While making datasets publicly available is a trend that will help further the ML/DL field, these public datasets are associated with limitations. Most importantly, the quality of public data is not optimal. The variety in dataset size, availability of metadata (DICOM headers), and clinical information is substantial. Moreover, datasets are oftentimes based on relatively old trials, resulting in images acquired on older hardware. Labeling images is a time-intensive and expensive process, and therefore, many datasets lack expert labels. Sample sizes of these public datasets are generally relatively small, which is not problematic for academic research projects. However, if an ML/DL model is intended to be made commercially available or clinically applied, public datasets are oftentimes not sufficient. Moreover, public datasets are often not allowed to be used for commercial applications, and the competitive advantage of public datasets is limited.

Another option is to gather fully de-identified datasets by partnering with multiple institutions. While this is a time-intensive process, there are platforms in development where a variety of hospitals and imaging clinics share fully de-identified datasets, which allows for affordable, high-quality, and heterogeneous datasets [20].

In the remainder of this chapter, the process of preparing cardiothoracic imaging data within the researcher's own hospital or clinic is described.

Ethical Approval

The first step that is necessary before cardiovascular imaging data can be accessed for training, validation, and testing of ML/DL models is to gain ethical approval. For each involved hospital, approval from the local institutional review board (IRB) is required. First, an IRB proposal needs to be written, which is evaluated by the IRB committee. The proposal needs to describe what the risks and benefits of the proposed project entail, and the committee will approve the study if the benefits outweigh the risks. Most often, researchers design a retrospective study, which means that existing data is used for ML/DL model development. Patients who participate in retrospective studies do not need to undergo additional exams or procedures because the data was already collected before. Therefore, explicit informed consent is usually waived by the IRB committee for retrospective studies. In contrast, if data is going to be collected in the future—in other words, the study has a prospective design—the IRB committee will require informed consent from each study participant.

After the IRB committee approves the study, the next steps are to access, query, de-identify, transfer, quality control, structure, and label the data. This is needed to structure the data into machine-readable formats [21].

Data Access

Generally, AI engineers are located outside the hospital, resulting in limited or no access to medical imaging data stored in picture archiving and communication systems (PACS). This is especially the case for AI engineers who work at commercial companies. In contrast, only accredited professionals generally have access to PACS. These professionals include radiologists and other physicians (e.g., cardiologists, oncologists, etc.), radiology technicians, PACS managers, and clinical researchers. Permitting AI engineers to access medical imaging data can be challenging and requires a multiple step approach. Ideally, there should be a collaborative environment in which clinical professionals and AI engineers work together on premises (within the hospital) or with a research agreement allowing to share data.

Querying Data

After all essential members of the AI development team have gained access to the data, the next step is to identify the needed data to solve the problem. Current clinical systems were built with clinical practice in mind. In clinical practice, images obtained from imaging equipment end up in PACS and Vendor neutral archive (VNA) systems and are destined to be accessed several times in the lifetime of an imaging study. These systems provide a limited level of searchability because doctors usually pull data from a system based on protected health information (PHI) features such as a name or last name of a patient. In turn, the level of searchability required for the purposes of assembly of an ML/DL dataset is outside of the specifications of any clinical data system. Obtaining data is hindered by PACS/VNA vendors too. Their solutions for clinical practice often prohibit programmatic access to the images, which make data export operation difficult or impossible.

Limited search strategies are available to find medical imaging and clinical data. PACS and/or radiology information systems (RIS) generally allow for basic search (e.g., patient name, date of birth, or medical record number). However, systematic searching and data extraction from PACS and electronic medical records (EMR) are often limited. Queries for identifying relevant data for ML/DL model development usually include more advanced strings (words or short sentences), current procedural terminology (CPT) codes, and international classification of disease codes (ICD-10). Some commercially available PACS systems allow their users to search through metadata, which can include annotations, number of series, number of images, and acquisition parameters.

Identifying relevant data for ML/DL model development may thus be difficult. Specific techniques are being evaluated and developed, including natural language processing (NLP) techniques, which will be discussed later in this chapter.

After identifying the correct information, data can often be exported and subsequently managed with other systems [22]. If PACS or RIS search engines are not sufficient, commercial and noncommercial software packages are available that allow for a simplified data querying process [23–25].

De-identification

Independent whether a prospective or retrospective study design is used, it is recommended both by the US Health Insurance Portability and Accountability Act (HIPAA) and the General Data Protection Regulation (GDPR) in Europe that medical imaging data are fully de-identified before they are used to train, validate, or test DL/ML models. The aim of de-identification is to make it impossible to reidentify the specific patient based on the provided data and to not taint the model gradients with PHI features. In order to do this, sensitive information, which is also referred to as PHI, needs to be removed from the data. PHI includes the following [26]:

- Patient name
- Patient address (all geographic subdivisions smaller than state, including street address, city, county, and zip code)
- All elements (except years) of dates related to an individual (including date of birth, hospital admission date, hospital discharge date, date of death, and exact age if older than 89 years)
- Telephone and fax numbers
- E-mail address
- Social Security number
- Medical record number
- Health plan beneficiary number
- Account number
- Certificate or license number
- Any vehicle or other device serial number
- Device identifiers and serial numbers
- Web URL
- Internet Protocol (IP) address
- Finger- or voice print
- Photographic image (not limited to the face)
- Any other characteristic that could uniquely identify the individual

Some of these PHI parameters are commonly present in the headers (or metadata) of DICOM files. Removing PHI parameters from DICOM headers is relatively easy. Multiple open source and commercial tools are available to remove PHI from DICOM headers [27, 28]. The specific DICOM tags that include sensitive information (such as the earlier mentioned PHI features) could be fully removed, or the information could be changed. For example, a medical record number could be changed to "studyname_patient_001." The Radiological Society of North America Clinical Trial Processor and the Cancer Imaging Archive defined profiles for de-identification of DICOM headers for multiple applications [29]. Unfortunately, PHI can also be present in other parts of medical imaging data. While it is relatively easy to remove sensitive information from DICOM metadata, it is much more difficult to remove this if embedded (or burned) into the images or if the metadata is stored in the wrong DICOM tag. This may, for example, be the case with echocardiography exams or scanned non-digital radiographs. Although this is not specifically a substantial problem for cardiovascular imaging, this problem may still occur in these data types. In order to remove this embedded PHI from the images, more advanced methods of de-identification are needed. More advanced methods include optical character recognition (OCR) [30] and evaluation of human observers to recognize handwritten information (which often is not recognized by automatic OCR methods). One must be cautious if mixing different data sets since the potential risk of reidentification increases with multiple data types by cross linking of unrelated data [31]. A potential solution is de-identification of medical data through k-anonymity methods. These are more advanced methods that transform original data sets which contain PHI into anonymous datasets, allowing for protection of the identity of patients [32]. To be fully sure that no PHI is present in DICOM headers, the full metadata information is often removed. This is essential for data that is made publicly available. In these cases, the DICOM headers are commonly completely removed, or the DICOM files are converted to other file formats including Neuroimaging Informatics Technology Initiative (NIFTI) files. With these files, the pixel/voxel information and patient position are retained, but otherwise no PHI is present. One should keep in mind that removing DICOM headers is beneficial in terms of patient privacy and potential data breaches; however, the value of the data does reduce since DICOM metadata contains information that could have been used as input for DL/ML models.

PHI can be present in ways other than in DICOM metadata and embedded into images. A frequently overlooked form of PHI includes photographs of specific identifiable body parts such as the face, as well as other parameters such as biometric information (e.g., a scan of the retina or fingerprints). In radiology, it is important to realize that a three-dimensional reconstruction of a head and neck CT exam may contain facial characteristics that may allow reidentification of the patient. One should thus be careful with specific body parts, especially if data is made publicly available. In cardiothoracic imaging, this is not as big of a problem since reidentification of the chest and abdomen is much harder than for other body parts such as the face.

Data Transfer and Storage

After imaging data are properly de-identified, the next step is to transfer and store the images. Data transfer can be done either to a local data storage or to an external data storage. For single-center studies, mostly a local data storage is used since only local researchers need access to the data. Local data are generally stored at an on-premise server, which has the advantage of relatively safe data storage (if encrypted properly) and availability of the data. However, sharing images with external institutions or researchers is limited. For multicenter and commercial ML/DL model development, data are usually transferred to an external data storage to allow multiple researchers and ML/DL developers to work with the data. Oftentimes, cloud-based storage is used, which is becoming more and more secure, and allows for sharing data between researchers at different locations, and it also provides a secure backup opportunity. The major disadvantages of cloud-based storage include the need for expertise in cloud-environment configuration and relatively high costs, and a fast Internet connection is needed.

Quality Control

Generally, medical data are known for being unstructured. In that sense, medical imaging data are not different from other medical data. Once the data is transferred and stored, the next step is to evaluate the quality of the data. It is important to evaluate quality to better understand the data and the influence of the quality on potential DL/ML model performance. For example, if the aim is to develop an algorithm to automatically segment the left ventricle on coronary CT angiography exams, it is essential to know whether the images are acquired with electrocardiography (ECG) synchronization, and if so, whether a retrospectively gated or prospectively triggered protocol was applied. Also, it would be good to randomly assess the image quality of some images, to evaluate both the objective image quality (e.g. noise and contrast-to-noise ratio) and subjective image quality (e.g., the presence of cardiac motion artifacts). Quality control is often done in a randomized way and on a case-by-case basis. This makes quality control an expensive process. To do quality control at scale, more advanced (machine learning) algorithms are needed.

Another aspect of quality is the diversity of the dataset. To improve the generalizability of the developed ML/DL model, it is essential to have a diverse dataset in terms of geography, population (race, ethnicity, gender), and scanner/machine types. By using a diverse dataset, the risk of inducing bias in the developed ML/DL model will be reduced.

Structure Data

Medical imaging and clinical data are quite abundant, but in their native sources, they are mostly heterogeneous, unstructured, and unlabeled. Unstructured data pose a challenge for AI development since current supervised and semi-supervised machine learning techniques operate on structured data [21]. Therefore, dealing with unstructured data is a fundamental part of data preparation for ML/DL model development.

In healthcare, unstructured data is found in clinical texts such as radiology reports, pathology reports, and electronic health records. It is estimated that over 40% of the data in healthcare record systems are text [33]. Clinical text contains non-word tokens, abbreviations, domain-specific acronyms, and jargon, all of which makes it difficult to process this type of text with standard automatic tools. Clinical narratives intended for internal use and written under time pressure, such as clinical notes, contain substantial amounts of noise, including misspellings and incomplete sentences. Additionally, physicians' notes reflect their clinical reasoning that speculates possible diagnosis, or findings that cannot be excluded (e.g., "Possible myocardial infarction," "Neoplasia is suspected"). Negations are also very common for signs, symptoms, and diagnoses (e.g., "No history of cough," "Consolidation is absent"). Special attention should be given when extracting negated terms from clinical text, since false-positive labels can inadvertently be created.

Radiology reports are more carefully written than clinical notes because they are intended for an external audience. They are organized in a standard fashion, which includes a heading for the study modality and protocol, semi-headings for the anatomic structure being described, and an impression or conclusion at the end. This semi-structured format can be helpful when extracting data from radiology reports.

Natural language processing (NLP) can be used to automate clinical text classification by extracting structured information from the narratives. NLP is a computer-based approach that analyzes free-form text or speech with a set of theories and technologies, including linguistics and statistical methods, to convert the text into a structured format of hierarchically itemized elements [34]. The text becomes more easily queried and manipulated. Rule-based classification is then applied to extract information such as the presence or stage of a disease. The simplest approach is to apply a logic rule that resolves "true" when a report contains a combination of clinical findings. For example, if an NLP system identifies a significant stenosis in a cardiac computed tomography angiography report, the exam may be classified positive for myocardial infarction. These clinical rules are developed manually on the basis of expert knowledge. As such, they are labor intensive and cumbersome to generate, since they must comprise a multitude of concepts and their combinations [35, 36].

Rule-based algorithms are usually based on keywords. Word embeddings can significantly leverage the use of keywords. Embeddings project semantically similar terms into nearby points in a vector space [37]. For instance, an initial term is expanded into multiple terms, and any of the expanded terms is then used to classify the data. Clinical ontologies systems such as SNOMED CT [38] and Unified Medical Language System (UMLS) [39] integrate and distribute key terminology, classification, and coding standards that can be applied for queries and data classification. Therefore, deep representation using word embeddings enables ML methods to learn extra patterns from weakly labeled data, and it has been shown to outperform rule-based NLP systems when extracting structure data from clinical narratives [36].

More advanced techniques like GloVe [40] and word2vec [41] rely on unsupervised machine learning models to cluster semantic terms. Such models learn word associations and create a semantic dictionary from the text they are trained on. A hybrid method combining semantic-dictionary mapping and word2vec achieved high accuracy in classifying chest CT reports. Their target was to extract pulmonary embolism information from the free text. The hybrid method classified the reports in pulmonary embolism present or absent, acute or chronic pulmonary embolism, and central or subsegmental pulmonary embolism with a precision of over 97% for each task [42].

Label Data

Most currently developed ML/DL models for cardiovascular imaging are based on supervised learning. With supervised learning, ML/DL models are trained, validated, and tested with a ground truth that is linked to the medical imaging data. True ground truth information is based on the reference (or gold) standard for a specific disease. For example, for an algorithm that tries to automatically determine the relevance of a coronary luminal stenosis on a coronary CT angiography exam, the ground truth could be the fractional flow reserve as determined by invasive angiography. The ground truth may also be based on annotations performed by medical experts (e.g., radiologists or cardiologists). For certain diagnoses, medical imaging alone is considered the ground truth, such as for aortic dissection that is diagnosed on CT angiography. However, many diseases need more information than can be found in just imaging exams. If a true ground truth is not available, oftentimes other kinds of labels are used. Most commonly, images are labeled or segmented by medical experts. This can be done either prospectively (with clinical information being present) or retrospectively (only limited information is present); see Fig. 4.2. Selecting the right label for each ML/DL algorithm requires choosing the right balance between identifying appropriate discriminating categories (e.g., normal versus abnormal) and relevant clinical granularity (e.g., a specific type of cardiomyopathy). While only using medical images (without clinical information or labels) may be sufficient for the development of

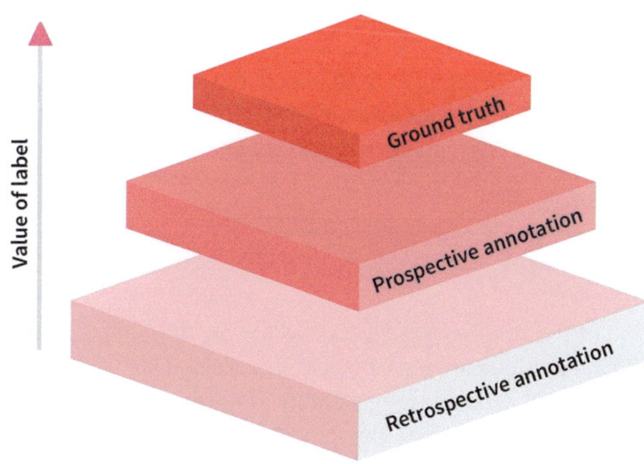

Fig. 4.2 Value of labels ranges from low for retrospective annotations, to medium for prospective annotation, to high for labels based on ground truth information

ML/DL models that improve image quality, the development of diagnostic models generally requires a consensus diagnosis from experts, image-based segmentations of organs or lesions, or a label based on imaging features or clinical information [1]. Gathering clinical information for many patients is known as electronic phenotyping [6, 10].

One way to (semi)automatically extract clinically relevant labels is by using natural language processing on the text in radiology reports. One of the most used natural language processing methods is topic modeling. With topic modeling, data set insights are provided by creating a summary of a dataset consisting of a large amount of text, for example, the radiology reports of coronary CT angiography may be associated with keywords such as "CTA," "cardiac," "coronary," and "stenosis." Recurrent neural networks are another architecture class that is used often for radiology report data extraction. These are models based on neural networks that are trained on a relatively small set of reports, while performances are similar to more traditional natural language processing methods [43, 44]. The strength of recurrent neural networks is that negative words (e.g., "No") do not have to be in close proximity to the target word in a sentence. For example, "No evidence can be found on this exam for significant coronary stenosis," the "no" is relatively far away from the target "stenosis." While picking up the relevant information in this example may be difficult for traditional natural language processing methods, recurrent neural networks perform better in these circumstances. One should note, however, that error rates of both natural language processing techniques as well as in the original radiology reports may decrease the quality of these (semi)automatically extracted labels. Radiology reports are usually unstructured and not created for developing ML/DL models. This may result in relatively low quality (or noisy) labels. This is an important issue since the estimated demonstrable error rate of radiology reports is approximately 2–20%. A solution could be the implementation of structured reporting, which is gaining interest in the medical imaging community. An example of structured reporting in cardiovascular imaging includes the Coronary Artery Disease Reporting and Data System (CAD-RADS) [45, 46].

Conclusion

One of the most important hurdles for the development and clinical implementation of machine learning (ML) and deep learning (DL) models is availability of medical imaging data. This chapter describes the process of preparing medical imaging data for ML/DL development, which consists of eight steps: ethical approval, data access, querying data, data de-identification, data transfer, quality control, structure data, and label data.

References

1. Langlotz CP, Allen B, Erickson BJ, et al. A roadmap for foundational research on artificial intelligence in medical imaging: from the 2018 NIH/RSNA/ACR/The Academy Workshop. Radiology. 2019;291:781–91.
2. Zhang N, Yang G, Gao Z, et al. Deep learning for diagnosis of chronic myocardial infarction on nonenhanced cardiac cine MRI. Radiology. 2019;291:606–17.
3. Tao Q, Yan W, Wang Y, et al. Deep learning–based method for fully automatic quantification of left ventricle function from cine MR images: a multivendor, multicenter study. Radiology. 2019;290:81–8.
4. Ngo TA, Lu Z, Carneiro G. Combining deep learning and level set for the automated segmentation of the left ventricle of the heart from cardiac cine magnetic resonance. Med Image Anal. 2017;35:159–71.
5. de Vos BD, Wolterink JM, Leiner T, de Jong PA, Lessmann N, Isgum I. Direct automatic coronary calcium scoring in cardiac and chest CT. IEEE Trans Med Imaging. 2019;38:2127–38.
6. Willemink MJ, Koszek WA, Hardell C, Wu J, Fleischmann D, Harvey H, Folio LR, Summers RM, Rubin DL, Lungren MP. Preparing medical· imaging data for machine learning. Radiology. 2020;295:4–15.
7. Soffer S, Ben-Cohen A, Shimon O, Amitai MM, Greenspan H, Klang E. Convolutional neural networks for radiologic images: a radiologist's guide. Radiology. 2019;290:590–606.
8. Park SH, Han K. Methodologic guide for evaluating clinical performance and effect of artificial intelligence technology for medical diagnosis and prediction. Radiology. 2018;286:800–9.
9. Xi P, Shu C, Goubran R. Abnormality detection in mammography using deep convolutional neural networks. In: 2018 IEEE international symposium on medical measurements and applications (MeMeA). Rome, Italy: IEEE. 2018. p. 1–6.
10. Lee RS, Gimenez F, Hoogi A, Miyake KK, Gorovoy M, Rubin DL. A curated mammography data set for use in computer-aided detection and diagnosis research. Sci Data. 2017;4:170177.
11. Bakas S, Akbari H, Sotiras A, Bilello M, Rozycki M, Kirby JS, Freymann JB, Farahani K, Davatzikos C. Advancing the cancer genome atlas glioma MRI collections with expert segmentation labels and radiomic features. Sci Data. 2017;4:170117.
12. Di Martino A, Yan C-G, Li Q, et al. The autism brain imaging data exchange: towards a large-scale evaluation of the intrinsic brain architecture in autism. Mol Psychiatry. 2014;19:659–67.
13. Jack CR Jr, Bernstein MA, Fox NC, et al. The Alzheimer's disease neuroimaging initiative (ADNI): MRI methods. J Magn Reson Imaging. 2008;27:685–91.
14. Mennes M, Biswal BB, Castellanos FX, Milham MP. Making data sharing work: the FCP/INDI experience. NeuroImage. 2013;82:683–91.
15. Menze BH, Jakab A, Bauer S, et al. The multimodal brain tumor image segmentation benchmark (BRATS). IEEE Trans Med Imaging. 2015;34:1993–2024.
16. Van Essen DC, Smith SM, Barch DM, Behrens TEJ, Yacoub E, Ugurbil K, WU-Minn HCP Consortium. The WU-Minn Human Connectome project: an overview. NeuroImage. 2013;80:62–79.
17. Wang X, Peng Y, Lu L, Lu Z, Bagheri M, Summers RM. ChestX-Ray8: hospital-scale chest X-ray database and benchmarks on weakly-supervised classification and localization of common thorax diseases. In: 2017 IEEE conference on computer vision and pattern recognition (CVPR). 2017. https://doi.org/10.1109/cvpr.2017.369.
18. Irvin J, Rajpurkar P, Ko M, et al. CheXpert: a large chest radiograph dataset with uncertainty labels and expert comparison. 2019. arXiv 1901.07031.

19. Bien N, Rajpurkar P, Ball RL, et al. Deep-learning-assisted diagnosis for knee magnetic resonance imaging: development and retrospective validation of MRNet. PLoS Med. 2018;15:e1002699.
20. Segmed. In: Segmed. https://www.segmed.ai/. Accessed 29 Nov 2020.
21. Harvey H, Glocker B. A standardised approach for preparing imaging data for machine learning tasks in radiology. In: Ranschaert ER, Morozov S, Algra PR, editors. Artificial intelligence in medical imaging: opportunities, applications and risks. Cham: Springer International Publishing; 2019. p. 61–72.
22. Goyal N, Apolo AB, Berman ED, Bagheri MH, Levine JE, Glod JW, Kaplan RN, Machado LB, Folio LR. ENABLE (Exportable Notation and Bookmark List Engine): an interface to manage tumor measurement data from PACS to cancer databases. J Digit Imaging. 2017;30:275–86.
23. Illuminate. In: Illuminate. Instant access to actionable data. https://goilluminate.com/solution/insight/. Accessed 28 Nov 2020.
24. Improved outcomes with mPower clinical analytics. In: Nuance communications. https://www.nuance.com/content/dam/nuance/en_us/collateral/healthcare/data-sheet/ds-mpower-clinical-analytics-en-us.pdf. Accessed 28 Nov 2020.
25. STAnford Research Repository (STARR). In: Stanford Research Informatics Center. https://med.stanford.edu/starr-tools.html. Accessed 28 Nov 2020.
26. The Health Insurance Portability and Accountability Act (HIPAA). 2004.
27. Aryanto KYE, Oudkerk M, van Ooijen PMA. Free DICOM de-identification tools in clinical research: functioning and safety of patient privacy. Eur Radiol. 2015;25:3685–95.
28. Segmed Conphidence. In: Segmed Conphidence. https://www.segmed.ai/segmed-deid. Accessed 5 Dec 2020.
29. Moore SM, Maffitt DR, Smith KE, Kirby JS, Clark KW, Freymann JB, Vendt BA, Tarbox LR, Prior FW. De-identification of medical images with retention of scientific research value. Radiographics. 2015;35:727–35.
30. De-identifying DICOM data. In: Google Cloud. 2019. https://cloud.google.com/healthcare/docs/how-tos/dicom-deidentify. Accessed 29 Nov 2020.
31. Price WN 2nd, Cohen IG. Privacy in the age of medical big data. Nat Med. 2019;25:37–43.
32. El Emam K, Dankar FK. Protecting privacy using k-anonymity. J Am Med Inform Assoc. 2008;15:627–37.
33. Dalianis H. Clinical text mining: secondary use of electronic patient records. Springer Nature: Switzerland; 2018.
34. Cai T, Giannopoulos AA, Yu S, Kelil T, Ripley B, Kumamaru KK, Rybicki FJ, Mitsouras D. Natural language processing technologies in radiology research and clinical applications. Radiographics. 2016;36:176–91.
35. Wang Y, Mehrabi S, Sohn S, Atkinson EJ, Amin S, Liu H. Natural language processing of radiology reports for identification of skeletal site-specific fractures. BMC Med Inform Decis Mak. 2019;19:73.
36. Wang Y, Sohn S, Liu S, Shen F, Wang L, Atkinson EJ, Amin S, Liu H. A clinical text classification paradigm using weak supervision and deep representation. BMC Med Inform Decis Mak. 2019;19:1.
37. Ye C, Fabbri D. Extracting similar terms from multiple EMR-based semantic embeddings to support chart reviews. J Biomed Inform. 2018;83:63–72.
38. Willett DL, Kannan V, Chu L, et al. SNOMED CT Concept hierarchies for sharing definitions of clinical conditions using electronic health record data. Appl Clin Inform. 2018;9:667–82.
39. Bodenreider O. The Unified Medical Language System (UMLS): integrating biomedical terminology. Nucleic Acids Res. 2004;32:D267–70.
40. Pennington J, Socher R, Manning CD. Glove: global vectors for word representation. In: Proceedings of the 2014 conference on empirical methods in natural language processing (EMNLP). 2014. aclweb.org. p. 1532–43.
41. Mikolov T, Chen K, Corrado G, Dean J. Efficient estimation of word representations in vector space. arXiv [cs.CL]. 2013.
42. Banerjee I, Chen MC, Lungren MP, Rubin DL. Radiology report annotation using intelligent word embeddings: applied to multi-institutional chest CT cohort. J Biomed Inform. 2018;77:11–20.
43. Banerjee I, Ling Y, Chen MC, et al. Comparative effectiveness of convolutional neural network (CNN) and recurrent neural network (RNN) architectures for radiology text report classification. Artif Intell Med. 2019;97:79–88.
44. Choi E, Schuetz A, Stewart WF, Sun J. Using recurrent neural network models for early detection of heart failure onset. J Am Med Inform Assoc. 2017;24:361–70.
45. Cury RC, Abbara S, Achenbach S, et al. CAD-RADSTM Coronary Artery Disease – Reporting and Data System. An expert consensus document of the Society of Cardiovascular Computed Tomography (SCCT), the American College of Radiology (ACR) and the North American Society for Cardiovascular Imaging (NASCI). Endorsed by the American College of Cardiology. J Cardiovasc Comput Tomogr. 2016;10:269–81.
46. Clunie DA. DICOM structured reporting. PixelMed Publishing: Bangor, PA; 2000.

Data Storage, Cloud Usage and Artificial Intelligence Pipeline

5

Peter M. A. van Ooijen, Erfan Darzi, and Andre Dekker

Introduction

It is a well-known fact that artificial intelligence (AI) performance depends heavily on the availability of data and the corresponding annotations or labels that define the ground truth about the (clinical) question at hand. To obtain this data, they need to be made available by multiple institutions geographically distributed all over the world. One option is to centralize data, which not only requires de-identification of this data but also an informed consent that includes the possibility of distribution and sharing of the acquired data [1]. A second option is to apply federated learning principles in which data does not have to move but the AI application and computing resources must be distributed [2]. In both options, the gathering of large collections of imaging data of the same pathology or disease and of a pre-defined population is a challenging task, and many projects suffer from the limitations of a small dataset, not only because of the limited availability of data but also because of limited willingness of healthcare institutes to share medical data.

To tackle this problem and to enable the collection of large imaging databases, careful technical considerations are required concerning the IT infrastructure. Three important parts of this IT infrastructure that can help driving AI forward are data storage, cloud usage and AI pipeline implementation. This chapter will dive into these three larger topics by addressing more specific topics such as imaging biobanking, cloud storage and compute, federated learning and different implementation versions of the AI pipeline in medical imaging.

Data Storage

In 2010, the Quantitative Imaging Network (QIN) performed a questionnaire among their members to explore the field of informatics methods in imaging research [3]. One of their goals was to share data among institutes in order to accelerate quantitative imaging research. Important findings were a large variation in tools used for the de-identification, local image file storage varying from XNAT and (commercial) Picture Archiving and Communication System (PACS) solutions to open consumer platforms such as Dropbox and local image meta-data databases varying from dedicated tools like REDCap to simple spreadsheets on a local hard drive or USB drive.

Imaging Biobanking

According to the European Society of Radiology (ESR) position paper on imaging biobanks, a biobank is an 'organised database of medical images and associated imaging biomarkers (radiology and beyond) shared among multiple researchers and linked to other biorepositories' [4]. The key points resulting from this work were the following:

- Imaging biobanks are 'shared databases of imaging biomarkers, linked to biorepositories'.
- Exploitation of traditional and imaging biobanks is meaningful for 'personalized medicine'.
- A European imaging biobank network would significantly boost research in the imaging domain.

The immediate purpose of an imaging biobank is to allow the generation of imaging biomarkers for use in research

P. M. A. van Ooijen, MSc, PhD, CPHIMS (✉) · E. Darzi, MSc
Department of Radiation Oncology and Data Science Center in Health, University Medical Center Groningen, Groningen, The Netherlands
e-mail: p.m.a.van.ooijen@umcg.nl; e.darzidehkalani@umcg.nl

A. Dekker, MSc, PhD
Department of Radiation Oncology (MAASTRO), GROW School for Oncology and Developmental Biology, Maastricht University Medical Centre+, Maastricht, The Netherlands
e-mail: andre.dekker@maastro.nl

C. N. De Cecco et al. (eds.), *Artificial Intelligence in Cardiothoracic Imaging*, Contemporary Medical Imaging,
https://doi.org/10.1007/978-3-030-92087-6_5

studies (using 'conventional' techniques or AI/deep learning) and to support biological validation of existing and novel imaging biomarkers. The long-term scope of imaging biobanks is the creation of a network/federation of such repositories.

An imaging biobank can exist in different scenarios. First, an imaging biobank could contain clinical research data gathered in clinical research/trials. Second, it could contain disease-specific data with data from clinical practice or screening programmes (e.g. breast, lung and colon cancer) based on disease characteristics. These data collections are not necessarily directly connected to a clinical research question. Third, an imaging biobank can contain general population data. In this case, data is collected from the general population (not only patients or population at risk), with no specific goal or disease-oriented approach. This usually involves the collection of long-term longitudinal data.

Imaging biobanks can exist as a single entity with centralized data collection or storage, but federations of biobanks are also possible. Such a federated setup of imaging biobanks requires a centralized database or catalogue of data collections present at different local imaging biobanks [4] preferably using Findable, Accessible, Interoperable and Reusable (FAIR) data principles [5]. Utilization of the data in such a federated environment could involve collecting the imaging data at the site where they are needed when needed, but also to have the data remain at the site of acquisition or collection and allowing software tools to access that data to perform analysis with only returning the analysis results [6].

To allow the merging of (imaging) data collected from multiple biobanks, a common FAIR data model is required. This common data model should include common data schemes, standard nomenclatures, reference to common ontologies, etc. Furthermore, access policies should be implemented to request and grant access to data collections for specific research projects.

The ESR Position Paper on Imaging Biobanks [4] lists four requirements for the appropriate implementation and use of imaging biobanks. First, the aim should be to achieve an ecosystem with a combination of central and federated approach where query, analysis and retrieval across multiple data repositories should be possible. Second, data access should be secure and permission based. Third, proper de-identification of both imaging and meta-data should be in place. And finally, standard information models and terminologies should be used.

To achieve part of this standardization, the Quantitative Imaging Network proposed a system architecture to enable data sharing, collaborative experimentation and translation of methods to clinical practice [3]. This system architecture proposes a four-layer design (Fig. 5.1). It includes informatics tools to support data repositories in a data storage layer (in blue) based on standard information models and shared semantics (in red). The data repositories in the storage layer can be accessed by different processing and analysis in the research methods layer. Nowadays, this layer is of course extended by the training, validation and deployment of AI systems. Finally, the clinical systems layer provides the clin-

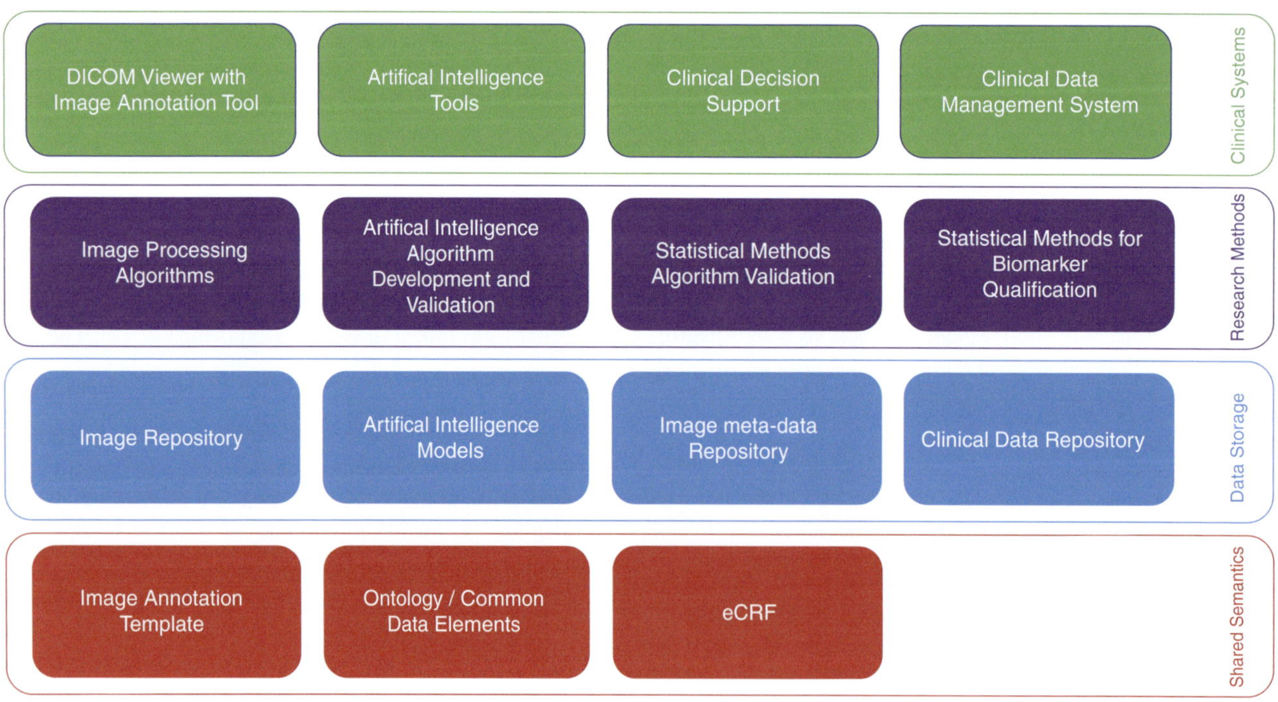

Fig. 5.1 Quantitative Imaging Network (QIN) system architecture expanded with AI-related elements [3]

ical users with the tools to get access to the data in the underlying layers including the results from the algorithms in the research methods layer.

Quite a large body of work exists on the design and implementation of data environments for medical imaging, both for research and clinical practice [6–8]. Commonly used open source tools are XNAT (imaging) and REDCap (meta data), but also other environments and implementations both commercial and open source [6, 7] exist. One common denominator of the environments is that they can all operate in the 'cloud' of the World Wide Web. Often mentioned advantages of cloud usage are economy of scale, improved performance, data portability, increased and flexible storage capacity, data migration and patient-centric connected systems [9].

Data Storage Challenges and Considerations

In order for AI pipelines to work properly, data must be annotated, which introduces the challenge of obtaining a proper ground truth. Ground-truth images in imaging biobanks are discrepant most of the times as medical experts are not fully concordant in their annotations.

Also, the quality of the data collection is vital, and several aspects have to be considered when collecting and storing data. In the medical imaging domain, numerous scanners, imaging protocols and parameter choices exist, which results in images of significantly different distributions. It is important to store the provenance of the images, i.e. by which protocol, scanners, parameters they were obtained, whether they contain missing slices or artefacts, etc., to enable AI algorithms to decide what data to query and to avoid improper samples. As an example, motion-corrupted MR images cause substantial problems in AI algorithms for diagnosis or segmentation [10], whereas they are useful for motion-correction AI models.

Cloud Usage

The National Institute of Standards and Technology (NIST) defines cloud computing as follows:

> Cloud computing is a model for enabling ubiquitous, convenient, on-demand network access to a shared pool of configurable computing resources (e.g., networks, servers, storage, applications, and services) that can be rapidly provisioned and released with minimal management effort or service provider interaction [11].

In the NIST special publication on cloud computing, five essential characteristics, three service models and four deployment models are defined (Fig. 5.2) [9, 11].

Essential Characteristics

The first part of the NIST cloud model are the Essential Characteristics, which are on-demand self-service, broad network access, resource pooling, rapid elasticity and measured service. A cloud implementation should include all of these characteristics.

On-demand self-service is about the ability of a user to provision the required computing capabilities (such as server time or network storage) by themselves on-demand and automatically without requiring human intervention from the server provider side.

Next, *broad network access* means that easy access should be provided through network access by using standard mech-

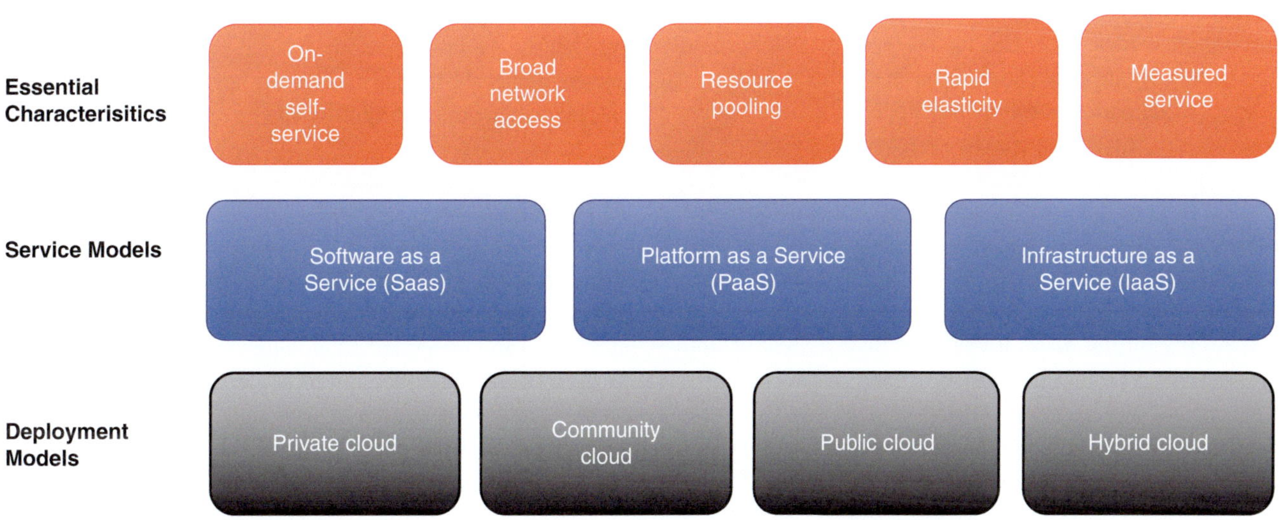

Fig. 5.2 Summary of the NIST cloud model

anisms. This broad access also refers to the requirement that it should be accessible through a wide variety of different thin or thick client platforms ranging from smartphones and tablets to laptops and workstations.

Resource pooling refers to the fact that the provider is running pooled computing resources that can be used to serve multiple customers using a so-called multi-tenant model. The assignment of virtual resources is dynamically executed based on the requirements of the consumer. This also means that the user is not knowledgeable about the exact location of the provided resources (e.g. which server or rack is providing the resources). However, because of legal restrictions that might occur, most providers do allow a user to select a designated location on a higher abstraction level to limit the resource location to, for example, a certain country, state or datacenter. The resources that can be provided and dynamically assigned by the cloud provider are multiple and include storage capacity, CPU and GPU processing, memory and network bandwidth.

Finally, *rapid elasticity* is used to describe the characteristic of the cloud that rapid on-demand scaling of resources is possible within the virtual environment of the consumer. This scaling could even be done automatically based on certain triggers when additional resources are needed. This kind of scaling gives a sense of unlimited resources available to the user.

Service Models

The service models describe three different variations of cloud services that provide software, platform or infrastructure through cloud access.

Software as a Service (SaaS)

In short, SaaS deals with running specific applications through a cloud service. This means that a provider provides access to a single application through the cloud service. All management and control of the underlying infrastructure such as the servers, operating system and storage is fully controlled by the provider of the service without any influence on this by the user. A typical example is a web-based e-mail service such as Gmail.

Platform as a Service (PaaS)

Expanding on the SaaS, a PaaS provides a suite of applications, programming languages and other user tools through a cloud service. This means that a user is able to deploy required applications, either own or acquired, to a cloud service. The underlying cloud infrastructure is still fully controlled by the cloud provider, but the user has influence on what applications should be deployed in the environment.

Infrastructure as a Service (IaaS)

Finally, IaaS provides the most flexible solution providing access to fundamental computing resources. In this service model, the underlying cloud infrastructure is provided by the cloud provider, but the user can control and configure the operating system, storage and application deployment. Also limited control over selected networking component, for example, hosting a firewall, could be granted to the user.

Deployment Models

The Deployment Models proposed by NIST range from Private, via Community to Public cloud and also allow for Hybrid solutions combining private and public cloud technology.

The *private cloud* is the most closed – and assumed to be the most secure – deployment model. In this model, a single organization will be granted exclusive use for multiple consumers belonging to that organization. This does not mean it needs to be owned, managed and operated by that organization and all hardware must exist on-premise. Third parties could be involved in one or multiple of these points.

In case of a *community cloud*, the use is not exclusive to one organization but to multiple organizations that are part of a community. In most cases, such a community will exist of a group of organizations with shared concerns such as a group of hospitals in a region or country. Again, ownership, management and operation can be shared with a third party, and the actual hardware may be on- or off-premises.

A *public cloud* is a cloud infrastructure that is open for use by the general public. This will, in most cases, physically exist on-premise with the cloud provider, which can be single or combination of a number of companies, universities and/or government organizations.

In a *hybrid cloud*, the cloud infrastructure is deployed consisting of a combination of cloud models. The different environments are unique entities but have the ability to share and exchange data and applications.

AI Pipeline

Because of the complex nature of the process of AI and the different steps involved, research is ongoing to develop more automated and integrated AI pipelines that support the whole process from data collection to deployment [8]. Depending on the situation, each step in such an AI pipeline is prone to automation, thus eliminating as many of the manual steps as possible.

There is a distinction between a development and a deployment pipeline. The development pipeline consists of the steps of data collection, data annotation or labelling, data cleansing, training and validation. In a deployment pipeline, one or more trained networks will be included to receive (imaging) data and produce a final prediction, which needs to be integrated into a (clinical) database [8].

Local Implementation

When implementing AI locally, it can be part of the current PACS or EMR environment or run as a private cloud or on-premise service.

Networking

Local networks consist of data storage systems, processors and deployment systems. These components are interdependent; that is, each system is unable to operate unless it receives response from other systems. This interdependency makes communication a crucial factor in developing AI pipelines. The ultimate goal of a local network should be to minimize latency and to synchronize the processing among different nodes. If communication in a network is sub-optimal, the network with its costly hardware resources becomes under-utilized and inefficient.

Several techniques can be considered to enhance communication efficiency in a locally implemented network. A first effective technique in high-performance computing is reducing model precision. In many cases, data and model parameters are stored with double precision, which could be converted to single floating point or less. Since medical data are not required to have double floating-point precision, this conversion does not hurt the model performance. Removing additional integers could help saving bandwidth and reduces model size and network burden [12].

Another useful technique to improve data exchange speed is compression of data transferred between different nodes. This is especially important in (medical) infrastructures where network bandwidths are limited. Some compression techniques utilize lossless methods, i.e. data is fully recoverable after decompression, but have limited capacity to save bandwidth usage. Instead, lossy methods are utilized more frequently. One method in deep learning-based AI applications to perform compression is to limit the values of gradient updates to binary values, this method ensures gradient updates in the correct direction and transferred data will be as low as just one bit. Another technique is to neglect insignificant, small gradient update values and convey only significant gradients. Tao et al. implemented this method for federated systems, which is applicable in medical AI pipelines [13].

An AI pipeline consisting of multiple components requires each component to participate actively, exchange data and allow access to other components when necessary. But most PACSs are unable to operate within an active environment. They might, for example, fail when changing IP, hostname and DICOM attributes, since these are hardcoded to work on a pre-defined situation with limited options and minimum flexibility [14].

GPU and CPU

Early AI pipelines and deep learning deployments used CPUs to perform computations and depended on clusters of CPUs to parallelize computing and improve model efficiency. However, state-of-the-art deep learning pipelines nowadays rely on GPUs instead. For many medical institutes, acquiring local or cloud-based GPUs is a crucial step in deploying AI pipelines.

To build an AI pipeline, both CPU and GPU nodes are needed, and tasks are divided between them to reach the optimal cost efficiency. Since GPUs maximize performance, not latency, they have worse latency than CPUs. Hence, GPU nodes are mostly used in the training phase, and CPU nodes are mostly used in the deployment phase when the latency becomes an important factor. Thus, when building large local sites for AI in healthcare, a combination of GPU and CPU devices is preferred.

Data Management

Having high volumes of data requires careful data preparation, storage, processing and exchange between systems when developing local AI pipelines. Data should also be well integrated into existing hospital IT systems in both development and deployment stages.

Developing DL models on existing hospital image archiving systems requires a good integration. This interoperability may be hampered by the co-existence of multiple imaging databases (PACS) in the hospital environment. During development, the DL model can be trained on a data dump of DICOM images to avoid using PACSs in the process. After deployment, it could be needed to ensure all systems within a local/cloud network have the same PACS version, or that PACSs are connected with an intermediary web-based protocol, which allows to integrate data from different PACSs.

AI systems, similar to clinical experts, require various types of patient data to obtain comprehensive knowledge about a medical situation. For example, in radiology, additional patient EMR data might be required, and AI models cannot be trained properly until they integrate all relevant data. This requires data exchange between different departments within the same hospital. Protocols and data type standardizations should thus be developed for all the relevant departments to facilitate information exchange.

AI Models

Trained AI models should also be stored in the medical IT environment. AI researchers might need future access to the trained models for testing, deployment, enhancement and migration to a new framework. Thus, models have to be accessed, queried and analysed easily through hospital systems. In larger networks, model interoperability is another concern. Each system might have its own DL framework, which is a burden to develop an AI pipeline. Research is being done to facilitate the interoperability of DL models trained on different frameworks by introducing standardized exchange formats. One popular framework is ONNX [15], which enables various DL frameworks, including PyTorch, TensorFlow, Caffe, MXNet and CNTK to share their model properties and cooperate within the same network.

For AI pipelines implemented locally, there is a risk for AI models to be prone to various kinds of bias, including demographic bias (gender, age) or data bias (annotation, equipment, acquisition), thus having limited capacity for generalization. Solutions include using distributed datasets and transfer learning. Current DL models might be designed to work with limited data types (e.g. one modality or annotation protocol). However, with current pace in imaging techniques, any change has to be expected in model design. Models are required to handle new data formats, with minimal interruption. Thus, it is better to avoid static AI models for medical usages and design flexible models.

Cloud Implementation

In the *development phase* of the AI pipeline, the cloud can be employed to provide compute power (cloud-based learning), data science workspaces, crowd-sourced annotation or distributed learning.

The process of annotation or labelling of imaging data can be quite time-consuming and difficult to organize because of the low availability of busy healthcare professionals that are needed for expert annotation. Cloud implementations could help in such cases to provide an online annotation environment where experts from all over the world can provide their annotations on the imaging data [7]. Important in such a process is to have a transparent annotation procedure in place, which is well documented and uses guidelines to ensure the annotation from different users is uniform [1].

With cloud-based learning, the cloud is used to train the deep learning network utilizing cloud-provisioned CPU or GPU computation power. The programming and implementation of the deep learning network are done locally, and the High-Performance Computing (HPC) environment in the cloud is used to perform the iterative learning process.

Data science workspaces provide access to a full data science environment and allow all development steps to be performed in the cloud. In this case, the full programming environment is provided through a virtual machine in the cloud, and access to the HPC cloud facilities is also provided.

Because of the move to the cloud, it has also become feasible to not limit the learning phase in the development to a single location but to distribute the work over multiple locations and even with different databases at those different locations. This distributed or federated learning is a novel area that could solve issues concerning the limited sharing of data and data privacy; it will be described in more detail separately in the next section.

The *deployment phase* introduces possibilities such as a single AI algorithm in the cloud, compute power in the cloud, federative deployment of AI and AI platforms [16].

Many AI applications are provided by their vendor as a single AI algorithm in the cloud. This means that the imaging data will be sent to a cloud-based DICOM receiver from the PACS or an upload through a web interface is done. After processing of the data, a report or other generated output (e.g. segmentation files, processed imaging data, etc.) will be returned to the source. In a 2020 report, Mehrizi et al. showed that of 269 AI applications on the market, 32% were offered as a cloud-only solution and 46% offer a choice to be either cloud-based or on-premise [17]. Besides commercial implementations, these kinds of cloud-based solutions for online AI applications are also available from research institutions. The RECOMIA platform is an example of such a research-based AI application provider that also aims to expand and function as a research marketplace for AI applications developed by other research groups [7]. In the deployment phase, compute power in the cloud could also be used if the required HPC facilities are not available on-premise.

Several federative deployments of AI can be envisioned. One possible solution is proposed by the Early Lung Imaging Confederation (ELIC) [6] that proposed and tested a federative environment where imaging data is distributed over the world at the locations where the data were obtained. A central database is updated on the content of these different systems. Software tools (AI or other) that perform tasks on the decentralized images will be distributed to the relevant nodes in the federative network where automated image analysis is performed. All resulting quantitative measurements are collected on the central HUB where further analysis can be done on the aggregated database.

AI platforms can also provide a centralized environment to manage and run multiple applications that can be accessed by the user through some sort of online marketplace [16]. In such a cloud-based marketplace of AI tools, developers can distribute their tools (after approval by the marketplace holder) to a large customer base without the requirement of their own sales and deployment team [16]. The deployment only needs to be done in the environment of the marketplace, saving the costly and tedious in-hospital connectivity challenges. Also, all workflow and user interaction are covered by the platform, ensuring that the AI tool developer can focus on the core technology and the API connection to the platform.

For the user, such platforms remove the burden of installing a multitude of different AI applications all performing their own task; application selection and implementation of AI are also simplified to a large extent. The platform will handle the data transfer and ensures the right data is sent to the right application and ensures the data transfer security. The organization using the platform only has to deal with the configuration and implementation of the required data connections once. When connecting to the platform, all AI tools will rely on that single data connection to obtain data. Furthermore, maintenance and future changes will also be limited to that single platform connection (e.g. when migrating to a new PACS or changes in imaging modalities), and updates and upgrades of the AI tools themselves will be handled by the platform provider. The AI tools provided can either be from one specific vendor or from a variety of suppliers including scientific institutions that provide access to research outcome. The platform provider will select AI tools based on pre-defined criteria concerning the legal status of the tools and the quality of the results. A variety of these marketplaces already exist; in their technography study, Mehrizi et al. reported ten of such marketplaces that provide access to other applications in 2019 [17].

Distributed/Federated Learning

Training deep learning models requires finding optimal values for millions of parameters, which is time-consuming. Sometimes, it is important to distribute the processing on parallel machines, to reduce the training time and improve network efficiency. Besides, there might be privacy considerations and challenges regarding data governance. In such cases, distributed/federated deep learning allows researchers to develop an AI pipeline, without having direct access to data from other institutions.

Parallelization Methods

In *data parallelization*, each worker (e.g. GPU machine) is given an identical copy of a DL model and part of the data. To avoid duplication of tasks, data should be split into non-overlapping batches (Fig. 5.3). After each model finished its processing, the DL parameters for all workers will be updated. Hence, a strong synchronization among workers is required.

In *model parallelism*, processors are parallelized to perform operations of a certain part of a deep neural network (Fig. 5.4). For example, a neural network can be divided into multiple sections, each processor assigned to one section, and processors exchange information in both forward and backward propagation. A major concern in model parallelism is how to split the network into multiple sections so that the processors work together properly.

Pipeline parallelism is a combination of model and data parallelism and has the benefits of both methods. In pipeline parallelism, data is divided into non-overlapping mini-batches, and neural network is divided into sections and each section is assigned to a processor (Fig. 5.5). In backpropagation, the gradient of a certain mini-batch is propagated through layers, and gradient processing is performed on GPUs, associated to those layers.

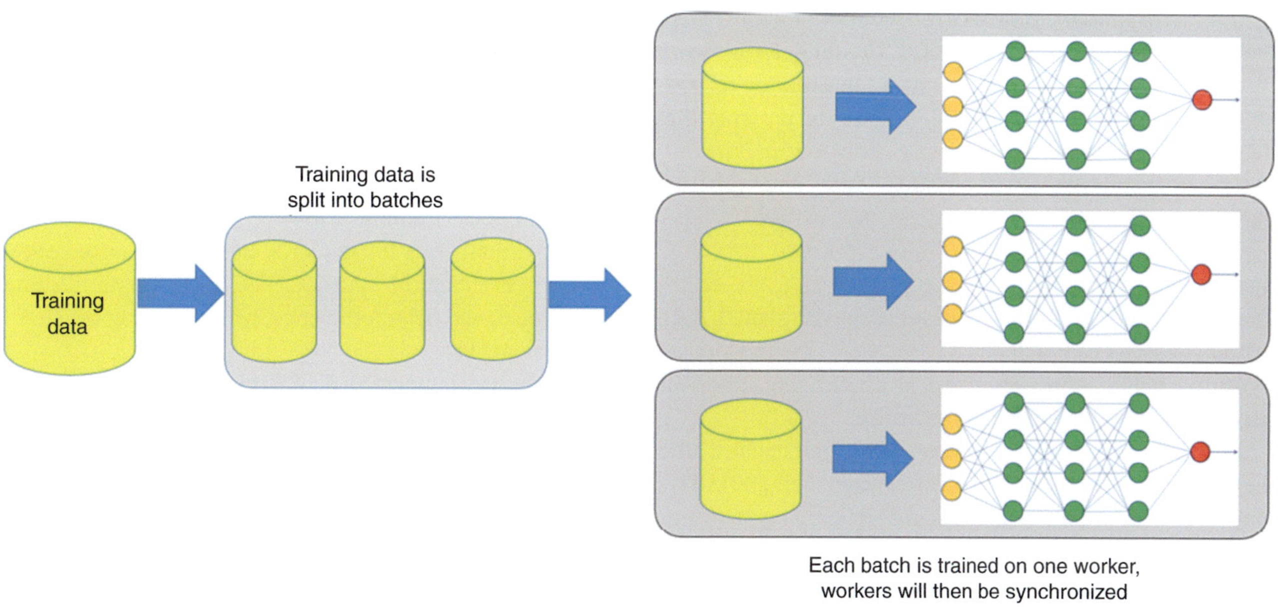

Fig. 5.3 Data parallelism [18]

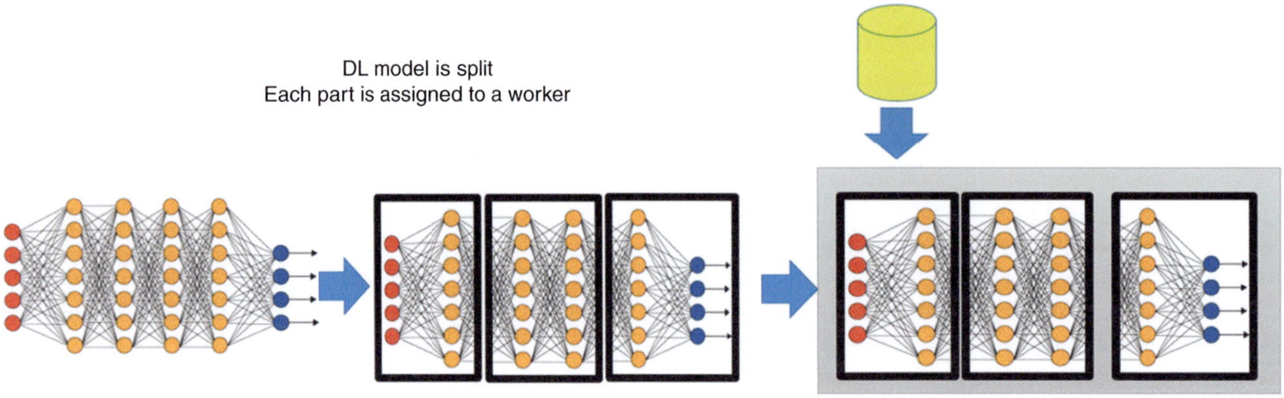

Fig. 5.4 Model parallelism [18]

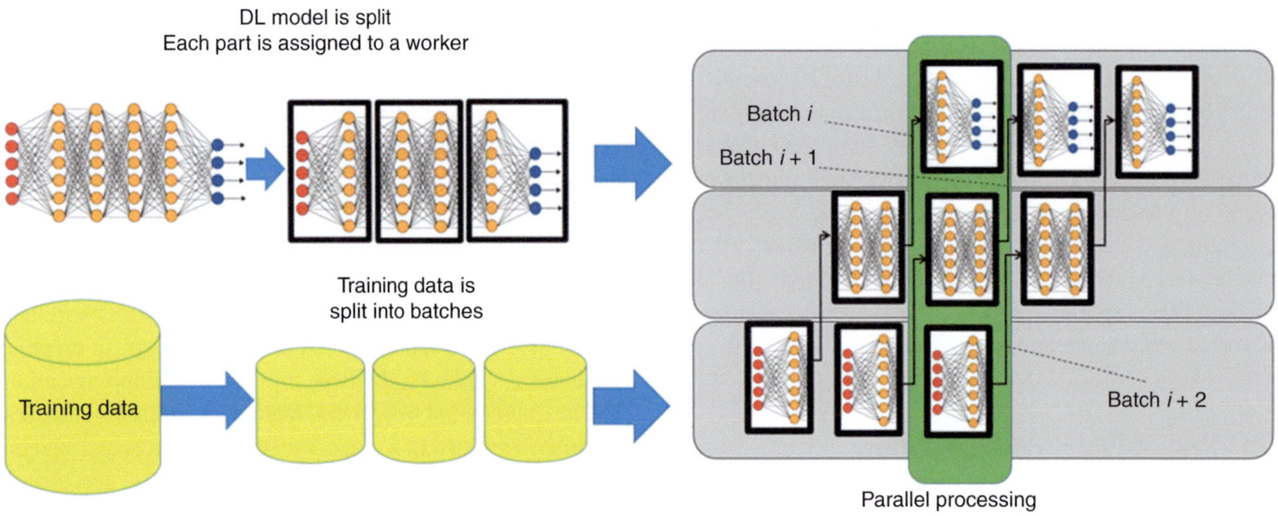

Fig. 5.5 Pipeline parallelism [18]

For more complex networks that consist of many layers and complex network architectures, dividing the network or data to distinct parts might not be feasible or reasonable. Thus, large distributed deep learning projects that deal with complex networks mostly apply *hybrid parallelism* – a combination of model, data and pipeline parallelism.

Synchronization

One of the most important questions in distributed deep learning is *when* to synchronize parameters among workers. Synchronization strategies exert a challenging trade-off between network speed and performance.

In *synchronous training*, workers share their updates after they processed one batch (i.e. after each iteration). This method is widely used in distributed deep learning platforms and has better convergence that other synchronization paradigms. However, synchronous training has the *straggler problem*; the network speed will be determined by the speed of the slowest worker, and other workers have to wait until the last worker finishes its processing.

In *bounded synchronous training*, workers train on stale parameters, and parameters resulting from bounded-synchronous training are an approximation of the parameters of synchronous training. However, to prevent that the approximation harms the model accuracy and convergence, the staleness should be bounded. This allows more freedom of the model, and better efficiency, while avoiding the straggler problem [19].

Another way to update a model is by updating parameters independently or *asynchronous*; that is, the model is updated once one worker finishes its batch and sends the gradients to the network, regardless of other workers. This approach might cause problems in convergence. However, the model will be considerably more flexible, and training proceeds faster.

System Architectures

Having a large number of workers, another major challenge in designing a distributed deep learning architecture is *how* to synchronize parameters among different workers. Many inter-connected workers exchange considerable amounts of information. The performance of each processors is dependent on the parameters it receives from other processors. Thus, if the system architecture is not designed properly, failure in one worker causes interruption of the whole system. Different system architectures will be discussed in this section.

Centralized architectures are architectures in which every node or worker reports its parameters to a central node (or nodes), called parameter server (PS). One approach is to divide the model parameters into a few chunks and send parameters belonging to each chunk to a PS, thus letting model processors and PSs work in parallel. Notable systems using PS architecture are GeePS [20], DistBelief [21] and TensorFlow [22].

Processors in *decentralized networks* communicate directly with one another (in a fully connected network without a PS) or communicate through other processors. In a fully connected network, in which every single worker is connected to all other workers, communication is a major concern. However, alternative topologies exist. For example, a ring topology is implemented in the widely used Horovod [23] framework from Uber. The major drawback of all topologies other than fully connected topology is that communication between nodes might require involvement of the other nodes and processing time is substantially increased.

Decentralized topologies are much easier to deploy than centralized topologies. There is no need to set up a PS, and complexities of PS planning are avoided. Another advantage is that decentralized topologies are more robust to failure since there is no central hub on which the existence of the network depends. Instead, in decentralized networks, other workers can easily take over other failed workers' duties, and the network goes on without interruption. Decentralized architectures also have disadvantages. Communication is a major problem in decentralized networks. Changing topology from fully connected also introduces other complexities and trade-offs.

Both centralized and decentralized topologies assume that data is available for all workers, and the network data and model parameters are being controlled, either by a central server or by individual nodes. However, in some scenarios, especially in the medical domain, data and model parameters might not be visible to other workers or PS.

In such cases, a *federated learning* topology is used. In federated learning, data is kept locally on each worker, and a global network is trained based on the data stored in each server. Each worker reports the updated model parameters based on its dataset to the whole network. This topology is also beneficial for networks with limited bandwidth because in federated learning, heavy training data is not exchanged in network and only parameters are propagated.

Common topologies of federated learning are the *aggregation server method, peer-to-peer method*, and *sequential methods*.

In the *aggregation server method*, a server initializes the model between different workers, and each worker computes its gradients and sends them back to the central server. After all of the workers computed their gradients, the model is aggregated and updated from the aggregation server, and the new model is sent back to continue training the next iteration.

The *peer-to-peer topology* avoids using a server to save the whole model. Instead, a model is initialized from one node, and each worker starts training based on its own data. After each node computed its gradients, it reports the calculated parameters to all other nodes. The model is then updated after all of the workers reported their own updates.

In *sequential methods*, a model is trained on data from one institution and is then adapted to new institutions, with different scanners and protocols. Two forms of sequential methods are domain adaptation and lifelong learning. In domain adaptation, a model is trained on a source domain with rich data. It then will be trained again (fine-tuned) on new samples from the target domain to learn the new distribution. Since the goal of domain adaptation is maximizing performance on the new domain, the model might not be able to preserve its performance on the source domain. Lifelong learning is another variant of sequential methods, aiming to solve this issue. In lifelong learning, a pre-trained model sees a few samples from the new domain and learns the new distribution while maintaining the model's capability on previous data. This can be done by learning batch normalization parameters for different domains and sharing the convolutional filters [24].

Discussion

Although very promising in healthcare data exchange, cloud solutions still have to cope with fear and unease about the technology by hospital IT leadership. On the level of performance, this fear is about image latency because of low bandwidth, delay in image access and cloud service disruption by downtime. But also, security issues such as DDoS or hacking attacks and confidential data leakage are major concerns.

That this is still an issue in the current cloud environments of medical imaging was shown by the Health IT Security report in November 2019: about 1.19 billion images were accessible through a very large number of PACSs that were connected to the cloud and easily accessed by unauthorized users [25].

Security issues prominent in the cloud are secure transfer – including, for example, data encryption – privacy, confidentiality and integrity of the (imaging) data. The cloud design and implementation should be such that it takes these four points into careful consideration.

Besides security, cloud implementations should also consider safety by providing backup or redundant storage to avoid data loss, high availability with low downtime and restricted and tracked access by implementation of role-based access and extensive user activity tracking and audit trails.

Deep learning models trained on large-scale datasets ensure better clinical performance and generalizability and allow to make less biased decisions. Federated learning helps to provide access to high-quality diagnosis and treatment even in remote locations and the benefit of using data from other institutions. This advantage is significant, especially when dealing with rare diseases. Furthermore, hospitals retain control over their own data, limiting concerns about data leakage or data misuse by third parties, although some concerns remain such as what one might learn from the updates to the parameter server. For researchers, federated learning helps them to train their models based on a vast amount of diverse data from multiple institutions. This is especially important since even the strongest DL models fail when trained on inadequate data.

However, heterogeneity of data might also have major consequences. For example, if an FL framework is trained at multiple institutions, it converges to an optimal point for all parties. But the global optimal point might not be the optimal point for each institution, since each institution has a particular group of patients and has some bias in favour of that group.

Federated learning training ensures some levels of privacy, but it does not guarantee full security of the model.

FL models are also prone to information leakage, even though they do not share direct information from training data. For example, techniques like model inversion, gradient leakage and adversarial attacks can extract confidential data from the model. If adversaries can track the gradient updates, for example, the values of gradients of a single institute, data from that institute can be stolen. Some techniques can be applied, but they all add their own complexities to the model and cause trade-offs. Hence, when designing a federated learning paradigm, the desired level of security and performance should always be considered, and an optimal trade-off should be designed based on the level of trust in other institutions, legal limitations, etc.

A high level of safety, reproducibility and traceability is critical in federated networks. In centralized and local DL models, all the data and systems are in control of a master system. This means that model history, hardware configurations and hyperparameters are all accessible. As a consequence, faults can be debugged and tracked easily. However, in large-scale federated set-ups, not all of the above properties are trackable. Each institution has its own settings, software, network and infrastructure. One solution to ensure model traceability and integrity is to compel all parties to declare their hyperparameters and training settings.

Finally, in federated topologies, secure data transmission is a necessity. For most strict cases, an additional operator might be required as a 'trusted broker' to transmit data between nodes. It exerts an extra cost on the system, which sometimes is undesirable. Encryption of transmitted data is also crucial. Secure data transmission prevents third parties to access network parameters.

The implementation of data sharing using imaging biobanking and cloud solutions still has to cope with technical, legal and societal challenges. To overcome these, a number of conditions have to be met. One of these is the standardization of communication, data format and lexicons or terminologies, which is essential to achieve environments with a high level of interoperability. Interchanging data between cloud solutions and standardization of APIs is still limited [9]. In medical imaging, common data standards like DICOM and HL7 could help in this, together with workflow definitions as provided by the IHE.

Conclusion

AI solutions are a step towards solving many existing problems in the area of healthcare. They provide a strong tool for healthcare experts. Distributed AI solutions, especially federated learning, have the capability to provide accurate, safe, privacy-preserving and unbiased models for clinical usage. However, when designing distributed AI pipelines, many considerations should be taken into account. Proper infrastructure, data preparation and AI model design are necessary for accurate training. How to perform parallelization and how to enable efficient and secure communication among workers is another challenge which should be addressed.

We need to enable sharing within an institution, between institutions and with patients. To realize this, the cloud plays an important role in fostering better models for fluent exchange of images and information and cloud-based medical image sharing and multicentre databases have many advantages. It can be cost effective because of the economy of scale and can improve performance. Furthermore, with online patient health records, it is easier to access and share data between patients and doctors and between doctors. Cloud also offers an increased and more flexible storage capacity. PACS independent storage in the cloud could remove the necessity of tedious data migration projects when moving to another PACS vendor. And finally, consolidating and storing medical image information in single centralized repository in the cloud instead of multiple PACS in different sites means healthcare providers can quickly access and share images across various departments and organizations, resulting in a more patient-centric environment.

References

1. He J, Baxter SL, Xu J, Xu J, Zhou X, Zhang K. The practical implementation of artificial intelligence technologies in medicine. Nat Med. 2019;25(1):30–6.
2. Shi Z, Zhovannik I, Traverso A, Dankers FJWM, Deist TM, Kalendralis P, Monshouwer R, Bussink J, Fijten R, Aerts HJWL, Dekker A, Wee L. Distributed radiomics as a signature validation study using the personal health train infrastructure. Sci Data. 2019;6:218.
3. Levy MA, Freymann JB, Kirby JS, Fedorov A, Fennessy FM, Eschrich SA, Berglund AE, Fenstermacher DA, Tan Y, Guo X, Casavant TL, Brown BJ, Braun TA, Dekker A, Roelofs E. Informatics methods to enable sharing of quantitative imaging research data. Magn Reson Imaging. 2012;30:1249–56.
4. European Society of Radiology. ESR position paper on imaging biobanks. Insights Imaging. 2015;6(4):403–10.
5. Wilkinson MD, Dumontier M, Aalbersberg IJ, et al. The FAIR Guiding Principles for scientific data management and stewardship. Sci Data. 2016;3:160018. Erratum in: Sci Data. 2019;6(1):6.
6. Mulshine JL, Avila RS, Conley E, Devraj A, Ambrose LF, Flanagan T, Henschke CI, Hirsch FR, Janz R, Kakinuma R, Lam S, McWilliams A, van Ooijen PM, Oudkerk M, Pastorin U. The International Association for the study of lung cancer early lung imaging confederation. JCO Clin Cancer Inform. 2020;4:89–99.
7. Trägårdh E, Borrelli P, Kaboteh R, Gillberg T, Ulén J, Enqvist O, Edenbrandt L. RECOMIA – a cloud-based platform for artificial intelligence research in nuclear medicine and radiology. EJNMMI Phys. 2020;7:51.
8. González G, Evans CL. Biomedical image processing with containers and deep learning: an automated analysis pipeline. BioEssays. 2019;41:e1900004.
9. Kagadis GC, Kloukinas C, Moore K, Philbin J, Papadimitroulas P, Alexakos C, Nagy PG, Visvikis D, Hendee WR. Cloud computing in medical imaging. Med Phys. 2013;40(7):070901.
10. Mathai TS, Wang Y, Cross N. Assessing lesion segmentation bias of neural networks on motion corrupted brain MRI. In: MICCAI BrainLes. Springer, Lima, Peru 2020.
11. Mell P, Grance T. The NIST definition of cloud computing. NIST Special Publication, no. 800-145. 2011.
12. Gupta S, Agrawal A, Gopalakrishnan K, and Narayanan P. Deep learning with limited numerical precision. In Proceedings of the 32nd International Conference on International Conference on Machine Learning, Lille, France - 2015 Volume 37. JMLR.org, 1737–46.
13. Tao Z, Li Q. "esgd: Communication efficient distributed deep learning on the edge." USENIX Workshop on Hot Topics in Edge Computing (HotEdge 18), USENIX Association. 2018.
14. Alhajeri M, Ghulam S, Shah S. Limitations in and solutions for improving the functionality of picture archiving and communication system: an exploratory study of PACS professionals' perspectives. J Digit Imaging. 2019;32:54–67.
15. "ONNX," [Online]. Available: https://onnx.ai.
16. Blackford Analysis Ltd. Adopting a platform strategy: simplify the deployment and management of medical imaging applications and AI algorithms. Edinburgh: Blackford Analysis Ltd.; 2019.
17. Mehrizi MHR, van Ooijen P, Homan M. Applications of artificial intelligence (AI) in diagnostic radiology: a technography study. Eur Radiol. 2021;31(4):1805–11.
18. Mayer R, Jacobsen HA. Scalable deep learning on distributed infrastructures: challenges, techniques, and tools. ACM Comput Surv. 2021;53(3):1–37.
19. Cipar J, Ho Q, Kim J, Lee S, Ganger G, Gibson G, Keeton K, Xing E. Solving the straggler problem with bounded staleness. In: Proceedings of the 14th USENIX conference on Hot Topics in Operating Systems (HotOS' 13). USENIX Association, USA, 22.
20. Cui H, Zhang H, Ganger G, Gibbons P, Xing E. Scalable deep learning on distributed GPUs with a GPU-specialized parameter server. EuroSys '16: Proceedings of the Eleventh European Conference on Computer Systems, London, UK, April 2016, Article No.: 4, 1–16.
21. Dean J, Corrado G, Monga R, Chen K, Devin M, Mao M, Senior A, Tucker P, Yang K, Le Q. Large scale distributed deep networks. NIPS'12: Proceedings of the 25th International Conference on Neural Information Processing Systems - Volume 1, December 2012, pp. 1223–31.
22. Abadi M, Barham P, Chen J, Chen Z, Davis A, Dean J, Devin M, Ghemawat S, Irving G, Isard M. Tensorflow: a system for large-scale machine learning. In: In Proceedings of the 12th USENIX conference on Operating Systems Design and Implementation (OSDI'16). USENIX Association, USA, 265–283. 2016.
23. Sergeev A, Balso M. Horovod: fast and easy distributed deep learning in tensorflow. CoRR abs/1802.05799. 2018.
24. Karani N, Chaitanya K, Baumgartner C, Konukoglu E. A lifelong learning approach to brain MR segmentation across scanners and protocols. In: MICCAI: medical image computing and computer-assisted intervention; Springer, Cham. Granada, Spain. pp 476–84, 2018.
25. Davis J. Health IT Security, Xtelligent Healthcare Media. 19 November 2019. [Online]. Available: https://healthitsecurity.com/news/number-of-exposed-pacs-medical-images-increasing-us-biggest-culprit. Accessed 27 Oct 2020.

6 How to Build Artificial Intelligence Algorithms for Imaging Applications

Lewis Hahn, Evan Masutani, and Kyle Hasenstab

Introduction

Building algorithms based on radiologic imaging data is fundamentally a problem in computer vision, the field that seeks to allow computers to "see" and understand digital images. As a result, most of the algorithms used for purposes of cardiothoracic radiology are applications of computer vision techniques. The field of computer vision is broad, and it is impossible to describe the construction of all relevant algorithms in a single chapter. We will instead focus on deep learning methods since they are now the most commonly used methods applied to radiology and computer vision at large. These methods have led to vast improvements in performance of many computer vision tasks, putting clinical implementation within reach.

We will divide the process of building an algorithm for imaging purposes into the following steps: (1) identify your imaging task; (2) determine the appropriate algorithm(s) to use for your imaging task; (3) determine the loss function; (4) set training parameters; (5) train your algorithm. We will briefly discuss data preparation, but this will be covered in more depth in Chap. 5. Algorithm testing will be covered in Chap. 12. In addition, we cover several more advanced approaches that may be useful for developing sophisticated algorithms that go beyond basic tasks of computer vision. We close with a discussion of machine learning library and hardware selection.

L. Hahn, MD (✉)
Division of Cardiothoracic Imaging,
Department of Radiology, UC San Diego School of Medicine,
La Jolla, CA, USA
e-mail: lehahn@health.ucsd.edu

E. Masutani, CPhil
Department of Bioengineering, UC San Diego, La Jolla, CA, USA

K. Hasenstab, PhD
Department of Mathematics and Statistics, San Diego State University, San Diego, CA, USA

Identify Your Imaging Task

Most recent problems in cardiothoracic radiology that have been addressed with artificial intelligence (AI) fall into several main categories: classification, localization, segmentation, reconstruction, and postprocessing (Fig. 6.1). In classification, an image is analyzed by an algorithm to determine to which of several predefined classes it belongs. Examples might include whether a particular pulmonary nodule is malignant versus benign, or whether pulmonary edema is present on a chest X-ray. In localization, the problem is determining the location of an object within a 2D image or 3D volume. An example of a localization task would be to draw a bounding box around pulmonary nodules in a CT of the chest. In segmentation, an image or volume is partitioned into different classes—for instance, a chest CT might be segmented into voxels representing lung, soft tissue, bones, vessels, and objects external to the body. A reconstruction problem is one in which images are generated from measured data such as k-space sampling for MRI or sinograms for CT. A postprocessing algorithm is one in which images are further enhanced. One example would be reduction of streak artifact in CT.

Design/Select Your Algorithm

In the following sections, we discuss common deep neural network components and architectures used for each imaging task. This guide is in no way comprehensive, and the reader is invited to read the original papers and examine source code online for in-depth guidance.

C. N. De Cecco et al. (eds.), *Artificial Intelligence in Cardiothoracic Imaging*, Contemporary Medical Imaging,
https://doi.org/10.1007/978-3-030-92087-6_6

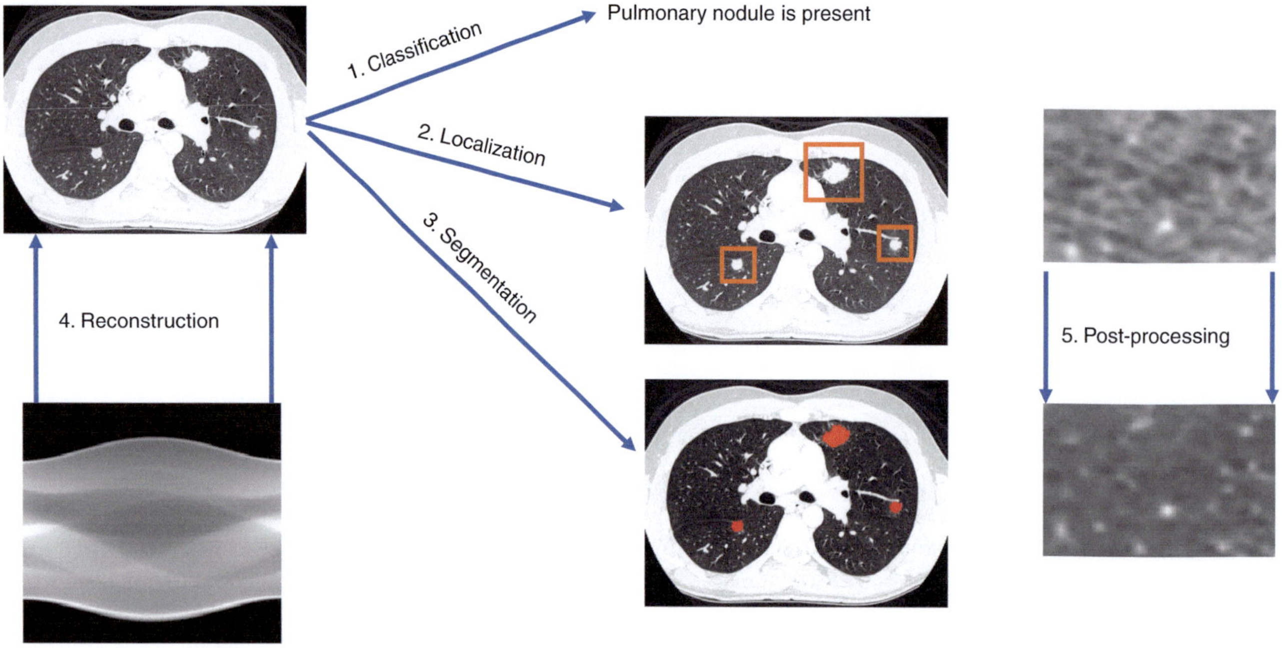

Fig. 6.1 Common AI algorithm applications applied to CT chest: 1. Classification of image to determine whether pulmonary nodule is present. 2. Localization of pulmonary nodules on image if present. 3. Segmentation of image into pulmonary nodules versus background. 4. Reconstruction of CT sinogram data into image. 5. Postprocessing removal of streak artifact from low-dose CT chest; images are zoomed in on lung parenchyma

Basic Components of Convolutional Neural Networks

Many of the recent advances in computer vision are due to the widespread adoption of deep convolutional neural networks (CNNs), in turn facilitated by the development of large image datasets and Graphics Processing Unit (GPUs). In order to discuss CNN design, it is useful to first describe their key components.

On a basic level, a neural network is a biologically inspired network of interconnected nodes (neurons) that process multiple inputs (analogous to dendrites), perform simple computations, and propagate a single calculated output to subsequent nodes (analogous to axons and synapses). For imaging purposes, nodes in the input layer of a network can be considered the pixel or voxel intensity values of a 2D or 3D image array; for color images, input nodes would comprise the red, blue, or green pixel values. For CT data, input nodes may represent voxel-wise density measured in Hounsfield units. Graphically, neural networks comprise multiple sequential layers of parallel nodes, such that each layer receives as input the outputs of its preceding layer. In traditional artificial neural networks, each node receives a weighted sum of the outputs of *all* nodes in its preceding layer and is said to be *fully connected*. The node itself then evaluates a nonlinear *activation function* using this weighted sum as input, producing a single output value passed onto *all* nodes in the subsequent layer. These weights are continually updated throughout the training process and constitute the learned parameters of all neural networks. As an example case, for two input values x_1 and x_2, the output of a node would be $f(w_1x_1 + w_2x_2 + b)$ where f is the nonlinear activation function (Fig. 6.2a). The constants w_1, w_2, and b are the learnable weights, which are optimized to match a desired output. The most common activation function f is the rectified linear unit (ReLU), defined as $g(x) = \max(0, x)$ (Fig. 6.2b). Other examples include the sigmoid function, tanh, and leaky ReLU. Neural networks are a powerful method and theoretically can approximate any continuous function (Universal Approximation Theorem).

Due to the *fully connected* structure of traditional artificial neural networks, the algorithm's memory requirements and computational demands rapidly increase with model complexity, rendering them largely impractical for medical imaging purposes. *Convolutional* neural networks have been developed to address these shortcomings. As with artificial neural networks, nodes in convolutional neural networks are arranged in layers. However, instead of taking as input *all* the outputs of the preceding layer, nodes in convolutional neural networks instead leverage a *receptive field*, where, given a 2D image, each node will receive as input a weighted sum from a subsampled 2D patch. To analyze the entire image, each node's receptive field (itself a 2D array of weights) slides over the 2D image, evaluating the activation function

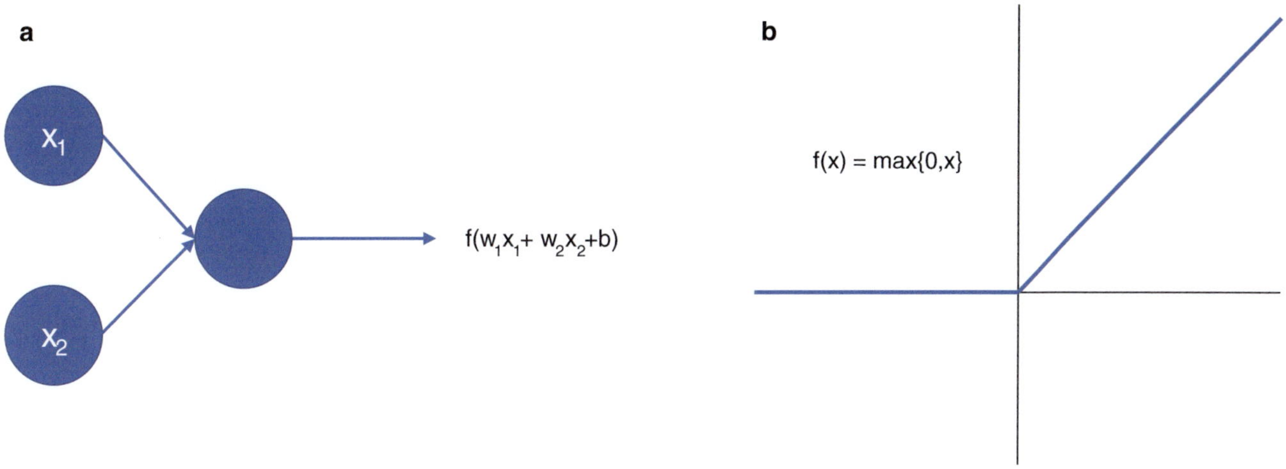

Fig. 6.2 (**a**) Basic neural network node performs a nonlinear function f on a linear combination of inputs, x_1 and x_2. w_1 and w_2 are weights, and b is the bias term. (**b**). f is a nonlinear function, most often the rectified linear unit (ReLU)

at every location and effectively generating a 2D output—this is known mathematically as *convolution*. Thus, convolutional neural networks comprise ordered, sequential convolutional layers.

A *convolutional layer* (Fig. 6.3a) is so named because it consists of multiple *convolutional filters* (also called *kernels*), which are 2D or 3D arrays of weights. For instance, for a 2D CT image input, the first layer's filters might have dimensions of 3 × 3 × 1. For a color image, the filter might have dimension 3 × 3 × 3, with the third dimension expanded to account for each color channel of the input. These kernels are slid over the input image, and the dot product between the filter and all local patches is obtained; this measures the response of the filter at every possible position of the input (Fig. 6.3b, c). The result is called an activation map.[1] For the above example, if the input was $n \times n \times 1$ and we had ten filters, the result would be an $n{-}2 \times n{-}2 \times 10$ activation map, which would then be passed to the next layer.[2] Thus, convolutional layers extract local information based on all filter responses from the activation maps of the previous layer.

Another critical component of CNNs is *max pooling layers* (Fig. 6.4a). The max pooling layers examine a small patch of pixels known as the pooling kernel and take the maximum value. This has several effects: the next layer will be smaller because of the pooling function, reducing the number of trainable parameters in the network and memory usage. Max pooling preserves the strongest feature responses so that less important features are ignored in subsequent layers. It also has the effect of making the output invariant to small translations. Average pooling is an alternative that performs a similar downsampling operation but instead averages values within the pooling kernel. However, average pooling generally leads to weaker results than max pooling.

Fully connected layers (Fig. 6.4b) are layers in which every single input is connected to a node and are hence analogous to traditional artificial neural network layers. Because of this, the number of parameters used in fully connected layers can be very large.

Upsampling layers start with a layer of a certain size and generate a result with larger dimensions, often in a learnable way. One commonly used example of an upsampling layer is a *transposed convolutional layer*. This operation is equivalent to adding zeros to an input and then performing a convolution (Fig. 6.4c). These layers are used in conjunction with *max pooling* for 2D-to-2D tasks such as image segmentation to produce pixel-wise outputs at input-image spatial resolution.

CNN Architectures by Task

Classification

Visual classification tasks are now commonly performed using convolutional neural networks (CNNs). Traditional computer vision algorithms required the researcher to develop handcrafted imaging features useful for accomplishing the classification task. A major benefit of CNNs over these traditional approaches is their ability to automatically learn features relevant for visual classification—specifically, the filter weights in convolutional layers are tunable; that is, they are updated during the training process to better perform the classification task. This differs from prior approaches in which the filters were prespecified manually.

[1] Also called a feature map.

[2] While this is the original formulation of a convolutional layer, in many cases, a padding operation is now performed, for instance, by adding zeros on the edges of the input images, so that the output has the same dimensions as the input.

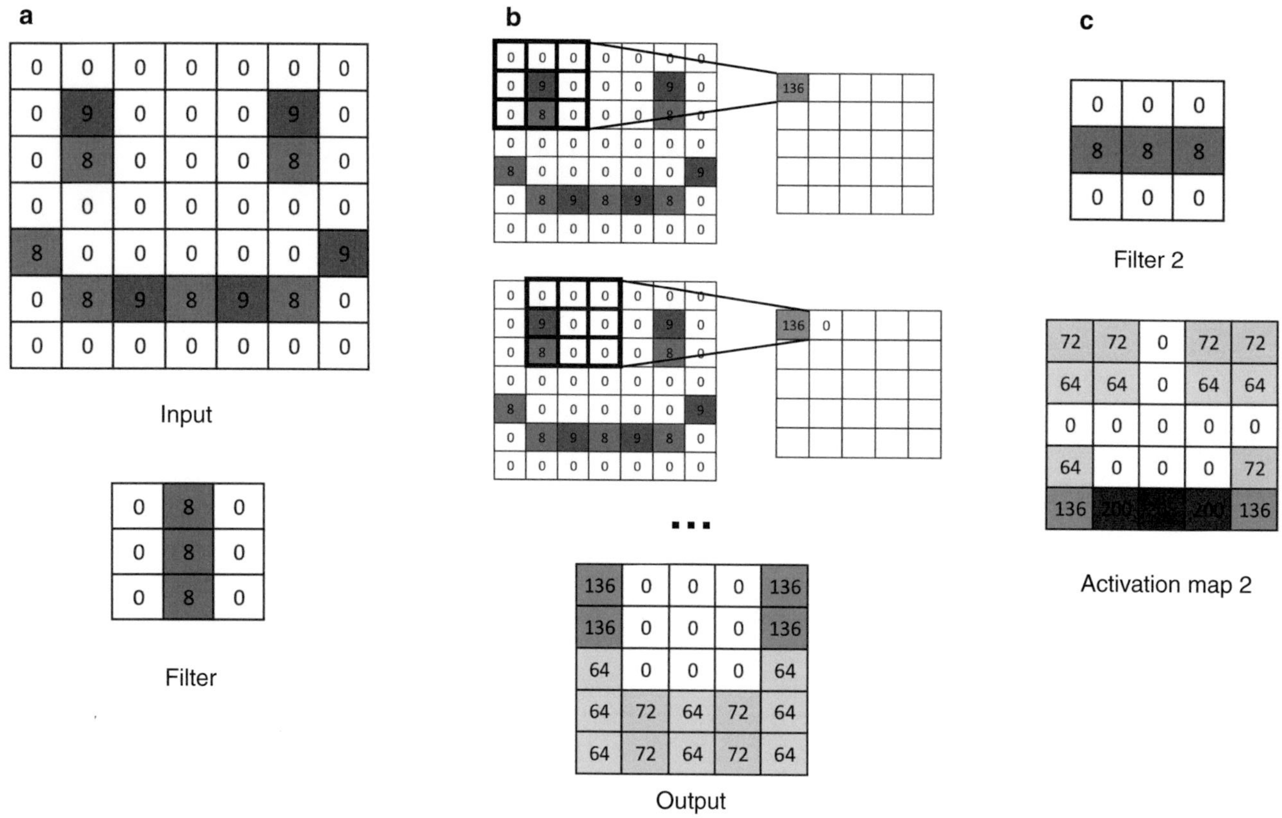

Fig. 6.3 (**a**) A convolutional filter measures local response of an image to arbitrary patterns of a small size. In this example, a 7 × 7 input image is displayed along with a 3 × 3 filter. Pixel shading is scaled to the numeric values. (**b**) By sliding the filter across an image, local responses to the filter are measured, forming an activation map for that particular filter. At the end of this process, a 5 × 5 activation map is produced that records the local responses at all locations of the image. This activation map can then be used for the subsequent layer. (**c**) Example of a different output for a different layer. Note how this horizontally oriented filter has a greater response at the mouth of the smiley face, whereas the first vertically oriented filter had a greater response at the eyes

Classification CNNs often consist of multiple convolutional layers separated by pooling layers. The first convolutional layer records local information (e.g., edges, texture, brightness) about image features; the next combines those bits of local information and so on such that each successive layer identifies an increasingly complex synthesis of visual information. The final layers are usually fully connected and provide the network output/classification. An important distinction of classification CNNs is that they perform dimensionality reduction: they condense information from a 2D or 3D input image to a 1D vector of output classes.

A prototypical example of this type of architecture is LeNet-5 [1], which was created in 1998 and consisted of three convolutional layers separated by average pooling layers. This algorithm was successfully used for recognition of handwritten digits on the MNIST dataset.

The widely known AlexNet [2], which won the 2012 ImageNet competition, similarly consists of five convolutional and three max pooling layers (Fig. 6.5a). One reason this algorithm performed better was the addition of dropout and data augmentation techniques, which improved generalizability. These are further discussed below. Subsequent state-of-the-art architectures remain fundamentally based on CNNs, with various architectural tricks and improvements. Notable examples include GoogLeNet (aka Inception v1) [3], VGG [4], ResNet [5], DenseNet [6], ResNeXt [7], and SENet [8].

CNNs have been applied to numerous applications in thoracic imaging. Lahani and colleagues used GoogLeNet and ResNet to classify chest X-rays as positive or negative for tuberculosis [9]. A five-layer CNN was used to classify interstitial lung disease on 32 × 32 voxel patches [10]. Tang et al. used AlexNet, VGG, ResNet, Inception, and DenseNet to classify chest X-rays as normal versus abnormal with excellent performance [11].

Object Detection

Object detection adds onto classification by finding the location of an object[3] in addition to its identity. A variety of strat-

[3]This is known as a regression problem, in which the output is a number rather than a class.

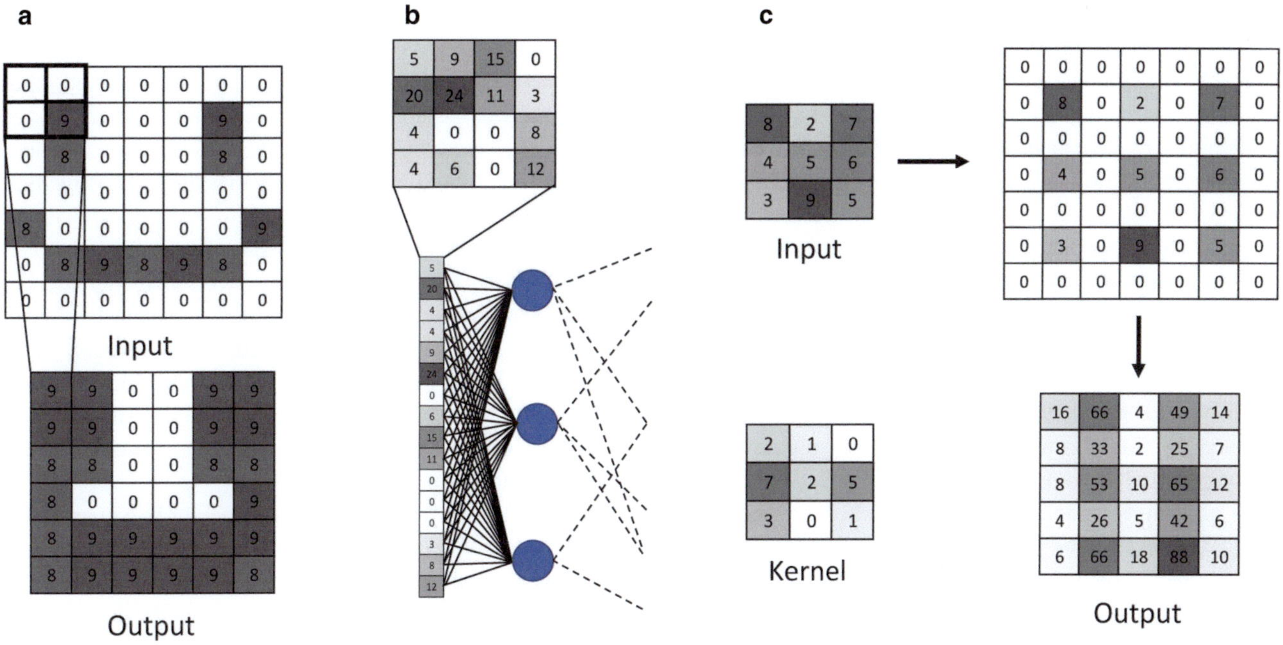

Fig. 6.4 Common layer types used in neural networks. (**a**) Max pooling. For a 2 × 2 kernel, maximum values are obtained within every 2 × 2 block. (**b**) Fully connected layer. Each neuron in a fully connected layer is connected to every input. (**c**) Transposed convolution. This operation is equivalent to zero-padding an input and then performing a convolution, enabling an output with larger dimensions than the input

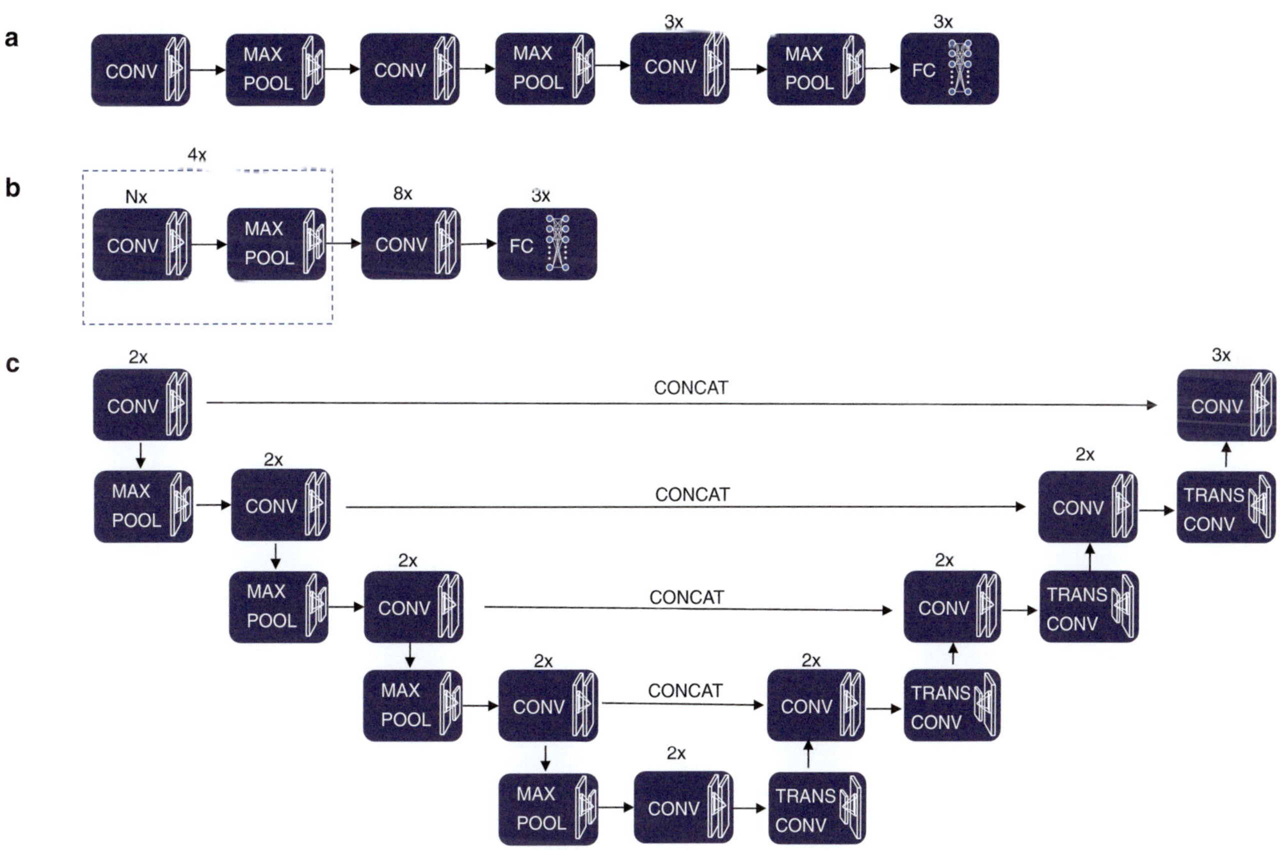

Fig. 6.5 Examples of CNN architectures. (**a**) AlexNet. This is a typical CNN containing alternating convolutional and max pooling layers followed by fully connected layers. (**b**) YOLO. Convolutional and max pooling layers are again alternated before fully connected layers. C. U-Net. Symmetric upsampling and downsampling layers are alternated with convolutional layers. CONCAT stands for concatenation. Note that no fully connected layers are used

egies have been created for this purpose, and we review two classes of approaches here.

R-CNN [12] and its successors, Fast R-CNN [13] and Faster R-CNN [14], are a popular class of object detection methods containing (1) a pretrained feature extractor derived from a classification algorithm (e.g., the first layers from VGG) that derives features from candidate bounding boxes, (2) a region proposal algorithm that searches for potential objects of interests (i.e., bounding boxes with specific locations), and (3) a classifier that uses the extracted features to determine the object identity. R-CNN and Fast R-CNN used a separate algorithm for region proposal, but Faster R-CNN built region proposal into a single neural network that could be trained end to end. The first step was the feature extractor, which then was used to train the region proposal network. The output of the region proposal network undergoes a pooling operation that is then used to train the classifier. Training is alternated between the region proposal network and the remainder of components. This led to a first-place finish in the 2015 ImageNet Large Scale Visual Recognition (ILSVRC) object detection challenge.

Another popular type of object detection is You Only Look Once (YOLO, Fig. 6.5b) [15]. YOLO divides an image into grid cells; for each grid cell, multiple bounding boxes are proposed along with "confidence," the predicted overlap of each bounding box with ground truth bounding boxes. In addition, a prediction of the likelihood that the grid represents an object is generated. The network design consists of multiple convolutional/max pooling layers followed by fully connected layers before generating the aforementioned outputs. This approach has the benefit of speed at relatively modest costs in accuracy relative to other methods such as Faster R-CNN. Updated versions of this architecture [16, 17] have led to incremental improvements.

Faster R-CNN and YOLO have been used for multiple applications in thoracic imaging including detection of foreign bodies on chest X-rays [18], pulmonary nodules on CT chest [19, 20], and other abnormalities on chest X-ray [21].

Segmentation

Most segmentation architectures now take advantage of fully convolutional neural networks, which do not incorporate fully connected layers. Fully convolutional networks (FCNs) [22, 23] are adaptations of CNNs used for image classification applied to segmentation. The insight of the original work describing FCNs in 2015 was that fully connected layers are equivalent to convolutional layers. For instance, if the final convolutional layer of a CNN has j activation maps and has size $k \times k$ with final dense layer of a CNN consisting of n neurons, then the output of the CNN is a weighted sum of the $j \times k \times k$ activations for each of the n neurons; however, this is equivalent to the output of a convolutional layer with n filters of size $k \times k$.

The benefit of this conversion is that the network can now be applied to images of arbitrary size since unlike fully connected layers, convolutional layers do not have a fixed input size. If the FCN is applied to a larger image than the image size it was trained on, the result is a low-resolution segmentation of the original image rather than a single classification for the entire image.

A refined segmentation map at the original resolution can be obtained by adding upsampling layers that increase the size of the output activation map. In FCNs, the upsampling is performed by using a transposed convolutional layer (Fig. 6.3c). Furthermore, through skip connections, the segmentations can be further refined by adding information from more shallow layers, which retain finer structural information of the original image.

Similar ideas are employed in the popular U-Net architecture [24]. A set of convolutions/downsampling layers are followed by a set of upsampling layers. Compared to FCN, the downsampling layers and upsampling layers demonstrate full symmetry, and the skip connections used perform concatenation rather than addition operations. These skip connections also have the critical property of countering *vanishing gradient*, in which weights of layers are updated inefficiently due to the depth of the architecture. The symmetric appearance of downsampling and upsampling layers leads to a U-shape, hence U-Net. Such architectures are also called encoder-decoder architectures.

The Mask R-CNN [25] architecture is an adaptation of Faster R-CNN as described for purposes of object detection. This adds an FCN branch for each proposed region that predicts segmentations in parallel with classification.

U-Nets have been used for many applications including left ventricular size and function from cardiac MRI [26] and segmentation of true and false lumen in CT of aortic dissection [27]. A 3D U-Net style architecture was used to quantify myocardial delayed enhancement of hypertrophic cardiomyopathy patients [28]. Mask R-CNN has been used for lung cancer detection and segmentation on PET-CT [29].

Reconstruction

Reconstruction algorithms that convert raw CT or MRI data usually require specialized knowledge to develop. Such reconstruction algorithms are often framed as minimization problems with known solutions; however, deep learning methods can be used to speed up the process by determining specific hyperparameters. For instance, in one of the first examples of this method, Yang and colleagues [30] reframed the Alternating Direction Method of Multipliers (ADMM) algorithm for compressed-sensing MRI as a deep neural network. This resulted in superior image quality with low reconstruction times.

Postprocessing

Another class of algorithms takes data that has already been transferred to the image domain and then tries to perform some operation such as artifact reduction, noise reduction, or other processes that enhance the image. Architectures of this type usually use many of the same building blocks already discussed. For instance, a denoising algorithm for CT used an encoder-decoder type of architecture in addition to skip connections and residual connections [31]. Jin and colleagues similarly used a U-Net with skip/residual connections for improving quality of low-dose CT [32]. Masutani and colleagues used two architectures—one with three convolutional layers and the other a U-Net style architecture—to generate "super-resolution" cardiac MRI images based on images reconstructed from a fraction of k-space sampling.

Other Common Architectural Components

Dropout

Dropout layers are a useful method for preventing overfitting by removing neurons randomly during training. Prior to training, a dropout probability p is selected, and each neuron is randomly switched off with probability p. Because neurons are randomly shut off, the neural network tends to not rely on any single neuron's output, building redundancy into the network. This has the effect of decreasing overfitting, improving robustness of the model, and improving generalizability. Using dropout lengthens training time, but the results are usually better.

Batch Normalization

One issue of training deep neural networks is that the process of gradient descent (used to optimize weights) has a tendency to lead to smaller and smaller gradients (the vanishing gradient problem) or larger and larger gradients (the exploding gradient problem). Because of this, weights of the network do not change at all or their magnitude becomes large/unstable, making it impossible to train a good model. In brief, the reason for this relates to the tendency of the variance of outputs to increase for deeper layers but activation functions potentially saturating for extreme input values (e.g., 0–1 in the case of the sigmoid function), resulting in small gradients. There are several solutions that have been proposed such as nonsaturating activation functions, but one popular method to address this is batch normalization, which essentially normalizes the input in order to control the variance of any specific layer. Because of this, batch normalization is now often performed between convolutional layers of deep neural networks.

Pretrained Versus De Novo Networks

Neural networks can either be developed from scratch or repurposed from the work of others by taking advantage of open access libraries. For rapid prototyping, it is usually faster to start with a tried and true existing network architecture rather than developing a new one. In many cases, pretrained networks exist for use from online repositories in which the weights of the network have been initialized by training on a separate dataset. Starting with a pretrained neural network can reduce training time and amount of data required when compared to starting from scratch; this process is known as transfer learning. It is ideal to have a network pretrained on a dataset similar to the one that is going to be used for new algorithm development; for example, a pretrained model for identifying pulmonary nodules on CT would be a good starting point for developing a model that identifies consolidation. However, even in the absence of directly relevant features, using pretrained networks can still be useful. For instance, starting with a CNN used for classifying colorized images of objects such as boats and planes from the ImageNet dataset would still be useful for radiology applications. This is because many of the earlier layers of neural networks identify primitive features that are universally relevant for visual recognition and can still be applied to other modalities. In most cases, it is beneficial to start from a pretrained network, though in some cases a relevant architecture may not exist.

Determine the Loss Function

As with any optimization problem, it is necessary to specify a *loss function* (also known as a cost or objective function) which is what the algorithm seeks to minimize. An important property of the loss function is that it be differentiable, as this is necessary to perform the backpropagation process that optimizes weights.

For classification problems with N classes, the loss function is often cross entropy loss, defined as

$$-\sum_{k=1}^{N} \mathrm{c}_k \log\left(p_k\right)$$

where c_k is the true label (1 if it is the true class, 0 otherwise).

The intuition for this loss function is that it amounts to the log probability of predicting the true class. For instance, if the true class is a for $1 \leq a \leq N$, then the loss is simply $-\log(p_a)$; that is, for low probability p_a, the loss will be high, and for a high probability, the loss will be low.

For two classes, we obtain binary cross entropy or

$$-\left[c \log p + (1-c)\log(1-p)\right]$$

where p is the probability for class $c = 1$.

For object detection problems, the loss function will incorporate a classification loss for determining the true class in addition to a separate regression loss for determining the adequacy of the bounding box.

The most common regression losses are known as the mean square error loss and mean absolute error.

The mean square error loss (L2 loss) for N predicted values $\hat{y}_k$ and a true quantity of y_k is

$$\frac{1}{N}\sum_{k=1}^{N}\left(y_k - \hat{y}_k\right)^2$$

The mean absolute error (L1 loss) is

$$\frac{1}{N}\sum_{k=1}^{N}\left|y_k - \hat{y}_k\right|$$

As an example, Faster RCNN uses a loss function composed of a weighted sum of cross entropy and a modified L1 loss called smooth L1 loss.

The loss function for segmentation problems can also be binary cross entropy. However, it is useful to use other loss functions in order to account for class imbalance. The dice coefficient is often used to evaluate the results of two sets A and B defined as twice the intersection between two sets divided by the sum of their number of elements. To make the function differentiable, a small modification is made to dice loss in which it is defined as $1-\frac{2A \cap B+\varepsilon}{|A|+|B|+\varepsilon}$ where ε is a small number. Some segmentation loss functions combine this with binary cross entropy.

Loss functions for reconstruction problems include L2 loss and functions incorporating the structural similarity index (SSIM) [33].

SSIM between two images x and y is defined as

$$\frac{2\mu_x\mu_y + C_1}{\mu_x^2 + \mu_y^2 + C_1} \cdot \frac{2\sigma_{xy} + C_2}{\sigma_x^2 + \sigma_y^2 + C_2}$$

where μ_x is the average value of x, μ_y is the average value of y, σ_{xy} is the covariance of x and y, σ_x^2 is the variance of x, and σ_y^2 is the variance of y. C_1 and C_2 are chosen on the basis of the dynamic range of x and y.

Set Training Parameters

Prior to actually training, there are several additional considerations to make prior to starting. We briefly discuss these, as they are more general issues of training neural networks rather than being specific to building algorithms for imaging purposes.

Learning Rate and Optimizers

The learning rate is the parameter that determines how much to update the weights at a time based on the gradient of the loss function and its intermediaries. If too high, weights will change too quickly, and convergence to a minimum loss value will not occur. A learning rate that is too low may result in a local minimum of the loss rather than a more optimal minimum. Furthermore, it will take longer to obtain convergence. As such, the learning rate can have significant effects both on the performance of an algorithm and training time. A set of learning rate optimizer algorithms have been developed to improve this process by taking into account the size of the gradient at previous steps. Commonly used examples include AdaGrad, RMSProp, and Adam. Nevertheless, it is good practice to train your algorithm using learning rates at multiple orders of magnitude—finding the "sweet spot" for the learning rate often makes all the difference in model convergence!

Batch Size

The batch size is the number of training samples examined at once for purposes of updating weights. For many imaging applications, the batch size is constrained by the amount of GPU memory, and the largest batch size should be used.

Augmentation

During training time, it is common to use augmentation methods to effectively enlarge the size of the training set. The concept of augmentation is that many operations should not fundamentally change the content of an image; for example, if a pulmonary nodule is rotated, then it is still a pulmonary nodule. Therefore, a rotated image of a pulmonary nodule along with its label can serve as a valid training example. Common augmentation techniques include brightness/contrast adjustment, blurring, flipping, displacement, rotation, shearing, cropping, and zoom. Similar to dropout, augmentation helps filter out spurious signals and has the effect of making algorithms more generalizable.

Training Your Algorithm/Hyperparameter Tuning

A Note on Data Preparation

One must take special care in data curation prior to algorithm selection and training, as ultimately the strength and accuracy of any machine learning algorithm is entirely dependent on the quality and quantity of provided training data. While the quantity of training data required for convergence scales with the complexity of the desired task (e.g., segmentation of the heart chambers on chest CT is likely to require less training data than segmenting them in patients with congenital heart disease), at a minimum, one should have a few hundred datasets sourced from unique patients. Additionally, one must also consider what annotations are necessary and available for these images—if one were trying to simply identify patients with congenital heart disease, obtaining this diagnosis from clinical notes is likely trivial, but the segmentation of heart chambers requires substantial *manual* annotation. Lastly, it is exceedingly important to carefully partition into independent training and testing sets. For the example of cardiac chamber segmentation on chest CT, which itself is a stack of 2D slice, you should *not* allow slices from the same patient to appear in both training *and* testing sets. This leads to *overfitting*, where the algorithm becomes exceptionally good at its task on the training dataset—at the expense of performance on other independent datasets, i.e., *generalizability*. Thus, failure to appropriately partition datasets will likely lead to over-inflated estimates of model performance, as the algorithm will have previously "seen" similar images during training and render these analyses invalid. Readers should refer to Chap. 5 of this text for additional details and recommendations on preparation and curation of imaging data for cardiothoracic AI algorithms.

Hyperparameter Tuning

With data preparation, algorithm development, and training parameters setup complete, the next step is to train the algorithm. During training, various parameters such as the learning rate, batch size, degree of regularization, degree of dropout, and augmentation options are adjusted to obtain optimal results. This process is called hyperparameter tuning.

Hyperparameter tuning can be a daunting task due to the potentially large search space of hyperparameters. The most basic way to examine hyperparameters is to pick several possible values for each of the hyperparameters and then try all combinations of the hyperparameters; this is known as grid search. While this search is exhaustive, it is also the most time-consuming. In randomized search, a range of values for each hyperparameter is specified, from which a random set of hyperparameters is selected. For a large set of values, randomized search is preferred over grid search due to its ability to find a reasonable solution faster than grid search, potentially outperforming grid search due to its lack of constraint on hyperparameter values.

However, randomized search still only captures a relatively small amount of a search space. A more methodical approach would be to try various sets of hyperparameters but use the information obtained to direct the selection of the next set of hyperparameters. For instance, if we found that runs with a learning rate of 0.1 led to divergence, we would no longer want to try learning rates this large. This optimization problem can be addressed with the process of Bayesian optimization. Briefly, this process consists of defining a surrogate model that models loss as a function of hyperparameters. A separate function called the acquisition function is used to determine the next set of hyperparameters. Examples of surrogate models include Random Forest Regressions, Gaussian Processes, and Tree-structured Parzen Estimators (TPE). Examples of acquisition functions include expected improvement (EI) and upper confidence bound (UCB). Many optimization methods already have publicly available implementations, for instance, Scikit Optimize.

After training, the next step is to validate and test your algorithm, which will be further discussed in Chap. 12.

Advanced Approaches

Ensemble Networks

Ensemble networks, specifically stacked ensemble networks, are a popular approach for improving algorithm performance by simultaneously leveraging the predictive power of multiple component networks to increase algorithm flexibility. Rather than using a single network to accomplish a predictive task, several networks are simultaneously developed to accomplish the same task. Predictions from each of these networks are then consolidated using a voting or averaging procedure and, in some cases, more complex fusion approaches using a separate network. Component networks in the ensemble can have dramatically different architectures, capturing diverse sets of features that help boost algorithm performance. Ensemble components may also be completely different classes of machine learning algorithms, such as generalized additive models, random forests, and support vector machines.

Although the extended training time and computational complexity of deep learning algorithms prevent the implementation of large ensemble networks, smaller ensemble algorithms, comprising two or three carefully chosen network architectures, can offer substantial performance gains. For example, Bahrami et al. [34] proposed an ensemble deep learning algorithm, comprising only two component networks, for automated selection of myocardial inversion time. The first component network had a VGG19 architecture, which captured spatial imaging features. The second component network was a bidirectional LSTM and was included to capture temporal information across the sequence of images. Output features from both networks were then used for myocardial inversion time selection using a smaller fully connected network. The ensemble achieved greater accuracy (92.1%) than each of its component networks (VGG19, 83.9%; LSTM, 81.9%), when compared to inversion time expert-annotated ground truths.

Cascaded Networks

Radiologists implicitly perform imaging tasks in multiple stages. For example, to characterize pulmonary nodules on CT, a radiologist may first detect the presence of a nodule candidate by scrolling through a CT series. In a second stage, the radiologist may then subcategorize the nodule candidate as malignant or benign using its imaging features.

Cascaded deep learning algorithms, a subclass of ensemble learning, explicitly emulate this multistage process by dividing a complex imaging task, such as nodule detection, into simpler tasks performed by separately trained networks. These separately trained networks are then sequentially concatenated.

Several cascaded approaches have been developed for a variety of cardiothoracic imaging applications, including pulmonary nodule detection on CT and imaging plane prescription for cardiac MRI. Cui et al. and Tan et al. [35, 36] both used cascaded approaches for the task of lung nodule detection. In a first stage, a network was used for localization of lung nodule candidates. Nodule candidates were then cropped and propagated through a second network for nodule classification. Tan et al. additionally applied a lung segmentation network, prior to the localization of nodule candidates, to ensure nodule detection within the lung areas.

Blansit et al. [37] developed a cascaded deep learning algorithm to prescribe imaging planes for cardiac MRI. They divided the overarching task of automated plane prescription into three smaller tasks performed by three separately trained networks: a mitral valve slice (MVS) localization network, a cardiac bounding box (BB) network, and a third network for valve localization. The MVS slice from the MVS localization network was cropped using the BB network and subsequently propagated through the final network for valve localization, which was then used to prescribe imaging planes.

Multitask Networks

Deep learning algorithms in cardiothoracic imaging are typically designed to accomplish a singular overarching imaging task (e.g., nodule detection, cardiac segmentation, pneumonia detection). Through training, networks are able to learn imaging features useful for automating the given task. However, by focusing on a single imaging task, networks may ignore imaging features that could further improve algorithm performance. Multitask networks can be used to leverage underutilized imaging features by forcing the deep learning algorithm to perform multiple related tasks simultaneously. As a result, imaging features learned by the network are synergistically shared across each of the related tasks, which often improves algorithm performance.

Spatial Transformation Layers and Image Registration

Spatial transformation networks (STNs) are typically embedded within larger networks and learn to spatially manipulate images to make algorithms robust to spatial variability (e.g., patient positioning in the scanner). In the field of radiology, STNs are most often used to standardize image views using fast automated affine and deformable image registration [38].

Customized Architectures

The advanced approaches described above can be combined in a multitude of ways, allowing for increasingly flexible algorithm architectures for a variety of imaging tasks. One might first use a spatial transformer network to standardize an image view, which then contributes to a cascade of stacked ensemble networks, each with their own multitask objectives, but where does this end? The development of overly complex architectures is typically limited by computing power or the amount of training data available. Therefore, in the context of cardiothoracic imaging, it is important to leverage the knowledge of domain experts to gain an understanding of the mechanisms behind the desired task when designing more complex network architectures.

Deep Learning Libraries and Hardware

Software

Python is usually the programming language of choice for machine learning—it is the most commonly used and the simplest to learn.

A variety of software libraries are available to use for deep learning. A brief discussion of each follows.

TensorFlow is Google's open source deep learning library and currently the most widely used. It has excellent documentation, and a majority of applications to radiologic applications have been implemented in TensorFlow. Adopters of TensorFlow have the benefit of accessing a large number of pretrained models. TensorFlow is suited to deployment/production, and TensorFlow users also have the advantage of more easily using Tensor Processing Units (TPUs), a custom Google application-specific integrated circuit chip that can be used for acceleration of machine learning tasks.

Keras is a library that sits on top of other deep learning libraries. It is excellent for use by inexperienced programmers due to its ease of use and excellent documentation. Keras can be used with TensorFlow, Theano, and other deep learning backends and has recently been fully integrated into TensorFlow 2 due to its popularity. While Keras is generally high level and may lack certain aspects of customizability, this can be supplemented by the versatility of TensorFlow.

PyTorch is an open source library developed by Facebook's AI Research group (FAIR). As implied by the name, PyTorch retains syntax of Python, allowing for easy adoption by those who are already familiar with Python. PyTorch is less commonly used compared to TensorFlow but is preferred by many AI researchers due to the ability to prototype quickly. Whereas TensorFlow previously required a fixed computation graph, PyTorch employs dynamic computation graphs that can be adjusted at any time, for instance, to accommodate inputs of varying sizes. It was initially developed as a Python version of Torch, also a machine learning library, that is no longer in active development.

Caffe is a library developed at Berkeley that is geared toward computer vision applications. It was popular in academic communities, and many early works on application to cardiothoracic radiology were written using Caffe. Caffe has now been succeeded by Caffe2, which in turn has been merged into PyTorch. Caffe2's emphasis is on scalability and production purposes such as mobile device applications.

Other frameworks include Microsoft Cognitive Toolkit, MXNet, and Theano. While all have their advantages and disadvantages, we recommend that beginners start with Keras/TensorFlow or PyTorch due to their documentation and overall ease of use.

Hardware

Hardware requirements will vary widely by application. Shallow 2D CNNs with few layers can be expected to train in a reasonable time on CPU. Practically speaking, however, the enormous size of medical images requires a substantial amount of memory for many applications. We would recommend a graphics card with at least 11 GB memory (the size of a Nvidia GTX 1080 Ti) and more if one's budget can handle it. Any network employing 3D convolutions, e.g., 3D U-Nets, is likely to be resource hungry, and larger amounts of memory are a necessity.

An important consideration for machine learner practitioners is deciding on buying/building a workstation versus using cloud-based services such as Amazon Web Services, Google Cloud, and Microsoft Azure. For low levels of utilization or light applications, cloud-based services are more cost-effective, but for sustained use (e.g., more than a few months of continuous GPU use), an on-site solution will be cheaper for equivalent builds. Cloud-based services do give one the flexibility of spinning up an instance at any time with varying hardware requirements depending on the application. They also are very reliable; building one's own workstation implies that the user will have to address any hardware failures. A middle ground is a prebuilt workstation, in which warranties and technical support are usually part of the purchase, though these are more expensive than assembling the components yourself. Finally, cloud-based solutions are susceptible to cyberattacks, while on-site solutions are usually more secure.

Conclusion/Further Reading

In this chapter, we have outlined the process of building an AI algorithm for imaging purposes from defining the problem type to common architectures and basic concepts of algorithm training. We invite the reader to further explore these topics in greater depth through resources produced by experts in the field. *Computer Vision: Algorithms and Applications* [39] provides a comprehensive overview of classic computer vision methods; an updated edition is anticipated for 2021. *Deep Learning with Python* is written by the creator of Keras, Francois Chollet [40], and provides excellent guidance on getting started with writing deep neural networks. Online courses include Andrew Ng's Deep Learning course on the Coursera platform and Stanford's CS231n: Convolutional Neural Networks for Visual Recognition, the lectures and notes for which are freely available online. Finally, it likely goes without saying but much of building imaging algorithms simply comes with experience. The best way to learn is to program, and this chapter is just a start.

References

1. Lecun Y, Bottou L, Bengio Y, Haffner P. Gradient-based learning applied to document recognition. Proc IEEE. 1998;86(11):2278–324. https://doi.org/10.1109/5.726791.
2. Krizhevsky A, Sutskever I, Hinton GE. ImageNet classification with deep convolutional neural networks. In: Proceedings of the 25th international conference on neural information processing systems, vol. 1. Lake Tahoe, Nevada: Curran Associates Inc.; 2012. p. 1097–105.
3. Szegedy C, Liu W, Jia Y, Sermanet P, Reed S, Anguelov D, Erhan D, Vanhoucke V, Rabinovich A, editors. Going deeper with convolutions. In: Proceedings of the IEEE conference on computer vision and pattern recognition. 2015.
4. Simonyan K, Zisserman A. Very deep convolutional networks for large-scale image recognition. arXiv preprint arXiv:14091556. 2014.
5. He K, Zhang X, Ren S, Sun J, editors. Deep residual learning for image recognition. In: Proceedings of the IEEE conference on computer vision and pattern recognition. 2016.
6. Huang G, Liu Z, Van Der Maaten L, Weinberger KQ, editors. Densely connected convolutional networks. In: Proceedings of the IEEE conference on computer vision and pattern recognition. 2017.
7. Xie S, Girshick R, Dollár P, Tu Z, He K, editors. Aggregated residual transformations for deep neural networks. In: 2017 IEEE Conference on Computer Vision and Pattern Recognition (CVPR). 2017. 21–26 July 2017.
8. Hu J, Shen L, Sun G, editors. Squeeze-and-excitation networks. 2018 IEEE/CVF Conference on computer vision and pattern recognition. 2018. 18–23 June 2018.
9. Lakhani P, Sundaram B. Deep learning at chest radiography: automated classification of pulmonary tuberculosis by using convolutional neural networks. Radiology. 2017;284(2):574–82. https://doi.org/10.1148/radiol.2017162326. Epub 2017/04/25. PubMed PMID: 28436741.
10. Anthimopoulos M, Christodoulidis S, Ebner L, Christe A, Mougiakakou S. Lung pattern classification for interstitial lung diseases using a deep convolutional neural network. IEEE Trans Med Imaging. 2016;35(5):1207–16. https://doi.org/10.1109/TMI.2016.2535865.
11. Tang Y-X, Tang Y-B, Peng Y, Yan K, Bagheri M, Redd BA, Brandon CJ, Lu Z, Han M, Xiao J. Automated abnormality classification of chest radiographs using deep convolutional neural networks. NPJ Digit Med. 2020;3(1):1–8.
12. Girshick R, Donahue J, Darrell T, Malik J, editors. Rich feature hierarchies for accurate object detection and semantic segmentation. In: 2014 IEEE conference on computer vision and pattern recognition. 2014. 23–28 June 2014.
13. Girshick R, editor. Fast R-CNN. 2015 IEEE International conference on computer vision (ICCV). 2015. 7–13 Dec 2015.
14. Ren S, He K, Girshick R, Sun J, editors. Faster r-cnn: towards real-time object detection with region proposal networks. Adv Neural Inf Process Syst. 2015;28:1–9.
15. Redmon J, Divvala S, Girshick R, Farhadi A, editors. You only look once: unified, real-time object detection. In: 2016 IEEE Conference on computer vision and pattern recognition (CVPR). 2016. 27–30 June 2016.
16. Redmon J, Farhadi A, editors. YOLO9000: better, faster, stronger. In: 2017 IEEE Conference on computer vision and pattern recognition (CVPR). 2017. 21–26 July 2017.
17. Redmon J, Farhadi A. Yolov3: an incremental improvement. arXiv preprint arXiv:180402767. 2018.
18. Santosh KC, Dhar MK, Rajbhandari R, Neupane A, editors. Deep neural network for foreign object detection in chest X-rays. In: 2020 IEEE 33rd International symposium on computer-based medical systems (CBMS). 2020. 28–30 July 2020.
19. Sindhu Ramachandran S, George J, Skaria S, Varun VV. "Using YOLO based deep learning network for real time detection and localization of lung nodules from low dose CT scans," Proc. SPIE 10575, Medical Imaging 2018: Computer-Aided Diagnosis, 105751I (27 February 2018); https://doi.org/10.1117/12.2293699. Event: SPIE Medical Imaging, 2018, Houston, Texas, United States.
20. Traoré A, Ly AO, Akhloufi MA, editors. Evaluating deep learning algorithms in pulmonary nodule detection*. In: 2020 42nd Annual International Conference of the IEEE Engineering in Medicine & Biology Society (EMBC). 2020. 20–24 July 2020.
21. Cho Y, Lee SM, Cho YH, Lee JG, Park B, Lee G, Kim N, Seo JB. Deep chest X-ray: detection and classification of lesions based on deep convolutional neural networks. Int J Imaging Syst Technol. 2021;31(1):72–81.
22. Shelhamer E, Long J, Darrell T. Fully convolutional networks for semantic segmentation. IEEE Trans Pattern Anal Mach Intell. 2017;39(4):640–51. https://doi.org/10.1109/TPAMI.2016.2572683.
23. Long J, Shelhamer E, Darrell T, editors. Fully convolutional networks for semantic segmentation. In: Proceedings of the IEEE conference on computer vision and pattern recognition. 2015.
24. Ronneberger O, Fischer P, Brox T, editors. U-net: convolutional networks for biomedical image segmentation. In: International conference on medical image computing and computer-assisted intervention. Springer; New York, 2015.
25. He K, Gkioxari G, Dollar P, Girshick R. Mask R-CNN. In: International Conference on Computer Vision (ICCV). 2017.
26. Tao Q, Yan W, Wang Y, Paiman EH, Shamonin DP, Garg P, Plein S, Huang L, Xia L, Sramko M. Deep learning–based method for fully automatic quantification of left ventricle function from cine MR images: a multivendor, multicenter study. Radiology. 2019;290(1):81–8.
27. Hahn LD, Mistelbauer G, Higashigaito K, Koci M, Willemink MJ, Sailer AM, Fischbein M, Fleischmann D. CT-based true-and false-lumen segmentation in Type B aortic dissection using machine learning. Radiol Cardiothorac Imaging. 2020;2(3):e190179.
28. Fahmy AS, Neisius U, Chan RH, Rowin EJ, Manning WJ, Maron MS, Nezafat R. Three-dimensional deep convolutional neural networks for automated myocardial scar quantification in hypertrophic cardiomyopathy: a multicenter multivendor study. Radiology. 2020;294(1):52–60.
29. Zhang R, Cheng C, Zhao X, Li X. Multiscale mask R-CNN–based lung tumor detection using PET imaging. Mol Imaging. 2019;18:1536012119863531.
30. Yang Y, Sun J, Li H, Xu Z. ADMM-CSNet: a deep learning approach for image compressive sensing. IEEE Trans Pattern Anal Mach Intell. 2020;42(3):521–38.
31. Chen H, Zhang Y, Kalra MK, Lin F, Chen Y, Liao P, Zhou J, Wang G. Low-dose CT with a residual encoder-decoder convolutional neural network. IEEE Trans Med Imaging. 2017;36(12):2524–35. https://doi.org/10.1109/TMI.2017.2715284. Epub 2017/06/18. PubMed PMID: 28622671; PMCID: PMC5727581.
32. Jin KH, McCann MT, Froustey E, Unser M. Deep convolutional neural network for inverse problems in imaging. IEEE Trans Image Process. 2017;26(9):4509–22.
33. Zhao H, Gallo O, Frosio I, Kautz J. Loss functions for image restoration with neural networks. IEEE Trans Comput Imaging. 2017;3(1):47–57. https://doi.org/10.1109/TCI.2016.2644865.
34. Bahrami N, Retson T, Blansit K, Wang K, Hsiao A. Automated selection of myocardial inversion time with a convolutional neural network: spatial temporal ensemble myocardium inversion network

(STEMI-NET). Magn Reson Med. 2019;81(5):3283–91. https://doi.org/10.1002/mrm.27680. Epub 2019/02/05. PubMed PMID: 30714197.

35. Cui S, Ming S, Lin Y, Chen F, Shen Q, Li H, Chen G, Gong X, Wang H. Development and clinical application of deep learning model for lung nodules screening on CT images. Sci Rep. 2020;10(1):13657. https://doi.org/10.1038/s41598-020-70629-3. Epub 2020/08/14. PubMed PMID: 32788705; PMCID: PMC7423892.
36. Tan J, Huo Y, Liang Z, Li L. Expert knowledge-infused deep learning for automatic lung nodule detection. J Xray Sci Technol. 2019;27(1):17–35. https://doi.org/10.3233/XST-180426. Epub 2018/11/20. PubMed PMID: 30452432; PMCID: PMC6453714.
37. Blansit K, Retson T, Masutani E, Bahrami N, Hsiao A. Deep learning–based prescription of cardiac MRI planes. Radiol Artif Intell. 2019;1(6):e180069. https://doi.org/10.1148/ryai.2019180069.
38. de Vos BD, Berendsen FF, Viergever MA, Sokooti H, Staring M, Isgum I. A deep learning framework for unsupervised affine and deformable image registration. Med Image Anal. 2019;52:128–43. https://doi.org/10.1016/j.media.2018.11.010. Epub 2018/12/24. PubMed PMID: 30579222.
39. Szeliski R. Computer vision: algorithms and applications. Springer Science & Business Media; New York, 2010.
40. Chollet F. Deep learning with Python. Manning Publications Company; Shelter Island, NY, 2017.

Radiomics: Technical Background

7

Bettina Baessler

Introduction

'Images are more than pictures, they are data' [15]. With this statement, the basic idea behind radiomics becomes clear: to use the data of pixel grey levels being encoded in digital medical images (and having a certain spatial relationship) to extract more information about tissue structure and even genetic phenotypes through quantitative image analysis. By means of statistical and mathematical algorithms, the digitally encrypted information in medical images, which is hidden to the human eye [23] and thus not accessible through traditional visual inspection of an image, can be revealed [15, 17, 19]. Differences in image intensity, shape or texture [9, 28] can be quantified by means of radiomics, thus overcoming the subjective nature of image interpretation. The extracted information is then used to enhance the existing clinical data for improved diagnosis, prognosis or assessment of treatment response, paving the way towards precision medicine.

Innumerable quantitative features can now be extracted using high-throughput computing from medical images of all modalities [18]. Since radiomics represents 'big data', analysis methods from the field of artificial intelligence such as machine learning are usually used to generate knowledge out of these data. As a consequence, radiomics is of high interest in order to enhance existing diagnostic processes with additional, quantitative data. In addition, radiomics – combined with advanced modelling – might be a valuable tool in providing prognostic information in various diseases.

Consequently, a steady increase in publications related to the field of radiomics could be observed over the past few years (Fig. 7.1). While the vast majority of these publications have been focused on the field of oncological imaging, first applications in cardiac imaging have been shown over the past few years, that radiomics and especially texture analysis might represent an interesting field of research with high potential in the cardiac imaging domain as well. An increasing number of publications have appeared within the past 3 years (Fig. 7.1), and an exponential rise is to be expected for the next 10 years.

This chapter summarizes the technical basics of the emerging field of radiomics with a special focus on the concepts behind texture analysis and texture features, which are especially important when it comes to cardiovascular imaging.

The Radiomics Workflow: Overview

The principle of radiomics is based upon a step-wise workflow, beginning with patient scheduling and image acquisition/reconstruction, continuing with image segmentation and image processing and finally leading to the extraction of a large number of radiomic features from different feature matrices, consecutive data analysis and building of predictive models for improved diagnostic or prognostic assessment. Figure 7.2 shows an exemplary radiomics workflow for cardiac MRI.

While this chapter mainly focuses on the technical basics of radiomic feature extraction, the following sections are intended to give a short overview over the basics of each step required in the radiomics workflow after image acquisition and reconstruction.

Image Segmentation

Definition of the region of interest (ROI) in two-dimensional (2D) or of the volume of interest (VOI) in three-dimensional (3D) approaches (i.e. definition of the region in the image, where radiomic features will be calculated) is

B. Baessler, MD (✉)
Institute of Diagnostic and Interventional Radiology, University Hospital Würzburg, Würzburg, Germany

Institute of Diagnostic and Interventional Radiology, University Hospital Zurich, Zurich, Switzerland
e-mail: Baessler_B@ukw.de

C. N. De Cecco et al. (eds.), *Artificial Intelligence in Cardiothoracic Imaging*, Contemporary Medical Imaging,
https://doi.org/10.1007/978-3-030-92087-6_7

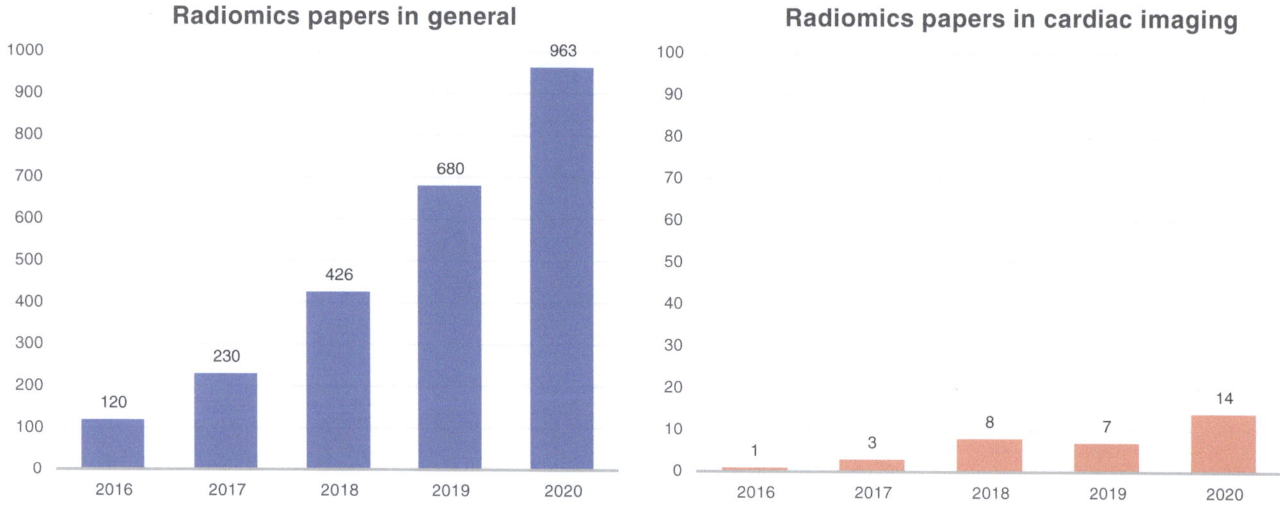

Fig. 7.1 Radiomics studies in medical and cardiac imaging. Number of radiomics studies in all fields of imaging (left) and in the field of cardiac imaging (right) according to a PubMed search (as of the end of November 2020)

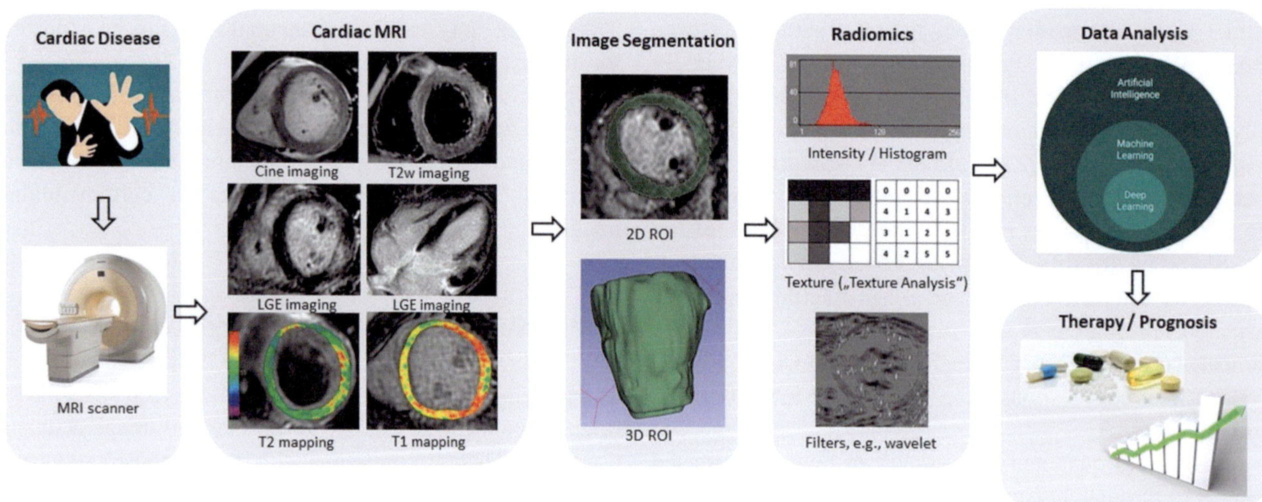

Fig. 7.2 Exemplary radiomics workflow for cardiac MRI. Schematic illustration of the patient journey including image acquisition, image analysis using radiomics and derived patient-specific therapy and prognosis. Symptomatic patients undergo cardiac MRI, where a multiparametric examination is performed. After image segmentation and image processing, radiomic features are extracted. High-level statistical modelling involving machine learning is applied for disease classification, patient clustering and individual risk stratification

the first step in the radiomics workflow after images have been acquired and reconstructed. ROI/VOI definition might be achieved by manual, semi-automated or fully automated methods, for each of which a variety of different software solutions are available (either open source or commercial).

It has to be noted that image segmentation requiring user interaction (as for manual and semi-automated methods) leads to potential observer bias in the extracted radiomic features and thus has to be taken into account during data analysis. For a more comprehensive discussion and practical advice on the image segmentation step, please refer to the recently published 'Radiomics how to' guide [30].

Image Processing

After image segmentation, image processing is the next crucial step before radiomic features can be extracted. In practice, image processing and feature extraction usually are performed in combination, but the image processing step has to be discussed separately because of its important implications for reproducible research and potential translatability of radiomics.

Image processing aims at homogenization of the images prior to extraction of radiomic features with respect to pixel spacing, grey-level intensities or bins of the grey-level histogram, aiming at an improved robustness of the extracted radiomic features [1, 7, 25]. Interpolation to isotropic voxel spacing is necessary for most texture features to become rotationally invariant and to increase reproducibility [31]. After an interpolation algorithm has been applied to the image, also the delineated ROI/VOI should be interpolated [31]. Range re-segmentation and intensity outlier filtering (i.e. normalization) are performed to remove pixels/voxels from the ROI/VOI, which fall outside of a pre-specified range of grey levels [31]. While range re-segmentation usually is feasible for CT and PET data, it is not possible for data with arbitrary intensity units such as MRI, where intensity outlier filtering is commonly applied [10, 29, 31]. Image discretization aims at grouping the original pixel/voxel grey-level values according to pre-defined range intervals (i.e. bins), a procedure that is conceptually comparable to the creation of a histogram. Three parameters characterize discretization: the range of the discretized quantity, the number of bins and their width (size).

For a detailed description of image interpolation and different interpolation algorithms, please refer to Zwanenburg et al. [32]. A discussion on optimal image processing settings can be found in van Timmeren et al. [30]. The most important message of this section is that the image processing step is one of the most crucial parts of a radiomics analysis and should be performed with care. Image processing settings hugely influence not only the robustness and reproducibility but also the bare values of the extracted features. Image processing settings thus should be reported in the methods sections of each radiomics study and adhere to the guidelines of the Image Biomarker Standardization Initiative (IBSI) [31, 32].

Feature Extraction

After thoughtful image processing, the step of radiomic feature extraction is finally reached. Feature extraction refers to the final processing step, where various feature descriptors are calculated, which quantify the characteristics of the grey levels within the defined ROI/VOI. The basis for feature extraction is the underlying structure of a medical image, which consists of a matrix of pixels/voxels with a limited number of grey levels. In digital images, the number of grey levels is limited, consisting of integer numbers ranging from 0 to $2^b - 1$, with b standing for the number of bits of the image [9]. For most digital images, 8 bits are sufficient, thus yielding a grey-level range from 0 to 255. MRI usually uses 12 bits with a grey-level range of 0–4095. Figure 7.3 shows an example of a 3-bit digital image with 5 × 5 pixels. The convention is that dark grey levels are attributed with lower values (i.e. black being attributed to 0) and lighter grey levels with higher values.

Many different ways and mathematical definitions of those features exist, leading to substantial variations in the radiomics literature and sometimes poor reproducibility of radiomics studies. Adherence to the IBSI guidelines [31, 32] thus is highly recommended.

Different families or matrices of radiomic features exist, the most often encountered ones being shape features, intensity (histogram)-based features, texture features and model-based features. In addition, different types of filters (e.g. wavelet or Gaussian filters) can be applied during the feature extraction step.

Shape Features

Shape or morphological features describe geometric aspects of an ROI/VOI, such as area and volume [31]. Besides such

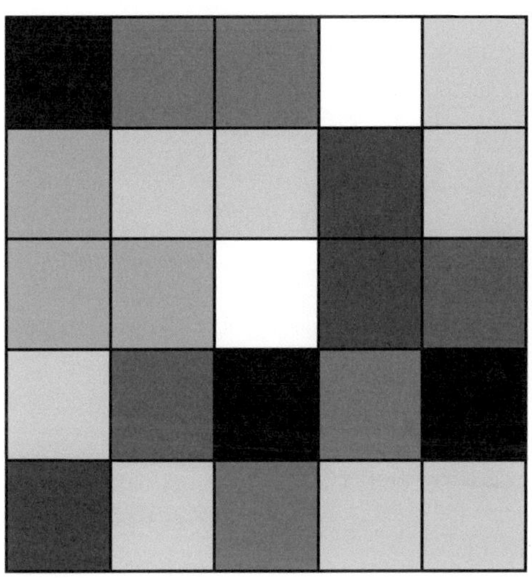

1	4	4	7	6
5	6	6	2	6
5	5	7	2	3
6	3	1	4	1
2	6	4	6	6

Fig. 7.3 Example of a digital image. Pixel matrix with 5 × 5 pixels and grey-level values ranging from 0 (black) to 7 (white). The right side shows the numerical representation of the image

relatively simple descriptors, shape features are also used to reflect the complex structural surface of a certain ROI/VOI, such as its compactness or sphericity. These features are mainly applied in the field of oncological imaging, where some tumours have been described as having a more spiculated appearance or 'ill-defined borders', indicating potential invasiveness and aggressiveness [12, 22]. Shape features have not been reported to be useful in cardiac imaging so far, since most applications used the entire myocardium as ROI/VOI input to radiomic feature extraction. Although it cannot be excluded that shape feature will become of interest while more and more cardiac radiomics studies will come out, this chapter focuses on feature categories currently used in cardiac imaging. Please refer to Zwanenburg et al. [31] for further discussion on computation of shape features.

Intensity (Histogram) Features

Intensity-based features are derived from the histogram of the pixel matrix, which is why these features are also called histogram features. The histogram of an image displays the count of how often each pixel value occurs in the image. Figure 7.4 shows an example of a conversion of a cardiac MR image to a pixel matrix and to a histogram; the *x*-axis thereby displays the grey-level value, and the *y* axis the respective pixel count.

Radiomic parameters derived from the histogram usually are easier and more intuitive to understand as compared to the more complex features from the higher-order statistics as further discussed below. Table 7.1 summarizes various histogram features, which can be computed. For example, the

Table 7.1 Intensity/histogram features with corresponding feature names

Feature family	Feature name
Intensity-based statistical (histogram) features	Mean (discretized) intensity
	(Discretized) intensity variance
	(Discretized) intensity skewness
	(Excess) (discretized) intensity kurtosis
	Median (discretized) intensity
	Minimum (discretized) intensity
	10th (discretized) intensity percentile
	90th (discretized) intensity percentile
	Maximum (discretized) intensity
	(Discretized) intensity interquartile range
	(Discretized) intensity range
	(Discretized) intensity-based mean absolute deviation
	(Discretized) intensity-based robust mean absolute deviation
	(Discretized) intensity-based median absolute deviation
	(Discretized) intensity-based coefficient of variation
	(Discretized) intensity-based quartile coefficient of dispersion
	(Discretized) intensity-based energy
	Root mean square (discretized) intensity
Intensity-volume histogram features	Volume at intensity fraction
	Intensity at volume fraction
	Volume fraction difference between intensity fractions
	Intensity fraction difference between volume fractions
	Area under the IVH curve

Intensity/histogram features for different feature categories. For mathematical definitions of all features, please refer to the recommendations of the Image Biomarker Standardization Initiative (IBSI) [31, 32].

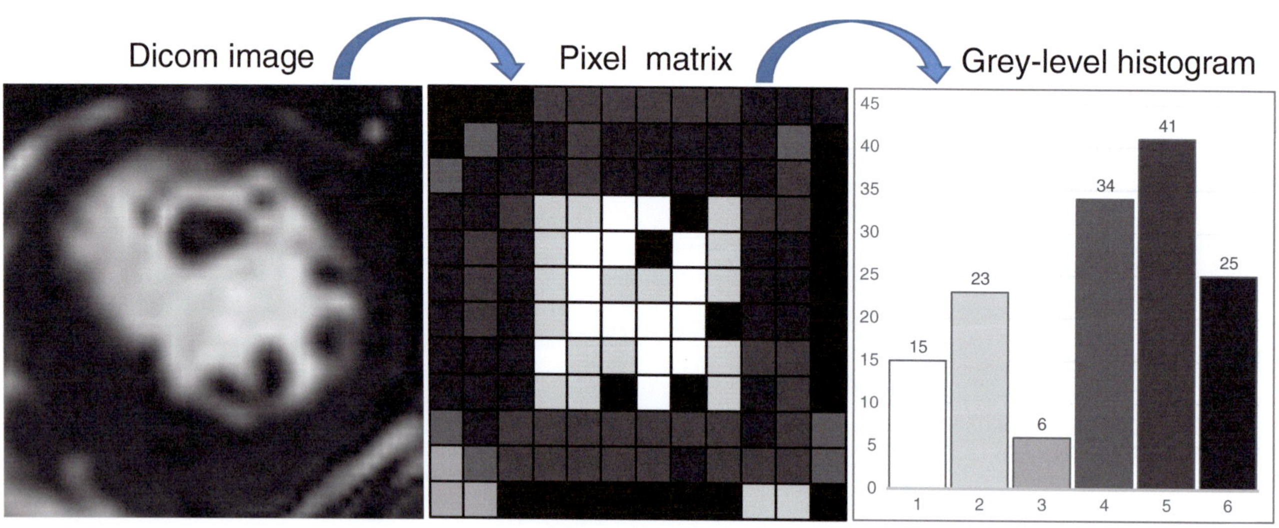

Fig. 7.4 From medical image to histogram. A digital image in DICOM format (e.g. a cardiac MR cine image) is a matrix of pixels (2D) or voxels (3D) with different grey-level values. The histogram displays the count (*y*-axis) of how often each pixel value (*x*-axis) occurs in the image

mean of the histogram represents the mean grey-level value of the image. The variance is a measure of how far the grey levels in the image are distributed relative to the mean.

Features that are also commonly encountered and derived from the histogram are skewness and kurtosis. Figure 7.5 illustrates the concept of positive vs. negative skew and kurtosis, respectively. Skewness measures the asymmetry of the distribution of values around the mean value. Depending on where the tail is elongated and the mass of the distribution is concentrated, this value becomes positive or negative. Kurtosis is a measure of the 'peakedness' of the distribution of values in the histogram. A positive kurtosis implies that the mass of the distribution is concentrated towards a spike near the mean (leptokurtic), whereas a negative kurtosis implies that the mass of the distribution is concentrated towards the tail(s) rather than towards the mean (platykurtic).

Texture Features/Texture Analysis

Moving beyond simply counting the number of pixels yielding a certain grey level for histogram-based analyses, texture analysis focuses on the quantification of the spatial distribution and relationship of pixel/voxel grey levels in the image. The most comprehensible description of image texture might be the more homogeneous or heterogeneous visual appearance of a certain tissue. Figure 7.6 shows an example of two different grey-level distributions within a pixel matrix, one appearing more heterogeneous (A) and the other one appearing rather homogeneous (B). While the histogram of the two matrices is identical (because the pure number of pixel grey levels is the same), the corresponding so-called co-occurrence matrices (GLCM), which are calculated based on the spatial relationship of neighbouring pixels (for an explanation of the calculation of the co-occurrence matrix, please also refer to Figs. 7.7 and 7.8), look completely different. Texture analysis thus enables the quantification of tissue homo-/heterogeneity, with coarse textures yielding larger and fine textures yielding smaller groups of pixels/voxels with similar grey levels [8]. Texture analysis consequently is perceived as the most interesting radiomic feature class for cardiac imaging, and different texture features have been demonstrated to have additional diagnostic value in myocardial infarction [6, 20, 21], hypertrophic cardiomyopathy [5, 24] or myocarditis [3–5].

Different feature families, also called matrices, are known, from which texture features can be computed: the GLCM, the grey-level run length matrix (GLRLM), the grey-level size zone matrix (GLSZM), the grey-level distance zone matrix (GLDZM), the neighbourhood grey tone difference matrix (NGTDM) and the neighbouring grey-level dependence matrix (NGLDM). Table 7.2 summarizes the available features for each of these matrices as recommended by the IBSI [32].

The above mentioned GLCM is also called a 'second-order histogram' and reflects how combinations of neighbouring pixel/voxel grey levels are distributed along different image directions [16] (Figs. 7.7 and 7.8). In general, the neighbourhood for GLCM has eight directions for 2D and 26

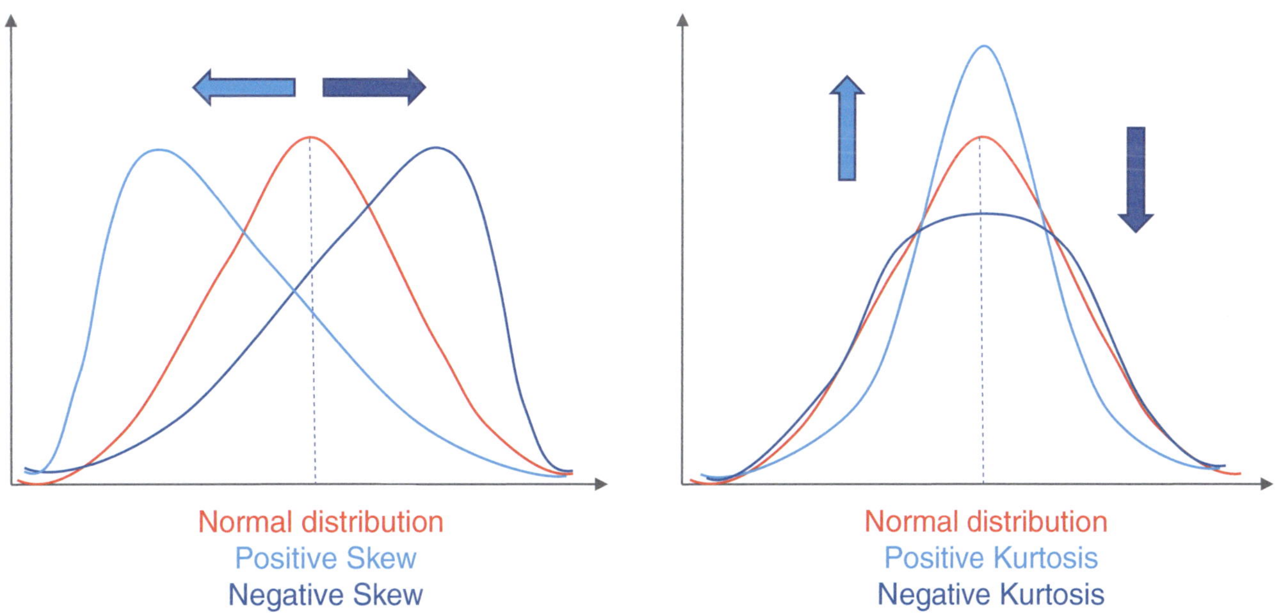

Fig. 7.5 Illustration of the concept of skew and kurtosis. Illustration of the concept of positive and negative skew (left) and positive and negative kurtosis (right) in comparison to the normal distribution. Skewness measures the asymmetry of the distribution of values around the mean value. Kurtosis is a measure of the 'peakedness' of the distribution of values in the histogram

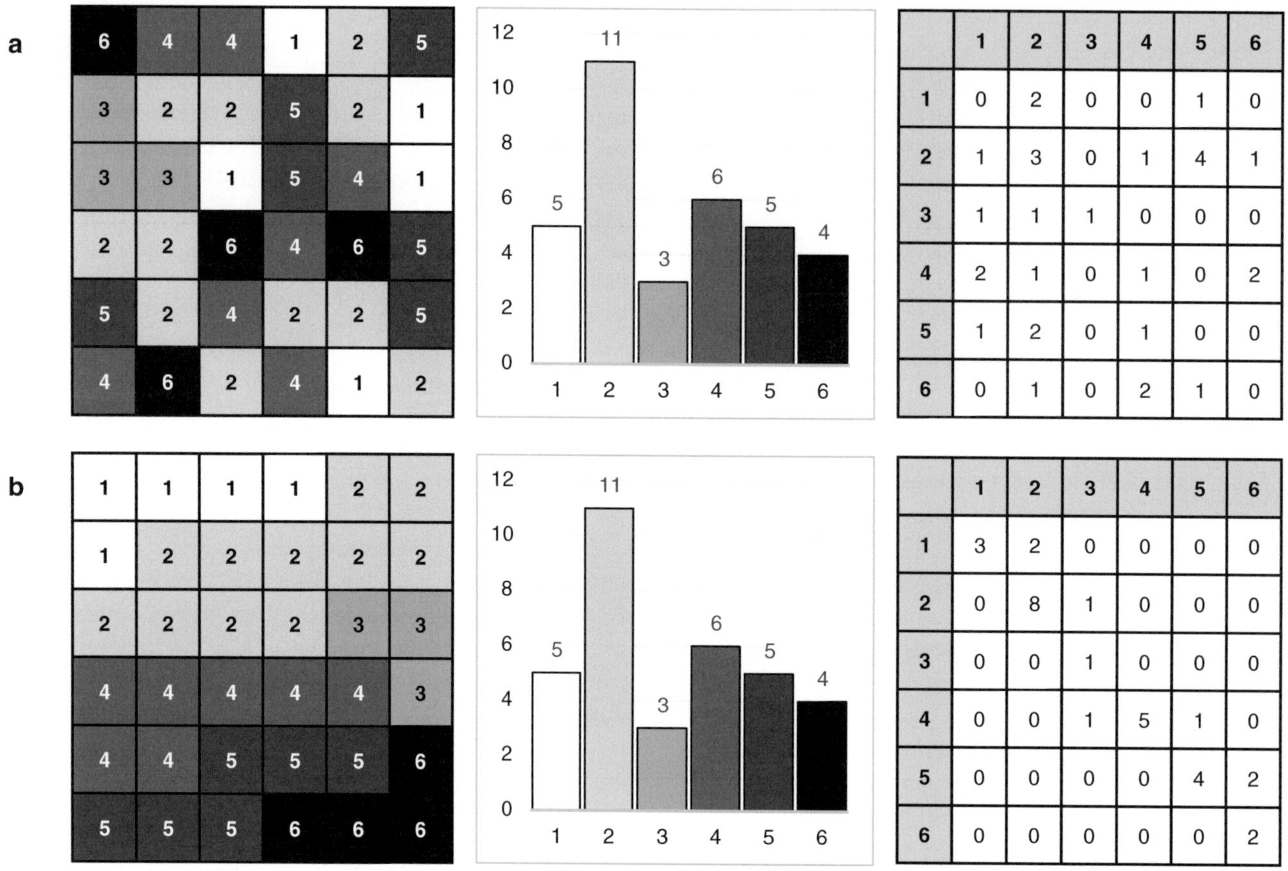

Fig. 7.6 Comparison of histogram and grey-level co-occurrence matrix. Pixel matrices with identical numbers of certain grey-level values were rearranged to simulate more heterogeneous (**a**, left) and more homogeneous (**b**, left) tissue. The central figure shows identical histograms (with count on the *y*-axis and grey-level value on the *x*-axis). Computed grey-level co-occurrence matrices (GLCMs) on the right. Row and column numbers represent grey-level values; cells contain the number of times the corresponding grey-level value occurred adjacent to each other. The GLCMs show that despite identical histograms, the spatial distribution of the pixel grey levels is completely different in the two images. Thus, the GLCM is one way to reflect tissue homo-/heterogeneity

directions for 3D data (Fig. 7.7) [32]. Since the GLCM is symmetry invariant, only one direction without its inverse direction usually is computed [14], resulting in four (2D) and 13 (3D) unique direction vectors, respectively [32]. To improve rotational invariance, GLCM feature values are often computed by aggregating information from the different underlying directional matrices [11]. Different methods can be used to aggregate GLCMs in order to obtain at a single feature value. Please refer to Zwanenburg et al. [31] for further details. Besides using the neighbourhood of 2 pixels (i.e. a 1-pixel distance) as shown in Fig. 7.8, other pixel distances can be used for computation of GLCM features. Usually, a set of 20 co-occurrence matrices is computed for distances ranging from 1 to 5 pixels [9]. Table 7.2 shows features that can be computed from the GLCM.

In contrast to GLCM features, which assess the co-occurrence of grey levels within neighbouring pixels/voxels, the GLRLM [13] assesses run lengths (Fig. 7.9). A run length is defined as 'the length of a consecutive sequence of pixels or voxels with the same grey level' along a certain direction [31]. This means, that the run length matrix is a means to search the image for 'runs' of 2, 3, 4, 5 and so on pixels/voxels with the same grey level value in a given direction (whereas directions are identical to the GLCM, Fig. 7.7). Similar to the GLCM, four (2D) or 13 (3D) unique directions are usually computed [9, 31]. As for GLCM, different methods can be used to aggregate GLRLMs in order to obtain at a single feature value. Please refer to Zwanenburg et al. [31] for further details. As an example, the feature called short runs emphasis is meant to show the proportion of runs in the image with a short run length [9].

The grey-level size zone matrix (GLSZM) counts the number of groups (or zones) of linked pixels/voxels [27], i.e. pixels/voxels with an identical grey level. In a 2D approach, a so-called 8-connectedness is considered, which indicates that a centre pixel is linked to all of the eight neighbouring pixels with the same grey level [31]. Conversely, a 26-connectedness is considered for a 3D approach. Table 7.2 shows features that can be computed from the GLSZM.

The grey-level distance zone matrix (GLDZM) reflects the relationship between a grey level and its location in the image by counting the number of groups (or zones) of linked pixels/voxels that share a specific grey level and has the same distance to the margin of the ROI/VOI [27, 31]. Table 7.2 shows features that can be computed from the GLDZM.

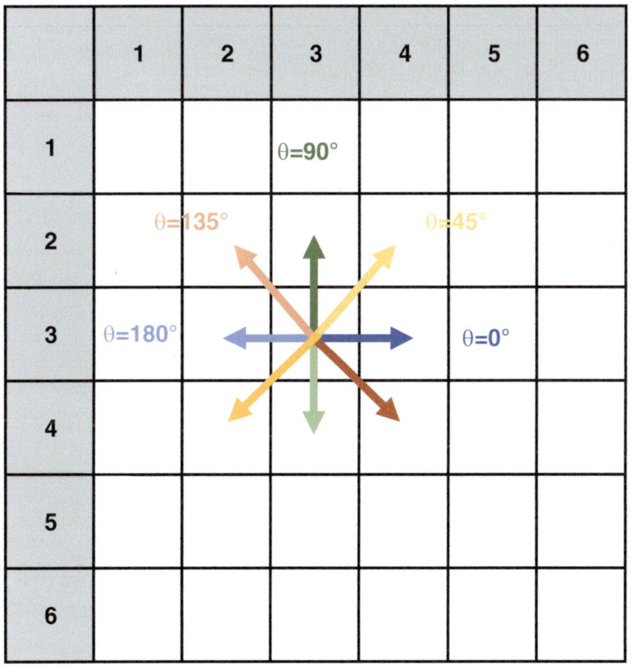

Fig. 7.7 Directions in a digital image. The neighbourhood of pixel grey levels in a digital image has eight directions for 2D data (and 26 directions for 3D data; not shown). Θ is the angle between neighbouring pixels in the image

The neighbourhood grey tone difference matrix (NGTDM) represents an alternative to the GLCM and contains the sum of grey-level differences of pixels/voxels with a certain grey level and the average grey level of neighbouring pixels/voxels within a given distance [2, 31]. A second, rotationally invariant alternative to the GLCM is the neighbouring grey-level dependence matrix (NGLDM) [26]. Table 7.2 shows features that can be computed from the NGTDM and NGLDM.

Filters

Radiomic features can be calculated from different sets of images. The basis is formed by the digital image derived from the PACS. Further, these images can be transformed using different types of filters such as wavelet or Gabor filters and features than can be calculated based on those transformed images. This leads to the high number of radiomic features usually encountered in radiomics studies.

Wavelet filters are an example for image filters, which are very commonly used in radiomics studies. Wavelets represent a technique that analyses the frequency content of an image within different scales of that image [9]. Each pixel in the original image is associated to a set of numbers (i.e. the wavelet coefficients), which characterize the frequency

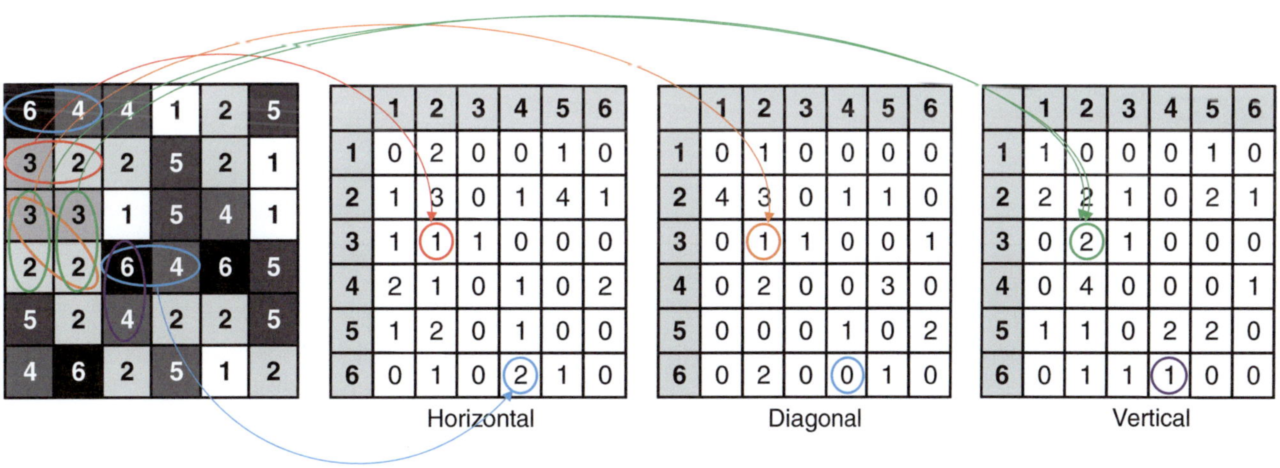

Fig. 7.8 Computation of the grey-level co-occurrence matrix. Grey scale digital image and computed grey-level co-occurrence matrices (GLCMs) in three directions: horizonal, diagonal and vertical. Numbers in the grey-level matrix represent their grey levels (here from 1 (white) to 6 (black), which does not represent the standard definitions). Row and column numbers in the GLCMs represent grey-level values; cells contain the number of times the corresponding grey-level value occurred adjacent to each other. The red circle (left) indicates that grey-level values 3 and 2 occur adjacent to each other once in horizontal direction. This frequency of co-occurrence (i.e. 1) is then mapped onto the corresponding cell of the horizontal GLCM. The same has been done for the diagonal (orange) and vertical directions (green, purple)

Table 7.2 Texture feature families with corresponding feature names

Feature family	Feature name
Grey-level co-occurrence matrix (GLCM)	Joint maximum
	Joint average
	Joint variance
	Joint entropy
	Difference average
	Difference variance
	Difference entropy
	Sum average
	Sum variance
	Sum entropy
	Angular second moment
	Contrast
	Dissimilarity
	Inverse difference
	Normalized inverse difference
	Inverse difference moment
	Normalized inverse difference moment
	Inverse variance
	Correlation
	Autocorrelation
	Cluster tendency
	Cluster shade
	Cluster prominence
	Information correlation 1
	Information correlation 2
Grey-level run length matrix (GLRLM)	Short runs emphasis
	Long runs emphasis
	Low grey-level run emphasis
	High grey-level run emphasis
	Short run low grey-level emphasis
	Short run high grey-level emphasis
	Long run low grey-level emphasis
	Long run high grey-level emphasis
	Grey-level non-uniformity
	Normalized grey-level non-uniformity
	Run length non-uniformity
	Normalized run length non-uniformity
	Run percentage
	Grey-level variance
	Run length variance
	Run entropy
Grey-level size zone matrix (GLSZM)	Grey-level size zone
	Large zone emphasis
	Low grey-level zone emphasis
	High grey-level zone emphasis
	Small zone low grey-level emphasis
	Small zone high grey-level emphasis
	Large zone low grey-level emphasis
	Large zone high grey-level emphasis
	Grey-level non-uniformity
	Normalized grey-level non-uniformity
	Zone size non-uniformity
	Normalized zone size non-uniformity
	Zone percentage
	Grey-level variance
	Zone size variance
	Zone size entropy
Grey-level distance zone matrix (GLDZM)	Small distance emphasis
	Large distance emphasis
	Low grey-level zone emphasis
	High grey-level zone emphasis
	Small distance low grey-level emphasis
	Small distance high grey-level emphasis
	Large distance low grey-level emphasis
	Large distance high grey-level emphasis
	Grey-level non-uniformity
	Normalized grey-level non-uniformity
	Zone distance non-uniformity
	Normalized zone distance non-uniformity
	Zone percentage
	Grey-level variance
	Zone distance variance
	Zone distance entropy
Neighbourhood grey tone difference matrix (NGTDM)	Coarseness
	Contrast
	Busyness
	Complexity
	Strength
Neighbouring grey-level dependence matrix (NGLDM)	Low dependence emphasis
	High dependence emphasis
	Low grey-level count emphasis
	High grey-level count emphasis
	Low dependence low grey-level emphasis
	Low dependence high grey-level emphasis
	High dependence low grey-level emphasis
	High dependence high grey-level emphasis
	Grey-level non-uniformity
	Normalized grey-level non-uniformity
	Dependence count non-uniformity
	Normalized dependence count non-uniformity
	Dependence count percentage
	Grey-level variance
	Dependence count variance
	Dependence count entropy
	Dependence count energy

Texture features for different feature categories. For mathematical definitions of all features, please refer to the recommendations of the Image Biomarker Standardization Initiative (IBSI) [31, 32].

content of the image. All of the above-described radiomic features can then be computed from the different wavelet-transformed images.

Data Analysis

The resulting dataset after feature extraction consists of hundreds or thousands (in theory unlimited) features, what can be subsumed under the notion 'big data'. As a consequence, analysis techniques from the machine learning spectrum are usually applied for data analysis in order to make predictions about diagnoses or prognoses.

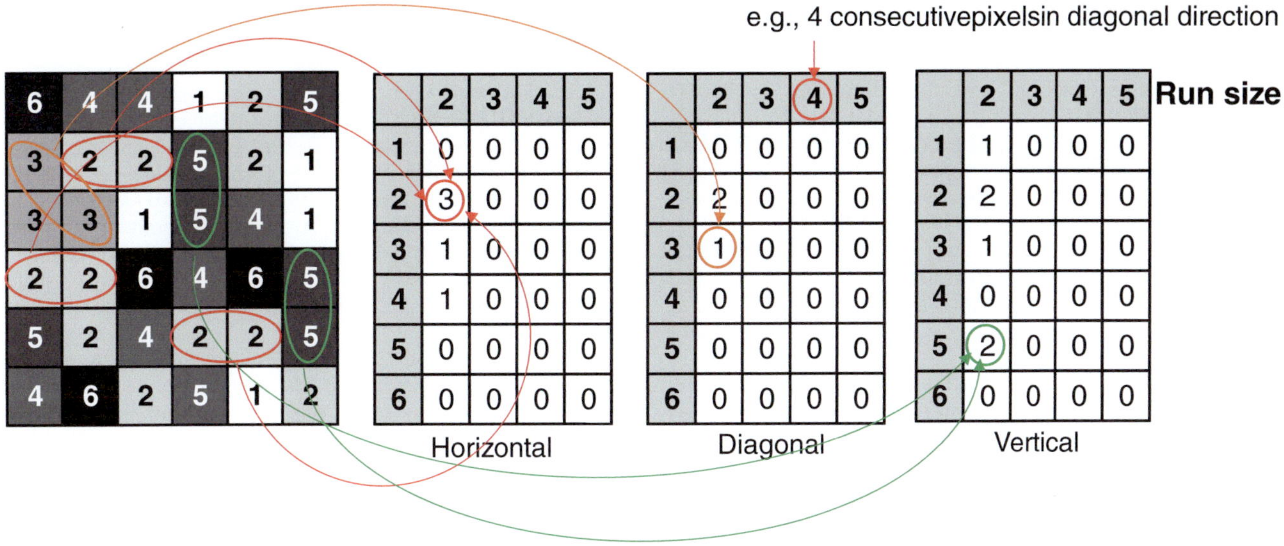

Fig. 7.9 Computation of a grey-level run length matrix (GLRLM) in three directions. Grey scale digital image and computed grey-level run length matrices (GLRLMs) in three directions: horizonal, diagonal and vertical. Numbers in the grey-level matrix represent their grey levels (here from 1 (white) to 6 (black), which does not represent the standard definitions). Row numbers in the GLRLMs represent grey-level values; column numbers represent the run size (i.e. number of adjacent pixels in a run); cells contain the number of times the corresponding grey-level value occurred in the corresponding run size (note that a run size of 2 is comparable to the GLCM)

The higher the number of features in a model and the smaller the sample size of the included patient groups, the higher the risk of model overfitting. Thus, a critical step in a radiomics data analysis is the reduction of the number of features (also called feature selection or dimension reduction) in order to achieve more reliable and generalizable results. Dimension reduction can be done in multiple ways, including intra- and inter-observer analysis and exclusion of all non-reproducible features (thus accounting for potential biases in manual or semi-automated ROI/VOI definition), application of feature selection algorithms such as LASSO or Boruta algorithms, correlation matrices, hierarchical clustering and so forth. An exemplary data analysis workflow is described in the 'Radiomics how to' guide [30], and many more have been applied so far throughout the radiomics literature.

It has to be noted, however, that the selection of the analysis pipeline and the consecutive reporting of data analysis should be undertaken with care and follow predefined quality guidelines [18] in order to make radiomics research more reproducible and translatable to clinical routine practice.

Conclusions and Outlook

Radiomics has potential to become an integral part of cardiovascular imaging research with high likelihood for translation into clinical routine. Many of the abovementioned technical basics, however, require a standardized and validated approach and careful use and reporting including adherence to certain quality standards. Current limitations have to be addressed, which are hampering the generalizability of trained models, either on the technical image acquisition side or on the image processing and feature extraction side. Recently published guidelines and checklists aim to improve the quality of future radiomics studies, but transparency has been recognized as the most important factor for reproducibility. Understanding the technical basics of radiomics as presented in this chapter will enable a better understanding of the underlying concepts and hopefully motivate further research in the field of radiomics in cardiac imaging, finally contributing towards the concept of precision cardiovascular medicine.

References

1. Altazi BA, Zhang GG, Fernandez DC, Montejo ME, Hunt D, Werner J, Biagioli MC, Moros EG. Reproducibility of F18-FDG PET radiomic features for different cervical tumor segmentation methods, gray-level discretization, and reconstruction algorithms. J Appl Clin Med Phys. 2017;18:32–48. https://doi.org/10.1002/acm2.12170.
2. Amadasun M, King R. Textural features corresponding to textural properties. IEEE Trans Syst Man Cybern. 1989;19:1264–74. https://doi.org/10.1109/21.44046.
3. Baessler B, Luecke C, Lurz J, Klingel K, Das A, Roeder M, Waha-Thiele S, Besler C, Rommel K-P, Maintz D, Gutberlet M, Thiele H, Lurz P. Cardiac MRI and texture analysis of myocardial T1 and T2 maps in myocarditis with acute versus chronic symptoms of heart failure. Radiology. 2019;292:608–17. https://doi.org/10.1148/radiol.2019190101.
4. Baessler B, Luecke C, Lurz J, Klingel K, Roeder M, Waha S, Besler C, Maintz D, Gutberlet M, Thiele H, Lurz P. Cardiac MRI texture analysis of T1 and T2 maps in patients with infarctlike acute myocarditis. Radiology. 2018;289:357–65. https://doi.org/10.1148/radiol.2018180411.

5. Baeßler B, Mannil M, Maintz D, Alkadhi H, Manka R. Texture analysis and machine learning of non-contrast T1-weighted MR images in patients with hypertrophic cardiomyopathy-preliminary results. Eur J Radiol. 2018;102:61–7. https://doi.org/10.1016/j.ejrad.2018.03.013.
6. Baessler B, Mannil M, Oebel S, Maintz D, Alkadhi H, Manka R. Subacute and chronic left ventricular myocardial scar: accuracy of texture analysis on nonenhanced cine MR images. Radiology. 2017:170213. https://doi.org/10.1148/radiol.2017170213.
7. Bailly C, Bodet-Milin C, Couespel S, Necib H, Kraeber-Bodéré F, Ansquer C, Carlier T. Revisiting the robustness of PET-based textural features in the context of multi-centric trials. PLoS One. 2016;11:e0159984. https://doi.org/10.1371/journal.pone.0159984.
8. Bashir U, Siddique MM, Mclean E, Goh V, Cook GJ. Imaging heterogeneity in lung cancer: techniques, applications, and challenges. Am J Roentgenol. 2016;207:534–43. https://doi.org/10.2214/AJR.15.15864.
9. Castellano G, Bonilha L, Li LM, Cendes F. Texture analysis of medical images. Clin Radiol. 2004;59:1061–9. https://doi.org/10.1016/j.crad.2004.07.008.
10. Collewet G, Strzelecki M, Mariette F. Influence of MRI acquisition protocols and image intensity normalization methods on texture classification. Magn Reson Imaging. 2004;22:81–91. https://doi.org/10.1016/j.mri.2003.09.001.
11. Depeursinge A, Fageot J. Biomedical texture operators and aggregation functions. In: Biomedical texture analysis. Elsevier; 2017. p. 55–94. https://doi.org/10.1016/B978-0-12-812133-7.00003-X.
12. Edge SB, Compton CC. The American Joint Committee on Cancer: the 7th edition of the AJCC cancer staging manual and the future of TNM. Ann Surg Oncol. 2010;17:1471–4. https://doi.org/10.1245/s10434-010-0985-4.
13. Galloway MM. Texture analysis using gray level run lengths. Comput Graph Image Process. 1975;4:172–9. https://doi.org/10.1016/S0146-664X(75)80008-6.
14. Gao Y, Shi Y, Cao W, Zhang S, Liang Z. Energy enhanced tissue texture in spectral computed tomography for lesion classification. Vis Comput Ind Biomed Art. 2019;2:16. https://doi.org/10.1186/s42492-019-0028-3.
15. Gillies RJ, Kinahan PE, Hricak H. Radiomics: images are more than pictures, they are data. Radiology. 2016;278:563–77. https://doi.org/10.1148/radiol.2015151169.
16. Haralick RM, Shanmugam K, Dinstein I. Textural features for image classification. IEEE Trans Syst Man Cybern. 1973;SMC-3:610–21. https://doi.org/10.1109/TSMC.1973.4309314.
17. Kumar V, Gu Y, Basu S, Berglund A, Eschrich SA, Schabath MB, Forster K, Aerts HJWL, Dekker A, Fenstermacher D, Goldgof DB, Hall LO, Lambin P, Balagurunathan Y, Gatenby RA, Gillies RJ. Radiomics: the process and the challenges. Magn Reson Imaging. 2012;30:1234–48. https://doi.org/10.1016/j.mri.2012.06.010.
18. Lambin P, Leijenaar RTH, Deist TM, Peerlings J, de Jong EEC, van Timmeren J, Sanduleanu S, Larue RTHM, Even AJG, Jochems A, van Wijk Y, Woodruff H, van Soest J, Lustberg T, Roelofs E, van Elmpt W, Dekker A, Mottaghy FM, Wildberger JE, Walsh S. Radiomics: the bridge between medical imaging and personalized medicine. Nat Rev Clin Oncol. 2017;14:749–62. https://doi.org/10.1038/nrclinonc.2017.141.
19. Lambin P, Rios-Velazquez E, Leijenaar R, Carvalho S, van Stiphout RGPM, Granton P, Zegers CML, Gillies R, Boellard R, Dekker A, Aerts HJWL. Radiomics: extracting more information from medical images using advanced feature analysis. Eur J Cancer. 2012;48:441–6. https://doi.org/10.1016/j.ejca.2011.11.036.
20. Larroza A, López-Lereu MP, Monmeneu JV, Gavara J, Chorro FJ, Bodí V, Moratal D. Texture analysis of cardiac cine magnetic resonance imaging to detect nonviable segments in patients with chronic myocardial infarction. Med Phys. 2018;45:1471–80. https://doi.org/10.1002/mp.12783.
21. Larroza A, Materka A, López-Lereu MP, Monmeneu JV, Bodí V, Moratal D. Differentiation between acute and chronic myocardial infarction by means of texture analysis of late gadolinium enhancement and cine cardiac magnetic resonance imaging. Eur J Radiol. 2017;92:78–83. https://doi.org/10.1016/j.ejrad.2017.04.024.
22. Limkin EJ, Reuzé S, Carré A, Sun R, Schernberg A, Alexis A, Deutsch E, Ferté C, Robert C. The complexity of tumor shape, spiculatedness, correlates with tumor radiomic shape features. Sci Rep. 2019;9:4329. https://doi.org/10.1038/s41598-019-40437-5.
23. Mannil M, von Spiczak J, Manka R, Alkadhi H. Texture analysis and machine learning for detecting myocardial infarction in noncontrast low-dose computed tomography: unveiling the invisible. Investig Radiol. 2018;53:338–43. https://doi.org/10.1097/RLI.0000000000000448.
24. Neisius U, El-Rewaidy H, Nakamori S, Rodriguez J, Manning WJ, Nezafat R. Radiomic analysis of myocardial native T1 imaging discriminates between hypertensive heart disease and hypertrophic cardiomyopathy. JACC Cardiovasc Imaging. 2019. https://doi.org/10.1016/j.jcmg.2018.11.024.
25. Shafiq-Ul-Hassan M, Zhang GG, Latifi K, Ullah G, Hunt DC, Balagurunathan Y, Abdalah MA, Schabath MB, Goldgof DG, Mackin D, Court LE, Gillies RJ, Moros EG. Intrinsic dependencies of CT radiomic features on voxel size and number of gray levels. Med Phys. 2017;44:1050–62. https://doi.org/10.1002/mp.12123.
26. Sun C, Wee WG. Neighboring gray level dependence matrix for texture classification. Comput Vis Graph Image Process. 1983;23:341–52. https://doi.org/10.1016/0734-189X(83)90032-4.
27. Thibault G, Angulo J, Meyer F. Advanced statistical matrices for texture characterization: application to cell classification. IEEE Trans Biomed Eng. 2014;61:630–7. https://doi.org/10.1109/TBME.2013.2284600.
28. Tourassi GD. Journey toward computer-aided diagnosis: role of image texture analysis. Radiology. 1999;213:317–20. https://doi.org/10.1148/radiology.213.2.r99nv49317.
29. Vallières M, Freeman CR, Skamene SR, Naqa IE. A radiomics model from joint FDG-PET and MRI texture features for the prediction of lung metastases in soft-tissue sarcomas of the extremities. Phys Med Biol. 2015;60:5471–96. https://doi.org/10.1088/0031-9155/60/14/5471.
30. van Timmeren JE, Cester D, Tanadini-Lang S, Alkadhi H, Baessler B. Radiomics in medical imaging—"how-to" guide and critical reflection. Insights Imaging. 2020;11:91. https://doi.org/10.1186/s13244-020-00887-2.
31. Zwanenburg A, Leger S, Vallières M, Löck S. Image biomarker standardisation initiative. 2016.
32. Zwanenburg A, Vallières M, Abdalah MA, Aerts HJWL, Andrearczyk V, Apte A, Ashrafinia S, Bakas S, Beukinga RJ, Boellaard R, Bogowicz M, Boldrini L, Buvat I, Cook GJR, Davatzikos C, Depeursinge A, Desseroit M-C, Dinapoli N, Dinh CV, Echegaray S, Naqa IE, Fedorov AY, Gatta R, Gillies RJ, Goh V, Götz M, Guckenberger M, Ha SM, Hatt M, Isensee F, Lambin P, Leger S, Leijenaar RTH, Lenkowicz J, Lippert F, Losnegård A, Maier-Hein KH, Morin O, Müller H, Napel S, Nioche C, Orlhac F, Pati S, Pfaehler EAG, Rahmim A, Rao AUK, Scherer J, Siddique MM, Sijtsema NM, Fernandez JS, Spezi E, Steenbakkers RJHM, Tanadini-Lang S, Thorwarth D, Troost EGC, Upadhaya T, Valentini V, van Dijk LV, van Griethuysen J, van Velden FHP, Whybra P, Richter C, Löck S. The image biomarker standardization initiative: standardized quantitative radiomics for high-throughput image-based phenotyping. Radiology. 2020. https://doi.org/10.1148/radiol.2020191145.

Biobanks and Artificial Intelligence

8

Musa Abdulkareem, Nay Aung, and Steffen E. Petersen

Introduction

The applications of artificial intelligence (AI) are becoming ubiquitous in the modern society. Similar to other areas, medicine and healthcare are beginning to witness the rapid growth of AI-based techniques and tools that are addressing complex healthcare problems such as optimising healthcare pathways [1, 2], identifying latent relationships in patient phenotypes [3], improving accuracy of medical decision making [4, 5] and standardising clinical diagnosis [6, 7]. Although AI-based technologies in healthcare are still relatively new, biobanks, which represent infrastructure for collecting lifestyle and healthcare information, biological samples, imaging and clinical outcomes of consented participants with the purpose of advancing scientific research, will play a crucial role as a source of data to realise the full potential of AI-based applications.

The term "AI" describes the concept of developing computer algorithms with human-like intelligence to solve specific tasks. Machine learning (ML) methods are a set of techniques designed to achieve AI and include, among others, supervised [8], unsupervised [9], semi-supervised [10, 11] and reinforcement learning [12]. Some of these methods and other terms often encountered in AI literature are briefly defined in Box 8.1.

The data analysis and exploration possible with data from biobanks is a consequence of digitisation – that is, having healthcare data in formats that can be easily processed by the computers. Taking full advantage of the scope and scale of biobank data will require going beyond the limits of traditional statistical methods; this is where advanced AI techniques display their true potentials.

Firstly, biobank data are often large in terms of volume and highly multidimensional due to the depth of information collected from each participant. Conventional statistical methods often do not perform well with such datasets. Moreover, with the widespread use of electronic health records (EHR), the amount of data currently available for biomedical research is growing exponentially through linkage to biobanks. AI techniques are highly versatile due to their ability to learn from voluminous and diverse data types [13], making them suitable for interrogating numerous research questions related to healthcare. Secondly, many research findings in cardiovascular medicine are reported for an 'average patient', but these insights may be limited by the complexity and heterogeneity of human pathophysiology [14]. AI techniques can be used to address this problem by enabling patient-specific decision support tools because of their inherent capability to generalise [13, 15, 16]. Thirdly, when biobank data are linked to EHR of participants, they create opportunity for longitudinal studies which provide the means to test multiple epidemiological hypotheses [17–19] that would otherwise be impossible. Thus, research findings from biobank data analysis can be used to inform, monitor and improve the quality of public health policies [20]. AI also provides novel methods to investigate the attributes and comorbidities of various diseases that lead to different outcomes [21–25]. Fourthly, AI techniques can be used to explore biobank data and develop applications, such as algorithms for identification of biomarkers that will aid early detection and treatments of many diseases [26].

M. Abdulkareem, MSc, PhD (✉) · N. Aung, PhD
National Institute for Health Research (NIHR) Barts Biomedical Research Centre, William Harvey Research Institute, Queen Mary University of London, London, UK

Barts Heart Centre, St Bartholomew's Hospital, Barts Health National Health Service (NHS) Trust, London, UK
e-mail: musa.abdulkareem@nhs.net; n.aung@qmul.ac.uk

S. E. Petersen, MSc, MPH, MD, DPhil
Barts Heart Centre, St Bartholomew's Hospital, Barts Health National Health Service (NHS) Trust, London, UK

National Institute for Health Research (NIHR) Barts Biomedical Research Centre, William Harvey Research Institute, Queen Mary University of London, London, UK

The Alan Turing Institute, London, UK
e-mail: s.e.petersen@qmul.ac.uk

C. N. De Cecco et al. (eds.), *Artificial Intelligence in Cardiothoracic Imaging*, Contemporary Medical Imaging,
https://doi.org/10.1007/978-3-030-92087-6_8

Box 8.1 Some terms and methods commonly used in AI

- **Artificial Intelligence (AI)**: The concept of developing computer algorithms with human-like intelligence to solve specific tasks.
- **Machine Learning (ML)**: A subset of AI and consists of a collection of techniques to achieve AI.
- **Supervised Learning**: A set of ML algorithms for developing mathematical models using data that consists of both the input and the desired output data.
- **Unsupervised Learning**: A set of ML algorithms for finding underlying structures or patterns in datasets using only the input data.
- **Reinforcement Learning**: A set of ML algorithms that is based on the interaction between an agent and its environment. In general, the agent seeks to take actions in the environment by maximizing a cumulative reward.
- **Deep Learning** (also referred to as **Deep Neural Network**): A set of ML algorithms that are based on neural network (NN) that are used for feature learning. The term 'deep' refers to the fact that they have multiple layers between the input and the output layers.
- **Convolutional Neural Network (CNN)**: A set of DL algorithms that are particularly efficient in developing AI-based applications involving images. CNN acts as the backbone of many well-known neural network architectures (such as VGG-16 and U-net) used in image processing.
- **Support Vector Machines (SVM)**: A set of supervised learning algorithms that constructs hyperplanes in a high-dimensional space. These algorithms are often used for classification tasks, regression analysis, and other problems. In a classification problem, for instance, out of the many hyperplanes, the one that has the largest distance to the data point of any class is considered the 'optimal' classifier.
- **Random Forests (or Random Decision Forests) Method**: A set of learning algorithms involving several decision trees and whose output is the class that is the statistical mode (in classification tasks) or statistical mean (in regression tasks) of each of the decision trees. These algorithms are often used for classification tasks, regression analysis, and other problems.
- **Dice Similarity Coefficient (DSC**, or **Dice metric)**: An evaluation metric that uses spatial overlap between two segmentations (e.g. an overlap between the predicted output segmentation and the ground truth segmentation).
- **Receiver Operating Characteristic (ROC)**: A graphical plot that shows the performance of a classification model as its threshold is varied.
- **Area Under the ROC Curve (AUC)**: A measure of a model's performance across all its possible classification threshold.
- **Sensitivity**: A measure of the extent to which true positives are not overlooked (i.e. correctly identified) by a classification model.
- **Specificity**: A measure of the extent to which true negatives are not overlooked by a classification model.

In the remainder of this chapter, we will present some examples of biobanks and discuss AI-based applications that have explored and used biobank data for their development. Practical issues, challenges and opportunities presented by the use of biobank data are also highlighted.

Biobanks

The first appearance of the term 'biobank' in scientific literature occurred in 1996 [27]. It has been defined as 'an organised biological sample collections with associated personal and clinical data' [28] and as 'an organized collection of human biological material and associated information stored for one or more research purposes' [29]. Several definitions of biobanks exist, and although early definitions have limited biobanks to human-based collections, some literature have extended their definitions further to include collections of non-human materials such as animals, plants, environments and microbes [30]. According to the response of 303 individuals in a survey of people that are involved in the managing of biobank collections [27], there is a consensus that the term should only apply to collections that are managed according to professional standards – be it human, animal, plant or microbial samples. There was no consensus, however, on the size (number of participants and features of each participant), the level of access (private or public, national or international, and so on) or the purpose of collection of a biobank. Accordingly, as a recommendation, the following general definition was proposed: 'A biobank is a facility for the collection, preservation, storage and supply of biological samples and associated data, which follows standardised operating procedures and provides material for scientific and clinical use' [27], and for our purpose in this chapter, we use this definition and limit it to human population-based collections.

Biobanks represent or provide infrastructure for collecting and storing biomedical data and data related to health records and lifestyle of participants with the purpose of advancing scientific research and improving healthcare.

They are often large databases that can store, among others, imaging data, text data from EHR and lifestyle information (such as activities and diet) and numerical data obtained by physical measurements (including those from medical measurement devices) of consented participants. Several types of biobanks with different population sizes exist around the world including genetic banks, blood banks and tissue banks. Also, there are disease-specific and population-wide biobanks as well as private and public (national) biobanks. Furthermore, they can be classified into general or project-driven biobanks.

Biobanks contain valuable data that can provide insights into how the health of a population develops over years. It is a powerful tool that puts data resources in the hands of researchers that can be used to improve the diagnosis and treatment of common and complex diseases that will inevitably occur in sub-groups of the biobank population. It also provides opportunities to uncover the relationships between different phenotypic features and human diseases. Biobanking is particularly powerful for its concept of a unified data repository with mostly standardised data collecting protocols compared to the real-world healthcare data. In contrast, the hospital data are often termed 'messy' due to the ad hoc nature of data collection, storage across multiple repositories and limited interconnectivity between legacy systems, limiting data integration.

An alternative to biobanks is population-based cohort studies where a specific set of data of a sample or a whole of a population is selected for assessment of exposure-outcome relationships in order to evaluate single or multiple hypoth eses (e.g. estimation of the prevalence of a disease or its risk factors). The major disadvantage is the comparative high cost and logistic complexity of setting this up as only a relatively small group in a population will have particular conditions of interest for a given study [31].

For common and complex diseases, such as heart diseases and dementia, that affect a large proportion of the population, biobanks present great opportunities for research. Biobanks offer opportunities to study pathophysiological and health impacts of diseases including drivers of health and health outcomes. They provide a rich source of data that can be harnessed to unveil complex relationships among variables (such as environmental [32, 33], lifestyle choice [34, 35], genetics [36, 37] and so on) that are associated with heart diseases [38], cancer [39–41] and other diseases. They can help us understand sex- and age-specific variations of determinants of health in a specific population or a population across several regions [42–44]. Biobanks provide a platform for storing and sharing large amount of data for the use of the research community at large, enormously increasing the advancement and collaboration among research teams.

Examples of biobanks include the UK Biobank with 500,000 participants [45], Maastricht Study with 10,000 participants [46], German National Cohort (GNC) with 30,000 participants [47], Rhineland Study with 30,000 participants [48], Biobank of Vanderbilt University Medical Centre (BioVU) with over 1.4 million participants [49], Kaiser Permanente's Research Program on Genes, Environment and Health (RPGEH) with 200,000 participants [50], China Kadoorie Biobank with 500,000 participants [51, 52], India's Chennai biobank with 500,000 participants [53] and Multi-ethnic Study of Atherosclerosis (MESA) biobank with 6814 participants [54, 55]. The UK Biobank is one of the largest currently in the world in terms of data volume and depth with multi-organ imaging, and we discuss it further in the paragraphs that follow.

UK Biobank is a cohort study of about 500,000 voluntary participants aged between 40 and 69 at recruitment (mean age, 56.5 years; 54.4% female). The recruitment took place at one of 22 centres across England, Scotland and Wales. UK Biobank makes its data accessible to researchers worldwide (both academic research and commercial purposes) subject to approval of an access application. Physical measurements of participants were taken, and samples for genetic-related analysis (i.e. blood, urine and saliva) of participants were collected. In addition, each participant answered an extensive questionnaire about aspects of health, medical history and lifestyle. The recruitment and collection of participants' data for the UK Biobank ran between 2006 and 2010. By 2014, it has begun the process of inviting back these participants for heart, brain and body MRI with a target of reaching 100,000 participants by 2023. The imaging data of this cohort are already accessible to researchers [56, 57]. One of the unique attributes of UK Biobank stems from its access to the UK's National Health Service (NHS) electronic health records of the participants – which gives researchers the potential to find biomarkers for different diseases. The participants are also linked to the national death and cancer registries [45]. According to [58], up to 1800 and 8000 of UK Biobanks participants are expected to develop stroke and diabetes, respectively, by 2022; these figures will rise to 4000 and 14,000, respectively, by 2027. More details and reviews on UK Biobank data can be found in [58–61].

AI-Based Applications Using Biobank Data

Generally, recent popularity of the use of AI in many applications is driven by the advances and accessibility to high-performance scalable computing equipment. This advancement has also prompted an expansion of research into new AI techniques and algorithms. Biobanks have the ability to collect and integrate biomedical and healthcare data. AI algorithms have the potential to interpret these data particularly for tasks where conventional statistical methods are less efficient. The algorithms are even more suitable for elaborate cardiovascular biobank data as these are often of varying scale and high dimension. The algorithms can, as such, be used to solve problems related to identifying relationships in patient phenotypes, optimising care pathways, standardising clinical diagnosis and developing predictive models [62]. While AI-based methods can be used to solve many of these problems, the success of an AI project often depends on the choice of the method, data quality and context associated with the way data is used. For example, deep learning (DL) algorithms are particularly well suited for computer vision problems such as image segmentation [63].

In the subsections that follow, we describe areas in which AI-based applications have been used to tackle different challenges in cardiovascular medicine using data from biobanks.

Cardiac Imaging

Imaging data obtained using different modalities such as echocardiography, computed tomography (CT), magnetic resonance imaging (MRI), single-photon emission computed tomography (SPECT) or others in cardiovascular medicine are of high dimension and therefore contain very rich information that can be used for AI and big data analysis. Cardiac images from biobanks can be used to generate many image-derived phenotypes that are obtained via qualitative and quantitative assessment of structural changes (which characterises the volumetric, structural and functional properties of the heart) [64–66]. Moreover, these can be combined with non-imaging data from the biobank or elsewhere for identifying biomarkers and predicting disease risk factors [26]. Automated and faster reading and interpretation of cardiovascular image workflow can be achieved using AI-based tools [67–69], and the biobank data can help in developing these tools.

Medical images are often affected by noise, artefacts and other uncertainties associated with imaging, making image segmentation useful. Medical image segmentation is the process of contouring a medical image into biologically relevant structures (e.g. sub-group of organs, tissues and so on). It therefore helps to quantify biological structures and functions and produce measurements that act as biomarkers (i.e. quantities that are used to diagnose, monitor or prognosticate diseases). AI-based automatic image segmentation tools are particularly beneficial as they encourage standardisation, eliminating variability that would have been introduced by manual human segmentation. In cardiac magnetic resonance (CMR) imaging, for example, it is common to segment the left ventricle (LV) and the right ventricle (RV) from short-axis images and the left atrium (LA) and the right atrium (RA) from long-axis images in order to compute clinically relevant measures when assessing cardiac structures and functions such as the LV end-diastolic and end-systolic volumes (LVEDV and LVESV, respectively), the RV end-diastolic and end-systolic volumes (RVEDV and RVESV, respectively) and the LV mass (LVM). Indeed, in [70], a type of convolutional neural network (CNN) [71] that can predict the label class of each pixel of a given input image that was based on the VGG-16 architecture [15] was used to develop a DL model for automatically contouring the LV, LA, RV and RA using CMR imaging data of 4875 UK Biobank participants. The performance of the model using the Dice metric for measuring the accuracy on short-axis image test set of 600 participants achieves 0.94 for the LV cavity (i.e. endocardium), 0.88 for the LV myocardium (i.e. epicardium) and 0.90 for the RV cavity. The corresponding Dice metric for the long-axis image test set for the same number of participants achieves 0.96 for the RA cavity (four-chamber view), 0.93 for the LA cavity (two-chamber view) and 0.95 for the LA cavity (four-chamber view). Moreover, the mean absolute difference between prediction and manual measurement is 6.1 mL for LVEDV, 5.3 mL for LVESV, 8.5 mL for RVEDV, 7.2 mL for RVESV and 6.9 g for LVM. The DL-based model therefore has the ability to automate the analysis and derivation of clinically relevant measures, achieving a performance that is comparable to human experts. For comparison with this DL model, a recent research with the similar goal of performing automatic multi-view image segmentation and analysis of CMR images using UK Biobank data is presented in [72]. In this case, the number of participants is 20,000 – with 4620 of these used as the test set. Importantly, a 3D-based Active Shape Model (ASM) technique [73], known as SPASM [74], was used (rather than a DL-based model such as the 2D-based CNN architecture used in [70]). The Dice metric on short-axis image test set achieves 0.93 for the LV cavity, 0.87 for the LV myocardium and 0.87 for the RV cavity.

Risk and Outcome Prediction

AI-based risk prediction models can be used for primary prevention of cardiovascular disease (CVD) by, for example, identifying asymptomatic patients that may benefit from preventive actions. Some of the main approaches to assess CVD risk include the current US guidelines based on American College of Cardiology/American Heart Association (ACC/AHA) Pooled Cohort Equations Risk Calculator [75], the European Society of Cardiology guidelines [76] and the Adult Treatment Panel III guidelines [77]. Similar to many other guidelines and risk calculators, these approaches measure common risk factors and predict events over a specific

Table 8.1 Some AI-based CVD risk prediction models

Authors	Biobank	No. of predictors	Definition of outcomes	Prediction horizon	Algorithms
Ambale-Venkatesh et al. [82]	MESA	735	All CVD and death considered as part of the MESA	12	Random forest method
Alaa et al. [26]	UK Biobank	473	All CVD considered as vascular dementia (ICD-10 codes [84] F01), coronary and ischemic heart diseases (I20–I25), heart failure events (I50), cerebrovascular diseases (I60–I69), ischemic heart disease (ICD-9 codes [85] 410–414), cerebrovascular disease (436–438) and ICD-9 codes 430–434	5	A model involving automatic tuning of an ensemble of several ML algorithms
Shen et al. [83]	China Kadoorie Biobank	14	Arrhythmia, ischemia, and hypertrophy	5	Kernel density estimation and SVM methods

time horizon (e.g. 5 years [26], or 10 years [78]) or a lifetime. Studies have shown that these approaches underestimate the risk of cardiovascular events in certain high-risk individuals and overestimate the risk in others (e.g. in women and certain ethnic groups) [79–81]. ML methods may offer a more accurate risk prediction that can tackle this challenge. In [78], the data of 6459 participants with a follow-up of 13 years from MESA biobank were used to develop an ML model for risk prediction using support vector machine (SVM) method. Twofold cross validation was used by splitting the data set into two equally sized samples in order to assess the model's generalisation ability. The participants were CVD-free at baseline. The model considered nine risk factors, namely, age, sex, ethnicity, total cholesterol, high-density lipoprotein cholesterol, systolic blood pressure, treatment for hypertension, history of diabetes mellitus, and smoking status. The 'Hard CVD' events (i.e. outcomes) defined for the modelling process are myocardial infarction (MI), coronary heart disease (CHD) death, stroke, and stroke death. Based on 7.5% 10-year risk threshold and using ACC/AHA Risk Calculator, statin was recommended to 46.0%, whereas from the actual events (the ground truth), only 23.8% of the 480 'Hard CVD' events actually occurred in those not recommended statin (i.e. recommended statin for 46% out of 6459 but misses 23.8% out of 480 that actually occurred). That gives a sensitivity of 0.76, a specificity of 0.56, and an AUC of 0.71. However, using the ML model, statin was recommended to 11.4%, missing only 14.4% of the 480 'Hard CVD' events that actually occurred in those not recommended statin (i.e. recommended statin for 11.4% out of 6459 but misses only 14.4% out of 480 that actually occurred), corresponding to a sensitivity of 0.86, a specificity of 0.95, and an AUC of 0.92. It is clear that the ML model outperformed the ACC/AHA risk calculator and also has lower number of misses.

Other AI-based CVD risk prediction models developed using biobank data also exist, such as the models presented in [26, 82] and [83] that use MESA biobank data, the UK Biobank data and the China Kadoorie Biobank data, respectively. As shown in Table 8.1, these models mainly differ in the number of risk factors, biomarkers and other phenotypes used as parameters for the model, the number of CVD events or outcomes considered, the prediction horizon (i.e. outcomes predicted within a specific time of baseline) and the ML method used for developing the model. In general, ML models (regardless of the complexity of the algorithm) with large number of parameters increase the accuracy of the cardiovascular risk prediction models.

Imaging Genomics

Variations in cardiovascular structure and function are modulated by the individual genetic predisposition, non genetic factors and their complex interactions. The effects of modifiable cardiovascular risk factors (e.g. physical activity level, obesity, smoking) and non-modifiable risk factors such as age, sex and ethnicity on cardiac structure and function have been studied extensively. However, even taken altogether, these known risk factors explain between 6.7% and 65.5% of individual differences in LV and RV measurements [86]. A large proportion of unexplained phenotypic variation is thought to be determined by the genetic factors as highlighted by a high degree of heritability observed in family and twins studies [87–99]. The genomic machinery that controls phenotypic expression is remarkably elaborate due to the intricate interplay between causal and modifier genes, epigenetics and regulators of transcription and translation such as microRNAs and protein modifiers [100]. By strategically leveraging on the expanding genome-wide genotype data in large-scale population studies, it has become possible to delve into the genetic drivers of cardiac remodelling. In April 2003, an international initiative to sequence the entire human genome consisting of approximately three billion nucleotide base pairs was completed at the cost of ~2.7 billion US dollars [101]. The per-sample genotyping cost has since plunged exponentially (~1000 US dollars for whole genome sequencing and <100 US dollars for microarrays), enabling large-scale genotyping in the national biobanks.

The most widely used study design that capitalises on the availability of whole-genome genotype data is a statistical association analysis known as genome-wide association study (GWAS). Although the human genome is 99.9% identical between individuals, each individual genome differs from the reference human genome at four to five million sites, a majority of which are single nucleotide polymorphisms (SNPs) [102]. GWASs systematically examine these genetic variants across the genome in order to identify regions (loci) associated with a particular trait or disease. There is a multitude of potential benefits from the downstream investigations of GWAS findings, which include but not limited to (i) estimation of heritability of a trait, (ii) examination of genetic correlations across different traits to understand their shared genetic basis, (iii) identification of candidate causal genes that explain the biology and may lead to novel therapies and drug repurposing opportunities and (iv) creation of genetic instruments for Mendelian randomisation studies to evaluate causal relationships. More recently, the genetic variants identified by GWASs are used to build polygenic risk scores that can be integrated into advanced cardiovascular risk stratification strategies [103, 104]. Because each SNP usually has very small effect on the phenotype, well-powered GWASs typically require sample size of at least several thousands. Automatic segmentation algorithms powered by deep learning, therefore, have a major role in permitting high-throughput extraction of reproducible cardiovascular measurements suitable for genetic association analyses.

One of the first imaging genomics studies that applied deep learning used a modified U-Net [70] to segment ~17,000 CMR studies from the UK Biobank [105]. It reported 14 loci (regions) in the genome associated with variation in LV structure and function. These loci harbour some noteworthy genes including (i) titin (*TTN*) involved in sarcomere assembly and stretch sensing with its truncating variants found to be causal in 10–20% of dilated cardiomyopathy (DCM) cases [106]; (ii) Bcl-2-Associated Athanogene 3 (*BAG3*) that regulates Z-disc integrity and also implicated in DCM [107]; (iii) Alpha Kinase 3 (*ALPK3*) that modulates cardiomyocyte differentiation [108]; and (iv) Matrix Metallopeptidase 11 (*MMP11*) involved in extracellular matrix homeostasis [109]. Polygenic risk scores constructed from the LV GWASs were predictive of incident heart failure supporting the role of imaging phenotypes (specifically, their genetic risk) as intermediate biomarkers for hard outcomes. On the whole, the technical breakthrough in image segmentation enabled by deep learning allows large-scale implementation of imaging-genomics studies to identify genetic underpinning of imaging phenotypes, which play a major role in the pathogenesis of cardiovascular diseases.

Automated Quality Control

Quality control tasks can be highly challenging if done manually due to the scale of imaging data in biobanks. Researchers have therefore proposed several AI-based automated quality control tools for identifying images with problems that resulted from the acquisition process, the image reconstruction algorithm or even in a step of data preprocessing pipeline [67, 110, 111]. AI-based automated quality control models are built on the supervised learning paradigm in which ground truth images are images classified into categories of different possible problems these images might have by manual inspection. Categories of the problems could be defined, for example, as poor and good. Based on the image artefact, an image could be considered as having a 'poor' quality if it will make results from subsequent processes or processing impossible or unreliable, and as 'good' otherwise.

An example of using image segmentation for quality control of CMR images and using biobank data can be found in [112] where the Reverse Classification Accuracy technique [113] – which does not need the ground truth information on segmentation quality – is used to determine the accuracy of the prediction as it compares the input image and the predicted image. This accuracy estimate is then used to classify whether an image is accepted (high quality) or rejected (low quality). The predicted contours were produced by a CNN algorithm [114] trained with the UK Biobank data.

Practical Issues on Using Biobank Data for AI-Based Applications

Using biobank data for developing AI application is not necessarily straightforward. In the subsections that follow, we briefly outline some of the issues to be considered when applying AI techniques and developing AI applications using data from biobanks.

Image Data Pre-processing Pipeline

Cardiac imaging data, like many other medical imaging data, are mostly not immediately usable for analysis in their raw formats. Several image processing and optimisation tools, usually in the form of software or programming scripts, are required in order to transform the raw images into formats that are suitable for extracting meaningful information from the images. These pre-processing tools, often referred to as pre-processing pipelines, are used to reorganise and rename the image files in specific forms for easy accessibility in project-specific processing steps. Also, pipelines are often designed for specific needs defined by the characteristics of the projects such as for image segmentation tasks, CVD risk prediction tasks and so on.

A typical pipeline involves (i) final format conversion, for example, from the Digital Imaging and Communications in Medicine (DICOM) format to the Neuroimaging Informatics Technology Initiative (NIfTI) format; (ii) data organisation and quality control (checking for completeness of the dataset and handling missing or repeated files); and (iii) defining a naming scheme for the final output files. Conversion to NIfTI (or any other) format is often useful as the format puts several separate DICOM files into a small number of files with consistent naming style, although the final NIfTI files may become larger than the combination of the raw DICOM files [115].

Data Cleaning and Feature Engineering Considerations

In general, not all data collected in a biobank are as accurate or complete as they should be. In practice, general data science cleaning methods (such as methods to handle missing data or repeated readings with different values, methods to handle unrealistic values, data transformation methods, quality control methods and so on) need to be performed rigorously, and the methods used need to be properly documented. There are many methods, such as the Rubin's rules [116], that can be used for addressing these data cleaning challenges. Descriptions and survey of some of these methods can be found in [117–119].

In many machine learning problems, the performance of the learning algorithms can be significantly improved by extracting features that could be useful or relevant in the model training process and for solving the problem at hand from the raw (often, cleaned) data. This feature extraction or data transformation process, often referred to as feature engineering, may require domain knowledge of the problem (e.g. the manual tracing of the LV endocardial and epicardial borders and the RV endocardial borders by experts as described in [70] in order to serve as the ground truth for the image segmentation problem). In other problems, domain knowledge may not be required (such as the principal component analysis and the singular value decomposition methods [120, 121], among others). Some advantages of feature engineering in addition to performance and predictive accuracy improvements include dimensionality reduction of the feature space, noise reduction, reduction in computational memory cost and improved speed and convergence of the learning algorithms [122–124].

Model Performance Validation and Evaluation

In order to validate the performance of AI models, common approaches for prediction-related problems in the literature include area under the receiving operating characteristic curve (AUC), sensitivity and specificity. For image segmentation problems, they include Dice similarity coefficient metric (or F_1 score) and the Jaccard similarity coefficient or index (or Intersection over Union). Whichever evaluation method is used, it is important that performance of a model is externally evaluated in order to assess the generalisability of the predictions on independent datasets; that is, for a model to be acceptable, the evaluation of its performance with external data set (i.e. test dataset that is not used during the training process) must only degrade negligibly. For a model that has good performance index, model validation ensures that the model has learnt the underlying features or structure of the process that produces the data rather than 'memorising' the features of a particular set of data. One of the most popular techniques used for validation is the cross-validation methods (such as the leave-one-out exhaustive cross-validation method [125] and the k-fold non-exhaustive cross-validation method [126]).

Figure 8.1 shows the steps in developing models using AI algorithms and data from biobanks.

Challenges and Future Opportunities

Generally, in order to aid the development of comprehensive personalised medicine using AI-based applications, the following are some useful properties that biobanks should have: (i) the capacity to collect data longitudinally, (ii) the inclusion of participants' complete health record from external EHR (such as the EHR from the NHS in a biobank based in the UK), (iii) the diverse scope of the data collected from the participants and (iv) the inclusion of both healthy (free of known disease) and diseased participants. The limitations of many biobanks are as a result of the lack of one or more of these properties. Although EHR are increasingly being linked to the biobanks around the world [127], there are some challenges in linking biobank to EHR data. These challenges include different data formats, regulatory processes and data anonymisation schemes that are involved across different centres where EHR are stored [128].

Importantly, while many biobanks contain vast amount of information, analysis and models based on them do not necessarily generalise to the whole population (e.g. UK Biobank is biased towards white Caucasians as they constitute majority of the participants: 94.4% White, 1.9% Asian/Asian British, 1.6% Black/Black British [129]). The implication is that most ML models based on them will be significantly biased [130], which can reduce the performance of the models as these models will

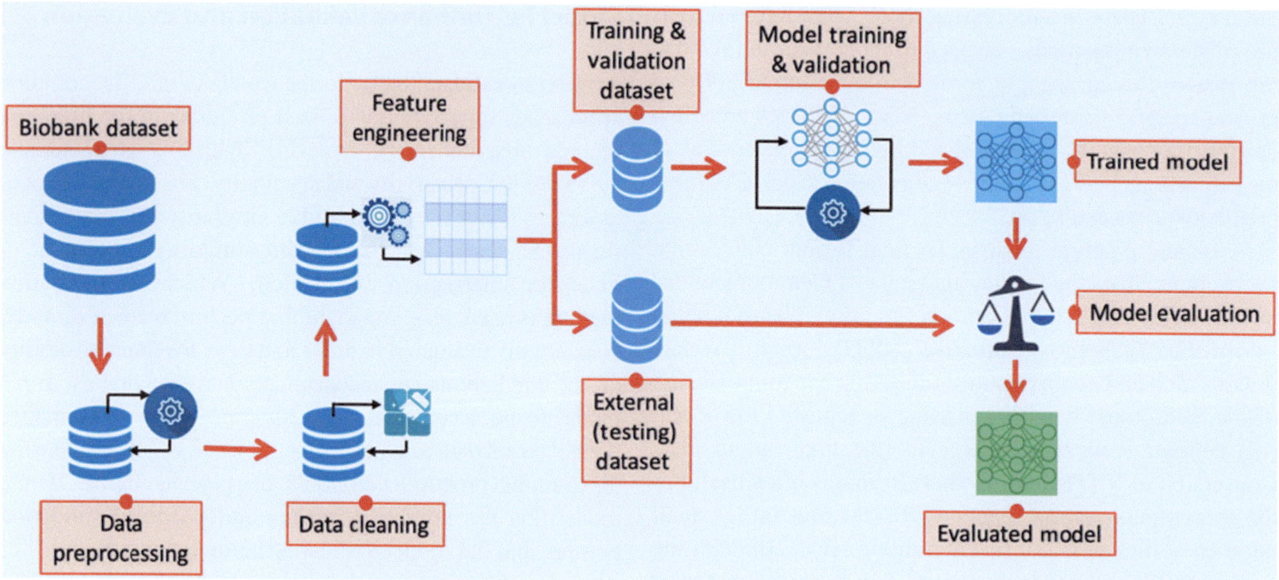

Fig. 8.1 Steps in developing models using AI algorithms and data from biobanks

favour the majority class at the expense of the minority class [131]. As noted in [132], many mainstream ML algorithms for classification problems, including decision trees, nearest neighbour and SVM, were developed based on the assumption that the dataset has balanced class distribution [133]. This therefore results in significant error when classifying the minority class. Algorithms that have been developed to overcome this challenge deal with this problem algorithmically or at data level [130]. Algorithmic methods, such as those proposed in [134, 135], modify the existing algorithms (e.g. by giving the minority class greater weight than the majority class) to improve performance of models around the minority class, but this approach requires expert-level knowledge of the algorithms and the domain in which the application is to be applied. The algorithms related to data-level approach modify (pre-process) the dataset – either by over-sampling [132, 136] or under-sampling [137, 138] – independent of the ML algorithms. This data-level approach can cause loss of important information in the data (in the under-sampling case) or overfitting (in the over-sampling case) [132]. On deciding which method to use to address this data imbalance problem, one may try a number of methods and choose the one that has the highest accuracy for the minority class but with negligible reduction in the accuracy of the majority class. Newer methods are also needed as data stored in biobanks continue to grow.

Furthermore, ML models can only be as good as the quality of the data used for their training. Thus, it is important for published research findings using biobank data to report the pre-processing, the cleaning and the feature engineering steps applied to the data used as well as the structure and amount of the data used for model training, validation and evaluation. All other information that is important for replication of the results will be critical (even if it means releasing the source codes in public repository). The importance of transparency also extends to the learning algorithms used for training ML models. The algorithms will need to be described in a manner that will ensure reproducibility of the results. There is also a need to develop validation and evaluation methods and guidelines for the ML models developed using data from biobanks.

The process of transforming biobank data into uniform common formats, or data format standardisation, that researchers can easily understand and use will be important in the future of AI-based applications. Data format standardisation encourages transparency of the AI algorithms, interoperability of their models for solving several problems and objectivity in interpreting their results. It also simplifies the process of improving the accuracy and performance of the algorithms when more data becomes available (often necessary to optimise performance and evaluate models) and across different biobanks and hardware equipment.

With the advent of digital healthcare and advancement in healthcare technologies (such as wearable and mobile health monitoring devices) [139–147], healthcare data are only going to increase. Infrastructure and technologies, such as the Internet of Things (IoT) [148, 149], that will allow real-time life-course-oriented healthcare, lifestyle and behavioural data to be stored in biobanks will be relevant primarily because of the cost associated with each hospital having to store different logs of IoT data from participants' wearable sensors. Harnessing the large volume of data will require new AI techniques given the large size of attributes (features) that can be collected for each patient. IoT will therefore bring unprecedented research opportunities. To tap the full potential of these opportunities, however, will require multi-disciplinary research efforts such as research projects involving collaborations among mathematicians, AI engineers, computer scientists, data scientists, ethicists and experts from other disciplines. Of course, advances in the development of AI-based tools and their adoption in cardiovascular healthcare will only be achieved with the involvement of clinicians, imagers, patients and other stakeholders.

Summary

This chapter presents some areas in which AI-based applications have been used to tackle different challenges in cardiovascular medicine using the data from biobanks. Drawing from applications in cardiac imaging, risk and outcome prediction, imaging genomics and automated quality control, the main conclusions are that AI techniques are well suited for dealing with the large and multidimensional biobank data and can therefore be used to develop healthcare applications for precision medicine. In addition, the techniques can be used to carry out exploratory data analysis that could be useful in informing, monitoring and improving the quality of public health policies. Data pre-processing, data cleaning and feature engineering and model performance validation and evaluation are practical issues that should be given due consideration when developing AI applications. While data from biobanks offer enormous future opportunities for AI research and applications that will assist humans and improve their abilities to provide healthcare, interdisciplinary research efforts will be necessary in order to tackle some of the most important challenges.

Acknowledgements MA and SEP acknowledge support from the CAP-AI programme (led by Capital Enterprise in partnership with Barts Health NHS Trust and Digital Catapult and funded by the European Regional Development Fund and Barts Charity) and Health Data Research UK (HDR UK; www.hdruk.ac.uk). SEP acknowledges support from the National Institute for Health Research (NIHR) Biomedical Research Centre at Barts and from the "SmartHeart" EPSRC programme grant (www.nihr.ac.uk; EP/P001009/1). SEP has received funding from the European Union's Horizon 2020 research and innovation programme under grant agreement No. 825903 (euCanSHare project). NA acknowledges the NIHR Integrated Academic Training Programme for supporting his Clinical Lectureship.

References

1. Lu H, Wang M. RL4health: crowdsourcing reinforcement learning for knee replacement pathway optimization. ArXiv Prepr ArXiv190601407. 2019.
2. Blasiak A, Khong J, Kee T. CURATE. AI: optimizing personalized medicine with artificial intelligence. SLAS Technol Transl Life Sci Innov. 2020;25:95–105.
3. Shivade C, Raghavan P, Fosler-Lussier E, Embi PJ, Elhadad N, Johnson SB, et al. A review of approaches to identifying patient phenotype cohorts using electronic health records. J Am Med Inform Assoc. 2014;21:221–30.
4. Bennett CC, Hauser K. Artificial intelligence framework for simulating clinical decision-making: a Markov decision process approach. Artif Intell Med. 2013;57:9–19.
5. Shortliffe EH, Sepúlveda MJ. Clinical decision support in the era of artificial intelligence. JAMA. 2018;320:2199–200.
6. Wang Y, Yan F, Lu X, Zheng G, Zhang X, Wang C, et al. IILS: intelligent imaging layout system for automatic imaging report standardization and intra-interdisciplinary clinical workflow optimization. EBioMedicine. 2019;44:162–81.
7. Hagiwara A, Fujita S, Ohno Y, Aoki S. Variability and standardization of quantitative imaging: monoparametric to multiparametric quantification, radiomics, and artificial intelligence. Investig Radiol. 2020;55:601.
8. Kotsiantis SB, Zaharakis I, Pintelas P. Supervised machine learning: a review of classification techniques. Emerg Artif Intell Appl Comput Eng. 2007;160:3–24.
9. Barlow HB. Unsupervised learning. Neural Comput. 1989;1:295–311.
10. Chapelle O, Scholkopf B, Zien A. Semi-supervised learning (Chapelle, O. et al., eds.; 2006) [book reviews]. IEEE Trans Neural Netw. 2009;20:542.
11. Zhu XJ. Semi-supervised learning literature survey. Department of Computer Sciences, University of Wisconsin-Madison. 2005;1530: 1–38.
12. Sutton RS, Barto AG, et al. Introduction to reinforcement learning, vol. 135. Cambridge: MIT Press; 1998.
13. Bzdok D, Altman N, Krzywinski M. Points of significance: statistics versus machine learning. 2018:1–7.
14. Shameer K, Johnson KW, Glicksberg BS, Dudley JT, Sengupta PP. Machine learning in cardiovascular medicine: are we there yet? Heart. 2018;104:1156–64.
15. Simonyan K, Zisserman A. Very deep convolutional networks for large-scale image recognition. ArXiv Prepr ArXiv14091556. 2014.
16. Vidyasagar M. Learning and generalisation: with applications to neural networks. London, UK: Springer Science & Business Media; 2013.
17. Flint E, Webb E, Cummins S. Change in commute mode and body-mass index: prospective, longitudinal evidence from UK Biobank. Lancet Public Health. 2016;1:e46–55.
18. Macfarlane GJ, Barnish MS, Jones GT. Persons with chronic widespread pain experience excess mortality: longitudinal results from UK Biobank and meta-analysis. Ann Rheum Dis. 2017;76:1815–22.
19. Xu L, Jiang CQ, Lam TH, Zhang WS, Cherny SS, Thomas GN, et al. Sleep duration and memory in the elderly Chinese: longitudinal analysis of the Guangzhou Biobank Cohort Study. Sleep. 2014;37:1737–44.
20. Cullen B, Newby D, Lee D, Lyall DM, Nevado-Holgado AJ, Evans JJ, et al. Cross-sectional and longitudinal analyses of outdoor air pollution exposure and cognitive function in UK Biobank. Sci Rep. 2018;8:1–14.
21. Uzuner Ö. Recognizing obesity and comorbidities in sparse data. J Am Med Inform Assoc. 2009;16:561–70.
22. Sheth VM, Guo Y, Qureshi AA. Comorbidities associated with vitiligo: a ten-year retrospective study. Dermatology. 2013;227:311–5.
23. Wang X, Wang F, Hu J. A multi-task learning framework for joint disease risk prediction and comorbidity discovery. In: 2014 22nd Int. Conf. Pattern Recognit. New York, USA: IEEE; 2014. p. 220–5.

24. Osakunor DNM, Sengeh DM, Mutapi F. Coinfections and comorbidities in African health systems: at the interface of infectious and noninfectious diseases. PLoS Negl Trop Dis. 2018;12:e0006711.
25. Hsieh N-C, Hung L-P, Shih C-C, Keh H-C, Chan C-H. Intelligent postoperative morbidity prediction of heart disease using artificial intelligence techniques. J Med Syst. 2012;36:1809–20.
26. Alaa AM, Bolton T, Di Angelantonio E, Rudd JHF, van der Schaar M. Cardiovascular disease risk prediction using automated machine learning: a prospective study of 423,604 UK Biobank participants. PLoS One. 2019;14:e0213653.
27. Hewitt R, Watson P. Defining biobank. Biopreserv Biobank. 2013;11:309–15.
28. Cambon-Thomsen A, Rial-Sebbag E, Knoppers BM. Trends in ethical and legal frameworks for the use of human biobanks. Eur Respir J. 2007;30:373–82.
29. Kauffmann F, Cambon-Thomsen A. Tracing biological collections: between books and clinical trials. JAMA. 2008;299:2316–8.
30. Hewitt RE. Biobanking: the foundation of personalized medicine. Curr Opin Oncol. 2011;23:112–9.
31. Szklo M. Population-based cohort studies. Epidemiol Rev. 1998;20:81–90.
32. Hall MA, Dudek SM, Goodloe R, Crawford DC, Pendergrass SA, Peissig P, et al. Environment-wide association study (EWAS) for type 2 diabetes in the Marshfield Personalized Medicine Research Project Biobank Biocomput. World Sci. 2014:200–11.
33. Wright AF, Carothers AD, Campbell H. Gene--environment interactions—the BioBank UK study. Pharmacogenomics J. 2002;2:75–82.
34. Said MA, Verweij N, van der Harst P. Associations of combined genetic and lifestyle risks with incident cardiovascular disease and diabetes in the UK Biobank Study. JAMA Cardiol. 2018;3:693–702.
35. Rutten-Jacobs LCA, Larsson SC, Malik R, Rannikmäe K, Sudlow CL, Dichgans M, et al. Genetic risk, incident stroke, and the benefits of adhering to a healthy lifestyle: cohort study of 306 473 UK Biobank participants. BMJ. 2018;363:k4168.
36. Wang H, Zhang F, Zeng J, Wu Y, Kemper KE, Xue A, et al. Genotype-by-environment interactions inferred from genetic effects on phenotypic variability in the UK Biobank. Sci Adv. 2019;5:eaaw3538.
37. Arnau-Soler A, Macdonald-Dunlop E, Adams MJ, Clarke T-K, MacIntyre DJ, Milburn K, et al. Genome-wide by environment interaction studies of depressive symptoms and psychosocial stress in UK Biobank and Generation Scotland. Transl Psychiatry. 2019;9:1–13.
38. Tikkanen E, Gustafsson S, Ingelsson E. Associations of fitness, physical activity, strength, and genetic risk with cardiovascular disease: longitudinal analyses in the UK Biobank Study. Circulation. 2018;137:2583–91.
39. Sachs N, de Ligt J, Kopper O, Gogola E, Bounova G, Weeber F, et al. A living biobank of breast cancer organoids captures disease heterogeneity. Cell. 2018;172:373–86.
40. van de Wetering M, Francies HE, Francis JM, Bounova G, Iorio F, Pronk A, et al. Prospective derivation of a living organoid biobank of colorectal cancer patients. Cell. 2015;161:933–45.
41. Bruna A, Rueda OM, Greenwood W, Batra AS, Callari M, Batra RN, et al. A biobank of breast cancer explants with preserved intra-tumor heterogeneity to screen anticancer compounds. Cell. 2016;167:260–74.
42. Ritchie SJ, Cox SR, Shen X, Lombardo MV, Reus LM, Alloza C, et al. Sex differences in the adult human brain: evidence from 5216 UK Biobank participants. Cereb Cortex. 2018;28:2959–75.
43. Chen J, Campbell TC, Li J, Peto R. Diet, lifestyle and mortality in China: a study of the characteristics of 65 Chinese Counties 1990. Oxford: Oxford University Press; 2015.
44. Chen K, Jin M. Mortality, biochemistry, diet and lifestyle in rural China. Geographical study of the characteristics of 69 counties in mainland China and 16 areas in Taiwan. J Epidemiol Community Health. 2007;61(3):271.
45. Biobank UK. About UK Biobank. Available https://www.ukbiobank.ac.uk. 2014.
46. Schram MT, Sep SJS, van der Kallen CJ, Dagnelie PC, Koster A, Schaper N, et al. The Maastricht Study: an extensive phenotyping study on determinants of type 2 diabetes, its complications and its comorbidities. Eur J Epidemiol. 2014;29:439–51.
47. German National Cohort (GNC) Consortium. The German National Cohort: aims, study design and organization. Eur J Epidemiol. 2014;29:371–82. geschaeftsstelle@ nationalekohorte. de GNC (GNC) C 49-62-213152.
48. Breteler MMB, Stöcker T, Pracht E, Brenner D, Stirnberg R. IC-P-165: MRI in the Rhineland study: a novel protocol for population neuroimaging. Alzheimers Dement. 2014;10:P92.
49. Roden DM, Pulley JM, Basford MA, Bernard GR, Clayton EW, Balser JR, et al. Development of a large-scale de-identified DNA biobank to enable personalized medicine. Clin Pharmacol Ther. 2008;84:362–9.
50. Kaiser Permanente: research program on genes, environment and health. n.d. https://divisionofresearch.kaiserpermanente.org/genetics/rpgeh/rpgehabout. Accessed 1 Nov 2020.
51. Chen Z, Chen J, Collins R, Guo Y, Peto R, Wu F, et al. China Kadoorie Biobank of 0.5 million people: survey methods, baseline characteristics and long-term follow-up. Int J Epidemiol. 2011;40:1652–66.
52. Chen Z, Lee L, Chen J, Collins R, Wu F, Guo Y, et al. Cohort profile: the Kadoorie study of chronic disease in China (KSCDC). Int J Epidemiol. 2005;34:1243–9.
53. Gajalakshmi V, Peto R, Kanimozhi VC, Whitlock G, Veeramani D. Cohort profile: the Chennai prospective study of mortality among 500 000 adults in Tamil Nadu, South India. Int J Epidemiol. 2007;36:1190–5.
54. Bild DE, Bluemke DA, Burke GL, Detrano R, Diez Roux AV, Folsom AR, et al. Multi-ethnic study of atherosclerosis: objectives and design. Am J Epidemiol. 2002;156:871–81.
55. MESA. Multi-ethnic study of atherosclerosis (MESA). 2020. https://www.mesa-nhlbi.org/. Accessed 21 Nov 2020.
56. Petersen SE, Matthews PM, Francis JM, Robson MD, Zemrak F, Boubertakh R, et al. UK Biobank's cardiovascular magnetic resonance protocol. J Cardiovasc Magn Reson. 2015;18:8.
57. Petersen SE, Matthews PM, Bamberg F, Bluemke DA, Francis JM, Friedrich MG, et al. Imaging in population science: cardiovascular magnetic resonance in 100,000 participants of UK Biobank-rationale, challenges and approaches. J Cardiovasc Magn Reson. 2013;15:46.
58. Sudlow C, Gallacher J, Allen N, Beral V, Burton P, Danesh J, et al. UK biobank: an open access resource for identifying the causes of a wide range of complex diseases of middle and old age. PLoS Med. 2015;12:e1001779.
59. Elliott P, Peakman TC. The UK Biobank sample handling and storage protocol for the collection, processing and archiving of human blood and urine. Int J Epidemiol. 2008;37:234–44.
60. Allen N, Sudlow C, Downey P, Peakman T, Danesh J, Elliott P, et al. UK Biobank: current status and what it means for epidemiology. Health Policy Technol. 2012;1:123–6.
61. Littlejohns TJ, Holliday J, Gibson LM, Garratt S, Oesingmann N, Alfaro-Almagro F, et al. The UK Biobank imaging enhancement of 100,000 participants: rationale, data collection, management and future directions. Nat Commun. 2020;11:2624. https://doi.org/10.1038/s41467-020-15948-9.
62. Johnson KW, Shameer K, Glicksberg BS, Readhead B, Sengupta PP, Björkegren JLM, et al. Enabling precision cardiology through

multiscale biology and systems medicine. JACC Basic Transl Sci. 2017;2:311–27.
63. Shen D, Wu G, Suk H-I. Deep learning in medical image analysis. Annu Rev Biomed Eng. 2017;19:221–48.
64. Suinesiaputra A, Sanghvi MM, Aung N, Paiva JM, Zemrak F, Fung K, et al. Fully-automated left ventricular mass and volume MRI analysis in the UK Biobank population cohort: evaluation of initial results. Int J Cardiovasc Imaging. 2018;34:281–91. https://doi.org/10.1007/s10554-017-1225-9.
65. Petersen SE, Aung N, Sanghvi MM, Zemrak F, Fung K, Paiva JM, et al. Reference ranges for cardiac structure and function using cardiovascular magnetic resonance (CMR) in Caucasians from the UK Biobank population cohort. J Cardiovasc Magn Reson. 2017;19:18.
66. Mauger C, Gilbert K, Lee AM, Sanghvi MM, Aung N, Fung K, et al. Right ventricular shape and function: cardiovascular magnetic resonance reference morphology and biventricular risk factor morphometrics in UK Biobank. J Cardiovasc Magn Reson. 2019;21:41.
67. Robinson R, Valindria VV, Bai W, Oktay O, Kainz B, Suzuki H, et al. Automated quality control in image segmentation: application to the UK Biobank cardiovascular magnetic resonance imaging study. J Cardiovasc Magn Reson. 2019;21:1–14. https://doi.org/10.1186/s12968-019-0523-x.
68. Bai W, Suzuki H, Huang J, Francis C, Wang S, Tarroni G, et al. A population-based phenome-wide association study of cardiac and aortic structure and function. Nat Med. 2020:1–9.
69. Petersen SE, Abdulkareem M, Leiner T. Artificial intelligence will transform cardiac imaging--opportunities and challenges. Front Cardiovasc Med. 2019;6:133.
70. Bai W, Sinclair M, Tarroni G, Oktay O, Rajchl M, Vaillant G, et al. Automated cardiovascular magnetic resonance image analysis with fully convolutional networks. J Cardiovasc Magn Reson. 2018;20:1–12. https://doi.org/10.1186/s12968-018-0471-x.
71. Long J, Shelhamer E, Darrell T. Fully convolutional networks for semantic segmentation. Proc IEEE Conf Comput Vis Pattern Recognit. 2015:3431–40.
72. Attar R, Pereañez M, Gooya A, Albà X, Zhang L, de Vila MH, et al. Quantitative CMR population imaging on 20,000 subjects of the UK Biobank imaging study: LV/RV quantification pipeline and its evaluation. Med Image Anal. 2019;56:26–42.
73. Cootes TF, Edwards GJ, Taylor CJ. Active appearance models. IEEE Trans Pattern Anal Mach Intell. 2001;23:681–5.
74. van Assen HC, Danilouchkine MG, Frangi AF, Ordás S, Westenberg JJM, Reiber JHC, et al. SPASM: a 3D-ASM for segmentation of sparse and arbitrarily oriented cardiac MRI data. Med Image Anal. 2006;10:286–303. https://doi.org/10.1016/j.media.2005.12.001.
75. Goff DC, Lloyd-Jones DM, Bennett G, Coady S, D'agostino RB, Gibbons R, et al. 2013 ACC/AHA guideline on the assessment of cardiovascular risk: a report of the American College of Cardiology/American Heart Association Task Force on Practice Guidelines. J Am Coll Cardiol. 2014;63:2935–59.
76. Piepoli MF, Hoes AW, Agewall S, Albus C, Brotons C, Catapano AL, et al. 2016 European Guidelines on cardiovascular disease prevention in clinical practice: the Sixth Joint Task Force of the European Society of Cardiology and Other Societies on Cardiovascular Disease Prevention in Clinical Practice (constituted by representatives of 10 societies and by invited experts) Developed with the special contribution of the European Association for Cardiovascular Prevention & Rehabilitation (EACPR). Eur Heart J. 2016;37:2315–81.
77. Grundy SM, Cleeman JI, Merz CNB, Brewer HB, Clark LT, Hunninghake DB, et al. Implications of recent clinical trials for the national cholesterol education program adult treatment panel III guidelines. J Am Coll Cardiol. 2004;44:720–32.
78. Kakadiaris IA, Vrigkas M, Yen AA, Kuznetsova T, Budoff M, Naghavi M. Machine learning outperforms ACC/AHA CVD risk calculator in MESA. J Am Heart Assoc. 2018;7:e009476.
79. Muntner P, Colantonio LD, Cushman M, Goff DC, Howard G, Howard VJ, et al. Validation of the atherosclerotic cardiovascular disease Pooled Cohort risk equations. JAMA. 2014;311:1406–15.
80. DeFilippis AP, Young R, McEvoy JW, Michos ED, Sandfort V, Kronmal RA, et al. Risk score overestimation: the impact of individual cardiovascular risk factors and preventive therapies on the performance of the American Heart Association-American College of Cardiology-Atherosclerotic Cardiovascular Disease risk score in a modern mult. Eur Heart J. 2017;38:598–608.
81. Kavousi M, Leening MJG, Nanchen D, Greenland P, Graham IM, Steyerberg EW, et al. Comparison of application of the ACC/AHA guidelines, Adult Treatment Panel III guidelines, and European Society of Cardiology guidelines for cardiovascular disease prevention in a European cohort. JAMA. 2014;311:1416–23.
82. Ambale-Venkatesh B, Yang X, Wu CO, Liu K, Hundley WG, McClelland R, et al. Cardiovascular event prediction by machine learning: the multi-ethnic study of atherosclerosis. Circ Res. 2017;121:1092–101.
83. Shen Y, Yang Y, Parish S, Chen Z, Clarke R, Clifton DA. Risk prediction for cardiovascular disease using ECG data in the China Kadoorie Biobank. In: 2016 38th Annu. Int. Conf. IEEE Eng. Med. Biol. Soc. New York, USA: IEEE; 2016. p. 2419–22.
84. International statistical classification of diseases and related health problems: instruction manual, vol. 2. 10th ed. Geneva, Switzerland: World Health Organization; 2004.
85. Rogers G, editor. International classification of diseases, 9th revision--clinical modification. 1996.
86. Petersen SE, Sanghvi MM, Aung N, Cooper JA, Paiva JM, Zemrak F, et al. The impact of cardiovascular risk factors on cardiac structure and function: insights from the UK Biobank imaging enhancement study. PLoS One. 2017;12:e0185114.
87. Post WS, Larson MG, Myers RH, Galderisi M, Levy D. Heritability of left ventricular mass: the Framingham Heart Study. Hypertension. 1997;30:1025–8.
88. Garner C, Lecomte E, Visvikis S, Abergel E, Lathrop M, Soubrier F. Genetic and environmental influences on left ventricular mass: a family study. Hypertension. 2000;36:740–6.
89. Fox ER, Klos KL, Penman AD, Blair GJ, Blossom BD, Arnett D, et al. Heritability and genetic linkage of left ventricular mass, systolic and diastolic function in hypertensive African Americans (From the GENOA study). Am J Hypertens. 2010;23:870–5.
90. Jin Y, Kuznetsova T, Bochud M, Richart T, Thijs L, Cusi D, et al. Heritability of left ventricular structure and function in Caucasian families. Eur J Echocardiogr. 2011;12:326–32.
91. Noh H-M, Lee SC, Park SW, Sung J, Song Y-M. Genetic influence on left ventricular structure and function: a Korean twin and family study. Twin Res Hum Genet. 2015;18:281–9.
92. Arnett DK, Hong Y, Bella JN, Oberman A, Kitzman DW, Hopkins PN, et al. Sibling correlation of left ventricular mass and geometry in hypertensive African Americans and whites: the HyperGEN study. Am J Hypertens. 2001;14:1226–30.
93. Palatini P, Krause L, Amerena J, Nesbitt S, Majahalme S, Tikhonoff V, et al. Genetic contribution to the variance in left ventricular mass: the Tecumseh Offspring Study. J Hypertens. 2001;19:1217–22.
94. Swan L, Birnie DH, Padmanabhan S, Inglis G, Connell JMC, Hillis WS. The genetic determination of left ventricular mass in healthy adults. Eur Heart J. 2003;24:577–82.
95. Bella JN, MacCluer JW, Roman MJ, Almasy L, North KE, Best LG, et al. Heritability of left ventricular dimensions and mass in American Indians: the Strong Heart Study. J Hypertens. 2004;22:281–6.

96. Juo S-HH, Di Tullio MR, Lin H-F, Rundek T, Boden-Albala B, Homma S, et al. Heritability of left ventricular mass and other morphologic variables in Caribbean Hispanic subjects: the Northern Manhattan Family Study. J Am Coll Cardiol. 2005;46:735.
97. Chien K-L, Hsu H-C, Su T-C, Chen M-F, Lee Y-T. Heritability and major gene effects on left ventricular mass in the Chinese population: a family study. BMC Cardiovasc Disord. 2006;6:37.
98. Sharma P, Middelberg RPS, Andrew T, Johnson MR, Christley H, Brown MJ. Heritability of left ventricular mass in a large cohort of twins. J Hypertens. 2006;24:321–4.
99. Busjahn CA, Schulz-Menger J, Abdel-Aty H, Rudolph A, Jordan J, Luft FC, et al. Heritability of left ventricular and papillary muscle heart size: a twin study with cardiac magnetic resonance imaging. Eur Heart J. 2009;30:1643–7.
100. Marian AJ. Genetic determinants of cardiac hypertrophy. Curr Opin Cardiol. 2008;23:199.
101. NIH. The cost of sequencing a human genome. Natl Hum Genome Res Institute, Natl Institutes Heal; 2020. https://www.genome.gov/about-genomics/fact-sheets/Sequencing-Human-Genome-cost. Accessed 21 Nov 2020.
102. Consortium 1000 Genomes Project, et al. A global reference for human genetic variation. Nature. 2015;526:68–74.
103. Khera AV, Chaffin M, Aragam KG, Haas ME, Roselli C, Choi SH, et al. Genome-wide polygenic scores for common diseases identify individuals with risk equivalent to monogenic mutations. Nat Genet. 2018;50:1219–24.
104. Damask A, Steg PG, Schwartz GG, Szarek M, Hagström E, Badimon L, et al. Patients with high genome-wide polygenic risk scores for coronary artery disease may receive greater clinical benefit from alirocumab treatment in the odyssey outcomes trial. Circulation. 2020;141:624–36.
105. Aung N, Vargas JD, Yang C, Cabrera CP, Warren HR, Fung K, et al. Genome-wide analysis of left ventricular image-derived phenotypes identifies fourteen loci associated with cardiac morphogenesis and heart failure development. Circulation. 2019;140:1318–30.
106. Herman DS, Lam L, Taylor MRG, Wang L, Teekakirikul P, Christodoulou D, et al. Truncations of titin causing dilated cardiomyopathy. N Engl J Med. 2012;366:619–28.
107. Villard E, Perret C, Gary F, Proust C, Dilanian G, Hengstenberg C, et al. A genome-wide association study identifies two loci associated with heart failure due to dilated cardiomyopathy. Eur Heart J. 2011;32:1065–76.
108. Hosoda T, Monzen K, Hiroi Y, Oka T, Takimoto E, Yazaki Y, et al. A novel myocyte-specific gene Midori promotes the differentiation of P19CL6 cells into cardiomyocytes. J Biol Chem. 2001;276:35978–89.
109. Li YY, McTiernan CF, Feldman AM. Interplay of matrix metalloproteinases, tissue inhibitors of metalloproteinases and their regulators in cardiac matrix remodeling. Cardiovasc Res. 2000;46:214–24.
110. Biasiolli L, Hann E, Lukaschuk E, Carapella V, Paiva JM, Aung N, et al. Automated localization and quality control of the aorta in cine CMR can significantly accelerate processing of the UK Biobank population data. PLoS One. 2019;14:e0212272.
111. Tarroni G, Bai W, Oktay O, Schuh A, Suzuki H, Glocker B, et al. Large-scale quality control of cardiac imaging in population studies: application to UK Biobank. Sci Rep. 2020;10:1–11.
112. Robinson R, Valindria VV, Bai W, Oktay O, Kainz B, Suzuki H, et al. Automated quality control in image segmentation: application to the UK Biobank cardiovascular magnetic resonance imaging study. J Cardiovasc Magn Reson. 2019;21:18.
113. Valindria VV, Lavdas I, Bai W, Kamnitsas K, Aboagye EO, Rockall AG, et al. Reverse classification accuracy: predicting segmentation performance in the absence of ground truth. IEEE Trans Med Imaging. 2017;36:1597–606.
114. Bai W, Sinclair M, Tarroni G, Oktay O, Rajchl M, Vaillant G, et al. Human-level CMR image analysis with deep fully convolutional networks. Department of Computing, Imperial College London. 2017. p. 1–11.
115. Li X, Morgan PS, Ashburner J, Smith J, Rorden C. The first step for neuroimaging data analysis: DICOM to NIfTI conversion. J Neurosci Methods. 2016;264:47–56.
116. Rubin DB. Multiple imputation for nonresponse in surveys, vol. 81. New Jersey, USA: Wiley; 2004.
117. Barnard J, Rubin DB. Miscellanea. Small-sample degrees of freedom with multiple imputation. Biometrika. 1999;86:948–55.
118. Marshall A, Altman DG, Holder RL, Royston P. Combining estimates of interest in prognostic modelling studies after multiple imputation: current practice and guidelines. BMC Med Res Methodol. 2009;9(57). https://doi.org/10.1186/1471-2288-9-57.
119. Van Buuren S. Flexible imputation of missing data. Boca Raton, FL, USA: CRC Press; 2018.
120. Deka A, Sarma KK. SVD and PCA features for ANN based detection of diabetes using retinopathy. In: Proc. CUBE Int. Inf. Technol. Conf. New York, USA: ACM; 2012. p. 38–41.
121. Cateni S, Vannucci M, Vannocci M, Colla V. Variable selection and feature extraction through artificial intelligence techniques. Multivar Anal Manag Eng Sci. 2012:103–18.
122. Ladha L, Deepa T. Feature selection methods and algorithms. Int J Comput Sci Eng. 2011;3:1787–97.
123. Khalid S, Khalil T, Nasreen S. A survey of feature selection and feature extraction techniques in machine learning. In: 2014 Sci. Inf. Conf. New York, USA: IEEE; 2014. p. 372–8.
124. Liu H, Motoda H. Feature extraction, construction and selection: a data mining perspective, vol. 453. Norwell, MA, USA: Springer Science & Business Media; 1998.
125. Molinaro AM, Simon R, Pfeiffer RM. Prediction error estimation: a comparison of resampling methods. Bioinformatics. 2005;21:3301–7.
126. McLachlan GJ, Do K-A, Ambroise C. Analyzing microarray gene expression data, vol. 422. New Jersey, USA: Wiley; 2005.
127. Krittanawong C, Bomback AS, Baber U, Bangalore S, Messerli FH, Tang WHW. Future direction for using artificial intelligence to predict and manage hypertension. Curr Hypertens Rep. 2018;20:75.
128. Adamska L, Allen N, Flaig R, Sudlow C, Lay M, Landray M. Challenges of linking to routine healthcare records in UK Biobank. Trials. 2015;16:1.
129. Thompson SG, Willeit P. UK Biobank comes of age. Lancet. 2015;386:509–10.
130. He H, Garcia EA. Learning from imbalanced data. IEEE Trans Knowl Data Eng. 2009;21:1263–84.
131. Chawla NV, Bowyer KW, Hall LO, Kegelmeyer WP. SMOTE: synthetic minority over-sampling technique. J Artif Intell Res. 2002;16:321–57.
132. Almogahed BA, Kakadiaris IA. NEATER: filtering of over-sampled data using non-cooperative game theory. Soft Comput. 2015;19:3301–22.
133. Chen JJ, Tsai CA, Young JF, Kodell RL. Classification ensembles for unbalanced class sizes in predictive toxicology. SAR QSAR Environ Res. 2005;16:517–29.
134. Barandela R, Sánchez JS, Garca V, Rangel E. Strategies for learning in class imbalance problems. Pattern Recogn. 2003;36:849–51.

135. Oh S-H. Error back-propagation algorithm for classification of imbalanced data. Neurocomputing. 2011;74:1058–61.
136. Kubat M, Matwin S, et al. Addressing the curse of imbalanced training sets: one-sided selection. ICML. 1997;97:179–86.
137. Hart P. The condensed nearest neighbor rule (Corresp.). IEEE Trans Inf Theory. 1968;14:515–6.
138. Laurikkala J. Improving identification of difficult small classes by balancing class distribution. Conf Artif Intell Med Eur. 2001:63–6.
139. Sarwar CMS, Vaduganathan M, Anker SD, Coiro S, Papadimitriou L, Saltz J, et al. Mobile health applications in cardiovascular research. Int J Cardiol. 2018;269:265–71.
140. Piette JD, List J, Rana GK, Townsend W, Striplin D, Heisler M. Mobile health devices as tools for worldwide cardiovascular risk reduction and disease management. Circulation. 2015;132:2012–27.
141. Jatoba LC, Grossmann U, Kunze C, Ottenbacher J, Stork W. Context-aware mobile health monitoring: Evaluation of different pattern recognition methods for classification of physical activity. In: 2008 30th Annu. Int. Conf. IEEE Eng. Med. Biol. Soc. New York, USA: IEEE; 2008. p. 5250–3.
142. Kumar S, Nilsen WJ, Abernethy A, Atienza A, Patrick K, Pavel M, et al. Mobile health technology evaluation: the mHealth evidence workshop. Am J Prev Med. 2013;45:228–36.
143. Wang X, White L, Chen X, Gao Y, Li H, Luo Y. An empirical study of wearable technology acceptance in healthcare. Ind Manag Data Syst. 2015;115(9);1704–23.
144. Pentland A. Healthwear: medical technology becomes wearable. Computer (Long Beach Calif). 2004;37:42–9.
145. Schüll ND. Data for life: wearable technology and the design of self-care. BioSocieties. 2016;11:317–33.
146. Lmberis A, Dittmar A. Advanced wearable health systems and applications-research and development efforts in the European Union. IEEE Eng Med Biol Mag. 2007;26:29–33.
147. Park S, Jayaraman S. Enhancing the quality of life through wearable technology. IEEE Eng Med Biol Mag. 2003;22:41–8.
148. Lee I, Lee K. The Internet of Things (IoT): applications, investments, and challenges for enterprises. Bus Horiz. 2015;58:431–40.
149. Baker SB, Xiang W, Atkinson I. Internet of things for smart healthcare: technologies, challenges, and opportunities. IEEE Access. 2017;5:26521–44.

Biostatistics and Artificial Intelligence

9

Lance A. Waller

Introduction

We live in an increasingly data-rich world. Multiple, linked devices track our location and put us into the context of the world around us. We post and comment on our activities, our photos, and our friends. Our constantly connected world provides benefits (real-time driving directions) and risks (a loss of privacy). In the world of clinical medicine and biomedical research, rapid expansion in measurement technology generates data in volumes and at speeds previously unimaginable. Detailed medical images are created, collated, and stored across a wide range of patients every day. Data, formerly only associated with scientific inquiry, now surround us and drive our daily decisions.

Not only is the nature and availability of data changing, but our approaches to managing, analyzing, and understanding data are shifting to accommodate novel data settings. The discipline of *data science* includes familiar elements of mathematics, statistics, and computing but places these ideas in new settings and scenarios. This expanded framework extends the data analytic toolbox to include *machine learning* and other artificial intelligence approaches building on newly available data, newly available computational platforms, and newly available storage capacities.

How do new data types, new computational platforms, and new analytic techniques fit into biomedical imaging research? In this chapter, we provide a brief overview of traditional and emerging data types and outline how tools, algorithms, and ideas from the fields of biostatistics and machine learning, separately and together, enhance the analytic toolbox available in cardiothoracic imaging research.

L. A. Waller, BS, PhD (✉)
Department of Biostatistics and Bioinformatics, Rollins School of Public Health, Emory University, Atlanta, GA, USA
e-mail: lwaller@emory.edu

Shifting Data Paradigms and Analytic Paradigms

Many years ago, researchers viewed scientific data as expensive, particularly biomedical data from clinical settings. In this *traditional data paradigm*, each research project collected its own relevant data with a goal of gaining the most information from the smallest sample size that provided a prespecified level of statistical accuracy. In contrast, the rapid growth of biomedical measurement technology, computational processing power, and computational storage provide researchers ready access to large sets of measurements. In this *emerging data paradigm*, available data may not include *exactly* what a biomedical investigator wishes to collect, but there are large amounts of related measurements, similar to what is desired. For instance, clinical settings often now routinely store and retain large numbers of digitized images (scanned from historical film images or collected directly in a digital format), thereby providing a collection of images far greater than can be collected within the typical budgetary constraints of a single research project. From an investigator's perspective, the traditional and emerging paradigms reflect a difference in focus between "What specific data should I gather?" and "What relevant data can I find?" The rapid increase in the availability of and access to such data repositories motivates investigators to wonder: At what point does the volume of available-but-imperfect available data outweigh the focused design of investigator-based collection of data specifically tailored to address a research question?

Accompanying this changing data paradigm is a shift in the data analysis paradigm from a primary focus on *estimation* of associations between interventions and outcomes to *prediction* of outcomes given a set of observations (including interventions). Both estimation and prediction have been present in thinking about data analysis for some time [4], but as greater amounts of data become more available and accessible, we find an increasing focus on prediction. The

C. N. De Cecco et al. (eds.), *Artificial Intelligence in Cardiothoracic Imaging*, Contemporary Medical Imaging,
https://doi.org/10.1007/978-3-030-92087-6_9

emerging data paradigm, coupled with large-scale cloud computing, allows the development of data-hungry prediction algorithms exploring and classifying massive data sets with impressive results. Familiar examples include crowd-sourced calculations of expected travel times utilizing volunteered location data from millions of mobile phones to online translators matching phrases in one language to their best match in another. Looking further, image classifiers can identify facial features or potential malignancies, and autonomous vehicles are "driven" by algorithms that rapidly classify the input from multiple sensors to predict the best course of action. Networks of finely tuned prediction algorithms can learn from large-scale collections of data and form the basis of many current artificial intelligence (AI) systems controlling everything from our household thermostats to complex communications systems.

The success of AI systems, particularly those based on variants of *machine learning* algorithms, prompts some to propose that we are headed toward "hypothesis-free science" or to boldly state that all fields of science will be branches of computer science in the near future [3]. However, while such statements typically reflect self-promotional hyperbole, it is important to assess whether artificial intelligence based on machine learning is replacing or simply is adding to the analytic options open to the biomedical investigator. In order to explore this question, we will compare brief overviews of the two data paradigms and accompanying data analytic paradigms mentioned above.

The Traditional Data Paradigm and Biostatistical Analysis

While probability calculations had been developed (in part to understand games of chance) in the eighteenth and nineteenth centuries, the twentieth century saw a detailed development of disciplined *experimental design* wherein data were purposefully collected in ways to explore predefined hypotheses taking into account observed variation in measurements. The traditional data paradigm (data are expensive, so focus collection on what is needed to best answer the question at hand) drove the development of statistical techniques focused on comparisons of intervention and nonintervention groups adjusting for (and attempting to minimize) the variances in measurements in both groups. The mathematical rules of probability defining the distributions of observations provided the ingredients for estimation of and inference about distributional parameters (e.g., means, variances, correlations) from observations generated from these distributions. Statistically independent observations provided the most information per observation, and sample size calculations allowed experimenters to define how many independent observations would be required to provide estimates within a given level of precision. Regression-based methods and models (e.g., linear regression, generalized linear models) provided analytic tools for estimating associations between covariates and outcomes. Independence assumptions were relaxed, allowing longitudinal correlations between observations from the same patient over time, correlations between different patients evaluated at the same clinic, or spatial correlations between observations taken at nearby locations (e.g., neighboring voxels in a medical image). The statistical toolbox is large and offers tools as simple as comparing mean values between two groups and as complex as identifying regions of significant difference between resting and active states in brain and heart images. Importantly, the biostatistical toolbox is not complete but rather grows to address the challenges that arise when traditional assumptions are violated.

The field of *biostatistics* focuses on building and expanding this traditional data toolbox; specifically, biostatistics involves the development, application, interpretation, and evaluation of statistical methods for application to biomedicine and public health. To illustrate, two general areas of biostatistical methodology research focus include clinical trials and epidemiology.

Clinical trials are defined by the US National Institutes of Health as:

> A research study in which one or more human subjects are prospectively assigned to one or more interventions (which may include placebo or other control) to evaluate the effects of those interventions on health-related biomedical or behavioral outcomes. (https://grants.nih.gov/policy/clinical-trials/definition.htm)

Several key aspects arise in this definition. First, clinical trials involve experimentation with human subjects, where interventions are prospectively assigned and outcomes are evaluated. Ethical and safety concerns require regulation and clearly designed protocols for participant recruitment, intervention assignment, measurement of outcomes, and evaluation of differences in outcomes by intervention groups.

In the clinical trial setting, experimental design is of utmost importance, and biostatistical issues play critical roles. Investigators must summarize past knowledge, define clear hypotheses in terms of anticipated intervention effects, evaluate measurement uncertainty, predefine analytic plans, and calculate appropriate sampling plans and sample sizes to recruit participants, assign interventions, collect data, and evaluate results. Central elements include summaries of measurements within groups, assessment of variation in these measurements, and comparisons of summaries between intervention groups. Comparisons are often assessed via statistical hypothesis testing or through the calculation of confidence interval estimates.

Statistical hypothesis testing and its summary of statistical significance, the p-value, have received critical consideration in recent years [1]. The p-value represents the chance of observing a summary measure at least as extreme as that observed in the data, if the null hypothesis of no intervention effect is true. That is, if we were to repeat the experiment under identical conditions and there was no difference between intervention groups, what proportion of the time would we see an observed difference in summaries at least as large as that we observed in our observed data? Note, the definition of the p-value is different than simply representing the probability that the null hypothesis is true (as many of us were reminded frequently in our statistics courses!). Much of the recent criticism of the use of *p*-values to determine whether experimental findings are important is based on the overreliance of a fixed (usually 0.05) threshold for statistical significance and using this threshold to define whether an investigator has a publishable finding. In today's data-rich world, blindly applying a p-value threshold to a large number of tests ("p-hacking") will invariably lead to a result that is statistically significant but may only be due to chance [7]. In addition, in the case of very large sample sizes, statistically significant differences may be of such small magnitude as to be clinically irrelevant.

In contrast to the experimental setting of clinical trials, the field of epidemiology often involves the analysis of observational (i.e., non-experimental) data wherein an investigator compares data from individuals with and without the health outcome of interest with respect to factors that may contribute to differences in risk. Such observational studies can be based on prospective data wherein cohorts of individuals are followed over time to observe which individuals develop the outcome of interest and which do not or can be based on retrospective data wherein investigators identify individuals with and without the outcome of interest and look back in time to evaluate past exposures that may relate to risk.

Relevant biostatistical issues of measurement variability, estimation of contrasts between groups, and assessments of similarity between intervention (or, more generally, exposure) groups remain key biostatistical issues in epidemiologic data analysis. In addition, the observational setting includes a reduction in the amount of control an investigator has over the settings and experiences of research subjects, and as a result, issues of bias, confounding, and interactions can occur between risk factors and influence (bias) estimated associations between risk factors and outcomes, an issue of increased importance in epidemiology compared to the more controlled setting of clinical trials.

The transition from the traditional data paradigm where investigators collect their own data to the emerging data paradigm where investigators both collect and seek out existing data relevant to the questions of interest has a clear impact on both clinical trials and epidemiology. In clinical trials, the availability of past clinical (and nonclinical) information can rapidly increase identification and enrollment of potential participants meeting eligibility criteria. In epidemiology, the rapid access of administrative data can, for example, reveal past patterns in housing type, environmental exposures, traffic volumes, and clinic location. Such examples suggest potential opportunities for emerging data analytic tools to better incorporate larger volumes of available and accessible data. Before considering how one might combine traditional biostatistical thinking and tools with modern data access, we first provide a brief overview of machine learning approaches to analyzing data in the emerging data paradigm.

The Emerging Data Paradigm and Machine Learning

In the emerging data paradigm, large volumes of data are available and can be accessed for analysis. In addition, this paradigm also encourages data sharing to allow reproducible research wherein results may be verified, adapted, and extended by other investigative teams. To support this ideal, increasingly, many fields of science aim to follow the FAIR data principles, i.e., making data Findable, Accessible, Interoperable, and Reusable [13]. Scientific journals increasingly require data associated with publications to be available as a condition of publication. While data sharing can be complicated with biomedical data, particularly clinical data that often fall under federal privacy regulations, in some cases, the development of clearly defined data use agreements can allow sharing of data at some level of aggregation. Simply put, the curation, storage, and citation of data sets are a growing and dynamic part of today's biomedical research environment, and the creation and curation of citable data sets are becoming a critical component of a researcher's scholarly output [11]. The broad and growing universe of generally accessible data motivates many new approaches to data analyses, including the broad field of machine learning.

As noted above, machine learning algorithms form the general basis of much of today's artificial intelligence applications in biomedicine and other fields. Such algorithms explore large, complex data sets seeking ways to classify information and "learn" how to classify the next sets of observed data. While machines do not really "learn" in the same way as living creatures, algorithms can be very efficient in classifying patterns within large data sets to build computational and statistical *models* linking input data (e.g., clinical records, images) into output labels and classifications (e.g., diagnostic categories of healthy, moderate disease, and severe disease).

In most machine learning applications, each data observation includes values for a large (sometimes *very* large) number of variables. The *models* mentioned above are typically mathematical functions that, roughly speaking, weight observed input variable to provide a summary score as output. This summary score can be a single value or a collection of values (e.g., a scorecard) but is typically of much smaller dimension than the original data. For example, in a cardiothoracic imaging study, the data from each patient may include a high-resolution image (or series of images), patient demographics, chart history, etc. The collection of input data can be heterogeneous and contain numerical values, voxel-specific readings from images, and text information from clinical notes.

Continuing the example, for *output*, we may be interested in identifying image-based predictors associated with the identification and diagnoses of a specific physiological anomaly, something that traditionally would be diagnosed by a human reader from diagnostic imaging in consultation with clinical visits. The function translating input to output will be a summary of all of the information in patient images and charts giving high weight to data elements related to the anomaly of interest and low (or zero) to data elements unassociated with the anomaly. These weights could be assigned by an expert or, in the case of machine learning, calculated by evaluating which input values are most strongly associated with the output diagnostic classification across a very large number of images. The goal is to define the function (set of weights) that can best classify new data inputs (say, new images) that do not have associated diagnosis information. In other words, we focus on *prediction* and seek to define the function that best predicts the outcome based on the input. This shift from the traditional analysis goal of *estimation* of associations between interventions and outcomes to *prediction* of outcomes given interventions is a key ingredient in the rise of *data science*. This idea is eloquently described in an overview of the "two cultures" of statistical modeling described in Breiman [4] and expanded in historical context by Donoho [6].

Machine learning builds on the input-to-function-to-output idea where our goal is to use an algorithm to identify the ingredients of our function that optimize our ability to provide the best output. Differing details defining optimization and what defines the "best" predictions lead to different flavors of machine learning, and we briefly define two general classes of algorithms below. For readers interested in broader overviews, Shane [9] provides a very readable and entertaining introduction to the intuition driving what machine learning does (and does not) do well, while Burkov's [5] text provides a more technical (but still very readable) summary of specific families of machine learning approaches.

To motivate our discussion, suppose we continue our example above: we have a large set of cardiac images and we want to build an algorithm to scan and identify the images indicating the presence of a particular anatomical defect. Such an algorithm, if perfect, would remove the need for human review of images. While no classification system (even an expert human reader) is perfect, even a system that could identify and classify the subset of images worth a more careful look by a human expert could save a great deal of time and effort in processing large numbers of images in clinical practice.

Typical machine learning algorithms will split the full set of images into a *training set* and a *validation set*. We use the training set to develop and refine our algorithm and then apply the algorithm to the validation set to see how well it does. *Supervised machine learning* begins with a set of images in the training set labeled by an expert (or set of experts) as containing the anomaly or not. The algorithm will then seek to identify which features in the labeled images have in common with each other in order to identify what information in the images represents signal related to the desired classification and what information represents noise. The algorithm optimizes the definitions of weights in the function linking input data to predicted outcomes based on the labeled images in the training set. In some settings, all images in the training set will be prelabeled, but, more commonly, the training data include both labeled and unlabeled images. If this is the case, the algorithm next applies the features identified as signal in the labeled images to the unlabeled images in the training set and begins to classify these as well. The algorithm picks up additional features from the unlabeled images that appear to contain the defect and examines whether these features are also present in the labeled features. After this classification exercise with the data in the training set, the algorithm will have a set of rules (the weights in the function) to classify images. Note that this set of rules has been developed and tested on the training set. Next, to assess whether the rules apply to data not included in the process of fine-tuning the algorithm, we apply the algorithm with the optimized weights to the data in the validation set to evaluate which images the algorithm identifies as containing the anomaly. Having human experts review the algorithm's diagnostic predictions for the validation data allows the user to assess how well the algorithm will behave on new data.

In contrast to supervised learning, *unsupervised learning* follows much the same process (develop the algorithm on the test data set and then apply to the validation set), but without the initial expert labels. In this case, the algorithm seeks to classify images by common features. Typically, unsupervised machine learning will not have a single goal in mind (e.g., identifying images containing evidence of the anomaly) but rather seeks to identify groups (often multiple groups) of images with common features. These groups of classified images will then be reviewed by subject matter experts to assess the diagnostic utility of the groups, perhaps leading to a subsequent round of supervised learning.

Extending these ideas further, if one includes multiple steps in machine learning (i.e., "learning" from the output of previous machine learning results), one may extend the ideas into the area of *deep learning* [2]. Multiple layers of optimization and evaluation can provide additional levels of precision in classification problems, much the same way that a biopsy and more detailed testing can provide additional specificity in diagnosis following a cancer screening test. Each step refines the previous step.

Discussion: Analytic Toolboxes with Both Types of Approaches

The brief descriptions above sweep many details under the rug but highlight a key difference in goals between the traditional biostatistical and the machine learning approaches to biomedical data analysis. At the risk of oversimplifying, we contrast the motivations of the two data analytic paradigms as follows:

- Statistics begins with describing how the data were collected using probability distributions and then uses the data observed to estimate the defining characteristics (parameters) of those distributions. The distributions define the expected observations (and their variability) under different intervention settings in order to assess differences in outcomes between intervention settings.
- Machine learning begins with large quantities of data and evaluates these data to optimize prediction of patterns within the data. In our examples, we place special emphasis on patterns relating to health outcomes and diagnoses. Importantly, while causal associations are often of interest, by default, patterns found in machine learning predictions need not be causal in nature to be useful for prediction; they are simply based on correlations. For instance, an increase in Internet searches for high school basketball scores is not directly causally related with increased risk of influenza, but both basketball searches and flu cases increase in the fall. While banning basketball may not measurably impact the transmission of influenza, including the temporal pattern of basketball searches may improve our predictions of influenza transmission each year.

Machine learning algorithms power much of current commercially available AI, and there is a large volume of research exploring their application to human healthcare and biomedical research. The first wave of such research often focuses on showing one *can* apply machine learning approaches to high-volume human health data, but interesting and important work on how and whether one *should* apply such approaches is starting to appear. In one example, Vollmer et al. [10] raise a set of critical questions specifically for assessing patient benefits of machine learning and AI research. These fall into six categories, briefly summarized here:

- Study inception (What information/hypotheses motivated the study?)
- Study (How do data related to the question of interest? How are patients involved?)
- Statistical methods (What analytic approaches drive study conclusions?)
- Reproducibility (Are data available to other researchers? If so, in what form?)
- Impact evaluation (How do study results generalize to the full population?)
- Implementation (Is the AI model cost effective for practical use in patient care?)

These and the full list of questions in Vollmer et al. [10] outline a principled discussion of how and where machine learning algorithms can benefit patient-based biomedical research and highlight different decisions in different dimensions of the research cycle.

In addition to these important questions across the patient-based research cycle, it is also important to recognize that while the traditional and emerging analytic paradigms are different [8], they need not be mutually exclusive. In fact, it is important to use tools from biostatistics to assess performance of machine learning, and it is important for biostatistics to adopt some of the concepts, capacity, and capability of machine learning and the emerging data paradigm.

The field of biostatistics can benefit from the possibilities enabled when one considers widely available data of different types, and the field of machine learning can benefit from traditional biostatistical understanding aggregate behavior of diagnostic decisions. To illustrate an example of the later, suppose the outcome of a machine learning algorithm is to identify the presence of a specific cardiac anomaly in biomedical imaging and that we have a very large number of historical images. Machine learning is well-suited to this problem, and once our algorithm is defined, we can input large number of new images and receive a binary (anomaly present/absent) classification for each. As noted above, no diagnostic tool (algorithm or expert) is perfectly accurate. Note that there are two types of correct diagnoses: an image from a patient who has the anomaly can be diagnosed with anomaly present (a *true positive* result), and an image from a patient who is anomaly-free is diagnosed as anomaly-free (a *true negative* result). In biostatistics, the term *sensitivity* denotes the probability of the algorithm diagnosing an anomaly present when the patient indeed has the anomaly, the probability of a true positive result. In biostatistics, the *specificity* denotes the probability of the algorithm diagnosing the absence of the anomaly when, in fact, the patient does not have the anomaly, the probability of a true negative result. Sensitivity (diagnosing presence when the anomaly is indeed present) and specificity (diagnosing absence when the anomaly is indeed not present) are two related but different measures of diagnostic performance from the biostatistical literature on diagnostic testing. Note that there are also two types of mistaken diagnosis: an image from a patient who does indeed have the anomaly can be diagnosed as anomaly-free (a *false-negative* result), and an image from an anomaly-free patient can be diagnosed as having the anomaly (a *false-positive* result).

These definitions contain two sets of related probabilities:

- If sensitivity is high, the probability of a false-negative result is low (these probabilities represent a proportion of the population of *individuals with the anomaly*). In individuals with the anomaly, the algorithm diagnoses one of two options, so the sensitivity and the probability of a false-negative result add to one.
- Similarly, if the specificity is high, the probability of a false positive is low (these probabilities represent proportions of the population of *individuals without the anomaly*). If individuals do not have the anomaly, the algorithm diagnoses one of two options, so the sum of specificity and the probability of a false-positive result is one.

It is important to note sensitivity and specificity are properties of the same diagnostic tests, but they represent proportions of *different groups of patients* and cannot be added or directly compared to each other.

Suppose we have a very large number of images available, and we have a machine learning algorithm with high sensitivity (say, 0.99) and high specificity (say, 0.95). The emerging data paradigm suggests we apply the algorithm to the set of images and collect the diagnoses. However, past biostatistical experience suggests that we may find some confusing results, depending on how common the anomaly is within our large number of images. Let us take a closer look.

For every 100 images from individuals with the anomaly, the sensitivity of 0.99 suggests we will receive, on average, one false-negative result. For every 100 images from individuals without the anomaly, the specificity of 0.95 suggests that we will receive, on average, five false-positive results. Across the 200 images combined, we will observe (on average) 104 positive results (99 true positives + five false-positive results). The *positive predictive value* (the proportion of anomaly diagnoses that are true will be 99/104 = 95.19%, a good value). If we maintain an equal balance of images from individuals with and without the anomaly, we will maintain this same high value of the positive predictive value. (To see this, note that the same result happens if we have 100,000 images with the anomaly and 100,000 without and the same with 100,000,000 images in each category.)

However, suppose the anomaly is rare in our set of images, say, only one image has the anomaly out of every ten images without the anomaly. In this case, we say the *prevalence* of the anomaly is 1/10. If we apply the algorithm to 100 images with the anomaly, we will again, on average, receive 99 true positive results and one false-negative result. The prevalence of 1/10 means that for our 100 images with the anomaly, we apply the algorithm to 1000 images without the anomaly. Based on the specificity of 0.95, we will, again, diagnose (on average) 5% of these images as false positives. Five percent of 1000 images corresponds to 50 false-positive diagnoses. In case where prevalence of the anomaly in our total set of images is 1/10, we observe, on average, 149 positive results (99 true positives and 50 false positives). In this case, the positive predictive value is 99/149 = 66.44%, a considerable reduction from the positive predictive value when half of our images were from patients with the anomaly.

If we continue to test 100 images that truly contain the anomaly but test more and more images without the anomaly (i.e., we further reduce the prevalence of images with the anomaly within the set of all images tested), we note that even though the *proportion* of false-positive diagnoses stays constant with a specificity of 95%, the *number* of false-positive results increases with decreasing prevalence, for instance:

- With 10,000 anomaly-free images, we expect 500 false-positive diagnoses.
- With 100,000 anomaly-free images, we expect 5000 false-positive diagnoses.
- With 1,000,000 anomaly-free images, we expect 50,000 false-positive diagnoses.

If we only have 100 images with anomalies in each case, we see we will soon have more false-positive diagnoses than true positive diagnoses.

This association between prevalence and positive predictive value is well-known in biostatistics and is often used to motivate the use of Bayes' theorem to link the concepts of sensitivity, specificity, prevalence, and positive predictive value. Despite its familiarity, the associations can be confusing, and multiple press reports relating to the performance of mass testing for COVID19 often expressed exasperation that a diagnostic test with high sensitivity and specificity could have such low positive predictive value [12]. The machine learning community rediscovered the association and refers to it a problem of *unbalanced design* [9]. However, sometimes, the situation is viewed as a signal to revise the algorithm with improved weights rather than recognizing that the problem is, in a sense, baked into diagnostic systems. Rather than adjusting a single algorithm, providing multiple layers of diagnoses and testing, similar to follow-up clinical testing following a screening diagnosis, offers more control of the positive predictive value and is, roughly speaking, the basis of the deep learning approaches mentioned above.

The diagnostic testing example illustrates that even in a relatively straightforward setting, both machine learning and biostatistics have much to learn from each other. A traditional data approach of only analyzing images collected in the current study would miss the opportunity to gain information from the full set of available images, while a machine-learning-only approach applied to all available images could result in very poor positive predictive performance of an automated diagnostic procedure potentially resulting in unnecessary treatment for patients.

Conclusion

In conclusion, we note that we are working in a transitional time. Amounts of and access to data are changing rapidly, and our analytic tools should both adapt to new settings and take advantage of lessons learned in the past. The evolution of data science in the biomedical research arena requires expertise from both analytic paradigms in order to gain advantage of today's data resources. The data analysis toolbox is not static, nor is it complete, and the savvy investigator will work closely with data scientists, statisticians, computer scientists, and mathematicians in order to gain the most information from the available data and minimize chances for erroneous conclusions.

In an interview with a *Saturday Evening Post* writer, bank robber Willie Sutton famously answered the question "Why do you rob banks?" with "Because that's where the money is" [14]. The data analytic parallel is our recommendation advocating the informed use of all tools available in data analysis. This allows us to answer the question "Why do you analyze data?" "Because that's where the information is."

References

1. Amrhein V, Greenland S, McShane B. Scientists rise up against statistical significance. Nature. 2019;567:305–7.
2. Baraniuk R, Donoho D, Gavish M. The science of deep learning. Proc Natl Acad Sci USA. 2020;117:30029–32. https://doi.org/10.1073/pnas.2020596117.
3. Barker ED, Roberts S, Walton E. Hidden hypotheses in 'hypothesis-free' genome-wide epigenetic associations. Curr Opin Psychol. 2019;27:13–7.
4. Breiman L. Statistical modeling: two cultures. Stat Sci. 2001;16:199–215.
5. Burkov A. The hundred-page machine learning book. Andriy Burkov. 2019.
6. Donoho D. 50 years of data science. J Comput Graph Stat. 2017;26:745–66.
7. Head ML, Holman L, Lanfear R, Kahn AT, Jennions MD. The extent and consequences of p-hacking in science. PLoS Biol. 2015;13(3):e1002106. https://doi.org/10.1371/journal.pbio.1002106.
8. Li JJ, Tong X. Statistical hypothesis testing versus machine learning binary classification: distinctions and guidelines. Patterns. 2020;1:100115.
9. Shane J. You look like a thing and i love you: how artificial intelligence works and why it's making the world a Weirder place. New York: Little, Brown, and Company; 2019.
10. Vollmer S, Mateen BA, Bohner G, Kiràly FJ, Ghani R, Jonsson P, Cumbers S, Jonas A, McAllister KSL, Myles P, Grainger D, Birse M, Branson R, Moons KGM, Collins GS, Ioannidis JPA, Holmes C, Hemingway H. Machine learning and artificial intelligence research for patient benefit: 20 critical questions on transparency, replicability, ethics, and effectiveness. Br Med J. 2020;368:169297. https://doi.org/10.1136/bmj.16927.
11. Waller LA, Miller GW. More than manuscripts: reproducibility, rigor, and research productivity in the big data era. Toxicol Sci. 2016;149:275–6. https://doi.org/10.1093/toxsci/kfv330.
12. Waller L, Levi T. Building intuition regarding the statistical behavior of mass medical testing programs. Harvard Data Science Review; 2021. Retrieved from https://hdsr.mitpress.mit.edu/pub/hodep31o.
13. Wilkinson MD, Dumontier M, Aalbersberg IJ, Appelton G, Azton M, Baak A, Blomberg N, Boiten J-W, da Silva Santos LB, Bourne PE, Bouwman J, Brookes AJ, Clark T, Crosas M, Dillo I, Dumon O, Edmunds S, Evelo CT, Finkers R, Gonzalez-Beltran A, Gray AJG, Groth P, Goble C, Grethe JS, Heringa J, Hoen PAC, Hooft R, Kuhn T, Kok R, Kok J, Lusher SJ, Martone ME, Mons A, Packer AL, Persson B, Rocca-Serra P, Roose M, van Schaik R, Sansone S-A, Schultes E, Sengstag T, Slater T, Strawn G, Swertz MA, Thompson M, van der Lei J, van Mulligen E, Velterop J, Waagmeester A, Wittenberg P, Wolstencroft K, Zhao J, Mons B. The FAIR guiding principles for scientific data management and stewardship. Sci Data. 2016;3:160018. https://doi.org/10.1038/sdata.2016.18.
14. Yoder RM. Someday they'll get slick Willie Sutton. The Saturday Evening Post. 1951;223(30). Saturday Evening Post Society, Indianapolis.

Part II

Artificial Intelligence: General Approaches and Applications

Structured Reporting in Medical Imaging: The Role of Artificial Intelligence

10

Peter D. Filev and Arthur E. Stillman

Definition and Benefits of Structured Reporting

A major strategy for improving the value of radiology services has been innovation of radiology reporting. The radiology report is a critical component of any imaging procedure. Its most important purpose is to communicate diagnostic information to the referring physicians. This should be done using clear and unambiguous language [1]. Historically, radiology reports consisted of freestyle text in prose format. The use of nonstandard terminology often caused ambiguity and inaccurate interpretation [2]. Over the past decade, structured reporting has emerged as a strategy to improve the clarity and effectiveness of radiology reports. The first section of this chapter will provide a general introduction to structured reporting and discuss its major benefits. Following sections will examine specific applications within cardiothoracic imaging. Lastly, there will be a focus on the integration of structured reporting with artificial intelligence.

Structured reporting refers to the utilization of predefined templates and formats to generate an imaging report [1]. There are three fundamental levels of structured reporting. The first and most basic consists of a structured format of paragraphs with subheadings. Separate sections are assigned to describe the examination protocol, clinical history, radiology findings, and overall impression. The second level requires a more consistent organization of the report, such as based on relevant anatomic regions. For example, the body of a chest CT report would have separate sections dedicated to describing the mediastinum, lungs and pleura, and bones and soft tissues. The third level adds an additional layer of sophistication, which is the required use of a standardized lexicon. A common lexicon enables more unambiguous interpretation of reporting terminology. A notable example of this is RadLex, which was developed and distributed by the Radiological Society of North America (RSNA) with the support of more than 30 specialty societies [1]. RadLex is a machine-accessible controlled terminology that consists of a comprehensive list of terms and relationships used to describe imaging. It also provides a standard nomenclature for naming of imaging procedures [3]. RadLex evolved into an ontological system that bridged the gap between several previously developed radiologic lexicons. A comprehensive controlled terminology such as RadLex allows for computer applications to recognize multiple synonymous terms referring to the same entity. This enhances structured reporting to facilitate data mining and query. This also gives developers capabilities to create diversity of applications such as radiology-coded teaching files and decision support [4].

The RSNA has developed an online library (www.radreport.org) containing more than 270 report templates. The templates are indexed by RadLex vocabulary terms [5]. Users can search for a specific template by keyword, specialty, or participating organization. Some of the templates in the RSNA library allow capture of coded and/or quantitative information that can then facilitate the incorporation of guideline-based recommendations directly into the report. Additionally, captured data can be seamlessly sent into patient registries [5].

Structured reporting can bring multiple benefits to radiologists, referring providers, and ultimately patients. Perhaps the most important of these is improvement in overall report quality that is manifest in several ways. First, a structured template can function as a "checklist" to ensure that the critical elements of a particular examination have been addressed in the report [6]. This ensures that clinically significant information is not omitted. Second, structured reporting can significantly decrease the number of textual errors and diagnostic discrepancies in radiology reports [7]. Third, structured reporting allows for easier comparison with prior reports that in many cases are composed by different radiologists and sometimes are even performed at different institutions.

P. D. Filev, MD (✉) · A. E. Stillman, MD, PhD
Department of Radiology and Imaging Sciences, Emory University School of Medicine, Atlanta, GA, USA
e-mail: peter.dimitrov.filev@emory.edu; aestill@emory.edu

C. N. De Cecco et al. (eds.), *Artificial Intelligence in Cardiothoracic Imaging*, Contemporary Medical Imaging,
https://doi.org/10.1007/978-3-030-92087-6_10

Lastly, structured reporting improves overall quality by facilitating adherence to consensus guidelines. For example, guidelines for a low-dose lung cancer screening program mandate that results are reported using a structured reporting system, such as ACR Lung-RADS. This allows for direct communication of pertinent findings and provides clear management recommendation based on risk of malignancy [8]. Ultimately, this minimizes variation in pulmonary nodule management strategies and can improve patient outcomes.

Structured reporting also helps ensure appropriate coding and reimbursement for radiology reports. Many radiologists are not completely aware of the complex processes that are required to generate appropriate claims and reimbursement. Traditional free-text radiology reports can omit pertinent billing information and lead to inaccurate coding. This may require that a different and more limited code, usually associated with lower reimbursement, is assigned to the imaging study. In the end, this can contribute to the current trend of declining reimbursement for imaging services [9]. Structured reporting addresses this problem by facilitating a standardized and complete report that ensures appropriate reimbursement [9].

Structured Reporting in Cardiothoracic Imaging

In the following sections, we will review several of the most significant structured reporting systems used in cardiothoracic imaging. These include Lung Reporting and Data System (Lung-RADS), Coronary Artery Disease Reporting and Data System (CAD-RADS), Thyroid Imaging Reporting and Data System (TI-RADS), Interstitial Lung Disease Reporting and Data System (ILD-RADS), and COVID-19 Reporting and Data System (CO-RADS). These systems are loosely modeled after the Breast Imaging Reporting and Data System (BI-RADS) used in mammography. The central aim is to standardize reporting and recommendations for management of abnormal imaging findings.

Lung-RADS

CT lung cancer screening can reduce lung-cancer-specific mortality as was demonstrated by the National Lung Screening Trial (NLST) [10]. Based on the results of this trial, the US Preventive Services Task Force recommended low-dose CT (LDCT) lung cancer screening for high risk patients with significant smoking history. However, a major concern associated with such screening was a high false-positive rate of detected pulmonary nodules. An additional initial concern was the lack of a standardized reporting system [11]. As a response, the ACR developed a standardized reporting system called Lung-RADS (Reporting and Data System), which is in many ways analogous to the use of Breast Imaging Reporting and Data System (BI-RADS) for mammography.

The major function of Lung-RADS is to clearly define a positive lung cancer screening result and to describe the appropriate management recommendations based on the degree of risk. The classification system consists of seven categories (0, 1, 2, 3, 4A, 4B, and 4X) (Table 10.1) [12]. Cases assigned to Lung-RADS 1 are considered "negative" with less than 1% chance of malignancy. At the opposite end of the spectrum, those in Category 4B and Category 4X are considered "suspicious" with greater than 15% chance of malignancy. Each of these categories is coupled with an associated management recommendation, which may range from "return to annual LDCT screening" (Category 1) to "PET-CT and/or tissue sampling" for Category 4B and Category 4X [11].

Lung-RADS was successful in decreasing the false-positive rate of NLST. The size threshold for a positive pulmonary nodule seen on screening increased from a transverse diameter of 4 mm to 6 mm [11]. Pinsky et al. performed a retrospective study in which they applied the Lung-RADS criteria to 26,722 LDCT participants. They found that at baseline screening, the false-positive rate of 12.8% with Lung-RADS was significantly lower compared to 26.6% that was observed in NLST [13]. Similarly, after baseline, Lung-RADS achieved a lower false-positive rate compared to NLST, 5.3% versus 21.8%. As expected, the sensitivity decreased when Lung-RADS was applied, from 93.5% to 84.9% at baseline and from 93.8% to 78.6% after baseline [13].

Similar overall findings were made in a different retrospective study of 2180 high-risk patients who had undergone

Table 10.1 The ACR Lung-RADS assessment categories [12]

Category descriptor	Lung-RADS score	Management
Incomplete	0	Additional screening CT images and/or comparison to prior chest CT are needed
Negative	1	Continue annual screening with LDCT in 12 months
Benign appearance or behavior	2	Continue annual screening with LDCT in 12 months
Probably benign	3	6 months LDCT
Suspicious	4A	3 months LDCT or PET/CT when nodule >8 mm
Very suspicious	4B/4X	CT versus PET/CT and/or tissue sampling
Other	S	As appropriate to the specific clinical findings

LDCT lung cancer screening. The application of Lung-RADS resulted in a reduction of the false-positive rate from 27.6% to 10.6% [14]. Also notably, no false negatives were found among the 152 patients with 12-month follow-up, which were reclassified as benign by Lung-RADS. Lastly, Lung-RADS increased the positive predictive value for diagnosis of lung cancer from 6.9% to 17.3% [14]. These studies seemed to confirm the low likelihood of malignancy in pulmonary nodules measuring from 4 to 6 mm in diameter. Reporting with Lung-RADS can result in less interval scans for monitoring such low-risk nodules and increase the cost-effectiveness of CT lung cancer screening [14]. Over the past several years, the field of radiomics has gained momentum as it applies to lung cancer screening. The extraction of quantitative and subvisual image features from a large database of pulmonary nodules has allowed for the development of models that can be used to predict malignancy. Mao et al. developed a predictive model for assessing solitary pulmonary nodules by extracting 385 quantitative radiomic features, from a training set of 156 benign and 40 malignant nodules [15]. Their model for malignancy differentiation achieved a sensitivity of 81% and a specificity of 92%, which were high than those of ACR Lung-RADS [15]. While this study was limited to small solitary pulmonary nodules, it highlights the interest in comparing the performance of radiomic predictive models to ACR Lung-RADS.

Ti-RADS

Indeterminate thyroid nodules are an extremely prevalent finding on cross-sectional imaging. For example, about 50% of women older than 70 are expected to have at least one thyroid nodule [16]. Similar to small pulmonary nodules, the vast majority of thyroid nodules are benign [17]. The ACR Thyroids Imaging Reporting and Data System (TI-RADS) was developed to provide an easy method for radiologist to determine the appropriate management for such nodules. In brief, the TI-RADS score is based on the evaluation of US features in five categories: composition, echogenicity, shape, margin, and echogenic foci [17]. Features within these categories are assigned a score ranging from 0 to 3 points. The overall point total determines the risk level that ranges from TR1 (benign) to TR5 (highly suspicious) [17, 18] (Table 10.2). Again, similar to the Lung-RADS, the assigned risk category is used to guide the management recommendation. For cases assigned to TR1 and TR2, no additional follow-up or fine needle aspiration (FNA) is indicated. Nodules falling in the TR3–TR5 categories may require invasive sampling, depending on their size. One of the ACR's goals was to increase the threshold of "moderately suspicious" nodules (TR3 and TR4), which would decrease the number of unnecessary biopsies of benign thyroid nodules [17]. The ACR was aware that this may, however, also potentially result in fewer biopsies of malignant nodules. To compensate, additional recommendations were put in place for follow-up of suspicious nodules (TR3–TR5) that do not meet a size criteria for FNA [17].

Table 10.2 ACR TI-RADS assessment categories [18]

Category descriptor	Points	TI-RADS category	Management
Benign	0	TR1	No FNA
Not suspicious	2	TR2	No FNA
Mildly suspicious	3	TR3	FNA if >2.5 cm; follow if >1.5 cm
Moderately suspicious	4–6	TR4	FNA if >1.5 cm; follow if >1 cm
Highly suspicious	7 or more	TR5	FNA if >1 cm; follow if >0.5 cm

ACR TI-RADS was only recently developed in 2017; however, it has already been validated by several studies. Middleton et al. observed a total of 3422 thyroid nodules, 352 of which were proven to be malignant by cytology. Their risk for malignancy was also retrospectively assessed using TI-RADS by radiologists blinded to the cytologic analysis. The study found that more than 85% of the studied nodules were within 1% of their corresponding TI-RADS risk thresholds [19]. The rising incidence of thyroid nodules requires for an accurate and organized risk stratification methodology that also minimizes overdiagnosis and unnecessary invasive procedures. TI-RADS helps accomplish this through a standardized assessment of thyroid nodules leading to appropriate management recommendations. Artificial intelligence may play an important role in optimizing the TI-RADS scoring system such that its specificity is improved. Wildman-Tobriner et al. recently developed a genetic algorithm trained on a data set of 1325 thyroid nodules that had already been assigned a TI-RADS score [20]. The TI-RADS score combined with the pathologic data (benign or malignant) for each training nodule was used to create a more optimized scoring system, AI TI-RADS [20]. The diagnostic performance of AI TI-RADS was then compared to that of ACR TI-RADS on a test set of 100 thyroid nodules. AI TI-RADS was able to achieve similar sensitivity while achieving a significantly improved specificity [20].

ILD-RADS

Many radiologists, particularly those not subspecialty trained in thoracic imaging, often find cases of interstitial lung disease (ILD) challenging. It is, however, of utmost importance to accurately distinguish certain diagnoses, such as usual interstitial pneumonia (UIP), from other fibrotic lung disease. A confident recognition of a UIP pattern of fibrosis on CT can be used to diagnose idiopathic pulmonary fibrosis (IPF), which has a significantly worse prognosis compared to many other ILDs [21]. This can in turn obviate the need for surgical lung biopsies. Incorrect or nonspecific diagnoses are also undesirable. For example, misclassification of a case of hypersensitivity pneumonitis as UIP/IPF can have significant prognostic and therapeutic implications [21]. The main goal of ILD-RADS, introduced in 2019, is to elucidate the distinction between a UIP and non-UIP diagnosis as much as possible. It consists of a standardized reporting template based on an established algorithm used for diagnosis of ILD. The template requires the reporting of a number of specific imaging features such as traction bronchiectasis, honeycombing, mosaic attenuation, reticulation, and zonal and axial distribution of fibrosis. The combination of features selected in the template guides the radiologist to choose one of five ILD-RADS categories. These range from ILD-RADS 1 (typical UIP pattern) to ILD-RADS 4 (CT features most consistent with non-IPF diagnosis). ILD-RADS 0 corresponds to an incomplete or nondiagnostic exam [21]. Following its recent introduction, the template was piloted at a single academic institution over a period of 8 weeks. Feedback was obtained from the radiologists who used the template as well as from referring pulmonologists [21]. Surveyed pulmonologists saw ILD-RADS as a significant improvement over previous reporting methodology, which they often found inconsistent. Similarly, radiologists found that ILD-RADS improved compliance with established ILD CT reporting guidelines [21]. Structured reporting, as applied to ILD, can decrease potential variability in reporting and improve the likelihood of arriving at a specific diagnosis. Furthermore, such a system can help familiarize general radiologists and radiology trainees in the appropriate High resolution computed tomography (HRCT) reporting of ILD. There are currently many initiatives to develop AI algorithms that can provide accurate automated classification of fibrotic lung disease and can be used in conjunction with ILD-RADS structured reporting.

CAD-RADS

A standardized reporting system for patients undergoing coronary computed tomography angiography (CTA) was introduced in 2016 by an expert multidisciplinary consensus involving both major radiology and cardiology societies [22]. The main purpose of CAD-RADS (Coronary Artery Disease Reporting and Data System) is to provide a consistent structure for reporting the final assessment of the coronary CTA and help guide selection of the appropriate management. The reporting system requires the selection among one of seven CAD-RADS categories that are based on the degree of coronary artery stenosis (Table 10.3). For example, CAD-RADS 0 corresponds to no stenosis, and CAD-RADS 1 corresponds to 1–24% stenosis. At the other end of the spectrum, CAD-RADS 4 consists of severe stenosis (>70% or > 50% in the left main), while CAD-RADS 5 is reserved for total occlusion [22]. As would be expected, to each of these categories is assigned a clear recommendation for further management. The recommendations range from "no further evaluation" (for CAD-RADS 0) to "expedited invasive coronary angiography" (CAD-RADS 5 acute setting). To address potential reporting pitfalls, several modifiers are available to complement the CAD-RADS categories. Two key modifiers are "N" (e.g., CAD-RADS 3 N) and "V" (e.g., CAD-RADS 3 V), which respectively indicate a nondiagnostic study and the presence of a vulnerable high-risk plaque [22]. A single-center prospective study of 287 patients reported sensitivity, specificity, and accuracy ranging between 96.8% and 100% for CAD-RADS for prediction of significant CAD. Additionally, CAD-RADS was described as "quite helpful" or "completely helpful" for clinical decision-making by 87% of referring providers in the same study [23]. CAD-RADS should eliminate reporting ambiguity, improve communication between interpreting and referring physicians, and streamline recommendation for further management. Recently, work has been done to investigate the application of machine learning for automated assessment of coronary CT angiography (CCTA) based on CAD-RADS. Muscogiuri et al. developed and evaluated a deep convolutional neural network (CNN) that classified CCTA studies in the appropri-

Table 10.3 CAD-RADS assessment categories [22]

Degree of maximal coronary stenosis	CAD-RADS category	Interpretation	Further cardiac investigation
0%	0	Documented absence of CAD	None
1–24%	1	Minimal non-obstructive CAD	None
25–49%	2	Mild non-obstructive CAD	None
50–69%	3	Moderate stenosis	Consider functional assessment
70–99%	4A	Severe stenosis	Consider ICA[a] or functional assessment
Left main >50% or 3 vessel obstructive >70% disease	4B	Severe stenosis	ICA is recommended
100% (total occlusion)	5	Total coronary occlusion	Consider ICA and/or viability assessment
Nondiagnostic study	N	Obstructive CAD cannot be excluded	Additional or alternative evaluation

[a]*ICA* invasive coronary angiography

ate CAD-RADS category [24]. The study included 288 patients undergoing clinically indicated CCTA. The developed CNN was tested on this dataset, and the results were compared to the reference on site readings by experienced cardiac imagers. Diagnostic accuracies ranging from 60% to 86% were achieved by the CNN. The authors were able to demonstrate that an AI algorithm can reliably differentiate between CAD-RADS 0 and CAD-RADS >0 [24].

COVID-19

By March of 2020, COVID-19, the disease caused by SARS-CoV-2, was spreading rapidly throughout the community and had reached a pandemic stage. Most major radiology societies do not recommend the use of CT to screen for the disease; however, regardless, a very high number of persons under investigation (PUI) undergo CT for various reasons. The CT imaging features of COVID-19, resembling a pattern of organizing acute lung injury, can in many situations distinguish it from certain other pneumonias. However, nearly identical imaging features are also commonly encountered in other disease process such as inhalational exposures, acute exacerbations of ILD, drug toxicities, or other infections [25]. This overlap makes CT interpretation challenging; however, an accurate diagnosis is paramount, given the significant morbidity and mortality associated with COVID-19. For this reason, shortly after the outbreak of the pandemic, a structured reporting system for CT reporting of COVID-19 was devised by an expert panel. Four major categories for COVID-19 imaging classifications are offered to describe the imaging findings. The categories include "typical appearance," "indeterminate appearance," "atypical appearance," and "negative for pneumonia" [25]. Each of these categories is accompanied by a suggested structured reporting lexicon. A listing of the associated CT findings for each category is also included in the template to help guide the radiologist. Unlike other described structured systems, this one does not offer an exact likelihood of pneumonia for each category, as this is thought to also be dependent on additional factors such as prevalence in the community, degree of exposure, and other risk factors [25]. The aim of this reporting system is to reduce variability and uncertainty in reporting findings and improve subsequent clinical decision-making [25]. In April 2020, a categorical system was introduced to assess suspicion of lung involvement by COVID-19 on chest CT. The COVID-19 Reporting and Data System (CO-RADS) differs in that it was designed for patients presenting with moderate to severe symptoms of COVID-19. It offers five categories [1–5], each indicating increasing suspicion for pulmonary involvement (Table 10.4) [26]. CO-RADS 1 corresponds to "very low" level of suspicion, while CO-RADS 5 and 6 correspond to "very high" suspicion and "proven"

Table 10.4 CO-RADS assessment categories [26]

CO-RADS category	Level of suspicion for pulmonary involvement of COVID-19	Summary
0	Not interpretable	Scan technically insufficient
1	Very low	Normal or noninfectious
2	Low	Typical for other infection but not COVID-19
3	Equivocal/unsure	Features compatible with COVID-19 but also other diseases
4	High	Suspicious for COVID-19
5	Very high	Typical for COVID-19
6	Proven	RT-PCR positive for SARS-CoV-2

COVID-19, respectively. The system was then evaluated on 105 chest CTs of patients who had presented with COVID-19 like symptoms and who had also received the RT-PCR test [26]. The scans were read by eight observers using CO-RADS. The study demonstrated that CO-RADS had high discriminatory power for RT-PCR results (mean area under the ROC curve of 0.91) [26]. To date, multiple AI-based systems have been developed since the onset of the epidemic, which differentiate COVID-19 pneumonia from other causes of pneumonia on chest CT. COVNet is one such deep learning model that is trained on a data set of 4356 chest CTs achieving a remarkable sensitivity and specificity of 90% and 96% for differentiation of COVID-19 from other community-acquired pneumonias [27]. There also, however, significant limitations associated with such models, and they have yet to be implemented in clinical practice.

Integration of Artificial Intelligence with Structured Reporting

Data Mining

In parallel to the paradigm shift toward structured reporting, there has been tremendous advancement in the application of artificial intelligence in medical imaging. Machine learning algorithms are developed and fine-tuned using multiple train-test iterations. This requires an enormous amount of training data. Seemingly, prior radiology reports can serve as a large reservoir from which such data can be mined. However, data mining from unstructured reports can be challenging [28]. This can be further examined by reviewing a simplified model of the development of a machine learning algorithm (Fig. 10.1). In this example, a hypothetical classification algorithm is trained to distinguish between images of usual interstitial pneumonia (UIP) and sarcoidosis. A

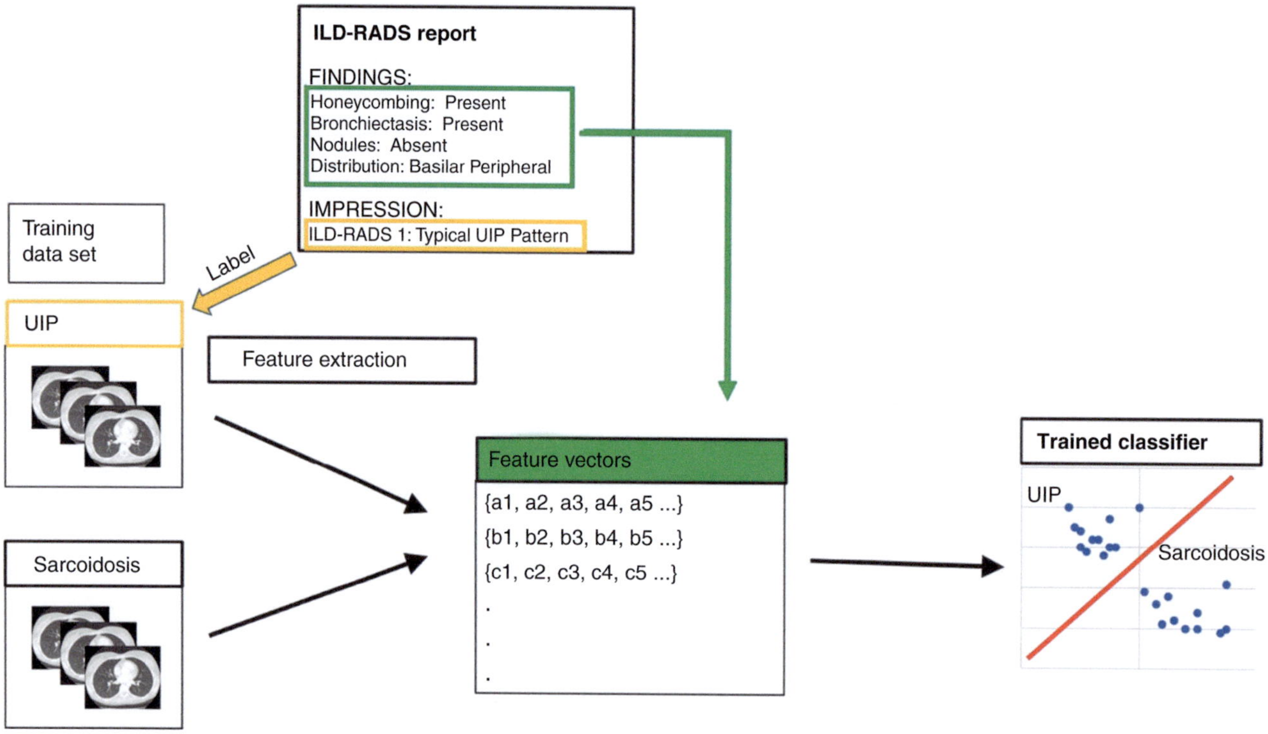

Fig. 10.1 Schematic illustrating training of a hypothetical AI algorithm. The function of this algorithm is to distinguish between CT images of UIP and sarcoidosis. An ILD-RADS report is structured such that the diagnosis (orange) is clearly defined, allowing for easy labeling of training images. Also, the presence or absence of important features (features) useful for training is systematically included in the report

large set of input images (training set) is required. First, it is imperative that the training images contain an appropriate set of features. More specifically, these features (i.e., "bronchiectasis," "honeycombing," "nodules") should be representative of the different disease classes, such that the AI system can learn to distinguish between them. Second, each training case must be accurately and unambiguously labeled as belonging to one of the diagnostic classes (in this case, either UIP or sarcoidosis). The importance of accurate and clear labeling cannot be understated. It serves as the "ground truth" for training, and errors in labeling would inherently result in training a faulty classifier. Moreover, ambiguous labels such as "nonspecific fibrosis, possibly UIP versus sarcoidosis" also offer little value to training the algorithm.

Such an example brings to light the clear advantages that structured reporting offers for AI data mining when compared to non-structured reports. In a structured reporting system, such as ILD-RADS, the presence or absence of critical imaging features is indicated in a clear binary way. This remarkably streamlines the process of collecting an appropriate set of training images containing suitable features. Additionally, ILD-RADS requires that each case be assigned a final ILD-RADS categorical diagnosis (i.e., ILD-RADS 1 – typical UIP). This serves as an unambiguous label, shall that case be selected for training.

Unfortunately, however, the vast majority of radiology reports are unstructured and consist of narrative text. Critical data elements are scattered haphazardly throughout the report. Data mining for thousands of accurately labeled cases containing the right set of features from a trove of such reports can be a laborious endeavor. This can put excessive strain on workflow and result in delays. Structured reporting is clearly a superior platform for future development of AI in medical imaging.

Enhancing Workflow

A structured reporting system is also easier to assimilate with already developed highly practical AI algorithms. This can be further examined through the lens of cardiac MRI reporting. There are currently very effective deep learning algorithms that provide accurate automatic segmentation of the cardiac chambers at the click of a mouse button. This in turn allows for very fast computation of a multitude of important clinical parameters such as cardiac chamber diameters, volumes, and ejection fraction. This already saves significant time compared to the traditional method of manually segmenting the ventricles. However, structured reporting also offers significant incremental value in this setting. The body of a typical structured cardiac MRI report includes a section of standardized fields where each of these measurements is to be reported. The AI algorithm can thus be synched to auto-populate these data elements. This eliminates the need to individually dictate each measurement into the report, saving significant time. Similarly, AI postprocessing can be applied to the assessment of late gadolinium enhancement. AI systems, when integrated with a structured template, can produce an auto-populated section of the report describing LGE by the standardized 17-segment model. This concept is of course easily expanded to other modalities such as CT. For example, CT calcium scores can be automatically entered into a structured report in their assigned data fields, eliminating the need for dictation.

Clinical Decision Support

With the continued shift of healthcare, there is increased demand for value-for-care. Clinical decision support (CDS) is a software designed to help doctors decide on the most appropriate management that is aligned with this paradigm. The main value of CDS for radiologists is in helping to provide the appropriate guidance through their reporting. More specifically, the ACR has sponsored the development of a computer-assisted reporting and decision support (CAR/DS) framework intended to be embedded with the reporting environment [29]. CAR/DS again highlights the importance of integrating AI with structured reporting. In a classic CAR/DS system, the radiologist inputs data elements into a structured report. For example, in a report for lung cancer screening, the radiologist would fill in the data elements for nodule size, nodule location, and nodule type (i.e., solid versus ground glass). The next level in evolution of CAR/DS is a hybrid CDS and AI system. In such a system, the report software would take a combination of input from the AI algorithm and from the radiologist. For example, an automatic AI nodule detector can locate and measure the pulmonary nodules; however, the radiologist may be required to assess the radiodensity of the nodules. The most advanced system would be full CDS-AI integration. In such a system, all data elements of a report would be filled out automatically using the AI input. The radiologist would be required to review the report prior to signing it [29]. Furthermore, with its continuing evolution, AI can be used to significantly improve CDS as it applies to clinical imaging.

Summary

Structured reporting offers many important benefits that are in keeping with the current trend toward value-based healthcare. Various studies have shown that structured reporting systems improve the overall quality of radiology reports. There is a decrease in report ambiguity, which improves communication between radiologists and referring providers. Additionally, structured reporting facilitates an adherence to consensus guidelines in both classification of important findings and providing appropriate management recommendations. Specifically, within cardiothoracic imaging, several impactful structured reporting data systems have been introduced such as Lung-RADS, TI-RADS, CAD-RADS, ILD-RADS, and CO-RADS. The design of these systems allows for integration of AI algorithms, such as automatic lung nodule detectors, to auto-populate the appropriate data elements within the structured reports. Furthermore, structured reporting serves as a platform for development of new AI systems. Structured reporting systems can provide clearly labeled data as inputs for further training of AI algorithms. Lastly, clinical decision support (CDS) tools have taken an important role in the drive to improve quality and affordability of healthcare. The combination of structured reporting with ever-evolving AI algorithms can be expected to generate powerful CDS tools. Structured reporting is an invaluable platform for the emerging integration of AI in medical imaging.

References

1. Kahn CE Jr, Langlotz CP, Burnside ES, Carrino JA, Channin DS, Hovsepian DM, et al. Toward best practices in radiology reporting. Radiology. 2009;252(3):852–6.
2. Goldberg-Stein S, Chernyak V. Adding value in radiology reporting. J Am Coll Radiol. 2019;16(9 Pt B):1292–8.
3. Langlotz CP. RadLex: a new method for indexing online educational materials. Radiographics. 2006;26(6):1595–7.
4. Rubin DL. Creating and curating a terminology for radiology: ontology modeling and analysis. J Digit Imaging. 2008;21(4):355–62.
5. Morgan TA, Helibrun ME, Kahn CE Jr. Reporting initiative of the Radiological Society of North America: progress and new directions. Radiology. 2014;273(3):642–5.
6. European Society of R. ESR paper on structured reporting in radiology. Insights Imaging. 2018;9(1):1–7.
7. Rosskopf AB, Dietrich TJ, Hirschmann A, Buck FM, Sutter R, Pfirrmann CW. Quality management in musculoskeletal imaging: form, content, and diagnosis of knee MRI reports and effectiveness of three different quality improvement measures. AJR Am J Roentgenol. 2015;204(5):1069–74.
8. Mazzone P, Powell CA, Arenberg D, Bach P, Detterbeck F, Gould MK, et al. Components necessary for high-quality lung cancer screening: American College of Chest Physicians and American Thoracic Society Policy Statement. Chest. 2015;147(2):295–303.
9. Pysarenko K, Recht M, Kim D. Structured reporting: a tool to improve reimbursement. J Am Coll Radiol. 2017;14(5):662–4.
10. National Lung Screening Trial Research T, Aberle DR, Adams AM, Berg CD, Black WC, Clapp JD, et al. Reduced lung-cancer mortality with low-dose computed tomographic screening. N Engl J Med. 2011;365(5):395–409.
11. Mehta HJ, Mohammed TL, Jantz MA. The American College of Radiology lung imaging reporting and data system: potential drawbacks and need for revision. Chest. 2017;151(3):539–43.

12. Lung CT. Screening Reporting & Data System (Lung-RADS). 2019. Available from: https://www.acr.org/-/media/ACR/Files/RADS/Lung-RADS/LungRADSAssessmentCategoriesv1-1.pdf.
13. Pinsky PF, Gierada DS, Black W, Munden R, Nath H, Aberle D, et al. Performance of lung-RADS in the National Lung Screening Trial: a retrospective assessment. Ann Intern Med. 2015;162(7):485–91.
14. McKee BJ, Regis SM, McKee AB, Flacke S, Wald C. Performance of ACR lung-RADS in a clinical CT lung screening program. J Am Coll Radiol. 2015;12(3):273–6.
15. Mao L, Chen H, Liang M, Li K, Gao J, Qin P, et al. Quantitative radiomic model for predicting malignancy of small solid pulmonary nodules detected by low-dose CT screening. Quant Imaging Med Surg. 2019;9(2):263–72.
16. Tappouni RR, Itri JN, McQueen TS, Lalwani N, Ou JJ. ACR TI-RADS: pitfalls, solutions, and future directions. Radiographics. 2019;39(7):2040–52.
17. Tessler FN, Middleton WD, Grant EG. Thyroid imaging reporting and data system (TI-RADS): a user's guide. Radiology. 2018;287(3):1082.
18. ACR. Thyroid Imaging Reporting & Data System (TI-RADS). 2017. Available from: https://www.acr.org/-/media/ACR/Files/RADS/TI-RADS/TI-RADS-chart.pdf?la=en.
19. Middleton WD, Teefey SA, Reading CC, Langer JE, Beland MD, Szabunio MM, et al. Multiinstitutional analysis of thyroid nodule risk stratification using the American College of Radiology Thyroid Imaging Reporting and Data System. AJR Am J Roentgenol. 2017;208(6):1331–41.
20. Wildman-Tobriner B, Buda M, Hoang JK, Middleton WD, Thayer D, Short RG, et al. Using artificial intelligence to revise ACR TI-RADS risk stratification of thyroid nodules: diagnostic accuracy and utility. Radiology. 2019;292(1):112–9.
21. Berkowitz EA, Bernheim A, Little BP. Introducing ILD-RADS: a pilot study of an interstitial Lung disease standardized reporting template. J Am Coll Radiol. 2019;16(9 Pt A):1169–72.
22. Cury RC, Abbara S, Achenbach S, Agatston A, Berman DS, Budoff MJ, et al. Coronary artery disease - reporting and data system (CAD-RADS): an expert consensus document of SCCT, ACR and NASCI: endorsed by the ACC. JACC Cardiovasc Imaging. 2016;9(9):1099–113.
23. Basha MAA, Aly SA, Ismail AAA, Bahaaeldin HA, Shehata SM. The validity and applicability of CAD-RADS in the management of patients with coronary artery disease. Insights Imaging. 2019;10(1):117.
24. Muscogiuri G, Chiesa M, Trotta M, Gatti M, Palmisano V, Dell'Aversana S, et al. Performance of a deep learning algorithm for the evaluation of CAD-RADS classification with CCTA. Atherosclerosis. 2020;294:25–32.
25. Simpson S, Kay FU, Abbara S, Bhalla S, Chung JH, Chung M, et al. Radiological Society of North America expert consensus statement on reporting chest CT findings related to COVID-19. Endorsed by the Society of Thoracic Radiology, the American College of Radiology, and RSNA - secondary publication. J Thorac Imaging. 2020;35(4):219–27.
26. Prokop M, van Everdingen W, van Rees VT, Quarles van Ufford J, Stoger L, Beenen L, et al. CO-RADS - a categorical CT assessment scheme for patients with suspected COVID-19: definition and evaluation. Radiology. 2020;296:201473.
27. Li L, Qin L, Xu Z, Yin Y, Wang X, Kong B, et al. Using artificial intelligence to detect COVID-19 and community-acquired pneumonia based on pulmonary CT: evaluation of the diagnostic accuracy. Radiology. 2020;296(2):E65–71.
28. Pinto Dos Santos D, Baessler B. Big data, artificial intelligence, and structured reporting. Eur Radiol Exp. 2018;2(1):42.
29. Bizzo BC, Almeida RR, Michalski MH, Alkasab TK. Artificial intelligence and clinical decision support for radiologists and referring providers. J Am Coll Radiol. 2019;16(9 Pt B):1351–6.

Artificial Intelligence: Clinical Relevance and Workflow

11

William Moore and Jane Ko

Introduction

Artificial intelligence (AI) refers to an overarching term that covers many different computational science disciplines designed to mimic humanlike intelligence. Machine learning (ML) is an area of significant interest within medicine and more specifically within medical imaging. In medical imaging, ML utilizes data sets that can be test images, although in workflow applications, differing types of data can serve as input. Regardless of the type, data to be analyzed are run through a series of computations depending on the type of ML learning being applied. There are various ML systems; some include artificial neural networks (ANNs), support vector machines, k-nearest neighbors, and random forest [1–3].

AI systems are common outside of the medical field with impact seen or in development for many aspects of life including finance [4]; marketing; manufacturing; tourism [5]; entertainment; weather forecasting; geological sciences, energy utilization, and exploration [6, 7]; social and population studies; and science and engineering. Adoption of technology in medicine often lags behind other fields; however, the need to adapt to modern patient requirements is pushing the use of AI in many areas.

ML algorithms have many far-reaching applications extending beyond image recognition and into clinical decision-making, optimal scheduling, efficient resource allocation, image acquisition, reporting guidance and follow-up, quality improvement, and many more potential functions. The use of ML algorithms is applicable to many different systems, including pattern recognition, natural language processing, as well as workflow management. These application do not necessarily require dedicated networks, and the use of generic system such as GoogLeNet (Inception v1) or AlexNet has been used in medical applications [8]. The objective of this chapter is to review the current status of AI in radiology with a focus on cardiothoracic imaging applications and discuss how AI can aid the patient at multiple steps in their imaging experience.

W. Moore, MD (✉) · J. Ko, MD
Department of Radiology, New York University Grossman School of Medicine, New York, NY, USA
e-mail: william.moore@nyulangone.org

Machine Learning in Exam Ordering

Clinical Decision Support (CDS) systems have been available for many years. The first were created by academic medical centers [9]. Commercial versions of CDS systems are now available, and many of these systems leverage matching rules, where there are large number of indications that require the referring clinician to specifically pick one. There is essentially no flexibility in this type of system leading to the potential of selection of only partially correct clinical indications.

With more robust natural language processing (NLP), a new paradigm can be explored. NPL is a form of machine learning where free text can be interpreted by an ML algorithm and connect the indication entered in free text by the clinician with the most appropriate specific indication and provide the suggested examination for the indication [8, 10]. NLP systems may provide improved consistency in ordering of exams. For example, if a clinician writes in "acute pleuritic chest," the NLP program might suggest computed tomography angiogram (CTA) exam for pulmonary embolism and could launch a series of questions pertinent to the ordered exam. The Wells Criterion, or another institutional agreed-upon screening criterion, can be a potential input provided by the clinician. This can then provide guidance to the clinician during the ordering process. For example, if the institutional policy was to do a low-dose perfusion-only ventilation perfusion (V/Q) scan for pregnant patients, the CDS could direct the clinician to this study rather than a CT pulmonary angiogram.

C. N. De Cecco et al. (eds.), *Artificial Intelligence in Cardiothoracic Imaging*, Contemporary Medical Imaging,
https://doi.org/10.1007/978-3-030-92087-6_11

An even more sophisticated application of ML, one can imagine an NLP system that interrogates a clinical note and automatically suggests the most appropriate imaging study based on the current data including lab values, past medical history, clinical history, and physical exam within the note. This is particularly interesting in teaching scenarios where variation in ordering could be a function of level of training [11].

ML Enable Protocoling

Protocoling cases is an essential part of imaging and is one of the times that radiologists are able to interact with the patient prior to an imaging study being performed. All practices for the need for careful consideration of imaging protocols is essential. In cardiothoracic imaging, an order for a CTA of the aorta may need very different protocols. For example, a postoperative aorta is a very different protocol from a preoperative transcatheter aortic valve replacement (TAVR). Studies [12, 13] have shown that using demographic data and free text, an ML system can reliably (95% accuracy) predict the correct protocol in MRI studies. Systems like this could help to streamline the process of protocoling rather than replacing the radiologist in this task. There are two reasons that the radiologist is not replaced by these systems: (1) The radiologist is responsible for the establishment of the specific protocols, and (2) a radiologist would still be responsible to validate all protocols.

ML in Improving Scanner Utilization and Decreasing Wait Time

ML systems can enable scheduling of imaging exams with variable goals in mind. For example, with the recent pandemic, minimizing the time a patient is in a waiting room is critically important as a driver of patient satisfaction while enabling continuous efficient utilization of imaging resources. Other potential objectives include maximal scanner utilization and minimizing no-shows and/or late-arriving patients. Understanding factors that contribute to high probability of late arrivals and failures to appear for a scheduled appointment have been a focus of ML systrems [14].

Efficient Utilization of Imaging Resources and Appointment Scheduling

Reduction of patient wait times has taken on new meaning in the last year related to the need for social distancing in waiting rooms [15]. In part, wait times depend on optimizing scanner and staff utilization; this can be accomplished by understanding factors such as length of exam and preparation of the patient for the exam. With the use of ML algorithms, predicting patient wait time can be accomplished by analyzing currently available data within the EMR. In one study, Curtis et al. [16] used a series of 40 standard parameters within the EMR to create an ML algorithm system to predict patient wait times. In this study, prediction of ultrasound wait time was accurate approximately 60% of the time. This is one of the first attempts to perform these types of predictions and, as such, is a significant move in understanding patient wait times.

Understanding when delays occur allows for actions to be taken to potentially avoid crowding. Muelly et al. [17] evaluated parameters such as MR scan protocol, patient age, contrast usage, and number of unplanned repeat imaging sequences and were able to predict the amount of time that the patient would occupy a scanner. This knowledge could aid in predicting image appointment length from dressing, preparation and imaging duration, and post procedure observation. Optimization of the time the patient is in the imaging center results in several downstream effects, including increased scanner utilization, appropriate staffing levels, minimized patients delays, and avoidance of overcrowding.

An important concept in imaging is AI algorithm fragility. This basic concept is that when an algorithm is put into a new setting, for example, a new hospital, the algorithm fails to perform in the same manner as it did in other locations. The reasons behind these failures are often poorly understood but may be related to minor variations in the imaging data which have profound changes in the algorithm output.

Decreasing Late and Missed Appointments

In the medical imaging, missed appointments can lead to potential loss of revenue, given the [18] current pay-for-service model. For example, Mieloszyk et al. estimated that a midsize academic practice could lose $700,000 per year due to no-show patients [18]. Given this, Deceunick et al. [14] were able to predict patients who would not come to their appointments or would come late using an ML algorithm. The analysis required significant data farming, and they identified that factors such as physician lateness, service interruption, and walk-ins were the primary causative factors for late patients. No specific predictors were given for no-show patients. However, other studies have pointed to transportation issues as one of the drivers for patient failure to show up for appointments [19]. With this knowledge, ML can potentially be used to schedule to minimize late arrivals and no-show patients.

ML Optimize Image Acquisition and Assessing Quality

ML systems are well suited for the task of assessing quality. The overarching concept is if a system is given a strict rule that is determined to be a quality metric, the system can assess the difference between the output of a system and the quality metric. For example, accurate patients centering is an important quality metric within CT imaging since accurate isocentering minimizes radiation dose [20]. Booij et al. [21] used a 3D camera and ML algorithm to assess and potentially improve patient positioning and table location relative to the scanner gantry during CT exams. This study included 432 patients and compared standard radiology technologist workflow with the use of a 3D camera/ML system to aid the technologist determine the isocenter. The 3D camera/ML system attained a 5.6–9.5 mm variance from isocenter compared to 12–17.6 mm for CT technologists (using typical workflow) ($P < 0.001$). Also, a system like this could alert the radiology technologist prior to scan acquisition that the patients is not at optimal isocenter, giving the technologist the opportunity to intervene as appropriate.

Image quality has historically relied solely on the radiology technologist. However, lack of uniformity in training and understanding of quality metrics leads to the potential for inhomogeneous image quality due to overexposure and underexposure in addition to positioning. The retake rate in radiography is a quality metric that serves as a measure of quality and is reported to be around 5% [22]. Automated methods can aid in improving image acquisition in terms of the quality factors measured, such as automatic exposure control in addition to automated patent positioning as discussed. These techniques could minimize retake rates and improve homogeneity in diagnostic image quality. This can be used for radiography, CT, MR, and any imaging modality. ML techniques could allow evaluation of large volumes of imaging studies for quality assessment and improvement. Currently, such processes are limited often to samplings of imaging studies.

Studies have used ML systems to assess MRI image quality related to motion artifact during scanning [23]. These types of ML systems aim to objectively assess motion on all series and give instant feedback to the technologist so they can determine if additional images are needed and for which sequence. In cardiothoracic imaging, cardiac MR could significantly benefit from this technology. In both MRI and CT imaging of the heart, reducing motion artifact is of crucial importance. Often, the degree of motion is not fully appreciated until the study is completed, especially in the cardiac MR. While not currently available, these tools should become a reality for most vendors in the next several years.

An additional objective of ML is to decrease image acquisition time, which is particularly important when performing longer studies such as MRI of the heart [24]. Recently, ML algorithms have been explored to further increase image acquisition rates via undersampling without degradation of image quality [25–27]. To this purpose, ML algorithms have been applied to undersampled images (with low signal-to-ratio (SNR), low contrast, etc.) to improve image quality after image acquisition [28] resulting in near identical image quality to standard images. Recently, Recht et al. [29] showed, in 108 MR studies, a theoretical net of 3.5 times increase in image acquisition time without degradation of image quality [30]. In fact, in this study, image quality of the ML images was judged to be superior to standard clinical images by all 6/6 blinded readers.

While the focus of MRI is on decreasing image acquisition time, the focus of CT especially in thoracic imaging is to decrease radiation dose. ML has been used for some time to accomplish this task [31–33]. Each of these ML has shown similar abilities as the MR to maintain image quality by removing image noise, which is created when imaging at lower radiation-dose protocols compared to standard-dose protocols. The most common applications for this technique include low-dose chest CT (LDCT) images, coronary CT angiography [34, 35], and aortic CTA [36]. As in Recht et al. [29], Shan et al. [32] showed a preference of the reader for the ML images over the standard clinical images in low-dose abdominal and chest CT images. In this study, the group trained the ML algorithm on low-dose CT from a lung cancer screening trial and then applied the algorithm to low-dose CT of the chest and abdomen from a separate location. The blinded readers in this study favored the ML algorithms reconstructed images to the best commercially available iterative reconstructed images. ML algorithms that are developed must be translatable to a busy clinical practice so the amount of time it takes to perform the reconstructions is of significant interest. Potentially, ML systems may prove faster than current commercially available iterative reconstruction methods, as reported by Chen et al. [34].

Finally, ML systems may potentially decrease the volume of intravenous contrast used in both MR and CT examinations. Studies have shown similar image quality ratings for standard volumes of intravenous contrast compared with simulated reduced contrast volumes with the application of ML algorithms [37]. Gong et al. [38] showed a ten-fold decrease in contrast volumes with no change in the image quality rating in brain MRI.

ML-Assisted Reorganization of Reading Priority

Currently, reading worklists which contains cases to be interpreted/reported are typically organized typically based on a time and some priority chosen by a clinician. ML systems have been designed and are now commercially available that move away from the traditional paradigm to a workflow that prioritizes and organizes a worklist based on the results on an ML system in real time. Clearly, a critical aspect to this functionality is the accuracy of the ML systems; however, other chapters will focus on these areas. ML algorithms may aid underresourced areas where there are significant delays in the interpretation of imaging studies. Annarumma et al. [39] developed a CNN and were able to analyze the system to understand potential changes in turnaround time (TAT). This study focused on 15 categories of abnormalities on chest radiographs similar to others [40] including airspace opacification/consolidation. Each category was mapped into one of four priority levels of normal, nonurgent, urgent, and critical. An automated language mapping system used NLP algorithm to extract findings from reports for annotation of radiographs for ML algorithm development. Then an ML algorithm for extracting imaging findings on CXRs and automatically mapping the finding to a priority category was tested and validated. The actual TAT of the interpretation was compared to the simulated TAT utilizing the ML prioritization, with a projected decrease in TAT for abnormal chest radiographs from 11.2 days to 2.7 days. The Food and Drug Administration (FDA) has approved several ML tools which identify abnormal imaging studies and change the priority of the exam on worklists. Some of the first radiology-related ML algorithms were first approved by the FDA for the indication of image prioritization.

ML in Structured Reporting and Improved Follow-up Recommendations

Radiology reports are subject to significant interobserver and intraobserver variation in both the reporting and the interpretation of the reporting. Attempts have been made to create consistent verbiage in imaging reports, such as RadLex/RadReport [41]. Further, vocabulary terms have been put forth but major societies, and in thoracic radiology the Fleischner Society, have taken a clear leadership position with its glossary of terms [42]. Despite these efforts, there continues to be significant variance in reporting. This variance can result in challenges in the interpretation of the report by clinicians and especially by patients.

Given the recent legislation [43] planned to be released in 2020 which requires all notes and all reports (including radiology imaging reports) from medical encounters to be immediately released, this issue has become particularly prescient. Studies have assessed the use of natural language processing (NLP) as a method to analyze radiology reports and output the contents in meaningful text for either a health-care provider and potentially for a layperson. Spandorfer et al. [44] found that NLP systems could correctly differentiate positive versus negative results in reports from CTA performed for pulmonary embolism correctly in 96% of free text reports. Kang et al. [45] used open-source NLP systems to identify the word "lung nodule" in unstructured CT chest reports and were able to show high sensitivity and specificity (91.1% and 82.2%). These results suggest the potential for robust interpretation of imaging reports using NLP. A future application would be the use of NLP to automatically suggest the appropriate follow-up as recommended by guidelines for a finding such as a nodule. Such technology may improve consistency in reporting and recommendations. Kang et al. [45] found in their study that the interpreting radiologist followed Fleischner Society guidelines in only 75.0% of the reported lung nodules. This low compliance could potentially be mitigated with NLP systems that suggest the structured follow-up and thus allowing the radiologist the opportunity to adjust their recommendations. A system that could accomplish this could improve patient safety [46].

Many health-care systems and now Federal law mandate the release of imaging report directly to patients. NLP can potentially help patients understand the meaning of these imaging reports. A meta-analysis of current NLP systems [47] shows very high sensitivity (>90%) and positive predictive value (>80%). One potential application of NLP would be the creation of a patient-facing report; they explained the meaning of an imaging report. Despite excellent NLP results, there are still many concerns about the release of limited report to patients given that these systems are still not perfect; even in the best-case scenario, there is no one who will be explaining the meaning of the results to the patients, let alone have a plan for the next steps.

ML System Development (Issue Around Fragility and System Integration)

Implementation of ML systems in a health-care system can be fraught with issues. First and foremost is the concept of algorithm fragility. This term refers to the concept that when a new set of data is added to an already existing algorithm, potentially the algorithm will not perform at the same level as it did on the initial data set [48]. Research is now focused on mitigating these risks. Studies are now focusing on what the ML system is using within the image to make determination of the ML output. For example, Besse et al. [49] assessed a classic ML challenge, the differentiation of a wolf from a husky. One algorithm was unusually robust, and the team was able to determine the features that the ML system was using the background of the image rather than the animal in the image to make the decision.

There is the need to closely monitor ML results when using ML systems. As presented by Lui et al. [50], a system designed to find intracranial hemorrhage identified a hemorrhage in the left axilla of a chest CT. Despite the best attempts for companies who are currently selling AI systems to control images sent to the algorithm, there is always the potential for "outliers" to cause unexpected outcomes. Companies are using different approaches to control the flow of images into an ML algorithm. At first, there was a focus on using the Digital Imaging and Communications in Medicine (DICOM) standard to route images to the correct algorithms; however, it became evident quickly that this would not be a reasonable solution. The high variation in DICOM labels among institutions can result in significant variance in outcomes of a computer-based system [51]. Thus, most AI companies have now pivoted and have developed ML algorithms to be the gatekeepers. So, for example, algorithms to assess for pulmonary emboli might be deployed in an environment where all CTs are sent to a server that detects whether the anatomy is present in the image that would be assessed for pulmonary embolism, irrespective of the naming convention used. So in the scenario, the inferiormost images of a contrast-enhanced CT of the neck would be assessed, as would the superiormost images of an abdominal CT, thus allowing for assessment of pulmonary embolism in any study with contrast. While these systems have been shown to be robust, errors can occur as described [50].

As ML systems become deployed into large practices, workflow considerations include turnaround time (TAT) of the results, variance reports, and how the results are displayed. First, TAT for ML results will vary widely depending on the design of the system. For example, a chest radiographic system that only analyzes one image and returns a numerical score for prioritization would be much faster than a system expected to assess more than 1000 CT images and return a heat map result to the Picture Archiving and Communication Systems (PACS) . An additional consideration when assessing an ML system is how positive and negative results are handled. Most ML systems have a very high negative predictive value, partially related to prevalence of disease; however, these systems will often have a lower positive predictive value (PPV) as presented by Yoo et al. [52]. Companies have created strategies to address these lower positive predictive values. One strategy to minimize false positives is once a positive result is returned by the ML systems, the data set can be sent to a second algorithm and sometimes a third to increase the probability of returning a true positive result. In large data sets, this can result in slow return of results, sometimes on the order of 10 s of minutes. In an emergency department setting, this could result in delayed interpretation or potentially interpretation without the benefit of the ML result.

Assessment of the ML algorithm in clinical practice can be monitored by creating a variance report that assesses the difference between a radiology report and an ML algorithm result. These reports require robust NLP systems integrated into the voice dictation systems. There are some systems in place currently that could allow for a variance report from the ML result and the imaging report to be automatically sent to either the interpreting physician or a supervising radiologist. Experiences with these systems are variable and highly dependent on the positive and negative predictive values (NPV) or the ML result and on accuracy of the NLP system.

Finally, the decision on how to display the results of an ML system is hotly debated. Some favor the idea of a heat map (Fig. 11.1), showing the radiologist a region of interest. Heat maps are generated by the ML algorithm by highlighting the highest probability regions that gave the ML result (a.k.a., the area of interest on the chest radiograph in Fig. 11.1 was the primary area that the ML system used to determine that the patient had a high probability of pneumothorax). Studies of computer-aided detection (CAD) systems prior to the widespread use of ML algorithms for the use in the diagnosis of PE [53] have shown high false-positive rates, precluding wide application of these systems, as the false-positive rate was too high. The potential bias, especially in less well-trained individuals, is high. Although these results are from a CAD, the observations are applicable to ML algorithms also. However, as the PPV and NPV continue to improve, this risk will be mitigated. Another display strategy used by ML companies is the reordering of the worklist without a heat map display. This alerts the radiologist that there is a finding to be

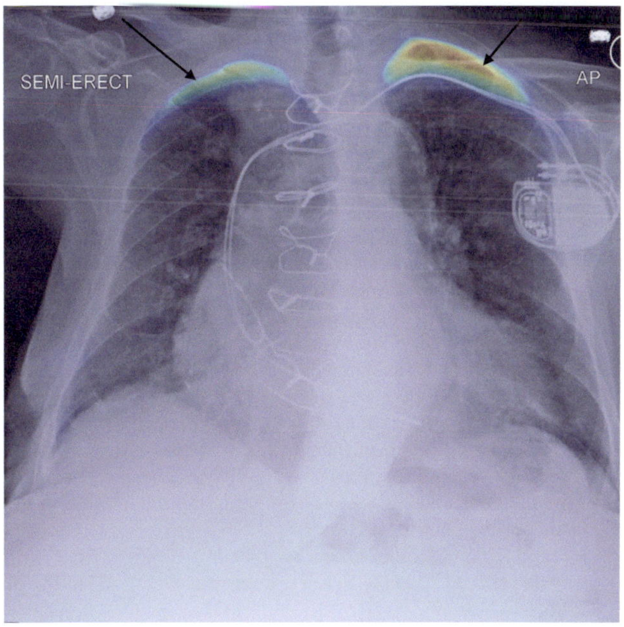

Fig. 11.1 Chest radiograph posterior anterior view showing an overlay of a heat map. In this example, the heat map is displayed as a color map with darker areas representing the areas where the AI system predominantly used to determine the output, in this particular case areas concerning for pneumothorax

dealt with without the added bias of a heat map. So the system will go to the next step and hold the heat map result until the radiologist asks for the result. The choice of these displays will be a local preference as there has been little guidance from regulatory agency to this point.

Conclusion

Artificial intelligence algorithms are in development, in refinement, and deployed for many applications within radiology and cardiothoracic imaging. Although many systems have been designed as computer-aided detection/diagnosis systems, there are many workflow options that are available to improve all aspects of the radiology experience from ordering to final interpretation of the imaging report. The back-end design of these systems has a significant impact on how and where these systems can be deployed. The future of ML in imaging is clearly robust, however perhaps not only for image interpretation but also for workflow optimization.

References

1. Kotsiantis SB, Zaharakis I, Pintelas P. Emerging artificial intelligence applications in computer engineering. In: Maglogiannis IG, Karpouzis K, Wallace M, Soldatos J, editors. Supervised machine learning: a review of classification techniques. Amsterdam: IoS Press; 2007.
2. Liaw A, Wiene M. Classification and regression by random forest. R news. 2002;2/3:18–22. Published online.
3. Rosenblatt F. The perceptron: a probabilistic model for information storage and organization in the brain. Psychol Rev. 1958;65:386.
4. Nassirtoussi AK, Aghabozorgi S, Wah TY, Ngo DCL. Text mining for market prediction: a systematic review. Expert Syst Appl. 2014;41(16):7653–70.
5. Liu H, Liu Y, Wang Y, Pan C. Hot topics and emerging trends in tourism forecasting research: a scientometric review. Tour Econ. 2019;25(3):448–68.
6. Reichstein M, Camps-Valls G, Stevens B, Jung M, Denzler J, Carvalhais N. Deep learning and process understanding for data-driven earth system science. Nature. 2019;566(7743):195–204.
7. Deo RC, Şahin M, Adamowski JF, Mi J. Universally deployable extreme learning machines integrated with remotely sensed MODIS satellite predictors over Australia to forecast global solar radiation: a new approach. Renew Sust Energ Rev. 2019;104:235–61.
8. Zhang Y, Trepp R, Wang W, Luna J, Vawdrey DK, Tiase V. Developing and maintaining clinical decision support using clinical knowledge and machine learning: the case of order sets. J Am Med Inf Assoc. 2018;25(11):1547–51. https://doi.org/10.1093/jamia/ocy099.
9. Khorasani R. Clinical decision support in radiology: what is it, why do we need it, and what key features make it effective? JACR. 2006;3:142–3.
10. Lisboa PJ, Taktak AF. The use of artificial neural networks in decision support in cancer: a systematic review. Neural Netw. 2006;19:408–15. https://doi.org/10.1016/j.neunet.2005.10.007.
11. Dunneck NR, Applegate KE, Arenson RL. The inappropriate use of imaging studies: a report of the 2004 intersociety conference. J Am Coll Radiol. 2005;2:401–6.
12. Hardy M, Harvey H. Artificial intelligence in diagnostic imaging: impact on the radiography profession. Br J Radiol. 2020;93(1108):20190840.
13. Brown AD, Marotta TR. Using machine learning for sequence-level automated MRI protocol selection in neuroradiology. J Am Med Inf Assoc. 2018;25:568–71.
14. Deceunick M, Fiems D, De Vuysta S. OutPatient scheduling with unpunctual patients and no-shows. E J Oper Res. 2018;265:195–207.
15. Salazar G, Quencer K, Aran S, Abujudeh H. Patient satisfaction in radiology: qualitative analysis of written complaints generated over a 10-year period in an academic medical center. J Am Coll Radiol. 2013;10(7):513–7. https://doi.org/10.1016/j.jacr.2013.03.013.
16. Curtis C, Liu C, Bollerman TJ, Pianykh OS. Machine learning for predicting patient wait times and appointment delays. J Am Coll Radiol. 2018;15:1310–6.
17. Muelly M, Vasanawala SS. MRI schedule optimization through discrete event simulation and neural networks as a means of increasing scanner productivity. In: Iology Society of North America, 102nd scientific assembly and annual meeting; 2019.
18. Mieloszyk RJ, Rosenbaum JI, Hall CS, Raghavan UN, Bhargava P. The financial burden of missed appointments: uncaptured revenue due to outpatient no-shows in radiology. Curr Probl Diagn Radiol. 2018;45(5):285–6.
19. Syed ST, Gerber BS, Sharp LK. Traveling towards disease: transportation barriers to health care access. J Community Health. 2016;38(5):976–93. https://doi.org/10.1007/s10900-013-9681-1.
20. Habibzadeh MA, Ay MR, Asl AR, Ghadiri H, Zaidi H. Impact of miscentering on patient dose and image noise in x-ray CT imaging: phantom and clinical studies. Phys Med. 2012;28:191–9.
21. Booij R, Budde RP, Dijkshoorn ML, et al. Accuracy of automated patient positioning in CT using a 3D camera for body contour detection. Eur Radiol. 2019;29:2079–88.
22. Hoffman B, Rosanowsky TB, Jensen C, Wah KHC. Image rejects in general direct digital radiography. Acta Radio Open. 2015;4(10):1–6.
23. Esses SJ, Lu X, Zhao T, et al. Automated image quality evaluation of T2-weighted liver MRI utilizing deep learning architecture. J Magn Reson Imaging. 2017;47:723–8. https://doi.org/10.1002/jmri.25779.
24. Ben-Eliezer N, Sodickson DK, Shepherd T, Wiggins GC, Block KT. Accelerated and motion-robust in vivo T mapping from radially undersampled data using bloch-simulation-based iterative reconstruction. Magn Reson Med. 2016;75(3):1346–54. https://doi.org/10.1002/mrm.25558.
25. Hammernik K, Klatzer T, Kobler E, et al. Learning a variational network for reconstruction of accelerated MRI data. arXiv. Published 2017. Accessed 19 Sept 2019. https://arxiv.org/abs/1704.00447.
26. Golkov V, Dosovitskiy A, Sperl JI, et al. q-space deep learning: twelve-fold shorter and model-free diffusion MRI scans. IEEE Trans Med Imaging. 2016;35:1344–51.
27. Dalca AV, Bouman KL, Freeman WT, et al. Population based image imputation. In: International conference on information processing in medical imaging. New York: Springer; 2017. p. 659–71.
28. Basha TA, Akçakaya M, Liew C, Tsao CW, Delling FN, Addae G, et al. Clinical performance of high-resolution late gadolinium enhancement imaging with compressed sensing. J Magn Reson Imaging. 2017;46:1829–38.
29. Recht MP, Zbontar J, Sodickson DK, Knoll F, Yakubova N, Sriram A, Murrell T, Defazio A, Rabbat M, Rybak L, Kline M, Ciavarra G, Alaia EF, Samim M, Walter WR, Lin DJ, Lui YW, Muckley M, Huang Z, Johnson P, Stern R, Zitnick CL. Using deep learning to accelerate knee MRI at 3 T: results of an interchangeability study. AJR. 2020;14(1–9):1421–9.
30. Zhontar J, Knoww F, Sriram A, Muckley M, et al. An open dataset and benchmarks for accelerated MRI. arXiv. Published 2018. Accessed 21 Nov 2018. arxiv:1181.08839v1.

31. Retson TA, Besser AH, Sall S, et al. Machine learning and deep neural networks in thoracic and cardiovascular imaging. J Thorac Imaging. 2019;34(3):192–201.
32. Shan H, Padole A, Homayounieh F, Kruger U, Khera RD, Nitiwarangkul C, Kalra MK, Wang G. Competitive performance of a modularized deep neural network compared to commercial algorithms for low-dose CT image reconstruction. Nat Mach Intell. 2019;1:269–76.
33. Chen H, Zhang Y, Zhang W, et al. Low-dose CT via convolutional neural network. Biomed Opt Express. 2017;8:679–94.
34. Chen H, Zhang Y, Kalra MK, et al. Low-dose CT with a residual encoder-decoder convolutional neural network (RED-CNN). arXiv. Published 2017. Accessed 10 Sept 2019. arxiv:1702.00288. 2017.
35. Tatsugami F, Higaki T, Nakamura Y, Yu Z, Zhou J, Lu Y, Fujioka C, Kitagawa T, Kihara Y, Iida M, Awai K. Deep learning-based image restoration algorithm for coronary CT angiography. Eur Radiol. 2019;29(10):5322–9. https://doi.org/10.1007/s00330-019-06183-y.
36. Iyama Y, Nakaura T, Kidoh M, Oda S, Utsunomiya D, Sakaino N, Tokuyasu S, Osakabe H, Harada K, Yamashita Y. Submillisievert radiation dose coronary CT angiography: clinical impact of the knowledge-based iterative model reconstruction. Acad Radiol. 2016;23(11):1393–401. https://doi.org/10.1016/j.acra.2016.07.005.
37. Green M, Marom EM, Konen E, Kiryati N, Mayer A. A.3-D neural denoising for low-dose coronary CT angiography (CCTA). Comput Med Imaging Graph. Published online 2018. https://doi.org/10.1016/j.compmedimag.2018.07.004.
38. Gong E, Pauly JM, Wintermark M, Zaharchuk G. Deep learning enables reduced gadolinium dose for contrast-enhanced brain MRI. J Magn Reson Imaging. 2018;48(2):330–40. https://doi.org/10.1002/jmri.25970.
39. Annarumma M, Withey SJ, Bakewell E, Pesce E, Goh V, Montana G. Automated triaging of adult chest radiographs with deep artificial neural networks. Radiology. 2019;291:196–202. https://doi.org/10.1148/radiol.2018180921.
40. Rajpurkar P, Irvin J, Zhu K, Yang B, Mehta H, Duan T, et al. CheXNet: radiologist-level pneumonia detection on chest X-rays with deep learning. arXiv. Published 2017. Accessed 7 Jan 2020. https://arxiv.org/abs/1711.05225.
41. Morgan TA, Helibrun ME, Kahn CE Jr. Reporting initiative of the Radiological Society of North America: progress and new directions. Radiology. 2014;273:642–5.
42. MacMahon H, Naidich DP, Goo JM, et al. Guidelines for management of incidental pulmonary nodules detected on CT images: from the Fleischner society 2017. Radiology. 2017;284(1):228–53. https://doi.org/10.1148/radiol.2017161659.
43. (ONC) O of the NC for HIT, (HHS) D of H and HS. 21st Century Cures Act: interoperability, information blocking, and the ONC Health IT. Federal Register. Published 2020. Accessed 1 Oct 2020. https://www.healthit.gov/sites/default/files/cures/2020-03/ONC_Cures_Act_Final_Rule_03092020.pdf.
44. Spandorfer A, Branch C, Sharma P, et al. Deep learning to convert unstructured CT pulmonary angiography reports into structured reports. Eur Radiol Exp. 2018;3(1):37. https://doi.org/10.1186/s41747-019-0118-1.
45. Kang SK, Garry K, Chung R, Moore WH, Iturrate E, Swartz JL, et al. Natural language processing for identification of incidental pulmonary nodules in radiology reports. J Am Coll Radiol. 2019;16(11):1587–94. https://doi.org/10.1016/j.jacr.2019.04.026.
46. Carrodeguas E, Lacson R, Swanson W, Khorasani R. Use of machine learning to identify follow-up recommendations in radiology reports. J Am Coll Radiol. 2016;16(3):336–43.
47. Pons E, Braun LM, Hunink M, Kors JA. Natural language processing in radiology: a systematic review. Radiology. 2016;279(2):329–43.
48. Xie H, Yi J, Xu W, Mudumbai R. An information-theoretic explanation for the adversarial fragility of AI classifiers. IEEE Int Symp Inf Theory. Published online 2019:1977–1981. https://doi.org/10.1109/ISIT.2019.8849757.
49. Besse P, Castets-Renard C, Garivier A, Loubes JM. Can everyday AI be ethical? Machine learning algorithm fairness. arXiv. Published 2020. Accessed 20 Oct 2020. https://doi.org/10.13140/RG.2.2.22973.31207.
50. Lui YW, Geras K, Block KT, Parente M, Hood J, Recht MP. How to implement AI in the clinical enterprise: opportunities and lessons learned. J Am Coll Radiol. 2020;17(11):1394–7. https://doi.org/10.1016/j.jacr.2020.09.039.
51. Talati RK, Dunkin J, Parikh S, Moore WH. Current methods of monitoring radiation exposure from CT. J Am Coll Radiol. 2013;10(9):702–7. https://doi.org/10.1016/j.jacr.2013.03.002.
52. Yoo H, Kim KH, Singh R, Digumarthy SR, Kalra M. Validation of a deep learning algorithm for the detection of malignant pulmonary nodules in chest radiographs. JAMA Netw Open. 2020;3(9):e2017135. https://doi.org/10.1001/jamanetworkopen.2020.17135.
53. Wittenberg R, Peters JF, Sonnemans JJ, Bipat S, Schaefer-Prokop CM. Impact of image quality on the performance of computer-aided detection of pulmonary embolism. AJR. 2011;196(1):95–101. https://doi.org/10.2214/AJR.09.4165.

Patient Selection and Scan Preparation Optimization: The Role of Artificial Intelligence

12

Matthias Eberhard, Bettina Baessler, and Hatem Alkadhi

Introduction

Artificial intelligence (AI) refers to a general field of computer science dedicated to the creation of learning schemes to perform tasks that usually require human intelligence [1]. The majority of AI applications is designed to support image processing, image recognition, and image interpretation. In contrast, only a minority of AI algorithms have been designed so far to support patient selection and scan preparation [2].

In the past 20 years, ordering an imaging study, scheduling the patient, and selecting a proper image acquisition protocol has shifted from paperwork to a paperless, fully digital process. The electronic health record represents an overwhelming source of information, including ordering information, patient history, laboratory parameters, and results from previous imaging studies. Reading and sorting all this information is a time-consuming, yet important task, with some potential to miss relevant information. On the basis of knowledge about each patient, the radiologist must appropriately select or create study protocols. There are several tasks where AI algorithms could assist in patient selection and scan preparation [3].

Image Ordering

Ordering diagnostic imaging is the first step in a chain (Fig. 12.1) involving not only the identification of the appropriate imaging modality for patients' symptoms but is also meant to ensure, where possible, that the selected imaging examination is performed safely and effectively. Clinical decision support (CDS) systems may support care providers in selecting and ordering the appropriate imaging for a given patient [4]. On the basis of preexisting conditions and current symptoms, CDS systems may suggest the most effective or most cost-effective imaging modality and imaging examination. For example, the European Society of Radiology offers an online Web portal which is called "iGuide" that requires patient data as user input and accordingly displays which imaging tests are suggested together with their appropriateness level, estimated cost, and expected radiation exposure [5, 6]. Therefore, CDS systems may guide the cost-effectiveness for imaging in patients with lower back pain, calculate the effectiveness of lung cancer screening for a long-term smoker, and support the clinician in judging the appropriateness to screen for lung fibrosis and/or pulmonary hypertension in a patient with systemic sclerosis [4]. In patients with lower back pain, Chen et al. evaluated the efficacy of an electronic medical record best practice alert [7]. This CDS tool decreased imaging and magnetic resonance imaging rates by 10% and 15%, respectively [7]. In clinicians overruling the best practice alert, almost 60% entered a non-guideline-supported rationale to legitimate their decision [7], showing the capabilities of such algorithms to reduce potentially unnecessary examinations.

Patient Scheduling

Scheduling of imaging examinations and selection of optimal imaging protocols may be hampered by insufficient or incomplete clinical information [8]. In this case, CDS alerts could remember the referring physician that information needed for choosing an optimal imaging protocol is missing. On the other hand, AI-assisted automated extraction of clinical information from notes to prepopulate imaging order requisitions may improve communication between ordering physicians and radiologists and enhance time-efficient and

M. Eberhard, MD · H. Alkadhi, MD, MPH (✉)
Institute of Diagnostic and Interventional Radiology, University Hospital Zurich, Zurich, Switzerland
e-mail: matthias.eberhard@usz.ch; hatem.alkadhi@usz.ch

B. Baessler, MD (✉)
Institute of Diagnostic and Interventional Radiology, University Hospital Zurich, Zurich, Switzerland

Institute of Diagnostic and Interventional Radiology, University Hospital Würzburg, Würzburg, Germany
e-mail: matthias.eberhard@usz.ch; baessler_b@ukw.de; hatem.alkadhi@usz.ch

C. N. De Cecco et al. (eds.), *Artificial Intelligence in Cardiothoracic Imaging*, Contemporary Medical Imaging, https://doi.org/10.1007/978-3-030-92087-6_12

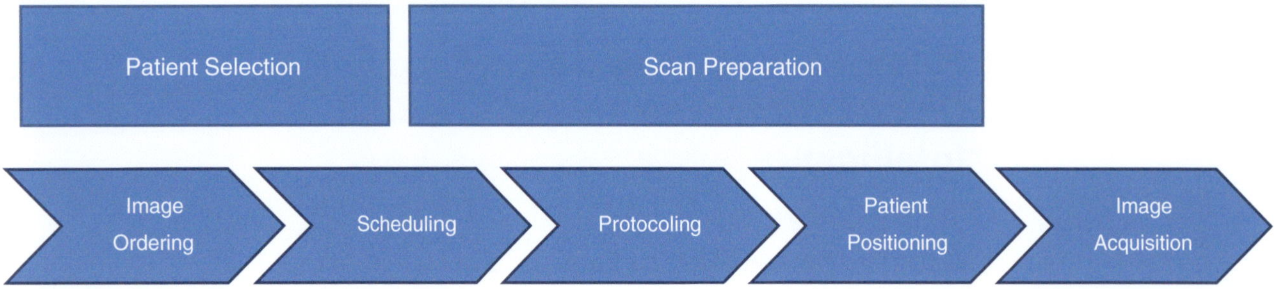

Fig. 12.1 Patient selection and scan preparation

complete imaging orders [9]. Natural language processing, translating any free text into the closest matching indication, could here be beneficial for ordering clinicians as well as radiology departments. NLP uses feedback loops and contextual features within text to interpret its meaning [10]. Closer information of natural language processing can be found in Chap. 10 of this book. More complete and accurate clinical information will most likely improve the quality of image examination protocoling and image interpretation [8].

Protocoling

Once the clinically appropriate imaging is ordered, AI applications may also be able to ensure patient safety during imaging. For instance, a rule-based AI algorithm could check for inaccuracies in patient ordering or image protocol selection, such as duplicate examination orders or protocol selection with contrast media application in patients with a history of allergic reaction after contrast media application or severe kidney dysfunction. Here, the AI algorithm could reduce exposition of patients to unnecessary radiation and help avoiding contrast media-related complications [4].

While initial results provided an optimistic perspective for future application of CDS systems, currently. The number of software solutions which are ready for clinical application is still limited [11].

Arrows showing the clinical workflow from (1) image ordering, (2) patient scheduling, (3) protocol selection, (4) patient positioning to (5) image acquisition. Artificial intelligence-driven clinical decision support algorithms can enhance each of these steps to improve effectiveness of diagnostic imaging and to increase patient safety.

Patient Positioning

AI can influence scan preparation by optimizing patient centering in computed tomography (CT) imaging. Vertical patient off-centering of only 20 mm above or below the isocenter may cause significant radiation dose changes in chest organs because of overestimation or underestimation of the patient size from the localizer radiograph [12]. In pediatrics, Euler et al. could show that vertical patient positioning has a substantial impact on organ radiation dose and image noise with differences between body regions [13]. Impact of patient off-centering on radiation dose and noise was mainly affected by the bowtie filter in head CT and affected by both the automatic tube current modulation and the bowtie filter in thoracoabdominal CT [13].

A combined color/depth 3D camera enabling consistent automatic table positioning in the isocenter of the scanner was recently introduced (Siemens Healthineers, Forchheim, Germany) [14]. The 3D depth sensor of the camera employs infrared light and the time-of-flight principle to measure the distance of objects to the camera. Afterward, a machine learning algorithm detects anatomic landmarks in the camera data and fits a model of the most likely virtual patient avatar to the 3D data, with the virtual patient avatar being based on data from a training population [14, 15]. To set the vertical table position, the geometric center of the avatar hull is computed for the selected scan range, and the table height at which the 3D camera planning image was taken is then adjusted such that the virtual patient avatar is aligned in the isocenter of the CT scanner. Saltybaeva et al. [14] found a significant improvement in patient centering (5 ± 3 mm) using the automatic positioning algorithm with the 3D camera compared to manual positioning (19 ± 10 mm) in patients undergoing chest or abdomen CT. Boji et al. [15] showed that for CTs of the head, chest, and abdomen, the 3D camera was able to attain a significantly lower median variance of 5 to 10 mm from the isocenter (as determined by measuring the anterior and posterior skin surface on axial CT images and determining the center point), which was significantly lower compared to the median variance of 12 to 15 mm for CT technologists [15]. Also in the pediatric population, the 3D camera outperformed radiographers in positioning pediatric patients without a fixation aid in CT with improvement of positioning especially in head CTs with a median table height deviation of 4 mm compared to 16 mm for radiographers [16].

Saltybaeva et al. [14] showed that this clinically used, AI-based application of individualized and automatic patient positioning using the 3D camera allows for more accurate patient centering as compared with manual positioning by technologists, which improves radiation dose utilization and image quality. On the basis of the detected anatomic landmarks, the operator may be warned in case of patient positioning inconsistent with the selected scan protocol (e.g., head first instead of feet first), and scan ranges (e.g., for scans of the chest) may be proposed. Future directions of the application of a 3D camera in cardiothoracic radiology may include virtual guidance for ECG electrode placement implementing virtual fusion of prior scans on the basis of acquired patient body landmarks and needle guidance for lung biopsy by virtual fusion of body landmarks with the planning scan. To perform a virtual topogram, obviating the acquisition and radiation dose of a conventional localizer radiograph, the system has to learn to correctly identify the position of internal organs to allow for a reasonable radiation dose modulation considering the unique patient anatomy [3]. The 3D camera is commercially available and is already in clinical use in many institutions (please see Chap. 21).

Summary

While so far only a few algorithms have been developed to support the patient selection and scan preparation process, AI has huge potential in these important fields in medical imaging, mainly because to its potential to analyze large and complex data sets in a fast manner. Future AI-based algorithms may enable increases in efficiency with time-saving, more cost-effective, and safe patient-centered imaging.

References

1. Samuel AL. Some studies in machine learning using the game of checkers. IBM J Res Dev. 1959;3:210–29.
2. Rezazade Mehrizi MH, van Ooijen P, Homan M. Applications of artificial intelligence (AI) in diagnostic radiology: a technography study. Eur Radiol. 2020;31:1805–11.
3. Eberhard M, Alkadhi H. Machine learning and deep neural networks: applications in patient and scan preparation, contrast medium, and radiation dose optimization. J Thorac Imaging. 2020;35(Suppl 1):S17–20.
4. Kapoor N, Lacson R, Khorasani R. Workflow applications of artificial intelligence in radiology and an overview of available tools. J Am Coll Radiol. 2020;17(11):1363–70.
5. Gabelloni M, Di Nasso M, Morganti R, Faggioni L, Masi G, Falcone A, et al. Application of the ESR iGuide clinical decision support system to the imaging pathway of patients with hepatocellular carcinoma and cholangiocarcinoma: preliminary findings. Radiol Med. 2020;125(6):531–7.
6. European Society of R. Methodology for ESR iGuide content. Insights Imaging. 2019;10(1):32.
7. Chen D, Bhambhvani HP, Hom J, Mahoney M, Wintermark M, Sharp C, et al. Effect of electronic clinical decision support on imaging for the evaluation of acute low Back pain in the ambulatory care setting. World Neurosurg. 2020;134:e874–e7.
8. Lacson R, Laroya R, Wang A, Kapoor N, Glazer DI, Shinagare A, et al. Integrity of clinical information in computerized order requisitions for diagnostic imaging. J Am Med Inform Assoc. 2018;25(12):1651–6.
9. Rousseau JF, Ip IK, Raja AS, Valtchinov VI, Cochon L, Schuur JD, et al. Can automated retrieval of data from emergency department physician notes enhance the imaging order entry process? Appl Clin Inform. 2019;10(2):189–98.
10. Zhang Y, Trepp R, Wang W, Luna J, Vawdrey DK, Tiase V. Developing and maintaining clinical decision support using clinical knowledge and machine learning: the case of order sets. J Am Med Inform Assoc. 2018;25(11):1547–51.
11. He J, Baxter SL, Xu J, Xu J, Zhou X, Zhang K. The practical implementation of artificial intelligence technologies in medicine. Nat Med. 2019;25(1):30–6.
12. Saltybaeva N, Alkadhi H. Vertical off-centering affects organ dose in chest CT: evidence from Monte Carlo simulations in anthropomorphic phantoms. Med Phys. 2017;44(11):5697–704.
13. Euler A, Saltybaeva N, Alkadhi H. How patient off-centering impacts organ dose and image noise in pediatric head and thoracoabdominal CT. Eur Radiol. 2019;29(12):6790–3.
14. Saltybaeva N, Schmidt B, Wimmer A, Flohr T, Alkadhi H. Precise and automatic patient positioning in computed tomography: avatar Modeling of the patient surface using a 3-dimensional camera. Investig Radiol. 2018;53(11):641–6.
15. Booij R, Budde RPJ, Dijkshoorn ML, van Straten M. Accuracy of automated patient positioning in CT using a 3D camera for body contour detection. Eur Radiol. 2019;29(4):2079–88.
16. Booij R, van Straten M, Wimmer A, Budde RPJ. Automated patient positioning in CT using a 3D camera for body contour detection: accuracy in pediatric patients. Eur Radiol. 2020;31:131–8.

13 Artificial Intelligence for Image Enhancement and Reconstruction in Magnetic Resonance Imaging

Kerstin Hammernik and Mehmet Akçakaya

Introduction

The physics of the data acquisition process in magnetic resonance imaging (MRI) cause a substantial slowdown compared to other medical imaging modalities leading to prolonged scan times. This is further exacerbated in cardiac MRI (CMR), where additional considerations due to cardiac and respiratory motions further increase the scan durations. Therefore, acceleration of MRI acquisitions remains an active topic of research, with many clinical applications. This is typically achieved by acquiring fewer data, i.e., subsampling, and using image reconstruction or enhancement strategies that exploit redundancies in the acquisition or the images of interest to produce high-quality images from these subsampled raw data.

Over the past two decades, numerous approaches, including parallel imaging (PI) [25, 60] and compressed sensing (CS) [50], have been proposed for accelerating MRI. These have also found many applications in cardiac MRI [2, 4–6, 8, 26, 53, 57, 58, 73–75, 80]. Recently, deep learning (DL) methods have received substantial interest due to their superior image quality. In this chapter, we will review DL-based image enhancement and reconstruction strategies for cardiac MRI, with a particular focus on fast imaging and artifact reduction.

K. Hammernik, PhD (✉)
AI in Healthcare and Medicine, Technical University of Munich, Munich, Germany

Department of Computing, Imperial College London, London, UK
e-mail: k.hammernik@tum.de

M. Akçakaya, PhD
Department of Electrical and Computer Engineering, University of Minnesota, Minneapolis, MN, USA

Center for Magnetic Resonance Research, University of Minnesota, Minneapolis, MN, USA
e-mail: akcakaya@umn.edu

Basics of Deep Learning for Image Enhancement and Reconstruction

The success of DL is based on recent advances in model architectures, the availability of large training databases, and the availability of powerful GPUs. In this chapter, we introduce the basic tools to build powerful reconstruction networks. An overview of different types of reconstruction networks are depicted in Fig. 13.1, which are further discussed in sections "Deep Learning for Image/K-Space Enhancement in CMR" and "Deep Learning with Algorithm Unrolling in CMR Reconstruction". The networks can be trained in a supervised, self-supervised, or unsupervised way with suitable training data, since it may be challenging to obtain fully sampled data for cardiac applications. In the following, we shortly outline important building blocks and base architectures for reconstruction networks and give an overview on training data and network training. For more details on these topics, we refer the interested reader to survey papers [21, 41, 49] and book chapters [27].

Network Types

The cornerstone of deep model architectures is deep convolutional neural networks (CNNs). CNNs are powerful feature extractors that perform sequential operations of convolutions and nonlinear activation functions. Further improvements can be achieved by analyzing the image in multiple scales as in UNets [64]. To downsample the image, building blocks such as strided or dilated convolutions and pooling layers are used. Skip connections are used to avoid the vanishing gradient problem during training. Upsampling is performed by using transposed convolutions and interpolation methods.

Convolution operations can be performed in N dimensions. However, the higher the dimensionality, the more memory is required. A solution to this issue is separable

C. N. De Cecco et al. (eds.), *Artificial Intelligence in Cardiothoracic Imaging*, Contemporary Medical Imaging,
https://doi.org/10.1007/978-3-030-92087-6_13

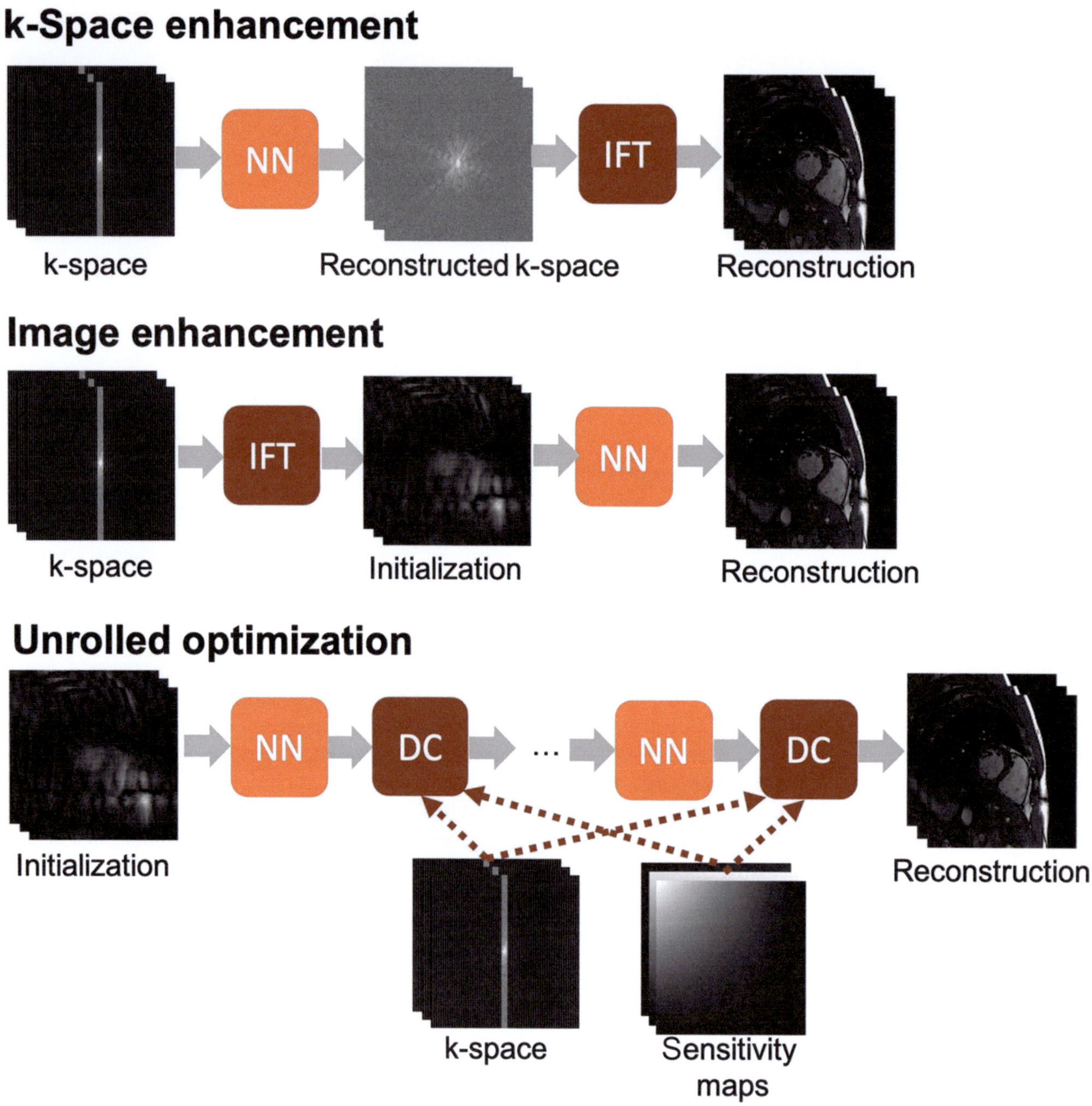

Fig. 13.1 Overview of different methods for cardiac image reconstruction. A neural network (NN) is trained to fill the missing k-space lines. The reconstructed k-space is then transformed to image space using an inverse Fourier transform (IFT) and coil combined. Enhancement can be also done in image domain on the IFT image. The third method combined NN building blocks and data consistency (DC) layers, where the NN acts in image domain, and data-related information is used in the physics-driven DC layer

convolutions. This not only overcomes the computational burden but also results in fewer parameters and improved performance compared to high-dimensional *N*-D convolutions [43, 45, 67]. In case of 2D+t, 2D convolutions might be first performed in spatial domain, followed by 1D convolutions in temporal domain.

Recurrent Neural Networks (RNNs) provide another way to process spatiotemporal sequences of arbitrary length. The individual frames are processed sequentially, and an additional variable termed *hidden unit* extracts and propagates information to later frames. Like CNNs, a number of RNN blocks can be sequentially applied to process the data.

Consistency to Acquired k-Space Data

The single network architectures are not the only important component to process the acquired MRI data accurately. The acquired k-space data contain lots of information that are beneficial to support the reconstruction process. Hence, consistency to acquired k-space data is added to many reconstruction approaches. This can be done by estimating nonlinear interpolation kernels from pairs of undersampled and fully sampled k-space data as in RAKI [7], similar to the estimation of linear GRAPPA kernels [25]. On the other hand, data consistency can be achieved similar to traditional optimization approaches by considering the data term D

$$D(\mathbf{Ax}, \mathbf{y}) = \| \mathbf{Ax} - \mathbf{y} \|_2^2 \quad (13.1)$$

in the optimization procedure. Here, $\mathbf{x}$ denotes the reconstruction, and $\mathbf{y}$ denotes the acquired raw k-space data. The linear MR operator $\mathbf{A}$ models the acquisition physics, i.e., sampling pattern, coil sensitivity maps, and the Fourier transform. In the case of non-Cartesian sampling, the operator $\mathbf{A}$ further includes the sampling trajectory and/or density compensation function. Inspired by classical optimization, various unrolled optimization schemes have been introduced, such as gradient descent [28], proximal gradient [3, 68], variable splitting [14], primal-dual [1], or ADMM [82]. Hence, data consistency layers can be defined that follow, e.g., a proximal mapping [3, 68] or a GD scheme [28] or are derived from other optimization schemes.

Training Data

To train an NN, suitable training data are required targeting the selected application. For MRI reconstruction or enhancement, ideally, fully sampled k-space data are available, which can then be retrospectively undersampled. While this is feasible to obtain for certain static 2D MRI applications, e.g., knee imaging [42], it is more challenging to acquire training data for numerous CMR applications, including both static and dynamic imaging. For static CMR scans, especially at high resolutions, such as whole-heart coronary MRI or late gadolinium enhancement (LGE), data are acquired with electrocardiogram (ECG) triggering in a k-space-segmented manner during the diastolic quiescence, which lasts approximately 100 ms. Thus, these large 3D volumetric acquisitions often require data acquisition well beyond a breath-hold duration, necessitating free-breathing acquisitions, which itself reduces acquisition efficiency by two- to threefold. Thus, for instance, a fully sampled whole-heart coronary MRI would require about 20 min of scan time, in which the image quality degrades due to respiratory drift. On the other hand, for many dynamic or quantitative CMR scans, including real-time cine imaging, perfusion imaging, 4D flow imaging, and quantitative parametric mapping, the trade-offs between coverage, spatial, and temporal resolutions make it impossible to acquire fully sampled data in the first place.

In these cases, where fully sampled data is unavailable, it is more challenging to define a suitable ground-truth. Thus, frequently, a surrogate reconstruction, e.g., based on PI at a lower acceleration rate or CS reconstruction at a similar rate, is used as reference data [17, 20, 45, 71]. However, this inherently hinders the performance benefits of DL methods since their performance is limited by the conventional surrogate method that is used to generate the reference data.

Another challenge in cardiac MRI is the availability of a high number of training samples. For musculoskeletal imaging and neuroimaging, more than thousands of raw datasets are made publicly available in the fast MRI dataset [42]. For cardiac imaging, only small databases are used for research purpose, which hinders the progress of reproducible research and the effectiveness of NNs. Recently, El-Rewaidy et al. [16] published a radial cine cardiac MRI dataset with 101 patients and 7 healthy subjects, constituting the first publicly available cardiac MRI raw dataset. Transfer learning or domain adaptation can be used to deal with limited training data [13, 32, 40, 85]. While this is mostly feasible for 2D applications, where the networks can be pretrained on, e.g., natural images, large databases are hardly available for high-dimensional applications. Another way to increase the robustness of NNs is to perform data augmentation in image domain. Image domain transformations are applied to generate a diverse dataset. In Computer Vision applications, transformations including translation, rotation, scaling, shearing, and nonrigid deformations are applied. However, these transformations cannot be directly applied to enhance the raw k-space data, requiring more realistic transformations. Oksuz et al. introduced physics-aware data augmentation by simulating motion [55]. Adversarial strategies to generate realistic datasets have been only introduced for CMR segmentation [11].

Training the Neural Network

Once the training data have been procured, and the NN architecture has been finalized, the tunable parameters of the network need to be learned from the database. The training procedure depends on two main components: the availability of a reference data and the choice of a function to evaluate the quality of the NN output. In the presence of such data, training is traditionally performed using supervision, where the output of the network is compared to the reference via a loss function, and the network parameters are updated during training to reduce this loss.

Loss Functions

A loss function (cost function, error) measures how well the NN is able to predict the reconstruction based on its network input, usually an image and/or k-space data. Several loss functions have been used in the literature [41], including pixel-wise measures, patch-based measures, or adversarial losses. Pixel-wise measures are simply quality measures, including mean-square error (or ℓ_2) loss and mean-absolute error (or ℓ_1 loss). However, pixel-wise measures are not able to represent the complex human perceptual system. Patch-based losses such as the structural similarity index [76, 84] or perceptual losses that are based on the extracted features of the VGG network [37, 47, 70] add more realistic information to the loss function. However, they are always used in combination with a pixel-wise loss function that is able to stabilize the training [31, 37, 70, 84]. Pixel-wise and perceptual losses are additionally equipped with adversarial losses to push the image quality toward realistic images [24, 47, 70]. However, in the field of medical imaging, it is still an open question if and how adversarial training strategies distort the real image content.

Supervised Learning

In case of supervised learning, the output of the NN is compared against a clean, artifact-free reference image [28, 68] or fully sampled k-space data. For many CMR exams, fully sampled data is difficult to acquire; thus, a surrogate reconstruction is used as reference data [17, 20, 45, 71]. Hybrid loss functions exist that add both a loss in image domain and k-space domain. This is typically used for image enhancement methods where data consistency is imposed only in the loss function [36].

Unsupervised and Self-Supervised Learning

An alternative line of training approaches, broadly falling under unsupervised learning, considers training NNs from unpaired data. Hence, no pairs of undersampled/fully sampled images or any other information about the measured k-space data are available. Self-supervised learning mitigates the absence of reference data by automatically generating training labels from the data itself and has found applications in many AI applications. For image reconstruction and enhancement, this is typically done by a masking operation, in which parts of the k-space are hidden from the NN and used as training labels, as proposed by Yaman et al. [77]. Then the network is trained to learn these parts of the k-space that are hidden from the NN. It has been shown that such methods can match the performance of supervised learning without significant differences [78] and have found applications in CMR [79]. Ke et al. proposed another semi-supervised learning strategy for CMR that relies on a view-sharing method to generate fully sampled references from time-interleaved samples [38].

Deep Learning for Image/k-Space Enhancement in CMR

Image/k-space enhancement techniques have been popular in CMR applications. One of the motivations for using such methods is the large size of multi-coil CMR data, which leads to large memory requirements for unrolled NNs and to slow processing times via traditional iterative methods. Additionally, non-Cartesian trajectories are utilized in many translational CMR scans, but the encoding operator is costly to implement for DL image reconstruction with algorithm unrolling, leading to a preference of enhancement methods for faster processing.

In image enhancement methods, the input to the NN is generated via an initial reconstruction, such as coil-combined zero-filling solution. The NN is designed and trained to enhance the solution to be similar to a reference solution. But this is often done without any knowledge about the acquisition physics. Several strategies to utilize additional information about the acquisition physics have been proposed to augment these methods, including enforcing data consistency after enhancement [36] and using a k-space data consistency term in the training loss function [81]. The NN for image enhancement methods is often trained with the residual, which may include noise, aliasing artifacts, and other obstacles in the data. This output is then subtracted from the input image to generate the final output.

In k-space enhancement, the input to the NN is typically the zero-filled k-space, and the goal is similarly to interpolate/enhance the solution to resemble the true solution. As in image enhancement, acquisition physics is not incorporated into the training explicitly, though dependencies among coils may be learned implicitly due to the use of multi-coil k-space data. Nevertheless, k-space consistency is given in contrast to image enhancement methods.

Next, several of these enhancement strategies that have been used in CMR applications will be outlined.

Dynamic/Quantitative CMR Applications

Image acceleration is critical for numerous dynamic and/or quantitative CMR scans where a series of images of the same anatomy is acquired over time and/or with different contrast weightings. Due to the need for acquiring multiple images over time, these methods have long scan times and often necessitate trade-offs between spatiotemporal resolution and coverage. Thus, improved reconstruction methods are critical for such acquisitions, making them an important application for DL methods. A further complication arises due to the large amount of data that is acquired in these scans, leading to large memory requirements. This is a challenge both for conventional iterative techniques and for DL methods based on algorithm unrolling. Thus, DL-based image enhancement methods have received attention in this setting.

Residual CNNs have been used to remove undersampling artifacts in cine imaging. Hauptmann et al. [33] reconstructed undersampled tiny golden angle radial SSFP data with a residual UNet architecture. The UNet was trained on the magnitude of pairs of gridded/reference reconstructions. The core of the UNet consisted of 3D convolutions. The UNet achieved 5× faster reconstruction times than conventional CS approaches. Assessment of biventricular volumes showed a superior reconstruction quality of the UNet reconstructions compared to CS.

Spatiotemporally Separated Convolutions for Dynamic Data

A drawback of UNets is the large number of network parameters, which makes it challenging to train networks on small training datasets. Kofler et al. proposed a residual UNet architecture for 2D radial cine MRI [44]. The convolutions in the UNet were implemented as a combination of *xt* and *yt*, i.e., 2D convolutions instead of 3D convolutions. This substantially reduced the number of network parameter and makes it easier to train on small training datasets.

Though cine imaging has received attention for DL-based image enhancement due to the availability of fully sampled reference datasets, several other important dynamic and quantitative applications also exist, often without such ground-truth data. One example is perfusion imaging where Fan et al. proposed a 2D+t UNet for reconstructing multi-slice non Cartesian myocardial perfusion MRI [20]. The conventional CS reconstruction was used as reference for supervised training with an MSE loss function. The results showed that the UNet reduced the reconstruction time by 14.4-fold, including the preprocessing and enhancement pipeline, while showing no visual difference to the CS reconstruction.

Another such application without ground-truth data is real-time cine imaging. Shan et al. [71] proposed a perceptual complex NN to accelerate the reconstruction times for 2D+t non-Cartesian real-time cine acquisitions. The core network was a UNet architecture with complex-valued building blocks, including complex convolutional layers. This complex UNet was trained using a combination of MSE loss and a perceptual VGG loss with the conventional CS reconstruction as reference. It yielded a reconstruction time of 24.5 s for 80 frames of a single image slice, including 23.7 s of preprocessing and 0.8 s of NN calculations. No significant difference in image quality and LV functional parameters were observed using the perceptual complex NN.

Combination with Pre-estimation of Temporal Basis Functions

For dynamic quantitative acquisitions using CMR multitasking [12], Chen et al. proposed a hybrid approach that combines conventional estimation of temporal features along with an NN approach for memory-efficient reconstruction of these massive imaging datasets [10]. In particular, they estimated the temporal features using a conventional principal component analysis-based method and combined this with the application of a dilated multilevel densely connected NN for enhancement in the corresponding spatial feature space. Using the conventional CS-type reconstruction as reference, the network was trained in a supervised manner with ℓ_1 loss. This approach sped up the calculation compared to the conventional iterative method, from 20 min to 0.4 s, while achieving similar image quality.

Superresolution Approaches

An alternative approach for the use of enhancement has been through superresolution. In such applications, instead of acquiring an undersampled dataset and trying to enhance the image by reducing residual aliasing artifacts, one acquires a low-resolution dataset and seeks to enhance its resolution retrospectively. In the context of dynamic CMR, Oktay et al. proposed a superresolution approach to map a stack of low-resolution short-axis images to high-resolution short-axis images using a residual NN [56]. The quality of the high-resolution volume is further improved by embedding additional long-axis scans in a Siamese multi-image superresolution network. Using CNNs, the quality of superresolution is highly improved compared to linear and cubic interpolation.

Another application of superresolution for cine imaging was explored by Masutani et al. [52]. This work used both single-frame and multi-frame CNNs based on the SRNet and UNet. The training data was generated by retrospectively downsampling standard cine acquisitions to lower resolutions by keeping the central part of the k-space from DICOM images without applying any ringing filters. A combination of ℓ_1 and SSIM loss was utilized. The CNNs outperformed zero padding and bilinear interpolation and yielded similar left ventricular volumes compared to full-resolution images for up to threefold downsampling.

Static CMR Applications

Image and k-space enhancement methods have also found utility in static CMR applications. Similar to the aforementioned dynamic CMR applications, one focus area has been to improve the computational speed for large volumetric datasets while matching the performance of conventional CS-type methods. Along these lines, El-Rewaidy et al. proposed a complex-valued UNet for undersampled 3D LGE imaging [17]. The network worked with 2D slices, generated by taking an inverse Fourier transform along the fully sampled frequency-encoding direction. It was trained using a CS-type reconstruction as reference with an MSE loss function. The results showed a 300-fold acceleration compared to

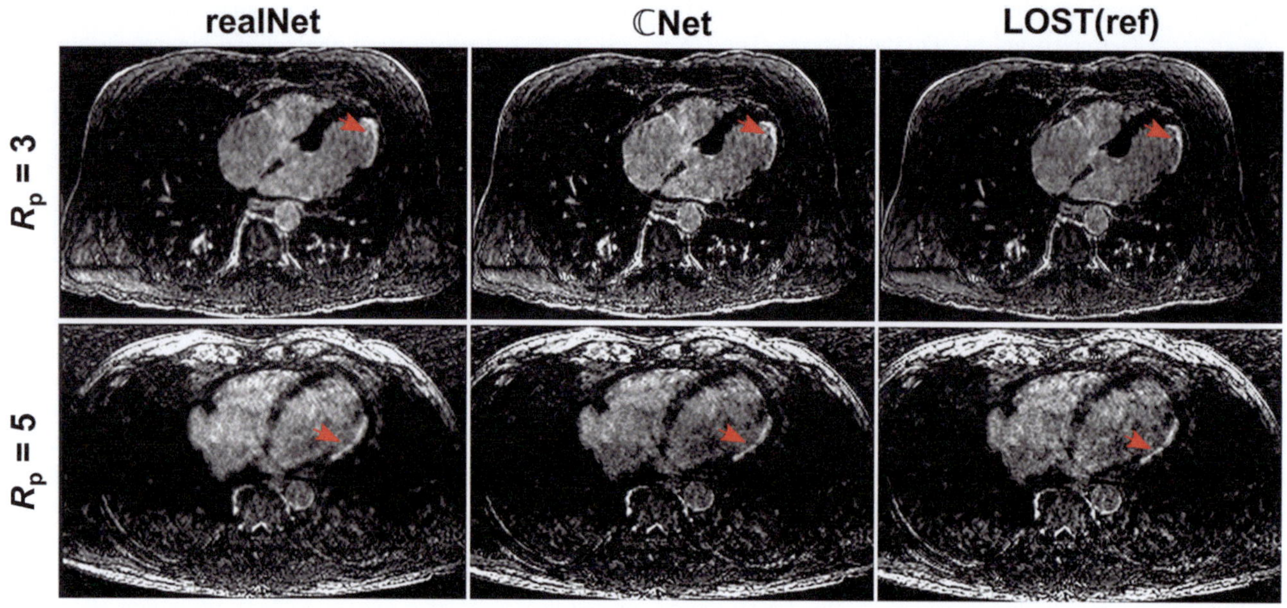

Fig. 13.2 Reconstruction results from 3D LGE imaging. The complex-valued NN from [17] matches the performance of compressed sensing, whereas its real-valued counterpart exhibits artifacts

the conventional reconstruction without a substantial change in image quality as depicted in Fig. 13.2.

An alternative line of work based on robust artificial-neural-networks for k-space interpolation (RAKI) explored the use of k-space enhancement in a scan-specific manner [7]. These methods use the calibration data to train a convolutional NN for k-space interpolation, extending the linear convolutional kernels used in conventional parallel imaging methods. Since the training is performed on calibration data, these methods do not rely on reconstructions from existing CS-type algorithms or acquisition of ground-truth data for training, improving its applicability to undersampled CMR datasets while potentially outperforming its conventional counterparts. For myocardial T_1 mapping, Akçakaya et al. showed that this approach outperforms its clinical parallel imaging counterpart calibrated on the same dataset in terms of noise reduction. An extension of this method, called self-consistent RAKI, was proposed by Hosseini et al. [34]. For coronary MRI, it was shown to outperform its conventional counterpart based on the SPIRiT formulation. One downside of these scan-specific methods is the longer reconstruction time due to the need for retraining for each scan.

Superresolution methods have also been used in the context of whole-heart CMR [72]. Steeden et al. trained a 3D residual UNet using synthetic downsampling by keeping 50% of the slice resolution and 50% of the phase resolution. Then using prospectively acquired data with threefold savings in scan time, the super-resolved images were shown to have better edge sharpness than low-resolution or high-resolution images and significantly better SNR than high-resolution data. However, a significant underestimation was found in the proximal left coronary artery diameter using the superresolution approach, with no other significant differences for measurements in other segments.

Deep Learning with Algorithm Unrolling in CMR Reconstruction

While image/k-space enhancement methods have received attention in CMR for their speed and lower memory requirements, more advanced reconstruction strategies may be developed by incorporating further information about the measured k-space data. Algorithm unrolling is a natural fit for such methods. Powerful regularization networks are alternately applied with data consistency layers, which allows one to exploit not only the available information in the raw measurement data but also redundant information in different domains. Various applications in static and dynamic CMR settings will be outlined in the following sections.

Static CMR Applications

Learned unrolled optimization schemes have been shown beneficial in a variety of reconstruction approaches for static CMR applications. Fuin et al. proposed a multi-scale variational network that uses a multi-scale fields-of-experts regularization [22, 28, 65], realized by filter kernels of different size for coronary magnetic resonance angiography (CMRA). Furthermore, applying the activation functions on magnitude and phase images further improved the reconstruction results. The overall reconstruction time is ~14 s for the multi-scale variational network, compared to ~5 min for the CS approach. The multi-scale variational network allows for up to ninefold accelerated acquisitions (2:34 min) with comparable image quality to the fully sampled reference scan (acquisition time: 18:55 min).

Malave et al. proposed a CNN with a proximal mapping step as data consistency layer for the reconstruction of 3D image navigators (iNAV) in a CMRA sequence [51]. The reconstructed 3D iNAV enables fast nonrigid motion estimation, without loss of quality compared to ℓ_1 ESPIRiT. Reported average reconstructions times per 3D iNAV are 0.53 s for the proposed network with data consistency and 1.55 s for ℓ_1 ESPIRiT using an NVIDIA Titan RTX graphics card.

Self-Supervised Learning

As training data is challenging to acquire for dynamic cardiac applications, self-supervised learning approaches have gained attention in the field of CMR reconstruction. Yaman et al. [79] proposed a physics-guided self-supervised learning approach for late gadolinium enhancement in cardiac MRI. The core of self-supervision lies in the sampling masks. Two masks are used to divide the acquired k-space locations into a training set and a set that is used during data consistency, embedded in an unrolled reconstruction algorithm. This approach for 6× undersampling outperforms clinically used CS with 3× acceleration [4] as depicted in Fig. 13.3.

A specific time interleaved sampling strategy serves as training data for semi-supervised learning in Ke et al. [38]. The training data is generated by using the acquired k-space data from adjacent temporal frames. The network consists of an ADMM-Net-III architecture and data consistency layers to reconstruct coil-by-coil images. A subsequent CNN block performs coil combination of the single-coil images to form the final reconstruction.

Dynamic/Quantitative CMR Applications

One of the first unrolled reconstruction approaches to accelerate dynamic single-coil cine reconstruction was proposed by Schlemper et al. in 2018 [68]. The data consistency CNN (DC-CNN) describes a proximal gradient scheme. The proximal mapping for the data consistency is solved in closed-form solution, and a 5-layer CNN is used as image regularization network. Average reconstruction time are reported with 8 s on an NVIDIA GeForce GTX 1080. In contrast, Dictionary Learning took 6.6 h per subject on the CPU.

Based on this work [68], Qin et al. proposed a recurrent convolutional neural network (CRNN) approach to exploit two types of recurrencies. First, a bidirectional convolutional recurrent unit is used to propagate information through time. Second, iteration recurrencies are used to propagate information across the unrolled iterations. While reducing the network parameters substantially (by a factor of 3), the image quality is improved compared to DC-CNN [68]. Additionally, runtime is reduced from 8 s (DC-CNN) to 6 s (CRNN).

ML for ungated cardiac multi-coil MRI and free-breathing was studied in Biswas et al. [9]. The proposed MoDL-StoRM network alternates between a denoising CNN, exploits nonlocal redundancies via smoothness regularization on manifolds, and solves the proximal mapping for multi-coil MRI using the conjugate gradient algorithm [3]. The

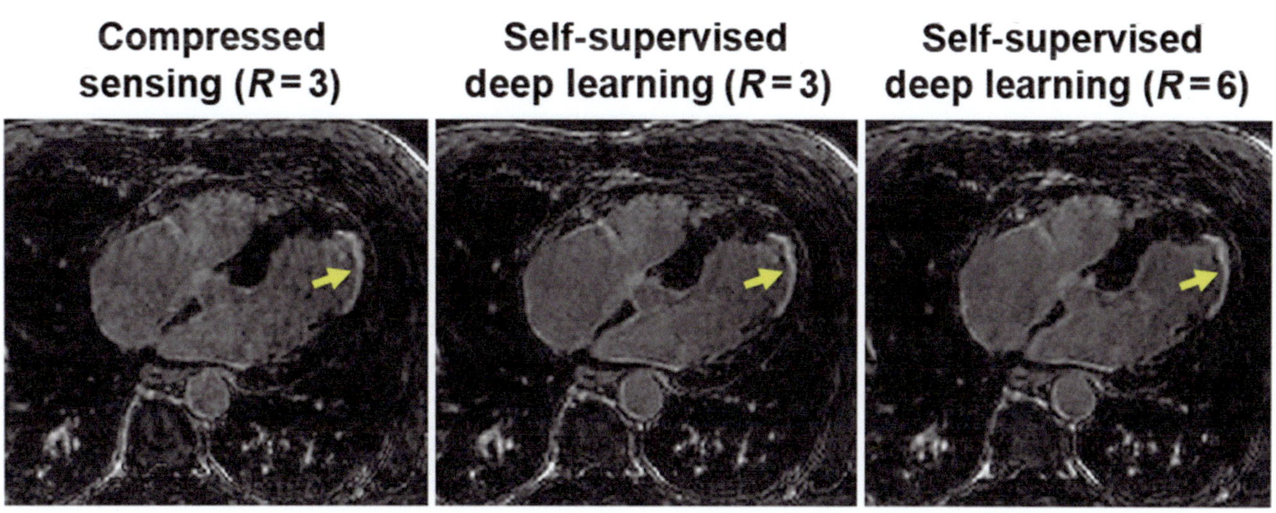

Fig. 13.3 Representative reconstruction results of a 3D LGE scan from a patient. The compressed sensing (CS) reconstruction has been used in clinical studies [5, 8]. The self-supervised deep learning approach at both $R = 3$ and 6 outperform CS reconstruction at $R = 3$ by suppressing noise and residual artifacts. All reconstruction methods successfully identify LGE shown with yellow arrows

manifold for smoothness regularization is estimated from a navigator signal [59].

High-Dimensional Cine Reconstruction with Separated Convolutions

Learning deep NNs is limited by the availability of data and resources, which makes it challenging to deal with high-dimensional data. Kuestner et al. proposed CINENet for the reconstruction of 3D+t data [45]. Unrolled optimization is performed with a multi-coil data consistency layer, and a complex-valued UNET as image prior network. To deal with the 3D+t data, the convolutions were separated into 3D spatial convolutions followed by 1D temporal convolutions. Results comparing single breath-hold CINENet to conventional multi-breath-hold 2D+t CINE acquisitions are depicted in Fig. 13.4. CINENet enables single breath-hold acquisitions, which not only reduces acquisition time but also minimizes slice misalignment and the impact of respiratory motion.

Separated convolutions not only reduce the number of parameters but also yield improved performance compared to 3D convolutions. This was further shown in Kofler et al. for image enhancement [43], and Hammernik et al. for non-Cartesian cine reconstruction using a Proximal Gradient Variational Network [30].

Sandino et al. [66] showed that separated 2D+t convolutions produced higher image quality measures for DL-ESPIRiT compared to 3D convolutions. Additionally, this network makes use of an extended set of coil sensitivity maps to overcome limited field-of-view issues. The coil sensitivity maps are embedded in the gradient-descent data consistency layer. Both data consistency layer and a 2D+t convolutional unit are applied iteratively. The proposed DL-ESPIRiT network does yield not only superior image quality measures but also more accurate functional cardiac parameters, such as left ventricular end-diastolic volume, end-systolic volume, stroke volume, and ejection fraction. Additionally, runtime decreases for the 3D approach (3.89 s) and 2D+t approach (4.89 s) compared to ℓ_1 ESPIRiT (5.36 s) for a single slice.

Exploiting Complementary Domains

Most of the approaches learn an NN in image domain. However, hybrid approaches make use of NN for both k-space interpolation and artifact reduction in image domain [19]. El-Rewaidy et al. use complex-valued subnetworks in k-space and image domain for the reconstruction of radial dynamic cardiac MRI data [18]. The re-gridded k-space is processed by a k-space network to interpolate the missing k-space data and exploits redundancies across different time frames. After an inverse Fourier transform, an image domain network is applied to remove remaining aliasing artifacts and to exploit information from multiple coils and different time frames in the finally reconstructed output frame. The networks themselves consist of complex-valued operations, radial batch normalization, and complex ReLUs (XReLUs).

Strong correlations between space, time, and frequency domain are exploited in [62, 63]. Inspired by k-t reconstruction, kt-NEXT [62] recovers signals in x-f domain, combined with an image domain network and data consistency layers. The complementary time-frequency domain networks [63] propagate information in x-t space and x-f space using a bidirectional and a unidirectional CNN, respectively. Multi-coil information is handled efficiently using a variable splitting scheme. Results show that imposing structure and exploiting all kinds of available information and redundancies is beneficial to reconstruct high-quality images from highly undersampled cardiac MRI data, as shown in Fig. 13.5.

Advanced Topics and Limitations

Apart from the enhancement and reconstruction approaches discussed earlier for handling subsampled data, there are several other venues in which DL may be useful for making CMR faster and more robust. We will overview new advances in motion correction as one such direction while also discussing challenges and future directions for DL-based CMR reconstruction and enhancement.

Deep Learning for Motion Correction in CMR

Motion-related artifacts distort images in a way that they become unusable for image analysis. Motion artifacts may occur when, e.g., the patient moves during the examination or when mis-triggering in the ECG occurs. In the following, we outline approaches that use machine learning to correct for motion artifacts in cardiac MR imaging.

Zhang et al. propose to correct CMR motion artifacts using adversarial training [83]. Generated motion artifacts serve as training data. A generator network, modeled by a residual architecture, tries to correct for the motion in image domain. The network is trained using a combination of Wasserstein loss, content loss, and edge loss to efficiently remove image blurring.

In Ghodrati et al., Variational Autoencoders (VAEs) were used for retrospective respiratory motion correction in free-breathing cine MRI [23]. The VAEs are trained on unpaired data of healthy volunteers and patients with suspected cardiovascular disease. While the encoder-decoder structure

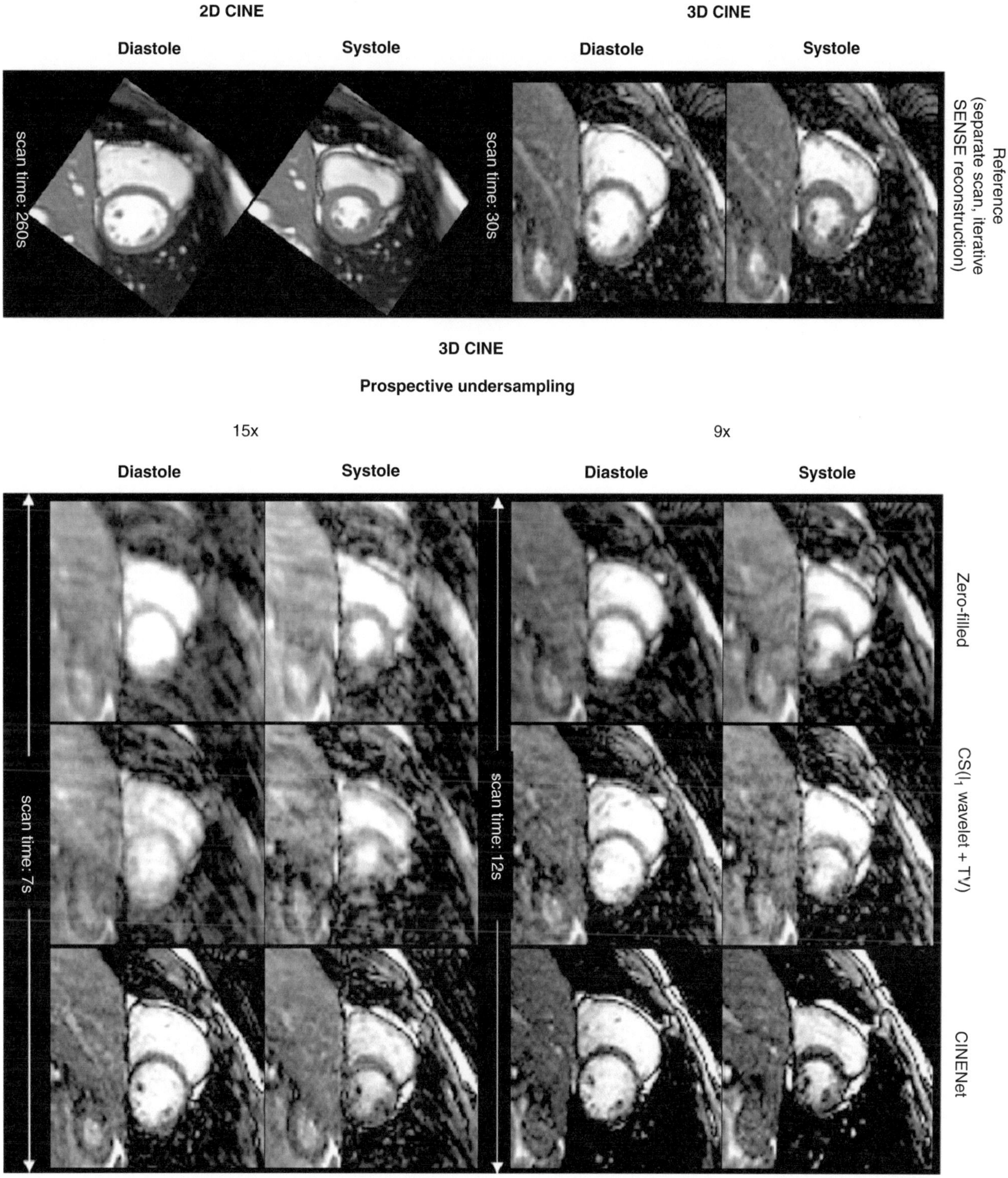

Fig. 13.4 Example reconstructions of CINENet [45]. As reference, an accelerated 3D single breath-hold CINE scan (acquisition time 31 s) and the clinical standard multi breath-hold scan (acquisition time 260 s) are shown. CINENet shows the least artifacts compared to zero-filling and compressed sensing for ninefold undersampling (acquisition time 12 s) and 15-fold undersampling (acquisition time 7 s)

preserves the general structure of the free-breathing images by learning an identity mapping, a discriminator network directs the encoder to remove artifacts.

Oksuz et al. address MR motion correction directly from k-space [54]. A generator network, motivated by Automap [85], transforms the k-space directly to image space. The

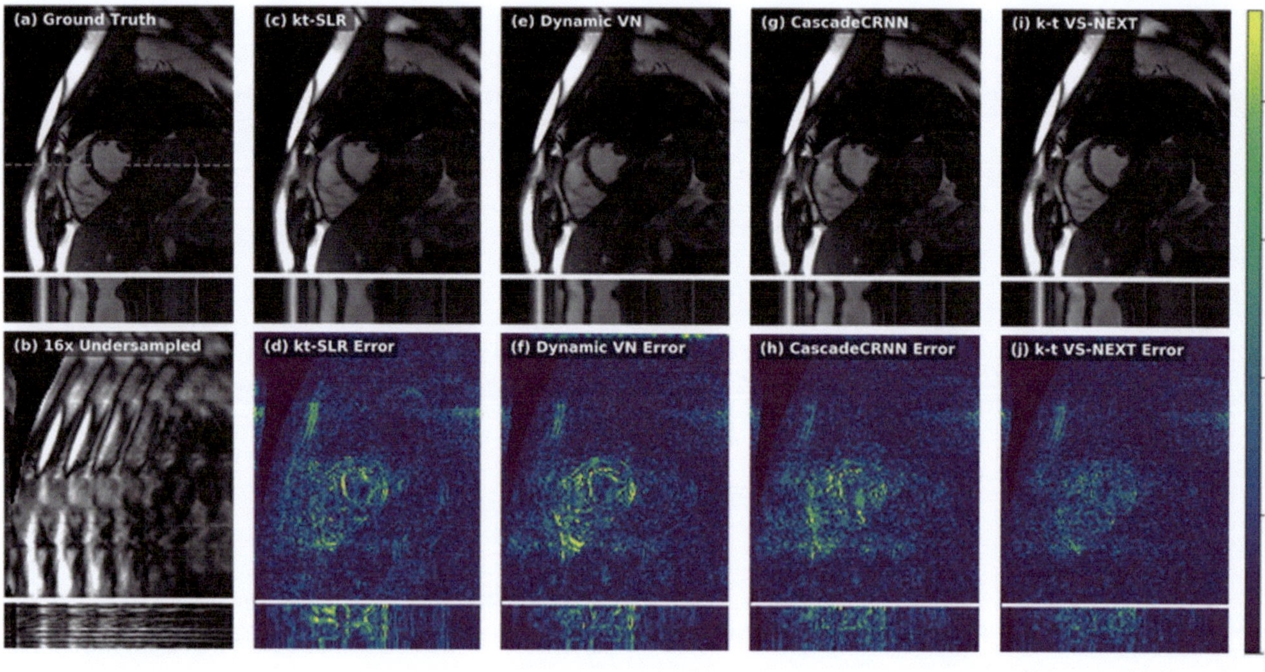

Fig. 13.5 Qin et al. [63]: Results are shown for undersampling rates R=16 (**b**) for different methods (**c**, **e**, **g** and **i**) on spatial and temporal dimensions and their respective error maps (**d**, **f**, **h** and **j**) compared to the ground truth image (**a**) (The proposed (**i**) k-t VS-NEXT exploits information in the complementary time-frequency domain. This outperforms traditional methods such as (**c**) kt-SLR [48], and learning-based methods such as the (**e**) variational network [29], and the (**g**) cascaded recurrent network [61]

network is trained with an adversarial training strategy on pairs of synthetically corrupted k-space data and uncorrupted images. The proposed network is able to correct the motion artifacts; however, textural information is lost.

NNs are used to detect and correct for cardiac MRI motion artifacts in Oksuz et al. [55]. A detection network is used to identify the corrupted k-space lines. The motion-corrected predicted sampling masks are fed into a data consistency layer. An additional CRNN is used to account for artifacts in image domain. For training, a reconstruction loss, i.e., mean-squared error, is combined with a detection loss, which is defined via cross-entropy of the binary mask and the probability of the predicted line being uncorrupted. This network outperforms the Automap-GAN [54] substantially.

Kuestner et al. proposed an end-to-end image reconstruction and motion-correction network in 4D magnetic resonance imaging of the body trunk [46]. A local all-pass network is deployed to estimate nonrigid deformation fields on motion-resolved k-spaces. These fields are directly fed into the data consistency layer for reconstruction. Both LAP net and the reconstruction network are trained jointly by minimizing a combined mean-squared error and end-point error as loss function.

Motion compensation is applied as a post-processing step for dynamic MRI in Huang et al. [35]. The reconstruction is performed in three steps. First, dynamic MRI reconstruction is addressed with a Convolutional-Gated Recurrent Units (ConvGRUs), followed by a data consistency layer. The reconstruction step is followed by a motion estimation step using a FlowNet with a Convolutional UNET architecture as backbone. The estimated motion is finally used to refine the reconstructed frames with the estimated motion. The proposed approach outperforms DC-CNN [68] and classical approaches such as kt-SLR [48].

Seegolam et al. embed motion estimation directly in a cascaded reconstruction approach [69]. A UNET architecture is used to estimate the motion fields. A novel data-consistent motion-augmented cine (DC-MAC) layer is presented that wraps an image using the estimated motion field to a consecutive frame to serve for data consistency. As all frames are consecutively processed, information is carried over the whole temporal axis. This approach allows for highly effective reconstruction of extremely accelerated data.

Challenges and Future Directions

In this chapter, we presented an overview of recent advances in using machine learning for cardiac MRI reconstruction and enhancement. While the presented methods hold a lot of promise, there are still some challenging open questions, which require further investigation.

In static CMR exams, one is often interested in the detection of subtle anatomical changes, such as stenoses in coronary MRI. Similarly, in dynamic CMR exams, the temporal dynamics are of utmost importance. Thus, in CMR, there is often a question about the degree of spatiotemporal blurring artifacts for regularized reconstruction methods. While DL methods tend to outperform compressed sensing methods for regularized reconstruction, more clinical studies are needed to establish that no artifact is introduced due to regularization. DL methods also face an additional challenge since they are trained on large databases. Thus, further investigations are also needed to assess how the methods will generalize to rare pathologies that are not prominent in the training databases [15] or adverse conditions like arrhythmia.

Several contemporary CMR scans are multidimensional in nature, often incorporating anatomical, dynamical, and quantitative information. While algorithm unrolling has proved to be very successful for DL reconstruction, their application to multidimensional data may be challenging. As these methods require enforcing consistency with acquired k-space data, as well as multidimensional NNs for regularization, the memory requirements may be prohibitive for typical GPU training. Thus, alternative methodologies for efficient training [39] and deployment strategies for multidimensional CMR data may be necessary.

CMR scans are often acquired in an undersampled manner. This is either due to acquisition constraints that make it impossible to fully sample data or due to time constraints in clinical workflow. Nonetheless, it is difficult or impossible to get fully sampled ground-truth data for most CMR scans. Early work in the field tackled this challenge by using surrogate reconstructions [17, 20, 45, 71], while later work has focused on using self-supervision with undersampled datasets [77] to achieve the full potential of DL methods. However, such techniques tend to rely on pixel-wise k-space losses, which are prone to blurring artifacts. The incorporation of more advanced loss functions, such as perceptual losses that align better with visual assessments, to such learning strategies is an open research problem.

A very important, yet less frequently studied area is motion compensation in cardiac MR imaging. The current available are very promising to improve image reconstruction substantially when incorporating motion into the reconstruction process. However, further investigations have to be made on multichannel MRI data used in a clinical setting and for applications such as perfusion and real-time imaging.

Finally, while large MR reconstruction data exists for musculoskeletal imaging, the availability of publicly available cardiac datasets is still under development with only one such example [16]. The sharing of larger training databases will help development for CMR reconstruction and enhancement.

References

1. Adler J, Öktem O. Solving ill-posed inverse problems using iterative deep neural networks. Inverse Problems. 2017;33(12):1–24.
2. Adluru G, Chen L, Kim SE, Burgon N, Kholmovski EG, Marrouche NF, Dibella EV. Three-dimensional late gadolinium enhancement imaging of the left atrium with a hybrid radial acquisition and compressed sensing. J Magn Reson Imaging. 2011;34(6):1465–71.
3. Aggarwal HK, Mani MP, Jacob M. Model based image reconstruction using deep learned priors (Modl). In: IEEE international symposium on biomedical imaging; 2018. p. 671–4.
4. Akçakaya M, Basha TA, Goddu B, Goepfert LA, Kissinger KV, Tarokh V, Manning WJ, Nezafat R. Low-dimensional-structure self-learning and thresholding: regularization beyond compressed sensing for MRI reconstruction. Magn Reson Med. 2011;66(3):756–67.
5. Akcakaya M, Rayatzadeh H, Basha TA, Hong SN, Chan RH, Kissinger KV, Hauser TH, Josephson ME, Manning WJ, Nezafat R. Accelerated late gadolinium enhancement cardiac MR imaging with isotropic spatial resolution using compressed sensing: initial experience. Radiology. 2012;264(3):691–9.
6. Akçakaya M, Basha TA, Chan RH, Manning WJ, Nezafat R. Accelerated isotropic sub-millimeter whole-heart coronary MRI: compressed sensing versus parallel imaging. Magn Reson Med. 2014;71(2):815–22.
7. Akçakaya M, Moeller S, Weingärtner S, Uğurbil K. Scan-specific robust artificial-neural-networks for k-space interpolation (RAKI) reconstruction: database-free deep learning for fast imaging. Magn Reson Med. 2019;81(1):439–53.
8. Basha TA, Akcakaya M, Liew C, Tsao CW, Delling FN, Addae G, Ngo L, Manning WJ, Nezafat R. Clinical performance of high-resolution late gadolinium enhancement imaging with compressed sensing. J Magn Reson Imaging. 2017;46(6):1829–38.
9. Biswas S, Aggarwal HK, Jacob M. Dynamic MRI using model-based deep learning and SToRM priors: MoDL-SToRM. Magn Reson Med. 2019;82(1):485–94.
10. Chen Y, Shaw JL, Xie Y, Li D, Christodoulou AG. Deep learning within a priori temporal feature spaces for large-scale dynamic MR image reconstruction: application to 5-D cardiac MR multitasking. Med Image Comput Comput Assist Interv. 2019;11765:495–504.
11. Chen C, Qin C, Qiu H, Ouyang C, Wang S, Chen L, Tarroni G, Bai W, Rueckert D. Realistic adversarial data augmentation for MR image segmentation. In: International conference on medical image computing and computer assisted intervention; 2020.
12. Christodoulou AG, Shaw JL, Nguyen C, Yang Q, Xie Y, Wang N, Li D. Magnetic resonance multitasking for motion-resolved quantitative cardiovascular imaging. Nat Biomed Eng. 2018;2(4):215–26.
13. Dar SUH, Özbey M, Çatlı AB, Çukur T. A transfer-learning approach for accelerated MRI using deep neural networks. Magn Reson Med. 2020;84(2):663–85.
14. Duan J, Schlemper J, Qin C, Ouyang C, Bai W, Biffi C, Bello G, Statton B, O'Regan DP, Rueckert D. VS-net: variable splitting network for accelerated parallel MRI reconstruction. In: International conference on medical image computing and computer-assisted intervention; 2019. p. 713–22.
15. Eldar YC, Hero AO III, Deng L, Fessler J, Kovacevic J, Poor HV, Young S. Challenges and open problems in signal processing: panel discussion summary from ICASSP 2017 [panel and forum]. IEEE Signal Process Mag. 2017;34(6):8–23.
16. El-Rewaidy H. Replication data for: multi-domain convolutional neural network (MD-CNN) for radial reconstruction of dynamic cardiac MRI. Harvard Dataverse. 2020;3. https://dataverse.harvard.edu/dataset.xhtml?persistentId=doi:10.7910/DVN/CI3WB6.
17. El-Rewaidy H, Neisius U, Mancio J, Kucukseymen S, Rodriguez J, Paskavitz A, Menze B, Nezafat R. Deep complex convolutional network for fast reconstruction of 3D late gadolinium enhancement cardiac MRI. NMR Biomed. 2020;33(7):e4312.
18. El-Rewaidy H, Fahmy AS, Pashakhanloo F, Cai X, Kucukseymen S, Csecs I, Neisius U, Haji-Valizadeh H, Menze B, Nezafat R. Multi-domain convolutional neural network (MD-CNN) for radial reconstruction of dynamic cardiac MRI. Magn Reson Med. 2021;85(3):1195–208.
19. Eo T, Jun Y, Kim T, Jang J, Lee HJ, Hwang D. KIKI-net: cross-domain convolutional neural networks for reconstructing

undersampled magnetic resonance images. Magn Reson Med. 2018;80(5):2188–201.
20. Fan L, Shen D, Haji-Valizadeh H, Naresh NK, Carr JC, Freed BH, Lee DC, Kim D. Rapid dealiasing of undersampled, non-Cartesian cardiac perfusion images using U-net. NMR Biomed. 2020;33(5):e4239.
21. Fessler JA. Optimization methods for MR image reconstruction (long version). arXiv Prepr. *arXiv:1903.03510*, 2019.
22. Fuin N, Bustin A, Küstner T, Oksuz I, Clough J, King AP, Schnabel JA, Botnar RM, Prieto C. A multi-scale variational neural network for accelerating motion-compensated whole-heart 3D coronary MR angiography. Magn Reson Imaging. 2020;70:155–67.
23. Ghodrati V, Bydder M, Ali F, Gao C, Prosper A, Nguyen K-L, Hu P. Retrospective respiratory motion correction in cardiac cine mri reconstruction using adversarial autoencoder and unsupervised learning. NMR Biomed. 2021;34(2):e4433. NBM-19-0275.R3.
24. Gong K, Guan J, Kim K, Zhang X, Yang J, Seo Y, El Fakhri G, Qi J, Li Q. Iterative PET image reconstruction using convolutional neural network representation. IEEE Trans Med Imaging. 2018;38(3):675–85.
25. Griswold MA, Jakob PM, Heidemann RM, Nittka M, Jellus V, Wang J, Kiefer B, Haase A. Generalized autocalibrating partially parallel acquisitions (GRAPPA). Magn Reson Med. 2002;47:1202–10.
26. Haji-Valizadeh H, Rahsepar AA, Collins JD, Bassett E, Isakova T, Block T, Adluru G, DiBella EVR, Lee DC, Carr JC, Kim D. Validation of highly accelerated real-time cardiac cine MRI with radial k-space sampling and compressed sensing in patients at 1.5T and 3T. Magn Reson Med. 2018;79(5):2745–51.
27. Hammernik K, Knoll F. Machine learning for image reconstruction. In: Rueckert D, Fichtinger G, Zhou SK, editors. Handbook of medical image computing and computer assisted intervention. Elsevier; 2020. p. 25–64.
28. Hammernik K, Klatzer T, Kobler E, Recht MP, Sodickson DK, Pock T, Knoll F. Learning a variational network for reconstruction of accelerated MRI data. Magn Reson Med. 2018;79(6):3055–71.
29. Hammernik K, Schloegl M, Kobler E, Stollberger R, Pock T. Dynamic multicoil reconstruction using variational networks. In: Proc. ISMRM 27th Annu. Meeting exhibit; 2019. p. 4656.
30. Hammernik K, Cruz G, Kuestner T, Prieto C, Daniel R. On the influence of prior knowledge in learning non-cartesian 2d cine image reconstruction. In: Proc. ISMRM Annu. Meeting exhibit; 2020. p. 0602.
31. Hammernik K, Schlemper J, Qin C, Duan J, Seegolam G, Ouyang C, Summers RM, Daniel R. Σ-net: Ensembled iterative deep neural networks for accelerated parallel mr image reconstruction. In: Proc. ISMRM annu. meeting exhibit; 2020. p. 0987.
32. Han Y, Yoo J, Kim HH, Shin HJ, Sung K, Ye JC. Deep learning with domain adaptation for accelerated projection-reconstruction MR. Magn Reson Med. 2018;80(3):1189–205.
33. Hauptmann A, Lucka F, Betcke M, Huynh N, Adler J, Cox B, Beard P, Ourselin S, Arridge S. Model-based learning for accelerated, limited-view 3-D Photoacoustic tomography. IEEE Trans Med Imaging. 2018;37(6):1382–93.
34. Hosseini SAH, Zhang C, Weingärtner S, Moeller S, Stuber M, Ugurbil K, Akçakaya M. Accelerated coronary MRI with sRAKI: a database-free self-consistent neural network k-space reconstruction for arbitrary undersampling. PLoS One. 2020;15(2):e0229418.
35. Huang Q, Yang D, Qu H, Yi J, Wu P, Metaxas D. Dynamic MRI reconstruction with motion-guided network. In: Cardoso MJ, Feragen A, Glocker B, Konukoglu E, Oguz I, Unal G, Vercauteren T, editors. Proceedings of the 2nd international conference on medical imaging with deep learning, volume 102 of Proceedings of Machine Learning Research. London, UK: PMLR, 08–10 Jul 2019. p. 275–84.
36. Hyun CM, Kim HP, Lee SM, Lee SM, Seo JK. Deep learning for undersampled MRI reconstruction. Phys Med Biol. 2018;63(13):135007.
37. Johnson J, Alahi A, Fei-Fei L, Assari SM, Idrees H, Shah M, Johnson J, Alahi A, Fei-Fei L. Perceptual losses for real-time style transfer and super-resolution. In: Proceedings of the European conference on computer vision, volume 9906 LNCS. Cham: Springer; 2016. p. 694–711.
38. Ke Z, Cheng J, Ying L, Zheng H, Zhu Y, Liang D. An unsupervised deep learning method for multi-coil cine MRI. Phys Med Biol. 2020;65(23):235041.
39. Kellman M, Zhang K, Markley E, Tamir J, Bostan E, Lustig M, Waller L. Memory-efficient learning for large-scale computational imaging. IEEE Trans Comput Imaging. 2020;6:1403–14.
40. Knoll F, Hammernik K, Kobler E, Pock T, Recht MP, Sodickson DK. Assessment of the generalization of learned image reconstruction and the potential for transfer learning. Magn Reson Med. 2019;81(1):116–28.
41. Knoll F, Hammernik K, Zhang C, Moeller S, Pock T, Sodickson DK, Akcakaya M. Deep-learning methods for parallel magnetic resonance imaging reconstruction: a survey of the current approaches, trends, and issues. IEEE Signal Process Mag. 2020;37(1):128–40.
42. Knoll F, Zbontar J, Sriram A, Muckley MJ, Bruno M, Defazio A, Parente M, Geras KJ, Katsnelson J, Chandarana H, Zhang Z, Drozdzalv M, Romero A, Rabbat M, Vincent P, Pinkerton J, Wang D, Yakubova N, Owens E, Zitnick CL, Recht MP, Sodickson DK, Lui YW. fastMRI: a publicly available raw k-space and DICOM dataset of knee images for accelerated MR image reconstruction using machine learning. Radiol Artif Intell. 2020;2(1):e190007.
43. Kofler A, Haltmeier M, Schaeffter T, Kachelrieß M, Dewey M, Wald C, Kolbitsch C. Neural networks-based regularization for large-scale medical image reconstruction. Phys Med Biol. 2020;65(13):135003.
44. Kofler A, Dewey M, Schaeffter T, Wald C, Kolbitsch C. Spatio-temporal deep learning-based undersampling artefact reduction for 2D radial cine MRI with limited training data. IEEE Trans Med Imaging. 2020;39(3):703–17.
45. Küstner T, Fuin N, Hammernik K, Bustin A, Qi H, Hajhosseiny R, Masci PG, Neji R, Rueckert D, Botnar RM, Prieto C. CINENet: deep learning-based 3D cardiac CINE MRI reconstruction with multi-coil complex-valued 4D spatio-temporal convolutions. Sci Rep. 2020;10(1):1–13.
46. Küstner T, Hepp T, Fischer M, Schwartz M, Fritsche A, Häring H-U, Nikolaou K, Bamberg F, Yang B, Schick F, Gatidis S, Machann J. Fully automated and standardized segmentation of adipose tissue compartments by deep learning in three-dimensional whole-body MRI of epidemiological cohort studies. arXiv Prepr. *arXiv:2008.02251*, 2020.
47. Ledig C, Theis L, Huszár F, Caballero J, Cunningham A, Acosta A, Aitken A, Tejani A, Totz J, Wang Z, Shi Twitter W. Photo-realistic single image super-resolution using a generative adversarial network. In: IEEE conference on computer vision and pattern recognition; 2017. p. 4681–90.
48. Lingala SG, Hu Y, DiBella E, Jacob M. Accelerated dynamic MRI exploiting sparsity and low-rank structure: k-t SLR. IEEE Trans Med Imag. 2011;30(5):1042–54.
49. Lundervold AS, Lundervold A. An overview of deep learning in medical imaging focusing on MRI. Z Med Phys. 2019;29:102–27.
50. Lustig M, Donoho D, Pauly JM. Sparse MRI: the application of compressed sensing for rapid MR imaging. Magn Reson Med. 2007;58(6):1182–95.
51. Malavé MO, Baron CA, Koundinyan SP, Sandino CM, Ong F, Cheng JY, Nishimura DG. Reconstruction of undersampled 3D non-cartesian image-based navigators for coronary MRA using an unrolled deep learning model. Magn Reson Med. 2020;84(2):800–12.

52. Masutani EM, Bahrami N, Hsiao A. Deep learning single-frame and multiframe super-resolution for cardiac mri. Radiology. 2020;295(3):552–61. PMID: 32286192.
53. Nagata M, Kato S, Kitagawa K, Ishida N, Nakajima H, Nakamori S, Ishida M, Miyahara M, Ito M, Sakuma H. Diagnostic accuracy of 1.5-T unenhanced whole-heart coronary MR angiography performed with 32-channel cardiac coils: initial single-center experience. Radiology. 2011;259(2):384–92.
54. Oksuz I, Clough J, Bustin A, Cruz G, Prieto C, Botnar R, Rueckert D, Schnabel JA, King AP. Cardiac MR motion artefact correction from k-space using deep learning-based reconstruction. In: Knoll F, Maier A, Rueckert D, editors. Machine learning for medical image reconstruction. Cham: Springer International Publishing; 2018. p. 21–9.
55. Oksuz I, Clough J, Ruijsink B, Puyol-Antón E, Bustin A, Cruz G, Prieto C, Rueckert D, King AP, Schnabel JA. Detection and correction of cardiac MRI motion artefacts during reconstruction from k-space. In: Shen D, Liu T, Peters TM, Staib LH, Essert C, Zhou S, Yap P-T, Khan A, editors. Medical image computing and computer assisted intervention – MICCAI 2019. Cham: Springer International Publishing; 2019. p. 695–703.
56. Oktay O, Bai W, Lee M, Guerrero R, Kamnitsas K, Caballero J, de Marvao A, Cook S, O'Regan D, Rueckert D. Multi-input cardiac image super-resolution using convolutional neural networks. In: Ourselin S, Joskowicz L, Sabuncu MR, Unal G, Wells W, editors. Medical image computing and computer-assisted intervention - MICCAI 2016. Cham: Springer International Publishing; 2016. p. 246–54.
57. Otazo R, Kim D, Axel L, Sodickson DK. Combination of compressed sensing and parallel imaging for highly accelerated first-pass cardiac perfusion MRI. Magn Reson Med. 2010;64(3):767–76.
58. Otazo R, Candès E, Sodickson DK. Low-rank plus sparse matrix decomposition for accelerated dynamic MRI with separation of background and dynamic components. Magn Reson Med. 2015;73(3):1125–36.
59. Poddar S, Jacob M. Dynamic mri using smoothness regularization on manifolds (storm). IEEE Trans Med Imaging. 2016;35(4):1106–15.
60. Pruessmann KP, Weiger M, Scheidegger MB, Boesiger P. SENSE: sensitivity encoding for fast MRI. Magn Reson Med. 1999;42(5):952–62.
61. Qin C, Bai W, Schlemper J, Petersen SE, Piechnik SK, Neubauer S, Rueckert D. Joint learning of motion estimation and segmentation for cardiac MR image sequences. In: Lecture notes in computer science (including subseries lecture notes in artificial intelligence and lecture notes in bioinformatics), vol. 11071 LNCS. Springer; 2018. p. 472–80.
62. Qin C, Schlemper J, Duan J, Seegoolam G, Price A, Hajnal J, Rueckert D. k-t next: dynamic MR image reconstruction exploiting spatio-temporal correlations. In: Shen D, Liu T, Peters TM, Staib LH, Essert C, Zhou S, Yap P-T, Khan A, editors. Medical image computing and computer assisted intervention – MICCAI 2019. Cham: Springer International Publishing; 2019. p. 505–13.
63. Qin C, Duan J, Hammernik K, Schlemper J, Küstner T, Botnar R, Prieto C, Price AN, Hajnal JV, Rueckert D. Complementary time-frequency domain networks for dynamic parallel MR image reconstruction. Magn Reson Med. 2021;86(6):3274–91.
64. Ronneberger O, Fischer P, Brox T. U-net: convolutional networks for biomedical image segmentation. In: International conference on medical image computing and computer assisted intervention; 2015. p. 234–41.
65. Roth S, Black MJ. Fields of experts. Int J Comput Vis. 2009;82(2):205–29.
66. Sandino CM, Cheng JY. Deep convolutional neural networks for accelerated dynamic magnetic resonance imaging. In: Stanford University CS231N, course project.
67. Sandino CM, Cheng JY, Chen F, Mardani M, Pauly JM, Vasanawala SS. Compressed sensing: from research to clinical practice with deep neural networks: shortening scan times for magnetic resonance imaging. IEEE Signal Process Mag. 2020;37(1):117–27.
68. Schlemper J, Caballero J, Hajnal JV, Price AN, Rueckert D. A deep Cascade of convolutional neural networks for dynamic MR image reconstruction. IEEE Trans Med Imaging. 2018;37(2):491–503.
69. Seegoolam G, Schlemper J, Qin C, Price A, Hajnal J, Rueckert D. Exploiting motion for deep learning reconstruction of extremely-undersampled dynamic MRI. In: Shen D, Liu T, Peters TM, Staib LH, Essert C, Zhou S, Yap P-T, Khan A, editors. Medical image computing and computer assisted intervention – MICCAI 2019. Cham: Springer International Publishing; 2019. p. 704–12.
70. Seitzer M, Yang G, Schlemper J, Oktay O, Würfl T, Christlein V, Wong T, Mohiaddin R, Firmin D, Keegan J, Rueckert D, Maier A. Adversarial and perceptual refinement for compressed sensing MRI reconstruction. In: Machine learning for medical image reconstruction. Cham: Springer International Publishing; 2018.
71. Shen D, Ghosh S, Haji-Valizadeh H, Pathrose A, Schiffers F, Lee DC, Freed BH, Markl M, Cossairt OS, Katsaggelos AK, Kim D. Rapid reconstruction of highly undersampled, non-Cartesian real-time cine k-space data using a perceptual complex neural network (PCNN). NMR Biomed. 2021;34(1):e4405.
72. Steeden JA, Quail M, Gotschy A, Mortensen KH, Hauptmann A, Arridge S, Jones R, Muthurangu V. Rapid whole-heart CMR with single volume super-resolution. J Cardiovasc Magn Reson. 2020;22(1):56.
73. Sudarski S, Henzler T, Haubenreisser H, Dösch C, Zenge MO, Schmidt M, Nadar MS, Borggrefe M, Schoenberg SO, Papavassiliu T. Free-breathing sparse sampling cine MR imaging with iterative reconstruction for the assessment of left ventricular function and mass at 3.0 T. Radiology. 2017;282(1):74–83.
74. Usman M, Prieto C, Schaeffter T, Batchelor PG. k-t Group sparse: a method for accelerating dynamic MRI. Magn Reson Med. 2011;66(4):1163–76.
75. Vincenti G, Monney P, Chaptinel J, Rutz T, Coppo S, Zenge MO, Schmidt M, Nadar MS, Piccini D, Chèvre P, Stuber M, Schwitter J. Compressed sensing single-breath-hold CMR for fast quantification of LV function, volumes, and mass. JACC Cardiovasc Imaging. 2014;7(9):882–92.
76. Wang Z, Simoncelli EP, Bovik AC. Multi-scale structural similarity for image quality assessment. In: IEEE Asilomar conference on signals, systems and computers, vol. 2. Pacific Grove: IEEE; 2003. p. 9–13.
77. Yaman B, Hosseini SAH, Moeller S, Ellermann J, Ugurbil K, Akcakaya M. Self-supervised learning of physics-guided reconstruction neural networks without fully-sampled reference data. Magn Reson Med. 2020;84(6):3172–91.
78. Yaman B, Hosseini SAH, Moeller S, Ellermann J, Uğurbil K, Akçakaya M. Ground-truth free multi-mask self-supervised physics-guided deep learning in highly accelerated MRI. In: 2021 IEEE 18th international symposium on biomedical imaging (ISBI). Nice: IEEE; 2021.
79. Yaman B, Shenoy C, Deng Z, Moeller S, El-Rewaidy H, Nezafat R, Akçakaya M. Self-supervised physics-guided deep learning reconstruction for high-resolution 3D LGE CMR. In: 2021 IEEE 18th international symposium on biomedical imaging (ISBI). IEEE; 2021.
80. Yang Y, Kramer CM, Shaw PW, Meyer CH, Salerno M. First-pass myocardial perfusion imaging with whole-heart coverage using L1-SPIRiT accelerated variable density spiral trajectories. Magn Reson Med. 2016;76(5):1375–87.
81. Yang G, Yu S, Dong H, Slabaugh G, Dragotti PL, Ye X, Liu F, Arridge S, Keegan J, Guo Y, Firmin D. DAGAN: deep de-aliasing generative adversarial networks for fast compressed sensing MRI reconstruction. IEEE Trans Med Imaging. 2017;37(6):1310–21.

82. Yang Y, Sun J, Li H, Xu Z. ADMM-net: a deep learning approach for compressive sensing MRI. Adv Neural Inf Proces Syst. 2016. https://papers.nips.cc/paper/2016/hash/1679091c5a880faf6fb5e6087eb1b2dc-Abstract.html.
83. Zhang Y, Zhang W, Zhang Q, Yang J, Chen X, Zhao S. CMR motion artifact correction using generative adversarial nets. CoRR. abs/1902.11121. 2019.
84. Zhao H, Gallo O, Frosio I, Kautz J. Loss functions for image restoration with neural networks. IEEE Trans Comput Imaging. 2016;3(1):47–57.
85. Zhu B, Liu JZ, Cauley SF, Rosen BR, Rosen MS. Image reconstruction by domain-transform manifold learning. Nature. 2018;555(7697):487–92.

Artificial Intelligence-Based Image Reconstruction in Cardiac Magnetic Resonance

14

Chen Qin and Daniel Rueckert

Introduction

Artificial intelligence (AI) and machine learning (ML), but in particular deep learning (DL), have been active and fast-moving areas of research in the field of medical imaging. These techniques have great potential for transforming clinical practice in the coming years [38]. DL-based methods have also led to significant improvement across various applications in cardiac imaging, such as cardiac image segmentation [3, 9], myocardial motion tracking [11, 41, 46] and image enhancement [34, 35]. Cardiac image reconstruction, as one of the key steps in cardiac imaging workflow, has also witnessed the important growth of the use of DL algorithms though the development of which is relatively new in comparison to other cardiac imaging applications.

In cardiac imaging, cardiac magnetic resonance (CMR) imaging is one of the most useful and important imaging modalities for the non-invasive assessment of morphology and function of the heart. It provides images with excellent soft tissue contrast as well as high spatial and temporal resolution and is therefore widely used for the assessment of cardiovascular diseases. However, the acquisition speed of CMR is limited, which is on account of the need of obtaining images of high temporal and spatial resolution, as well as the cardiac- and respiratory-induced motion that needs to be taken into consideration during the acquisition process [7].

To improve and accelerate the CMR acquisition process, several major advances have been made over the last few decades. Parallel imaging (PI) [15, 40, 54] is one of the techniques frequently used to accelerate the MR acquisition. In PI, the data is acquired using an array of multiple independent receiver coils, allowing for a reduction in the number of phase-encoding steps and enabling the combination of undersampled data from each receiver coil given the additional coil information. Particularly, for dynamic CMR imaging where substantial correlations in k-space and time exist, most PI-based imaging strategies have been designed to acquire part of the desired $k-t$ measurements and then reconstruct images by exploiting spatio-temporal redundancies in combination with coil sensitivity information [6, 20, 24]. Undersampled image reconstruction approaches such as compressed sensing (CS) have also been proposed for CMR image reconstruction. CS-based methods [30, 59] exploit signal sparsity with some sparse transforms such as finite differences or wavelet operators and recover original image from undersampled k-space data using non-linear reconstructions. For dynamic CMR image reconstruction, a common practice for CS-based approaches is to effectively exploit the spatio-temporal redundancies via enforcing the signal sparsity in spatio-temporal or its transform domain against the consistency of the undersampled acquired data, such as some state-of-the-art $k-t$ methods [23, 31, 37]. Combination of CS with low-rank Schemes [29, 36], spatio-temporal partial separability [61] and patch-based regularisation framework [33, 60] have also been proposed to exploit the spatio-temporal correlations or geometric similarities for the dynamic CMR image reconstruction.

Though CS-based methods have shown great potential for accelerated CMR imaging, they often impose strong assumptions on the data and require non-trivial manual adjustments of hyperparameters depending on the application. In addition, reconstruction speed of these methods is often slow due to the iterative optimisation used, and in the context of dynamic CMR imaging, the additional time domain further increases the computational demand. To enable progress beyond the limitations of conventional CS-based reconstruction methods,

C. Qin, B.Eng, MSc,PhD
Institute for Digital Communications, School of Engineering, University of Edinburgh, Edinburgh, UK
e-mail: Chen.Qin@ed.ac.uk

D. Rueckert, PhD (✉)
Department of Computing, Imperial College London, London, UK

Klinikum rechts der Isar, Technical University of Munich, Munich, Germany
e-mail: d.rueckert@imperial.ac.uk

C. N. De Cecco et al. (eds.), *Artificial Intelligence in Cardiothoracic Imaging*, Contemporary Medical Imaging,
https://doi.org/10.1007/978-3-030-92087-6_14

DL approaches have been proposed for CMR image reconstruction. These DL solutions can be roughly categorised as image post-processing techniques, model-driven image reconstruction methods or *k*-space interpolation approaches. Most of these approaches typically rely on large databases of MR scans as training data to exploit the prior knowledge. DL approaches have shown great performance in achieving high image reconstruction quality with extremely fast reconstruction speed, which is promising to further accelerate CMR acquisition as well as to improve the reconstruction.

In this chapter, we will first briefly introduce the problem formulation of CMR image reconstruction as an inverse problem, and then we will discuss the recent advances in DL for CMR image reconstruction with a major focus on supervised learning. Finally, current limitations, challenges and opportunities of DL for CMR reconstruction will be discussed.

Problem Formulation for Image Reconstruction

A general forward model for the MR imaging process can be formulated as

$$\mathbf{y} = \mathbf{E}\mathbf{x} + \mathbf{n}, \tag{14.1}$$

where $\mathbf{x} \in \mathbb{C}^{N_x}$ denotes the complex-valued MR images to be recovered, $\mathbf{y} \in \mathbb{C}^{N_y}$ represents the undersampled *k*-space measurements corrupted by additive Gaussian noise $\mathbf{n} \in \mathbb{C}^{N_y}$ and $\mathbf{E}: \mathbb{C}^{N_x} \to \mathbb{C}^{N_y}$ is a linear forward operator which describes the encoding process modelling the MR physics. Here, N_x and N_y define the dimensions of the reconstruction $\mathbf{x}$ and the *k*-space data $\mathbf{y}$ ($N_y \ll N_x$ in the undersampling scenario), and $\mathbf{E}$ includes the coil sensitivity maps (if available), Fourier transform as well as the undersampling mask according to the underlying multi-coil or single-coil setting. In dynamic CMR imaging, the measurements $\mathbf{y}$ are acquired in $k - t$ space with an additional temporal dimension NT, and $\mathbf{x}$ is the reconstructed image sequence.

Reconstructing image $\mathbf{x}$ from measurements $\mathbf{y}$ is an ill-posed inverse problem. To ensure that there exists a solution that is unique and plausible, the reconstruction problem is commonly formulated as a regularised optimisation problem of the form:

$$\hat{\mathbf{x}} = \operatorname{argmin}_{\mathbf{x}} \ \mathcal{R}(\mathbf{x}) + \lambda \| \mathbf{y} - \mathbf{E}\mathbf{x} \|_2^2 . \tag{14.2}$$

Here, R expresses the regularisation terms that act on $\mathbf{x}$, and $\hat{\mathbf{x}}$ is recovered via enforcing the regularisation against consistency with the acquired undersampled *k*-space data. For CS-based approaches, the regularisation terms R are often employed in some specific transform domain with sparse representations: Common choices are wavelet transforms [30] or total variation [5]. For low-rank-based methods, global or local low-rankness of the dynamic images is exploited via regularising the rank or nuclear norm of $\mathbf{x}$ to estimate the missing samples. Here, the model weight λ allows the adjustment of data fidelity based on the noise level of the acquired measurements $\mathbf{y}$.

To solve the inverse problem formulated as Eq. 14.2, various optimisation schemes can be employed [59], such as alternating directional method of multiplier (ADMM) [57], split Bregman iteration [13] and primal-dual algorithm [8]. A common practice to optimise Eq. 14.2 is to use variable splitting techniques [48], where an auxiliary variable $\mathbf{z}$ with the constraint $\mathbf{z} = \mathbf{x}$ is introduced to decouple the regularisation term from the data fidelity term. This reformulates Eq. 14.2 to minimise the following cost function via the penalty method:

$$\operatorname{argmin}_{\mathbf{x},\mathbf{z}} \ \mathcal{R}(\mathbf{z}) + \lambda \| \mathbf{y} - \mathbf{E}\mathbf{x} \|_2^2 + \mu \| \mathbf{x} - \mathbf{z} \|_2^2 . \tag{14.3}$$

Here, μ is a penalty parameter. By applying alternating minimisation over $\mathbf{x}$ and $\mathbf{z}$, Eq. 14.3 can be solved via the following iterative procedures:

$$\mathbf{z}^{(i+1)} = \operatorname{argmin}_{\mathbf{z}} \ \mathcal{R}(\mathbf{z}) + \mu \| \mathbf{x}^{(i)} - \mathbf{z} \|_2^2 \tag{14.4a}$$

$$\mathbf{x}^{(i+1)} = \operatorname{argmin}_{\mathbf{x}} \ \lambda \| \mathbf{y} - \mathbf{E}\mathbf{x} \|_2^2 + \mu \| \mathbf{x} - \mathbf{z}^{(i+1)} \|_2^2, \tag{14.4b}$$

where $\mathbf{x}^{(0)}$ is commonly a zero-filled reconstruction used as an initialisation, and $\mathbf{z}$ can be seen as an intermediate state of the optimisation process. For MRI reconstruction, Eq. 14.4b is often regarded as a data consistency (DC) step.

Deep Learning for CMR Image Reconstruction

Deep learning approaches have gained popularity for MRI reconstruction in recent years due to their excellent capabilities in reconstructing high-quality images at extremely fast reconstruction speeds. For CMR image reconstruction, most of the DL methods can be generally categorised into three main groups: (1) image reconstruction via DL-based image post-processing, (2) model-driven unrolled DL for iterative reconstruction and (3) *k*-space-based interpolation. Schematic illustrations of these DL techniques for CMR image reconstruction are shown in Fig. 14.1.

CMR Reconstruction Via DL-Based Image Post-Processing

The first group of methods for CMR reconstruction relies on image post-processing techniques for enhancement in the image domain. These approaches learn an end-to-end mapping from the zero-filled reconstructions to the fully sampled

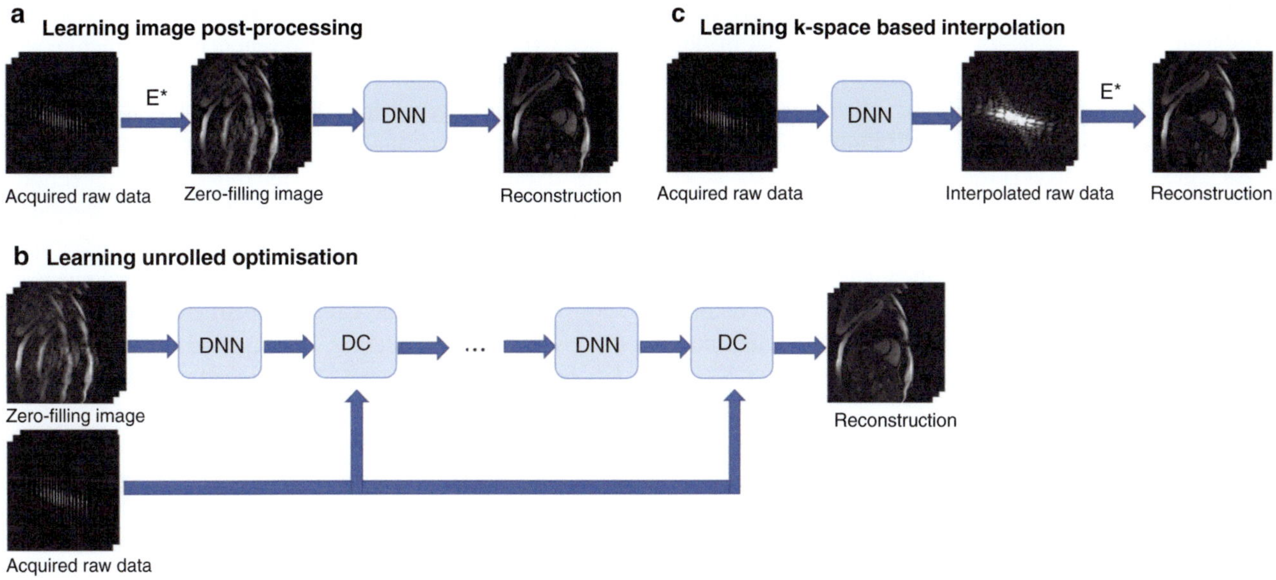

Fig. 14.1 Illustration of different types of DL-based approaches for CMR image reconstruction. (**a**) Learning image post-processing for CMR image reconstruction. (**b**) Learning unrolled optimisation for model-driven iterative reconstruction. (**c**) DL for k-space-based CMR reconstruction. DNN deep neural networks, DC data consistency

reference image without any requirement for prior knowledge about the image acquisition process. For instance, U-net architectures are commonly used for the CMR image post-processing to reduce noise-like image artefacts [19, 26]. They receive inputs in form of reconstructed, undersampled CMR sequences and learn to de-alias the images via multi-scale downsampling and synthesis paths with skip connections. To enforce temporal consistency between frames of cardiac cine sequences, the U-net can be equipped with either 3D convolutions to perform on the entire image sequences ($x - y - t$) [19] or 2D convolutions on the 2D spatio-temporal domain ($x - t$) for more efficient training [26]. These models [19, 26] showed better image quality and faster reconstruction speed recovered from undersampled 2D golden-angle radial cine CMR when compared to CS image reconstruction techniques.

Since these methods solely work on information from the initial zero-filling image data and information extracted from training samples, they can also be classified as purely data-driven approaches. Though these methods are simple and efficient in reconstructing images, one significant drawback is that they cannot guarantee the consistency of the reconstructed image with respect to the measured *k*-space data. This limits their performance in comparison to the model-driven approaches which will be discussed in the following.

Model-Driven DL for CMR Reconstruction

Another type of approaches for CMR image reconstruction are model-driven DL techniques based on unrolled schemes inspired by conventional iterative CS reconstruction, which also represents the majority of the work in this field. These methods utilise the physical domain knowledge with the incorporation of raw *k*-space data, combining the power of data-driven learning with the physics-derived model-based framework (Eq. 14.2). In contrast to CS-based methods where regularisation terms need to be specified manually beforehand, DL-based reconstruction approaches implicitly learn such prior information and regularisation from the routinely performed MR data.

In detail, model-driven DL-based solutions [1, 10, 16, 43, 49, 50] propose to learn the unrolled optimisation and embed the iterative reconstruction process in a learning setting based on Eq. 14.4. Specifically, Eq. 14.4a is commonly modelled via leveraging deep neural networks (DNNs) to learn the prior knowledge from the training data itself [1, 43, 50]. This allows the model to fully exploit the information contained in the population data for the regularisation and alleviates the need to explicitly predefine them based on certain assumptions. Accordingly, Eq. 14.4b can be derived as close-form solutions, which then can be embedded as DC layers in DNNs via exact update for DC [10, 43, 50] or through numerical optimisation such as conjugate gradient updates [1, 4, 32], depending on the way to solve Eq. 14.4b. Therefore, model-driven approaches based on Eq. 14.4 can be generally represented as the compact form:

$$\mathbf{z}^{(i+1)} = \mathrm{DNN}\left(\mathbf{x}^{(i)}\right), \tag{14.5a}$$

$$\mathbf{x}^{(i+1)} = \mathrm{DC}\left(\mathbf{z}^{(i+1)}; \mathbf{y}, \mathbf{E}, \lambda, \mu\right), \tag{14.5b}$$

which alternates the reconstruction process between image de-aliasing and DC steps for a predefined number of iterations. This represents the most commonly used scheme for DL-based CMR reconstruction. For other types of model-driven approaches (including applications not limited to CMR), please refer to [17] for details.

Based on types of deep-learned regularisation priors, we generally group these unrolled DL techniques into two classes: image-domain-regularisation and complementary-regularisation approaches. More specific network architectures and applied scenarios in cardiac imaging are introduced hereafter.

Learning Unrolled Optimisation with Image-Domain Regularisation

Unrolled Convolutional Neural Networks

Typical approaches for constructing Eq. 14.5a are to employ convolutional neural networks (CNNs) as regularisation operators in image domain. State-of-the-art methods such as DC-CNN [49, 50] and MoDL [1, 4] used five layers of CNN with a residual connection for 10 iterations. To exploit spatio-temporal redundancies, Schlemper et al. [50] proposed to incorporate a data sharing (DS) layer in a 3D ($x - y - t$) CNN cascade network, which allows to utilise similar information contained in neighbouring k-space samples. The method was performed on retrospectively undersampled single-coil cardiac cine MR images, where the single-coil setting enables solution to Eq. 14.4b to be analytically computed as an exact update for DC step. For multi-coil acquisition, variational network (VN) [16] proposed to embed a combined PI and CS reconstruction in a DL-based unrolled gradient descent scheme. An extension of it has also been applied for dynamic cine CMR via learning the complex spatio-temporal convolutions corresponding to spatio-temporal total variation regularisation [18]. Beyond applications on 2D dynamic cine CMR, Fuin et al. [12] has extended VN to a multiscale VN architecture for fast reconstruction of undersampled motion-compensated free-breathing whole-heart 3D ($x - y - z$) CMRA, and CINENet [27] was introduced for highly prospectively undersampled 3D Cartesian cardiac cine data via exploiting spatio-temporal redundancies by cascaded and complex-valued (3 + 1)D spatial and temporal convolutions.

Unrolled Convolutional Recurrent Neural Networks

Another type of representative approach for learning the deep priors in Eq. 14.5a is via recurrent architectures. Recurrent neural networks (RNNs) are known to be effective in processing sequential information with an internal state acting as "memory" and thus have been widely employed for modelling the iterative reconstruction steps [21, 43, 55, 62]. As one of the pioneering works in this direction, CRNN-MRI [43] proposed to embed the iterative optimisation scheme (Eq. 14.4a, b) into a recurrent network structure with hidden-to-hidden connections between each iteration step, which allows effective information propagation along iterations and avoids redundant computations. Furthermore, to fully exploit spatio-temporal redundancies, bidirectional RNNs were also designed to model the sequential dependencies along temporal axis together with recurrence over iteration dimension. An illustrative diagram of the model is shown in Fig. 14.2, where unfolded structures of each layer are given with more details. The method was validated on retrospectively undersampled single-coil cardiac cine MRI, which achieved better and more efficient reconstructions compared to CNN architectures with fewer number of network parameters.

Motion-Compensated Dynamic CMR Reconstruction

Due to the presence of motion patterns in dynamic CMR acquisition, combining motion estimation and motion compensation with model-driven DL-based reconstruction methods has also been explored. End-to-end motion-compensated reconstruction framework [21, 22, 51] commonly consists of DL-based motion estimation components [41] estimating motion information between frames within undersampled MRI sequences [51] or with respect to fully sampled reference frames [21]. The estimated motion then can be exploited to generate motion-compensated images to be infused into reconstruction process [21, 22] or to propagate k-space data along the full temporal dynamics via data consistency [51] for better reconstruction quality. These approaches have been validated on single-coil 2D cardiac cine MRI data with retrospective undersampling, and incorporating motion information into reconstruction process has shown to be effective in reconstructing aggressively accelerated data [51].

Learning Unrolled Optimisation with Complementary Regularisation

Similar to conventional CS-based approaches, model-driven DL for CMR reconstruction can also be learned with complementary regularisation. Typical $k - t$ methods [23, 31, 37] exploit signal sparsity and regularise the data in the combined spatial and temporal Fourier ($x - f$) domain for dynamic CMR reconstruction. This can also be similarly leveraged with DL by learning deep priors in complementary image and $x - f$ spaces. Qin et al. [44] proposed the $k - t$ NEXT approach along this direction, which alternates the learned DL-based regularisation between both image and $x - f$ domains in an iterative fashion for single-coil dynamic CMR reconstruction. Comparison results of $k - t$ NEXT against other model-driven DL approaches and CS-based method are shown in Fig. 14.3, where it can be seen that exploiting complementary domain knowledge can achieve

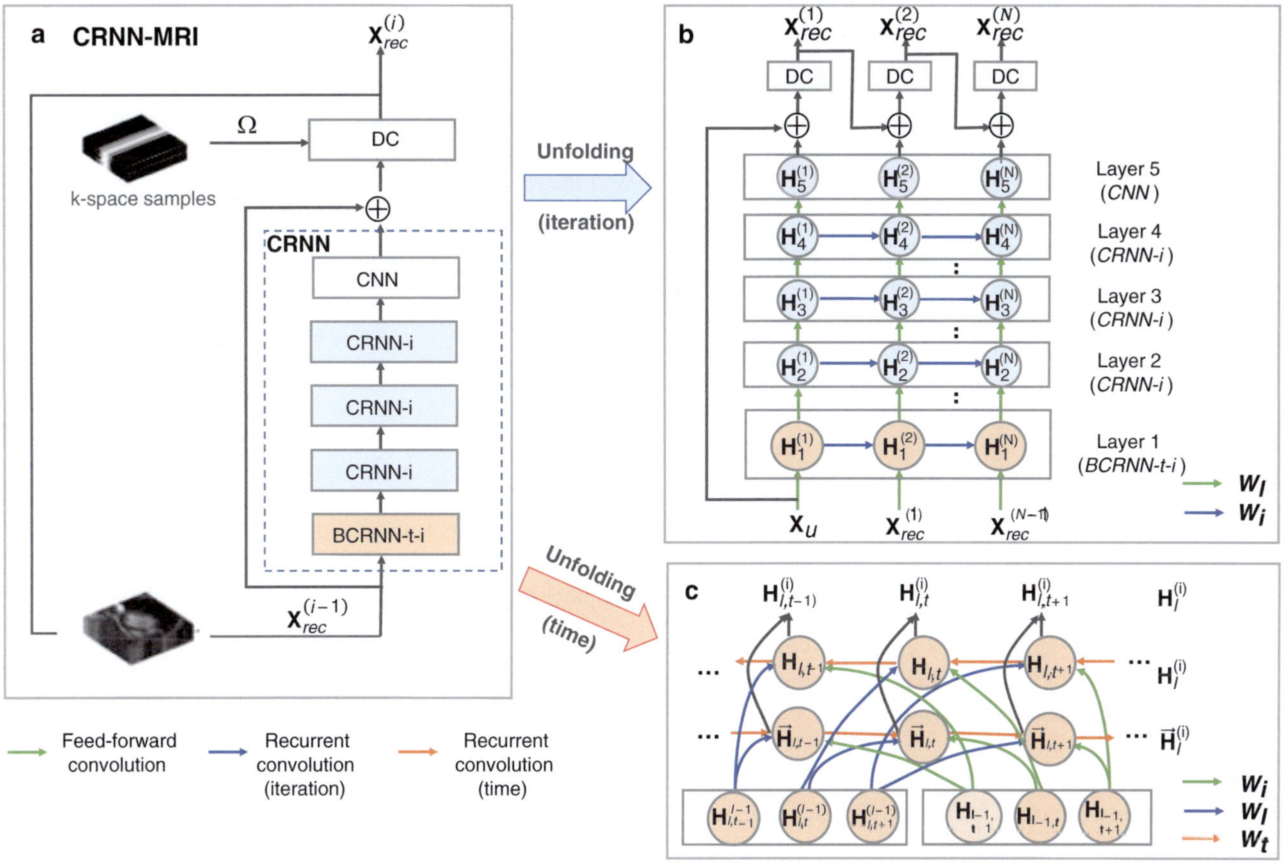

Fig. 14.2 (**a**) Architecture of CRNN-MRI network [43] for CMR image reconstruction. (**b**) The structure of CRNN-MRI when unfolded over iterative reconstruction steps. (**c**) The structure of bidirectional RNN layer (BCRNN-t-i) when unfolded over the time sequence. The method is able to jointly exploit spatio-temporal redundancies and iteration dependencies in a recurrent fashion with a single framework

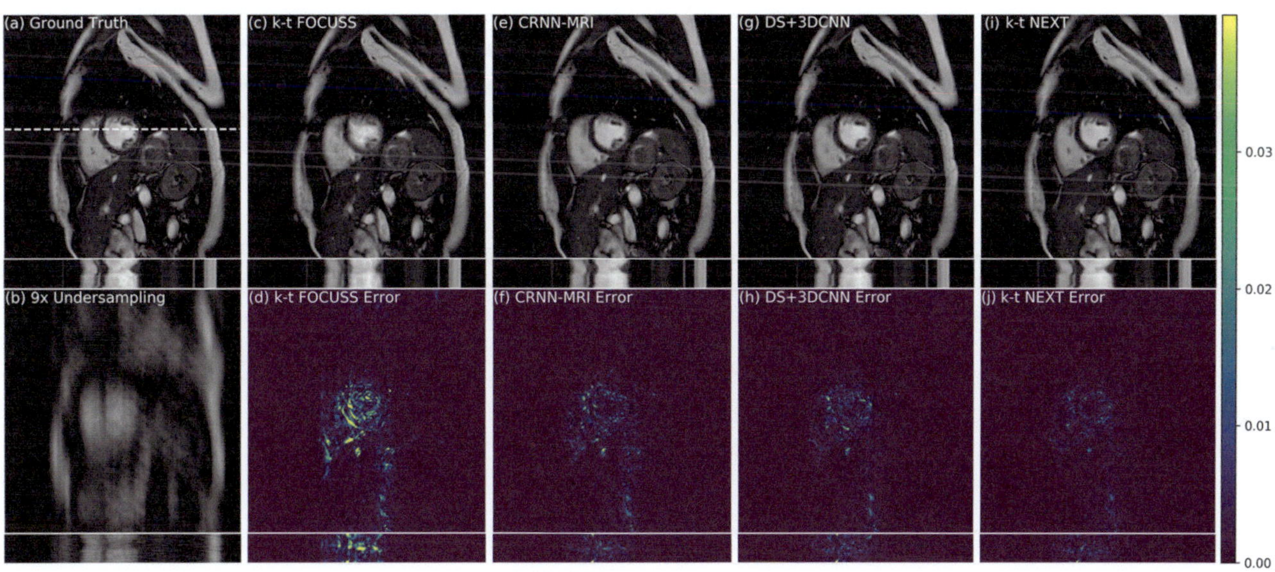

Fig. 14.3 CMR image reconstruction for nine-fold accelerated single-coil data along with their error maps. (**a**) Fully sampled reference. (**b**) 9× undersampled image. (**c**, **d**) $k-t$ FOCUSS [23]. (**e**, **f**) CRNN-MRI [43]. (**g**, **h**) DS + 3DCNN [50]. (**i**, **j**) $k-t$ NEXT [44]. Model-driven DL approaches outperform CS-based $k-t$ FOCUSS. Learning with complementary regularisation ($k-t$ NEXT) achieves better reconstruction than methods with single domain regularisation

better performance than single image-domain reconstructions, with better preservation of fine details and sharp structures. An extension of it has also been investigated for multi-coil dynamic CMR data with a complementary time-frequency domain network based on variable splitting technique in PI setting [42]. In addition to the $x-f$ regularisation, MoDL-SToRM [4] combines MoDL reconstruction [1] along with a complementary image regularisation penalty, i.e., SmooThness regularisation on manifolds (SToRM) prior [39], to recover free-breathing cardiac cine MR images. Similarly, this framework alternates between a learned regularisation of the image using CNN, an analytically defined SToRM prior and a conjugate gradient DC step for multi-channel measurements. Besides, the complementary information can also be exploited in both k-space and image space, and this has been shown in [56] where the frequency domain network and image-domain network were combined and trained with a multi-supervised technique for the single-coil 2D cardiac cine MR image reconstruction. All these above methods have demonstrated the benefits of combining complementary regularisation, achieving better performance than single image-domain approaches.

DL for K-Space-Based CMR Reconstruction

An alternative class of techniques for MRI reconstruction is based on k-space interpolation. This is represented by methods such as GRAPPA (generalised autocalibrating partially parallel acquisitions) [15] which recovers the missing data directly in k-space by employing autocalibrating signal (ACS) estimated for each subject. Similar to this, a CNN-based approach has also been proposed to improve the k-space interpolation for PI-based MRI reconstruction. The RAKI (robust artificial-neural-networks for k-space interpolation) reconstruction approach [2] enables non-linear estimation of missing k-space lines from acquired multi-coil data using CNNs trained on ACS data for k-space interpolation. This has been applied for reconstruction of retrospectively undersampled myocardial 2D T1 mapping data with improved noise resilience. Note that RAKI is a scan-specific and database-free DL approach, which does not require training datasets but relies on ACS data and separate CNN training for each scan.

Network Learning

In general, most of the aforementioned supervised DL methods rely on large databases of training data to learn the population-based prior information and the mapping between pairs of undersampled data and reference MRI scans. Due to the limited availability of the acquired images, most approaches consider retrospectively simulating the undersampled data from fully sampled raw k-space data, which are then used as input and target for DL models during the training process. To train these supervised models, metrics that measure the similarity between the reconstructed image $\mathbf{x}$ and the reference image $\mathbf{x}_{\text{ref}}$ are used as loss functions. One commonly used loss function is the mean-squared error (MSE) which measures the L2 distance between $\mathbf{x}$ and $\mathbf{x}_{\text{ref}}$ in the training set Ω:

$$\mathcal{L}_{\text{mse}}(\theta) = \frac{1}{n_\Omega} \sum_{(\mathbf{x},\mathbf{x}_{\text{ref}})\in\Omega} \left\|\mathbf{x}_{\text{ref}} - \mathbf{x}\right\|_2^2. \tag{14.6}$$

Here, θ is the network parameters, and n_Ω is the number of training samples. Though the MSE metric is easy to optimise, it often tends to generate blurry reconstructions due to the averaging effect. To remedy this, the L1 distance or structural similarity index measure (SSIM) are also often employed as the loss function to improve upon the sharpness of structures, such that:

$$\mathcal{L}_{\text{ssim}}(\theta) = \frac{1}{n_\Omega} \sum_{(\mathbf{x},\mathbf{x}_{\text{ref}})\in\Omega} \left(1 - \text{SSIM}\left(\mathbf{x},\mathbf{x}_{\text{ref}}\right)\right). \tag{14.7}$$

Additionally, adversarial loss functions [14] have also gained in popularity for reconstructing images with improved perceptual quality. Such a loss function has also been used for MRI reconstruction [47, 52, 58]. The adversarial approach works by learning a discriminator to discriminate whether a given sample is from a reconstruction network (generator) or from the reference distribution. The adversarial loss has shown to be effective in generating images with sharper textures and finer details compared to MSE. However, it is known to be unstable in training and is also prone to hallucinate unrealistic artefacts. This is problematic for MRI reconstruction in preserving the data fidelity and anatomical structures. Therefore, the adversarial loss is often combined with the content losses such as MSE and L1 norm to inform the reconstruction with image contents. An alternative way to balance the data fidelity and perceptual quality uses deep network interpolation [45] where these two effects can be trade off with an interpolation coefficient in parameter space. Finally, perceptual loss terms [28] have also been introduced to improve the reconstruction details based on feature representations of the VGG network [53], and this has also been applied for CMR reconstruction [52].

Discussion

Most of the current research shows exciting and promising developments of AI algorithms in image reconstruction for cardiac imaging. These are mostly attributed to their strong ability in recovering high-quality images with fast reconstruction speed, which therefore can further increase the acceleration capability. Current DL-based approaches, especially models learning an unrolled optimisation [4, 12, 27, 43, 50, 56], have shown to outperform conventional CS-based methods for CMR reconstruction, and their application in PI also indicates their potentiality in facilitating fast single-breath-hold 2D cardiac cine imaging. Though promising results have been achieved in recent developments, there are still some challenges yet to be solved for their use in clinical applications. One of the limitations of current studies for CMR image reconstruction is their limited validation in clinical practice. Most of the existing DL-based works focus on reconstructing images with retrospectively undersampling based on models trained on simulated undersampled data. Though such retrospective study can provide useful insights and initial validation of employed methods, it still remains unclear how well these methods can perform on prospectively undersampled data, which is a more clinically practical scenario. In addition, majority of current DL research for dynamic CMR image reconstruction works on simulated single-coil acquisition setting, whereas only a handful of works propose to address the more practical and commonly used multi-coil acquisitions. This is mainly due to the increased computational and model complexities introduced by the multi-coil data as well as the extra temporal dimension. Thus, efficient DL models for PI-based dynamic CMR image reconstruction are also highly desirable. Besides, as most work investigates reconstruction with Cartesian undersampling patterns, efforts towards non-uniform undersampling strategies such as radial sampling and golden angle sampling are also necessary, which represent the commonly used sampling strategies in acceleration of 2D cardiac MR imaging in practice.

Another issue with DL-based CMR image reconstruction methods is their generalisation ability when presented with data that looks different to the data used in training. It is not yet systematically evaluated how well DL models trained on MR scans with specific scanners, pulse sequences, imaging resolutions or acceleration factors can generalise to other MR scans with different acquisition parameters. Furthermore, the generalisation ability of these models on unseen pathologies still needs to be explored in detail. For instance, it will be interesting and useful to see if models trained on healthy cohorts can faithfully recover the pathological patterns of patients with cardiovascular diseases. Though a recent study [42] has made efforts towards this direction and shows promising generalisation potential of the DL-based approach, more thorough and systematic evaluations are still needed for a wider validation on this aspect including radiologists' evaluation to improve their translation into clinical practice.

Additionally, in comparison to conventional optimisation-based CS methods, training DL models normally requires large databases of training data. However, such large training database is not available for most of the CMR image reconstruction studies, and currently, most existing works rely on a small set of training samples with a great deal of data augmentations to remedy this. Though such strategy has shown to be effective, it could still limit the performance potential of such DL models as well as their validations due to the limited amount of available data. The FastMRI datasets [25] provide large databases of knee (~1000) and brain (~7000) MR images together with the corresponding k-space data, which brings a great opportunity for accelerating MR imaging with AI. However, such a large archive of images and their corresponding raw k-space data is still lacking in cardiac imaging, and efforts towards building a large CMR database will be helpful to further push the developments of the use of AI in this field. Besides, methods beyond supervised learning such as self-supervised learning and unsupervised learning will also be interesting to be explored to reduce the expensive need of fully sampled reference data for training, and models in transfer learning and domain adaptation can also be investigated to effectively exploit the large amount of available data in other domains for CMR reconstruction.

Conclusion

Based on recent advancements in AI technology, the field of cardiac image reconstruction also sees its exciting developments with the use of AI algorithms in recent years. This chapter provides an overview of these developments with a major focus on introducing the existing popular DL-based approaches for CMR image reconstruction as well as the current challenges. Though DL approaches for CMR image reconstruction are not yet established for clinical applicability and will require more thorough evaluation, they have already shown a huge potential for accelerating and improving the CMR image acquisition and reconstruction workflow.

References

1. Aggarwal HK, Mani MP, Jacob M. MoDL: model-based deep learning architecture for inverse problems. IEEE Trans Med Imaging. 2018;38(2):394–405.
2. Akçakaya M, Moeller S, Weingärtner S, Uğurbil K. Scan-specific robust artificial-neural-networks for k-space interpolation (RAKI) reconstruction: database-free deep learning for fast imaging. Magn Reson Med. 2019;81(1):439–53.
3. Bai W, Sinclair M, Tarroni G, Oktay O, Rajchl M, Vaillant G, Lee AM, Aung N, Lukaschuk E, Sanghvi MM, et al. Automated cardiovascular magnetic resonance image analysis with fully convolutional networks. J Cardiovasc Magn Reson. 2018;20(1):65.

4. Biswas S, Aggarwal HK, Jacob M. Dynamic MRI using model-based deep learning and SToRM priors: MoDL-SToRM. Magn Reson Med. 2019;82(1):485–94.
5. Block KT, Uecker M, Frahm J. Undersampled radial MRI with multiple coils. Iterative image reconstruction using a total variation constraint. Magn Reson Med. 2007;57(6):1086–98.
6. Breuer FA, Kellman P, Griswold MA, Jakob PM. Dynamic autocalibrated parallel imaging using temporal GRAPPA (TGRAPPA). Magn Reson Med. 2005;53(4):981–5.
7. Bustin A, Fuin N, Botnar RM, Prieto C. From compressed-sensing to artificial intelligence-based cardiac MRI reconstruction. Front Cardiovasc Med. 2020;7:17.
8. Chambolle A, Pock T. A first-order primal-dual algorithm for convex problems with applications to imaging. J Math Imaging Vis. 2011;40(1):120–45.
9. Chen C, Qin C, Qiu H, Tarroni G, Duan J, Bai W, Rueckert D. Deep learning for cardiac image segmentation: a review. Front Cardiovasc Med. 2020;7:25.
10. Duan J, Schlemper J, Qin C, Ouyang C, Bai W, Biffi C, Bello G, Statton B, O'Regan DP, Rueckert D. VS-net: variable splitting network for accelerated parallel MRI reconstruction. In: International conference on medical image computing and computer-assisted intervention. Cham: Springer; 2019. p. 713–22.
11. Duchateau N, King AP, De Craene M. Machine learning approaches for myocardial motion and deformation analysis. Front Cardiovasc Med. 2020;6:190.
12. Fuin N, Bustin A, Kuestner T, Botnar R, Prieto C. A variational neural network for accelerating free-breathing whole-heart coronary MR angiography. In: Proc. ISMRM 27th Annu. Meeting exhibit; 2019. p. 11–6.
13. Goldstein T, Osher S. The split Bregman method for L1-regularized problems. SIAM J Imag Sci. 2009;2(2):323–43.
14. Goodfellow I, Pouget-Abadie J, Mirza M, Xu B, Warde-Farley D, Ozair S, Courville A, Bengio Y. Generative adversarial nets. In: Advances in neural information processing systems; 2014. p. 2672–80.
15. Griswold MA, Jakob PM, Heidemann RM, Nittka M, Jellus V, Wang J, Kiefer B, Haase A. Generalized autocalibrating partially parallel acquisitions (GRAPPA). Magn Reson Med. 2002;47(6):1202–10.
16. Hammernik K, Klatzer T, Kobler E, Recht MP, Sodickson DK, Pock T, Knoll F. Learning a variational network for reconstruction of accelerated MRI data. Magn Reson Med. 2018;79(6):3055–71.
17. Hammernik K, Knoll F. Machine learning for image reconstruction. In: Handbook of medical image computing and computer assisted intervention. Elsevier; 2020. p. 25–64.
18. Hammernik K, Schloegl M, Kobler E, Stollberger R, Pock T. Dynamic multicoil reconstruction using variational networks. In: Proc. ISMRM 27th Annu. Meeting exhibit; 2019. p. 4656.
19. Hauptmann A, Arridge S, Lucka F, Muthurangu V, Steeden JA. Real-time cardiovascular MR with spatio-temporal artifact suppression using deep learning–proof of concept in congenital heart disease. Magn Reson Med. 2019;81(2):1143–56.
20. Huang F, Akao J, Vijayakumar S, Duensing GR, Limkeman M. k-t GRAPPA: a k-space implementation for dynamic MRI with high reduction factor. Magn Reson Med. 2005;54(5):1172–84.
21. Huang Q, Xian Y, Yang D, Qu H, Yi J, Wu P, Metaxas DN. Dynamic MRI reconstruction with end-to-end motion-guided network. Med Image Anal. 2020;68:101901.
22. Huang Q, Yang D, Qu H, Yi J, Wu P, Metaxas D. Dynamic MRI reconstruction with motion-guided network. In: International conference on medical imaging with deep learning. PMLR; 2019. p. 275–84.
23. Jung H, Ye JC, Kim EY. Improved k–t BLAST and k–t SENSE using FOCUSS. Phys Med Biol. 2007;52(11):3201.
24. Kellman P, Epstein FH, McVeigh ER. Adaptive sensitivity encoding incorporating temporal filtering (TSENSE). Magn Reson Med. 2001;45(5):846–52.
25. Knoll F, Zbontar J, Sriram A, Muckley MJ, Bruno M, Defazio A, Parente M, Geras KJ, Katsnelson J, Chandarana H, et al. Fastmri: a publicly available raw k-space and DICOM dataset of knee images for accelerated MR image reconstruction using machine learning. Radiol Artif Intell. 2020;2(1):e190007.
26. Kofler A, Dewey M, Schaeffter T, Wald C, Kolbitsch C. Spatio-temporal deep learning-based undersampling artefact reduction for 2D radial cine MRI with limited training data. IEEE Trans Med Imaging. 2019;39(3):703–17.
27. Küstner T, Fuin N, Hammernik K, Bustin A, Qi H, Hajhosseiny R, Masci PG, Neji R, Rueckert D, Botnar RM, et al. CINENet: deep learning-based 3D cardiac CINE MRI reconstruction with multi-coil complex-valued 4D spatio-temporal convolutions. Sci Rep. 2020;10(1):1–13.
28. Ledig C, Theis L, Huszár F, Caballero J, Cunningham A, Acosta A, Aitken A, Tejani A, Totz J, Wang Z, et al. Photo-realistic single image super-resolution using a generative adversarial network. In: Proceedings of the IEEE conference on computer vision and pattern recognition; 2017. p. 4681–90.
29. Lingala SG, Hu Y, DiBella E, Jacob M. Accelerated dynamic MRI exploiting sparsity and low-rank structure: k-t SLR. IEEE Trans Med Imaging. 2011;30(5):1042–54.
30. Lustig M, Donoho D, Pauly JM. Sparse MRI: the application of compressed sensing for rapid MR imaging. Magn Reson Med. 2007;58(6):1182–95.
31. Lustig M, Santos JM, Donoho DL, Pauly JM. kt SPARSE: high frame rate dynamic MRI exploiting spatio-temporal sparsity. Proc ISMRM 13th Annu Meeting Exhibit. 2006:2420.
32. Mardani M, Gong E, Cheng JY, Vasanawala SS, Zaharchuk G, Xing L, Pauly JM. Deep generative adversarial neural networks for compressive sensing MRI. IEEE Trans Med Imaging. 2018;38(1):167–79.
33. Mohsin YQ, Lingala SG, DiBella E, Jacob M. Accelerated dynamic MRI using patch regularization for implicit motion compensation. Magn Reson Med. 2017;77(3):1238–48.
34. Oktay O, Bai W, Lee M, Guerrero R, Kamnitsas K, Caballero J, de Marvao A, Cook S, O'Regan D, Rueckert D. Multi-input cardiac image super-resolution using convolutional neural networks. In: International conference on medical image computing and computer-assisted intervention. Springer; 2016. p. 246–54.
35. Oktay O, Ferrante E, Kamnitsas K, Heinrich M, Bai W, Caballero J, Cook SA, De Marvao A, Dawes T, O'Regan DP, et al. Anatomically constrained neural networks (ACNNs): application to cardiac image enhancement and segmentation. IEEE Trans Med Imaging. 2017;37(2):384–95.
36. Otazo R, Candès E, Sodickson DK. Low-rank plus sparse matrix decomposition for accelerated dynamic MRI with separation of background and dynamic components. Magn Reson Med. 2015;73(3):1125–36.
37. Otazo R, Kim D, Axel L, Sodickson DK. Combination of compressed sensing and parallel imaging for highly accelerated first-pass cardiac perfusion MRI. Magn Reson Med. 2010;64(3):767–76.
38. Pesapane F, Codari M, Sardanelli F. Artificial intelligence in medical imaging: threat or opportunity? Radiologists again at the forefront of innovation in medicine. Eur Radiol Experiment. 2018;2(1):35.
39. Poddar S, Jacob M. Dynamic MRI using smoothness regularization on manifolds (SToRM). IEEE Trans Med Imaging. 2015;35(4):1106–15.
40. Pruessmann KP, Weiger M, Scheidegger MB, Boesiger P. SENSE: sensitivity encoding for fast MRI. Magn Reson Med. 1999;42(5):952–62.

41. Qin C, Bai W, Schlemper J, Petersen SE, Piechnik SK, Neubauer S, Rueckert D. Joint learning of motion estimation and segmentation for cardiac MR image sequences. In: International conference on medical image computing and computer-assisted intervention. Springer; 2018. p. 472–80.
42. Qin C, Duan J, Hammernik K, Schlemper J, Küstner T, Botnar R, Prieto C, Price AN, Hajnal JV, Rueckert D. Complementary time-frequency domain networks for dynamic parallel MR image reconstruction. Magn Reson Med. 2021;86(6):3274–91.
43. Qin C, Schlemper J, Caballero J, Price AN, Hajnal JV, Rueckert D. Convolutional recurrent neural networks for dynamic MR image reconstruction. IEEE Trans Med Imaging. 2019;38(1):280–90.
44. Qin C, Schlemper J, Duan J, Seegoolam G, Price A, Hajnal J, Rueckert D. K-t NEXT: dynamic MR image reconstruction exploiting spatio-temporal correlations. In: International conference on medical image computing and computer-assisted intervention. Springer; 2019. p. 505–13.
45. Qin C, Schlemper J, Hammernik K, Duan J, Summers RM, Rueckert D. Deep network interpolation for accelerated parallel MR image reconstruction. In: Proc. ISMRM 28th Annu. Meeting exhibit; 2020.
46. Qin C, Wang S, Chen C, Qiu H, Bai W, Rueckert D. Biomechanics-informed neural networks for myocardial motion tracking in MRI. In: International conference on medical image computing and computer-assisted intervention; 2020. p. 296–306.
47. Quan TM, Nguyen-Duc T, Jeong WK. Compressed sensing MRI reconstruction using a generative adversarial network with a cyclic loss. IEEE Trans Med Imaging. 2018;37(6):1488–97.
48. Ramani S, Fessler JA. Parallel MR image reconstruction using augmented Lagrangian methods. IEEE Trans Med Imaging. 2010;30(3):694–706.
49. Schlemper J, Caballero J, Hajnal JV, Price AN, Rueckert D. A deep cascade of convolutional neural networks for MR image reconstruction. In: IPMI. Springer; 2017. p. 647–58.
50. Schlemper J, Caballero J, Hajnal JV, Price AN, Rueckert D. A deep cascade of convolutional neural networks for dynamic MR image reconstruction. IEEE Trans Med Imaging. 2018;37(2):491–503.
51. Seegoolam G, Schlemper J, Qin C, Price A, Hajnal J, Rueckert D. Exploiting motion for deep learning reconstruction of extremely-undersampled dynamic MRI. In: International conference on medical image computing and computer-assisted intervention. Springer; 2019. p. 704–12.
52. Seitzer M, Yang G, Schlemper J, Oktay O, Würfl T, Christlein V, Wong T, Mohiaddin R, Firmin D, Keegan J, et al. Adversarial and perceptual refinement for compressed sensing MRI reconstruction. In: International conference on medical image computing and computer-assisted intervention. Springer; 2018. p. 232–40.
53. Simonyan K, Zisserman A. Very deep convolutional networks for large-scale image recognition. In: International conference on learning representations; 2015.
54. Sodickson DK, Manning WJ. Simultaneous acquisition of spatial harmonics (SMASH): fast imaging with radiofrequency coil arrays. Magn Reson Med. 1997;38(4):591–603.
55. Wang P, Chen EZ, Chen T, Patel VM, Sun S. Pyramid convolutional RNN for MRI reconstruction. arXiv preprint arXiv:1912.00543 (2019).
56. Wang S, Ke Z, Cheng H, Jia S, Ying L, Zheng H, Liang D. DIMENSION: dynamic MR imaging with both k-space and spatial prior knowledge obtained via multi-supervised network training. NMR Biomed. 2019:e4131.
57. Wang Y, Yang J, Yin W, Zhang Y. A new alternating minimization algorithm for total variation image reconstruction. SIAM J Imaging Sci. 2008;1(3):248–72.
58. Yang G, Yu S, Dong H, Slabaugh G, Dragotti PL, Ye X, Liu F, Arridge S, Keegan J, Guo Y, et al. DAGAN: deep de-aliasing generative adversarial networks for fast compressed sensing MRI reconstruction. IEEE Trans Med Imaging. 2017;37(6):1310–21.
59. Ye JC. Compressed sensing MRI: a review from signal processing perspective. BMC Biomed Eng. 2019;1(1):1–17.
60. Yoon H, Kim KS, Kim D, Bresler Y, Ye JC. Motion adaptive patch-based low-rank approach for compressed sensing cardiac cine MRI. IEEE Trans Med Imaging. 2014;33(11):2069–85.
61. Zhao B, Haldar JP, Christodoulou AG, Liang ZP. Image reconstruction from highly undersampled (k, t)-space data with joint partial separability and sparsity constraints. IEEE Trans Med Imaging. 2012;31(9):1809–20.
62. Zhou B, Zhou SK. DuDoRNet: learning a dual-domain recurrent network for fast MRI reconstruction with deep T1 prior. In: Proceedings of the IEEE/CVF conference on computer vision and pattern recognition; 2020. p. 4273–82.

Artificial Intelligence-Based Image Enhancement and Reconstruction in Computed Tomography Imaging

15

Thomas Wesley Holmes and Amir Pourmorteza

Introduction

Computed tomography (CT) has become an important modality in diagnosis and monitoring of heart disease. Since its advent in the 1970s, there has been a steady rate of scientific publications on CT research (Fig. 15.1). Neural networks (NN) became popular in the late 1980s; however, it was not until the latter half of the 2010s that research in artificial intelligence (AI) and deep learning (DL) gained momentum.

This could be attributed to the recent developments in computer hardware, specifically graphics processing units (GPU), which made them more powerful and more affordable; in addition, several easy-to-use and mostly open-source software packages have been developed. The combination of these advances in software and hardware has led to the exponential growth of research articles in the fields of AI and deep learning.

The purpose of this chapter is to review applications of AI in CT image formation and image enhancement. It should be noted that many of the architectures shown in this chapter were trained and validated on a small number of datasets (Fig. 15.2). In addition, many of the proposed algorithms were trained and tested on nonclinical datasets (Fig. 15.3). These facts significantly limit the generalizability of the results, and we urge the readers to keep this point in mind and consider the results with caution. We hope that this review will inspire the readers to develop and utilize AI-based algorithms for CT imaging while being mindful of the limitation on the generalizability of these algorithms.

T. W. Holmes, PhD
Department of Radiology and Imaging Sciences and Winship Cancer Institute, Emory University, Atlanta, GA, USA
e-mail: thomas.wesley.holmes@emory.edu

A. Pourmorteza, PhD (✉)
Department of Radiology and Imaging Sciences and Winship Cancer Institute, Emory University, Atlanta, GA, USA

Department of Biomedical Engineering, Georgia Institute of Technology, Atlanta, GA, USA
e-mail: amir.pourmorteza@emory.edu

Image Enhancement and Image Reconstruction

When considering AI tasks with CT images, image enhancement and image reconstruction are two broad categories that it can be split into. The basic division between the two is centered on what the input to the AI algorithm is and what the desired output is. With image reconstruction, the input generally involves projection data in the form of a sinogram, and the output is the reconstructed CT image. With enhancement, the work is done after image reconstruction; therefore, the input is an image, and the output is something that improves your understanding of the input image.

Image Enhancement

There are several tasks that neural networks associated with CT image enhancement are designed to address. These include segmentation, material decomposition, image denoising, and image quality assessment.

Segmentation

Image segmentation is the process of partitioning a digital representation of an object into at least two or more characteristic objects. At its most basic level, this is assigning a logical operator of either a "yes" or "no" to each element of a two-dimensional (2D) or three-dimensional (3D) image. An accurate 3D geometrical representation of anatomical structures can facilitate and improve visualization, simulation, morphological assessment, and surgical planning [1]. For these geometrical representations to work correctly,

C. N. De Cecco et al. (eds.), *Artificial Intelligence in Cardiothoracic Imaging*, Contemporary Medical Imaging,
https://doi.org/10.1007/978-3-030-92087-6_15

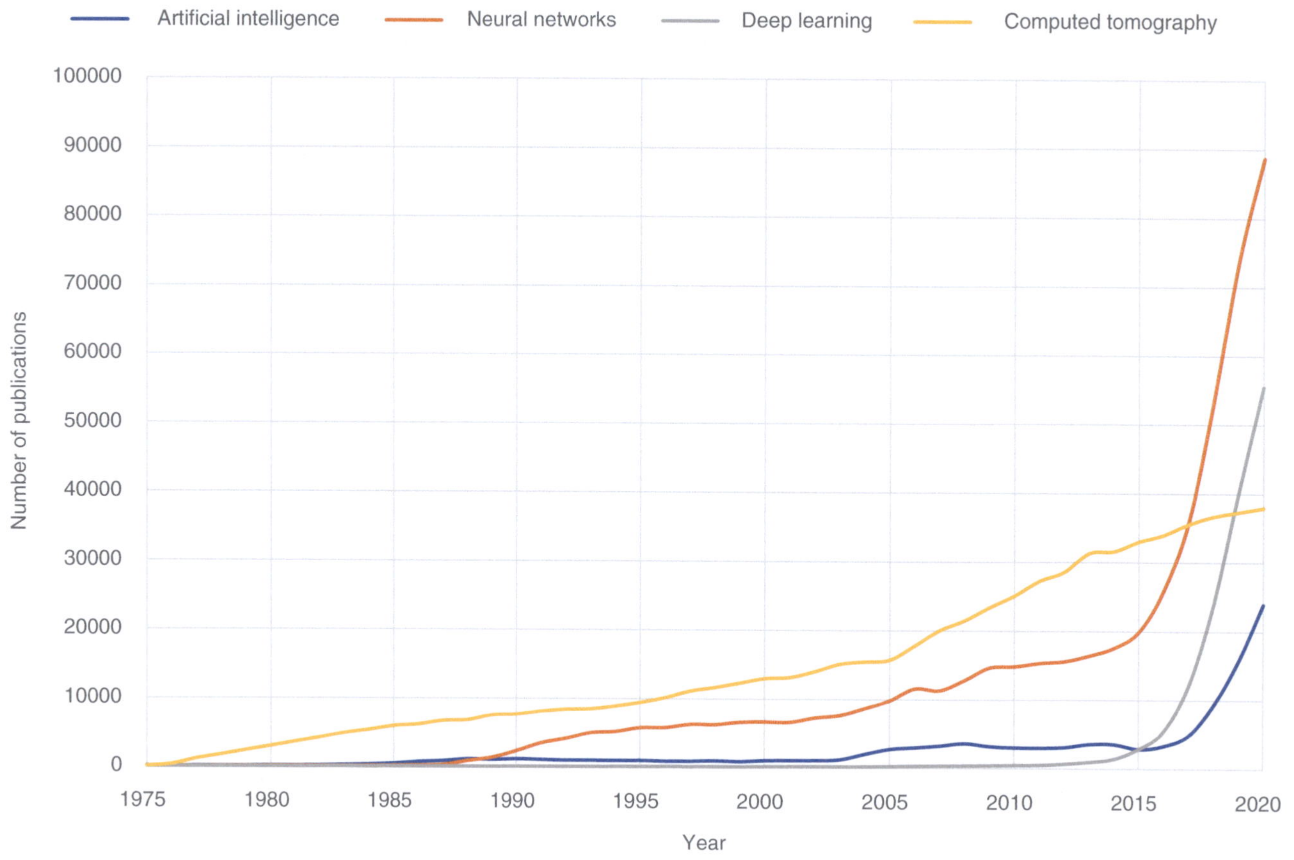

Fig. 15.1 Number of publications with the title or abstract containing the following keywords: artificial intelligence, neural networks, deep learning, and computed tomography. (https://app.dimensions.ai/discover/publication)

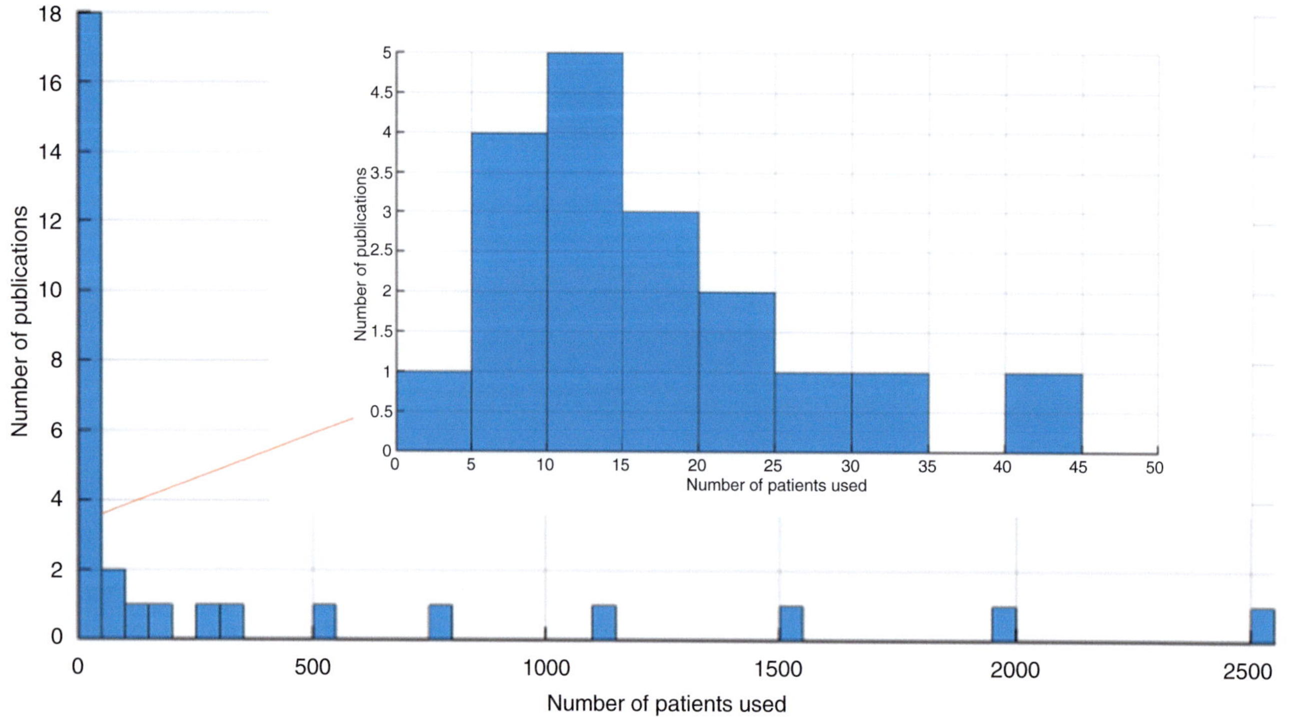

Fig. 15.2 The distribution of the number of patient cases used in each of the publications studied in this chapter

patient-specific image segmentation is necessary. This has traditionally required a significant amount of time by a trained radiologist to manually outline the desired anatomical structures and is inherently subject to human error. This time-intensive task results in a relatively low output rate, and as a result, some semiautomated threshold-based segmentations were developed. Regardless of the improvement with semiautomatic algorithms, segmentation has remained time-consuming and has intra- and interobserver variability [2]. This environment has facilitated the need to develop an accurate and reliable automatic method to perform segmentations quickly and consistently.

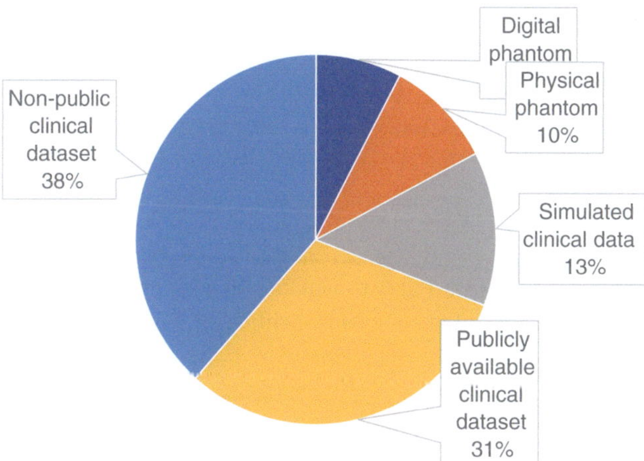

Fig. 15.3 Types of datasets used to train and test the AI algorithms. Digital phantoms are ideal and perfect shapes that are mathematically generated such as Shepp-Logan Phantom. A physical phantom is an object that is meant to mimic the human anatomy such as the COPDGENE phantom. Simulated clinical data is the case where a clinical dataset has been intentionally altered, for example, by adding quantum noise. Publicly available clinical datasets are a set of projections and/or reconstructed images that are publicly available online. Nonpublic clinical datasets are image obtained from a medical or research facility that are not available to the public

Lima et al. developed an NN that incorporated both PET and CT images to achieve a multimodal image segmentation of organ tumors within the abdomen [3]. They demonstrated that by incorporating the segmentation from both modalities, an improvement in the overall segmentation was achieved. Another interesting point about this NN was that the segmentation is used to assist the reconstruction of the PET image, and this newly reconstructed PET image is iteratively used to help the segmentation of the CT image. This pipeline and its resulting segmentation can be seen in Fig. 15.4. One of the challenges of this approach is the misregistration between the two modalities, which would cause the network to become unstable and produce unreliable outputs.

Another AI approach was developed to segment the left ventricular (LV) myocardium from CT images [2]. While this approach remains somewhat semiautomatic because it requires the input images to be put into short axis, it continues to be an interesting exploration on the utility of AI. While the proper alignment of the short axis remains a constraint to the successful segmentation of the LV, this poses a new possible AI development. An NN could be developed to automatically align the images in short axis and then be used in combination with this technique to achieve the desired result.

However, segmentation of the LV myocardium wall can be performed with a different perspective. The work done by Ye et al. produced an NN that utilizes a point cloud in the segmentation workflow [4]. The input image is passed through an NN to generate the point cloud which is then used to create the segmentation mask of the myocardial wall. The architecture for the segmentation NN can be seen in Fig. 15.5. This approach allows for an increase in the segmentation accuracy by incorporating the reconstructed point clouds prior and the encoder portion of the network into the segmentation branch.

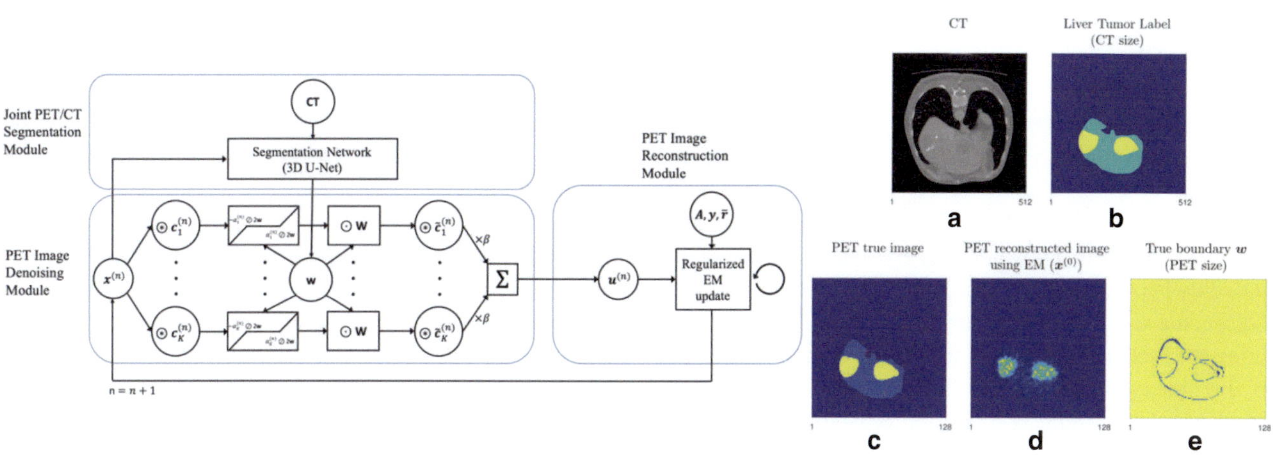

Fig. 15.4 Left: The block diagram of the overall pipeline for PET-CT segmentation. Right: Results from different segmentations. Segmentations (**a**) and (**b**) are the segmentation results and (**c**), (**d**), and (**e**) are the reconstructed images [3]

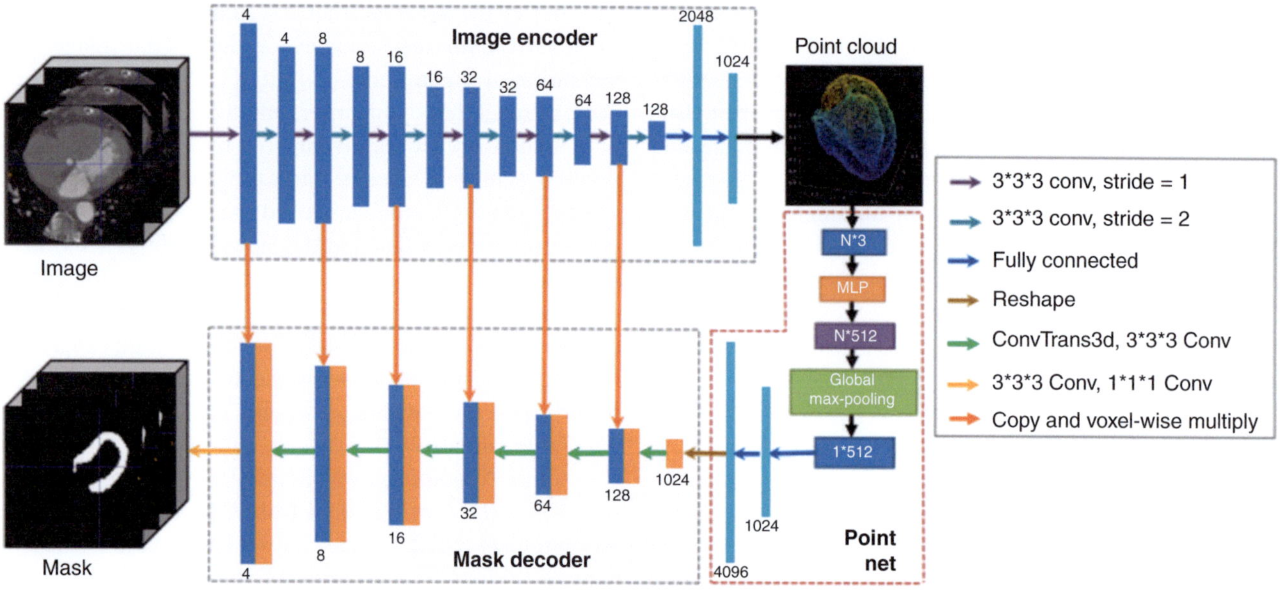

Fig. 15.5 Architecture for left ventricle myocardial wall segmentation: a U-Net CNN with a point cloud at the lowest encoding level [4]

In the previous segmentation applications, a specific feature of the cardiac structure was found, but the NN introduced by Kong et al. was developed to segment the surfaces of all four chambers and major vessels of the heart [1]. One unique feature about this approach is the implementation of a surface mesh from volumetric image data. This technique incorporates the basic structure of the heart to deform various spheres to fill the appropriate anatomical structures of the heart. Figure 15.6 shows the structure of the NN used by Kong. Utilizing this deformable mesh approach is different from the previous classification-based approaches in that it is more flexible and has the potential to be adapted to other anatomical structures or imaging modalities. The authors demonstrated some of this flexibility by showing its capabilities with both CT and MRI 4D cine cardiac data.

Material Decomposition

Material decomposition in x-ray CT imaging is the characterization of spectral CT images in order to estimate the expected elemental structures and composition of each voxel in the image [5, 6]. Spectral CT exploits the energy dependence of the linear attenuation coefficients of each of the materials [7]. In addition, it may be possible to decompose the spectral CT images into more material maps by incorporating the k-edge information, which is a sharp discontinuity in the linear attenuation coefficient of high-Z elements. These element specific k-edges are typically found within contrast agents, such as gadolinium, iodine, gold, and bismuth. Material decomposition is not only used to locate and characterize contrast agents as it can be used to quantify calcium and other elements found within the body. This capability allows for the assessment of bone mineral density, kidney stones, liver iron concentrations, blood perfusion, coronary artery calcifications and plaques, and breast cancer [8]. Several works have proposed AI and deep learning as possible solutions to generate and/or enhance spectral CT images and material decomposition maps.

One approach to utilizing material decomposition is using the technique within a larger pipeline. Lyu et al. take advantage of the considerable amount of redundant information in both the low- and high-energy images of dual-energy CT (DECT) [7]. While the DECT overlapping images do not provide substantially different anatomical information, Lyu proposes that a series of NNs can perform DECT imaging using a low-energy image and a single high-energy projection. The goal is to reduce the radiation dose to the patient and to allow conventional single-energy CT systems to produce DECT [7]. The material decomposition portion of the network found in Fig. 15.7 is essential for mapping the correct materials to the corresponding high-energy images. This is made possible by CNN's ability to learn complex nonlinear mappings.

Another interesting material decomposition implementation was developed by Absacal et al. The authors have proposed a technique that involves using only two different materials: bone and soft tissue. The method takes advantage of the spectral components of each material and incorporates both the reconstructed image and the individual projections to perform material decompositions [8]. Once the material decompositions with the projections were made, individual

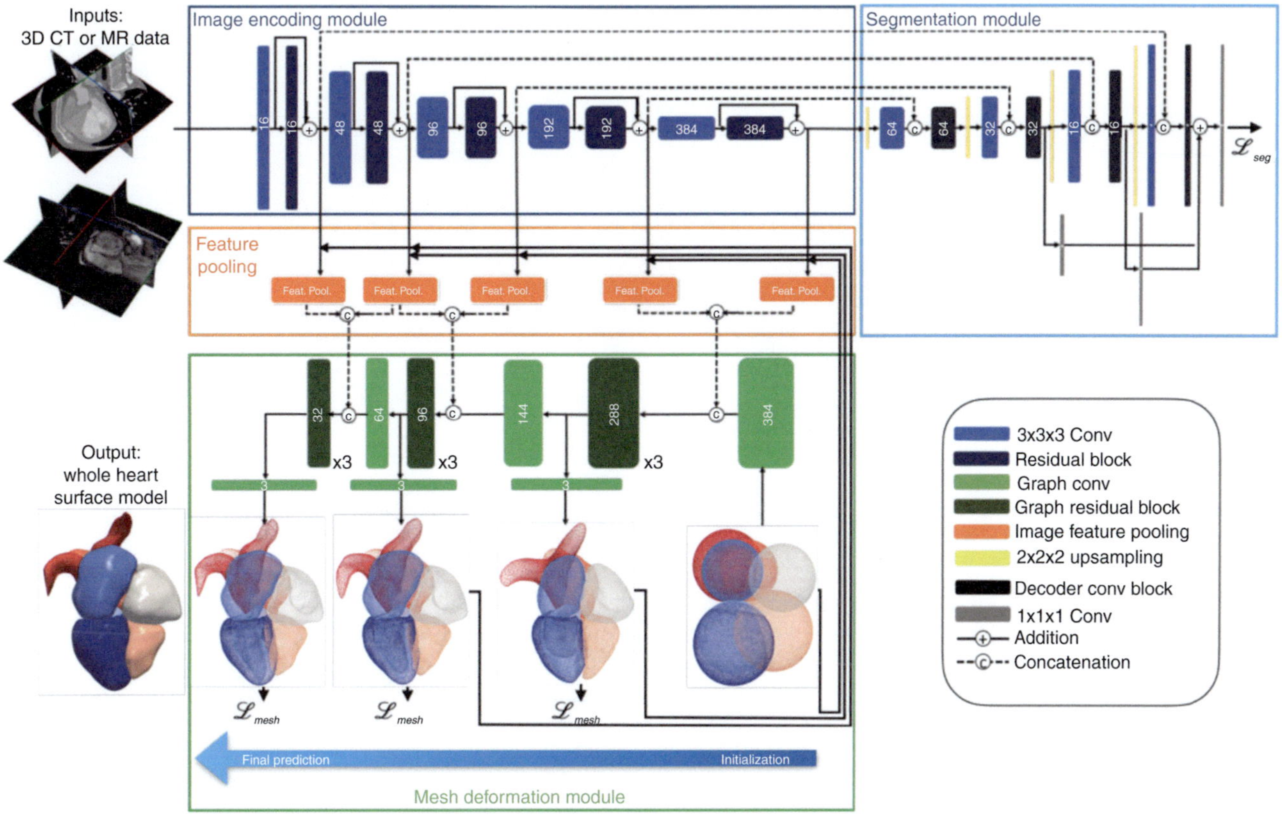

Fig. 15.6 The architecture of the NN used to segment four chambers and major vessels of the whole heart [1]

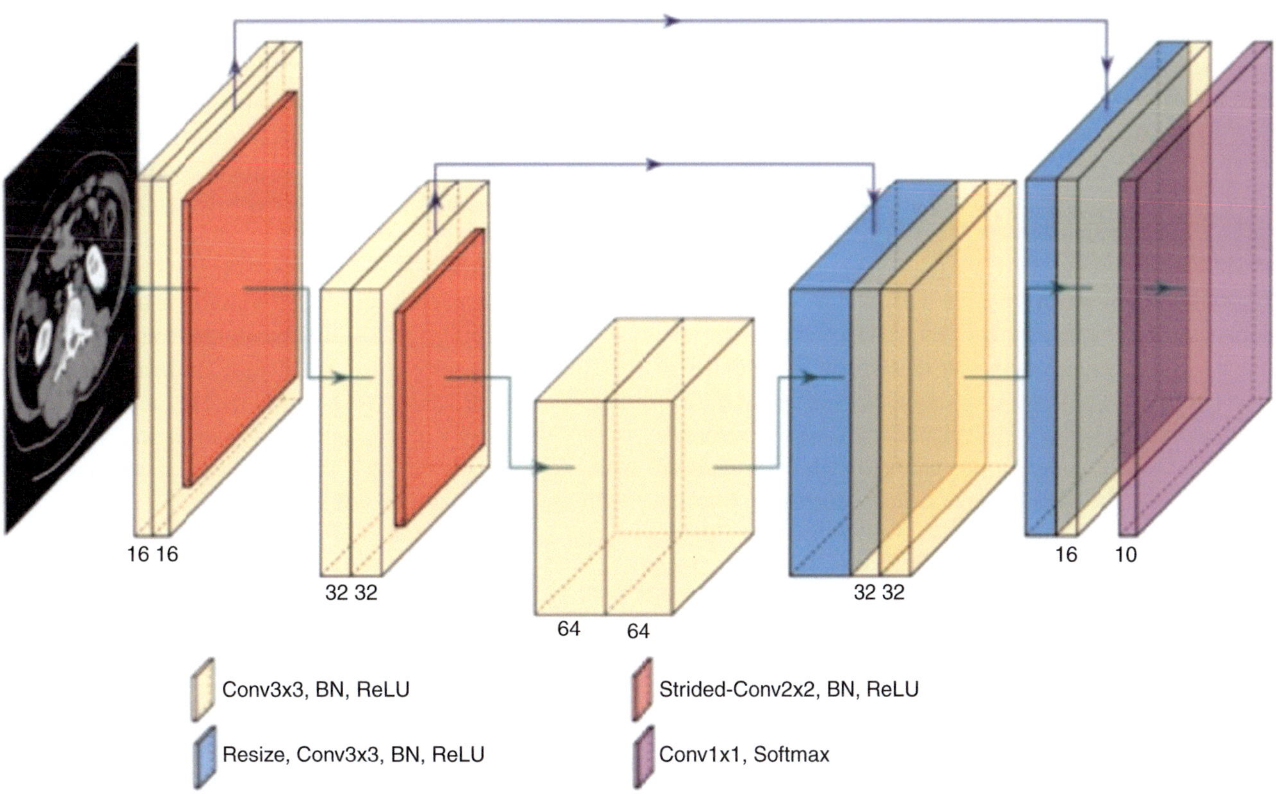

Fig. 15.7 The structure of the simplified U-Net CNN used for material decomposition [7]

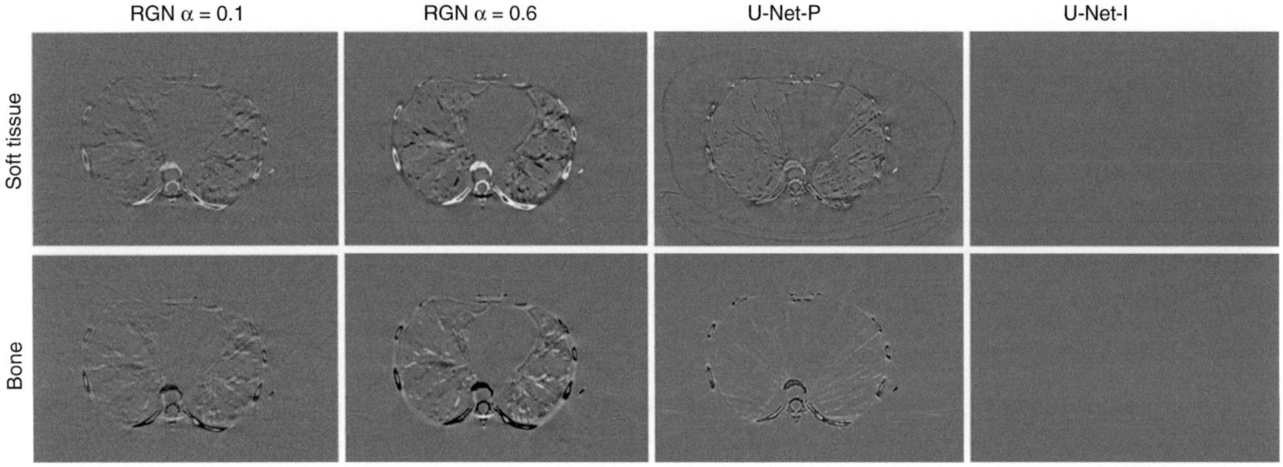

Fig. 15.8 The difference images of the ground truth and four different material-based reconstructions. Note the improved performance of the image-based reconstruction in U-Net-I [8]

reconstructions were performed to create material maps. The difference images between the known ground truth reconstructed images and those predicted from the NN are demonstrated in Fig. 15.8.

Image Denoising

Fundamentally, noise is unavoidable in CT; however, it can be reduced. At its core, noise is undesired variations in the pixel values of an otherwise homogenous image. It can be classified into two categories: quantum noise and detector noise. The quantum noise, which consists of photon generation, attenuation, and subsequent detection, can be modeled by the Poisson distribution, and the detector noise, which stems mostly from thermal fluctuations in electronic components, can be modeled by the Gaussian distribution [9]. The extant of noise is dictated by the number of detected photons. Some parameters responsible for noise are: patient size, slice thickness, x-ray tube current and voltage, and x-ray tube design. To reduce the noise, an increase in the number of detected photons is needed, but this comes at the cost of radiation dose to the patient. The balance is to find an acceptable amount of radiation dose to the patient that will produce an image that has the least amount of acceptable noise. In some instances, the dose to the patient outweighs the image noise, and the clinician is left to interpret a less-than-ideal image. In this case, a denoising algorithm could lead to better image interpretation.

A typical approach to denoising images in a post-processing fashion was demonstrated by Leuschner et al. where a noisy image is the input, and an image with reduced noise is the output of the AI algorithm. While this method can lead to overall improvements of the metrics used to evaluate the overall success of the network, it does produce artifacts in the resulting image, as seen in Fig. 15.9 [9]. These artifacts are manifested as a loss of details and blurring of edges, which could negatively affect image evaluation.

An interesting approach to denoising low-dose CT images involves wavelets. This was demonstrated by Kang et al. [10]. The idea behind incorporating directional wavelets into the NN is the assumption that it can detect the directional components of noise, and then the network can apply the appropriate transform to reduce the specific noise in that direction. The image is passed to the NN after some preprocessing, and the directional wavelet transform practically divides the NN into smaller sections which can be tuned to reduce noise in a specific direction [10]. The NN architecture used can be found in Fig. 15.10. The authors showed improved noise reduction with wavelet decomposition compared to a similar NN without wavelet decomposition.

It is also possible to train an NN to estimate the image noise as its output, which in turn can be subtracted from the noisy image in order to create an image with lower noise. Such an approach was used by Choe et al. where they trained a network to solve for the noise or residual image. The schematic of this implementation can be found in [11]. The authors demonstrated the success of this approach within similar reconstruction kernels but did note the limitation of the network's inability to move from a soft kernel to a sharp kernel.

Image Quality Assessment

The quality of an image is the overall level of accuracy that an imaging system can capture the true and unvaried object that is being digitally represented. The process of measuring the quality of an image falls into two categories: subjective measurements performed by humans and objective assessments performed by algorithms/machines which may be

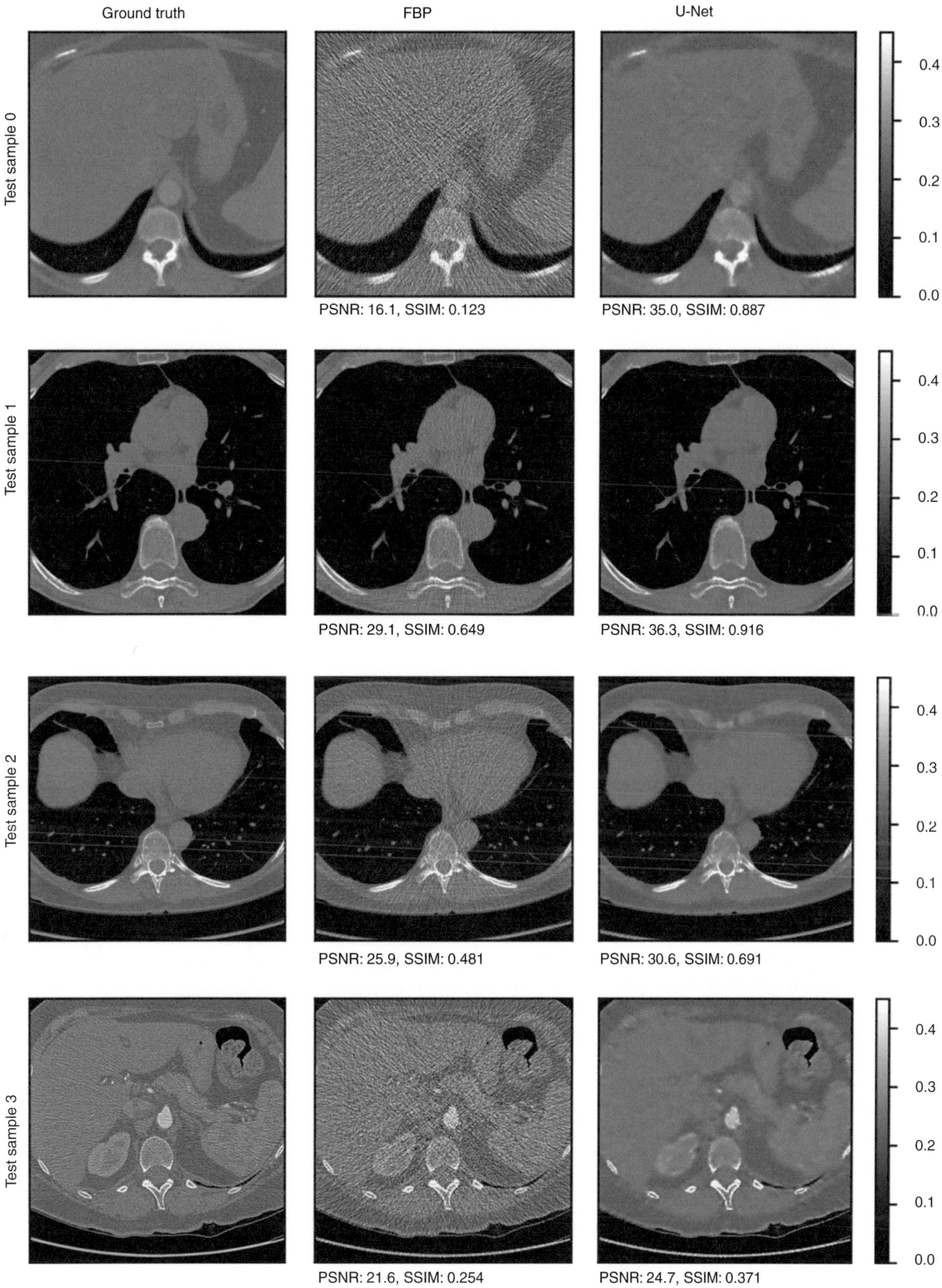

Fig. 15.9 Four different axial slices demonstrating the performance of the U-Net when compared with FBP to the ground truth. Note the improvement in the U-Net over the FBP but some residual streaking artifacts and oversmoothed soft tissues [9]

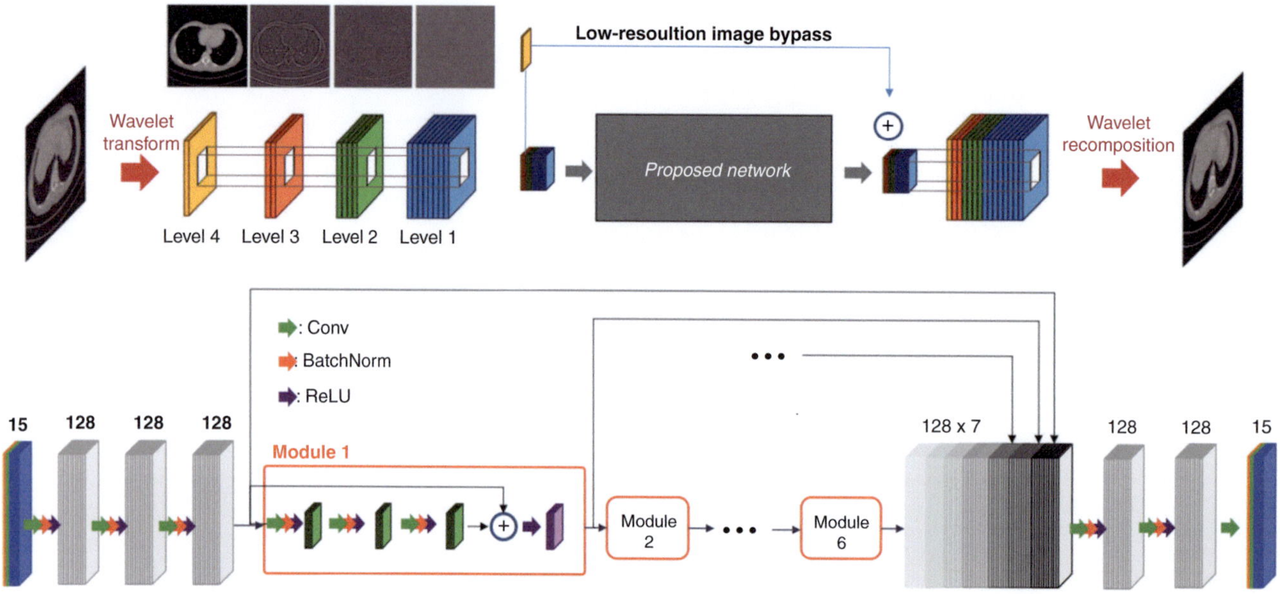

Fig. 15.10 The architecture of a network that utilizes directional wavelets to denoise images. This approach uses additional network layers which are placed after the wavelet sampling [10]

tuned to mimic human subjectivity. These types of machine objective measurements are suited for AI. In the previous section, we introduced NNs that were trained on a set of input/output pairs of images. Here, we introduce NNs that are designed to assess the quality of the input image and produce a map, a metric of image quality, or confidence as output. These algorithms have been previously applied to nonmedical photograph and video datasets and recently have been applied to medical CT images.

Automatic image quality assessment of an output of a CT reconstruction algorithm was explored by Patwari et al. The network architecture can be found in Fig. 15.11. They used a CNN to learn a similarity score between a reference image and a reconstructed image with a significant amount of quantum noise. The learned similarity could be considered as a quality reference score for the noisy image [12].

Another architecture that utilized a no-reference approach to assess the quality of an image was presented by Li et al. It utilized a common type of network, AlexNet, to perform image quality assessment at various levels of simulated acquisition radiation dose and image noise. The network structure is shown in Fig. 15.12. Specifically noted in this work was the explicit use of the whole image rather than patches of the image [13]. The driving reasoning behind this idea is that the image quality assessment is a holistic concept and that separate individual divisions of the image would not produce an adequate representation. The results of this research demonstrated that the NN was able to generate a reliable image quality assessment; however, it should be noted that a single image quality metric may not be a reliable substitute for the diagnostic value of an image.

Image Reconstruction

At its most basic interpretation, x-ray computed tomographic image reconstruction is the process of assembling many projections of an object, acquired at different angular locations, into a single cross-sectional (tomographic) image of the object. Tomographic techniques are some of the most popular clinical imaging modalities that are used to visualize various biological features, anatomical structures, and physiological functions [14]. As the number of CT exams has increased, the amount of radiation exposure to the population has increased, which is especially problematic for younger patients [15]. To address this issue, dose-reduction techniques have been developed, which include automatic exposure controls that modulate the tube current to account for patient size and organ-specific care. Additionally, an adjustable photon beam shaping filter can be used, as well as patient- and task-specific CT acquisition parameters can be optimized to reduce patient exposure.

These reconstruction techniques fall into two broad categories: filtered back projection (FBP) and iterative reconstruction (IR). The evolution of image reconstruction is very interesting and has been explored by previous authors [14, 15], but one of the more modern approaches to CT reconstruction, which does not always fall into the FBP or IR categories, employs AI. All reconstruction methods generate inexact results and attempt to reach a compromise between accuracy and computation time. The diagnostic performance of an x-ray CT acquisition should not be compromised by any reconstruction algorithm, AI based or not, as the reconstructed image directly impacts the ability of the clinician to

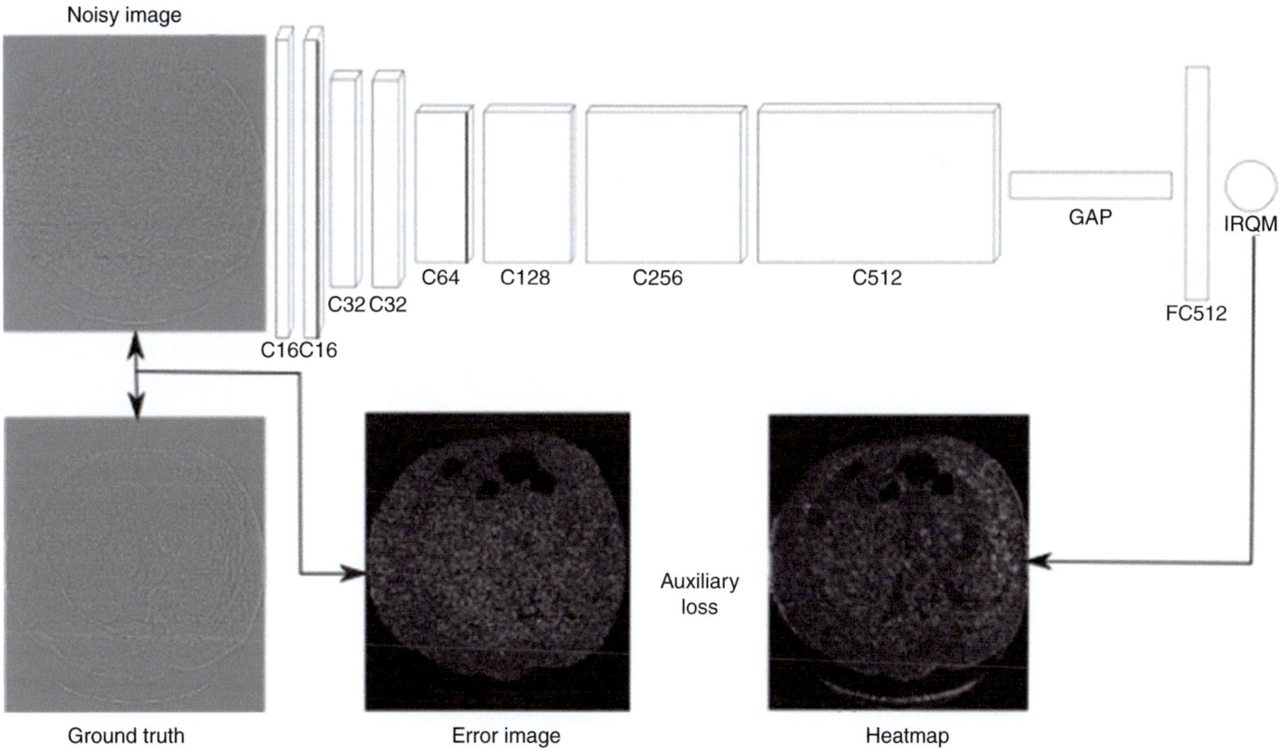

Fig. 15.11 CNN architecture to predict the image reconstruction quality metric score. *C* represents a convolutional layer with a respective number of filters, while *FC* represents a dense layer with respective number of neurons. The auxiliary loss generated with the heatmap and error map is also shown [12]

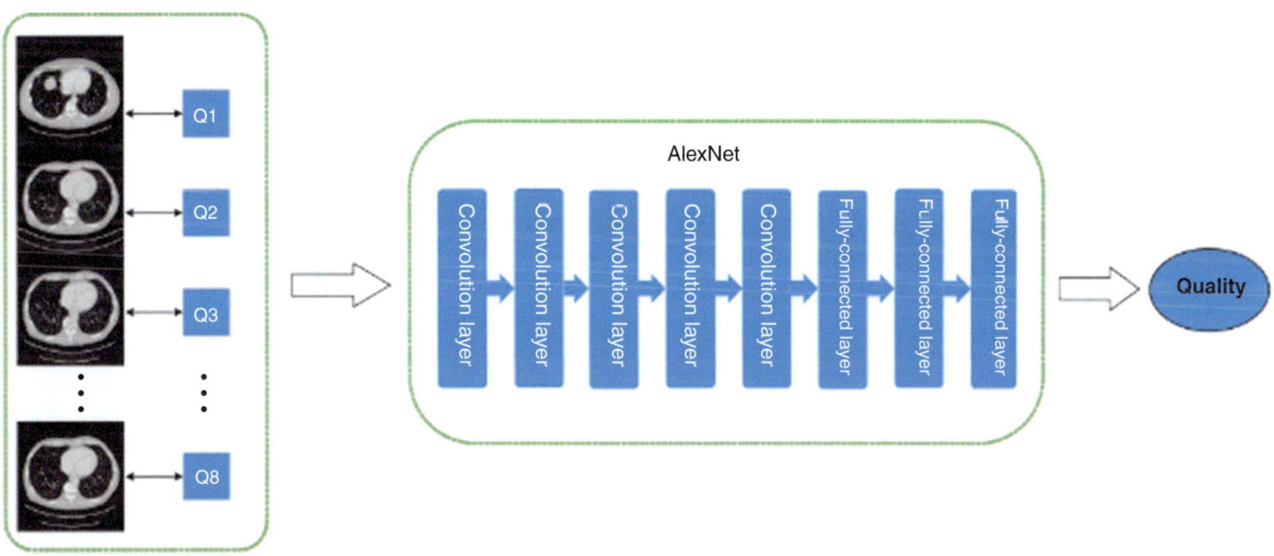

Fig. 15.12 AlexNet, a convolutional neural network architecture, is used to predict the image quality metric using different axial slices as input [13]

provide the most accurate answer to the question at hand [16]. Using AI to perform CT image reconstruction has a unique opportunity to outperform the previously developed methods by producing images in a fraction of the time required for IR algorithms.

It should be noted that any non-FBP reconstruction algorithm uses some form of prior knowledge or makes certain assumptions about the characteristics of the output image. While it might be relatively straightforward to understand what those assumptions are in the case of IR, it is more difficult to interpret what types of assumptions or prior knowledge is incorporated in NN-based algorithms. Therefore, NN-based algorithms should be considered with great caution. The task of AI-based image formation may be very attractive in a photo restoration task, in which damaged parts of a photograph are replaced (in-painted) with what the AI algorithm thinks should be there. However, the same task in CT, i.e., filling regions of a CT image that are contaminated by extreme noise or metal artifacts with what the AI assumes should be there, would be detrimental. Unfortunately, there are numerous AI-based CT reconstruction and artifact reduction algorithms which do exactly that.

We did not include any of those algorithms in this chapter. We firmly believe that an AI-based CT reconstruction algorithm should provide a "confidence map" that shows how much of the information used to create the image came from the measurements (i.e., projection data) and how much was based on the AI's expectation of what an image should look like. A good reconstruction algorithm should have a specific output where the value of the image voxels denotes "I do not know," i.e., the network cannot, with good confidence, estimate what the actual value of the voxel is.

The types of NNs used to perform CT image reconstruction can be broken down into several different categories. These reconstructions techniques are image-domain, projection-domain, hybrid-domain, and AI-driven iterative regularization.

Image-Domain Reconstruction

Machine learning reconstruction techniques that are image-domain-based are typically used to assist in denoising an image or reducing the impact of an artifact-corrupted image, but they can also be used to generate new images or further refine an image based on prior information. This process is complicated because the generation of new x-ray image data typically involves a nonlinear imaging model, which basically encompasses the various losses and changes due to photonic energy-dependent interactions. AI techniques are capable of accounting for a wide array of nonlinear mapping features that can approximate the resulting image of a different physical model.

One such image-domain reconstruction has been designed to learn a nonlinear transform to map the polychromatic CT image to a monochromatic sinogram at a prespecified energy level [17]. This technique was used to reconstruct energy-dependent attenuation images from a single polychromatic image. This method could be considered as learning an advanced beam hardening correction map that is able to transform a polychromatic image dataset into a virtual monochromatic image (VMI) dataset at a specific energy [17]. VMIs are traditionally generated from dual-energy CT (DECT) or photon counting CT (PCCT) images where multiple samplings along the material-specific photonic attenuation curves are used to produce a series of VMIs. VMIs can be useful in their ability to reduce beam hardening and small metal artifacts while also allowing for an increase in the separability of contrast agents. This NN could be useful in the scenario where their VMIs are needed, but only a traditional CT system is available because either DECT or PCCT are not at the clinical facility. One limitation of this approach is that each individual monochromatic sinogram would require an independent NN to be trained and validated.

Another image-domain reconstruction that uses AI with a modified DECT approach is designed to reduce the overall radiation exposure to the patient. This idea is centered on the assumption that a single fusion image can be generated from a half-scan range where the low- and high-energy projections each are acquired over nonoverlapping quarters. These two quarter projections are used in combination to create a limited-angle reconstruction that is fused together to produce a single CT image [18]. This procedure can be seen in Fig. 15.13. Once this fusion image is created, it then is passed to an NN which has a double branching U-Net structure where a single image is used as input and two

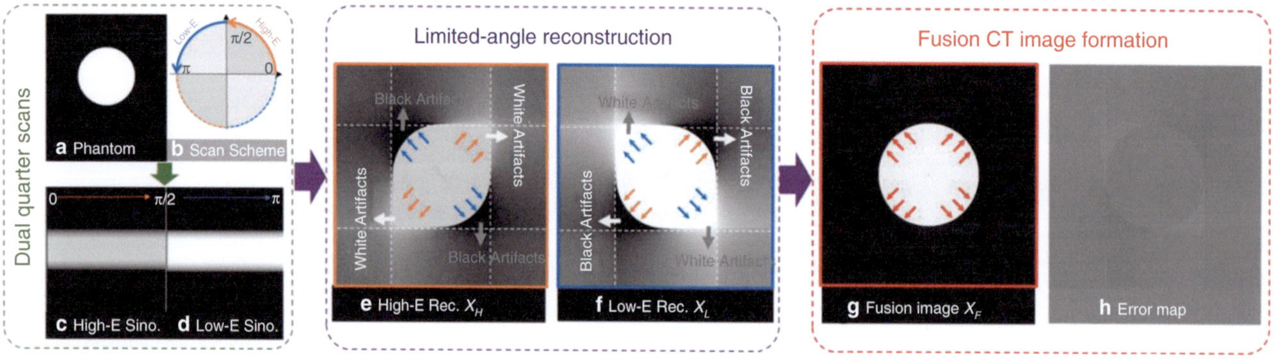

Fig. 15.13 A diagram demonstrating how two quarter projections taken at low and high energies can be used to create a single fused image. Panels (**a**) though (**d**) are demonstrating the phantom projection space acquisition, (**c**) and (**f**) are demonstrating the limited-angle reconstruction of the two energy acquisitions, and (**g**) and (**f**) are showing the fusion image and its corresponding error map (**h**) from the ground truth image [18]

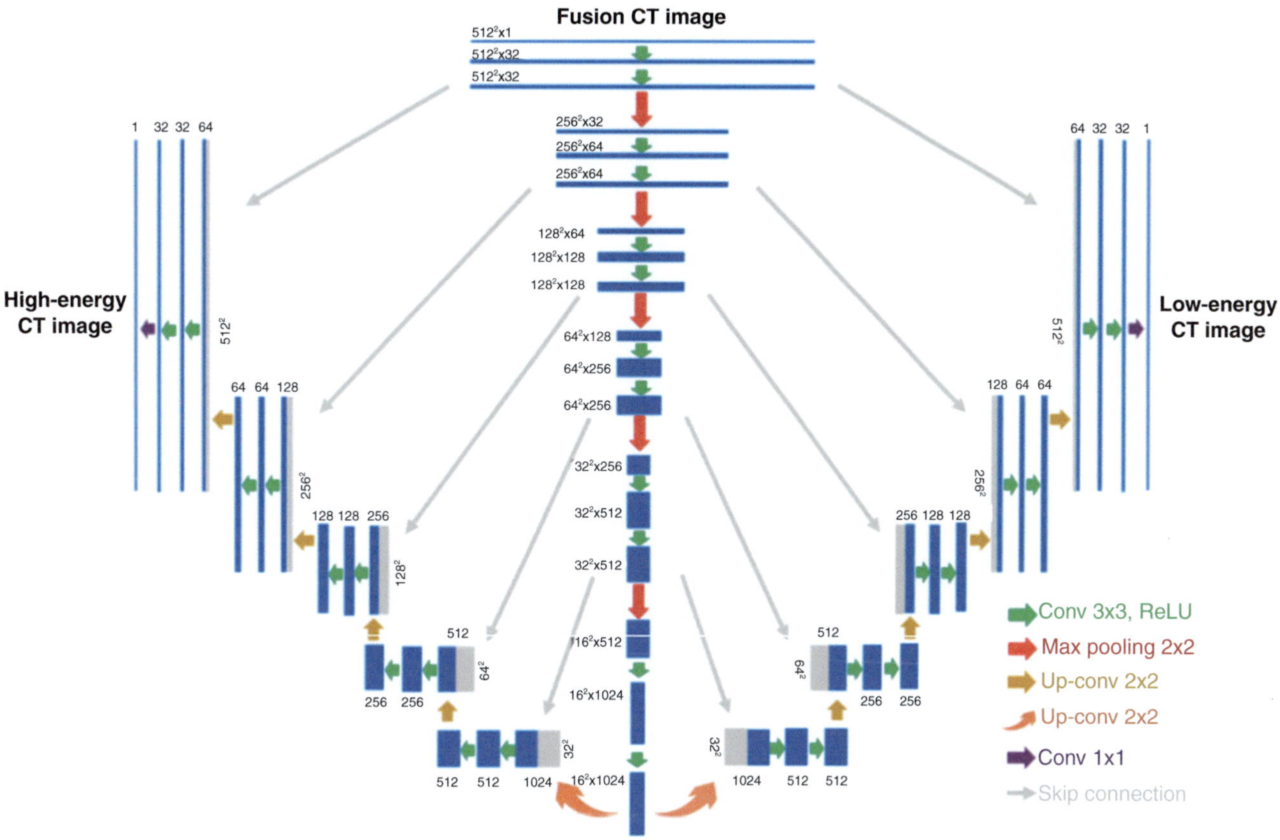

Fig. 15.14 The architecture of the double branching U-Net CNN type of network used to generate two separate DE images [18]

energy-dependent images are the output, one high-energy CT image and one low-energy CT image. The architecture for this NN design can be found in Fig. 15.14. While this idea and implementation are interesting, the technique requires a long training period as well as a large amount of computational power and memory. It is also dependent on the two low and high tube voltages remaining the same from training and testing as well as a successful generation of the fusion CT image. If the fusion image produces an image that is of low quality and contains reconstruction artifacts from the partial scan, then the NN prediction of the low- and high-energy images will also be plagued with a verity of artifacts.

Projection-Domain Reconstruction

Projection-domain image reconstructions performed by AI are designed to utilize the sinograms directly produced from the x-ray CT acquisition. Filtered back projection (FBP) is a mathematically accurate reconstruction algorithm when the projections have been acquired under the best data acquisition conditions. The NNs themselves are employing a data-driven ramp filter approach which is designed to minimize the losses in the image-domain. The design of the NN is to match the ideal image reconstructions that FBP can generate under ideal conditions but applied to less-than-ideal conditions. One such scenario that these types of reconstruction NNs are used involves sparse and truncated projection data. A representative idea that demonstrates how a sparse-view acquisition is different than a full-view CT acquisition can be found in Fig. 15.15 where the reduced number of projections can be easily seen [19]. These types of datasets are also known as compressed sensing and can be a way to reduce the radiation dose to the patient.

One such investigation involved the use a type of "in-painting" of missing data from a truncated projection dataset. This network was trained using projection data that had been removed as the input with the final reconstructed image from the full dataset as the target for the NN. If the truncated data set was used outright with FBP, the image would have artifacts induced by the reconstruction algorithm due to the incomplete sampling in the projection-domain. The network is designed to generate the missing projections and output the corrected sinogram which was then reconstructed with FBP [20]. To train the network, both fully sampled and incomplete projection data were used, which helped the network to recognize where the missing data was located that needed to be recovered. This type of approach is interesting in that the NN does not actually perform the

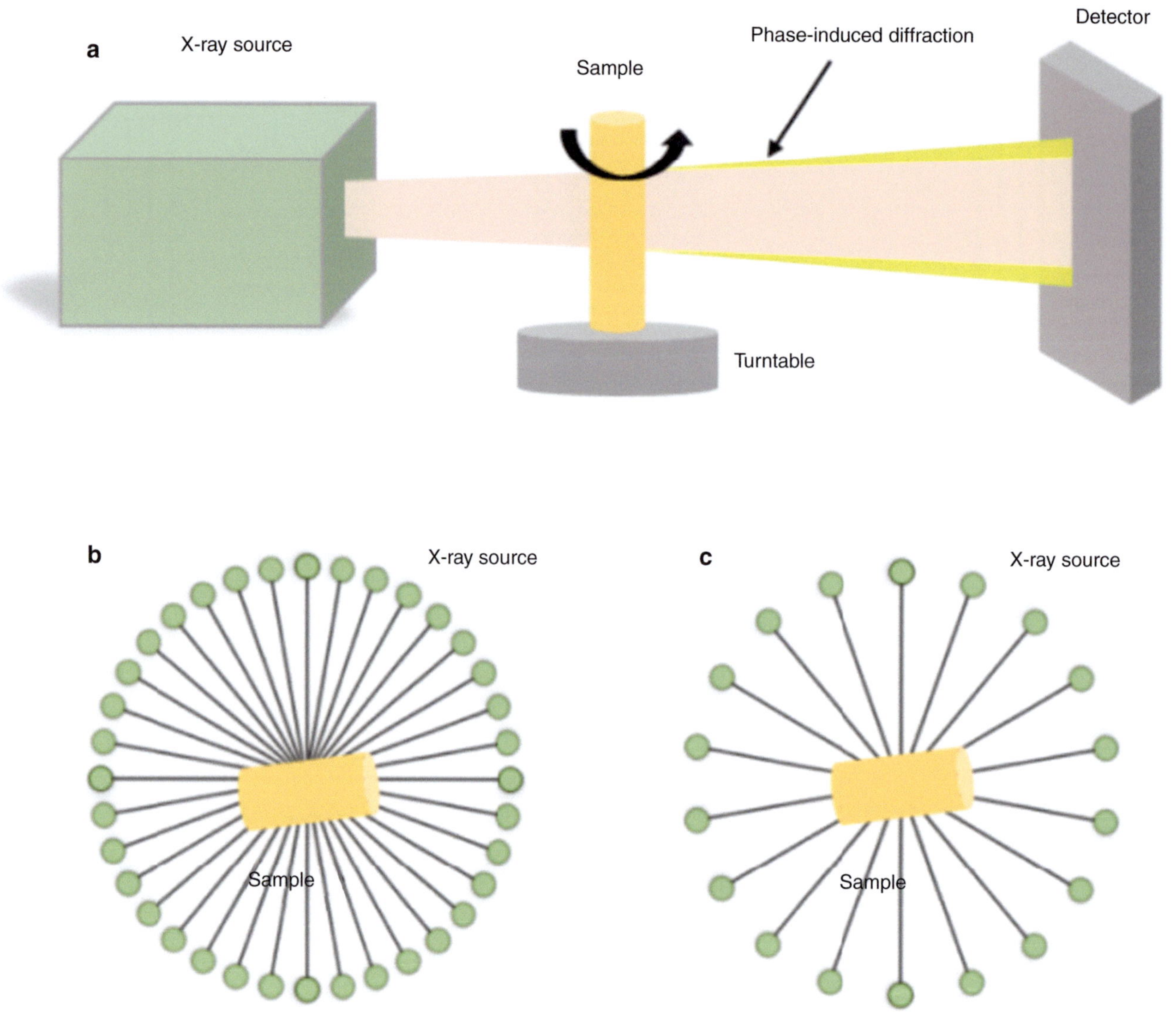

Fig. 15.15 A cartoon representation of an x-ray CT acquisition system (**a**) and a full-view CT (**b**) and the sparse-view CT (**c**) [19]

reconstruction itself but facilitates other reconstruction algorithms to generate a higher-quality image with less artifacts.

Another type of tactic to reduce image artifacts in the projection space was introduced by Lossau [21]. In this technique, there are three NNs in a pipeline to remove metal artifacts from implanted pacemakers and to reduce cardiac-included motion artifacts. The first NN is used to segment the metal shadows directly in the raw projection images. The second NN takes the metal segmentation mask and "in-paints" the metal-affected projection images with predicted line integrals. The third network determined the locations of the metal objects in the image-domain based on the segmented metal mask. This NN pipeline can be found in Fig. 15.16. To generate the necessary data to train this network, it required two different sets of clinical data, where the first set came from patients that had pacemakers where the metal pacemaker lead positions and pathways were extracted. These extracted pathways were then placed on top of the second dataset from patients that did not have a pacemaker. The combined overlaid image dataset served as the input to the network, and the pacemaker-free data served as the target for the network. This is an interesting approach to solving a complicated problem and one that probably would not have created a successful outcome if only a single NN had been used.

An NN was constructed to track tumors during therapy in near real time that utilized a full CT image from the planning phase and then created updated images based on a single projection. This approach uses a mask of the tumor from the planning 4D CT cine images to direct the network to neglect irrelevant pixels [22]. The schematic used to train and then apply the NN can be found in Fig. 15.17. After the network has been trained, the new projection image is passed into the

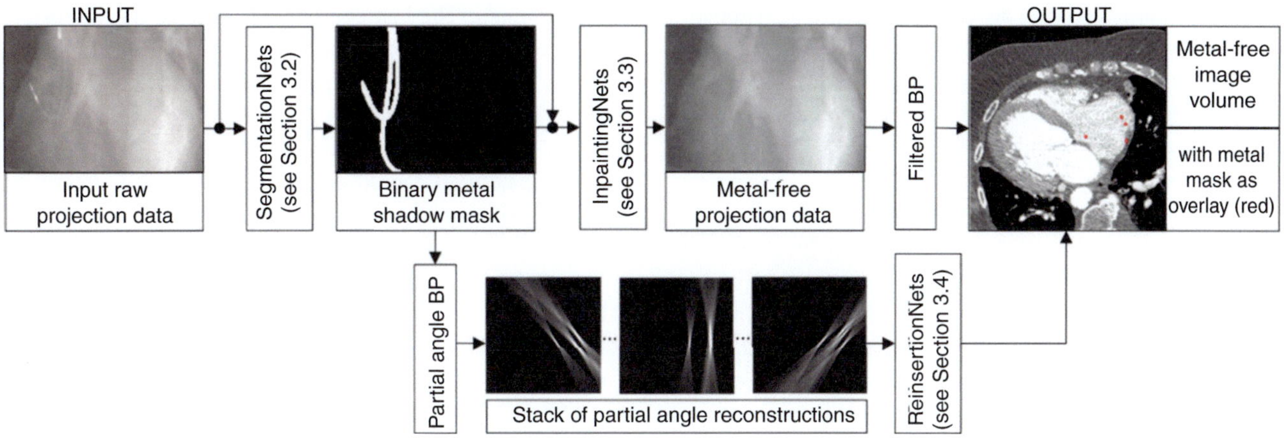

Fig. 15.16 The pipeline proposed that uses a series of NN that begins with the projection data, uses in-painting, and predicts a reconstructed image without metal leads [21]

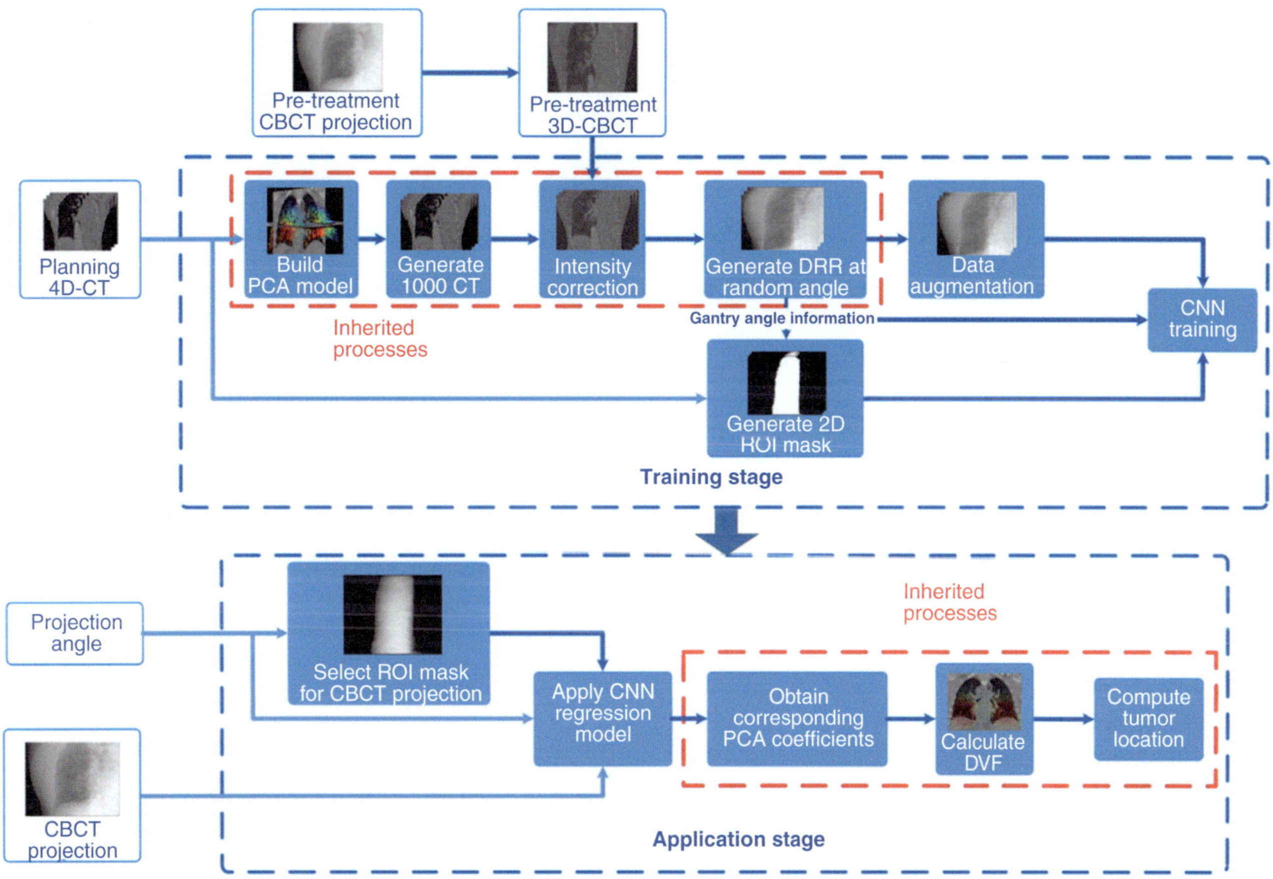

Fig. 15.17 The pipeline of the proposed method that demonstrates how the CNN is trained and then used [22]

network with the known projection angle, and an updated CT image is generated. Since the network included time-based images, it was able to predict and compensate for breathing and cardiac motion. This type of network could be very useful because the precise location of the tumor is very important during the treatment of patients, and being able to reduce the number of projections taken during the procedure will reduce the dose to the patient and to the surrounding clinicians. A limiting factor of this type of specific AI application is that each individual patient will require a separate NN to be trained and validated. This is because the individual locations of the tumor and other anatomical features are idiosyncratic to the patient and cannot be attributed to each patient the same way. This may also be true for the patient at different stages of treatment due to the change in size and composition of the tumor itself. Transfer learning from previously successful network weights may be a way to accelerate the training process and facilitate a stable network outcome.

Hybrid-Domain Reconstruction

Reconstruction techniques that are hybrid-domain incorporate a reconstructed image-domain prior from some other previous method along with the projection-domain sinogram. This approach allows the system to have an expectation of what the reconstructed image will be while still allowing the network to utilize the projection data to improve the image quality. One advantage of this type of reconstruction is that it can utilize the domain-specific information contained with either the image or projection-domain and allow the dual domain information to be supplementary.

An application of sparse-view projection data that used a hybrid-domain reconstruction technique was presented by Hu et al. [23]. This publication has several different steps to facilitate its hybrid-domain approach. It first "in-paints" or generates the missing projection data though an NN to produce the approximate full-view projection data. After this approximation, an initial reconstruction image is produced with reduced streaking artifacts. Finally, the initial reconstructions are used as input data to the final network to improve the feature details. The overall approach is in-painting the missing projection-domain data and then performing feature preservation in the image-domain. Figure 15.18 demonstrates the U-Net used and the overall flow of the reconstruction technique. One issue noted by the authors about this type of hybrid approach is that there are no feedback mechanisms to impose consistency between the reconstruction images and the initial projection data.

When considering data that was acquired from a limited-angle configuration, there are significant streaking artifacts. Employing a hybrid-domain reconstruction technique can be one such solution to reduce the artifacts because it takes advantage of both the projection- and image-domains simultaneously. The problem of limited-angle data comes from a situation in practical applications of CT where the data acquisition angle is limited by the size of the object, x-ray penetration, and the flexibility of the physical scan system. Some instances of this type of scenario are found in mammography and large-pitch helical CT. One possible solution to this problem consists of three components: an NN operating on the sinogram data, a domain transformation operation, and an NN operating in the image-domain [24]. The component focused on the sinogram data learns a weighted and filtered sinogram to generate the missing projections. The domain transformation operation consists of an analytical algorithm to exchange data between the projection to the image-domain. The last component, focused on the image-domain, is designed to reduce reconstruction and streaking artifacts. Each of these components can be found in Fig. 15.19. This approach shows promise, but there are some limitations with the geometric parameters of the CT system in that the network would need to be retrained if changes to the acquisition system were made.

AI-Driven Iterative Regularization Reconstruction

Iterative reconstruction (IR) techniques are based on a more complete model of the imaging system. It acts recursively and incorporates the imaging and sensor physics as well as the noise statistics to generate the best image possible. They attempt to improve the overall image quality by reducing noise and image artifacts. Sometimes, they are referred to as model-based image reconstruction (MBIR) or statistical image reconstruction (SIR) techniques where they incorporate a feedback portion of their algorithm to update the assumed prior information about the underlying object. These updates are based on minimizing a cost function and a set of penalty terms, which is referred to as the "regularizer". Using these type of iterative reconstruction techniques typically considers that the image reconstruction parameters lie within a linear manifold, but medical images tend to behave in a highly nonlinear fashion [25]. These inescapable inconsistencies between the mathematical model and various physical factors stem from nonlinear detector response functions, photonic scattering events, and electronic noise [26]. To account for this nonlinearity of the cost function and penalty terms, AI reconstruction approaches have been developed to adjust and fine-tune the parameters driving the regularization terms more accurately.

An implementation of iterative reconstruction where AI is used to assess and update the reconstruction has been applied to sparse data CT acquisitions. In this approach, the undersampled projection-domain data is fed directly into the NN without any preprocessing, and the regularization terms and balancing parameters are iteratively dependent [27]. This iterative dependency is important because with this technique, the number of iterations is fixed. This restriction in flexibility is based on the authors' understanding that the NN itself is not a black box and that it was selected based on physical, mathematical, and application-relevant knowledge [27]. The overall structure of the NN can be seen in Fig. 15.20 where each iteration block consists of an independent three-layer CNN. One of the advantages of this approach is that performing a limited number of iterations will reduce the computation time, but it may also reconstruct a poor-quality image if the input projection data is significantly dissimilar to the training images.

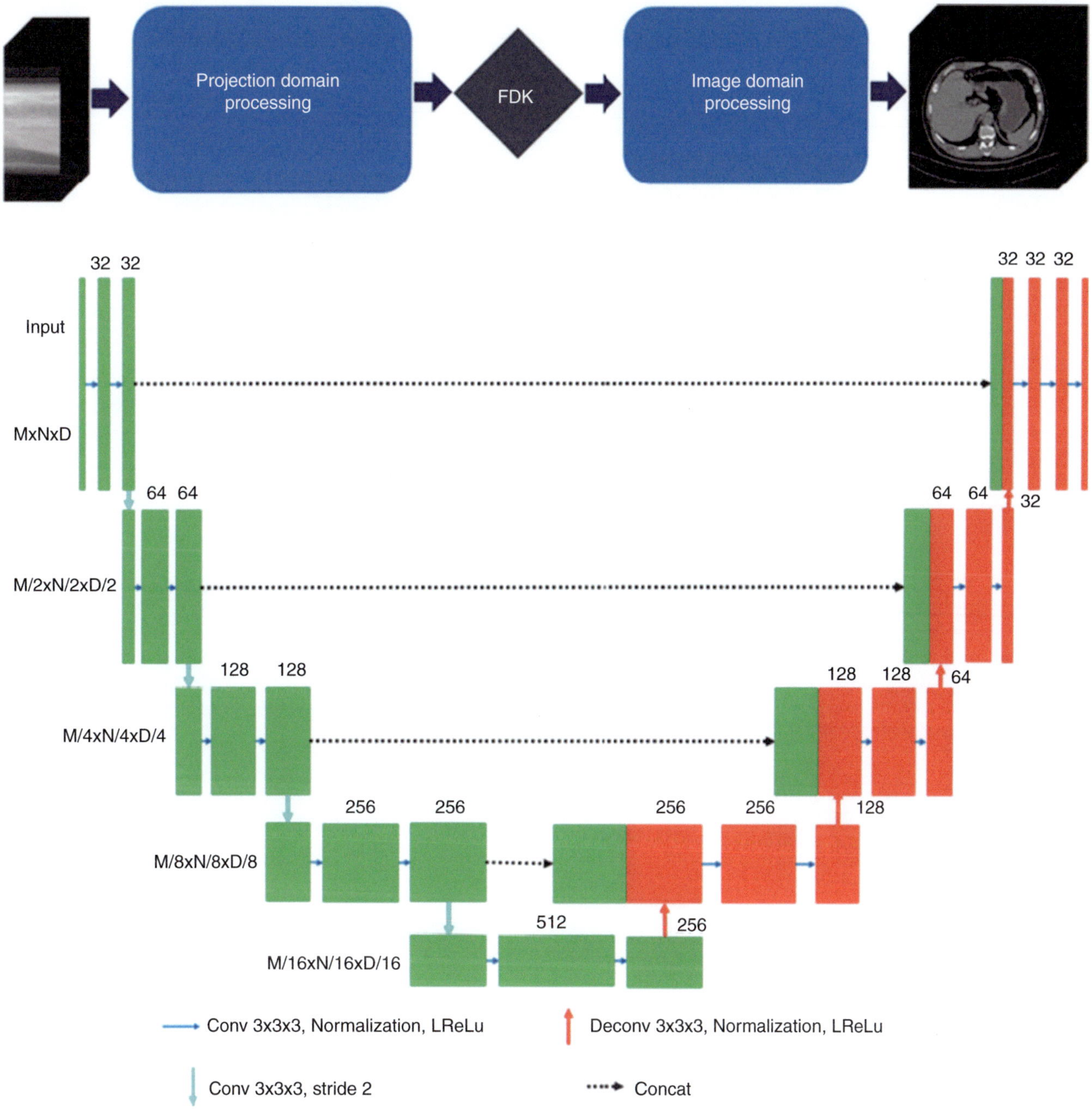

Fig. 15.18 The overall pipeline of the proposed technique is at the top of the figure and demonstrates the feed forward approach. The U-Net CNN structure used is at the bottom of the figure [23]

In an approach that allows for more flexibility, an AI technique has been developed by Shen et al. to tune parameters based on the output of the iterative reconstruction algorithm. This approach is using the total variation (TV) iterative reconstruction algorithm to perform the reconstructions and then allowing the network to analyze output patches to improve the reconstruction performance. The means by which the NN makes selections for image quality improvement implements a reinforcement learning strategy where the algorithm is allowed to make its own decisions and choices to obtain rewards based on the image patch and the desired outcome [28]. This architecture can be found in Fig. 15.21 where we can see the input is the image patch and the output are an action to be made by the TV reconstruction at its next iteration. One of the most limiting constraints with this approach is that the NN cannot adjust the reconstruction parameters until the iterative processes has finished which reduces the overall workflow efficiency and increases computation time.

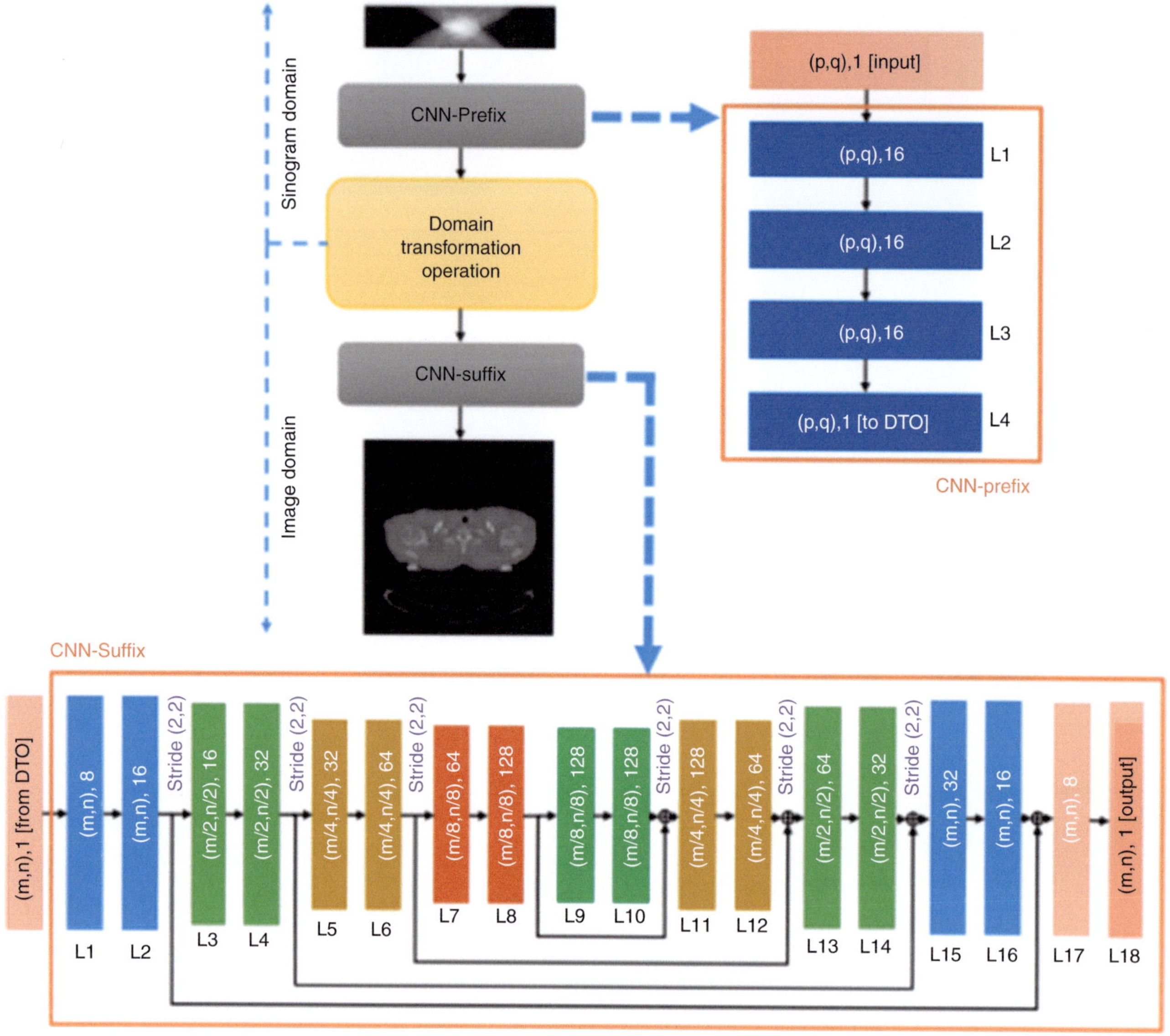

Fig. 15.19 The architecture of the NN that demonstrates where the projection-domain and image-domain NNs are located in the reconstruction process [24]

Applying a model-based iterative reconstruction approach to a low-dose projection dataset has also been explored, but He et al. have adopted the technique to include AI. This approach uses the NN to construct prior assumptions about the projection data and the reconstructed image to help with the MBIR. These NN are also updated upon each iteration to help the overall reconstruction task which implements a residual type of CNN block structure as seen in Fig. 15.22. In essence, the NN is used to help denoise and improve the image quality of the sinograms before being passed into the MBIR algorithm. Considering that the prior generation data by the NN is a very important factor for the MBIR, there are other iterative parameters that also need to be considered to have a successful reconstruction [29]. The authors noted that the number of residual CNN blocks used to generate the prior information must be determined before the reconstruction occurs. This specific number is directly correlated to the data and the amount of noise present, but the concern of overfitting is present if that number becomes too large.

Conclusion

The use of artificial intelligence in CT imaging is continuing to demonstrate its versatility and utility. This can clearly be seen in the variety of approaches and types of NN developed

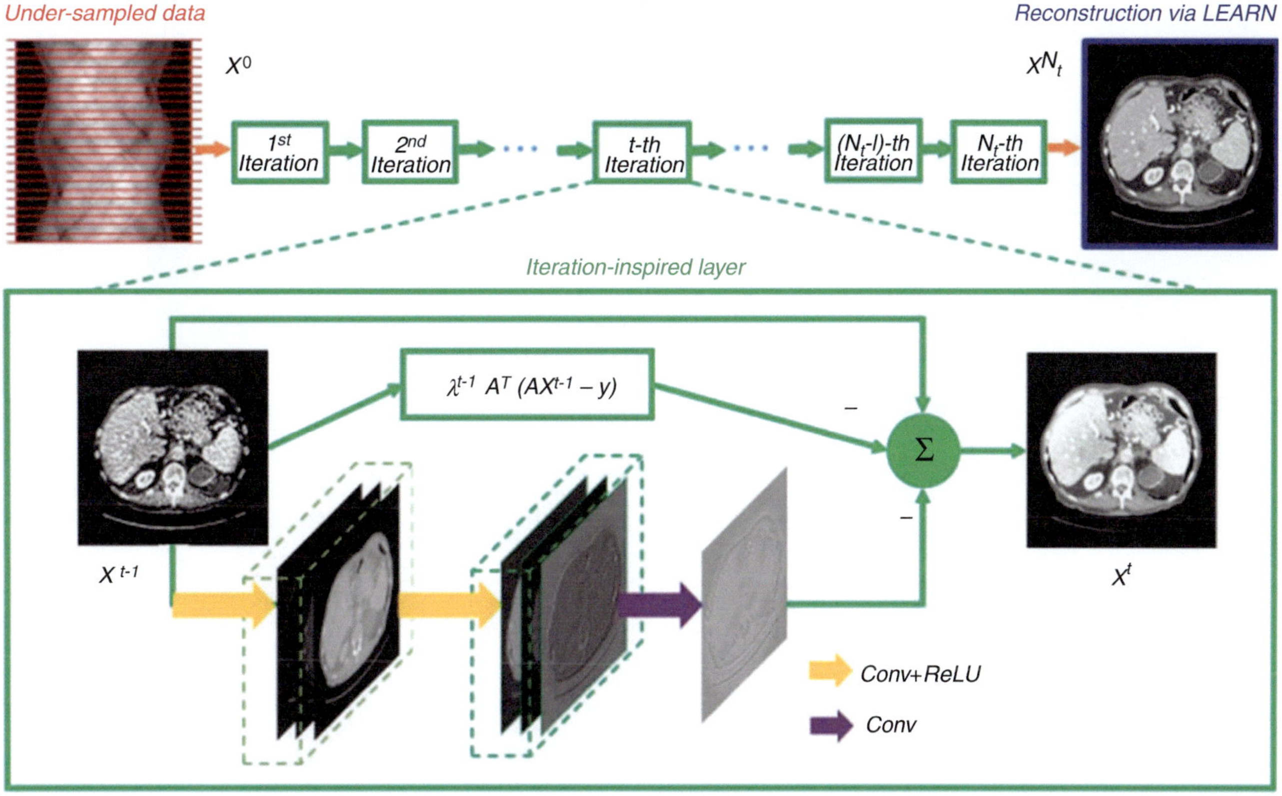

Fig. 15.20 The overall structure of the NN demonstrating how the undersampled input projection data is used to predict the reconstructed image [27]

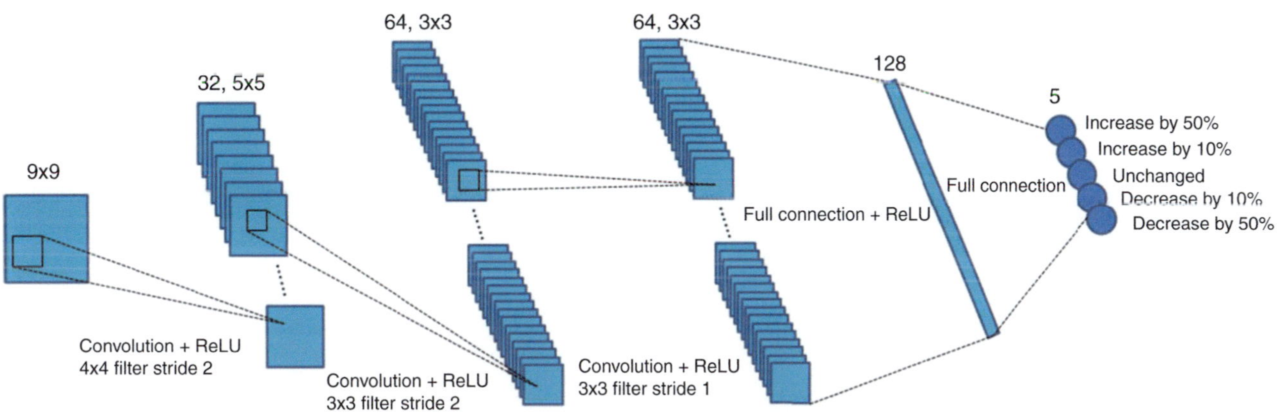

Fig. 15.21 The CNN style NN architecture used to generate predictions on the actions that the TV iterative reconstruction algorithm should perform [28]

for different applications of medical CT imaging. These approaches were split into two broad categories based on the input and output of the NN, image enhancement, and image reconstruction. NN-based image enhancement encompasses techniques that are designed to extract existing information about the current image and produce more meaningful results, whereas AI-based applications with image reconstruction are focused on producing a more meaningful image from a series of images. With either of these two applications and the specific task being solved, the approach requires a sufficient amount of preexisting knowledge about the initial information that will be used as input to the NN and the desired outcome. A warning should be given that while an NN may demonstrate its success, it may not provide enough testing and validation to prove that the NN is robust enough to adequately solve the problem.

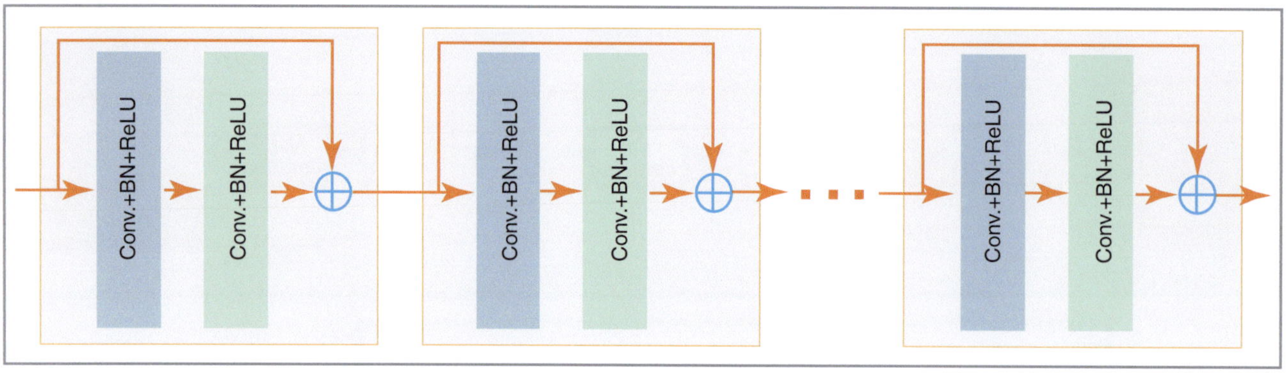

Fig. 15.22 Basic representation of a residual CNN block. Note the skip connection from the start to the finish of each individual block [29]

References

1. Kong F, Wilson N, Shadden SC. A deep-learning approach for direct whole-heart mesh reconstruction. arXiv Prepr. *arXiv2102.07899*, 2021.
2. Koo HJ, et al. Automated segmentation of left ventricular myocardium on cardiac computed tomography using deep learning. Korean J Radiol. 2020;21(6):660.
3. Lim H, Dewaraja YK, Fessler JA. Joint low-count PET/CT segmentation and reconstruction with paired variational neural networks. Med Imaging 2020 Phys Med Imaging. 2020;11312:113120U.
4. Ye M, et al. PC-U net: learning to jointly reconstruct and segment the cardiac walls in 3D from CT data. arXiv Prepr. *arXiv2008.08194*, 2020.
5. Symons R, et al. Dual-contrast agent photon-counting computed tomography of the heart: initial experience. Int J Cardiovasc Imaging. 2017:33(8). https://doi.org/10.1007/s10554-017-1104-4.
6. Willemink MJ, Persson M, Pourmorteza A, Pelc NJ, Fleischmann D. Photon-counting CT: technical principles and clinical prospects. Radiology. 2018;289(2):172656. https://doi.org/10.1148/radiol.2018172656.
7. Lyu T, et al. Estimating dual-energy CT imaging from single-energy CT data with material decomposition convolutional neural network. Med Image Anal. 2021;70:102001.
8. Abascal JFPJ, et al. "Material decomposition in spectral CT using deep learning: A Sim2Real transfer approach," IEEE Access. 2021;9:25632–47.
9. Leuschner J, Schmidt M, Baguer DO, Maaß P. The lodopab-ct dataset: a benchmark dataset for low-dose ct reconstruction methods. arXiv Prepr. *arXiv1910.01113*, 2019.
10. Kang E, Min J, Ye JC. A deep convolutional neural network using directional wavelets for low-dose X-ray CT reconstruction. Med Phys. 2017;44(10):e360–75.
11. Choe J, et al. Deep learning–based image conversion of CT reconstruction kernels improves radiomics reproducibility for pulmonary nodules or masses. Radiology. 2019;292(2):365–73.
12. Patwari M, Gutjahr R, Raupach R, Maier A. Measuring CT reconstruction quality with deep convolutional neural networks. In: International workshop on machine learning for medical image reconstruction. Cham: Springer; 2019. p. 113–24.
13. Li S, et al. Blind CT image quality assessment via deep learning strategy: initial study," in Medical Imaging 2018: Image Perception, Observer Performance, and Technology Assessment. Int J Opt Photonics. 2018;10577:44.
14. Ravishankar S, Ye JC, Fessler JA. Image reconstruction: from sparsity to data-adaptive methods and machine learning. Proc IEEE. 2019;108(1):86–109.
15. Willemink MJ, Noël PB. The evolution of image reconstruction for CT—from filtered back projection to artificial intelligence. Eur Radiol. 2019;29(5):2185–95.
16. Kambadakone A. Artificial intelligence and CT image reconstruction: potential of a new era in radiation dose reduction. J Am Coll Radiol. 2020;17(5):649–51.
17. Cong W, Xi Y, De Man B, Wang G. Monochromatic image reconstruction via machine learning. Mach Learn Sci Technol. 2021;2(2):025032.
18. Zhang W, et al. Dual-energy CT reconstruction from dual quarter scans. arXiv Prepr. *arXiv2012.11374*, 2020.
19. Wu Z, Yang T, Li L, Zhu Y. Hierarchical convolutional network for sparse-view X-ray CT reconstruction. Comput Imaging IV. 2019;10990:109900V.
20. Podgorsak AR, Shiraz Bhurwani MM, Ionita CN. CT artifact correction for sparse and truncated projection data using generative adversarial networks. Med Phys. 2021;48(2):615–26.
21. Lossau T, Nickisch H, Wissel T, Morlock M, Grass M. Learning metal artifact reduction in cardiac CT images with moving pacemakers. Med Image Anal. 2020;61:101655.
22. Wei R, et al. Real-time tumor localization with single x-ray projection at arbitrary gantry angles using a convolutional neural network (CNN). Phys Med Biol. 2020;65(6):65012.
23. Hu D, et al. Hybrid-domain neural network processing for sparse-view CT reconstruction. IEEE Trans Radiat Plasma Med Sci. 2020;5(1):88–98.
24. Zhang Q, Hu Z, Jiang C, Zheng H, Ge Y, Liang D. Artifact removal using a hybrid-domain convolutional neural network for limited-angle computed tomography imaging. Phys Med Biol. 2020;65(15):155010.
25. Wu D, Kim K, El Fakhri G, Li Q. Iterative low-dose CT reconstruction with priors trained by artificial neural network. IEEE Trans Med Imaging. 2017;36(12):2479–86.
26. Wang G, Ye JC, Mueller K, Fessler JA. Image reconstruction is a new frontier of machine learning. IEEE Trans Med Imaging. 2018;37(6):1289–96.
27. Chen H, et al. LEARN: learned experts' assessment-based reconstruction network for sparse-data CT. IEEE Trans Med Imaging. 2018;37(6):1333–47.
28. Shen C, Gonzalez Y, Chen L, Jiang SB, Jia X. Intelligent parameter tuning in optimization-based iterative CT reconstruction via deep reinforcement learning. IEEE Trans Med Imaging. 2018;37(6):1430–9.
29. He J, et al. Optimizing a parameterized plug-and-play ADMM for iterative low-dose CT reconstruction. IEEE Trans Med Imaging. 2018;38(2):371–82.

Artificial Intelligence-Based Contrast Medium Optimization

16

Bibi Martens, Babs M. F. Hendriks, Joachim E. Wildberger, and Casper Mihl

Background in Scan and Contrast Media Protocols

Coronary CT angiography (CCTA) has a very high negative predictive value for ruling out coronary artery disease (99%) [1]. Sufficient intravascular enhancement of the coronaries (>325 Hounsfield Units [HU]) is necessary to reach diagnostic accuracy [2]. The k-edge of iodine lies at 33 keV, and when the tube voltage approaches the k-edge, the attenuation of iodine increases [3]. This makes it possible to increase the vascular or parenchymal enhancement by decreasing the tube voltage of the scan acquisition. Different parameters can be adapted to reach sufficient enhancement of the coronaries in each patient on every occasion. First of all, the iodine delivery rate (IDR) is considered the most decisive parameter for attenuation of vascular structures [4, 5]. Second, a body weight-adapted CM injection protocol results in more homogeneous enhancement of the coronary arteries, compared to a one-size-fits-all protocol [6]. Lastly, the 10-to-10 rule optimises the CM application even further based on the tube voltage used: A 10 kV reduction should be followed by a 10% reduction in IDR and vice versa [7]. To optimise CM timing, a test bolus or bolus tracking technique can be used [8]. For the test bolus method, multiple low-dose axial image slices are acquired at one point on the z-axis after the injection of a small amount of CM. The test bolus is injected with the same flow rate and concentration as the main bolus. This creates a time-enhancement curve where the peak enhancement can be determined to find the optimal timing for the scan. The time to peak is used as an estimated scan delay for the scan with the main CM dose [9]. For bolus tracking, CM is injected and attenuation is measured in a predefined vessel until a threshold is reached. Once the attenuation reaches the threshold, the scan starts after a predefined fixed delay [10].

There are three different cardiac scan acquisition modes, ECG triggered or flash (high-pitch mode), prospective ECG gated (step and shoot) and retrospective ECG gating (helical). Based on heart rate and heart rhythm, a specific protocol is chosen [11].

Iterative Reconstruction (IR) techniques, automated tube current modulation (ATCM) and automated tube voltage selection (ATVS) are at present incorporated in daily clinical routine. These techniques are performed semi-automatically as they have to be approved by a radiographer and generally do not fall under the topic of AI. CM injectors that combine scanner protocol information (e.g., tube voltage and tube current selected by ATCM and ATVS) with the patient characteristics and clinical question are a promising tool for automatically optimising CM application but are yet to be developed and synchronised. To date, individualising CM injection protocols is still largely a manual and time-consuming action, which explains the preference for a standard "one-size-fits-all" protocol in many centres.

Artificial Intelligence for Contrast Media Optimisation

Because of technical developments, the cardiac CT scan duration nowadays is very short, ranging from several seconds to sub-second imaging. For imaging of the coronary arteries, a fast scan acquisition is beneficial as this makes imaging of the whole heart possible within one heartbeat, subsequently reducing radiation and CM dose. Faster scanners and shortened CM protocols result in more critical scan timing, as the chance of missing the peak enhancement increases, especially with respect to the vascular structures [9, 10, 12]. AI could improve coordination of scan and CM

B. Martens, MD · B. M. F. Hendriks, MD · J. E. Wildberger, MD, PhD
C. Mihl, MD, PhD (✉)
Department of Radiology and Nuclear Medicine, Maastricht University Medical Center, Maastricht, The Netherlands

CARIM School for Cardiovascular Diseases, Maastricht University, Maastricht, The Netherlands
e-mail: bibi.martens@mumc.nl; babs.hendriks@mumc.nl; j.wildberger@mumc.nl; casper.mihl@mumc.nl

C. N. De Cecco et al. (eds.), *Artificial Intelligence in Cardiothoracic Imaging*, Contemporary Medical Imaging,
https://doi.org/10.1007/978-3-030-92087-6_16

timing, resulting in optimised CM and radiation dose in each individual patient.

The possibility to perform thoracic scans in a single heartbeat reduces motion artefacts, and cardiac structures can nowadays often be assessed on a regular CT of the chest [12]. Image quality might be sufficient to evaluate the heart although on a regular chest CT, there might be not enough CM distribution in the cardiac chambers. Suboptimal cardiac enhancement is not surprising as a dedicated cardiac scan is performed later after start of CM injection than a regular CT of the chest [13]. As a result, information regarding cardiopathies and valvular changes stay hidden.

A triple rule out protocol has been advocated as a solution for better cardiac image quality on chest CTs [14]. AI however may bypass the additional CM volume of a triple rule out CM protocol, and it could bypass the need for CM entirely. A deep convolutional neural network (DCNN) has shown to be beneficial in these areas too [15]. Santini et al. developed a DCNN capable of producing contrast-enhanced CT (CECT) images out of a non-contrast image of the thorax by mimicking the human visual system with the created network [15]. The left cardiac ventricle was delineated by the software on the non-CECT images, leading to the synthesised CECT image. Non-contrast images were compared to real CECT images and the synthesised CECT images. A Normalized Mutual Information index (NMI) was used to quantify the capability of the model to create a synthesised CECT close to the real CECT. The Dice index is a statistical tool that compares the similarity between two datasets and was used to evaluate the estimation of the cardiac ventricles. The synthesised compared to the real CECT images gained a good similarity (NMI of 0.93 ± 0.03), and extraction of the left ventricle was possible (Dice = 0.88). Therefore, it was possible to subtract the left cardiac ventricle from a non-CECT image and, in addition, to provide volumetric information of the heart on a regular thoracic CT [15]. Mannil et al. used texture analysis and machine learning to detect a myocardial infarction on an unenhanced low radiation dose cardiac CT [16]. Both DCNN and machine learning turn out to be capable of retrieving latent information from a non-CECT image. As information about the cardiac ventricles can be subtracted from non-CECT images, it seems to be a small step to generate an optimal contrast-enhanced coronary image of a CT with reduced CM dosing or scans with alternative CM timing (such as chest CTs).

In current clinical practice, total CM volumes containing as little as 9 g of iodine can be used for CCTA with diagnostic image quality. Further reduction of CM might not be necessary for the protection of kidney function [17]. However, it should be pointed out that reducing the amount of CM also decreases health care costs. Furthermore, iodinated CM reaches the groundwater and has an influence on the environment as well [18]. AI could play a big role in aiding wide acceptance and implementation of individualised CM protocols by fully automating the process of CM individualisation. This individualisation might be beneficial for advanced data-characterisation algorithms, such as radiomics. Differences in, for example, cardiac output and CM injection protocols influence the distribution of the CM in tissue. In addition, differences in scan acquisition parameters might influence spatial analysis [19]. Therefore, differences in scan and CM protocols can influence features derived from radiomics algorithms. In order to optimally apply radiomics in the future, it seems vital that scan and injection protocols become comparable between hospital and countries.

Takumi et al. used bolus tracking data of previous CT scans of the same patient in dynamic liver imaging. The authors showed that a scan delay based on previous bolus tracking data resulted in a similar CM enhancement. Previous bolus tracking data could be used in following scans, shortening exam time and reducing radiation exposure [20]. However, this will be more challenging to apply in cardiac imaging as various different factors (e.g., medication, disease, patient stress level and time of the day) will influence cardiac output.

Uniformity of the CM protocol throughout the different hospitals in the world could lead to optimal (coronary) enhancement in each patient every time. In addition, by individualising and optimising CM injection protocols all around the world, attenuation of the targeted structures should become more uniform, which could be beneficial for future AI techniques.

Artificial Intelligence for Contrast Media Injection Protocol Selection

Scan duration and therefore the CM injection protocol for both the prospective and retrospective ECG-gated protocol are longer than for the ECG-triggered (flash) protocol to ensure optimal enhancement of the coronaries. Having three different cardiac scan protocols makes the individualisation of scan and CM protocols even more complex.

An irregular heartbeat can complicate the selection of the right protocol. Problems in synchronisation of ECG signal with data acquisition sometimes result in non-diagnostic image quality necessitating scan repetition, with no guarantee of the second scan being of diagnostic image quality. AI could learn to recognise specific heartbeat patterns and select the appropriate scan protocol. Moreover, while determining the best scan protocol for the individual patient, the AI model should be capable of selecting the appropriate CM injection protocol on the available scanner for the specific question at hand. Notably, bolus tracking with a fixed trigger delay could miss peak enhancement in patients with a very high or very low cardiac output because it does not take patient-specific cardiovascular parameters output into account [9, 10]. AI and machine learning algorithms could be applied to individualise trigger scan delay when using bolus tracking. Hinzpeter et al. proposed to use at least four bolus tracking enhancement values to evaluate the CM dynamics in the individual patient. This information can be used to match the data to the available enhancement curves in an online database containing different arterial blood circulation curves. Thereby, the optimal scan timing could be determined based on the best suited enhancement curve for each patient [10, 21].

Ideally, AI will suggest the most appropriate protocol, so suboptimal image quality and repeated scanning can be a thing of the past. In addition, it would be of great value if it were possible to predict whether a prospectively ECG-gated acquisition will be executed smoothly. For example, an AI algorithm capable of predicting that an extrasystole will lead to a longer scan time can adapt the CM bolus mid-scan to ensure sufficient enhancement throughout the whole scan duration.

AI-Based Image Reconstruction Techniques

As mentioned before, decreasing the tube voltage is advantageous for both radiation and CM dose. However, it comes at the expense of increased image noise. Noise reduction algorithms offer dedicated opportunities in this respect. A knowledge-based IR algorithm minimises the difference between measured raw CT data and the estimated image by a penalty-based cost function [22]. It decreases image noise and increases the contrast-to-noise ratio (CNR) [23]. Wang et al. evaluated an AI-based noise reduction algorithm based on a DCNN [24]. Their AI-based noise reduction algorithm is based on 40 CT scans of the aorta at normal dose and at a simulated low dose. The dedicated algorithm learned that the output was input minus noise and, in this way, was able to generate noise-reduced images. The algorithm improved image quality of the aorta, facilitating a 50% CM dose reduction [24].

Another possibility for radiation and CM reduction lies in the large portion of follow-up CT scans performed on a daily basis, for example, for oncological patients. These patients undergo repeated scanning of the same anatomical region. Therefore, shared anatomical information between those scans is available. This information can be used in an IR algorithm to significantly improve the diagnostic image quality [25]. In the future, it might become possible to use the anatomical information from scans performed for a different indication, for a scheduled cardiac scan of the same patient, thereby reducing both radiation and CM dose. This could lead to both scan and CM protocol optimisation as well as improvements in workflow.

Non-calcified and low-attenuating plaques are more prone to future events than calcified plaques as calcifications might stabilise the coronary plaque [26]. In addition, positive remodelling, spotty calcifications and the napkin-ring sign are indicators of a high-risk plaque [27]. Occasionally, some rather big differences in interpretation between readers can be present, and especially blooming artefacts hamper the interpretation of soft plaques. In that respect, subtraction techniques might be promising for reducing these blooming artefacts [28]. Differences in scan quality, CM application but also the experience of the reader and the subtlety of the findings will influence subjective evaluation of the CCTA [29]. AI techniques could be helpful in standardising plaque interpretation and might even go a step further in determining plaque characteristics [27, 30].

Workflow

Scheduling a CT or MRI scan is often a job done by the supportive staff in the radiology department. It is time-consuming and prone to errors. AI algorithms could be used to plan and schedule this medical care [31]. The selection of the correct imaging modality, scan and CM injection protocol, as well as the ideal study date (e.g., should the scan be performed within an hour or a month), is a parameter to keep in mind when scheduling an exam, a task that might be difficult and prone to changes but could be rather easy for an AI algorithm. This automated scheduling could involve prioritising patients and selecting the optimal imaging technique (e.g., ultrasound, CT or MRI) [31].

Information from previous studies could be taken into account. Anxious patients, known risk factors for CM-related unfavourable outcomes, difficulty with obtaining venous access or a known irregular heartbeat (with exception of paradoxical atrial fibrillation, which is often not predictable) could be known upfront. This information could be used to select specific time slots for the requested CT or MRI exam. Predicting the scan type and scan duration correctly will improve efficient use of scanners and staff [21]. Altogether, this optimised workflow will lead to improved patient care.

Red Flags

The minimal diagnostic vascular enhancement for the coronary arteries, the aorta and the pulmonary arteries is well studied [32]. An attenuation below the threshold might result in non-diagnostic image quality, but when the enhancement is too high, CM can lead to artefacts mimicking relevant findings, making image quality suboptimal as well. For each target (vascular structure), it is possible to define an attenuation range for each CT exam. In case the limit is not reached or if the diagnostic HU level is exceeded, the study is regarded as suboptimal. It might be possible to exclude gross pathologies on images with suboptimal attenuation of the designated structures, but there is an increased risk that significant findings might be missed or misinterpreted. Factors such as motion artefacts, irregular heartbeat and unintentional incorrect scanner and/or injector settings might result in an unanticipated insufficient image quality [33]. Ideally, an algorithm could approve image quality before the patient leaves the scanner room. The program should be capable of determining whether the coronary attenuation is sufficient and if artefacts are present that influence the interpretation significantly.

On some occasions, an outpatient CT or MRI scan might be in a worklist for several days, while the scan shows unexpected pathology requiring immediate attention. AI could be trained to recognise and "flag" a scan when unexpected clinically significant findings are indicated that should be reviewed right away. For example, a significant unstable coronary plaque, an aneurysm or dissection of the ascending aorta or an imminent cardiac tamponade could trigger an alarm signal notifying the radiologist to look at this exam immediately.

Summary

AI might be able to contribute to quality insurance by determining an individualised CM, scan and reconstruction technique in each patient. The scan could automatically be followed by an attenuation check of the targeted structure and a warning signal in case of any pathology present that is in need of immediate attention (Fig. 16.1). One step further, it would be valuable if AI could determine which parameters to adjust and to what extent to reach a sufficient image quality when the first or any previous scan was regarded as non-diagnostic.

AI could be useful in individualising CM protocols based on patient and scanner characteristics as well as on suspected clinical pathology to improve both daily clinical care and workflow although, in that respect, the question rises if this might be applicable in the near future because of legal considerations: Who is taking the responsibilities if something goes wrong? This leads to an ethical discussion that will have to take place before AI can become widely incorporated in medical imaging. The example of self-driving cars sets out the grey area clearly. Who is responsible when a bystander gets hurt, can the self-driving car be responsible? Compared to a human, the car will probably not be able to make a morally guided decision when an accident is about to happen. Because of these discussions, the introduction of self-driving cars did not happen yet [34]. AI taking over the radiologists' job is ethically not so easy either.

One frequently reappearing topic of discussion involves AI taking over the radiologists' job. According to Geoffrey Hinton, no more radiologists should be trained because deep learning would outperform the radiologist within 5 years, stated in 2016 in Toronto [35]. As long as AI is seen as a potential threat, we might miss all the opportunities it has in store for us. This chapter has pointed out the possibilities of

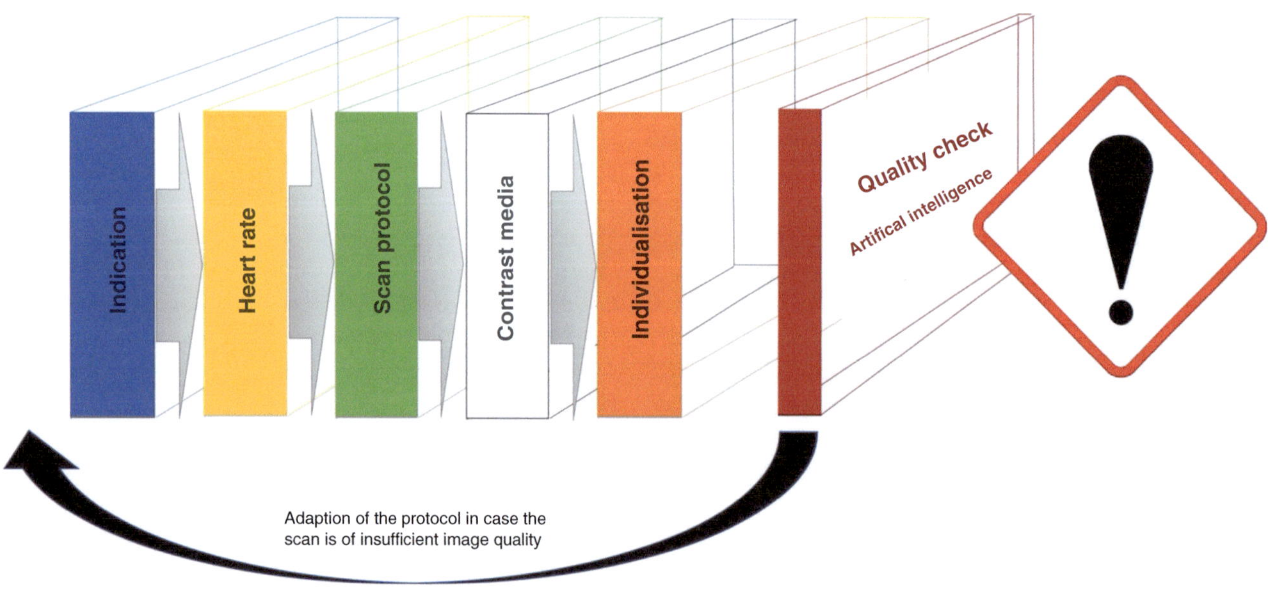

Fig. 16.1 The loop starts with the scan indication, followed by heart rate, which will influence the scan protocol regarded most appropriate. Next, the corresponding contrast media protocol will be selected and aligned with the individual patient parameters. The loop will end with a quality check. In case the quality is insufficient, the loop will iterate to improve the scan and contrast media protocol, based on errors and specific characteristics from previous exams. The loop is followed by an automated read for urgent findings in need of immediate attention

a DCNN, machine learning and deep learning as a tool for CM optimalisation in both CT and MRI. These kinds of applications could be used to improve workflow, image quality and even diagnostic capabilities. The future of radiology is bright, if we adopt the opportunities AI offers early.

References

1. Plank F, Friedrich G, Dichtl W, Klauser A, Jaschke W, Franz WM, et al. The diagnostic and prognostic value of coronary CT angiography in asymptomatic high-risk patients: a cohort study. Open Heart. 2014;1(1):e000096.
2. Eijsvoogel NG, Hendriks BMF, Nelemans P, Mihl C, Willigers J, Martens B, et al. Personalization of CM injection protocols in coronary computed tomographic angiography (people CT trial). Contrast Media Mol Imaging. 2020;2020:5407936.
3. Fleischmann U, Pietsch H, Korporaal JG, Flohr TG, Uder M, Jost G, et al. Impact of contrast media concentration on low-kilovolt computed tomography angiography: a systematic preclinical approach. Investig Radiol. 2018;53(5):264–70.
4. Kok M, Mihl C, Hendriks BM, Altintas S, Kietselaer BL, Wildberger JE, et al. Optimizing contrast media application in coronary CT angiography at lower tube voltage: evaluation in a circulation phantom and sixty patients. Eur J Radiol. 2016;85(6):1068–74.
5. Rengo M, Dharampal A, Lubbers M, Kock M, Wildberger JE, Das M, et al. Impact of iodine concentration and iodine delivery rate on contrast enhancement in coronary CT angiography: a randomized multicenter trial (CT-CON). Eur Radiol. 2019;29(11):6109–18.
6. Mihl C, Kok M, Altintas S, Kietselaer BL, Turek J, Wildberger JE, et al. Evaluation of individually body weight adapted contrast media injection in coronary CT-angiography. Eur J Radiol. 2016;85(4):830–6.
7. Martens B, Hendriks BMF, Mihl C, Wildberger JE. Tailoring contrast media protocols to varying tube voltages in vascular and parenchymal CT imaging: the 10-to-10 rule. Investig Radiol. 2020;55(10):673–6.
8. Cademartiri F, Nieman K, van der Lugt A, Raaijmakers RH, Mollet N, Pattynama PM, et al. Intravenous contrast material administration at 16-detector row helical CT coronary angiography: test bolus versus bolus-tracking technique. Radiology. 2004;233(3):817–23.
9. Bae KT. Intravenous contrast medium administration and scan timing at CT: considerations and approaches. Radiology. 2010;256(1):32–61.
10. Hinzpeter R, Eberhard M, Gutjahr R, Reeve K, Pfammatter T, Lachat M, et al. CT angiography of the aorta: contrast timing by using a fixed versus a patient-specific trigger delay. Radiology. 2019;291(2):531–8.
11. Machida H, Tanaka I, Fukui R, Shen Y, Ishikawa T, Tate E, et al. Current and novel imaging techniques in coronary CT. Radiographics. 2015;35(4):991–1010.
12. Lell MM, Wildberger JE, Alkadhi H, Damilakis J, Kachelriess M. Evolution in computed tomography: the Battle for speed and dose. Investig Radiol. 2015;50(9):629–44.
13. Frauenfelder T, Appenzeller P, Karlo C, Scheffel H, Desbiolles L, Stolzmann P, et al. Triple rule-out CT in the emergency department: protocols and spectrum of imaging findings. Eur Radiol. 2009;19(4):789–99.
14. Kidoh M, Nakaura T, Nakamura S, Namimoto T, Nozaki T, Sakaino N, et al. Contrast material and radiation dose reduction strategy for triple-rule-out cardiac CT angiography: feasibility study of non-ECG-gated low kVp scan of the whole chest following coronary CT angiography. Acta Radiol. 2014;55(10):1186–96.
15. Santini G, Zumbo L, Martini N, Valvano G, Leo A, Ripoli A, et al. Synthetic contrast enhancement in cardiac CT with deep learning 2018. Available from: https://arxiv.org/pdf/1807.01779.pdf.
16. Mannil M, von Spiczak J, Manka R, Alkadhi H. Texture analysis and machine learning for detecting myocardial infarction in noncontrast low-dose computed tomography: unveiling the invisible. Investig Radiol. 2018;53(6):338–43.
17. Nijssen EC, Rennenberg RJ, Nelemans PJ, Essers BA, Janssen MM, Vermeeren MA, et al. Prophylactic hydration to protect renal function from intravascular iodinated contrast material in patients at high risk of contrast-induced nephropathy (AMACING): a prospective, randomised, phase 3, controlled, open-label, non-inferiority trial. Lancet. 2017;389(10076):1312–22.
18. Kormos JL, Schulz M, Ternes TA. Occurrence of iodinated X-ray contrast media and their biotransformation products in the urban water cycle. Environ Sci Technol. 2011;45(20):8723–32.
19. Ibrahim A, Primakov S, Beuque M, Woodruff HC, Halilaj I, Wu G, et al. Radiomics for precision medicine: current challenges, future prospects, and the proposal of a new framework. Methods. 2020;188:20–9.
20. Takumi K, Fukukura Y, Shindo T, Kumagae Y, Tateyama A, Kamiyama T, et al. Feasibility of a fixed scan delay technique using a previous bolus tracking technique data for dynamic hepatic CT. Eur J Radiol. 2012;81(11):2996–3001.
21. Eberhard M, Alkadhi H. Machine learning and deep neural networks: applications in patient and scan preparation, contrast medium, and radiation dose optimization. J Thorac Imaging. 2020;35(Suppl 1):S17–20.
22. Yuki H, Utsunomiya D, Funama Y, Tokuyasu S, Namimoto T, Hirai T, et al. Value of knowledge-based iterative model reconstruction in low-kV 256-slice coronary CT angiography. J Cardiovasc Comput Tomogr. 2014;8(2):115–23.
23. Iyama Y, Nakaura T, Yokoyama K, Kidoh M, Harada K, Oda S, et al. Low-contrast and low-radiation dose protocol in cardiac computed tomography: usefulness of low tube voltage and knowledge-based iterative model reconstruction algorithm. J Comput Assist Tomogr. 2016;40(6):941–7.
24. Wang Y, Yu M, Wang M, Wang Y, Kong L, Yi Y, et al. Application of artificial intelligence-based image optimization for computed tomography angiography of the aorta with low tube voltage and reduced contrast medium volume. J Thorac Imaging. 2019;34(6):393–9.
25. Willemink MJ, Noel PB. The evolution of image reconstruction for CT-from filtered back projection to artificial intelligence. Eur Radiol. 2019;29(5):2185–95.
26. von Knebel Doeberitz PL, De Cecco CN, Schoepf UJ, Albrecht MH, van Assen M, De Santis D, et al. Impact of coronary computerized tomography angiography-derived plaque quantification and machine-learning computerized tomography fractional flow reserve on adverse cardiac outcome. Am J Cardiol. 2019;124(9):1340–8.
27. Kolossvary M, De Cecco CN, Feuchtner G, Maurovich-Horvat P. Advanced atherosclerosis imaging by CT: Radiomics, machine learning and deep learning. J Cardiovasc Comput Tomogr. 2019;13(5):274–80.
28. Duarte Conde MP, de Korte AM, Meijer FJA, Aquarius R, Boogaarts HD, Bartels R, et al. Subtraction CTA: an alternative imaging option for the follow-up of flow-diverter-treated aneurysms? AJNR Am J Neuroradiol. 2018;39(11):2051–6.
29. Saur SC, Alkadhi H, Stolzmann P, Baumuller S, Leschka S, Scheffel H, et al. Effect of reader experience on variability, evaluation time and accuracy of coronary plaque detection with computed tomography coronary angiography. Eur Radiol. 2010;20(7):1599–606.
30. van Assen M, Varga-Szemes A, Schoepf UJ, Duguay TM, Hudson HT, Egorova S, et al. Automated plaque analysis for the prognostication of major adverse cardiac events. Eur J Radiol. 2019;116:76–83.

31. Spyropoulos CD. AI planning and scheduling in the medical hospital environment. Artif Intell Med. 2000;20(2):101–11.
32. Scholtz JE, Ghoshhajra B. Advances in cardiac CT contrast injection and acquisition protocols. Cardiovasc Diagn Ther. 2017;7(5):439–51.
33. Ghekiere O, Salgado R, Buls N, Leiner T, Mancini I, Vanhoenacker P, et al. Image quality in coronary CT angiography: challenges and technical solutions. Br J Radiol. 2017;90(1072):20160567.
34. Lau A. The ethics of self-driving cars. Should cars determine if you live or die? 2020. Available from: https://towardsdatascience.com/the-ethics-of-self-driving-cars-efaaaaf9e320.
35. Mukherjee S. A.I Versus M.D. 2017. Available from: http://www.newyorker.com/magazine/2017/04/03/ai-versus-md.

Radiation Dose Optimization: The Role of Artificial Intelligence

17

Damiano Caruso, Domenico De Santis, Tiziano Polidori, Marta Zerunian, and Andrea Laghi

Introduction

Artificial intelligence (AI) is an emerging technique impacting the world we live in, including medical imaging. Its current massive popularity hinges on three intertwined pillars: big data availability, constant increase of computational power, and algorithms [1]. Among its various tasks, imaging denoising is the one holding the highest expectations for CT radiation dose optimization. AI is a generic term indicating a science that mimics cognitive human functions, aiming at performing tasks that are typical of human intelligence. Machine learning (ML) is a subset of AI in which algorithms build their own training data, requiring no explicit programming. Feature learning is a subset of machine learning in which the algorithm automatically selects the features useful to detect and classify data. Lastly, deep learning (DL) is a subset of representation whose architecture is formed by the composition of multiple-level mathematical equations, known as deep neural networks (DNNs), based on the demands of the specific task that must be accomplished in order to achieve what ML does.

Despite continuous technical advancements, CT radiation dose and the potential risk of induced carcinogenesis are still a matter of concern in terms of public health, both in the scientific community [2, 3] and in the lay press [4, 5]. In addition to the implementation of decision guidelines and the education of radiology personnel, referring clinicians, and patients [6, 7], CT scanning parameters such as tube voltage [8] and tube current modulation [9], prospective ECG gating in cardiac CTA (CCTA) [10], and high-pitch acquisition protocols [11] are determinant factors in radiation dose optimization. Among the CT technical parameters, image reconstruction plays a fundamental role in the final image quality and, consequently, in the management of radiation exposure.

D. Caruso, MD, PhD · D. De Santis, MD · T. Polidori, MD
M. Zerunian, MD · A. Laghi, MD (✉)
Department of Medical Surgical Sciences and Translational Medicine, Sapienza University of Rome - Sant' Andrea University Hospital, Rome, Italy
e-mail: damiano.caruso@uniroma1.it; marta.zerunian@uniroma1.it; andrea.laghi@uniroma1.it

Filtered Back Projection and Iterative Reconstruction

Filtered back projection (FBP) has been the main reconstruction algorithm applied to CT for three decades, mainly due to its time efficiency and its good performances in an "ideal setting." FBP is a robust analytic reconstruction algorithm that filters the acquired projection data to manipulate certain image features (such as edge smoothing or enhancement) and projects them back in the image space. This reconstruction technique is based on the assumption that images are ideal, namely, free of noise. On the contrary, CT images are intrinsically noisy, and the filtration process of the FBP itself amplifies the noise [12]. As a result, variables connected to the x-ray beam, the CT system, and the patient might result in low-quality images, eventually leading to radiation dose increase in order to keep the quality acceptable in clinical setting [13].

Iterative reconstruction (IR) techniques were commercially introduced in the late 2000s, aiming at overcoming FBP limitations and reducing patient's radiation exposure. However, it is worth noting that the very first CT scanners were equipped with a type of IR system, named algebraic reconstruction technique (ART) [14], soon abandoned in favor of FBP due to the lack of computational power of the computers of those years. IR techniques, either hybrid (combined with FBP) or model-based (pure IR) [15], are nowadays widely implemented in clinical practice, providing a good trade-off between image quality and radiation exposure [16]. Nevertheless, they might not be time effective and tend to impact noise magnitude and image texture, returning image datasets characterized by excessive smoothing and consequent "plastic" appearance compared to the standard

C. N. De Cecco et al. (eds.), *Artificial Intelligence in Cardiothoracic Imaging*, Contemporary Medical Imaging,
https://doi.org/10.1007/978-3-030-92087-6_17

FBP images radiologists are familiar with [17]. In clinical practice, such downside results in the avoidance of the highest levels of IR, eventually preventing a full exploitation of such technique's potential in terms of radiation exposure.

Artificial Intelligence in Imaging Reconstruction

AI has gained increasing interest for its potential to optimize image reconstructions [13]. A DL imaging reconstruction engine has to learn the specific properties of the ground truth image dataset, which works as training target. Such training dataset is formed by FBP- or IR-reconstructed images, characterized by a natural appearance in terms of noise and texture when acquired under ideal conditions and high radiation dose. Both phantom and actual patients' CT datasets have been used to train DL image reconstruction engines for them to be able to achieve the best results in terms of different body habitus, scan parameters, and clinical indications.

A DL image reconstruction engine needs to be trained, validated, and tested. To train the engine, two datasets are collected for each object of interest: a high-dose, low-noise dataset and a low-dose, high-noise dataset; the former is labeled as ground truth. The reconstruction engine is then applied to the low-dose dataset, aiming at generating output images. These images are subsequently compared to the ground truth to unveil differences in noise, texture, spatial resolution, etc. The DNN then learns how to make the low-dose images look as good as the high-dose dataset (ground truth). In other words, by training with pairs of images, a DNN learns the correlation between matching voxel values in a low-dose image and in a corresponding routine-dose image (Fig. 17.1). This process is repeated thousands of times, on different training data, until the engine is able to emulate ground truth images in various conditions. The validation and testing processes implement a large number of various datasets, not used in the training phase, that have to be accurately reconstructed by the DL engine to ensure its robustness.

Some major CT manufacturers have implemented DNN image reconstruction algorithms. In particular, GE Healthcare algorithm (TrueFidelity) is trained with FBP images, while model-based IR datasets are used to train Canon Medical algorithm (Advanced intelligent Clear-IQ Engine, AiCE) to differentiate signal from noise. AlgoMedica is another vendor that implemented its own vendor-agnostic DL reconstruction algorithm (PixelShine), proved to be effective in reducing image noise and improving image quality in pelvic arterial-phase CT images [18]. The performances of these DL-based imaging reconstruction algorithms have been tested with both phantoms and patients' CT images and are still currently under active investigation.

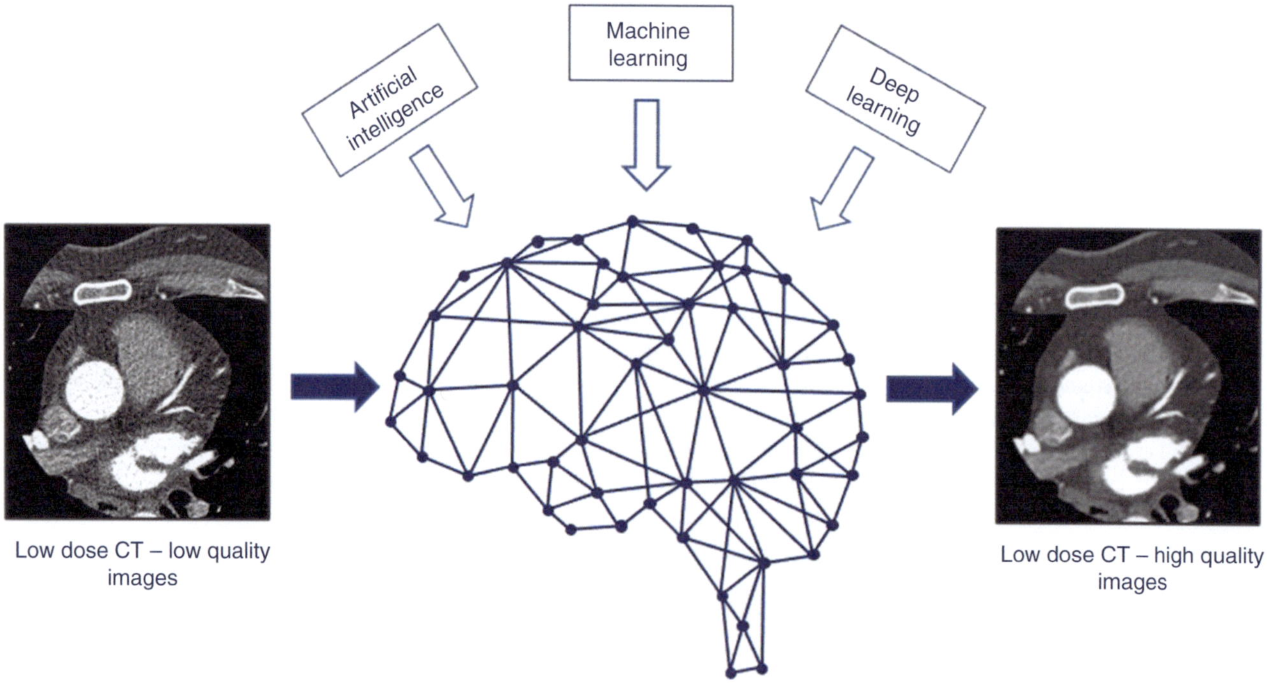

Fig. 17.1 Schematic representation of artificial intelligence influence on denoising and improvement of CT scans quality

Phantom Investigations

Higaki et al. [19] scanned a cylindrical phantom containing eight modules filled with contrast medium diluted at different concentrations, testing DL reconstruction technique performance compared to FBP and model-based IR. At high radiation doses, IR returned lower image noise, while at low radiation doses, DL reconstructed less noisy images. While IR outperformed DL in spatial resolution at both low- and high-dose setting, DL reconstruction provided the highest detectability at medium dose and reduced radiation dose settings. These characteristics are particularly useful in soft tissue examinations, such as abdominal CT, in which image contrast ranges from 50 to 200 HU. On the other hand, a higher spatial resolution can be fully exploited in chest CT imaging and CT angiography. Comparable results have been obtained by Shin et al. [20], both with a CT phantom and in clinical setting, proving DL reconstruction more effective than the other techniques in generating images with low image noise, leading however to a loss of spatial resolution.

Nevertheless, for a new technology to be fully exploitable in clinical practice, its denoising capabilities must be associated to improved diagnostic performances. Lesion detectability is indeed a key feature when assessing the performance of new reconstruction methods. A recent investigation, performed on a CT ACR 464 phantom, demonstrated that DL improves lesion detectability and reduces image noise compared to hybrid IR, without affecting image texture. As a consequence, radiation dose could be reduced from 9% to 56%, based on clinical task [21].

Despite enabling radiation dose reduction, AI could also be negatively affected by ultralow doses in performing other tasks, such as pulmonary nodule identification, as demonstrated by Fu et al. [22] in a recent investigation performed on a thorax anthropomorphic phantom. Therefore, AI-based software needs to be further optimized to be fully implemented in clinical work.

Clinical Investigations

DL reconstruction techniques have been also studied in clinical settings, attaining promising results. In 2007, Chen et al. [23] presented preliminary results with a lightweight DNN framework, trained with virtual low-dose CT datasets obtained by adding noise to the images of the teaching dataset. A deeper version of the DNN was subsequently presented, implementing directional wavelet specifically optimized to reduce image noise in low-dose CT [24]. Low-dose CT images are characterized by complex noise; by applying directional wavelets, the directional components of image noise are decomposed, allowing for an easier training of the DNN [25]. The proposed methods outperformed model-based IR, demonstrating a higher denoising power and a faster reconstruction time, achieving also the second place in the 2016 AAPM Low-Dose CT Grand Challenge [26].

A multicenter prospective trial including 22 patients who had undergone routine chest CT demonstrated that DL reconstruction outperformed low-dose and standard-dose IR images by generating images characterized by less noise and higher objective image quality. Additionally, DL allowed the identification of all nodules detectable with IR technique [27]. Favorable DL reconstruction results in terms of image quality have been additionally strengthened by a recent retrospective investigation performed on a population of 58 individuals who had undergone low-dose chest CT for lung cancer screening, as shown in Fig. 17.2 [28]. This study confirmed that DL outperformed adaptive statistical IR, providing less noisy images and higher objective image quality;

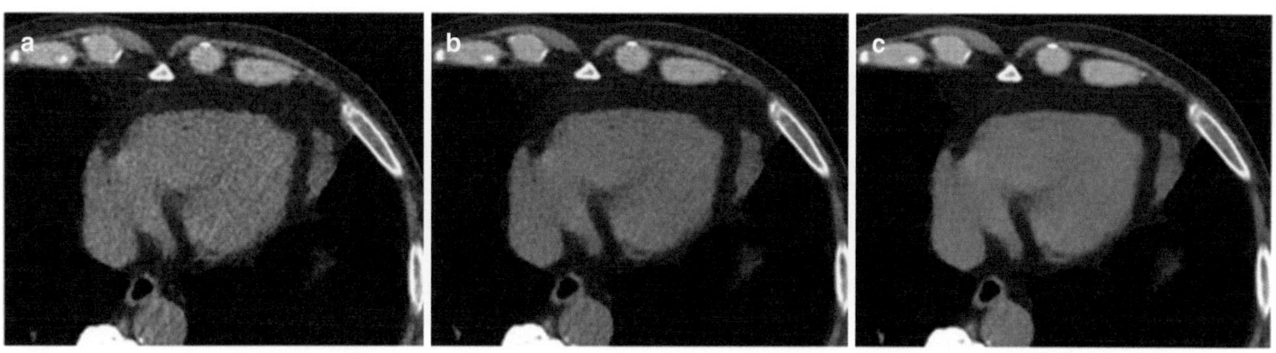

Fig. 17.2 Comparison of low-dose chest CT scan and axial soft tissue window images of mediastinum in a 73-year-old man. Reconstruction was performed with ASiR-V 30% (**a**), DLIR-M (**b**), and DLIR-H (**c**). Signal did not significantly vary across different reconstructions. However, image noise of DLIR images was lower than that of ASiR-V 30% images (ASiR-V 30% vs. DLIR-M, ASiR-V 30% vs. DLIR-H, and DLIR-M vs. DLIR-H, all $p < 0.001$). (Reprint from Kim et al. [28]; page 5, figure 2. (With permission) Author: Joo Hee Kim et al. [28], Publisher: Korean Society of Radiology , p. 1)

however, no lesion identification analysis has been performed.

DL reconstruction outperformed adaptive statistical IR also in contrast-enhanced CT exams in terms of overall image quality, lesion diagnostic confidence, artifacts, image noise, and image texture. It is worth noting that DL reconstruction progressively increases image blurring along with the generation of a denoised image dataset. Therefore, its strength must be carefully chosen based on clinical task, especially in oncologic settings, where the pretest probability of finding lesions is higher than in the general population [29].

Positive performances of DL reconstruction algorithm have been further confirmed in a recent investigation [30] which tested three strength levels of DL reconstruction versus adaptive statistical IR with high blending factors (80% and 100%). Nevertheless, it is worth nothing that similar to high blending factors in IR, excessive strength of DL reconstruction was accountable for more pronounced image blurring. However, images derived by DL reconstruction were always sharper than the ones obtained with IR.

Despite optimal results in terms of denoising, most DNN are trained to minimize the per-voxel mean squared error between the reference voxel and the predicted voxel. Therefore, the generated images might still be affected by edges over-smoothing and consequent loss of details. In the attempt of improving the performances in such task, some investigators developed denoising algorithms using generative adversarial network (GAN). A GAN is formed by two neural networks, namely, a generative network and a discriminator network, coupled and trained simultaneously. The generative network learns to produce low-dose realistic images, while the discriminator network is trained to tell real images from generated images, forcing the generator network to improve its performance by providing more realistic estimates of the routine-dose dataset. Wolterink et al. [31] applied a GAN to an anthropomorphic phantom and noncontrast-enhanced cardiac CT used to calculate coronary calcium scoring. This approach achieved a substantial noise reduction and generated images with a noise pattern similar to the reference routine-dose dataset. Additionally, this investigation proved DNN can learn to reduce noise even without voxel-wise spatially aligned training images, as might easily happen in cardiac imaging. It is noteworthy that the loss function of every algorithm has a major impact on the output images; the mean squared error (representing the square of the difference between pixel values in the low-noise image and the reduced-noise image) despite being quite used might not perform adequately in generating images for all clinical tasks. In fact, the universal loss function that works with all types of date does not exist. Hence, also the selection of the best loss function is a topic of ongoing research [32, 33].

The first study evaluating the effect of DL reconstruction on CCTA image quality was published in 2019 [34] and retrospectively enrolled 30 individuals with known or suspected coronary artery disease, proving DL effective in reducing image noise by 20%, obtaining significantly higher image quality and sharper coronary artery margins.

Promising results have been also obtained by a different DL-based denoising technique (specifically, a modified U-net model) trained with ultralow-dose CCTA scans to predict image noise from the given low-dose CCTA. This method reduce the overall noise by 70% and provided a pattern indistinguishable from that of real CCTA dataset [35]. This model, initially trained with 55,418 standard-dose CCTA images of 100 patients, has been subsequently tested in clinical setting by a retrospective single-center study, which documented CCTA images with 22% lower image noise, 40% higher quality, and no over-smoothing [36]. Nonetheless, diagnostic accuracy for coronary artery stenosis did not improve.

Benz et al. [37] proved a DL platform capable of improving image quality of CCTA by 138% and reduced image noise by 43% in comparison to adaptive statistical IR. Such considerable quality improvement allowed DL to generate images with 62% higher quality at IR-comparable levels of noise. More importantly, this investigation demonstrated that CCTA reconstructed with DL maintained comparable diagnostic accuracy of IR.

A recently published prospective study enrolled 70 patients who underwent CCTA, randomizing them into two groups: 80 and 100 kVp, both reconstructed with IR. The 80 kVp dataset was additionally used to degenerate a third, DL-based image dataset generated by a GAN trained with 500 sets of conventional dose CT images to which different proportion of noise were added, in order to simulate the CT images at various radiation dose. DL allowed for similar objective image quality of the 80 kVp dataset compared to IR-reconstructed 100 kVp images, a twofold increase in speed of reconstruction time, and a 55% radiation dose reduction compared to the IR-reconstructed 100 kVp [38].

Similar results have been obtained by a study performed on 289 patients with suspected stroke, which proved DL reconstruction technique effective in obtaining images of approximately 50% higher quality and 40% less effective dose compared to IR. Thus, DL techniques might allow for an even more significant dose reduction compared to standard algorithm if properly set to match the current image quality rather than outperforming it. Additionally, it is worth noting that such considerable dose savings have been achieved with patients laying on the CT table with their arms beside the torso, thus contributing to a higher radiation exposure than a standard CCTA-dedicated protocol [39]. Therefore, a DL-based CT protocol with proper patients' arms positioning and a prospective cardiac CT gating (responsible alone for a more than 80% dose reduction compared to retrospective acquisition [40]) holds promise for an optimal CCTA protocol characterized by low radiation dose and high image quality.

Besides good performance as concerns image quality and the consequent potential of further radiation dose savings compared to IR, the benefits of DL reconstruction algorithms are also significant in terms of time effectiveness. The main cost of computational time is in fact spent on the training phase of the reconstruction algorithms. IR do not require any training phase, but their operation time is much longer than DL reconstructions [23, 38].

The use of chest CT and CCTA will likely increase in the future, also driven by updated European and American guidelines [41, 42] and reimbursement policies in the United States commercial health insurer [43]. In such scenario, DL holds promises to be a breakthrough in radiation dose optimization (Fig. 17.3). Nevertheless, current available literature is limited due to the early stages of clinical investigations; therefore, further investigation is needed to fully assess its potential in clinical practice.

Sparse-View Sampling CT

A fascinating strategy to decrease CT radiation dose is sparse-view sampling, obtained by rapidly turning on and off the x-ray tube, obtaining few-view or reduced angular coverage. Unfortunately, image sparsity is not adequately exploitable by implementing IR approaches due to a large amount of image artifacts. Additionally, the minimal amount of data that need to be acquired to guarantee acceptable image quality varies based on clinical tasks and has to be carefully determined. The well-known limit of IR techniques in reconstruction time can also be a burden. Recent advancement in AI and DL-based approaches have been applied to image reconstruction in sparse-view sampling CT either in the sinogram domain [44] or in the image domain [45], proving that DNN-based interpolation of the sparsely sampled sinogram can effectively generate the missing data and reconstruct CT images characterized by similar quality to the ones derived from the fully sampled sinogram. Despite these promising results, the current CT acquisition principles do not support an easy implementation of sparse-view sampling; therefore,

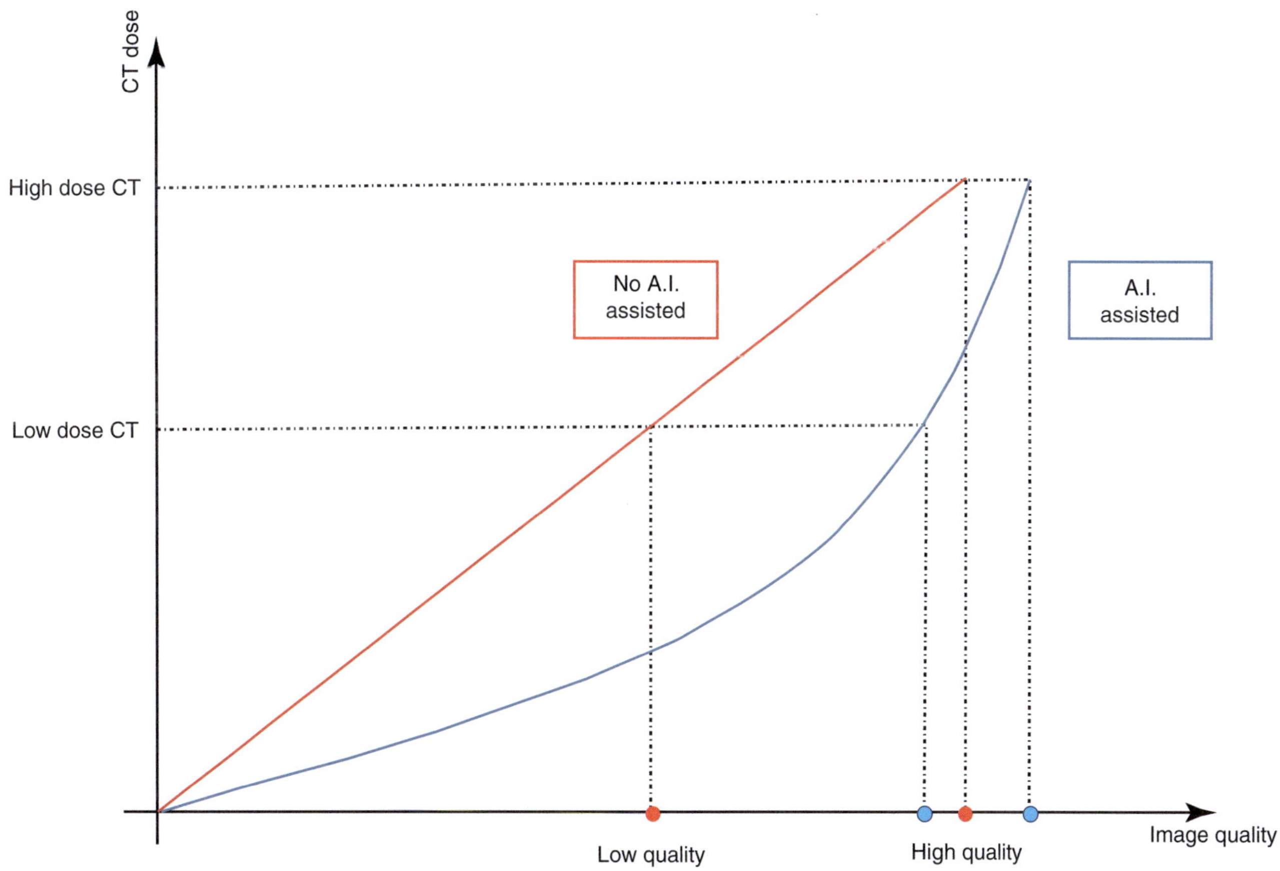

Fig. 17.3 Schematic plot of the correlation between radiation dose exposure and image quality. The graph shows how image quality is strictly related to radiation dose exposure in absence of artificial intelligence (AI) aid; meanwhile, the application of AI features helps to obtain high-quality images, even with low radiation dose levels

its implementation in the commercialized diagnostic CT scanners will not take place in the immediate future.

Artificial Intelligence in Patient Centering

A proper patient centering is a crucial step in radiation dose optimization since many technical solutions such as bow-tie filters and automatic tube current modulation work properly when the patient is correctly positioned at the isocenter [46]. Nevertheless, technical advances in patient positioning optimizations have been much overlooked, relying on radiographer's visual assessment. Patient mis-centering significantly reduces image quality and increases radiation exposure up to 51% in phantom scans and up 23% in patient examinations [47]. AI have been recently successfully applied in this task, allowing for automatic patient positioning (Siemens Healthineers).

A 3D camera mounted on the CT room ceiling above the patient obtains both a conventional 2D color image and a depth image. The latter is generated by means of infrared light and time-of-flight principle [48], containing distance information of all the objects included in the camera field of view. The camera is connected to the coordinate system of the CT scanner. A DL algorithm, trained with patients of different sizes, analyzes the images, detects the patient's anatomical landmarks, and deduces patient positioning, resulting in the generation of a patient avatar (a statistical shape model). These data are eventually used to set the optimal table position, in order that the anatomical center of the avatar lies at the scanner isocenter [49]. The implementation of such technology can lower the table vertical offset down to only 5 mm and keep it with the range of 15 mm, while manual positioning accounts for an average offset of 30 mm, with peaks of 60 mm [50]. This level of precision is critical since it is demonstrated that offsets lower than 20 mm do not significantly increase radiation dose [51, 52]. Automatic patient positioning proved effective in lowering radiation dose by 21–31% and significantly reduced the scan time of all CT protocols, helping standardize the workflow and speed up the scan routine, especially in a busy clinical practice [53].

Artificial Intelligence in Scan Range

Once the patient is correctly centered, the radiographer must acquire the scout view and select the proper scan field based on the specific clinical task. To date, no reliable automated system allows for a precise scan range selection. Therefore, the scan range is manually established by the radiographer and somehow influenced by their experience. However, there is a tendency to be somewhat cautious and extend the scan range beyond what is necessary to avoid excluding important anatomy by the field of view [54]. Patient over-scanning is responsible for significant radiation dose increase; hence, strategies to reduce it are beneficial for the patient [55]. AI has been proved effective in identifying the anatomical levels on chest CT and in estimating the over-scanning associated with inappropriate scan length in a time-effective manner [56]. These preliminary results might be translated into an AI tool that might actively assist the radiographer in the assessment of over-scanning or that might be able to select the proper scan range fully automatically, hence optimizing the radiation exposure.

Limitations

Routine CT dose has decreased by approximately a factor of four in the last 30 years [54], and AI will surely play a major role in further optimizing the radiation exposure, either denoising the already reconstructed images or reconstructing them itself. CT systems will, however, face a physical limitation due to the minimum amount of photons required to form images in which the reader can identify object with subtle contrast relative to the background [57]. Such limitation have been already demonstrated affecting IR and might have detrimental effect in clinical practice, increasing the probability of missing small lesions [58].

Conclusion

AI techniques can be applied to CT examinations to improve image quality, reduce radiation dose, and optimize the workflow. Despite holding the promise to be a major feature in further CT developments, active investigation must continue to further perfect such technology and robustly translate into clinical practice the current promising initial results. Prospective multicenter investigations will be essential to achieve results generalizability, which currently is the most challenging limitation to overcome, along with a clear definition of how AI should be trained and tested to exploit its full potentials.

References

1. van Assen M, Banerjee I, De Cecco CN. Beyond the artificial intelligence hype: what lies behind the algorithms and what we can achieve. J Thorac Imaging. 2020;35(Suppl 1):S3–S10.
2. Brenner DJ, Hall EJ. Computed tomography--an increasing source of radiation exposure. N Engl J Med. 2007;357:2277–84.
3. Fazel R, Krumholz HM, Wang Y, et al. Exposure to low-dose ionizing radiation from medical imaging procedures. N Engl J Med. 2009;361:849–57.
4. Brody JE. Medical radiation soars, with risks often overlooked. The New York Times. 2012.

5. Redberg RF, Smith-Bindman R. We are giving ourselves cancer. New York Times 30. 2014.
6. Hricak H, Brenner DJ, Adelstein SJ, et al. Managing radiation use in medical imaging: a multifaceted challenge. Radiology. 2011;258:889–905.
7. Mayo-Smith WW, Hara AK, Mahesh M, Sahani DV, Pavlicek W. How I do it: managing radiation dose in CT. Radiology. 2014;273:657–72.
8. Spearman JV, Schoepf UJ, Rottenkolber M, et al. Effect of automated attenuation-based tube voltage selection on radiation dose at CT: an observational study on a global scale. Radiology. 2016;279:167–74.
9. Herzog C, Mulvihill DM, Nguyen SA, et al. Pediatric cardiovascular CT angiography: radiation dose reduction using automatic anatomic tube current modulation. AJR Am J Roentgenol. 2008;190:1232–40.
10. Hausleiter J, Meyer TS, Martuscelli E, et al. Image quality and radiation exposure with prospectively ECG-triggered axial scanning for coronary CT angiography: the multicenter, multivendor, randomized PROTECTION-III study. JACC Cardiovasc Imaging. 2012;5:484–93.
11. Apfaltrer P, Hanna EL, Schoepf UJ, et al. Radiation dose and image quality at high-pitch CT angiography of the aorta: intraindividual and interindividual comparisons with conventional CT angiography. AJR Am J Roentgenol. 2012;199:1402–9.
12. Fleischmann D, Boas FE. Computed tomography--old ideas and new technology. Eur Radiol. 2011;21:510–7.
13. Willemink MJ, Noel PB. The evolution of image reconstruction for CT-from filtered back projection to artificial intelligence. Eur Radiol. 2019;29:2185–95.
14. Gordon R, Bender R, Herman GT. Algebraic reconstruction techniques (ART) for three-dimensional electron microscopy and x-ray photography. J Theor Biol. 1970;29:471–81.
15. Willemink MJ, de Jong PA, Leiner T, et al. Iterative reconstruction techniques for computed tomography part 1: technical principles. Eur Radiol. 2013;23:1623–31.
16. Tricarico F, Hlavacek AM, Schoepf UJ, et al. Cardiovascular CT angiography in neonates and children: image quality and potential for radiation dose reduction with iterative image reconstruction techniques. Eur Radiol. 2013;23:1306–15.
17. Geyer LL, Schoepf UJ, Meinel FG, et al. State of the art: iterative CT reconstruction techniques. Radiology. 2015;276:339–57.
18. Tian SF, Liu AL, Liu JH, Liu YJ, Pan JD. Potential value of the PixelShine deep learning algorithm for increasing quality of 70 kVp+ASiR-V reconstruction pelvic arterial phase CT images. Jpn J Radiol. 2019;37:186–90.
19. Higaki T, Nakamura Y, Zhou J, et al. Deep learning reconstruction at CT: phantom study of the image characteristics. Acad Radiol. 2020;27:82–7.
20. Shin YJ, Chang W, Ye JC, et al. Low-dose abdominal CT using a deep learning-based denoising algorithm: a comparison with CT reconstructed with filtered Back projection or iterative reconstruction algorithm. Korean J Radiol. 2020;21:356–64.
21. Greffier J, Hamard A, Pereira F, et al. Image quality and dose reduction opportunity of deep learning image reconstruction algorithm for CT: a phantom study. Eur Radiol. 2020;30:3951–9.
22. Fu B, Wang G, Wu M, et al. Influence of CT effective dose and convolution kernel on the detection of pulmonary nodules in different artificial intelligence software systems: a phantom study. Eur J Radiol. 2020;126:108928.
23. Chen H, Zhang Y, Zhang W, et al. Low-dose CT via convolutional neural network. Biomed Opt Express. 2017;8:679–94.
24. Kang E, Min J, Ye JC. A deep convolutional neural network using directional wavelets for low-dose X-ray CT reconstruction. Med Phys. 2017;44:e360–75.
25. Zhou J, Cunha AL, Do MN. Nonsubsampled contourlet transform: construction and application in enhancement. In: IEEE international conference on image processing 2005; 2005. p. I–469. ISBN:0-7803-9134-9.
26. McCollough CH, Bartley AC, Carter RE, et al. Low-dose CT for the detection and classification of metastatic liver lesions: results of the 2016 low dose CT grand challenge. Med Phys. 2017;44:e339–52.
27. Singh R, Digumarthy SR, Muse VV, et al. Image quality and lesion detection on deep learning reconstruction and iterative reconstruction of submillisievert chest and abdominal CT. AJR Am J Roentgenol. 2020;214:566–73.
28. Kim JH, Yoon HJ, Lee E, Kim I, Cha YK, Bak SH. Validation of deep-learning image reconstruction for low-dose chest computed tomography scan: emphasis on image quality and noise. Korean J Radiol. 2021;22:131–8.
29. Jensen CT, Liu X, Tamm EP, et al. Image quality assessment of abdominal CT by use of new deep learning image reconstruction: initial experience. AJR Am J Roentgenol. 2020;215:50–7.
30. Park C, Choo KS, Jung Y, Jeong HS, Hwang JY, Yun MS. CT iterative vs deep learning reconstruction: comparison of noise and sharpness. Eur Radiol. 2020. https://doi.org/10.1007/s00330-020-07358-8.
31. Wolterink JM, Leiner T, Viergever MA, Isgum I. Generative adversarial networks for noise reduction in low-dose CT. IEEE Trans Med Imaging. 2017;36:2536–45.
32. Yang Q, Yan P, Zhang Y, et al. Low-dose CT image denoising using a generative adversarial network with Wasserstein distance and perceptual loss. IEEE Trans Med Imaging. 2018;37:1348–57.
33. Kim B, Han M, Shim H, Baek J. A performance comparison of convolutional neural network-based image denoising methods: the effect of loss functions on low-dose CT images. Med Phys. 2019;46:3906–23.
34. Tatsugami F, Higaki T, Nakamura Y, et al. Deep learning-based image restoration algorithm for coronary CT angiography. Eur Radiol. 2019;29:5322–9.
35. Ahn CK, Jin H, Heo C, Kim JH. Combined low-dose simulation and deep learning for CT denoising: application of ultra-low-dose cardiac CTA. In: International Society for Optics and Photonics; 2019. p. 1094846.
36. Hong JH, Park EA, Lee W, Ahn C, Kim JH. Incremental image noise reduction in coronary CT angiography using a deep learning-based technique with iterative reconstruction. Korean J Radiol. 2020;21:1165–77.
37. Benz DC, Benetos G, Rampidis G, et al. Validation of deep-learning image reconstruction for coronary computed tomography angiography: impact on noise, image quality and diagnostic accuracy. J Cardiovasc Comput Tomogr. 2020;14:444–51.
38. Liu P, Wang M, Wang Y, et al. Impact of deep learning-based optimization algorithm on image quality of low-dose coronary CT angiography with noise reduction: a prospective study. Acad Radiol. 2020;27:1241–8.
39. Bernard A, Comby PO, Lemogne B, et al. Deep learning reconstruction versus iterative reconstruction for cardiac CT angiography in a stroke imaging protocol: reduced radiation dose and improved image quality. Quant Imaging Med Surg. 2021;11:392–401.
40. Earls JP, Berman EL, Urban BA, et al. Prospectively gated transverse coronary CT angiography versus retrospectively gated helical technique: improved image quality and reduced radiation dose. Radiology. 2008;246:742–53.
41. Knuuti J, Wijns W, Saraste A, et al. 2019 ESC guidelines for the diagnosis and management of chronic coronary syndromes. Eur Heart J. 2020;41:407–77.
42. Smith RA, Andrews KS, Brooks D, et al. Cancer screening in the United States, 2018: a review of current American Cancer Society guidelines and current issues in cancer screening. CA Cancer J Clin. 2018;68:297–316.

43. Coronary CTA Reimbursement Update (United Healthcare). 2020. Available via https://www.uhcprovider.com/en/resource-library/news/2020-network-bulletin-featured-articles/0520-coronary-cta-reimbursement.html.
44. Han YS, Yoo J, Ye JC. Deep residual learning for compressed sensing CT reconstruction via persistent homology analysis. arXiv preprint arXiv:161106391. 2016.
45. Lee H, Lee J, Kim H, Cho B, Cho S. Deep-neural-network-based Sinogram synthesis for sparse-view CT image reconstruction. IEEE Trans Radiat Plasma Med Sci. 2019;3:109–19.
46. Kaasalainen T, Palmu K, Reijonen V, Kortesniemi M. Effect of patient centering on patient dose and image noise in chest CT. AJR Am J Roentgenol. 2014;203:123–30.
47. Habibzadeh MA, Ay MR, Asl AR, Ghadiri H, Zaidi H. Impact of miscentering on patient dose and image noise in x-ray CT imaging: phantom and clinical studies. Phys Med. 2012;28:191–9.
48. Remondino F, Stoppa D. TOF range-imaging cameras. Heidelberg: Springer; 2013.
49. Booij R, Budde RPJ, Dijkshoorn ML, van Straten M. Accuracy of automated patient positioning in CT using a 3D camera for body contour detection. Eur Radiol. 2019;29:2079–88.
50. Saltybaeva N, Schmidt B, Wimmer A, Flohr T, Alkadhi H. Precise and automatic patient positioning in computed tomography: avatar Modeling of the patient surface using a 3-dimensional camera. Investig Radiol. 2018;53:641–6.
51. Ali Khawaja RD, Singh S, Padole A, et al. Point organ radiation dose in abdominal CT: effect of patient off-Centering in an experimental human cadaver study. Radiat Prot Dosim. 2017;175:440–9.
52. Saltybaeva N, Alkadhi H. Vertical off-centering affects organ dose in chest CT: evidence from Monte Carlo simulations in anthropomorphic phantoms. Med Phys. 2017;44:5697–704.
53. Dane B, O'Donnell T, Liu S, et al. Radiation dose reduction, improved isocenter accuracy and CT scan time savings with automatic patient positioning by a 3D camera. Eur J Radiol. 2021;136:109537.
54. McCollough CH, Leng S. Use of artificial intelligence in computed tomography dose optimisation. Ann ICRP. 2020;49:113–25.
55. Litmanovich DE, Tack DM, Shahrzad M, Bankier AA. Dose reduction in cardiothoracic CT: review of currently available methods. Radiographics. 2014;34:1469–89.
56. Colevray M, Tatard-Leitman VM, Gouttard S, Douek P, Boussel L. Convolutional neural network evaluation of over-scanning in lung computed tomography. Diagn Interv Imaging. 2019;100:177–83.
57. Rose A. Vision: human and electronic, vol. 197. New York: Springer; 1973.
58. Favazza CP, Ferrero A, Yu L, Leng S, McMillan KL, McCollough CH. Use of a channelized hotelling observer to assess CT image quality and optimize dose reduction for iteratively reconstructed images. J Med Imaging (Bellingham). 2017;4:031213.

Artificial Intelligence Integration into the Computed Tomography System

18

Michael Sühling, Stefan Großkopf, Ralf Gutjahr,
Max Schöbinger, Chris Schwemmer, Andreas Wimmer,
and Thomas Flohr

Introduction

Since its clinical introduction in the early 1970s, computed tomography (CT) has evolved into the backbone of radiological diagnosis. For many years, CT development has been driven by technical refinement of CT scanners to improve their performance, extend their clinical capabilities, and enable new applications such as CT angiography and electrocardiogram (ECG)-controlled imaging of the heart. The introduction of spiral CT in 1990 [26], the broad availability of multi-detector row CT in 1999 [35], and the introduction of advanced CT system concepts such as wide detector CT in 2004 [37] or dual source CT in 2005 [14] represented milestones in the technical progress of CT. Today, CT is a technically mature modality. The focus of CT development has shifted toward artificial intelligence (AI) supported improvement and automation of the scan workflow and approaches to enhance the clinical information of CT images. Modern CT scanners provide anatomy-aligned reconstructions and advanced visualizations as part of standard image reconstruction tasks, and even automated identification and quantification of pathological processes are routinely integrated into the CT workflow. In this chapter, we provide an overview of AI-supported approaches integrated into the CT system with a focus on cardiovascular imaging.

M. Sühling, PhD · S. Großkopf, PhD · R. Gutjahr, PhD
M. Schöbinger, PhD · C. Schwemmer, MS · A. Wimmer, PhD
T. Flohr, PhD (✉)
Siemens Healthcare GmbH, Computed Tomography, Forchheim, Germany
e-mail: michael.suehling@siemens-healthineers.com; stefan.grosskopf@siemens-healthineers.com; ralf.gutjahr@siemens-healthineers.com; max.schoebinger@siemens-healthineers.com; chris.schwemmer@siemens-healthineers.com; andreas.aw.wimmer@siemens-healthineers.com; thomas.flohr@siemens-healthineers.com

3D Camera-Based Patient Positioning, Characterization, and Scan Guidance

A source of error right at the beginning of each CT examination is positioning the patient. The radiographer needs to manually adjust the correct table height with the help of light markers, then the table is manually moved to the scan start position, and the scan range is set. If the table height is incorrect and the body region to be examined is not centered in the gantry, image quality may suffer and the applied radiation dose may be inappropriate. In a large study, a strong tendency by radiographers to position the patient too low was observed [1].

To address these challenges, automatic patient positioning supported by a 3D camera was introduced [3, 45]. The 3D camera is mounted on the ceiling and focuses on the table region of the CT system. It acquires color and depth images (see Fig. 18.1a, b). The depth measurements are obtained through the time-of-flight principle.

The camera images are continuously examined by AI algorithms [48]. Once a human is detected on the table in a stable position, the pose and body landmarks are determined. The landmarks (see Fig. 18.1b) are used to set the horizontal scan start position and propose the scan range, based on the scheduled examination and the individual physique of the patient. If there is a mismatch between the detected pose and the pose as specified in the scan protocol, the radiographer is warned. Then a virtual patient avatar is fitted to the camera data; see Fig. 18.1c. The avatar consists of a statistical shape model built from a large database of range scans of humans describing the skin surface. During the fitting of the model to the camera data, the avatar assumes the pose and the body proportions of the actual patient, within the limits permitted by the shape model. The avatar is helpful to separate clothes, blankets, or positioning aids like headrests from the patient. Once the avatar fit is complete, the isocenter of the model for the examination region is determined, and the table height is set accordingly; see Fig. 18.1d, e.

C. N. De Cecco et al. (eds.), *Artificial Intelligence in Cardiothoracic Imaging*, Contemporary Medical Imaging,
https://doi.org/10.1007/978-3-030-92087-6_18

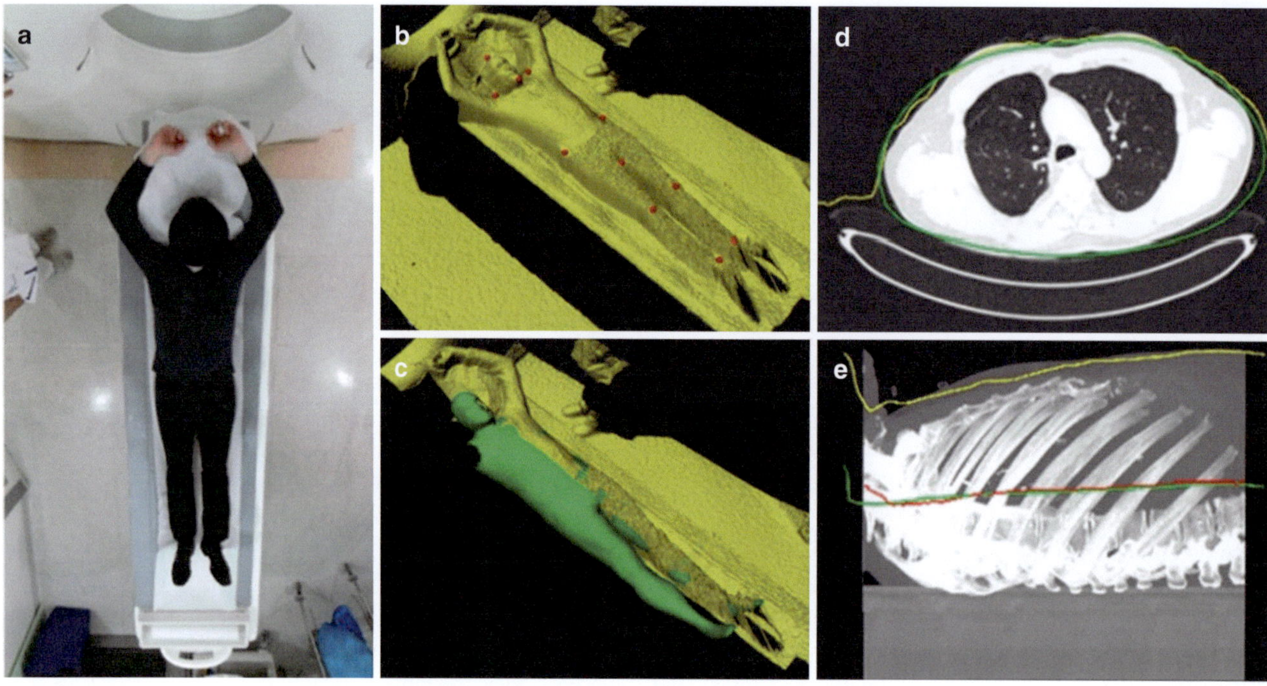

Fig. 18.1 (**a**) Color image. (**b**) Depth surface recovered from the measurements. Detected body landmarks are indicated as red dots. (**c**) Avatar model (green) fitted to the camera depth data. (**d**) Axial cross section with depth measurements (yellow) and fitted avatar (green). (**e**) Lateral projection with depth measurements (yellow), avatar isocenter curve (green), and ground truth isocenter curve (red) determined from the CT data. (CT data courtesy of Alec J. Megibow, NYU Langone Medical Center, New York, USA)

Several studies [3, 45] found 3D camera-based patient positioning to be more accurate and more consistent for routine examinations than manual positioning, even in a pediatric population [4]. Other investigators [8] observed radiation dose reduction (in terms of size-specific dose estimate, SSDE) by 1.0–2.4 mGy (21–31%) for the four most commonly performed protocols.

In addition to automatically setting the table height and determining the horizonal scan start position and scan range, a 3D camera can provide other relevant information, such as estimates for patient height and weight. These are important parameters, for example, to prescribe the right amount of contrast agent for a CT examination. The patient height can be determined directly from the avatar. The body volume can be derived from the avatar model representing the skin surface. Assuming a uniform density of human tissue leads to a coarse weight estimate. However, such a simple approach cannot accurately account for different body compositions. Instead, a linear regressor is determined on a training population consisting of 3D camera images and measured weights. The regressor takes the sub-volumes and the extents of parts of the avatar like head, torso, and legs as input to estimate the weight. Initial results show the potential of the method [16]: The correlation between the measured weight and the weight estimated by the 3D camera was more accurate ($R^2 = 0.89$) than the estimates of the radiologist ($R^2 = 0.78$) and the radiographer ($R^2 = 0.77$) but less accurate than the estimates of the well-informed patients ($R^2 = 0.99$). With further improvements patient-individual proposal of the amount of contrast agent for a specific examination may become possible.

When moving the patient into the gantry, the radiographer needs to ensure that no collisions happen between the patient, the scanner, and other objects in the scan room. Pertinent examples are elbows touching the gantry, medical equipment placed on or close to the patient, or very obese patients not adequately fitting into the gantry bore. With the use of the 3D camera, the dimensions of the patient and equipment moving with the table can be determined before the patient is moved into the gantry. This geometry can be intersected with a cylinder representing the gantry bore. If objects lie outside the cylinder or are close to its boundaries, the radiographer can be warned, for example, by highlighting the collision areas in the camera color image; see Fig. 18.2a and b.

Overlays on the camera color image can provide further guidance for less experienced radiographers. As an example, the ideal positions where to place ECG leads can be indicated on the live camera image of the patient based on the detected body landmarks and the selected scan protocol such that the electrodes are kept outside the scan range to avoid artifacts; see Fig. 18.2c.

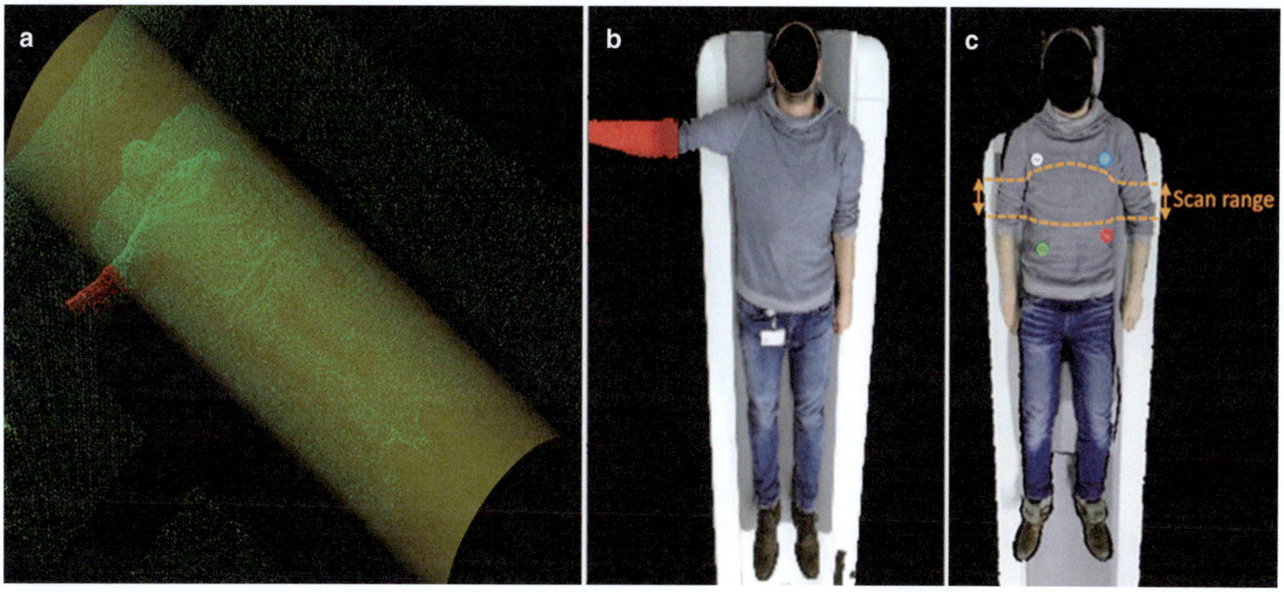

Fig. 18.2 (**a**) Collision detection. Intersection of the camera point cloud with the gantry bore cylinder (yellow). (**b**) The stretched-out arm is highlighted in red to indicate collision if the table is moved. (**c**) Color-coded overlay of suggested ECG electrode positions together with the planned scan range on the patient's camera image. The radiographer sees his hands in the live image and can match the real electrode positions and the suggested positions

Topogram-Based Automated Scan Range Definition

After patient positioning, a localizer radiograph (topogram) is usually acquired to plan the scan range or scan ranges (in case of multiple scans). The scan ranges need to cover the target anatomy of the planned examination as precisely as possible. Significant "over-ranging" leads to increased radiation dose to the patient and should be avoided especially if sensitive organs (e.g., eye lens) are irradiated unnecessarily. Cutoffs of relevant anatomy on the other hand may demand a partial or complete re-scan.

While the radiographer used to plan the scan ranges manually according to anatomical landmarks on the topogram, machine learning algorithms have been designed to take over this task in an automated way. The algorithm described in [40, 49, 55] is designed to calculate a rectangular or rhombic[1] reconstruction range on a topogram. It uses multi-scale Haar texture analysis, LEAP, and AdaBoost trees to learn annotated anatomical landmarks and target regions in an image-driven training; see Fig. 18.3. As a result, a rhomboid including all landmarks plus a safety margin is predicted as target. The algorithm can robustly predict extents of body regions even in difficult situations, for example, if the scanned topogram does not fully cover them, and results in increased consistency across operators [15].

[1] For head and spine scans the scan-region is a rhomboid, if the CT scanner gantry is tilted during acquisition.

Another aspect of scan preparation that can be supported by AI-driven algorithms is the detection of metal objects. Metal in the scan range may induce image artifacts. These artifacts can be reduced by intelligent postprocessing or image reconstruction algorithms. But still, the image quality of a CT scan is best if wearable metal objects (e.g., wrist watches) are removed beforehand.

A recently introduced algorithm screens the topogram for metals and alerts the radiographer to remove them from the patient. Unfortunately, the intensity of topogram pixels alone does not allow to conclude on metal. Therefore, a network was trained on about 3000 annotated images to learn shape and texture of metal objects [41]. The algorithm performs robustly with a sensitivity of 95% and specificity of 90% for the most frequently wearable metal objects left behind on a patient.

Patient-Specific Scan and Reconstruction Protocols

After patient positioning and scan range planning, the appropriate scan protocol needs to be selected for the individual patient and the planned examination. So far, the radiographer has chosen a scan protocol from a predefined protocol list and adapted certain scan and reconstruction parameters manually to the individual patient and the scan situation. A prominent example is the selection of the proper scan mode for ECG-controlled CT scans of the heart, which depends on the

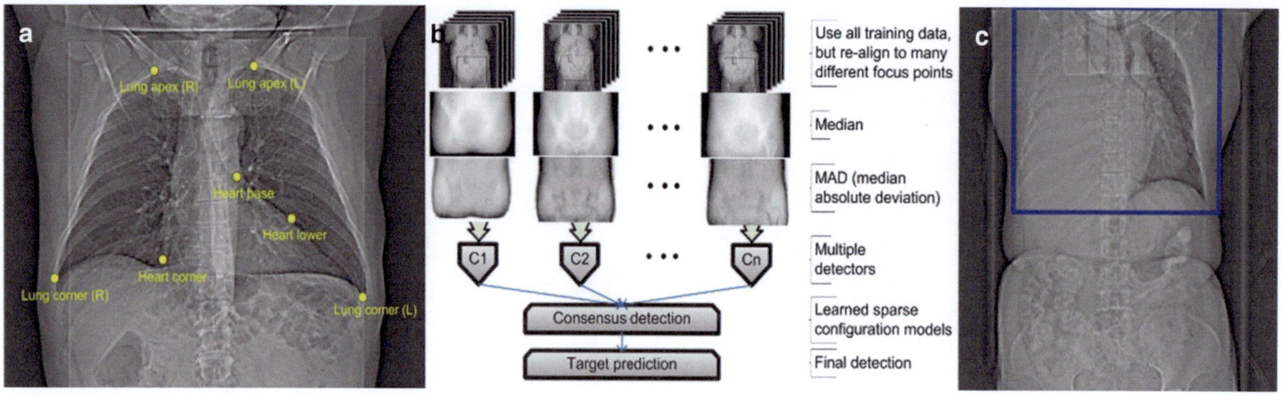

Fig. 18.3 (**a**) Anatomical landmarks on a thorax topogram. (**b**) LEAP framework that exploits redundancy in the training set and as a result predicts the target region. (**c**) Example target region for a thorax scan. (With permission from [55])

heart rate and heart rate variability of the patient. Manual selection of the scan mode and adaptation of parameters such as the adequate cardiac phase for image reconstruction are operator-dependent and error-prone. Recently, an approach has been presented that proposes optimal scan and reconstruction parameters based on clinical questions, patient age, gender, size and weight, lab values (if available), and online evaluation of physiological parameters such as heart rate and heart variability (myExam Companion, Siemens Healthcare, Germany). The approach is based on a large variety of preconfigured decision trees for routine and advanced examinations which are embedded in the scan protocols. The decision trees were derived from a large-scale analysis of scan and reconstruction protocols used by many different clinical sites. They can be modified according to site-specific preferences and also newly designed if needed for a specific clinical indication.

Assisted Contrast-Enhanced Scanning

The quality of CT angiographic (CTA) scans mainly depends on high and uniform contrast enhancement within the planned scan range. Finding the right scan timing after the contrast injection started remains a challenge. Typical approaches are the application of a (a) fixed scan delay; (b) the determination of contrast arrival using a small injection of contrast media (test bolus) while monitoring the contrast enhancement over time in a manually set Region of Interest (ROI), followed by a diagnostic CT scan; or (c) by applying bolus tracking. Bolus tracking comprises a single contrast injection, followed by a sequential monitoring of contrast enhancement within a vessel. As soon as the contrast enhancement exceeds a user-chosen threshold, a fixed delay is applied before the diagnostic scan starts. However, applying a fixed delay after contrast arrival does not account for factors influencing the patient's hemodynamics (such as altered cardiac output or peripheral resistance). Ultimately, using fixed delays can lead to missing the bolus. This becomes an even greater challenge the faster the CT scanners are. To facilitate the clinical workflow and improve the quality of CTAs, algorithmic support for bolus tracking has been developed.

With an algorithm based on landmark detection (similar to the one described in section "Topogram-Based Automated Scan Range Definition"), a circular ROI is automatically placed inside the ascending aorta, descending aorta, or pulmonary artery (depending on the clinical application and user preference) on a non-enhanced pre-monitoring slice. In a first step, the pre-monitoring slice is classified according to the z-location of its acquisition (at the aortic arch, above the coronary ostia, below the heart, etc. [54]). Then a specialized set of landmark detectors identifies four points (oriented to the patient's anterior, right, posterior, and left) on the contour of the target vessel to locate its center and to estimate its radius. Evaluation of 130 test series demonstrated accurate placement of the ROI in more than 95% of the cases. Interactive adaptions of ROI location and radius are still possible to handle more complex anatomies.

In an approach to personalize the scan delay in a CTA using bolus tracking, the slope of the contrast enhancement during the monitoring scans is analyzed [31]. Combining the slope with information about the contrast injection (iodine delivery rate over time), a patient-specific arterial impulse response function is derived, and further progression of the contrast enhancement (after exceeding the contrast enhancement threshold) is predicted. An ideal individualized scan delay is calculated while considering the scan direction and the scan duration.

The adapted scan delay may improve contrast opacification in the vessel while reducing the variance of contrast enhancement over the scan range [23]; see Fig. 18.4. As a

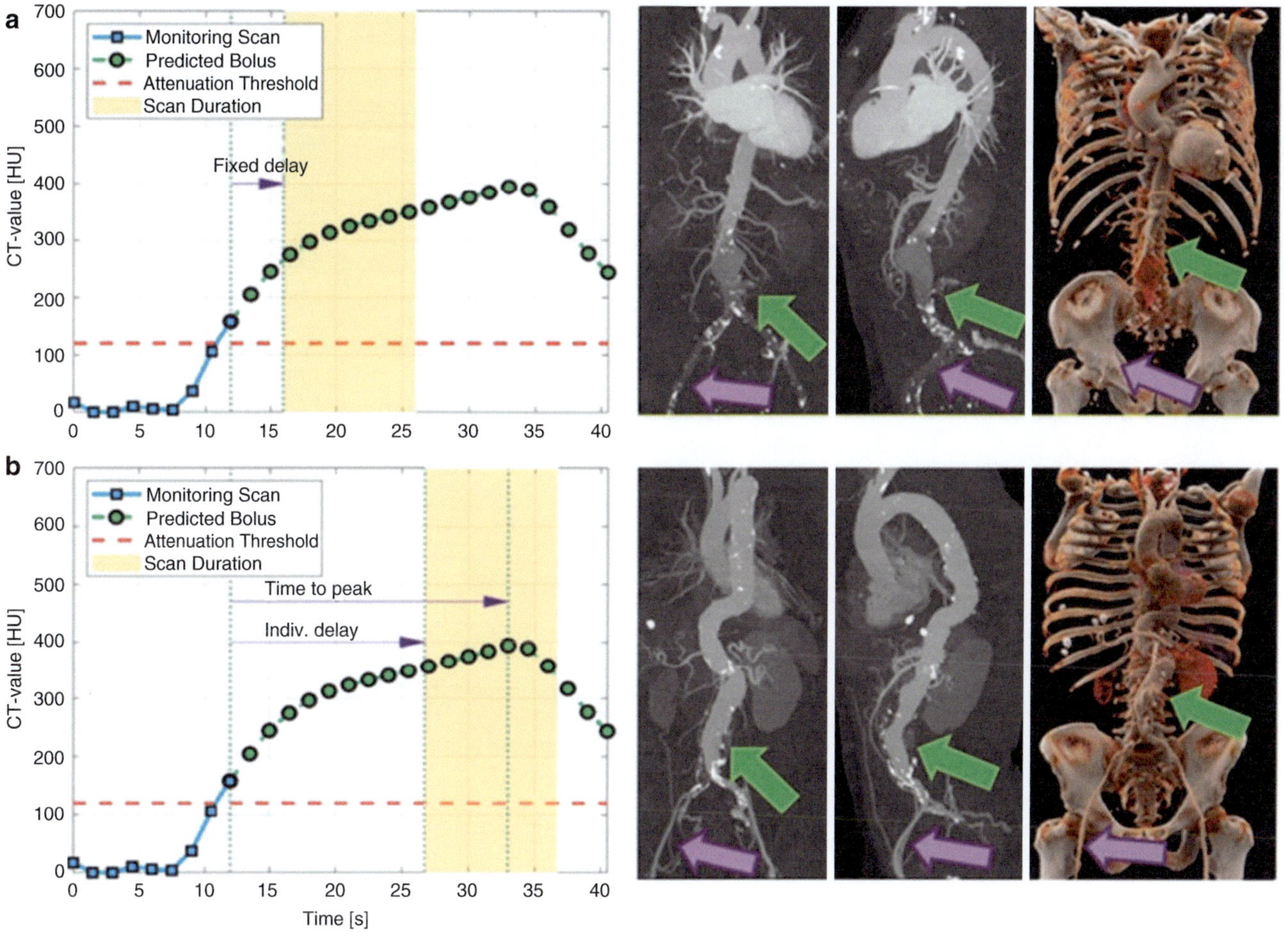

Fig. 18.4 (**a**) CTA with fixed delay of an 84-year-old patient with untreated infrarenal aortic aneurysm. The gradual decrease of contrast enhancement along the aorta indicates early start of the CT scan (see the arrows). (**b**) CTA with individualized delay of a 63-year-old patient with untreated infrarenal aortic aneurysm. Uniformly distributed CT enhancement along the aortic and iliac path was achieved. (CT data courtesy of Hatem Alkadhi, Universitätsspital Zürich, Switzerland)

consequence, CTAs with decreased contrast injection rates and/or smaller iodine loads (e.g., for patients with impaired kidney function) may be possible [21].

Initial Image Quality Assessment

Modern CT scanners use learning-based algorithms to assess certain quality criteria immediately after a CT scan, before the patient is released or the images are sent to the PACS or other reading stations. Two main criteria are automatically supervised: (a) Was the planned scan region completely covered? (b) Is there sufficient contrast enhancement in a CTA? (Check&Go, Siemens Healthcare, Germany).

For the coverage check, the 3D image of the scan after initial image reconstruction is back-projected into an artificial topogram. Anatomical landmarks are identified in both, the measured topogram and the artificial topogram, by detecting the landmarks trained for the scan range planning described in section "Topogram-Based Automated Scan Range Definition". For each landmark, the positions in both topograms are compared, and a relative distance of the positions is calculated. If significant distances are identified for any of the landmarks, the radiographer is informed about a potential difference between actual and planned scan range, and images suitable to quickly verify misalignments are rendered. The algorithm is particularly helpful when a patient was moving in the time between the topogram and the CT scan or even when the breathing pattern of the patient changed during this same period.

For the contrast enhancement check in CTAs, at least three slices in the scanned region (near the start, center, and last slice) are evaluated. These key slices are identified by an algorithm applying 3D landmark detection based on cascade AdaBoosting [54], which was trained with sample slices that were labeled according to their position throughout the body; see Fig. 18.5. On each slice, a landmark-based algorithm similar to the one described in section "Assisted

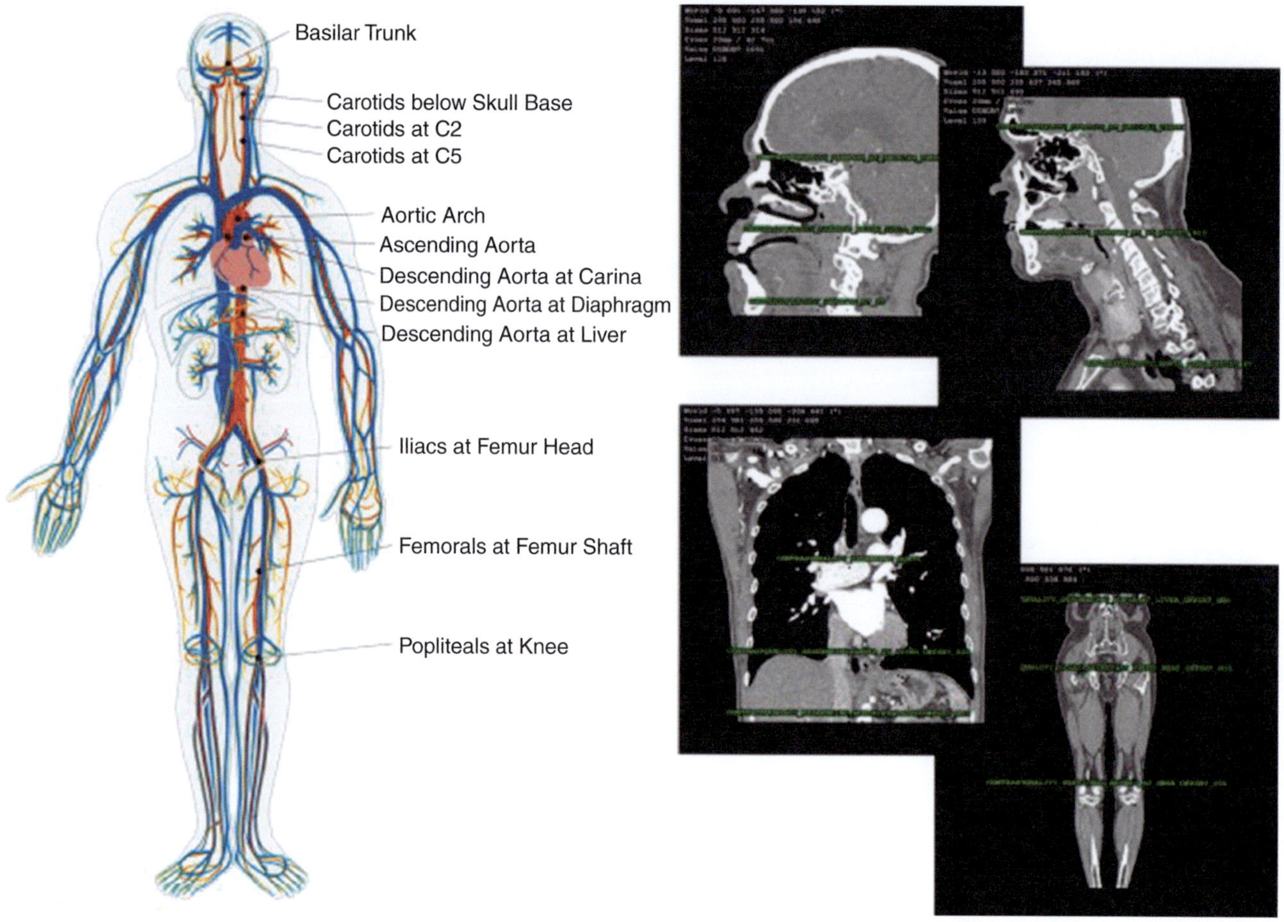

Fig. 18.5 Locations trained for the ROI-based automated measurement of contrast enhancement to alert the user in case of insufficient enhancement in a CTA

Contrast-Enhanced Scanning" for the detection of a monitoring ROI identifies up to two vascular ROI positions. Within the identified circular ROIs, the average CT number (in HU) and its standard deviation (in HU) are measured. If the average CT numbers fall below a predefined threshold, the user is informed about potentially insufficient contrast enhancement.

Automated Postprocessing and Reading Preparation

Upon completion of the CT image acquisition, AI plays a key role in preparing the data for reading. As described in section "Organ-Specific Reconstructions and Visualizations", AI-based augmentation of the original CT data by compact and intuitive reconstructions and visualizations generated directly at the CT scanner helps to reduce reading time and to increase expert reading sensitivity. Beyond advanced visualizations, the automated detection and quantification of abnormalities serves as a second reader, thereby increasing diagnostic confidence, efficiency, and precision. An overview of such AI algorithms is presented in section "Abnormality Identification and Quantification".

Organ-Specific Reconstructions and Visualizations

With the ever-increasing amount of high-resolution CT data generated with modern CT scanners, conventional reading of large series of planar images becomes more and more demanding. Oblique multiplanar reformations (MPRs) are commonly generated to represent planar image stacks centered around and rotated along desired orientations of anatomical structures of interest such as the ascending aorta [2]. Those MPRs allow, for example, to take appropriate size measurements within the rotated planes. Moreover, curved-planar reformations (CPRs) are routinely used to facilitate the tracing and analysis of vessels. However, CPRs do not

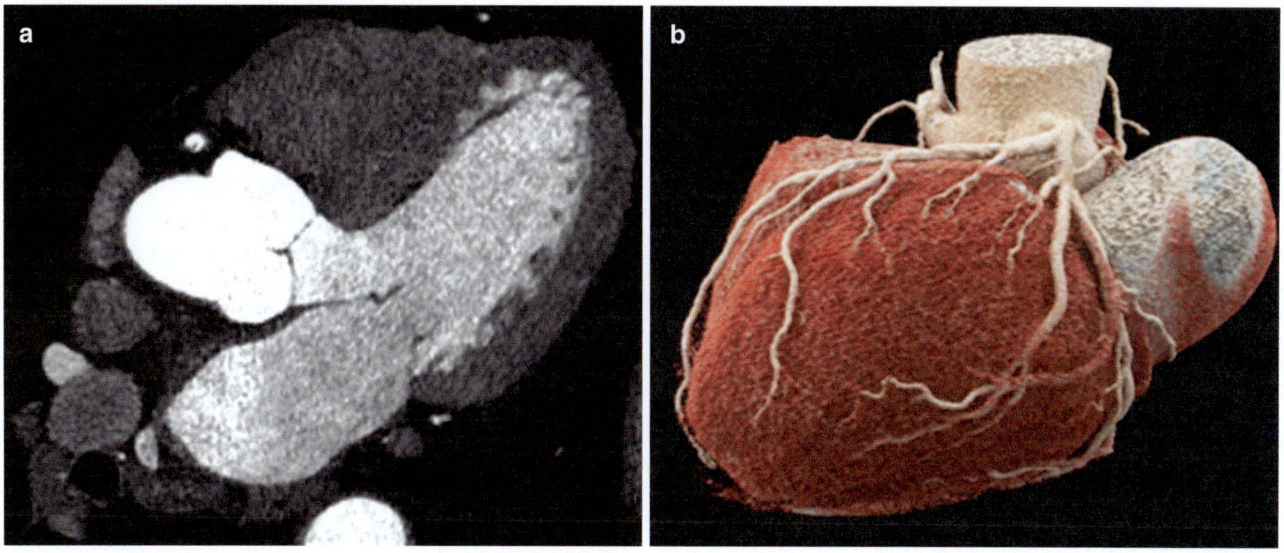

Fig. 18.6 Automated heart-specific reconstructions and visualizations: (**a**) cardiac three-chamber view. (**b**) Photorealistic Cinematic Rendering of isolated heart primarily suited as communication means to the referring cardiologist or patient. (CT data courtesy of Dr. Jones & Partners, Adelaide, Australia)

capture anatomical interrelations of the vessel tree morphology as individual vessel branches are displayed separately from each other. Until recently, in clinical routine, such MPR and CPR reformations have been generated semiautomatically on dedicated clinical workstations by technicians which is labor and time intensive and lacks standardization due to human operator dependency.

Recent advancements in AI technology [47] have put forth scanner-centric, fully automatic computation of anatomy-aligned reconstructions and advanced visualizations. Modern CT systems provide these anatomical ranges as part of standard reconstruction tasks (Recon & Go, Siemens Healthcare, Germany). The underlying AI technologies detect anatomical structures in the acquired images and create ready-to-read, standardized MPRs and CPRs for different body regions, joints, or vascular structures, which are automatically sent to the PACS or other reading stations. For instance, standardized cardiac imaging planes, including four-chamber, three-chamber, two-chamber, and short-axis views, are frequently used to assess cardiac morphology and function. Superseding the interactive step-by-step plane definition based on visual anatomical landmarks, these standardized imaging planes are automatically provided in an accurate and reproducible manner; see Fig. 18.6a. Besides 2D cardiac planes, 3D Cinematic Rendering visualizations [18] of the heart can be computed fully automatically; see Fig. 18.6b.

Reading and analysis of vascular structures is especially tedious on planar image planes. In Kanitsar [27], an untangled multipath CPR visualization was proposed. To reduce discontinuities in between distinct vessel branches and to maintain anatomical context, a novel vessel tree unfolding technique is used: Based on AI-driven vasculature detection, the vessel tree is automatically mapped to an as-rigid-as-possible, deformable projection geometry. Figure 18.7 demonstrates an unfolded view of the aorta and connected arteries ranging from the carotids to the lower extremities.

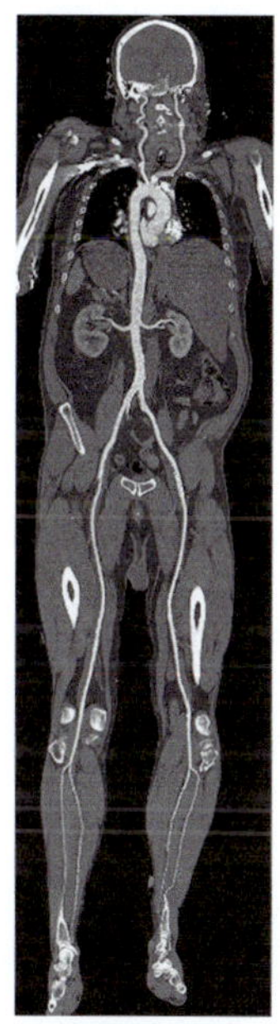

Fig. 18.7 Automated vessel unfolding. (CT data courtesy of T. Albrecht, Charité University Hospital Berlin, Campus Benjamin Franklin, Berlin, Germany)

This technique may substantially reduce the number of slices to be assessed for presurgical planning compared to maximum-intensity projections or standard coronal reconstructions [34].

CT bone reading also benefits from advanced visualizations; see Fig. 18.8 for an AI-driven projection of the entire rib cage onto a 2D plane ("rib unfolding"). In a recent study, higher sensitivity for rib fracture detection and reduction in reading time for trauma cases was reported when using rib unfolding [42]. Rib unfolding also resulted in improved bone metastasis detection compared with original chest CT reading at reduced reading time [22].

Overall, the described organ-specific reconstructions and visualizations facilitate reading by providing an intuitive and compact representation of the images. They reduce reading time and may improve the detection of findings. These views also facilitate the communication with referring physicians or even patients.

Abnormality Identification and Quantification

In the last decade, cardiac computed tomography has established its role as a noninvasive modality for the evaluation of coronary artery disease (CAD). As clinical progress is accompanied by increased technical demands, automated methods for the identification and quantification of pathological processes are subject of current research. This section presents recent contributions in the fields of AI-supported assessment of anatomical, functional, and morphological aspects of coronary artery disease. Again, modern CT scanners may provide these assessments automatically as part of standard reconstruction tasks.

Assessment of Coronary Calcium

Coronary artery calcium scoring (CACS) is an established and guideline-recommended method for the prediction of cardiovascular risk [19, 28]. CACS is performed using highly standardized CT protocols [36]. The calculation of calcium scores has so far been based on a manual selection of potential coronary calcifications exceeding a threshold of 130HU by the user (Agatston score). This is often not a difficult but tedious and time-consuming task. At the same time, due to the standardized image properties, calcium scoring is ideally suited for an AI-assisted approach. This could not only help to reduce user workload during reading but also allow for on-the-fly modifications to scanning strategies when the score is available directly at the scanner seconds after the calcium scoring acquisition has finished.

Several approaches to automatic CACS have been published so far, from traditional rule- or feature-based classification to modern deep learning methods [32]. The major challenge for an algorithm is the differentiation between coronary calcium and other high-density features within the heart region like valve calcifications, stents, or other implants. The assignment of calcifications to the individual coronaries is another challenge.

The method presented here relies on a combination of a Convolutional Neural Network (CNN) with image- and location-based features to decide whether a calcium candidate is a coronary calcification or not. First, the heart is identified, and further processing is limited to this region. A heart-centered coordinate system is set up, and a pre-learned coronary territory map is fit. For each candidate voxel (CT number > 130HU), an image patch around it is extracted and fed into the CNN. The location of the voxel in the heart-centered coordinates and local spatial characteristics are fed into a fully connected NN. The output of both networks is concatenated and used to predict

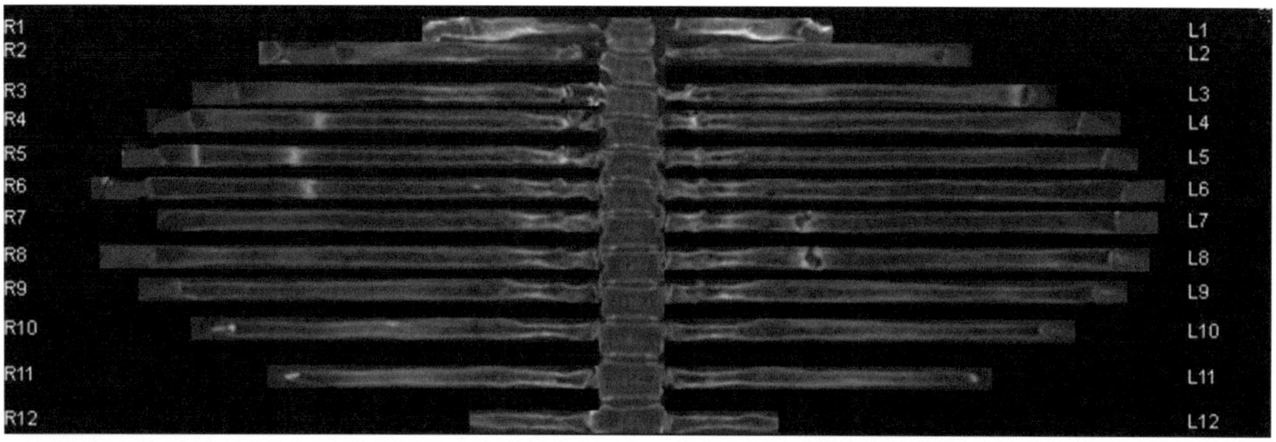

Fig. 18.8 Automated rib unfolding and labeling facilitates the assessment of right rib bone metastases and serial left rib fractures. (CT data courtesy of M. Horger, University Hospital Tübingen, Tübingen, Germany)

whether that voxel is coronary calcium. Finally, if the mean probability of a connected set of voxels exceeds a predefined threshold, that set is marked as a coronary calcification. An additional deep reinforcement learning algorithm detects the branching point between left main, left anterior descending, and left circumflex artery [17]. This landmark can be reliably extracted on non-contrasted acquisitions and is used to assign vessel labels to the calcifications with the aid of another fully connected network. Figure 18.9 gives an overview of the complete method. It has been successfully implemented both into on-scanner result preparation and postprocessing workstations. Sandstedt (2020) [46] compared the results with a routine expert read and found an intra-class correlation of 0.996 for the Agatston score while reducing the reading time by 39%.

Anatomical Assessment of Coronary Artery Disease

The anatomical assessment of the coronary arteries usually refers to an evaluation of the diameter course of their lumen. Computer-assisted methods try to detect abnormal narrowing in this course to identify potentially diseased sections. For most of these approaches, the explicit extraction of a model of the coronary arteries is a prerequisite. Several authors proposed different methods to detect and track the main and side branches of the coronary tree: CNNs [52], CNNs combined with information from automatic aorta and heart segmentation [43], and coronaries as optimal paths in a computed flow field combined with CNNs to remove erroneous detections [20]. The detection sensitivity of these methods ranges from 92% to 97%.

The description of the course of the coronary arteries is then input to lesion detection algorithms, as, for example, evaluated in Fischer [12] for the detection of calcified plaques in coronary CTAs. The authors employed a recurrent neural network with long-short-term-memory (LSTM) architecture, where 2D samples of cross-sectional images were used as temporal input to the LSTM network. In this approach, an overall accuracy of 90.3% was achieved. Similar approaches can also be combined with an additional step for lesion grading. For the detection and classification of significant (≥50%) and nonsignificant (<50%) lesions, an accuracy of 80% was demonstrated by employing a multitask recurrent CNN in a two-step approach combining feature extraction along the coronary artery and classification of the plaque type and the significance of the stenosis [56].

The approaches for detection and grading of CAD are not limited to individual coronary lesions. Alternatives have been published which attempt to classify CAD either on coronary segment level or on case level by classifying the case according to the CAD-RADs standard [7]. These approaches typically require algorithms that pre-classify the coronaries according to the 18-segment model as defined by the SCCT [33]. One example for such a method applies tree-structured LSTMs to combine the learned tree structures with global context information like, for example, the heart chambers. It achieved an average segment classification accuracy of 96%

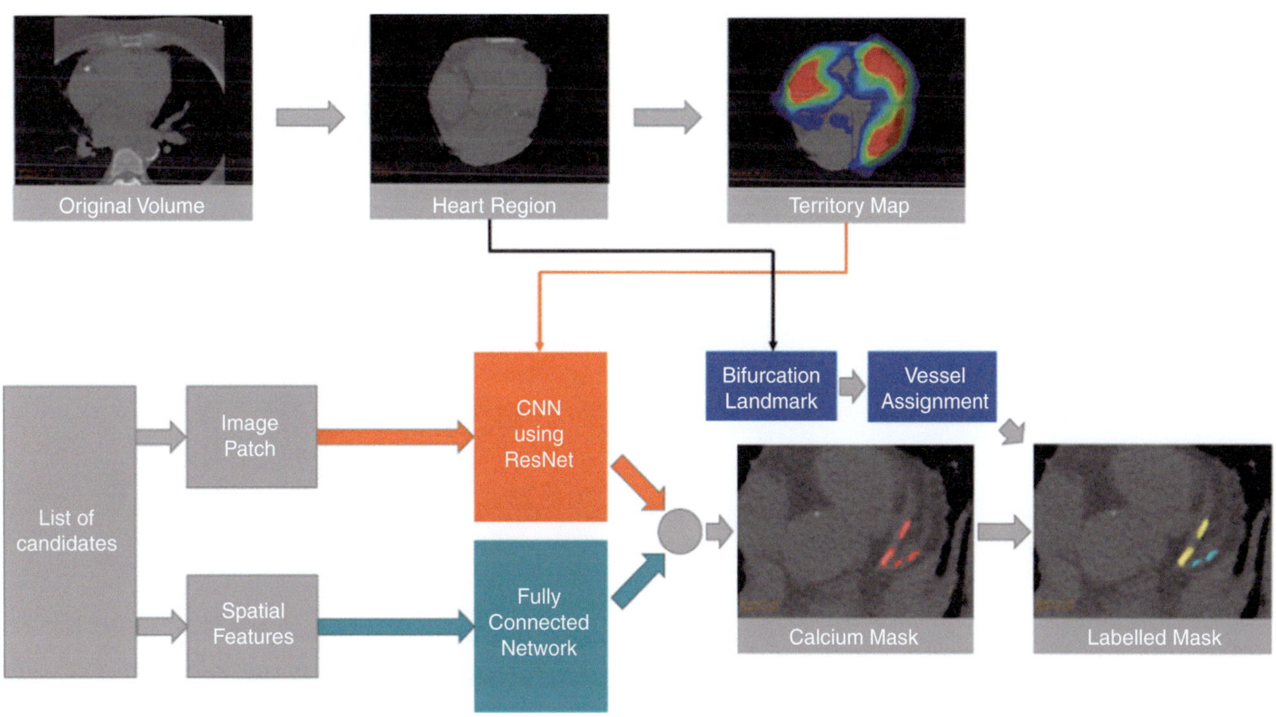

Fig. 18.9 Illustration of the automatic calcium scoring method

[13]. For automatic classification of the CAD-RADs category, a deep CNN was developed. Its accuracy for the rule-out and identification of obstructive CAD was found to be 86% and 71%, respectively [39]. An alternative approach [10] allows for the classification of the CAD-RADs score involving information from classifications of a segment-wise stenosis score and the calcification score. This approach also enables the prediction of the most significant lesion severity on case level. It achieved an accuracy of 88% and 86%, respectively, for rule-out (CAD-RADs 0 vs >0) and identification of obstructive disease (CAD-RADs 0–2 vs 3–5).

To appropriately visualize the results of lesion-, segment-, and case-level evaluations, approaches which combine the simultaneous display of all coronary arteries with traditional MPR and MIP viewing are beneficial. These visualizations (see Fig. 18.10 as an example) can be automatically provided by the CT scanner upon completion of the CTA scan.

Functional Assessment – CT-FFR

Anatomical assessment on CCTA has a high sensitivity but low specificity. In recent years, CT-derived fractional flow reserve (CT-FFR) has been established as a method for the hemodynamic assessment of coronary lesions. Compared to other methods for functional assessment, neither it requires an additional scan, modality, or stress agents, nor is it invasive. This makes CT-FFR very attractive for a comprehensive CT-based evaluation of coronary heart disease. Initially, the computation of CT-FFR was only possible using computational fluid dynamics (CFD) on supercomputers. By using reduced-order models, CFD can also be performed on regular desktop systems. Most recently, machine learning models that predict CT-FFR from coronary geometry have been employed to great success. They allow for the computation to be performed on site and within seconds instead of hours. If such a model was to be trained on invasive FFR results of real patients, the data collection and annotation effort would be tremendous. A recently presented approach ($cFFR_{ML}$) [25] uses a CFD solver ($cFFR_{CFD}$) to calculate CT-FFR values for an arbitrary amount of synthetic geometries and then train the ML model to predict the results of the CFD. Assuming the CFD is validated against invasive FFR, the resulting model should also predict the invasive FFR values well.

The synthetically generated geometries allow for a representative training set with any combination of coronary topologies and pathologies. Since the model works on geometric information only, its input are global and lesion-specific features (e.g., position of a stenosis, minimum radius, stenosis length, etc.) instead of image data. Its output are CT-FFR values for every position on the coronary tree which can be visualized by a color-coded overlay (Fig. 18.11).

A multicentric study [6] found excellent correlation of $cFFR_{ML}$ and $cFFR_{CFD}$ ($R = 0.997$). The per-patient diagnostic accuracy against invasive FFR improved from 71% (visual stenosis grading) to 85% ($cFFR_{ML}$), with a reduction of false-positive CTA results by 73%. Further studies have confirmed these findings with accuracies between 82% and 93% [24, 44, 53].

Plaque Morphology and Composition

The quantification of lipid-rich, fibrotic, and calcified plaques of the coronaries as well as the classification of vulnerable plaque features has gained more and more attraction in recent years. For the quantification of plaques in terms of plaque volume and total plaque burden, traditional approaches rely on semiautomatically generated segmentations of the vessel's lumen and outer wall with subsequent application of banded thresholding within the wall (e.g., [50]). Radiomics was proposed for the identification of vulnerable plaque characteristics, allowing the identification of napkin ring signs with an AUC of 0.91 [29, 30] or thin cap fibrous atheroma with an AUC of 0.952 [5]. In both approaches, radiomics was superior to visual inspection and HU-based assessment.

The large amount of information extracted from anatomical and morphological evaluation of lumen and plaques is used to train prediction models against clinical outcome for

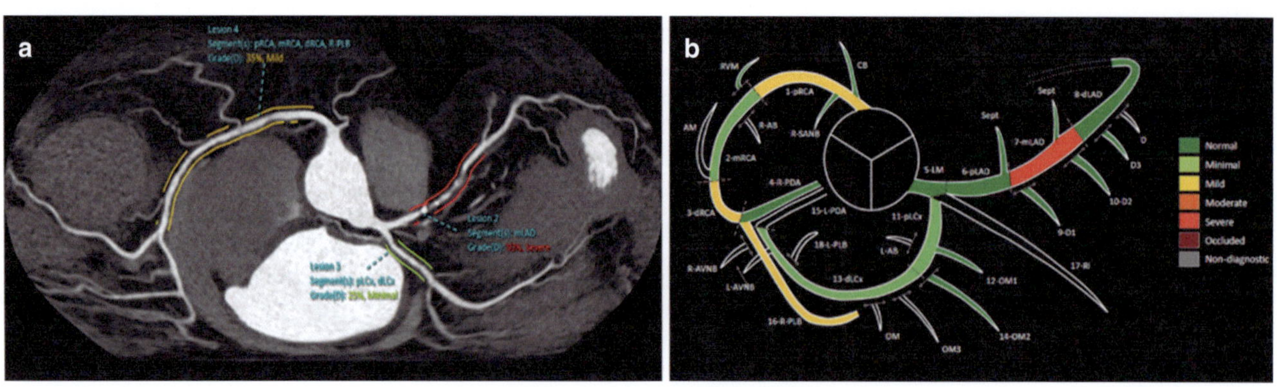

Fig. 18.10 (**a**) Unfolded view of the patient individual coronary anatomy. Automatically obtained lesion detection results are displayed as overlays. (**b**) Schematic overview image for the same patient. (CT data courtesy of J. Görich, Das Radiologische Zentrum, Heidelberg, Germany)

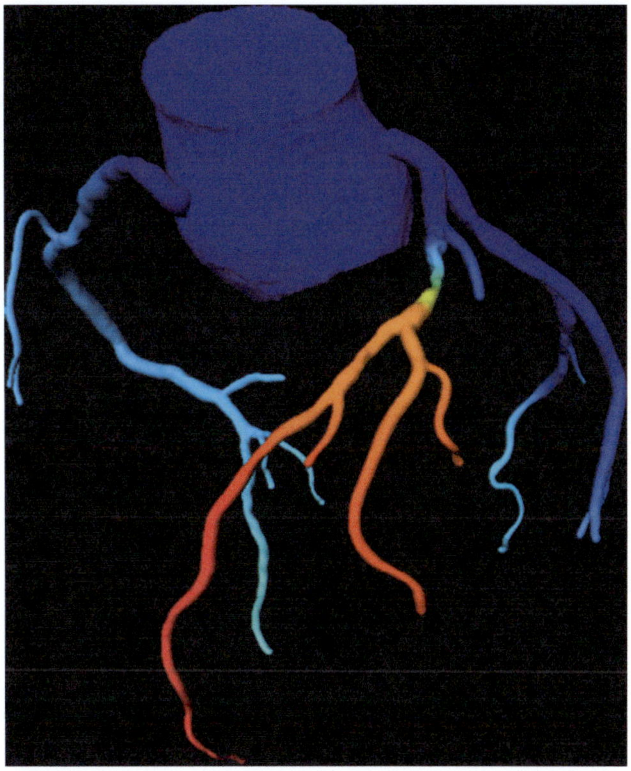

Fig. 18.11 Color-coded visualization of a CT-FFR result. Blue color represents normal flow ($cFFR_{ML} > 0.8$), while shades of yellow, orange, and red represent progressively reduced flow downstream of this mid-LAD stenosis. (CT data courtesy of Dr. Jones & Partners, Adelaide, Australia)

risk stratification and classification of the clinical relevance of lesions [11, 38, 51]. These models showed better performance than existing clinical variables and risk scores alone. In a recent approach [9], deep learning was fused with radiomics to predict if revascularization will be required. With an AUC of 0.88, this method showed an accuracy that is comparable to CT-FFR-based methods but with significantly less computational demands.

Conclusion

We have presented an overview on scanner-centric AI algorithms to simplify, streamline, and standardize the CT scan and image reconstruction workflow and to enhance and compress the clinical information of CT images. In the future, we will see further steps toward AI-supported workflow automation and standardization going hand in hand with refinement of image presentation and automated image evaluation. As a coveted goal, the CT scanner will directly provide relevant information about the clinical relevance of findings. It will therefore evolve from a mere imaging machine to a tool supporting the clinical decisions of radiologists and cardiologists.

References

1. Akin-Akintayo OO, Alexander LF, Neill R, Krupinksi EA, Tang X, et al. Prevalence and severity of off-Centering during diagnostic CT: observations from 57,621 CT scans of the chest, abdomen, and/or pelvis. Curr Probl Diagn Radiol. 2019;48(3):229–34.
2. Blanke P, Weir-McCall JR, Achenbach S, Delgado V, Hausleiter J, et al. Computed tomography imaging in the context of transcatheter aortic valve implantation (TAVI)/transcatheter aortic valve replacement (TAVR): an expert consensus document of the Society of Cardiovascular Computed Tomography. JACC Cardiovasc Imaging. 2019;12(1):1–24.
3. Booij R, Budde RPJ, Dijkshoorn ML, van Straten M. Accuracy of automated patient positioning in CT using a 3D camera for body contour detection. Eur Radiol. 2019;29(4):2079–88.
4. Booij R, van Straten M, Wimmer A, Budde RPJ. Automated patient positioning in CT using a 3D camera for body contour detection: accuracy in pediatric patients. Eur Radiol. 2021;31(1):131–8.
5. Chen Q, Pan T, Yin X, Xu H, Gao X, Tao X, Zhou L, Xie G, Kong X, Huang X, Gao N, Zhang JJ, Zhang LJ. CT texture analysis of vulnerable plaques on optical coherence tomography. Eur J Radiol. 2021;136:109551. https://doi.org/10.1016/j.ejrad.2021.109551. Epub ahead of print.
6. Coenen A, Kim YH, Kruk M, Tesche C, De Geer J, et al. Diagnostic accuracy of a machine-learning approach to coronary computed tomographic angiography-based fractional flow reserve: result from the MACHINE consortium. Circ Cardiovasc Imaging. 2018;11(6):e007217.
7. Cury RC, Abbara S, Achenbach S, Agatston A, Berman DS, et al. CAD-RADS(TM) Coronary Artery Disease Reporting and Data System. An expert consensus document of the Society of Cardiovascular Computed Tomography (SCCT), the American College of Radiology (ACR) and the North American Society for Cardiovascular Imaging (NASCI). Endorsed by the American College of Cardiology. J Cardiovasc Comput Tomogr. 2016;10(4):269–81.
8. Dane B, O'Donnell T, Liu S, Vega E, Mohammed S, et al. Radiation dose reduction, improved isocenter accuracy and CT scan time savings with automatic patient positioning by a 3D camera. Eur J Radiol. 2021;136:109537. https://doi.org/10.1016/j.ejrad.2021.109537. Online ahead of print.
9. Denzinger F, Wels M, Ravikumar N, Breininger K, Reidelshöfer A, et al. Coronary artery plaque characterization from CCTA scans using deep learning and radiomics. In: International conference on medical image computing and computer-assisted intervention. Cham: Springer; 2019. p. 593–601.
10. Denzinger F, Wels M, Breininger K, Gülsün MA, Schöbinger M, et al. Automatic CAD-RADS scoring using deep learning. In: Martel AL, et al., editors. Medical image computing and computer assisted intervention – MICCAI 2020, Lecture notes in computer science, vol. 12266. Cham: Springer; 2020.
11. Dey D, Gaur S, Ovrehus KA, Slomka PJ, Betancur J, et al. Integrated prediction of lesion-specific ischemia from quantitative coronary CT angiography using machine learning: a multicentre study. Eur Radiol. 2018;28(6):2655–64.
12. Fischer AM, Eid M, De Cecco CN, Gulsun MA, van Assen M, et al. Accuracy of an artificial intelligence deep learning algorithm implementing a recurrent neural network with long short-term memory for the automated detection of calcified plaques from coronary computed tomography angiography. J Thorac Imaging. 2020a;35(Suppl 1):S49–57.
13. Fischer A, Klein P, Radulescu P, Gulsun M, Ali AM, et al. Deep learning based automated coronary labeling for structured reporting of coronary CT angiography in accordance with SCCT guidelines. J Cardiovasc Comput Tomogr. 2020b;14(3):S21–2.

14. Flohr TG, McCollough CH, Bruder H, Petersilka M, Gruber K, et al. First performance evaluation of a dual-source CT (DSCT) system. Eur Radiol. 2006;16:256–68.
15. Fuld MK, Ramirez-Giraldo JC. Workflow design for CT of the thorax. In: Schoepf UJ, Meinel FG, editors. Multidetector-row CT of the thorax. Cham: Springer; 2016. p. 415–30.
16. Geissler F, Heiß R, Kopp M, Wiesmüller M, Saake M, et al. Personalized computed tomography - automated estimation of height and weight of a simulated digital twin using a 3D camera and artificial intelligence. Rofo. 2020. https://doi.org/10.1055/a--1253-8558. Epub ahead of print.
17. Ghesu FC, Georgescu B, Zheng Y, et al. Multi-scale deep reinforcement learning for real-time 3D-landmark detection in CT scans. IEEE Trans Pattern Anal Mach Intell. 2017;41(1):176–89.
18. Glemser PA, Engel K, Simons D. A new approach for photorealistic visualization of rendered CT images. World Neurosurg. 2018;114:e283–92. https://doi.org/10.1016/j.wneu.2018.02.174. Epub 2018 Mar 7
19. Grundy SM, Stone NJ, Bailey AL, Beam C, Birtcher KK, et al. 2018 AHA/ACC/AACVPR/AAPA/ABC/ACPM/ADA/AGS/APhA/ASPC/NLA/PCNA guideline on the management of blood cholesterol: a report of the American College of Cardiology/American Heart Association task force on clinical practice guidelines. Circulation. 2019;139:e1082–143.
20. Gülsün MA, Funka-Lea G, Sharma P, Rapaka S, Zheng Y. Coronary centerline extraction via optimal flow paths and CNN path pruning. In: International conference on medical image computing and computer-assisted intervention. Cham: Springer; 2016. p. 317–25.
21. Gutjahr R, Fletcher JG, Lee YS, Halaweish AF, Suresh V, et al. Individualized delay for abdominal computed tomography angiography bolus-tracking based on sequential monitoring: increased aortic contrast permits decreased injection rate and lower iodine dose. J Comput Assist Tomogr. 2019;43(4):612–8.
22. Ha JY, Jeon KN, Bae K, Choi BH. Effect of bone reading CT software on radiologist performance in detecting bone metastases from breast cancer. Br J Radiol. 2017;90(1072):20160809.
23. Hinzpeter R, Eberhard M, Gutjahr R, Reeve K, Pfammatter T, et al. CT angiography of the aorta: contrast timing by using a fixed versus a patient-specific trigger delay. Radiology. 2019;291(2):531–8.
24. Hu X, Yang M, Han L, Du Y. Diagnostic performance of machine-learning-based computed fractional flow reserve (FFR) derived from coronary computed tomography angiography for the assessment of myocardial ischemia verified by invasive FFR. Intl J Cardiovasc Imaging. 2018;34:1987–96.
25. Itu L, Rapaka S, Passerini T, Georgescu B, Schwemmer C, et al. A machine-learning approach for computation of fractional flow reserve from coronary computed tomography. J Appl Physiol. 2016;121:42–52.
26. Kalender W, Seissler W, Klotz E, Vock P. Spiral volumetric CT with single-breath-hold technique, continuous transport and continuous scanner rotation. Radiology. 1990;176:181–3.
27. Kanitsar A, Wegenkittl R, Fleischmann D, Groller ME. Advanced curved planar reformation: flattening of vascular structures. IEEE Visualization, 2003. VIS 2003, Seattle, 2003, p. 43–50. https://doi.org/10.1109/VISUAL.2003.1250353.
28. Knuuti J, Wijns W, Saraste A, Capodanno D, Barbato E, et al. 2019 ESC guidelines on the diagnosis and management of chronic coronary syndromes: the Task Force for diagnosis and management of chronic coronary syndromes of the European Society of Cardiology (ESC). Eur Heart J. 2020;41(3):407–77.
29. Kolossváry M, Karády J, Szilveszter B, Kitslaar P, Hoffmann U, et al. Radiomic features are superior to conventional quantitative computed tomographic metrics to identify coronary plaques with napkin-ring sign. Circ Cardiovasc Imaging. 2017;10(12):e006843.
30. Kolossváry M, Karády J, Kikuchi Y, Ivanov A, Schlett CL, et al. Radiomics versus visual and histogram-based assessment to identify atheromatous lesions at coronary CT angiography: an ex vivo study. Radiology. 2019;293(1):89–96.
31. Korporaal JG, Bischoff B, Arnoldi E, Sommer WH, Flohr TG, Schmidt B. Evaluation of a new bolus tracking-based algorithm for predicting a patient-specific time of arterial peak enhancement in computed tomography angiography. Investig Radiol. 2015;50(8):531–8.
32. Lee H, Martin S, Burt JR, Bagherzadeh PS, Rapaka S, et al. Machine learning and coronary artery calcium scoring. Curr Cardiol Rep. 2020;22(90):1–6.
33. Leipsic J, Abbara S, Achenbach S, Cury R, Earls JP, et al. SCCT guidelines for the interpretation and reporting of coronary CT angiography: a report of the Society of Cardiovascular Computed Tomography Guidelines Committee. J Cardiovasc Comput Tomogr. 2014;8(5):342–58.
34. May M, Wetzl M, Wust W, Heiss R, Treutlein C, et al. Advanced visualization of peroneal artery perforators prior to autologous transplantation in head and neck surgery by dual-energy CT and multiplanar vessel unfolding. Radiological Society of North America 2019 Scientific Assembly and Annual Meeting, December 1–December 6, 2019, Chicago. archive.rsna.org/2019/19012480.html
35. McCollough CH, Zink FE. Performance evaluation of a multi-slice CT system. Med Phys. 1999;26:2223–30.
36. McCollough CH, Ulzheimer S, Halliburton SS, Shanneik K, White RD, Kalender WA. Coronary artery calcium: a multiinstitutional, multimanufacturer international standard for quantification at cardiac CT. Radiology. 2007;243(2):527–38.
37. Mori S, Obata T, Nakajima N, Ichihara N, Endo M. Volumetric perfusion CT using prototype 256-detector row CT scanner: preliminary study with healthy porcine model. AJNR Am J Neuroradiol. 2005;26(10):2536–41.
38. Motwani M, Dey D, Berman DS, Germano G, Achenbach S, et al. Machine learning for prediction of all-cause mortality in patients with suspected coronary artery disease: a 5-year multicentre prospective registry analysis. Eur Heart J. 2017;38(7):500–7.
39. Muscogiuri G, Chiesa M, Trotta M, Gatti M, Palmisano V, et al. Performance of a deep learning algorithm for the evaluation of CAD-RADS classification with CCTA. Atherosclerosis. 2020;294:25–32.
40. Peng Z, Zhan Y, Zhou XS, Krishnan A. Robust anatomy detection from CT topograms. In: Medical imaging 2009: computer-aided diagnosis, vol. 7260. International Society for Optics and Photonics; 2009. p. 72603X.
41. Ren S, He K, Girshick R, Sun J. Faster R-CNN: towards real-time object detection with region proposal networks. IEEE Trans Pattern Anal Mach Intell. 2017;39(6):1137–49.
42. Ringl H, Lazar M, Töpker M, Woitek R, Prosch H, et al. The ribs unfolded-a CT visualization algorithm for fast detection of rib fractures: effect on sensitivity and specificity in trauma patients. Eur Radiol. 2015;25(7):1865–74.
43. Rjiba S, Urruty T, Boudon P, Fernandez-Maloigne C, Delepaule R, et al. CenterlineNet: automatic coronary artery centerline extraction for computed tomographic angiographic images using convolutional neural network architectures. In: 2020 tenth international conference on image processing theory, tools and applications (IPTA). IEEE; 2020. p. 1–6.
44. Röther J, Moshage M, Dey D, Schwemmer C, Tröbs M, et al. Comparison of invasively measured FFR with FFR derived from coronary CT angiography for detection of lesion-specific ischemia: results from a PC-based prototype algorithm. J Cardiovasc Comput Tomogr. 2018;12:101–7.
45. Saltybaeva N, Schmidt B, Wimmer A, Flohr T, Alkadhi H. Precise and automatic patient positioning in computed tomography: avatar Modeling of the patient surface using a 3-dimensional camera. Investig Radiol. 2018;53(11):641–6.

46. Sandstedt M, Henriksson L, Janzon M, Nyberg G, Engvall J, et al. Evaluation of an AI-based, automatic coronary artery calcium scoring software. Eur Radiol. 2020;30(3):1671–8.
47. Sharma P, Suehling M, Flohr T, Comaniciu D. Artificial intelligence in diagnostic imaging: status quo, challenges, and future opportunities. J Thorac Imaging. 2020;35:S11–6.
48. Singh V, Ma K, Tamersoy B, et al. DARWIN: deformable patient avatar representation with deep image network. In: Descoteaux M, et al., editors. Medical Image Computing and Computer-Assisted Intervention – MICCAI 2017: 20th International Conference, Quebec City, QC, Canada, September 11–13, 2017, Proceedings, Part II. Cham: Springer International Publishing; 2017. p. 497–504.
49. Tao Y, Peng Z, Krishnan A, Zhou XS. Robust learning-based parsing and annotation of medical radiographs. IEEE Trans Med Imaging. 2011;30(2):338–50.
50. Tesche C, De Cecco CN, Caruso D, Baumann S, Renker M, et al. Coronary CT angiography derived morphological and functional quantitative plaque markers correlated with invasive fractional flow reserve for detecting hemodynamically significant stenosis. J Cardiovasc Comput Tomogr. 2016;10(3):199–206.
51. van Rosendael AR, Maliakal G, Kolli KK, Beecy A, Al'Aref SJ, et al. Maximization of the usage of coronary CTA derived plaque information using a machine learning based algorithm to improve risk stratification; insights from the CONFIRM registry. J Cardiovasc Comput Tomogr. 2018;12(3):204–9.
52. Wolterink JM, van Hamersvelt RW, Viergever MA, Leiner T, Išgum I. Coronary artery centerline extraction in cardiac CT angiography using a CNN-based orientation classifier. Med Image Anal. 2019;51:46–60.
53. Xu PP, Li JH, Zhou F, Jiang MD, Zhou CS, Lu MJ, et al. The influence of image quality on diagnostic performance of a machine learning–based fractional flow reserve derived from coronary CT angiography. Eur Radiol. 2020;30:2525–34.
54. Zhan Y, Zhou XS, Peng Z, Krishnan A. Active scheduling of organ detection and segmentation in whole-body medical images. In: International conference on medical image computing and computer-assisted intervention. Berlin/Heidelberg: Springer; 2008. p. 313–21.
55. Zhou SX, Peng Z, Zhan Y, Dewan M, Jian B, et al. Redundancy, redundancy, redundancy: the three keys to highly robust anatomical parsing. In MIR '10: International conference on multimedia information retrieval, March 2010, p. 175–84. https://dl.acm.org/doi/10.1145/1743384.1743416.
56. Zreik M, van Hamersvelt RW, Wolterink JM, Leiner T, Viergever MA, Isgum I. A recurrent CNN for automatic detection and classification of coronary artery plaque and stenosis in coronary CT angiography. IEEE Trans Med Imaging. 2019;38(7):1588–98.

19 Artificial Intelligence Integration into the Magnetic Resonance System

Giuseppe Muscogiuri, Pablo Garcia-Polo, Marco Guglielmo, Andrea Baggiano, Martin A. Janich, and Gianluca Pontone

AI Approaches for Workflow Improvement

Automatic Slice Placement

Cardiac MR imaging allows for morphological, functional, and physiological assessment of the heart with high temporal and spatial resolution. However, precise and reproducible placement of the imaging planes is key for an accurate diagnostic reading. Dedicated training is needed for a technician to become familiar with the heart anatomy and to follow consistently the set of scans needed to acquire the standard views recommended by the SCMR guides: left ventricular short axis, two chambers, three chambers, four chambers, and, often in addition, right ventricular and valvular planes.

Regular CMR scanning workflow implies the acquisition of fast localizers, requiring breath holds, that are iteratively rotated and repositioned by the radiographer to acquire the full set of previously mentioned standard views. One view facilitates the accurate prescription of the next one, and therefore, any error may derive in re-scanning previous localizers with an impact in total scan time.

The high training need can impose a barrier for broader expansion of cardiac MRI, especially in smaller hospitals.

Some technical work focused on improving slice positioning has been developed in the last years. These advances have the final objective of improving exam workflow and optimizing exam time.

Giuseppe Muscogiuri and Pablo Garcia-Polo contributed equally with all other contributors.

G. Muscogiuri, MD, PhD (✉) · M. Guglielmo, MD
A. Baggiano, MD · G. Pontone, MD, PhD
Centro Cardiologico Monzino, IRCCS, Milan, Italy

P. Garcia-Polo, MSc
General Electric Healthcare, Madrid, Spain

M. A. Janich, PhD
General Electric Healthcare, Munich, Germany

Frick et al. [1] proposed a robust automatic scan planning which was entirely operator independent. This two-step-based method applied a segmentation and a deformation algorithm to delineate the major compartments of the heart, from which anatomical landmarks are extracted to, thereafter, used as a reference to position the scanning slices. Other works [3, 7, 8] proposed feature recognition and image classification to extract cardiac landmarks which may be later used to change the orientation of the acquisition planes.

Lu et al. [9] presented a fully automated method to prescribe short-axis, long-axis, two-chamber, three-chamber, and four-chamber views from a single 3D acquisition. In this work, a previously manually segmented 3D model of the left ventricle is co-registered and scaled to the actual patient heart through a tree-based classifier using probabilistic boosting trees. Then the 3D model is inflated or deflated to match the specific patient heart anatomy, and the slices can be prescribed.

In a recent study, e.g., Chow [10] used a machine learning based algorithm trained on hundreds of annotated datasets to identify the anatomical landmarks used for slice prescription. This work shows a high consistency for longitudinal studies and high reproducibility of slices positioning.

Blansit et al. [4] demonstrated that a deep learning-based (DL-based) algorithm trained on hundreds of annotated cardiac studies is a state-of-the-art strategy for planning cardiac MR planes. In this project, two-dimensional U-Nets were trained to predict the heatmaps that represent the probability of a specific landmark localization. The location of these landmarks (i.e., apex, mitral valve, tricuspid valve, aortic valve, and pulmonary valve) defined the angulations for the slice prescription and were compared against manual positioning. These works have been the basis of some vendor solutions or development efforts for automatic slice placement that are bringing improved exam workflow and reduced operator variability. The algorithm of automatic slice placement is shown in Fig. 19.1.

C. N. De Cecco et al. (eds.), *Artificial Intelligence in Cardiothoracic Imaging*, Contemporary Medical Imaging,
https://doi.org/10.1007/978-3-030-92087-6_19

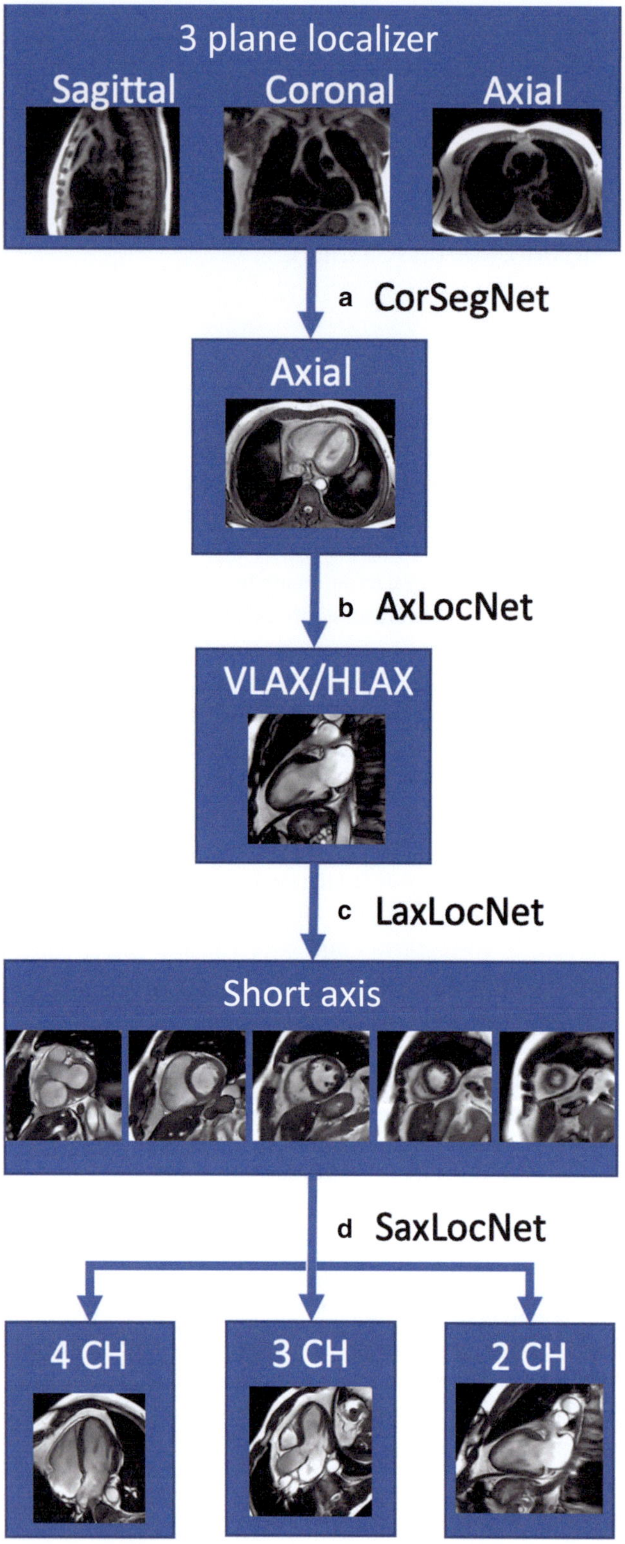

Fig. 19.1 Deep learning-based automatic slice prescription using U-Nets for landmark localization. (**a**) Prescription of axial stack based on three-plane localizer images. (**b**) Localization of vertical and horizontal long-axis planes using axial stack. (**c**) Short-axis prescription based on vertical and horizontal long-axis images. (**d**) Localization of landmarks in short-axis images leads to four-, three-, and two-chamber planes

Automatic Parameter Optimization

CMR image quality relies on several parameters that are dependent on patient anatomy and physiology. An interesting case of this is the delayed enhanced imaging to assess myocardial scar and viability. After contrast injection, the nulling point of background myocardial signal needs to be selected to optimize image contrast.

Bahrami et al. [11] suggest a new scope for deep learning and convolutional neural network (CNN) approaches to work in this sense. By introducing long short-term memory models (LSTM) and combining them with CNN, the new model has both temporal and spatial capabilities to solve for the nulling point automatically.

Image Quality

Magnetic resonance is considered one of the most flexible imaging modalities for clinical diagnosis, thanks to its soft tissue contrast and nonionizing radiation. Nevertheless, MRI acquisition protocols have to be carefully optimized to find the best tradeoffs between scan time, image resolution, and signal-to-noise ratio.

A natural approach to minimize these tradeoffs is moving to higher-field strengths where SNR and image resolution increase given the same scan time. However, certain artifacts such as field inhomogeneities and power deposition (SAR) begin to appear, affecting its simplicity of use and clinical adoption.

In parallel, new advances in low noise receiver chain, digitalization, coil design, and pulse sequences have kept improving MR examinations steadily.

There is currently a lot of effort to bring advances of deep learning to MRI, with a potential to break the tradeoff of SNR, image resolution, and scan time. The main approaches for AI-powered image quality improvements are described below.

Deep Resolve

Deep Resolve technology [12] brings deep learning and AI to the MR image reconstruction process. It is divided into Deep Resolve Gain and Deep Resolve Sharp.

Deep Resolve Gain makes use of specific noise maps extracted from the originally acquired raw data and feeds the reconstruction algorithm, which takes local noise variations into account and enables stronger denoising where noise would be most dominant when reconstructing with conventional methods.

Deep Resolve Sharp is a novel image reconstruction technology to generate images with increased sharpness. The deep neural network at the core of Deep Resolve Sharp generates a high-resolution image from low-resolution input data. The network was trained on a large number of pairs of low-resolution and high-resolution data. This solution can increase the matrix size by a factor of up to two along both in-plane axis, resulting in substantially increased image sharpness.

To ensure robust results, the acquired raw data is directly incorporated into the reconstruction and ensures consistency with the data from the scanner.

The inclusion of the cross-check with the acquired raw data is essential for the robustness of the reconstruction.

Advanced Intelligent Clear-IQ Engine (AiCE)

AiCE [13, 14] is a deep learning reconstruction method that is designed based on the knowledge of signal processing and MR physics, which allows AiCE's model to be interpretable and AiCE's performance to be explainable.

The AiCE DLR algorithm uses a deep convolutional neural network (DCNN) that was trained on a large dataset of examinations acquired on several subjects' brains and knees. These models included the analysis of a wide array of contrast weightings (T1, T2, FLAIR, PD), thus ensuring that AiCE DLR would be efficient and robust across multiple clinical contexts.

To perform this training, ideal high-SNR high-resolution datasets with 10 number of acquisitions were defined as "ground truth" and then mixed with Gaussian noise. This data was then processed by the neural network, which was built in such a way as to automatically define the noise level and to propose a denoising solution.

The resulting low noise images were then compared to native images. If they were different, the network learned adjusted the algorithm weights, and the denoising process was repeated. At the end of the training procedure, when the denoised images and the ground truth images were considered similar, algorithm weights were saved, and the trained database completed.

Denoising occurs in the spectral domain where only the high-frequency content is passed through the network. Adaptive activations automatically adjust to the input image noise level, producing high-quality images across all sequences without requiring any user interaction, thus efficiently optimizing the removal of noise while preserving key MR signals. After denoising, the low-frequency components containing the image-contrast information have remained untouched and are combined with the optimized results in order to maintain native contrasts. Interpolation and distortion/intensity corrections are finally applied following the DLR process, thus completing image reconstruction.

AIR™ Recon DL

AIR™ Recon DL is a feed-forward deep convolutional neural network (CNN) with a residual encoder architecture which was designed to achieve output images with higher signal-to-noise ratio (SNR), reduced truncation artifacts, and higher spatial resolution compared to standard non-DL image reconstruction [15]. The CNN is part of the standard reconstruction pipeline; takes as input data unfiltered complex-valued MR data and a user-defined noise reduction (NR) preference level of "low," "medium," or "high"; and produces improved output images. The resulting improved images have higher SNR, higher edge sharpness, and higher resolution. Low, medium, and high NR factors correspond to approximately $\sqrt{2}$, 2, and fourfold increased SNR, respectively.

The CNN was trained with a supervised learning approach, using pairs of near-perfect and lower-quality images. The latter images had higher noise levels, more truncation artifacts, and lower spatial resolution compared to the near-perfect images. A diverse set of training images spanning a broad range of image content were employed to enable generalizability of the CNN across all anatomies. The training database used millions of image pairs after applying data augmentation methods. The network was trained with gradient backpropagation and the ADAM optimizer. We would like to highlight a couple of recent clinical research publications in the field of cardiac MR that have used some of the algorithms described before.

Yaman et al. [16] extended a self-supervised learning approach to 3D LGE imaging and compares different acceleration rates with the clinical compressed sensing (CS) reconstruction algorithm. In this work, it is shown that CS-reconstructed images showed lower quality in form of noise amplification and incoherent aliasing artifacts when compared to the 3D physics-guided DL method.

Van der Velde et al. [5] showed the image quality improvements and sharpness gain impact in myocardial late gadolinium enhancements of myocardial fibrosis using GE Healthcare's AIR™ Recon DL. They also noted that care has to be taken when applying standard deviation-based scar quantification methods. They also showed that scar quantification based on full-width half-maximum (FWHM) was preferred as it was not sensitive to different levels of noise in the images compared to standard deviation-based scar quantification, and it corresponded best to manual scar segmentation. A representative case of late gadolinium enhancement reconstructed using AIRDL algorithm is shown in Fig. 19.2.

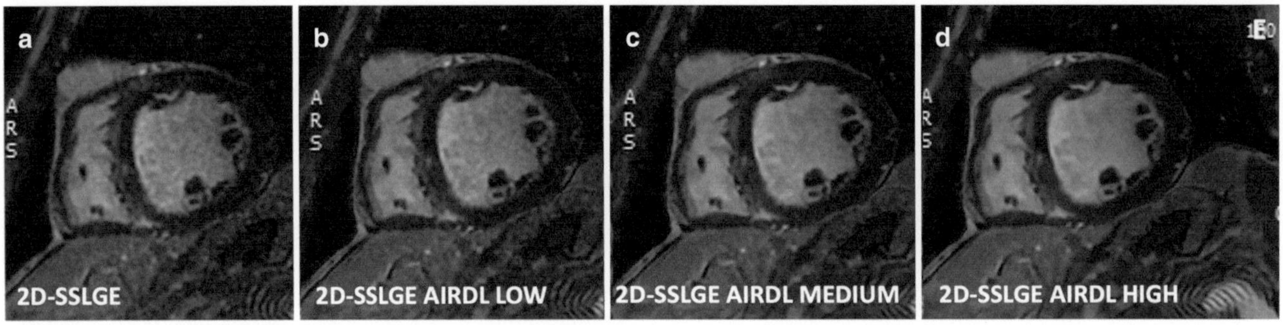

Fig. 19.2 A 65-year-old patient with dilated cardiomyopathy showing midwall fibrosis on basal septum in 2D standard segmented late gadolinium enhancement (2D-SSLGE) reconstructed in magnitude (**a**). Image noise reduction using AIRDL low, (**b**) AIRDL medium, and (**c**), AIRDL high (**d**)

Scan Speed

Cardiac magnetic resonance imaging (CMR) is considered the gold standard for measuring myocardial volume and function in a wide range of pathologies such as congenital heart disease, heart failure, pulmonary hypertension, and coronary artery disease. Typically, an ECG-gated 2D-balanced steady-state free precession (bSSFP)-based sequence is used to acquire cine images that permit the study of the heart with good temporal resolution (<45 ms) and high spatial resolution (<2 mm). Typical 2D cine imaging requires multiple breath holds of approximately 10–15 s in order to cover the full left ventricle (10–15 slices) in short-axis view. These repetitive breath holds may become difficult to a large number of patients and, if not performed consistently, can lead to slice misalignment [17] and incorrect assessment of left ventricular volume and function.

Some initial strategies to reduce total scan time come from the hand of reducing spatial resolution, limiting the number of slices, and decreasing temporal resolution but at the cost of limiting the clinical diagnostic value [18]. An early approach to the problem from Roifman et al. [19] compared a free breathing method with an accelerated spiral k-space readout trajectory against the conventional breath hold Cartesian k-space readout. Their new accelerated sequence provided a significant reduction in scan time and performed similarly to the traditional breath hold cine in the standard left ventricular function measurements.

Nowadays, in routine clinical scans, thanks to the multichannel array receiver coils, parallel imaging techniques such as SENSE, GRAPPA, ARC, or SPIRiT can be used and provide accelerated acquisition times up to 2–3×.

One important feature in cine images is their inherent temporal correlation information that has been exploited by certain acceleration algorithms as k-t SENSE [20], k-t BLAST [20], k-t GRAPPA [21], and k-t ARC, with the common final objective of reducing breath holds to a minimum [22].

Additional acceleration was reached with the inclusion of compressed sensing (CS) techniques [23], which take advantage of image sparsity and undersampled k-space in a sub-Nyquist-Shannon approach. These types of techniques are capable of single-breath hold acquisition or free breathing. CS reconstruction algorithms involve solving a regularized inverse problem under some assumptions (priors) that need to be carefully balanced in order to avoid over-regularization.

Very recently, deep learning-based solutions have been developed to resolve some of the CS scheme limitations. Schlemper et al. developed a convolutional neural network (CNN) reconstruction pipeline on highly undersampled cine Cartesian acquisitions [24]. Their CNN pipeline was trained on 10 fully sampled bSSFP datasets (with data augmentation) to reconstruct highly undersampled 2D cine images. The validation results outperform other CS methods although no validation was done on datasets with pathology.

Hauptmann et al. [25] trained a U-Net (multi-scale CNN) to remove aliasing artifacts from 13× accelerated cine images. The U-Net was trained on 250 high-quality, fully sampled bSSFP Cartesian cine images datasets and was evaluated against regular CS techniques on healthy volunteers and patients. Their results showed that higher accelerated artifact-free free breathing images could be achieved with this scheme, a reduced reconstruction time of images and an equal ventricular volume calculation compared to clinical standard techniques.

However, compared to other deep learning applications, it is very challenging to get a large training database. Sandino et al. [18] proposed a new method, named DL-ESPIRiT, to overcome the limitation. Unlike traditional end-to-end learning, they combined CNN-based reconstruction with conventional model-based reconstruction, alternatively updating the image based on CNN and ESPIRiT sensitivity model. This DL-ESPIRiT algorithm has proven to give improved results compared to regular CS algorithms (l1-ESPIRiT) and can reach acceleration factors of 12× with no image degradation, therefore being able to acquire one 2D cine slice within one heartbeat and during free breathing. Furthermore, Sandino [18] et al. also decomposed the 3D (x,y,t) convolution into 2D (x,y) and 1D (t) convolution operators in the CNN, which further improve the reconstructed image quality and left ventricular ejection fraction (LVEF) quantification and also speed up the convergence of the reconstruction model. Chen et al. [26] also proposed a faster reconstruction residual convolutional recurrent neural network (Res-CNN) for 2D cine images with ESPIRiT coil sensitivity model inclusion. Their solution achieved highly accelerated 12× cine data and higher expert scoring compared with L1-ESPIRiT techniques on noise reduction, artifacts, and motion depiction but slightly lower score on sharpness. A representative case using DL-ESPIRit is shown in Fig. 19.3.

Finally, Küstner et al. developed a 4D DL-based reconstruction algorithm for highly undersampled 3D Cartesian cine data, called CINENet [17]. Their proposed CINENet pipeline achieves single-breath hold 3D cine images with 1.9 mm^3 isotropic and LV coverage within 15 s, including less than 10s acquisition time and 5 s reconstruction time. They trained their CINENet with a set of 6500 4D retrospectively undersampled 3D cine datasets on a cascaded 3D spatial and 1D temporal convolution-based architecture that exploits the spatiotemporal redundancies. Results were compared against a 2D cine clinical gold standard acquisition and CS acquisition. Improved image quality was obtained with CINENet compared to CS, but decreased contrast was seen compared to 2D cine due to blood pool saturation effects which are common for 3D slab approaches. Nevertheless, quantitative results from LV function and qualitative image assessment were comparable between the conventional 2D cine and the proposed CINENet algorithm.

Besides the great improvements in accelerated cine imaging, Nath et al. applied deep learning reconstruction techniques to highly undersampled phase contrast imaging. Reconstruction times were improved, and velocity flow rates were closer to reference compared to regular CS techniques. Their work exemplifies that deep CNN can reconstruct not only magnitude images but phase information with high quality, allowing acceleration of 4D flow techniques [27].

Future Perspective

Application of AI to CMR, as described above, plays a key role in image prescription, acquisition, and reconstruction. Several vendors have adapted their MR system in order to facilitate images acquisition sparing time and improving image quality.

Further improvements with respect to automatization, acceleration, and ease-of-use are expected in the near future.

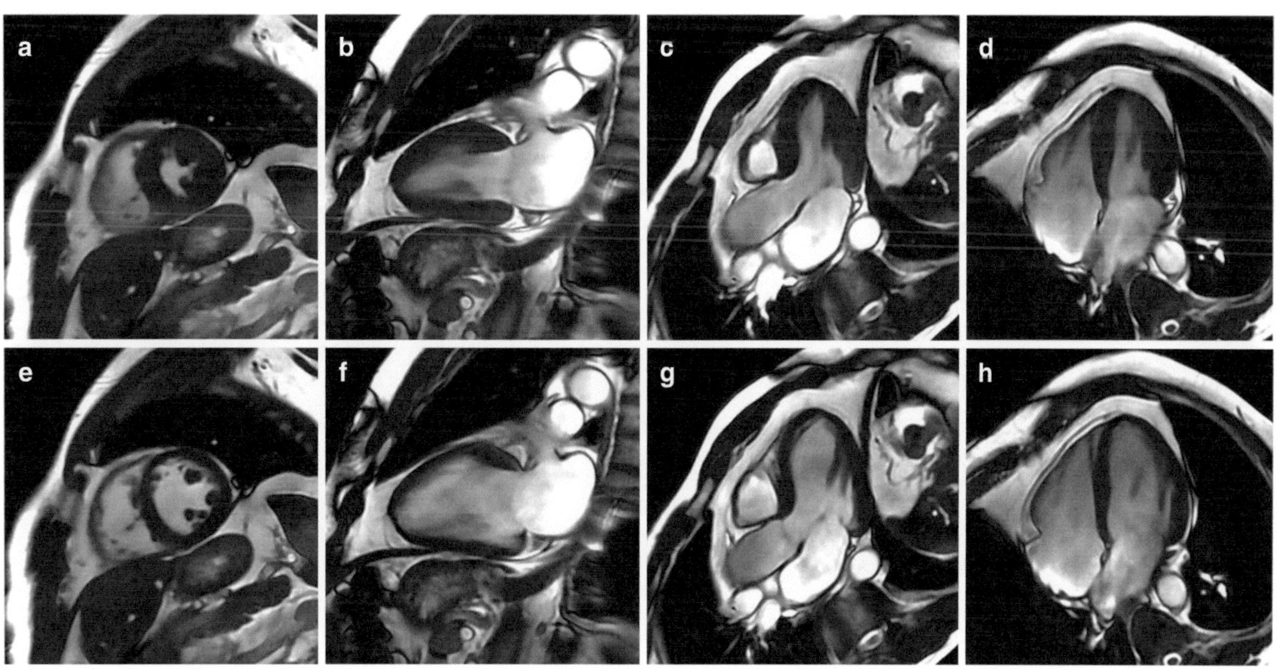

Fig. 19.3 Retrospectively gated bSSFP cine acquired on GE 3.0 T SIGNA Premier using DL-ESPIRiT Cine reconstruction. The real-time acquisition was performed in a single heartbeat per slice. Upper row shows images acquired in diastole (**a**, short axis; **b**, two chambers; **c**, three chambers; **d**, four chambers) and systole (**e**, short axis; **f**, two chambers; **g**, three chambers; **h**, four chambers)

References

1. Frick M, Paetsch I, den Harder C, Kouwenhoven M, Heese H, Dries S, Schnackenburg B, de Kok W, Gebker R, Fleck E, Manka R, Jahnke C. Fully automatic geometry planning for cardiac MR imaging and reproducibility of functional cardiac parameters. J Magn Reson Imaging. 2011;34:457–67.
2. Guaricci AI, Masci PG, Lorenzoni V, Schwitter J, Pontone G. CarDiac MagnEtic resonance for primary prevention implantable CardioVerter DebrillAtor ThErapy international registry: design and rationale of the DERIVATE study. Int J Cardiol. 2018;261:223–7.
3. Nitta S, Takeguchi T, Matsumoto N, Kuhara S, Yokoyama K, Ishimura R, Nitatori T. Automatic slice alignment method for cardiac magnetic resonance imaging. MAGMA. 2013;26:451–61.
4. Blansit K, Retson T, Masutani E, Bahrami N, Hsiao A. Deep learning-based prescription of cardiac MRI planes. Radiol Artif Intell. 2019;1:e180069.
5. van der Velde N, Hassing HC, Bakker BJ, Wielopolski PA, Lebel RM, Janich MA, Kardys I, Budde RPJ, Hirsch A. Improvement of late gadolinium enhancement image quality using a deep learning-based reconstruction algorithm and its influence on myocardial scar quantification. Eur Radiol 2021;31(6):3846-3855.
6. Moenninghoff C, Umutlu L, Kloeters C, Ringelstein A, Ladd ME, Sombetzki A, Lauenstein TC, Forsting M, Schlamann M. Workflow efficiency of two 1.5 T MR scanners with and without an automated user interface for head examinations. Acad Radiol. 2013;20:721–30.
7. Yokoyama K, Nitta S, Kuhara S, et al. Automatic slice-alignment method in cardiac magnetic resonance imaging for evaluation of the right ventricle in patients with pulmonary hypertension. AIP Adv. 2015;5:097182.
8. Oktay O, Bai W, Guerrero R, Rajchl M, de Marvao A, O'Regan DP, Cook SA, Heinrich MP, Glocker B, Rueckert D. Stratified decision forests for accurate anatomical landmark localization in cardiac images. IEEE Trans Med Imaging. 2017;36:332–42.
9. Lu X, Jolly MP, Georgescu B, Haye C, Speier P, Schmidt M, Bi X, Kroeker R, Comaniciu D, Kellman P, Mueller E, Guehring J. Automatic view planning for cardiac MRI acquisition. Med Image Comput Comput Assist Interv. 2011;14:479–86.
10. Chow K. 16 months of exercise–a case study of automated CMR with cardiac dot engine. MAGNETOM Flash SCMR Edition 2020. 2020.
11. Bahrami N, Retson T, Blansit K, Wang K, Hsiao A. Automated selection of myocardial inversion time with a convolutional neural network: spatial temporal ensemble myocardium inversion network (STEMI-NET). Magn Reson Med. 2019;81:3283–91.
12. https://www.siemens-healthineerscom/magnetic-resonance-imaging/technologies-and-innovations/deep-resolve.
13. Advanced intelligent Clear-IQ Engine (AiCE). https://global.medical.canon/products/magnetic-resonance/aice.
14. Deep Learning Reconstruction in Clinical MRI: a new realm combining ultra-high resolution and increased productivity. https://eu.medical.canon/publication/mr/Deep_Learning_Reconstruction_in_Clinical_MRI.
15. Lebel RM. Performance characterization of a novel deep learning-based MR image reconstruction pipeline. arXiv. 2008:06559.
16. Yaman B. Self-supervised physics-guided deep learning reconstruction for high-resolution 3D LGE CMR. arXiv. 2011:09414.
17. Kustner T, Fuin N, Hammernik K, Bustin A, Qi H, Hajhosseiny R, Masci PG, Neji R, Rueckert D, Botnar RM, Prieto C. CINENet: deep learning-based 3D cardiac CINE MRI reconstruction with multi-coil complex-valued 4D spatio-temporal convolutions. Sci Rep. 2020;10:13710.
18. Sandino CM, Lai P, Vasanawala SS, Cheng JY. Accelerating cardiac cine MRI using a deep learning-based ESPIRiT reconstruction. Magn Reson Med. 2021;85:152–67.
19. Roifman I, Gutierrez J, Wang E, Biswas L, Sparkes J, Connelly KA, Wright GA. Evaluating a novel free-breathing accelerated cardiac MRI cine sequence in patients with cardiomyopathy. Magn Reson Imaging. 2019;61:260–6.
20. Tsao J, Boesiger P, Pruessmann KP. k-t BLAST and k-t SENSE: dynamic MRI with high frame rate exploiting spatiotemporal correlations. Magn Reson Med. 2003;50:1031–42.
21. Huang F, Akao J, Vijayakumar S, Duensing GR, Limkeman M. k-t GRAPPA: a k-space implementation for dynamic MRI with high reduction factor. Magn Reson Med. 2005;54:1172–84.
22. Muscogiuri G, Gatti M, Dell'Aversana S, Pica S, Andreini D, Guaricci AI, Guglielmo M, Baggiano A, Mushtaq S, Conte E, Gripari P, Annoni A, Formenti A, Mancini ME, Rabbat MG, Pepi M, Pontone G. Reliability of single breath hold three-dimensional cine kat-ARC for the assessment of biventricular dimensions and function. Eur J Radiol. 2020;124:108820.
23. Bustin A, Fuin N, Botnar RM, Prieto C. From compressed-sensing to artificial intelligence-based cardiac MRI reconstruction. Front Cardiovasc Med. 2020;7:17.
24. Schlemper J, Caballero J, Hajnal JV, Price AN, Rueckert D. A deep cascade of convolutional neural networks for dynamic MR image reconstruction. IEEE Trans Med Imaging. 2018;37:491–503.
25. Hauptmann A, Arridge S, Lucka F, Muthurangu V, Steeden JA. Real-time cardiovascular MR with spatio-temporal artifact suppression using deep learning-proof of concept in congenital heart disease. Magn Reson Med. 2019;81:1143–56.
26. Chen EZ, Chen X, Lyu J, Zheng Y, Chen T, Xu J, Sun S. Real-time cardiac cine MRI with residual convolutional recurrent neural network. arXiv:200805044. 2020.
27. Nath R, Callahan S, Singam N. Accelerated phase contrast magnetic resonance imaging via deep learning. In: 2020 IEEE 17th international symposium on biomedical imaging (ISBI). 2020.

Magnetic Resonance Fingerprinting: The Role of Artificial Intelligence

20

Alexander Fyrdahl, Nicole Seiberlich, and Jesse I. Hamilton

Conventional Methods for CMR Parameter Mapping

The majority of clinical CMR scans collect qualitative images in which the image contrast is weighted by many different factors. The factors that determine the appearance of a tissue on an image include not only inherent properties of the tissue but also pulse sequence parameters and properties of the imaging system. Although quantitative metrics such as ejection fraction are often derived from qualitative images, intensities of the pixels in the image are arbitrarily scaled, and thus the image signal intensities are not a direct measurement of a single physical quantity. The aim of quantitative CMR is to calculate maps where the intensity of each image pixel directly corresponds to an inherent property of the underlying tissue [1]. Traditionally, quantitative maps are calculated by acquiring qualitative images where the image contrast is sensitized to a particular tissue property. Several qualitative images are acquired with different amounts of contrast weighting, and the signal intensity at each voxel is fit to a mathematical model to estimate the quantitative tissue property value. Most conventional methods assume a simplified mono-exponential model, such as exponential recovery when measuring T_1 or exponential decay when measuring T_2, and the tissue property values are calculated from the weighted images using nonlinear parametric fitting.

The following section will provide a brief overview of conventional quantitative CMR mapping techniques to provide a framework for understanding cardiac MRF. A schematic overview of several common conventional T_1 and T_2 mapping methods can be seen in Fig. 20.1. Although other properties are commonly measured in clinical CMR exams, such as T_2^*, this review will emphasize T_1 and T_2 mapping since much of the cardiac MRF literature has focused on these parameters.

A. Fyrdahl, PhD
Department of Radiology, University of Michigan,
Ann Arbor, MI, USA
e-mail: fyrdahl@med.umich.edu

N. Seiberlich, PhD · J. I. Hamilton, PhD (✉)
Department of Radiology, University of Michigan,
Ann Arbor, MI, USA

Department of Biomedical Engineering, University of Michigan,
Ann Arbor, MI, USA
e-mail: nse@med.umich.edu; hamiljes@med.umich.edu

T_1 Mapping

Quantitative maps of the longitudinal MRI relaxation time (T_1) are frequently collected in a clinical setting to assess a variety of conditions. An increase in myocardial T_1 values can be indicative of myocarditis [2], myocardial infarction [3], or amyloidosis [4], whereas a decrease may be linked to Fabry's disease [5]. T_1 mapping is also useful in the assessment of both focal and diffuse myocardial fibrosis. Compared to qualitative techniques like late gadolinium enhancement (LGE), T_1 mapping has advantages in the detection of diffuse disease since there is no requirement to have normal myocardial tissue in the image to serve as a reference. T_1 mapping can also be performed to assess the native (pre-contrast) myocardium or after the intravenous injection of a gadolinium-containing contrast agent. Because gadolinium is restricted to the extracellular space and cannot enter the myocyte, the acquisition of both pre-contrast and post-contrast T_1 maps can be used to quantify myocardial extracellular volume fraction (ECV), which also provides information about diffuse fibrosis [6]. Traditionally, T_1 is quantified by collecting several images that sample different time points along a T_1 recovery curve. To limit the T_1 mapping acquisition to a single-breath-hold and reduce cardiac motion artifacts, T_1-weighted images are typically acquired using a single-shot imaging readout with electrocardiogram (ECG) triggering, which yields one T_1-weighted image per heartbeat. A quantitative T_1 map is generated by performing a voxel-wise nonlinear fit of the T_1-weighted images to an

C. N. De Cecco et al. (eds.), *Artificial Intelligence in Cardiothoracic Imaging*, Contemporary Medical Imaging,
https://doi.org/10.1007/978-3-030-92087-6_20

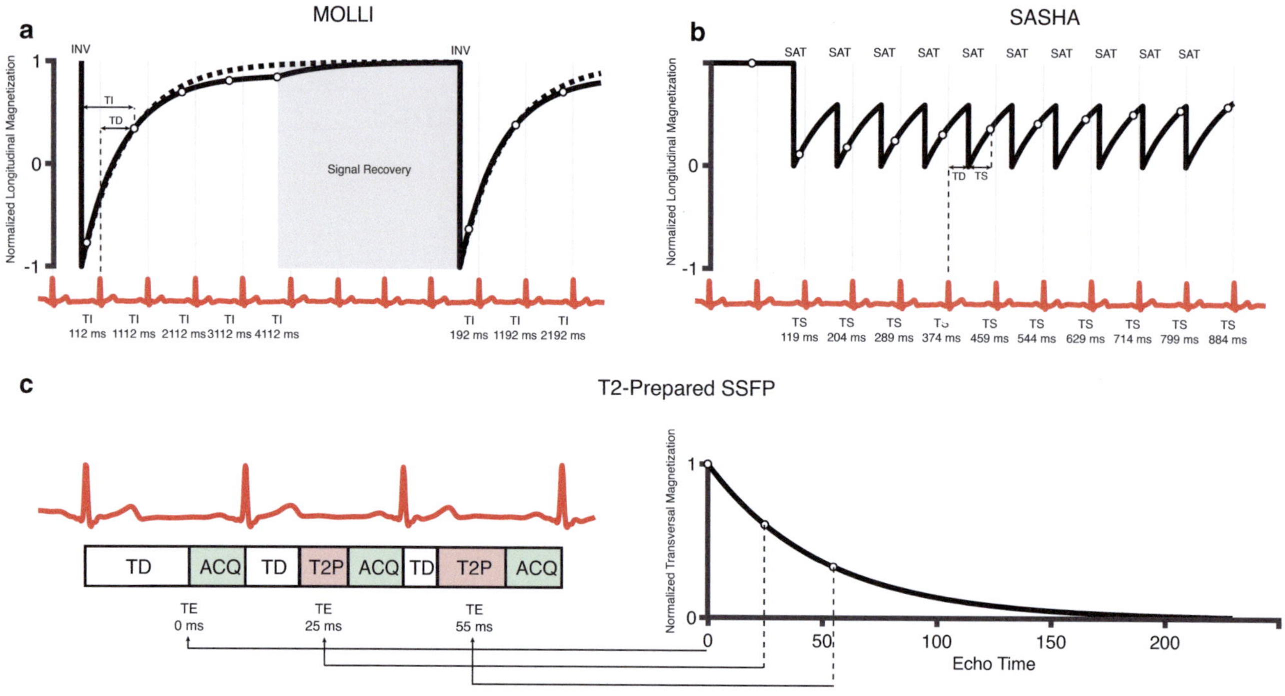

Fig. 20.1 (**a**) Schematic overview of the MOLLI 5(3)3 method. Single-shot images are acquired with varying inversion times (TI). The trigger delay (TD) is kept constant to ensure that the images are acquired in the diastolic phase of the cardiac cycle. The ideal signal recovery is indicated by the dashed line, and the apparent T_1 recovery due to influence from the readout (T_1^*) is indicated by the solid line. The gray box indicates the period during which the magnetization is allowed to return to equilibrium prior to the next inversion. (**b**) Schematic overview of the 10-point SASHA method. Single-shot images are acquired in every heartbeat following a saturation pulse that erases all transversal magnetization. The saturation time (TS) is varied to allow for a variable amount of T_1 recovery to happen prior to acquisition. The sum of TD and TS is kept constant to ensure that all images are acquired in the diastolic phase of the cardiac cycle. (**c**) A schematic overview of a prominent method for cardiovascular T_2 mapping, 3-point T_2-prepared SSFP. Multiple single-shot images are acquired following a T_2-preparatory (T2P) module varying echo times (TE) to induce a variable amount of T_2 decay prior to acquisition (ACQ). The sum of TD and TE is kept constant to ensure that all images are acquired in the diastolic phase of the cardiac cycle. Abbreviations: MOLLI Modified Look-Locker Inversion Recovery, SASHA Saturation Recovery Single-Shot Acquisition, INV inversion pulse, SAT saturation pulse, TI inversion time, TD trigger delay, TS saturation time, ACQ acquisition window, T2P T_2-preparation module, TE echo time

exponential recovery model. Conventional methods for cardiac T_1 mapping can be divided into two main categories that differ in the way the magnetization is prepared: inversion recovery (including MOLLI [7] and its variants [8]) and saturation recovery (such as SASHA [9]). Additional details about the MOLLI and SASHA acquisitions are shown in Fig. 20.1a, b, respectively.

T_2 Mapping

CMR T_2 mapping can provide information that is complementary to T_1 mapping. Assessment of myocardial T_2 is useful for identifying myocardial edema [10], sarcoidosis [11], and acute myocardial infarct [12], among other conditions. Several techniques have been proposed for the collection of quantitative T_2 maps during a single breath-hold, such as a steady-state free precession (SSFP) single-shot imaging readout preceded by a T_2-preparation (T_2-prep) module every heartbeat to enhance T_2 sensitivity. The T_2-prep module consists of a 90° tip-down excitation pulse, followed by a time delay during which T_2 dephasing occurs, and ending with a 90° tip-up excitation pulse. The amount of T_2 weighting is controlled by the time delay between the two excitation pulses (the T_2-prep time). Several images with different amounts of T_2 weighting are acquired by varying the T_2-prep times in different heartbeats, and T_2 maps are estimated by nonlinear fitting to an exponential decay model.

Joint T_1 and T_2 Mapping

Whereas most clinically deployed mapping methods only measure a single relaxation parameter, several techniques have been proposed to simultaneously quantify both T_1 and T_2. Such multi-parametric methods tend to be time efficient, and they produce maps that are anatomically co-registered because they are derived from a single acquisition. An overview of multi-parametric CMR T_1 and T_2 mapping methods is given below, which will eventually lead into a discussion of Magnetic Resonance Fingerprinting.

Interleaved Methods

Some approaches for multi-parametric mapping use sequences that interleave the acquisition of T_1 and T_2 information. One example is Cardiac Balanced-SSFP Inversion Recovery with Interleaved Acquisition (CABIRIA) in which single-shot images are collected after interleaved inversion recovery and T_2 preparation modules during an eight-heartbeat breath-hold. Quantitative maps are obtained by performing a voxel-wise nonlinear fitting of the image intensities to an analytical model of the inversion recovery bSSFP signal dynamics, including a correction for slice profile imperfections [13, 14]. Similar methods that interleave saturation recovery and T_2 preparation have also been proposed [15].

Model-Based Methods

Several methods have been introduced that combine Bloch equation signal modeling, rather than nonlinear fitting to an exponential model, with conventional CMR T_1 and T_2 mapping sequences [16]. Such model-based methods have the potential to provide accurate T_1 and T_2 maps because the parameter estimation incorporates a detailed simulation of the MRI physics during the scan, and fewer simplifying assumptions are made regarding the MRI signal behavior compared to methods that assume exponential regrowth or decay. Corrections for confounding variables that could potentially impact the T_1 and T_2 measurements, such as slice profile imperfections, can be included in the signal model to improve accuracy and reproducibility. BLESSPC [17] and SQUAREMR [18] are some examples of Bloch equation-based mapping methods. In addition to simultaneous T_1 and T_2 mapping, both BLESSPC and SQUAREMR have been used in combination with the conventional MOLLI sequence to improve the accuracy of the T_1 estimation [19]. One difficulty with this class of techniques is that performing Bloch equation simulations can be time-consuming, especially if additional physical effects are included in the signal model. The simulation times were reported to be up to 3 hours for BLESSPC; the reconstruction time can be shortened by using advanced hardware as SQUAREMR achieved a 6- to 7-minute reconstruction time using a multi-GPU system.

Magnetic Resonance Multitasking

Magnetic Resonance Multitasking enables the collection of joint T_1 and T_2 maps using a free-breathing and ungated acquisition that exploits correlations between images captured at multiple time points [20]. The image reconstruction is formulated as a low-rank tensor completion, with one dimension of the tensor capturing the spatial localization of the signal and the remaining tensors describing different contrast dynamics, such as T_1 and T_2 decay, and different motion dynamics, including cardiac and respiratory motion. This approach eliminates the need for respiratory and ECG triggering, and data are collected using a free-running radial golden angle spoiled gradient-echo sequence [21]. To simultaneously sensitize the signal to both T_1 and T_2 relaxation, a hybrid T_2 prep and inversion recovery (T_2IR) pulse is used with varying echo times interleaved with the imaging readouts. Basis functions for cardiac and respiratory motion and T_2 decay are derived from navigator readouts interleaved with the image acquisition, while basis functions for T_1 recovery are calculated from a Bloch equation simulation. Motion-resolved images are reconstructed at different time points along the T_1 and T_2 recovery curves, and quantitative maps are calculated by nonlinear fitting, with a median reconstruction time of 71 minutes.

Magnetic Resonance Fingerprinting

Magnetic Resonance Fingerprinting (MRF) encompasses a class of methods for rapid and simultaneous multi-parametric mapping that differ from conventional parameter mapping in several ways. First, MRF uses a pseudorandom or time-varying pulse sequence to produce transient signal evolutions that encode tissue property information. Much like a fingerprint, each signal evolution can be used to uniquely identify a set of tissue property values (e.g., T_1 and T_2). This is different from conventional mapping sequences, which often attempt to quantify relaxation properties by measuring the exponential recovery or decay of magnetization. Second, quantitative maps are obtained in MRF by comparing measured signal evolutions with a dictionary containing signals that have been simulated for many (typically thousands or more) different tissue property values. This "pattern matching" step makes use of the entire signal evolution rather than performing a nonlinear voxel-wise fit of single time points to an exponential model, as in conventional mapping methods. Third, most MRF implementations employ a highly accelerated non-Cartesian acquisition to sample the rapidly changing temporal dynamics of each fingerprint; this is different from typical CMR mapping approaches which often rely on Cartesian single-shot imaging. The following sections will describe the essential components of MRF in more detail, followed by a discussion of cardiac MRF in particular.

Overview of MRF

Pulse Sequence

Most conventional parameter mapping techniques acquire several images with different contrast weightings, and quantitative maps are obtained by a voxel-wise fitting of the signal intensities to an exponential model. In contrast, the sequence parameters in MRF are varied during the acquisition to produce distinguishable signal evolutions that are dependent on the underlying tissue property values. The most important requirement for an MRF sequence is that it is designed in such a way that maximizes sensitivity to the tissue properties of interest while maintaining a low sensitivity to undesirable effects, such as off-resonance or B_1^+ inhomogeneities, that may confound the measurements. MRF sequences for simultaneous T_1 and T_2 mapping commonly employ a schedule of time-varying flip angles and repetition times; magnetization preparation pulses, such as inversion pulses and T_2 preparation pulses, can also be used to further enhance the sensitivity for these tissue properties. A schematic overview of an MRF sequence is shown in Fig. 20.2. In the seminal MRF paper, a spiral balanced steady-state free precession (bSSFP) readout was used to jointly quantify T_1, T_2, proton spin density, and off-resonance frequency in the brain [22]. For cardiac MRF, gradient-spoiled fast imaging with steady-state precession (FISP) [23] is favored due to its insensitivity to off-resonance [24], which has also seen widespread use in abdominal [25] and prostate MRF [26]. Cardiac MRF has also been performed using a pseudo-balanced SSFP sequence, which combines the high SNR commonly associated with balanced SSFP and the off-resonance insensitivity of FISP [27], as well as RF-spoiled gradient-echo sequences [28].

Dictionary Generation

When subject to a well-designed MRF pulse sequence, different combinations of tissue properties will produce distinguishable MRI signals over time, often referred to as fingerprints. To reconstruct quantitative maps, fingerprints are simulated for many physiologically feasible combinations of tissue properties (primarily but not limited to T_1 and T_2) and are stored in a look-up table or dictionary. Dictionaries can be generated by either performing a Bloch equation simulation or using extended phase graphs [29]. To create the dictionary, it is necessary to know the pulse sequence parameters, including the schedule of time-varying flip angles, repetition times, and magnetization preparation pulses. In addition, a discrete set of tissue property values must be defined over which to simulate the MRF signal time courses. A typical dictionary for T_1 and T_2 mapping may contain several thousand signals corresponding to different combinations of T_1 and T_2 values; for applications that seek to quantify more than two properties, the dictionary size can be even larger. For many MRF applications, the dictionary can be precomputed for a fixed set of pulse sequence parameters and reused for all subsequent scans that employ the same settings. As will be discussed later, some cardiac MRF techniques have variable sequence timings that depend on the subject's heart rate and thus require a new dictionary to be simulated after every acquisition. One advantage of using a dictionary-based approach is the ability to include confounding effects in the MRF signal simulation to reduce their influence on the tissue properties of interest [30]. In the context of MRF, methods have been proposed to correct for slice profile imperfections [31], relaxation during inversion and T_2 preparation pulses, and B_0 and B_1^+ inhomogeneities [32, 33].

Spatial Encoding

In MRF, it is important to acquire data at a high temporal resolution in order to characterize the signal time courses and distinguish between different tissue property values. Non-Cartesian encoding methods are commonly used in MRF due to their speed, repeated sampling of the center of k-space, and incoherent aliasing properties when undersampled. Typically, a time series of non-Cartesian images are

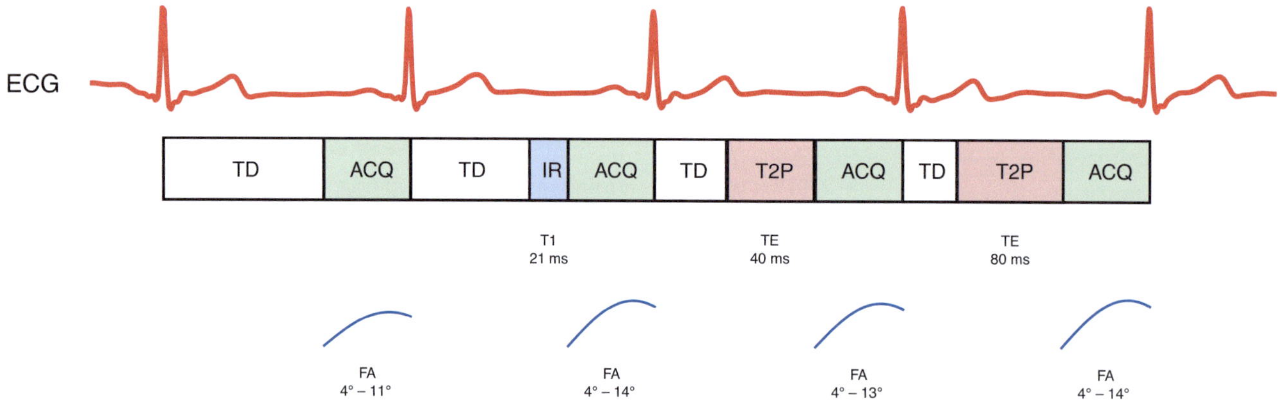

Fig. 20.2 Schematic overview of the cMRF pulse sequence. Here, only four heartbeats are shown, but the number is generally larger in real applications. Some heartbeats include an inversion pulse or T_2 preparation pulse before the image acquisition. During the diastolic readout period, a time-varying schedule of flip angles is applied, and the MRF data are collected along the selected trajectory. Abbreviations: TD trigger delay, ACQ acquisition window, IR inversion recovery, T2P T_2-preparation module, TE echo time, FA flip angle

acquired at a high temporal resolution and a high degree of undersampling. The seminal work on MRF proposed an interleaved variable density spiral trajectory [22], in which 1000 image frames were collected during a 12-second scan. Each image frame was highly undersampled at an acceleration factor of 48 using data acquired along just one spiral k-space interleaf during one repetition time, leading to a temporal resolution of 12 ms per image. In addition to spirals, other trajectories including radial [34], rosettes [35], and variable density Cartesian sampling [36] have all been deployed to impart different characteristics into the MRF signals. In addition to high sampling speed, the use of k-space trajectories that produces artifacts that are incoherent or "noise-like" can be beneficial in MRF. Such sampling enables successful pattern matching as it allows the temporal variation of the fingerprints to be separated from the aliasing that occurs due to the high acceleration rates. To ensure aliasing artifacts that are incoherent over time, the non-Cartesian k-space trajectories in MRF are rotated between successive image readouts, often using a golden angle rotation [21]. The choice of a suitable k-space sampling method has been investigated for different spiral undersampling patterns and has been shown to have a large effect on the resulting MRF maps [37]. Incoherent aliasing also enables the combination of MRF with sparsity-based reconstruction methods, such as low-rank methods or compressed sensing.

Pattern Matching

Pattern matching describes the process of estimating tissue property values from the measured MRF signal time courses. This step is performed by finding the entry in the dictionary that most closely matches the measured signal time course for each voxel in the dataset. The original MRF work employed template matching, in which the dot product is computed between the measured signal and all simulated signals in the dictionary. The best matching fingerprint is identified as the dictionary entry that maximizes the absolute value of the dot product (note that the dot product is computed using complex-valued signals). Because the tissue property combination (i.e., T_1 and T_2 value) that was used to generate the matching dictionary entry is known, these values can be assigned as the measured tissue property values for that voxel. By performing pattern matching at every voxel location, co-registered tissue property maps are reconstructed from a single MRF dataset. Dot product matching has the advantage of being fast, as matching can be performed on all voxels in parallel, at least when the number of tissue properties is limited, as is the case in simultaneous T_1 and T_2 mapping. Pattern matching is robust to sources of incoherent noise or errors in the measured signal evolutions, which enables the acceleration of MRF scans by choosing an appropriate k-space undersampling pattern that produces noise-like artifacts, as described above. However, there is a limit to the amount of noise and aliasing artifacts that can be tolerated by pattern matching. To address this limitation, more advanced iterative methods based on multi-scale approximation [38] or low-rank matrix completion [39, 40] have emerged to further improve the performance and precision of the dictionary matching, at the expense of increased reconstruction times.

Cardiac MRF

Although originally proposed for mapping in the brain, MRF has been successfully deployed to map tissue properties in other parts of the body, such as the abdomen [25] and the heart [41]. This section will provide an overview of cardiac Magnetic Resonance Fingerprinting (cMRF) for myocardial tissue property mapping. cMRF enables the rapid acquisition of T_1 and T_2 maps in a single breath-hold using an ECG-triggered data acquisition window during diastole [42]. As described in the original work, data are collected over a total of 16 heartbeats using variable flip angles. The flip angle range in cMRF is often restricted to small values (e.g., less than 25°) to reduce B_1^+ dependence. During some heartbeats, the data acquisition is preceded by an inversion pulse or T_2 preparation pulse with variable timings to increase the sensitivity to T_1 or T_2, respectively.

An overview of the cMRF reconstruction process is presented in Fig. 20.3. Unlike MRF applications in stationary organs that often use predetermined sequence timings, the sequence timings in cMRF are dependent on the patient's heart rate. Data are collected in a diastolic phase using ECG triggering to reduce cardiac motion. However, this triggered approach introduces pauses in the acquisition of up to one second between subsequent heartbeats. Therefore, a scan-specific cMRF dictionary must be generated after every acquisition that takes the patient's heart rate (derived from the ECG timings) into account for the Bloch equation simulation. The use of a patient-specific dictionary enables accurate cMRF T_1 and T_2 measurements despite heart rate variations. Figure 20.4 illustrates the importance of modeling the subject's heart rate when generating the dictionary using a simple example. A ground truth signal corresponding to $T_1 = 1200$ ms, $T_2 = 100$ ms, and a constant heart rate of 60 beats per minute (bpm) was simulated. This ground truth signal was then matched to a number of dictionaries generated using constant heart rates between 45 and 110 bpm. As shown in the figure, the T_1 and T_2 values deviate by as much as 54% for T_1 and 22% for T_2 when the dictionary is simulated using an incorrect heart rate, which highlights the importance of generating a scan-specific dictionary in cardiac MRF to obtain accurate T_1 and T_2 measurements. While the initial cMRF approach used the simple 16-heartbeat pulse sequence along with dictionary matching based on

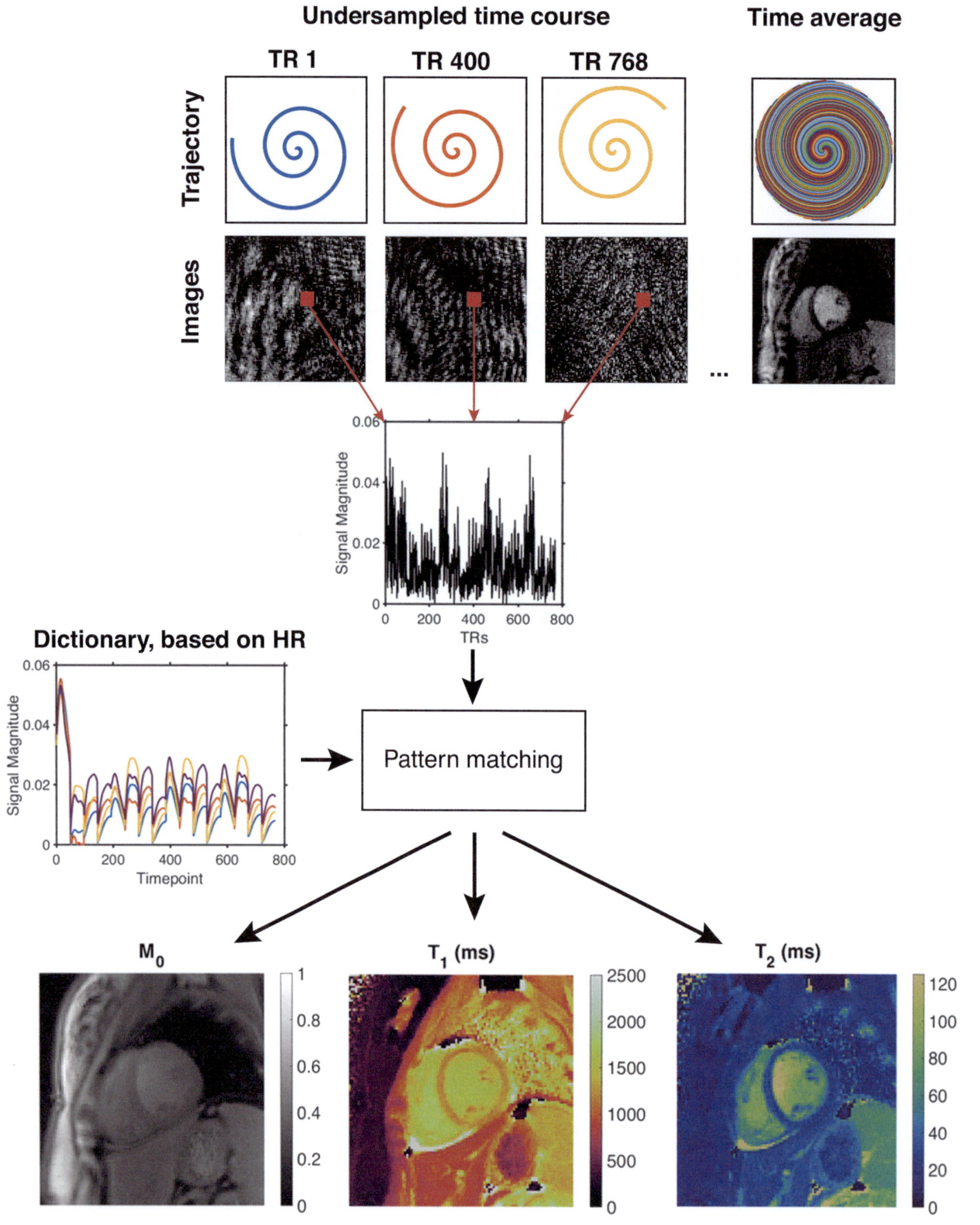

Fig. 20.3 Schematic overview of the cMRF technique. First, a time series of undersampled spiral images is acquired. Note that a time-averaged image (obtained by summing the undersampled images over time) is shown in the diagram to provide the reader with an anatomical reference, although this image is not used in the reconstruction. Next, at each voxel location, pattern matching is performed between the measured complex-valued signal evolution from the undersampled images and a dictionary of signals calculated from a Bloch equation simulation that incorporates the subject's heart rate (HR) timings obtained from an electrocardiogram. The result is a set of co-registered quantitative T_1 and T_2 maps. Proton density (M_0) is calculated as the complex-valued scaling factor between the measured signal evolution at each voxel and the best matching fingerprint from the dictionary

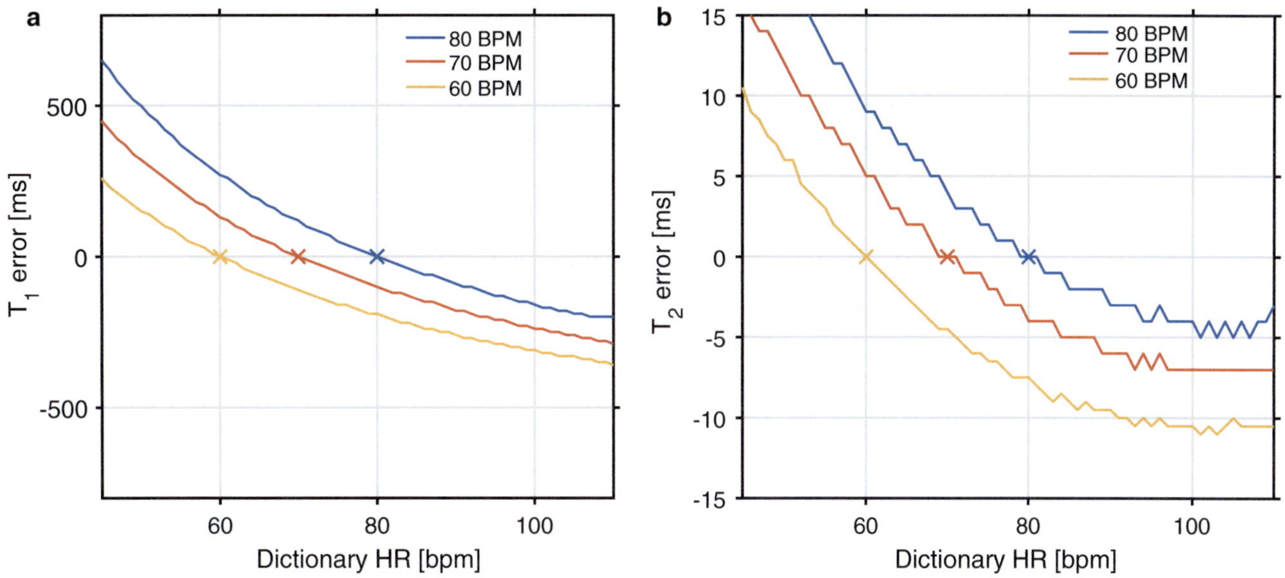

Fig. 20.4 A simple example demonstrating the importance of modeling heart rate in the cMRF dictionary to obtain accurate (**a**) T_1 and (**b**) T_2 measurements. Ground truth signals corresponding to $T_1 = 1200$ ms and $T_2 = 100$ ms were simulated using constant heart rates of 60, 70, and 80 beats per minute (BPM). Each ground truth signal was then matched to a number of dictionaries generated using incorrect heart rates, which ranged from 45 to 110 BPM. Note that when the ground truth signal is matched to a dictionary generated using the correct heart rate, the T_1 and T_2 values are matched accurately (indicated by the crosses). The steps in the curves are due to the discrete nature of the dictionary

Bloch equation simulations, a number of extensions to this original work have been proposed. For instance, it has been demonstrated that the accuracy of cMRF T_1 and T_2 mapping can be further improved by modeling additional pulse sequence-dependent factors in the dictionary, such as slice profile imperfections, inversion pulse efficiency, and B_1^+ inhomogeneities [30].

Cardiac MRF Beyond T_1 and T_2 Mapping

In addition to T_1 and T_2 mapping, extensions of cMRF have been proposed to quantify proton density fat fraction (PDFF) using rosette trajectories [35] or multi-echo Dixon methods [43]. Methods for joint T_1/T_2 mapping and cine imaging [44, 45] to quantify left ventricular ejection fraction have also been developed, which have the potential for considerable time savings compared to a standard CMR exam, where each acquisition typically only results in one kind of image. To further accelerate the acquisition, simultaneous multi-slice (SMS) approaches have been successfully used to enable acquisition of T_1 and T_2 maps from up to three slices during a single breath-hold. In addition, methods for whole-heart cMRF has also been developed [46]. Methods to accelerate CMR exams and reduce the number of breath-holds is beneficial as many cardiac patients often suffer from dyspnea or are otherwise unable to hold their breath for extended durations.

Challenges with Conventional Cardiac MRF

There are several technical challenges that are specific to cardiac implementations of MRF which may present opportunities for artificial intelligence research. First, cMRF requires frequent simulations to generate a heart rate-specific dictionary after every acquisition. This increases the computation time as the dictionary must be computed on-the-fly, in contrast to previous applications of MRF outside of the heart. The typical dictionary generation time has been reported to be approximately 12 seconds on a workstation [41]. Taking into account the time for non-Cartesian data gridding and pattern matching, the total reconstruction time may be as long as 8 minutes, making online reconstructions impractical in a clinical setting, especially when moving beyond 2D diastolic T_1 and T_2 mapping to cardiac phase-resolved or 3D mapping. Second, the correction of confounding variables in the dictionary can increase computation time and memory requirements. Preparation pulse efficiency and slice profile imperfections may be modeled in the cMRF dictionary by extracting the gradient and radiofrequency waveforms from the pulse sequence and performing Bloch simulations of the spin state with a short time step (such as 10 μs). This process increases the time needed to generate the dictionary but does not increase the time required for pattern matching or the size of the dictionary. Although many implementations of cMRF limit the flip angles to small values to reduce the B_1^+ sensitivity of the acquisition, B_1^+ can also be modeled in the dictionary as an additional parameter. However, B_1^+ corrections will increase the time needed to simulate the dictionary, the size of the dictionary, and the time needed for pattern matching. Whereas a simple dictionary simulation without corrections can be performed on the order of 10–20 seconds, including these sequence-dependent effects may increase the simulation time to several minutes [30]. Including other corrections or additional tissue properties will exacerbate this problem as the computation time and dictionary size will grow exponentially with the number of properties included in the dictionary. Third, pattern matching is in essence a brute force search, meaning that every combination of tissue property values must be compared to the measured signal to determine the best match. Applications that require large-scale dictionaries will thus also require long reconstruction times.

Several approaches that do not use artificial intelligence have been proposed to reduce computation time and memory requirements for dictionary generation and pattern matching. Advanced computing hardware could be used to shorten reconstruction times and enable online reconstructions, facilitating the use of cMRF techniques in a clinical setting [47]. The MRF dictionary can also be compressed along the time dimension to a low-dimensional temporal subspace using the singular value decomposition, which can reduce the memory needed to store the dictionary and the time needed for pattern matching [48]. A fast and memory-efficient method has also been developed for generating large-scale dictionaries using a low-rank approximation with polynomial fitting [49]. Novel algorithms, such as fast group matching, have also been developed to accelerate pattern matching by only searching a fraction of the MRF dictionary [50].

Artificial Intelligence in MRF

Artificial intelligence has emerged as a promising tool for solving many challenges associated with MRF. Many of the difficulties in MRF stem from the complexity of solving large nonlinear system of equations, and therefore training a neural network to learn this mapping can have a great benefit in terms of processing speed. A neural network can also be trained to implicitly learn correlations that otherwise have to be explicitly modeled in the dictionary generation or image reconstruction steps, as long as these effects can be included in the training data (i.e., slice profile correction in MRF). This section will provide an overview of several recent approaches which use of AI to address challenges in MRF associated with dictionary generation and tissue property quantification, including several methods specifically developed for cardiac MRF.

Dictionary Generation

One challenge that is well suited for deep learning approaches is MRF dictionary simulation. Recently, a Generative Adversarial Network (GAN) was proposed to accelerate the generation of MRF dictionaries. In general, the design of a GAN comprises two convolutional neural networks that are pitched against each other in a min-max game. A well-trained network is expected to result in an equilibrium between the two competing interests, known as the Nash equilibrium. The first network is known as the generator, and the second network is known as the discriminator [51]. In the context of dictionary generation for MRF, the network is trained on a set of simulated fingerprints generated using the Bloch equations. The input to the generator network is random noise, and it will output a fingerprint that mimics real fingerprints generated by a Bloch simulation. The discriminator network is tasked with distinguishing whether the fingerprints are from the training dataset (real) or created by the generator (fake). A recent application of this method is the "GAN-MRF" model (Fig. 20.5) [52]. The model was trained on a FISP sequence with slice profile correction and 1000 time points. The input layer of the discriminator network took three inputs—a fingerprint either from the training set or from the generator and a T_1 and T_2 value. The input layer was followed by three hidden layers with 128 nodes each, followed by a rectified linear unit (ReLU). The output layer used a sigmoid activation function, and the output was the probability that the fingerprint was "real." The GAN-MRF framework was able to generate MRF dictionaries much faster than conventional simulation methods, reducing the time to generate a dictionary of approximately 6 million entries from several hours using Bloch simulations to 0.3 seconds using the proposed method, representing an approximately 10,000-fold decrease in computation time. The relative root mean square error (RMSE) was reported to be 0.55% for T_1 maps and 2.66% for T_2 maps acquired in the brain. The GAN model architecture, however, has a number of known drawbacks. First, the min-max problem is not convex and convergence is not guaranteed. Second, a GAN is prone to what is known as mode collapse, where the generator learns a single fingerprint that always will fool the discriminator, thereby getting stuck in a local minimum.

Rapid Generation of Cardiac MRF Dictionaries

As mentioned above, a major challenge in cardiac MRF is the need for frequent scan-specific dictionary simulation, which must take individual variations in heart rate and sequence timing into account when the scan is ECG-triggered. To alleviate this problem, AI approaches have been developed specifically to accelerate the generation of dictionaries in cardiac MRF [53]. One approach uses a fully

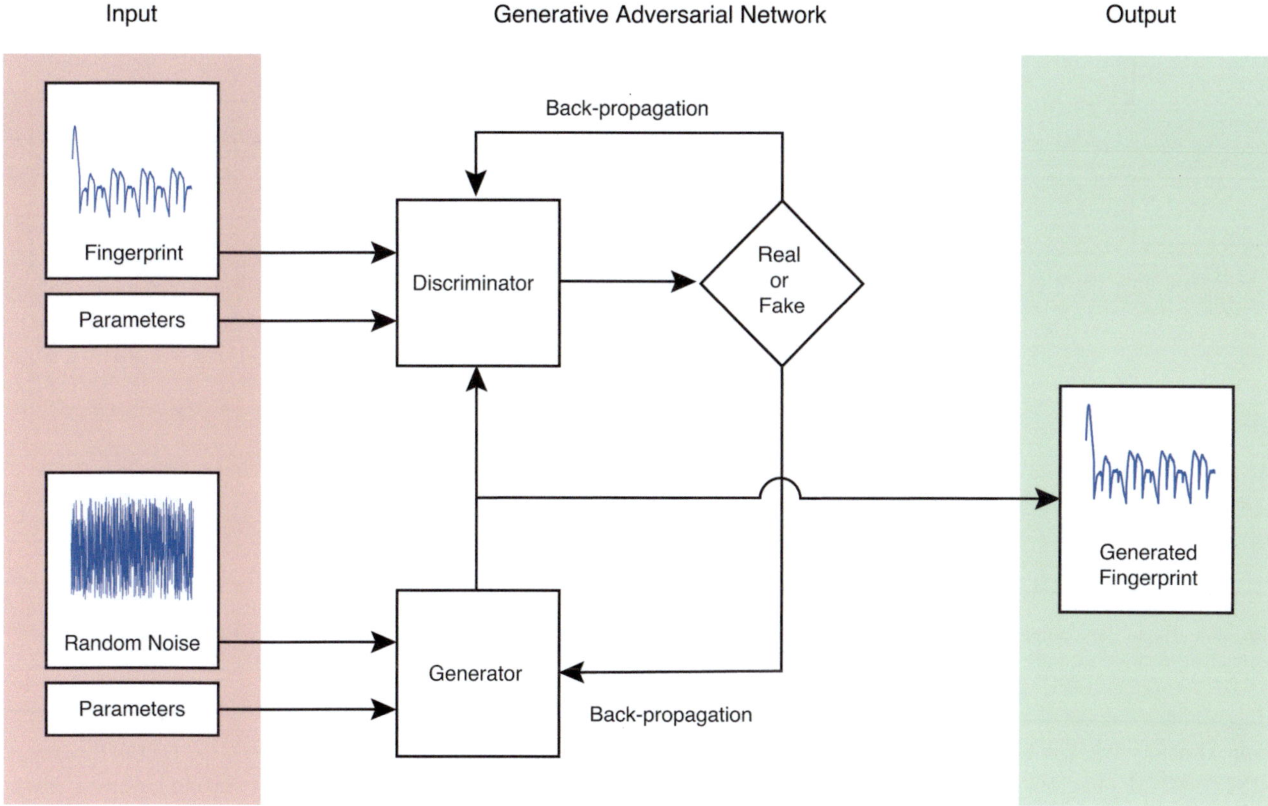

Fig. 20.5 Schematic overview of the GAN-MRF network architecture. A generation network and a discriminator network compete in a min-max game. The task of the discriminator is to determine whether the input signal is a real signal from a training dataset or a signal created by the generator network

connected feed-forward network where the input layer had 17 nodes, two for the T_1 and T_2 values and 15 for the timing between acquisition blocks (the heartbeat timing, or RR intervals). Note that although the cMRF scan duration was 16 heartbeats, only 15 RR intervals were needed since the signal was assumed to be at equilibrium before the first heartbeat. The input layer was followed by two fully connected hidden layers with 300 nodes each. The output of the network is the complex-valued cMRF signal time course; note that the number of nodes in the output layer is double the number of TRs in the scan to account for the real and imaginary parts of the signal. Figure 20.6 shows a diagram of the network architecture. The network was trained with signals simulated using the Bloch equations for randomly generated cardiac rhythms ranging from 40 to 120 beats per minute (bpm). For each average heart rate, 60 different rhythms were generated by applying Gaussian noise to each RR interval to introduce heart rate variability with standard deviations ranging from 0% to 50% of the average RR interval. In total, 1020 different heart rhythms were simulated. Corrections for slice profile and preparation pulse efficiency were included in the training data. A total of 4392 T_1 and T_2 combinations were simulated for each cardiac rhythm, resulting in a total of 4,177,920 simulated signals in the training dataset. To increase the robustness of the network, cMRF signals in the training dataset were simulated with a 5% probability of missed ECG triggers, a common occurrence in clinical CMR settings, by doubling the affected RR intervals. Generating the training data in MATLAB required 9 hours, and training the network required an additional 12 hours on a single CPU.

The robustness of the network to heart rate variations was tested using a Monte Carlo approach. A ground truth time course for a T_1/T_2 combination representing the myocardium (T_1 = 1400 ms, T_2 = 50 ms) was simulated using the Bloch equations for a heart rate between 40 and 120 bpm. Gaussian noise was applied to simulate different heart rate variations. Dot product matching was performed between the simulated time course and a dictionary generated by the network. The relative mean squared error (RMSE) was calculated between the matched T_1 and T_2 values and the corresponding reference values, and the maximum error was approximately 1.5% for T_1 and 3.5% for T_2. To validate robustness to missed triggers, a similar ground truth signal was simulated using the Bloch equation with 1 to 8 missing triggers. RMSE was used to calculate the error between the ground truth and the measured T_1 and T_2 values. The error increased with the number of missed triggers, and the maximum error was

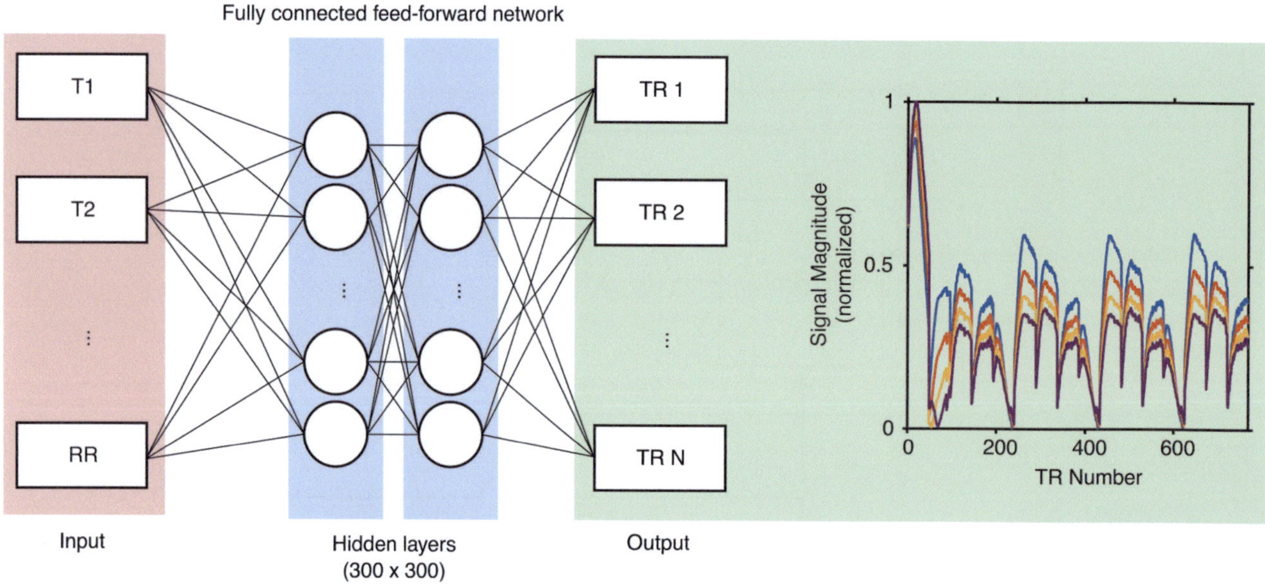

Fig. 20.6 Rapid generation of cMRF dictionaries using a fully connected feed-forward network. The input layer takes a T_1 and a T_2 value, as well as a vector containing all RR intervals. This is followed by two fully connected hidden layers (300 nodes each). The output is a cMRF fingerprint corresponding to the T_1/T_2 parameter combination and cardiac rhythm given in the input layer

approximately 2% for T_1 and 2.5% for T_2. In addition, the NIST/ISMRM phantom [54] was scanned using simulated heart rates ranging from 40 to 120 bpm. T_1 and T_2 maps were calculated both from precomputed dictionaries and dictionaries from the network. There was an excellent agreement between the two methods ($R^2 = 0.998$) and low bias. The time to generate a dictionary comprising 768 time points and 26,680 T_1/T_2 combinations was 0.8 seconds for the neural network and 158 seconds using Bloch equation simulation, an almost 200-fold decrease in time. The time for image gridding and pattern recognition was not affected.

Pattern Matching

In addition to accelerating the process of dictionary generation, AI approaches have also been investigated to replace pattern matching in MRF. Instead of performing an exhaustive search over the entire dictionary, a network can be trained to learn the nonlinear mapping from measured signals to the final maps. By bypassing the dictionary, the quantization error introduced by the discrete dictionary entries can be avoided, as the network will output tissue property values on a continuous spectrum and is not restricted to the discrete values used to populate the dictionary.

One example of a recent method using AI to replace dictionary-based pattern matching is the MRF Deep Reconstruction Network (DRONE) [55]. The network takes the magnitude of a measured MRF signal from one voxel location as input and produces an estimate of the T_1 and T_2 values. The network contains two fully connected hidden layers with 300 nodes each. Therefore, the DRONE network only requires 90,000 weights (300 × 300) to be saved, marking a large saving in memory when compared to storing the full dictionary. Two separate DRONE networks were designed to accommodate two different pulse sequences—an EPI sequence which required 25–50 input nodes and a spiral sequence with 48-fold undersampling, which was initially processed using a sliding window filter before the DRONE reconstruction, requiring a total of 571 input nodes. A schematic of the DRONE network can be seen in Fig. 20.7. The time to train the network was 10 minutes for EPI and 74 minutes for spiral MRF implementations. The network was tested in simulations, phantoms, and in vivo brain scans. Compared to conventional dictionary matching, DRONE reduced the time needed for tissue property quantification by a factor of 300 for EPI (10 ms vs. 3 s) and approximately 5000 for spiral (76 ms vs. 380 s) MRF implementations. One limitation of DRONE is that it does not directly account for non-Cartesian undersampling artifacts and instead relies on view sharing to mitigate these artifacts. Additionally, DRONE has thus far been limited to brain MRF applications with fixed sequence timings, which is not suitable for cardiac MRF where the scan timings vary with heart rate.

Deep Learning Parameter Map Reconstruction for Cardiac MRF

A deep learning approach for cardiac MRF has been proposed to bypass dictionary generation altogether and go directly from undersampled spiral cMRF images to quantitative T_1 and T_2 maps in less than half a second using a fully connected neural network with residual connections [56].

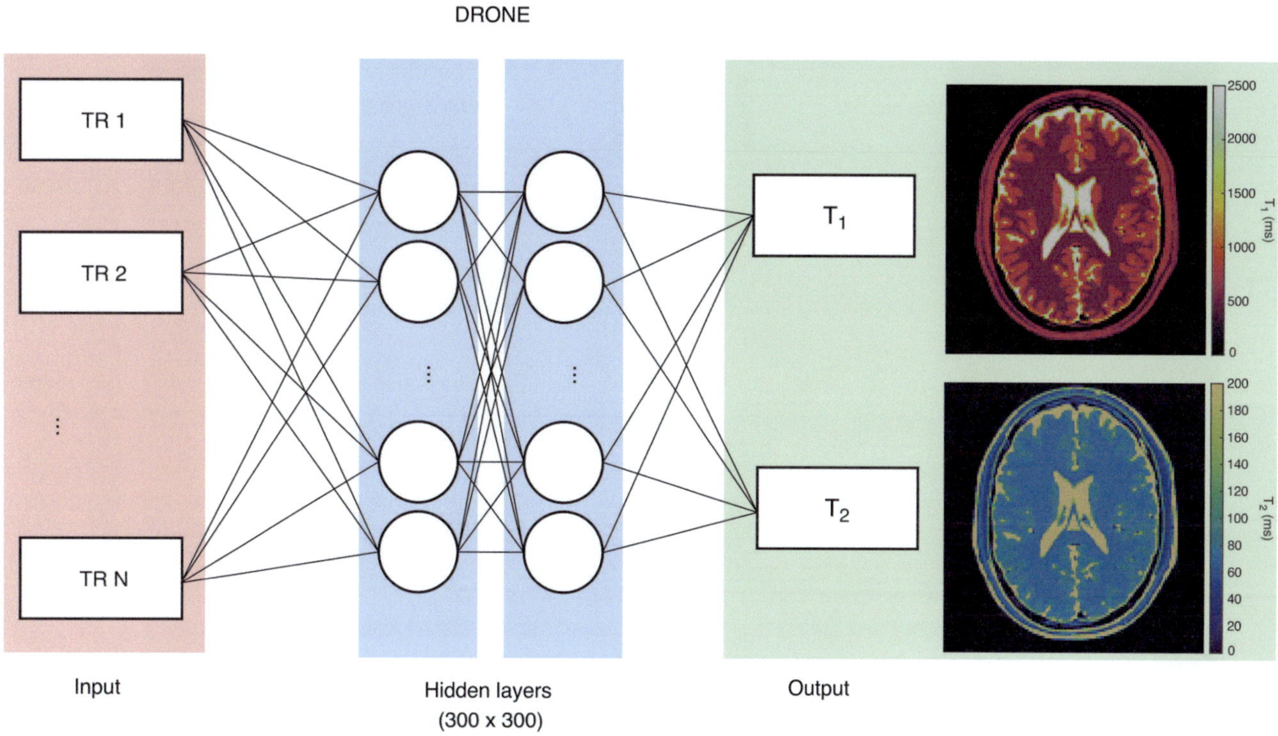

Fig. 20.7 Diagram of the DRONE network architecture. The input layer takes image input from each TR. The input layer is followed by two fully connected hidden layers with 300 nodes each. The output is T_1 and T_2 maps

The input to the network was the measured signal time course from a single voxel location, as well as the RR intervals from the patient's ECG. The network consisted of 18 hidden layers, including one fully connected layer, followed by 4 residual blocks each comprising 4 fully connected layers and a final fully connected layer. Skip connections were used between each residual block, and all layers had 300 nodes. The output layers had two nodes corresponding to the estimated T_1 and T_2 value for the given voxel. The pulse sequence was identical to the one described in the previous section, except in this work, only 10 heartbeats were used. The network was trained on time courses generated using Bloch equation simulations. A pseudo-noise function that mimicked the temporal aliasing due to the golden angle spiral acquisition was added to the time courses as well as a random phase shift. By including these effects in the training data, the robustness to non-Cartesian aliasing artifacts, varying coil sensitivities, and off-resonance effects could be improved. A random heart rate was used to generate the signals, and Gaussian noise was used to simulate heart rate variation within each simulated time course. In total, 2000 different heart rhythms were simulated together with 4000 T_1 and T_2 combinations. The numerical MRXCAT phantom [57] was used for evaluation of the final results. The cMRF pulse sequence was simulated on the phantom, and gridding was performed to yield images which were fed to the network along with the RR intervals. The mean values were calculated in the myocardium, left ventricular blood pool, and liver. Normalized relative mean squared error (nRMSE) was calculated between the cMRF maps and the ground truth values known from the numerical phantom. For all T_1 measurements, the nRMSE was below 1% independent of heart rhythm. For T_2 measurements, the nMRSE was below 4% for myocardium and liver and below 6% for blood. In vivo experiments were also performed in 58 healthy subjects. The same acquisition was used, and T_1/T_2 maps were reconstructed both using a Bloch simulated dictionary followed by dot product pattern match and the proposed network. Figure 20.8 shows an example of cMRF maps from one subject reconstructed using the deep learning approach and using the traditional dictionary matching reconstruction. There was a strong correlation for myocardial values (T_1: R^2 = 0.93, T_2: R^2 = 0.95). The processing time of the network was less than one second, which was achievable since the neural network removed the need to simulate a heart rate-dependent dictionary.

Future Applications

In this section, some future applications of cardiac MRF will be discussed, as well as open challenges that could be solved using AI.

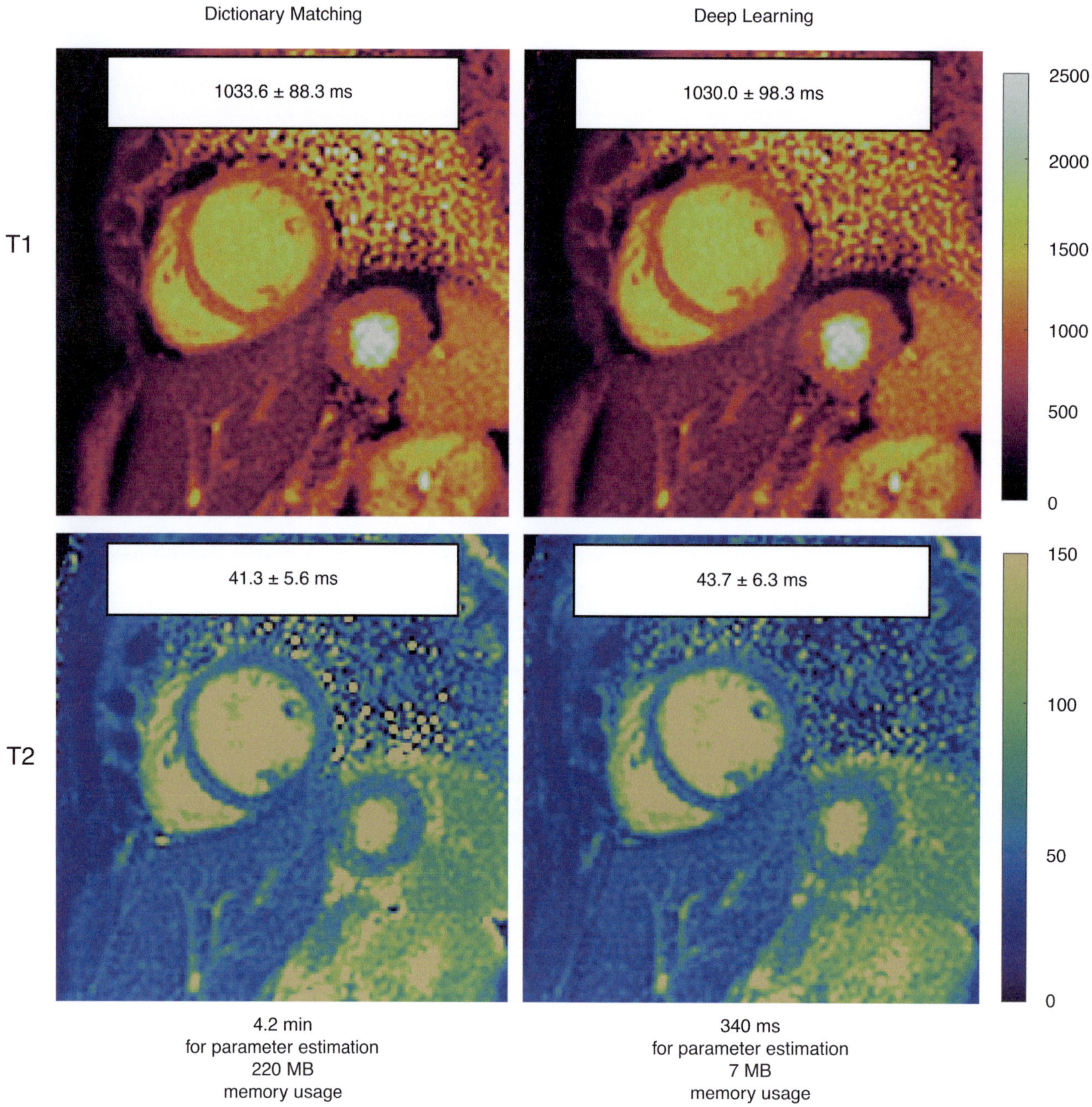

Fig. 20.8 Example of T_1 and T_2 maps acquired in a healthy volunteer at 1.5 Tesla and reconstructed using dot product dictionary matching (left column) and using the described deep learning approach (right column). The white boxes show the myocardial T_1 and T_2 values, respectively

Cardiac MRF with Multiple Parameter Dimensions

Although much of the initial work with cMRF focused on T_1 and T_2 mapping, there is a recent interest in extending the cMRF framework to quantify additional tissue and functional parameters. Cardiac cine MRF has been introduced to simultaneously obtain cardiac phase-resolved T_1 and T_2 maps, as well as qualitative (contrast-weighted) cine images for calculating left ventricular functional parameters, including ejection fraction [44, 45]. Cine MRF uses a free-running sequence as opposed to an ECG-triggered sequence, and MRF data are retrospectively binned into different cardiac phases using an ECG signal. Phase-resolved maps are obtained by performing a low-rank MRF reconstruction combined with nonrigid cardiac motion correction. The cardiac phase-resolved T_1, T_2, and M_0 maps obtained by dictionary matching can be used to generate synthetic cine images with adjustable image contrast. Thus, synthetic cine images with balanced SSFP can be obtained directly from the same MRF dataset. An alternative approach to obtaining contrast-weighted cine images from MRF is to select the subspace image which best represents the desired image contrast. A limitation of cine MRF is the relatively long reconstruction times. Typical times reported in the literature range from 3 hours for 8 cardiac phases [45] to 6 hours for 24 cardiac phases [44]. In addition, the degree of undersampling of the signal time course is also comparatively high. Previous cMRF methods for diastolic T_1 and T_2 mapping acquired 750–1000 undersampled images; however, a cine MRF acquisition with approximately 2000 undersampled images and 24 cardiac phases only corresponds to about 83 undersampled images per cardiac phase. Therefore, cine MRF may benefit from deep learning approaches to enable the rapid reconstruction of T_1 and T_2 maps over multiple cardiac phases.

Another emerging approach includes simultaneous T_1, T_2, and proton density fat fraction (PDFF) mapping. This can be achieved by combining the MRF framework with either a multi-echo radial trajectory [43] or a rosette trajectory that naturally crosses the k-space center multiple times per readout [35], enabling reconstruction of images with different echo times. By extracting images with different echo times, fat-water-separated images can be reconstructed, as well as B_0 maps which can be used to perform B_0 correction. The corrected fat-water-separated images can subsequently be used to produce PDFF maps that display the relative fat content in the tissue, leading to a more comprehensive diagnosis with uses both in the cardiac setting, but also in other anatomies such as the liver, where PDFF can be used for risk stratification in nonalcoholic fatty liver disease [58]. Other interesting avenues for research could include myocardial T_2^*, perfusion, or diffusion mapping. However, introducing multiple parameters increases the dictionary size and the time for pattern matching. Future extensions of cMRF that quantify many tissue properties simultaneously (beyond T_1 and T_2 mapping) may present an opportunity for novel deep learning methods, which can potentially avoid the long computation times and large memory requirements associated with a dictionary-based approach.

3D Cardiac MRF

Most of the methods discussed in this chapter have been two-dimensional, in which only a single slice is collected at a time. Whole-heart free-breathing T_1 and T_2 mapping using cMRF during a 7-minute acquisition has shown promising results [46], and other work has suggested that a whole-heart isotropic 3D cine acquisition can be performed in as little as 2 minutes [59], paving the way for other, highly accelerated methods in the future. A U-net reconstruction has recently been used to provide super-resolution for whole heart cardiac imaging [60] and 3D Cartesian cine imaging [61]. Such novel deep learning methods have the potential to dramatically shorten the reconstruction of large 3D cMRF datasets and enable shorter acquisitions with higher degrees of undersampling.

Short Reconstruction Times to Facilitate Clinical Translation

To ensure the successful translation of novel MRI technology, it is important that images can be acquired and reconstructed within a time frame that is acceptable in a clinical setting. Many methods discussed in this chapter demonstrate that cMRF maps can be reconstructed in a very short time, but for various reasons, many deep learning methods are still used offline. Performing image reconstruction on the scanner is often seen as a challenge to imaging researchers. However, image reconstruction can be performed in-line on the MRI scanner with relative ease using open-source software solutions. An implementation of cMRF has been developed for the Gadgetron platform to allow for the in-line reconstruction of T_1/T_2 maps [47, 62]. The advent of cloud-based services further enables researchers to utilize computing resources far beyond the capabilities of modern clinical scanners [63].

Conclusion

In conclusion, conventional methods for independent T_1 and T_2 mapping as well as methods for joint T_1/T_2 mapping have been discussed. The concept of Magnetic Resonance Fingerprinting (MRF) was introduced along with its benefits for rapid and simultaneous tissue property mapping. A number of methods have been presented that make use of deep learning to overcome some of the current limitations of MRF, including long dictionary generation times or matching approaches, including several methods specifically targeted for cardiac MRF. The potential for deep learning to dramatically reduce reconstruction times in MRF and pave way for clinical adoption has also been discussed. Finally, some future perspectives and open research questions in the context of deep learning methods for cardiovascular MRF have been put forward.

References

1. Seraphim A, Knott KD, Augusto J, Bhuva AN, Manisty C, Moon JC. Quantitative cardiac MRI. J Magn Reson Imaging. 2020;51(3):693–711.
2. Ferreira VM, et al. T1 mapping for the diagnosis of acute myocarditis using CMR: comparison to T2-weighted and late gadolinium enhanced imaging. JACC Cardiovasc Imaging. 2013;6(10):1048–58.

3. Messroghli DR, Niendorf T, Schulz-Menger J, Dietz R, Friedrich MG. T1 mapping in patients with acute myocardial infarction. J Cardiovasc Magn Reson. 2003;5(2):353–9.
4. Karamitsos TD, et al. Noncontrast T1 mapping for the diagnosis of cardiac amyloidosis. JACC Cardiovasc Imaging. 2013;6(4):488–97.
5. Sado DM, et al. Identification and assessment of anderson-fabry disease by cardiovascular magnetic resonance noncontrast myocardial T1 mapping. Circ Cardiovasc Imaging. 2013;6(3):392–8.
6. Ugander M, Oki A, Hsu L. Extracellular volume imaging by magnetic resonance imaging provides insights into overt and subclinical myocardial pathology. Eur Heart J. 2012;33(10):1268–78.
7. Messroghli DR, Radjenovic A, Kozerke S, Higgins DM, Sivananthan MU, Ridgway JP. Modified look-locker inversion recovery (MOLLI) for high-resolution T 1 mapping of the heart. Magn Reson Med. 2004;52(1):141–6.
8. Piechnik SK, et al. Shortened Modified Look-Locker Inversion recovery (ShMOLLI) for clinical myocardial T1- mapping at 1.5 and 3 T within a 9 heartbeat breathhold. J Cardiovasc Magn Reson. 2010;12:69.
9. Chow K, Flewitt JA, Green JD, Pagano JJ, Friedrich MG, Thompson RB. Saturation recovery single-shot acquisition (SASHA) for myocardial T 1 mapping. Magn Reson Med. 2014;71(6):2082–95.
10. Giri S, et al. T2 quantification for improved detection of myocardial edema. J Cardiovasc Magn Reson. 2009;11:56.
11. Crouser ED, Ono C, Tran T, He X, Raman SV. Improved detection of cardiac sarcoidosis using magnetic resonance with myocardial T2 mapping. Am J Respir Crit Care Med. 2014;189(1):109–12.
12. Abdel-Aty H, et al. Delayed enhancement and T2-weighted cardiovascular magnetic resonance imaging differentiate acute from chronic myocardial infarction. Circulation. 2004;109(20):2411–6.
13. Santini F, Kawel-Boehm N, Greiser A, Bremerich J, Bieri O. Simultaneous T1 and T2 quantification of the myocardium using cardiac balanced-SSFP inversion recovery with interleaved sampling acquisition (CABIRIA). Magn Reson Med. 2015;74(2):365–71.
14. Blume U, et al. Interleaved T1 and T2 relaxation time mapping for cardiac applications. J Magn Reson Imaging. 2009;29(2):480–7.
15. Akçakaya M, Weingärtner S, Basha TA, Roujol S, Bellm S, Nezafat R. Joint myocardial T1 and T2 mapping using a combination of saturation recovery and T2-preparation. Magn Reson Med. 2016;76(3):888–96.
16. Bloch F. Nuclear induction. Phys Rev. 1946;70:460.
17. Shao J, Rapacchi S, Nguyen K-L, Hu P. Myocardial T1 mapping at 3.0 tesla using an inversion recovery spoiled gradient echo readout and bloch equation simulation with slice profile correction (BLESSPC) T1 estimation algorithm. J Magn Reson Imaging. 2016;43(2):414–25.
18. Xanthis CG, et al. Simulation-based quantification of native T1 and T2 of the myocardium using a modified MOLLI scheme and the importance of Magnetization Transfer. Magn Reson Imaging. 2018;48:96–106.
19. Xanthis CG, Bidhult S, Kantasis G, Heiberg E, Arheden H, Aletras AH. Parallel simulations for QUAntifying RElaxation magnetic resonance constants (SQUAREMR): an example towards accurate MOLLI T1 measurements. J Cardiovasc Magn Reson. 2015;17:104.
20. Christodoulou AG, et al. Magnetic resonance multitasking for motion-resolved quantitative cardiovascular imaging. Nat Biomed Eng. 2018;2:215–26.
21. Winkelmann S, Schaeffter T, Koehler T, Eggers H, Doessel O. An optimal radial profile order based on the golden ratio for time-resolved MRI. IEEE Trans Med Imaging. 2007;26(1):68–76.
22. Ma D, et al. Magnetic resonance fingerprinting. Nature. 2013;495(7440):187–92.
23. Oppelt A, Graumann R, Barfuß H, Fischer H, Hartl W, Schajor W. FISP – a new fast MRI sequence. Electromedica. 1986;54:15–8.
24. Guzek B, Körzdörfer G, Mathias N, Pfeuffer J. Influence of off-resonance on FISP magnetic resonance fingerprinting (FISP-MRF). In: Proceedings of the Joint Annual Meeting ISMRM-ESMRMB; 2018. p. 4264.
25. Chen Y, et al. MR fingerprinting for rapid quantitative abdominal imaging. Radiology. 2016;279(1):278–86.
26. Yu AC, et al. Development of a combined Mr fingerprinting and diffusion examination for prostate cancer. Radiology. 2017;283(3):729–38.
27. Assländer J, Glaser SJ, Hennig J. Pseudo steady-state free precession for MR-fingerprinting. Magn Reson Med. 2017;77(3):1151–61.
28. Cruz G, et al. Comparing FLASH vs GRE for 2D cardiac MR fingerprinting. In: Proc. 28th Annu. Meet. ISMRM; 2020. p. 3761.
29. Weigel M. Extended phase graphs: dephasing, RF pulses, and echoes - pure and simple. J Magn Reson Imaging. 2015;41(2):266–95.
30. Hamilton JI, et al. Investigating and reducing the effects of confounding factors for robust T 1 and T 2 mapping with cardiac MR fingerprinting. Magn Reson Imaging. 2018;53:40–51.
31. Ma D, et al. Slice profile and B1 corrections in 2D magnetic resonance fingerprinting. Magn Reson Med. 2017;78(5):1781–9.
32. Körzdörfer G, et al. Magnetic resonance field fingerprinting. Magn Reson Med. 2019;81:2347–59.
33. Buonincontri G, Schulte RF, Cosottini M, Tosetti M. Spiral MR fingerprinting at 7 T with simultaneous B1 estimation. Magn Reson Imaging. 2017;41:1–6.
34. Cloos MA, et al. Multiparametric imaging with heterogeneous radiofrequency fields. Nat Commun. 2016;7:12445.
35. Liu Y, Hamilton J, Eck B, Griswold M, Seiberlich N. Myocardial T1 and T2 quantification and water–fat separation using cardiac MR fingerprinting with rosette trajectories at 3T and 1.5T. Magn Reson Med. 2021;85(1):103–19.
36. Buonincontri G, Sawiak SJ. MR Fingerprinting with Simultaneous B1 Estimation. Magn Reson Med. 2016;1135:1127–35.
37. Körzdörfer G, et al. Effect of spiral undersampling patterns on FISP MRF parameter maps. Magn Reson Imaging. 2019;62:174–80.
38. Pierre EY, Ma D, Chen Y, Badve C, Griswold MA. Multiscale reconstruction for MR fingerprinting. Magn Reson Med. 2016;75(6):2481–92.
39. Doneva M, Amthor T, Koken P, Sommer K, Börnert P. Matrix completion-based reconstruction for undersampled magnetic resonance fingerprinting data. Magn Reson Imaging. 2017;41:41–52.
40. Assländer J, Cloos MA, Knoll F, Sodickson DK, Hennig J, Lattanzi R. Low rank alternating direction method of multipliers reconstruction for MR fingerprinting. Magn Reson Med. 2018;79(1):83–96.
41. Hamilton JI, et al. MR fingerprinting for rapid quantification of myocardial T1, T2, and proton spin density. Magn Reson Med. 2017;77(4):1446–58.
42. Hamilton JI, et al. Simultaneous mapping of T1 and T2 using cardiac magnetic resonance fingerprinting in a cohort of healthy subjects at 1.5T. J Magn Reson Imaging. 2020;52(4):1044–52.
43. Jaubert O, et al. Water–fat Dixon cardiac magnetic resonance fingerprinting. Magn Reson Med. 2020;83(6):2107–23.
44. Hamilton JI, Jiang Y, Eck B, Griswold M, Seiberlich N. Cardiac cine magnetic resonance fingerprinting for combined ejection fraction, T1 and T2 quantification. NMR Biomed. 2020;33(8):e4323.
45. Jaubert O, et al. Free-running cardiac magnetic resonance fingerprinting: joint T1/T2 map and cine imaging. Magn Reson Imaging. 2020;68:173–82.
46. Cruz G, et al. 3D free-breathing cardiac magnetic resonance fingerprinting. NMR Biomed. 2020;33(10):1–16.
47. Ahad J, Lo W-C, Hamilton JI, Franson D, Jiang Y, Seiberlich N. Implementation of cardiac MRF in Gadgetron for online reconstruction. In: Proc. 26th Annu. Meet. ISMRM; 2018. p. 4789.
48. McGivney DF, et al. SVD compression for magnetic resonance fingerprinting in the time domain. IEEE Trans Med Imaging. 2014;33(12):2311–22.

49. Yang M, et al. Low rank approximation methods for MR fingerprinting with large scale dictionaries. Magn Reson Med. 2018;79(4):2392–400.
50. Cauley SF, et al. Fast group matching for MR fingerprinting reconstruction. Magn Reson Med. 2015;74(2):523–8.
51. Goodfellow I, et al. Generative adversarial nets. In: Advances in neural information processing systems; 2014. pp. 2672–2680.
52. Yang M, Jiang Y, Ma D, Mehta BB, Griswold MA. Game of learning bloch equation simulations for MR fingerprinting. arXiv; 2020.
53. Hamilton JI, Seiberlich N. Machine learning for rapid magnetic resonance fingerprinting tissue property quantification. Proc IEEE. 2020;108(1):69–85.
54. Russek SE, et al. Characterization of NIST/ISMRM MRI System Phantom. In: Proc. 20th Annu. Meet. ISMRM; 2012. p. 2456.
55. Cohen O, Zhu B, Rosen MS. MR fingerprinting Deep RecOnstruction NEtwork (DRONE). Magn Reson Med. 2018;80(3):885–94.
56. Hamilton JI, Currey D, Rajagopalan S, Seiberlich N. Deep learning reconstruction for cardiac magnetic resonance fingerprinting T1 and T2 mapping. Magn Reson Med. 2021;85(4):2127–35.
57. Wissmann L, Santelli C, Segars WP, Kozerke S. MRXCAT: Realistic numerical phantoms for cardiovascular magnetic resonance. J Cardiovasc Magn Reson. 2014;16:63.
58. Jaubert O, et al. Multi-parametric liver tissue characterization using MR fingerprinting: simultaneous T1, T2, T2*, and fat fraction mapping. Magn Reson Med. 2020;84(5):2625–35.
59. Küstner T, et al. Fully self-gated free-running 3D Cartesian cardiac CINE with isotropic whole-heart coverage in less than 2 min. NMR Biomed. 2021;34(1):1–13.
60. Steeden JA, et al. Rapid whole-heart CMR with single volume super-resolution. arXiv; 2019.
61. Küstner T, et al. CINENet: deep learning-based 3D cardiac CINE MRI reconstruction with multi-coil complex-valued 4D spatio-temporal convolutions. Sci Rep. 2020;10:1.
62. Hansen MS, Sørensen TS. Gadgetron: an open source framework for medical image reconstruction. Magn Reson Med. 2013;69(6):1768–76.
63. Xue H, Inati S, Sørensen TS, Kellman P, Hansen MS. Distributed MRI reconstruction using Gadgetron-based cloud computing. Magn Reson Med. 2015;73(3):1015–25.

Currently Available Artificial Intelligence Softwares for Cardiothoracic Imaging

21

Yasasvi Tadavarthi, Judy Wawira Gichoya, Nabile Safdar, Imon Banerjee, and Hari Trivedi

Introduction

The growth of commercially available artificial intelligence programs that aid in radiology workflow and diagnosis has been tremendous in the last 5 years. Initial targets of artificial intelligence applications included chest radiographs and mammograms due to the large availability of training data and the computational restraints. Since then, power of graphical processing units (GPUs) has grown exponentially along with advancements in deep learning architectures, and the ability to process three-dimensional imaging such as computed tomography became a target of interest for developers.

Regulatory Process

Regulatory approval of AI applications can vary based on the governing body and region, whether it's the US Food and Drug Administration (FDA), European Conformity (CE), South Korean Ministry of Food and Drug Safety (MFDS), or other national regulatory bodies. Current approval of AI-based algorithms requires that these algorithms are "frozen" in their current state and cannot be updated without re-approval; however this may change as the clinical impact of AI models and the risks associated with live "fine-tuning" or retraining of models are better understood.

Based on existing trends, CE approval frequently predicts FDA approval within 2 years, whether it be full FDA approval of pre-market 510k clearance for medical devices [1].

Y. Tadavarthi, MD
Department of Radiology, Washington University in St. Louis, St. Louis, MO, USA
e-mail: t.yasasvi@wustl.edu

J. W. Gichoya, MD · H. Trivedi, MD (✉)
Department of Radiology, Emory University, Atlanta, GA, USA

Department of Biomedical Informatics, Emory University, Atlanta, GA, USA
e-mail: judywawira@emory.edu; hari.trivedi@emory.edu

N. Safdar, MD
Department of Radiology, Emory University, Atlanta, GA, USA
e-mail: nabile.safdar@emory.edu

I. Banerjee, PhD
Department of Computer Science, University of Arizona, Tucson, AZ, USA
e-mail: ibanerj7@asu.edu

Current Application Offerings

There is a wide scope of current AI application offerings in cardiothoracic imaging which span all modalities and target various use cases such as decision support, exam acquisition and reconstruction, post-processing, diagnosis, or prognostication. In this chapter, we will discuss the various types of applications currently available for cardiothoracic applications including cardiac, pulmonary, and musculoskeletal applications. The current range of offerings vary widely and include quantification on cardiac MRI and echocardiography, disease detection and quantification on chest radiography and CT, disease progression on PET/CT, and fracture detection on both radiography and CT.

Note that all AI software offerings in this chapter are current as of September 2020 and are meant to present a representative sample of currently available AI tools. All claims of performance and software functionality are taken directly from conversations with company representatives or from online or print materials. These claims have not been independently verified, and the authors do not endorse the performance of any company or product.

Types of Integration

With hundreds of companies currently marketing AI applications, a major challenge in their adoption is implementation. While a few applications have been either purchased

C. N. De Cecco et al. (eds.), *Artificial Intelligence in Cardiothoracic Imaging*, Contemporary Medical Imaging,
https://doi.org/10.1007/978-3-030-92087-6_21

or developed directly by equipment vendors, most diagnostic applications perform optimally inside of their *own* platform. This results in a major challenge to integrate AI models into existing PACS software, a market that is dominated by approximately a half-dozen vendors. While all PACS software serves the same basic purpose, their ability for third-party integration of software modules, worklist management, or display of annotations can vary. There are groups such as the Data Standards Committee of the Society of Imaging Informatics (SIIM) (www.siim.org) that aim to standardize the data elements that can be passed between software applications for various applications; however these standards are not universally adopted. As a result, beyond algorithm performance, purchasers must also consider if an application under consideration will integrate with their existing PACS software and, if not, what impact that will have on user satisfaction and impact on any potential time savings.

Some software vendors circumvent the need for PACS integration by pushing all images to a cloud service where AI models are run, and the model results are then pushed back to the PACS. Although this implementation is PACS agnostic, it raises other challenges such as placing AI interpretations directly on images which are then permanently stored in PACS and in the patient's medical record. This can be less than ideal if the radiologist disagrees with the AI model's findings and could raise concerns over future medicolegal liability.

Other considerations are integration with the electronic health record (EHR) and/or reporting software. Applications that are able to pull additional information directly from the EHR (similar to what a radiologist would do) may have better diagnostic performance by incorporating clinical history; however this challenge is arguably even greater than that for PACS integration. Reporting integration is beneficial as it removes a step of manual reporting of results from the dictation software into the radiology report, and these integrations are considered desirable. The vast majority of radiology reporting software is made by one company, so this type of integration is easier than PACS and EHR integration which have more variability.

Lastly, there are several companies that serve as aggregators or marketplaces for radiology AI applications. Many of these companies offer multiple solutions for the same clinical problem (e.g., lung nodule detection) and allow the user to choose the algorithm that works best by offering free trial periods that allow an institution to pilot multiple models. However, the model implementation inside of these marketplaces can often be a diluted version of the original model with restricted feature sets since they must be standardized into a common platform.

Cardiac Imaging

Current cardiac AI applications apply to multiple modalities, including echocardiography, cardiac CT, and cardiac MR and target multiple steps along the imaging pathway from image acquisition, post-processing, and quantification. Of these, the majority target automated quantification and assist in performing quantitative measurements for physicians, allowing for quicker read-times and increased scan throughput.

Image Acquisition, Reconstruction, and Post-Processing

Image acquisition and quality assurance in echocardiography have been a topic of interest for AI vendors. Caption Guidance was one of the first companies to use AI to guide proper acquisition of echocardiograms [2]. The software functions on point-of-care ultrasound probes to provide real-time maneuvering suggestions to achieve adequate views, which may assist novice clinicians or sonographers [2, 3]. Some vendors go beyond this to assist in in automatic selection of key images with optimal image quality. Caption Guidance [3–5] and EchoGo [6–8] can automatically select good-quality images for EF calculation, whereas LVivo [9, 10] relies on the user to click a button on the ultrasound machine to perform analysis in real time. ContextVision [11] markets software for real-time US image enhancement, allowing for significant noise reduction to enhance soft tissue contrast. Companies like Caption Health demonstrate a decrease in acquisition time for novice clinicians or sonographers without prior training in echocardiography [5] and enabled registered nurses with no prior sonography experience to generate echocardiograms that were deemed acceptable by a team of cardiologists [2].

In cardiac CT acquisition, a primary target of novel deep learning-based techniques is reduction of radiation dose, which is often coupled with new reconstruction techniques to compensate for the resultant decreased signal-to-noise ratio. Examples include offerings by GE Healthcare which have successfully reduced radiation doses by up to 51% while reducing noise by up to 69% compared to similar full-dose CTs using filtered back projection (FBP) [12, 13] (Fig. 21.1a, b). GE healthcare has integrated this software in their Revolution CT scanner. Canon Medical Systems has implemented a similar reconstruction technology trained on model-based iterative reconstruction (MBIR) images and implements directly in certain CT scanners, achieving 3–5× faster reconstruction speeds than MBIR with improved noise reduction [14, 15] Other companies such as TeraRecon have provided AI-powered

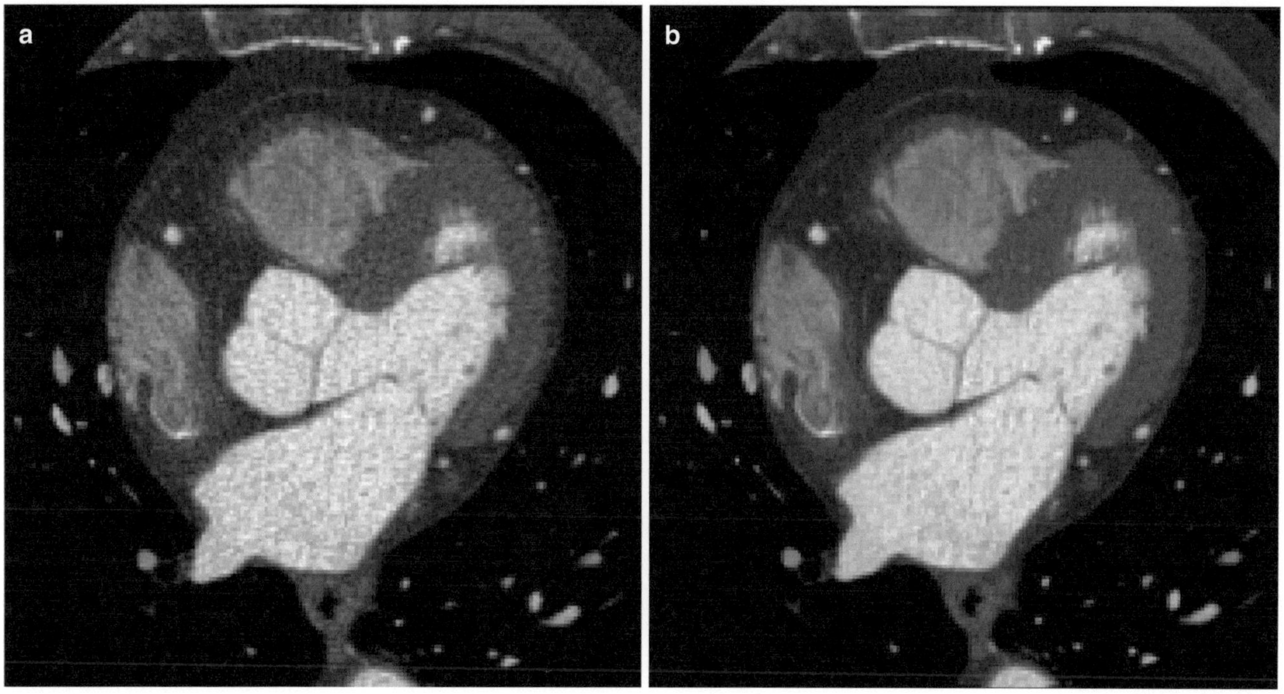

Fig. 21.1 (**a**, **b**) Offerings implemented by GE healthcare (**b**) show increased noise reduction with reduced effective radiation dosage compared to standard filtered back projection images (**a**) [12]

image reconstruction and visualization algorithms for automated valvular measurements before transcatheter aortic valve replacement (TAVR) [16].

Applications in cardiac MRI acquisition (CMR) can be complex due to heterogeneity of acquisition protocols, imaging planes, and the computational power required to analyze 3D images. Image quality is frequently affected by the technologist's experience and patient motion and resultantly has been the focus of several software solutions. HeartVista has enabled 6x faster acquisition of CMR and significantly reduced the number of required breath-holds by using a novel free-breathing accelerated CMR cine sequence [17]. They have also developed motion artifact reduction techniques to assist in imaging patients that are unable to breath-hold or have arrythmias [18]. This is currently being implemented in GE MRI scanners. Other targets include simulating multiple acquisitions using a randomized RF excitation and using AI algorithms to reconstruct multiple sequences in a much shorter time [18, 19].

Diagnostics and Quantification

Many quantifiable metrics can be extracted from echocardiograms, including left ventricular ejection fraction (LVEF), ventricular volumes, and myocardial strain. Several companies have software that is currently FDA approved for LVEF calculation but differ in the views required to do so. Some companies utilize the traditional apical four-chamber and apical two-chamber views used by human readers, whereas others are able to use non-traditional views such as the parasternal long axis (PLAX) view. This is useful because many patients who require echocardiography are limited in positioning (i.e., ICU patients) and therefore are more easily imaged using the PLAX view that does not require left lateral decubitus positioning. Reported performance of this software (Caption AI by Caption Health) is comparable to trained cardiologists while achieving a statistically significant lower variability than compared to trained cardiologists [20, 21]. This repeatability is important as LVEF can often be highly subjective and varies between readers.

Diagnostic software for cardiac CT has mainly targeted quantification of coronary artery disease, evaluation of plaques, measurement of stenosis, and measurement of chamber volumes [22]. Circle CVI, TeraRecon, Siemens, VoxelCloud, Zebra Medical, and Shukun all target one or more aspects of these measurements. The most common use case is automated calcified plaque segmentation based on a single click in the center of a plaque [23–25]. Siemens offers calculation of calcium scores based on total plaque burden [23]. Zebra Medical's solution automatically flags studies that have a moderate to severe coronary calcium score as part of the radiologists workflow [24].

Quantification software for cardiac MRI target measurements such as LV/RV chamber segmentation, quantitative perfusion, 2D and 4D valvular flow, valve stenosis measurement, and quantification of delayed enhancement. Arterys, Circle CVI, and Shukun semi-automate or automate many of the above measurements, leading to significant time savings. For example, Circle CVI reports up to 19 minutes saved per study for measurement calculations [26, 27]. Diagnostic software has also been developed, for example, by Galgo Medical who developed tools to aid in tissue characterization and help electrophysiologists visualize myocardial fibrosis for ablation planning [28]. Lastly, some companies have created post-processing algorithms to highlight zones of delayed myocardial enhancement which are overlayed on CMR images to assist radiologists in more easily identifying patterns of abnormal delayed enhancement to assist with diagnoses.

Thoracic Imaging

Acquisition, Reconstruction, and Post-Processing

Applications in CT acquisition target reduction of radiation dose and improving patient positioning. Siemens has developed software to automatically center patients in the gantry to optimize radiation dose and image quality [29, 30]. Similar to in cardiac CT, Canon has developed algorithms to reduce CT radiation dosage while still achieving regular-dose image quality through machine learning-assisted reconstruction [14]. Subtle Medical has similarly applied this technique to PET scans, enabling high-resolution PET scans with 1/200 of the standard dosage of radionuclide tracer while reducing scan time by up to 75% [31]. ClariPi and AlgoMedica enable ultra-low-dose CT by implementing a de-noising algorithms that can outperform FBP and iterative reconstruction (Fig. 21.2) [32–35].

A unique approach in image post-processing is to remove extraneous anatomy to make findings of interest more apparent. For example, Riverain uses artificial intelligence to remove bones from chest radiographs to make the lung parenchyma more visible [36, 37]. They also have an algorithm to remove pulmonary vasculature from chest CTs to make pulmonary nodules more visible [38, 39].

Diagnosis

Chest radiograph (CXR) is a major of area of focus for commercial AI algorithms due to the high volume of chest radiographs in practice, the abundance of public training data, and the finite scope of possible diagnoses. From a technical per-

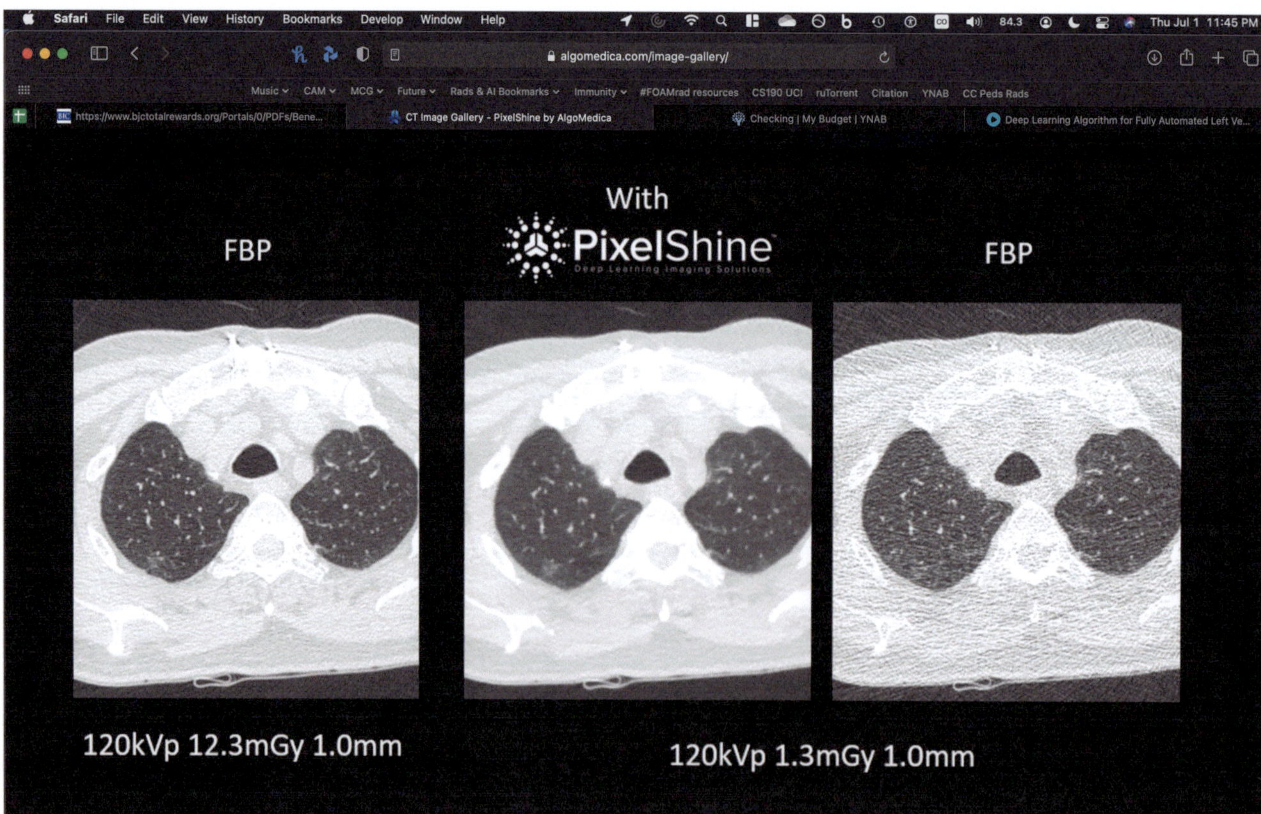

Fig. 21.2 AlgoMedica's PixelShine showing images reconstructed from 1.3 mGy dosage with machine learning assistance with comparable image quality of 12.4 mGy images reconstructed using filtered back projection. There is a significant decrease in image noise in PixelShine images when compared to a FBP-reconstructed image of the same radiation exposure

spective, 2D chest radiography is also less computationally expensive than 3D algorithms making it more efficient to apply in clinical settings. Many companies have targeted a range of diagnoses on chest radiograph, most frequently pneumonia and pneumothorax detection [1]. GE has interestingly incorporated a pneumothorax detection algorithm directly into a portable radiograph machine to provide instantaneous results at the point of care in the event of moderate or large pneumothorax [40]. Other common diagnostic targets include detection of cardiomegaly, rib fractures, and lung nodules. Less common algorithms include endotracheal tube and central line positioning offered by DeepTek, Oxipit, RADLogics, and Riverain.

Because chest radiographs can contain multiple simultaneous abnormalities, many vendors have applications that detect multiple pathologies simultaneously. Oxipit detects 75 of the most common chest x-ray diagnoses which encompasses over 90% of the abnormalities that may routinely be seen in chest radiography [41, 42]. If the algorithm has a high confidence for a study with no abnormality, it will also generate a preliminary report for the normal study for the radiologist to approve [41]. Enlitic similarly covers several chest radiograph diagnoses and is the first algorithm to be approved to be used in the Defense Health Agency (DHA) and Veterans Affairs (VA) Medical Treatment Facilities [43]. Qure.ai offers a detection of 29 different pathologies and automatically triages x-rays in the worklist [44]. They showed no statistical difference between Qure.ai's algorithm and a trained radiologist in detecting pulmonary opacities, pleural effusions, hilar prominence, and enlarged cardiac silhouette [45].

Many of these software offerings may increase study throughput or decrease read times in underserved areas both domestically and internationally. Qure.ai's qXR has been implemented in India as a screening tool for tuberculosis, as the prevalence of the disease is relatively high and there is a shortage of radiologists [46–48].This software has shown to have adequate sensitivity for screening based on prospective studies with sputum-culture-confirmed TB patients [49]. Other companies that have targeted tuberculosis screening include Thirona, 1Qbit (approved in Canada), DeepTek, PVMed, and Radisen.

CT imaging provides a bigger challenge compared to chest radiographs due to the 3D nature of scans which increases complexity and computational requirements and a higher number of possible pathologies which can be nuanced [1]. While several use cases of deep learning in chest CT are similar to those targeted in chest x-ray, one overwhelmingly predominant task of interest in chest CT is detection, measurement, and characterization of lung nodules. Lung nodule detection represents a tedious and repetitive task making it ideal to automate. Furthermore, training models for nodule detection does not require confirmation from patient follow-up or pathology, meaning that training data is easier to collect and annotate. Over 15 companies target one or more aspect of lung nodule management, including Aidoc, Arterys, Aidence, Infervision, Mindshare Medical, Mint Medical, Vuno, and Zebra Medical. Many of these companies go beyond lung nodule detection and assist with Lung-RADS scoring. This requires the ability to detect and track nodules across multiple exams so changes in nodule size and characteristics can be automatically assessed.

Several algorithms have also been created for the detection of pulmonary embolism on CT pulmonary angiograms. Aidoc currently received FDA clearance for pulmonary embolism detection and can triage positive scans for faster radiologist interpretation [50, 51]. They also offer a method to detect incidental pulmonary embolism found on routine chest CTs that are not acquired as pulmonary angiograms.

Lung disease quantification has been targeted by several companies. Specifically, analysis of lung parenchyma can help locate and quantify emphysematous changes through measurements of air trapping and airway morphology. Findings can often assist in pre-procedural planning. Thirona has developed such software that has been FDA approved. Other companies that target similar cases are Coreline Soft, Botkin.AI, ScanMed, TeraRecon, JLK inspection, Siemens, and VIDA. A novel application for lung disease visualization is from 4D Medical, which uses fluoroscopic cine sequences to assess regional lung function and ventilation during all phases of the breathing cycle [52]. The software then provides an overlay of ventilation quantification onto a preceding or concurrent chest CT (Fig. 21.3). The proposed benefit is increased granularity and sensitivity for chronic lung disease monitoring while decreasing radiation exposure.

Recently, due to the novel COVID-19 pandemic, many companies are developing chest radiograph and chest CT algorithms to diagnose and track the resolution of COVID-19 pneumonia. RADLogics has developed an investigational algorithm that calculates a "Corona score" based on CT features and uses it to detect the disease, quantify disease burden, and assess progression of COVID-19 [53]. Care Mentor AI has similarly developed a method to segment and assess disease burden and uses post-processing masks to delineate lung damage [54]. A similar scoring method has been developed by RADLogics for chest radiographs to assess COVID-19 disease severity [55].

Other non-parenchymal abnormalities such as vertebral compression fractures are detected by multiple companies, including Aidoc, Zebra Medical, and Siemens who all have regulatory approval for this use case. Companies have targeted this feature as compression fractures are largely underreported in spine-containing CT scans in the emergency setting. It is estimated that only one-third of vertebral fractures come to clinical attention [56, 57].

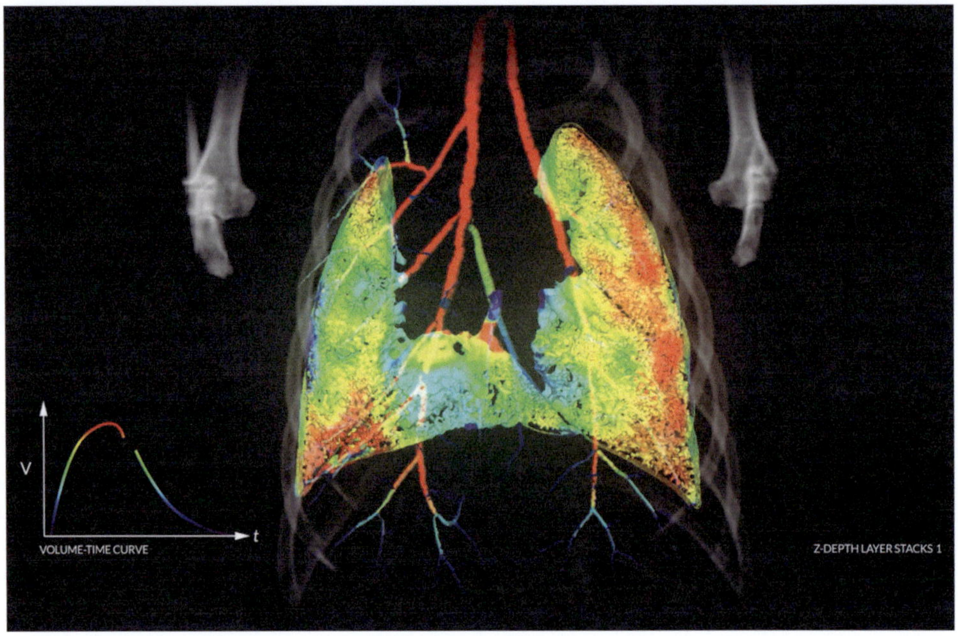

Fig. 21.3 4DMedical showing lung ventilation maps that are measured at all points of the breathing cycle. Red zones show regions of decreased air flow

Finally, PET/CT is a target for AI algorithms, although the number of companies working in this space is much smaller. 4Quant uses radiomic features on PET and CT to automatically stage non-small cell lung cancer (NSCLC) [58, 59]. Others such as MIM software detect and automatically detect, segment, and quantify hypermetabolic lesions.

Summary

Commercial radiology AI software offerings for cardiothoracic imaging continue to grow in both number and scope. The most common applications relate to the most common imaging exams – namely, chest radiographs, and chest CT – although many applications have been developed for more complex tasks related to cardiac imaging. Non-interpretive applications include image reconstruction to improve image quality or post-processing to ease interpretation. A major barrier to successful adoption of AI software remains the ability to tightly integrate models into existing workflows; however this should improve in the coming years as AI applications become more commonplace and vendors increase interoperability.

Bibliography

1. Tadavarthi Y, Vey B, Krupinski E, et al. The state of radiology AI: considerations for purchase decisions and current market offerings. Radiol Artif Intelligence. 2020;2(6):e200004. https://doi.org/10.1148/ryai.2020200004.
2. Narang A, Bae R, Hong H, Thomas Y, Surette S, Cadieu C, et al. Acquisition of diagnostic echocardiographic images by novices using a deep learning based image guidance algorithm. J Am Coll Cardiol. 2020;75(11):1564.
3. AI-Guided Ultrasound System | Caption Health. https://captionhealth.com/. Accessed 19 Nov 2020.
4. Main M, Bae R, Cadieu C, et al. Artificial intelligence guidance of novices to obtain diagnostic-quality echocardiographic images. J Am Soc Echocardiogr. 2020;33(6).
5. Schneider M, Bartko P, Geller W, et al. A machine learning algorithm supports ultrasound-naïve novices in the acquisition of diagnostic echocardiography loops and provides accurate estimation of LVEF. Int J Cardiovasc Imaging. 2020. https://doi.org/10.1007/s10554-020-02046-6.
6. EchoGo Suite | Ultromics. https://www.ultromics.com/echogo. Accessed 19 Nov 2020.
7. Beqiri A, Parker A, Mumith A, Hassanali N, Upton R. Fully automated quantification of contrast and non-contrast echocardiograms eliminates inter-operator variability.
8. Gao S, Stojanovski D, Parker A, Marques P, Heitner S. Automated view detection of contrast and non-contrast cardiac views in echocardiography; a multi-Centre, Multi-Vendor Study.
9. LVivo EF | DiA Imaging Analysis. https://www.dia-analysis.com/lvivo-ef. Accessed 19 Nov 2020.
10. Lai AC, Beerkens F, Bienstock S, Samtani R, Goldman ME. A novel artificial intelligence echocardiography software achieves equivalence to physician-read images with ultrasound enhancing agents in left ventricular volume determination. J Scientific Innov Med. 2020;3(3). https://doi.org/10.29024/jsim.72.
11. Ultrasound – ContextVision provides state-of-the-art image enhancement. https://www.contextvision.com/products/ultrasound/. Accessed 19 Nov 2020.
12. Hsieh J, Liu E, Nett B, Tang J, Thibault J, Sahney S. A new era of image reconstruction: TrueFidelityTM Technical white paper on deep learning image reconstruction; 2019.
13. Solomon J, Lyu P, Marin D, Samei E. Noise and spatial resolution properties of a commercially available deep learning-based CT reconstruction algorithm. Med Phys. 2020. https://doi.org/10.1002/mp.14319.
14. AiCE | Computed Tomography – CT Scanners | Canon Medical Systems USA. https://us.medical.canon/products/computed-tomography/aice/. Accessed 18 Nov 2020.
15. Higaki T, Nakamura Y, Zhou J, et al. Deep learning reconstruction at CT: phantom study of the image characteristics. Acad Radiol. 2020;27(1):82–7. https://doi.org/10.1016/j.acra.2019.09.008.

16. Product Overview | Single Solution for 3D and AI. https://www.terarecon.com/capabilities?locale=en. Accessed 18 Nov 2020.
17. Roifman I, Gutierrez J, Wang E, et al. Evaluating a novel free-breathing accelerated cardiac MRI cine sequence in patients with cardiomyopathy. Magn Reson Imaging. 2019;61:260–6. https://doi.org/10.1016/j.mri.2019.06.008.
18. For Physicians — HEARTVISTA. https://www.heartvista.ai/for-physicians. Accessed 18 Nov 2020.
19. Chen F, Taviani V, Malkiel I, et al. Variable-density single-shot fast spin-Echo MRI with deep learning reconstruction by using variational networks. Radiology. 2018;289(2):366–73. https://doi.org/10.1148/radiol.2018180445.
20. Asch FM, Poilvert N, Abraham T, et al. Automated echocardiographic quantification of left ventricular ejection fraction without volume measurements using a machine learning algorithm mimicking a human expert. Circ Cardiovasc Imaging. 2019;12(9):e009303. https://doi.org/10.1161/CIRCIMAGING.119.009303.
21. Poilvert N, Hong H, Martin R. Deep learning algorithm for fully automated left ventricular ejection fraction measurement. J Am Soc Echocardiogr. 2018;31(6):P2–45. https://doi.org/10.1016/j.echo.2018.04.010.
22. Selvarajah A, Bennamoun M, Playford D, Chow BJW, Dwivedi G. Application of artificial intelligence in coronary computed tomography angiography. Curr Cardiovasc Imaging Rep. 2018;11(6):12. https://doi.org/10.1007/s12410-018-9453-5.
23. syngo.CT CaScoring. https://www.siemens-healthineers.com/computed-tomography/options-upgrades/clinical-applications/syngo-ct-cascoring. Accessed 18 Nov 2020.
24. Zebra Medical Vision, Inc. Cardiac solution. https://www.zebra-med.com/cardiac-solution. Accessed 20 Nov 2020.
25. VoxelCloud. Accessible diagnoses http://www.voxelcloud.io/en/index.html. Accessed 5 July 2021.
26. Petersen SE. Hidden insights with machine learning: challenges and opportunities from UK BioBank. Presented at the: Euro CMR 2017; October 7, 2017; Prague, Czech Republic. https://www.youtube.com/watch?v=9zkbYeH0G3M. Accessed 1 Dec 2020.
27. Circle cardiovascular imaging. Cardiac MRI and CT Software - deep learning. https://www.circlecvi.com/cvi42/cardiac-mri/deep-learning/. Accessed 1 Dec 2020.
28. ADAS 3D LA: Technology. https://www.adas3d.com/en/adas-af-technology.html. Accessed 18 Nov 2020.
29. Eberhard M, Alkadhi H. Machine learning and deep neural networks: applications in patient and scan preparation, contrast medium, and radiation dose optimization. J Thorac Imaging. 2020;35 Suppl 1:S17–20. https://doi.org/10.1097/RTI.0000000000000482.
30. Saltybaeva N, Schmidt B, Wimmer A, Flohr T, Alkadhi H. Precise and automatic patient positioning in computed tomography: avatar modeling of the patient surface using a 3-dimensional camera. Invest Radiol. 2018;53(11):641–6. https://doi.org/10.1097/RLI.0000000000000482.
31. Xu J, Gong E, Pauly J, Zaharchuk G. 200x low-dose PET reconstruction using deep learning. arXiv preprint; 2017.
32. Hong JH, Park EA, Lee W, Ahn C, Kim JH. Incremental image noise reduction in coronary CT angiography using a deep learning-based technique with iterative reconstruction. Korean J Radiol. 2020;21(10):1165–77. https://doi.org/10.3348/kjr.2020.0020.
33. ClariPi. ClariCT.AI. ClariPi. http://www.claripi.com/eng/sub/sub02_01.php. Accessed 25 June 2020.
34. Hata A, Yanagawa M, Yoshida Y, et al. Combination of deep learning-based denoising and iterative reconstruction for ultra-low-dose CT of the chest: image quality and lung-RADS evaluation. AJR Am J Roentgenol. 2020;215(6):1321–8. https://doi.org/10.2214/AJR.19.22680.
35. PixelShine. What's that noise? How deep learning can elevate CT image quality, reduce dose exposure, and extend the life of older scanners. https://algomedica.com/wp-content/uploads/2020/11/PixelShine-White-Paper-2020-11-24.pdf. Accessed 6 June 2020.
36. ClearRead Xray Bone Suppress - Riverain Technologies. https://www.riveraintech.com/clearread-xray/xray-bone-suppress/. Accessed 18 Nov 2020.
37. Freedman MT, Lo S-CB, Seibel JC, Bromley CM. Lung nodules: improved detection with software that suppresses the rib and clavicle on chest radiographs. Radiology. 2011;260(1):265–73. https://doi.org/10.1148/radiol.11100153.
38. ClearRead CT Vessel Suppress - Riverain Technologies. https://www.riveraintech.com/clearread-ct/clearread-ct-vessel-suppress/. Accessed 18 Nov 2020.
39. Lo SB, Freedman MT, Gillis LB, White CS, Mun SK. JOURNAL CLUB: Computer-aided detection of lung nodules on CT with a computerized pulmonary vessel suppressed function. AJR Am J Roentgenol. 2018;210(3):480–8. https://doi.org/10.2214/AJR.17.18718.
40. Critical Care Suite on mobile and fixed x-ray systems | GE Healthcare | GE Healthcare. https://www.gehealthcare.com/products/radiography/mobile-xray-systems/critical-care-suite-on-optima-xr240amx. Accessed 18 Nov 2020.
41. ChestEye AI Chest X-Ray Radiology Suite | Oxipit | Request a demo today! https://oxipit.ai/products/chesteye/. Accessed 18 Nov 2020.
42. Ramanauskas N, Dementaviciene J, Bialopetravičius J, et al. Towards an end-to-end deep learning model for robust multiclass chest X-ray pathology classification; 2018.
43. Enlitic, Inc. awarded contract by the defense innovation unit to pilot advanced artificial intelligence platform for diagnostic imaging. https://www.globenewswire.com/news-release/2020/09/08/2090296/0/en/ENLITIC-INC-AWARDED-CONTRACT-BY-THE-DEFENSE-INNOVATION-UNIT-to-pilot-advanced-artificial-intelligence-platform-for-diagnostic-imaging.html. Accessed 18 Nov 2020.
44. Putha P, Tadepalli M, Reddy B, Raj T, Warier P. Can artificial intelligence reliably report chest X-rays? Radiologist validation of an algorithm trained on 1.2 million X-rays; 2018.
45. Singh R, Kalra MK, Nitiwarangkul C, et al. Deep learning in chest radiography: detection of findings and presence of change. PLoS One. 2018;13(10):e0204155. https://doi.org/10.1371/journal.pone.0204155.
46. Qure.ai | qXR for Tuberculosis screening. https://www.qure.ai/qxr-tuberculosis.html. Accessed 19 Nov 2020.
47. Nash M, Kadavigere R, Andrade J, et al. Deep learning, computer-aided radiography reading for tuberculosis: a diagnostic accuracy study from a tertiary hospital in India. Sci Rep. 2020;10(1):210. https://doi.org/10.1038/s41598-019-56589-3.
48. Engle E, Gabrielian A, Long A, Hurt DE, Rosenthal A. Performance of Qure.ai automatic classifiers against a large annotated database of patients with diverse forms of tuberculosis. PLoS One. 2020;15(1):e0224445. https://doi.org/10.1371/journal.pone.0224445.
49. Khan FA, Majidulla A, Tavaziva G, et al. Chest x-ray analysis with deep learning-based software as a triage test for pulmonary tuberculosis: a prospective study of diagnostic accuracy for culture-confirmed disease. Lancet Digital Health. 2020;2(11):e573–81. https://doi.org/10.1016/S2589-7500(20)30221-1.
50. Pulmonary Embolism Guidelines and the intersection with AI - Aidoc. https://www.aidoc.com/blog/pulmonary-embolism-guidelines-and-the-intersection-with-ai/. Accessed 19 Nov 2020.
51. Weikert T, Winkel DJ, Bremerich J, et al. Automated detection of pulmonary embolism in CT pulmonary angiograms using an AI-powered algorithm. Eur Radiol. 2020;30(12):6545–53. https://doi.org/10.1007/s00330-020-06998-0.
52. 4DMedical. XV LVAS. https://4dmedical.com/wp-content/uploads/2020/07/4DMedical_XVLVAS_Brochure_v1.pdf. Accessed 1 July 2021.

53. Gozes O, Frid-Adar M, Greenspan H, et al. Rapid AI development cycle for the coronavirus (COVID-19) pandemic: initial results for automated detection & patient monitoringusing deep learning CT image analysis. arXiv. https://arxiv.org/pdf/2003.05037.pdf. Accessed 5 Nov 2020.
54. Neural networks for operational diagnostics of COVID-19. https://carementor.me/covid-19. Accessed 19 Nov 2020.
55. Amer R, Frid-Adar M, Gozes O, Nassar J, Greenspan H. COVID-19 in CXR: from detection and severity scoring to patient disease monitoring. arXiv; 2020.
56. Fink HA, Milavetz DL, Palermo L, et al. What proportion of incident radiographic vertebral deformities is clinically diagnosed and vice versa? J Bone Miner Res. 2005;20(7):1216–22. https://doi.org/10.1359/JBMR.050314.
57. Ensrud KE, Schousboe JT. Clinical practice. Vertebral fractures. N Engl J Med. 2011;364(17):1634–42. https://doi.org/10.1056/NEJMcp1009697.
58. 4Quant | Lung Cancer Staging. https://www.lify.io/3p-products/lung-cancer-staging. Accessed 19 Nov 2020.
59. Sexauer R, Weikert T, Mader K, et al. Towards more structure: comparing TNM staging completeness and processing time of text-based reports versus fully segmented and annotated PET/CT data of non-small-cell lung cancer. Contrast Media Mol Imaging. 2018;2018:5693058. https://doi.org/10.1155/2018/5693058.

Part III

Artificial Intelligence: Cardiac Applications

22 Cardiac CT Guidelines and Clinical Applications: Where Does Artificial Intelligence Fit In?

Livia Marchitelli, Federica Catapano, Giulia Cundari, and Marco Francone

Introduction

In last the few years, a number of clinical guidelines, appropriateness criteria, and consensus documents on cardiac computed tomography (CCT) have been released by major national and international cardiovascular (CV) imaging societies in order to standardize scanning protocols and rationalize diagnostic workflows.

In a previous study, we identified 43 guidelines published in recent years by the European Society of Cardiology (ESC) and by the American College of Cardiology/American Heart Association (ACC/AHA) in which specific recommendations regarding the clinical use of CCT or cardiac magnetic resonance imaging were reported. Our analysis found 146 recommendations (ESC, n = 65; ACC/AHA, n = 81) of which 62 were made for CCT specifically (ESC, n = 28; ACC/AHA, n = 37) [1] (Fig. 22.1).

Those reports aimed to convey the expanding scientific literature into a single, consensus-, and/or evidence-based document drafted by a panel of experts and to produce a uniform guidance to support the role of CCT in clinical practice. Inappropriate CCT utilization can lead to increasing healthcare costs, unnecessary radiation exposure, and, finally, to the increased risk of legal repercussions related to clinical malpractice.

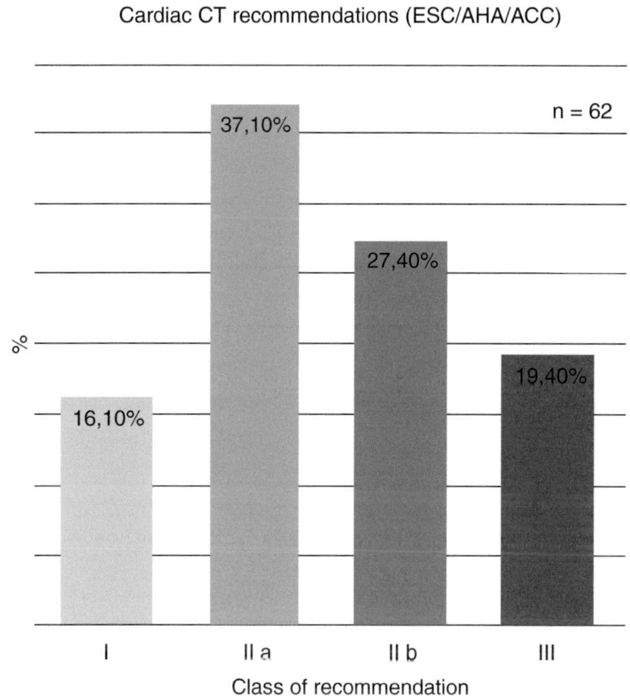

Fig. 22.1 Based on ESC (n = 28) and AHA/ACC (n = 37) clinical guidelines, the 62 cardiac CT recommendations were divided according to the classes of recommendation. (Class I = evidence that the procedure is clinically useful; Class IIa = weight of evidence in favor of efficacy; Class IIb = efficacy less well established; Class III = evidence that the procedure is not clinically useful). ESC European Society of Cardiology, AHA/ACC American Heart Association/American College of Cardiology, CT Computed tomography

However, appropriate guidelines and the adherence to them can be challenging in daily clinical routine considering the amount of recommendations and the complexity of mastering such a number of intricate recommendations in various clinical scenarios.

Artificial intelligence (AI)-based clinical decision-making can play a role in helping the clinician selecting the most appropriate imaging tests for the specific patient.

L. Marchitelli, MD · F. Catapano, MD · G. Cundari, MD
Department of Radiological, Oncological and Pathological Sciences, Sapienza University of Rome, Rome, Italy
e-mail: livia.marchitelli@uniroma1.it; giulia.cundari@uniroma1.it;

M. Francone, MD, PhD, EBCR (✉)
Department of Biomedical Sciences, Humanitas University, Via Rita Levi Montalcini, Pieve Emanuele (MI), Italy

IRCCS Humanitas Research Hospital, via Manzoni, Rozzano (MI), Italy
e-mail: federica.catapano@uniroma1.it; marco.francone@hunimed.eu

C. N. De Cecco et al. (eds.), *Artificial Intelligence in Cardiothoracic Imaging*, Contemporary Medical Imaging,
https://doi.org/10.1007/978-3-030-92087-6_22

AI-powered tools can also be helpful in identifying new diagnostic criteria that can be used to predict responses in different clinical settings.

The present chapter aims to review the emerging role of AI in preparation of supporting guidelines and helping with their application in clinical practice. Although limited material is available in the literature, this chapter will provide evidence on how the integration of AI and digital databases can be advantageous and provide new tools to facilitate the work of healthcare professionals and radiologist in specific.

Guidelines Development Process

Current Workflow

There is no consensus on how clinical practice guidelines' (CPGs) processes should be carried out, and therefore, each organization follows its own rules. Nevertheless, all the different development methodologies share basic principles and common features which progress through an extensive literature research and analysis of experimental evidence.

Taking into account the World Health Organization (WHO) handbook for guideline development [2], several key steps can be identified, as shown in Fig. 22.2. The development process usually starts with CPG's topic choice, which must reflect a global need of guidance in the selected area.A leading group is usually set up to establish the CPG's topic, which includes the definition of the content, clinical questions, and possible recommendations. The subject choice should be based on clinically actual problems, which drive the development. Potential subjects could emerge from the analysis of the most common cause of morbidity and/or mortality in a given population; unclear appropriateness criteria of a medical procedure, including imaging referral process; or the need to rationalize resources and avoid waste in providing care. Once a topic has been identified, a multidisciplinary CPG's development team needs to be recruited. The objective of this group is to set up a problem-solving analysis, through the formulation of a set of research questions that belong to three main categories: (1) definition/background, (2) facts/foreground, and (3) recommendation/decision. The next step of the process consists out of an extensive literature research aimed to find the best evidence available to answer the aforementioned question, usually performing a systematic review.

Once the studies have been identified, they must be assessed for relevance and quality. Several organizations adopt the Grading of Recommendations Assessment, Development and Evaluation (GRADE) approach for rating the quality of evidence. The GRADE approach has two steps, the evaluation of the quality of evidence and the summary of findings.

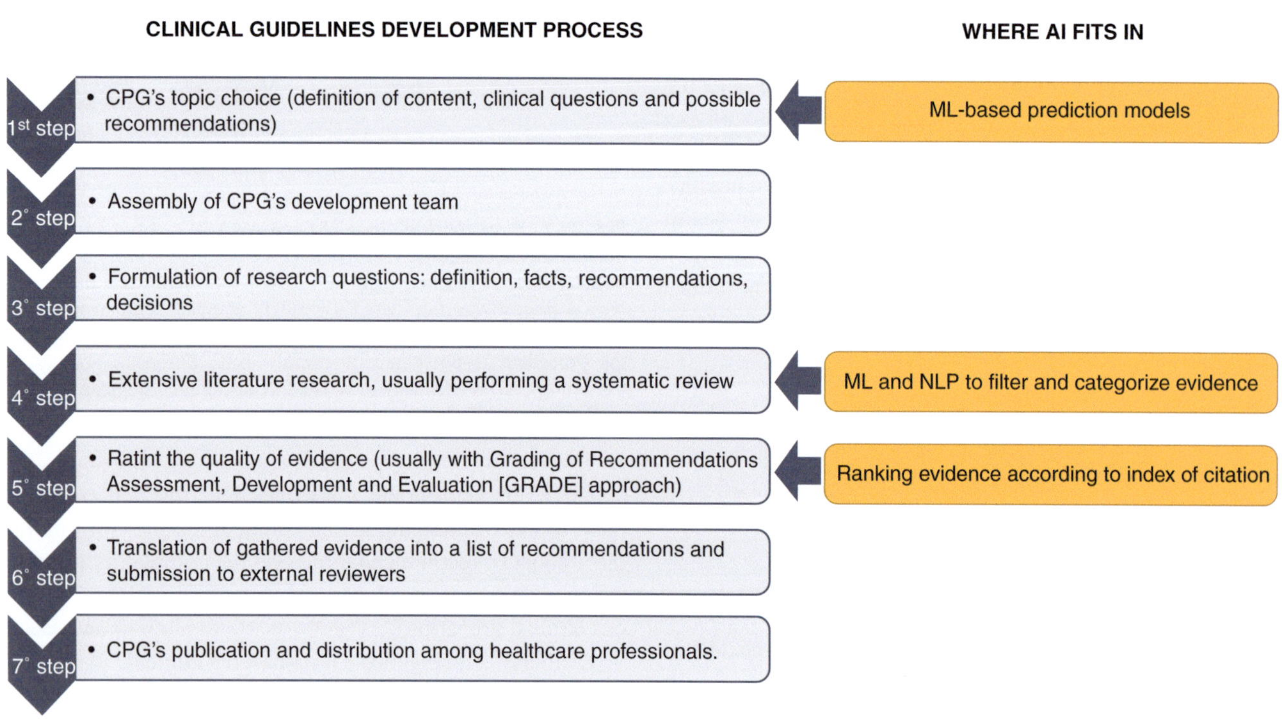

Fig. 22.2 CPG's development process, improved by the introduction of AI in topic choice, literature review, and quality assessment of the selected evidence. AI artificial intelligence, CPG clinical practice guidelines, ML machine learning, NLP Natural Language Processing

Collected evidence would therefore be translated into a list of recommendations, and a draft of the CPG should be written and submitted to external reviewers for final approval.

The final step consists in CPG's publication and distribution among healthcare professionals.

Artificial Intelligence Approaches

Taking into account the aforementioned flowchart, there are three crucial steps in which AI approaches could easily fit in and be of assistance: (1) topic choice, (2) literature review, and (3) quality assessment of selected evidence. As mentioned above, topic choice could emerge, for example, from the analysis of the most common causes of morbidity/mortality in a given population. For this purpose, machine learning (ML) techniques not only are able to analyze current morbidity/mortality causes but also can predict the morbidity/mortality rate of each cause in a given population. This can help clinicians to choose the area of interest for CPG's development. ML-based mortality prediction models have indeed been used in specific population settings, such as premature pediatric patients [3]; however, they can potentially be adopted in a larger population, as those referred in CPG.

As for evidence-based research, traditional literature review methods are based on human searches, which could be subject to bias and lack of reproducibility.

AI approaches, such as ML and natural language processing (NLP), could provide a more reliable process achieving more reproducible and accurate results in a more time-efficient way, allowing for periodically updates of the current literature. Nowadays, several AI-powered search tools exist worldwide. The algorithm behind such tools usually relies on two functions: (1) scientific content mining and (2) advanced services, including rating, filtering and categorizing. NLP techniques, a subfield of ML, which aims to comprehend human language, are typically adopted for extracting scientific evidence [4]. NLP-based tools are not just able to simplify literature research through the selection of the most relevant references but can also establish a connection among the extracted papers, detecting complex and nonlinear relationships between sets of an overwhelming amount of variables [5]. This aspect can be potentially relevant for the CCT guideline development process. Cardiac imaging recommendations are included in a wide spectrum of CPG or consensus papers by major national and international cardiological societies, and collecting all the recommendation can be challenging and time-consuming.

Concerning quality assessment, AI-powered tools can only rank evidence according to their relevance, estimated by using the citation index.

A team of the Massachusetts Institute of Technology (MIT, Cambridge MA, USA) has developed a neural network able to produce a brief and plain English summary of academic papers, which could help to speed up the CGP development process and keep them up to date [6].

Clinical Decision-Making

The use of AI in clinical decision-making, particularly in the field of cardiology, is widely increasing, both for diagnostic support to physicians (diagnosis, staging and prognosis) and for therapeutic planning. Clinical decision support systems aim to assist and not replace clinicians in their daily routine; ML algorithms rely on their transparency, efficiency, and simplicity and must be based on scientific evidence that confirms their reproducibility, safety, and validity [7].The use of ML algorithms can be based on as follows: (1) supervised learning, such as artificial neural network, support vector machine, or decision tree, mainly focused on discriminative learning and used to solve classification and regression problems; (2) unsupervised learning, in which the algorithm derives conclusions from unlabeled data; (3) reinforcement learning, based on reward and particularly used for robots or games [8]. While supervised learning has been used to solve problems in the diagnosis and treatment of cardiovascular diseases (CVD), unsupervised learning could help finding new risk factors or elaborate new predictive models [9].To date, studies investigating the use of AI as an aid in prognostic assessment in the field of CV imaging techniques have focused primarily on CCT and its role in coronary artery disease (CAD). The prognosis of CAD is determined by a multifactorial interplay between demographical, clinical, and laboratory patient indices with CCT-based parameters such as coronary anatomy, physiology, and plaque morphology. CCT is a widely used technique for the noninvasive assessment of CAD, as a one-stop-shop exam which allows to evaluate the degree of stenosis and its extent and the distribution and the composition of the plaques [10]. Multiple studies have demonstrated that CCT improves CAD risk stratification above patient's clinical risk defined by appropriate scores, such as the atherosclerotic cardiovascular disease risk score. As international guidelines have recently expanded the recommendation of CCT as a first-line investigation modality for patients with stable chest pain without known CAD, prognostic evaluation, such as survival analysis and assessment of response to atherosclerotic treatment, has become an important object of study in the field of CCT. More recently, in the ESC 2020 guidelines [11], the use of CCT extended to patients with non-ST elevation myocardial infarction and patients with low-intermediate pre-test probability of acute coronary syndrome. This further expanded the clinical arena of CCT use and triggers the development of appropriate diagnostic algorithms for patient selection.AI-based models have been applied for prognostic evaluation in CCT; in particular several ML-powered algorithms using CCT have been implemented in the last decade. Motwani et al. [12] used ML-based approach to predict a 5-year all-cause mortality in 10,030 patients with suspected CAD, combining 25 clinical variables with 44 CCT parameters. They demonstrated the feasibility of ML to improve prediction of death compared with the Framingham Risk Score, SSS, SIS, and Duke prognostic index (FRS, 0.61; SSS, 0.64; SIS, 0.64; DI, 0.62; P, 0.001). Van Rosendael et al. [13] created a similar prognostic model based on a ML algorithm that utilizes standard 16 coronary segment stenosis and plaque composition information (calcified, mixed, and non-calcified) derived from CCT. This model generated a risk score for adverse cardiac events among 8844 patients during a follow-up of >3 years and resulted in a greater prognostic accuracy (AUC 0.771) compared with current CCT-based risk scores (AUC ranging from 0.685 to 0.701). Assessing and integrating the multitude of risk predictors from a variety of sources for a single patient represent a challenge for clinicians, and drawing an overall conclusion about risk in a single patient becomes even more complex. The use of AI-based methods not only can help clinicians providing integration between CCT data (e.g., plaque volumes, stenosis severity, lesion length, contrast density difference, fractional flow reserve) and clinical data in performing risk assessment but also opens up a new perspective on traditional prognostic methods. Specifically, the ML method is not a "hypothesis-driven" approach and thus allows the exploration of all available data for nonlinear relationships that can predict the risk of a particular individual. This approach avoids overlooking important but unexpected predictor variables or interactions. Beyond the enthusiasm for exploring the potential of AI for decision support, several current limitations of the use of AI in the clinical setting must be taken into account. Some of these limitations are the need for larger datasets of patients with different characteristics (e.g., ethnicity, gender, age) in order to produce appropriate generalized models, as well as the problem of standardization and sharing of data and model settings [14]. The use of AI in CCT is a large and growing field of research, and in the context of clinical decision-making, it can be an additional step forward toward the realization of the personalized medicine process.

Conclusions

The recent development of numerous guidelines and consensus papers in the field of cardiac CT has certainly contributed to reach the goal of precision medicine. However, in both diagnostic and therapeutic strategies, the clinical approach can be blurred by the large amount of existing literature. In this scenario, AI techniques can contribute to the process of guidelines development as well as in their interpretation in the clinical decision-making.

Bibliography

1. Esposito A, Gallone G, Palmisano A, Marchitelli L, Catapano F, Francone M. The current landscape of imaging recommendations in cardiovascular clinical guidelines: toward an imaging-guided precision medicine. Radiol Med. 2020;125(11):1013–23. https://doi.org/10.1007/s11547-020-01286-9.
2. World Health Organisation. Handbook for guideline development. World Heal Organ. March, 2010.
3. Weng SF, Vaz L, Qureshi N, Kai J. Prediction of premature all-cause mortality: a prospective general population cohort study comparing machine-learning and standard epidemiological approaches. PLoS One. 2019;14(3):e0214365. https://doi.org/10.1371/journal.pone.0214365.
4. Extance A. How AI technology can tame the scientific literature. Nature. 2018;561(7722):273–4. https://doi.org/10.1038/d41586-018-06617-5.
5. Kricka LJ, et al. Artificial intelligence-powered search tools and resources in the fight against covid-19. Electron J Int Fed Clin Chem Lab Med. 2020;31(2):106–16.
6. Dangovski R, Jing L, Nakov P, Tatalović M, Soljačić M. Rotational unit of memory: a novel representation unit for RNNs with scalable applications. Trans Assoc Comput Linguist. 2019;7:121–38. https://doi.org/10.1162/tacl_a_00258.
7. Shortliffe EH, Sepúlveda MJ. Clinical decision support in the era of artificial intelligence. JAMA J Am Med Assoc. 2018;320(21):2199–200. https://doi.org/10.1001/jama.2018.17163.
8. Al'Aref SJ, et al. Clinical applications of machine learning in cardiovascular disease and its relevance to cardiac imaging. Eur Heart J. 2019;40(24):1975–86. https://doi.org/10.1093/eurheartj/ehy404.
9. Krittanawong C, Zhang HJ, Wang Z, Aydar M, Kitai T. Artificial intelligence in precision cardiovascular medicine. J Am Coll Cardiol. 2017;69(21):2657–64. https://doi.org/10.1016/j.jacc.2017.03.571.
10. Lim LJ, Tison GH, Delling FN. Artificial Intelligence in Cardiovascular Imaging. Methodist Debakey Cardiovasc J. 2020;16(2):138–45. https://doi.org/10.14797/mdcj-16-2-138.
11. Collet JP, et al. 2020 ESC guidelines for the management of acute coronary syndromes in patients presenting without persistent ST-segment elevation. Eur Heart J. 2020. https://doi.org/10.1093/eurheartj/ehaa575.
12. Motwani M, et al. Machine learning for prediction of all-cause mortality in patients with suspected coronary artery disease: a 5-year multicentre prospective registry analysis. Eur Heart J. 2017;38(7):500–7. https://doi.org/10.1093/eurheartj/ehw188.
13. van Rosendael AR, et al. Maximization of the usage of coronary CTA derived plaque information using a machine learning based algorithm to improve risk stratification; insights from the CONFIRM registry. J Cardiovasc Comput Tomogr. 2018;12(3):204–9. https://doi.org/10.1016/j.jcct.2018.04.011.
14. Siegersma KR, Leiner T, Chew DP, Appelman Y, Hofstra L, Verjans JW. Artificial intelligence in cardiovascular imaging: state of the art and implications for the imaging cardiologist. Neth Hear J. 2019;27(9):403–13. https://doi.org/10.1007/s12471-019-01311-1.

Natural Language Processing for Cardiovascular Applications

23

Amara Tariq, Thiago Santos, and Imon Banerjee

Introduction

Healthcare databases are growing exponentially, and the majority of the clinical information is embedded with clinical narratives, e.g., physician and nursing notes and radiology and pathology reports, since free text is the more natural and expressive method to document clinical events and facilitate communication among the care team in the healthcare environment. Text analytics and natural language processing (NLP) systems can turn this data into value. In the other words, developing computation models for understanding natural language data can help to unlock such wealth of data which has paramount value for advancing healthcare. However, extracting targeted information from free-text clinical narratives is a highly challenging task due to the ambiguity and subtlety of natural language and variations in syntactic style among different healthcare personnel and template variations among different organizations. NLP systems for clinical narratives are used to perform syntactic processing (e.g., tokenization, sentence detection), extract information (i.e., convert unstructured text into a structured form), capture meaning (i.e., assign a concept to a word or group of words), and detect relationships (i.e., assign relationships between concepts) from free text through the use of defined language rules and relevant domain knowledge and/or learning from the domain datasets. Due to the immense value of converting the wealth of clinical narratives into structured format, NLP applications in healthcare are one of the most popular areas of computational research and development from the 1970s up to the present.

Information extraction, (IE) which automatically extracts and encodes relevant clinical information from text, is one of the prominent NLP applications and serves as a critical component to facilitate the use of free-text data for clinical decision support, quality improvement, or clinical and translation research, e.g., extraction of gene-disease relations from scientific literature, extraction of patient's comorbidities, or medications history from clinic notes. Extraction of such patient characteristics from the large hospital database may also aid in automated cohort selection process for statistical analysis and clinical trial. Wide variety of NLP literature deals with extraction of such important pieces of information from free-flowing cardiovascular related text. For example, deep learning-based algorithm is used to identify 14 different radiographic findings from thoracoabdominal computed tomography (CT) reports of heart failure patients in the work done by Pandey et al. [54]. Rule-based approach was used to identify critical results from *radiology reports* [37]. Rule-based NLP approaches have been also used for automatic cohort selection through processing of patients' clinical records [19, 60, 62].

In addition to clinic notes, radiology and pathology reports are a rich resource for advancing machine learning applications in medicine by leveraging the large volume of imaging data continuously being updated, integrated, and shared. However, there are significant challenges as well, largely due to the unstructured nature of the free-form documentation of image findings. To effectively "mine" these large free-text data sets for hypotheses testing, a robust strategy for extracting the necessary information is needed. To unlock this rich source of medical data, several standard

A. Tariq, PhD
Department of Radiology, Mayo Clinic, Phoenix, Arizona, USA

T. Santos, MS
Department of Computer Science, Emory University, Atlanta, GA, USA
e-mail: thiago.pereira.maia.do.santos@emory.edu

I. Banerjee, PhD (✉)
Department of Radiology, Mayo Clinic, Phoenix, Arizona, USA

Department of Computer Engineering, SCAI, Arizona State University, Tempe, USA
e-mail: imon.banerjee@emory.edu

C. N. De Cecco et al. (eds.), *Artificial Intelligence in Cardiothoracic Imaging*, Contemporary Medical Imaging,
https://doi.org/10.1007/978-3-030-92087-6_23

NLP methods (rule-based, dictionary-based, supervised learning) have been successfully applied to radiology and pathology reports for extracting information and/or performing *automatic report classification and assigning labels according to the pre-defined coding criteria* [6, 7, 9, 47, 56, 66]. Such automated scoring/labeling of data may not only have many applications in machine learning work by providing accurate labeling of medical images on a large scale from the radiology report; these techniques may also be valuable for computing accurate diagnostic scoring while reducing inter-rater variability.

Finally, NLP also plays a crucial role in clinical outcome prediction which has a strong implication for health service delivery of clinical treatment processes (CTPs) and is important for both patients and healthcare providers. Previous studies typically use a priori knowledge, such as demographics or patient physical factors, to estimate clinical outcomes at early stages of CTPs (e.g., admission). Cardiology-related applications may include mortality risk prediction [22], treatment strategy prediction [31], etc. Even though clinic notes contain wealth of information, rarely prediction tasks include information from clinic notes due to complexity of IE. Some recent studies applied complex semantic NLP models to harness the power of temporal clinical encounter notes and showed tremendous performance improvement over structured only data [4, 32, 64].

The rest of the chapter is organized as follows – section "NLP Methodologies" introduces the timeline of NLP methodologies and briefly describes the rationale; section "Existing NLP Methods and Applications" presents the systematic survey of the state-of-the-art NLP tools introduced in the cardiovascular domain starting from the 1990s up to 2020; finally, we summarize the current advancements in field and share our views on future directions in section "Conclusion".

NLP Methodologies

Natural language processing was first introduced back in the early 1950s, as a step on research toward achieving an automatic translation of languages, led by John Hutchins and IBM [33]. Figure 23.1 presents the overall timeline of the appearance of NLP methodologies in generic, clinical and particularly in cardiology applications. NLP reached the medical domain only in the early 1970s with one of the first works from R. Wong et al. – an automated parsing routine for diagnostic statements of surgical pathology reports, which was used as a clinical decision support in hospitals [72]. Almost a decade later, we started to see NLP on cardiology specific tasks. K. Canfield et al. used NLP and Unified Medical Language System (UMLS) to create a patient database for echocardiography. In the following subsections, we briefly introduced the core methodologies and their advancement.

Rule-Based and Intelligent Systems

We define rule-based NLP as the techniques that do not require any training or learning phase (Fig. 23.2a). Decisions are made based on predefined rules set by domain experts

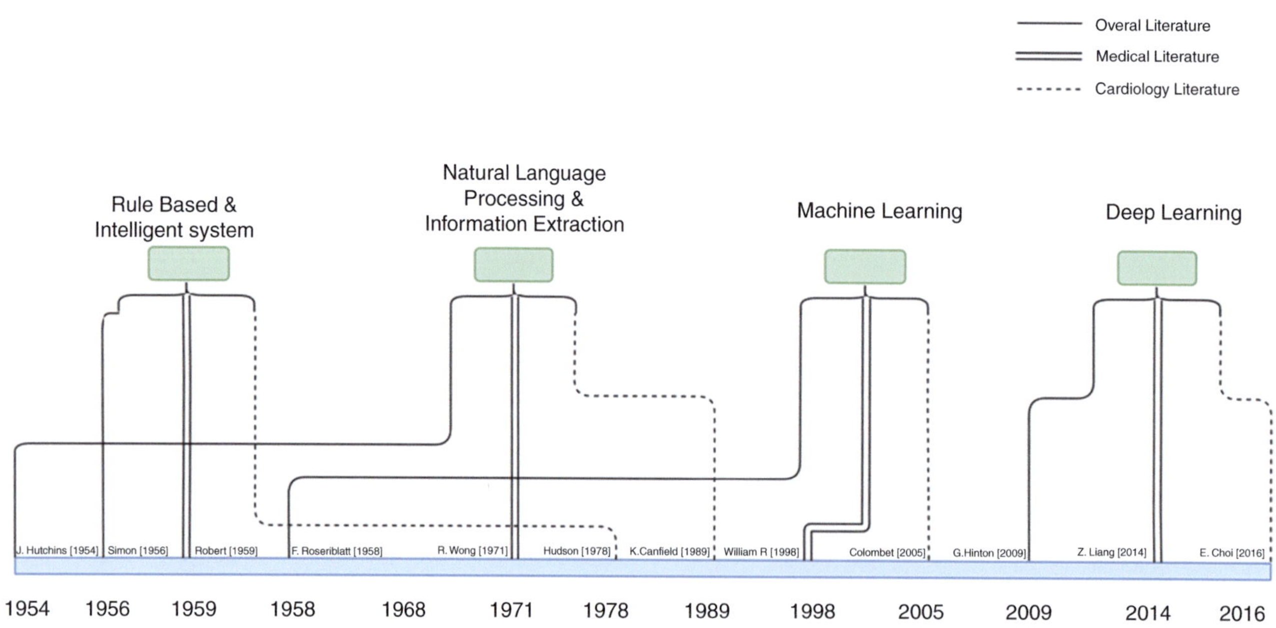

Fig. 23.1 Timeline of NLP methodologies, starting from traditional rule-based proposed in 1954 up to recent deep learning models. Applications also highlighted for generic clinical and cardiology domain (dashed line)

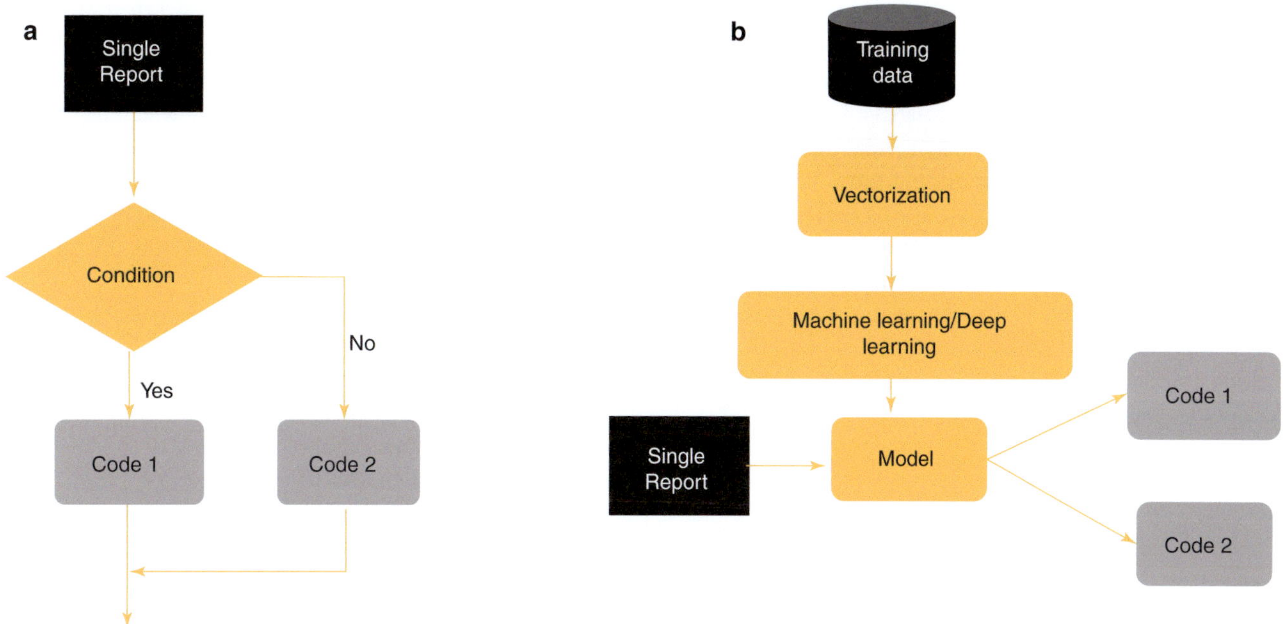

Fig. 23.2 Working principle of rule-based (**a**) and machine learning and deep learning systems (**b**)

using their prior knowledge. For example, a rule to identify birth dates of people from text is *{ (([{ PERSON }]) /was/ /born/ /on/ ([{ DATE }])) => "DATE_OF_BIRTH" }*. This simple rule is applied on Wikipedia text, and dates of birth of thousands of noted people can be identified automatically. Regular expressions are an important part of rule-based NLP technique that are used to describe text characteristics of interest or strings to be extracted from the text. A good example of rule-based NLP for biomedical data is provided on Chen, Hinote, and Chen [12] where rule-based NLP is being used to handle co-reference resolution.

Looking back at the history, "intelligent systems" in the form of rule-based were first introduced in the late 1950s, by Simon and Newell with their math theorems proof solver, named Logic Theorist [27]. They used a mix of symbolic logic and rule-based to create a program that could prove a given theorem. Their work was perhaps the first program that simulated some aspects of peoples' ability to solve complex problems. With the spread use of rule-based systems, it did not take long to be first introduced to the medical domain. A study in 1959 by Ledley et al. has shown how the use of computers and symbolic logic could be used to create a rule-based system to narrow down the options of the diagnoses, based on the given symptoms of the patient [39]. Although rule-based and intelligent systems were first introduced in the late 1950s, they were used for a cardiology-specific task as early as in 1978. Hudson et al. developed an expert system capable of helping doctors on clinical decision-making for chest pain analysis in the emergency room (Hudson, L. Donna, & Estrin, 1978). Similar to Ledley et al. study [39], the system was able to narrow down the options of the diagnosis based on patient symptoms and condition.

Machine Learning (ML)

We define machine learning-based NLP as all text processing algorithms that include learning mechanism to be trained from available data (Fig. 23.2b). Machine learning is a very promising field since the late 1950s. The first well-known project comes from Frank Rosenblatt in 1958, with the creation of perception, a type of artificial neural network that simulates human thought processes [59]. Due to the limitations of computer resources and advancements in the area of ML and its understandings, it was only in the late 1990s that medical research started to dive in the power that machine learning could bring. One of the first works proposed is from William R. Hersh et al. where they use machine learning and NLP to predict Trauma Registry Procedure Codes from emergency room patient notes [30]. To achieve their goal, they used only words and phrases from the dictated report by the initial ER physician to predict procedures that were performed during the first 24 hours after arrival to the ER. Not many years later, I. Colombet et al. proposed to use a multivariate ML approach for predicting cardiovascular disease risk which is a very complicated task [15].

Broadly ML approaches can be divided into two sets, i.e., (i) supervised and (ii) unsupervised. Supervised machine learning algorithms learn the mapping function f(x) from the input x to the output y. Supervised learning problems can be further grouped into regression and classification algorithms. Classification algorithms predict discrete labels out of a given labels set such as {`malignant', `benign'} or set of CAD-RADS scores [16] as labels, i.e., {0,1,2,3,4,5}. Popular classification algorithms include linear discriminator, random forest, maximum entropy, support vector machine (SVM), Gaussian Naive Bayes (NB), etc. [29]. On the other hand, regression algorithms predict continuous output value such as dollar amount of healthcare cost. Linear regression is the very basic regression algorithm, while more sophisticated regression approaches include regularization approach which applies some restriction on the coefficients of the trained algorithm, e.g., ElasticNet [77]. In contrast, unsupervised ML algorithms require no labeled training data; instead, it allows the model to work on its own to discover patterns and information from the data. Clustering algorithms like K-means are one example of unsupervised learning that identify groups of items in the training data that are similar to each other according to some similarity measure [29].

Importantly, getting any free-flowing textual input, such as radiology reports, into a machine learning algorithm needs to be converted to an appropriate numeric representation, known as feature vector. Bag-of-words (BoW) is the very basic featurization technique where common words from a training set of texts are placed in a vocabulary set and each text is converted to an N-dimensional vector. Corresponding element value indicates the presence/absence or the count of that word in the given input text. In this approach, order of words in a document is completely ignored, and different words with similar meaning are considered two distinct words with no link to each other. Advanced featurization techniques, such as Word2Vec [68], have been designed that can consider word order as well as semantic similarity between two distinct words.

Deep Learning (DL)

Deep learning is a category of machine learning algorithms (Fig. 23.2b) where the architecture consists of several nonlinear hidden layers with millions of tunable parameters. Large training datasets along with huge computational resources are needed to train such complex models. Although the term deep learning was first introduced back in the 1980s by Rina Dechter and with some work on some combinations of multilayer perceptron and convolutions, like Yann LeCun works for recognizing handwritten ZIP codes [38], we consider the start and the big hit of deep learning to be later in the late 2000s. With the advancement of computer technology, processing speed, and lower price computational hardware, DL emerged and filled a big gap that ML itself could not handle. One of the most important steps in this new era came from Geoffrey Hinton et al. in 2009, in his work "Deep Belief Networks for phone recognition" in which he created a new model architecture, named restricted Boltzmann machines [45]. This model is a composition of multiple hidden layers, and each layer contains various latent variables. Each layer would be connected to the next one, but no connections inside of each layer.

Since 2010, there has been tremendous development in the field of deep learning for various application areas including natural language processing in medical domains. One of the first deep learning works in NLP was led by Z. Liang et al. in 2014 [74], with a goal of applying a deep belief network for unsupervised text feature extraction from clinic notes and then performing a simpler supervised classification model to predict the diagnosis (ICD-10 code). A few years later, in 2016, E. Choi et al. conducted one of the first DL applied projects for a cardiology task where they explored the use of recurrent neural networks to model temporal relations among events in EHRs and predict initial diagnosis of heart failure (HF) [20]. Gridach et al. used bidirectional long short-term memory (LSTM) to extract entities from free-flowing text such as text of scientific literature [26].

Existing NLP Methods and Applications

In order to obtain a comprehensive capture of potentially relevant NLP articles in the cardiovascular domain, we employed three arm search strategies: literature databases and top journals and snowballing. First, the PubMed, Google Scholar, and Web of Science databases were searched from 1995 up to Sept. 2020. In our search strategy, we included the key terms [((cardiology) OR (cardiac) OR (cardiovascular) OR (mild cardiac) OR (heart) OR (coronary)) AND ((nlp) OR (Natural language processing))]. As a second search strategy, we searched among top 20 journals in biomedical informatics and top 10 journals in cardiology and cardiovascular medicine according to impact factors in 2020 by Google Scholar Metrics. Further hand searches (snowballing) were also conducted to survey literature regarding application of NLP in the field of cardiology and cardiovascular medicine.

State-of-the-Art Information Extraction

Table 23.1 lists the 32 relevant prior works starting from the mid-1990s focused on the task of information extraction from clinical text where we present the year of publication,

Table 23.1 Prior publications related to information extraction applied to the domain of cardiology

Citation	Year	Methodology	Extraction task	Data	Evaluation
[17]	2020	Deep Learning	Radiologic findings, anatomical location, descriptors	Radiology reports (chest X-ray, brain MRI, and Babygram from the MIMIC III clinical database)	BERT_large: F-score = 81.61, using gold spatial triggers F-score = 66.25, using predicted triggers
[54]	2020	Deep learning	Radiographic findings	CT reports	AUC = 0.97, F-score = 0.90
[40]	2020	Deep learning	Identify symptoms from patient notes	Patient notes (manually annotated)	Accuracy = 99.4%, recall = 66.8%, Precision = 77.6%, F1 score = 71.8
[63]	2019	Rule-based	Disease phenotyping	EMR – free-text reports	Inclusion of free-text information increased the sensitivity for detection and classification of the type of myocardial infarction (MI)
[46]	2019	Rule-based	Risk factors for sudden cardiac death	EMR – clinical narratives	Sensitivity = 0.96, 0.91, and 0.95; specificity = 0.90, 0.98, and 0.95; PPV = 0.90, 0.97, and 0.92; NPV = 0.96, 0.96, and 0.97 (syncope, FH-SCD, and FH-HCM, respectively)
[34]	2018	Rule-based	Asthma predictive indexing	EMR – Clinical notes	Sensitivity = 86%, specificity = 98%, PPV = 88%, NPV = 98% comparison between NLP and manual chart review: Kappa index = 0.86, agreement = 97%
[25]	2018	Rule-based, machine learning	Concept extraction for quality control for heart failure procedures	EMR – Free-text TIU reports	Patient level sensitivity = 98.9%, PPV = 98.7%; HF medication extraction: Recall = 97.8–99.7%, precision = 96–97.8% LVEF mention: recall = 97.8–98.6%, precision = 98.6–99.4% RNM extraction: accuracy = 31.1–40.4%, recall = 24.7–32.1%
[3]	2017	Rule-based	Peripheral arterial disease detection and surveillance	EMR – -all clinical notes	PPV = 0.93, sensitivity = 0.70, NPV = 0.80, specificity = 0.95
[8]	2017	Machine learning	Coronary artery disease	EMR – -all clinical notes	Naïve Bayes: F = score = 68.8%; ontology filter for feature extraction without PCA, F-score = 76.6% ML for feature extraction: F-score = 77.1%
[55]	2017	Rule-based	Electrocardiogram measures	EMR – -all clinical notes	27 measurements extracted: high precision for every extraction (>0.92) Low recall range (0.4)
[35]	2017	Rule-based, machine learning	Left ventricular ejection information	EMR – ECG reports, clinical notes	CHIEF EF: F-score = 80.7%, high accuracy CHIEF ADAHF: F-score = 69.1%, low accuracy
[2]	2017	Machine learning	Peripheral arterial disease	EMR – clinical notes	F1 NLP,91.8%; full model, 81.8%; simple model, 83%; P < 0.001; PPV NLP, 92.9%; full model, 74.3%, simple model, 79.9%; P < 0.001; and specificity NLP, 92.5%; full model, 64.2%; simple model, 75.9%; P < 0.001
[1]	2016	Rule-based	Peripheral arterial disease	EMR – clinical notes	PPV = 0.92, sensitivity = 0.96, NPV = 0.99, specificity = 0.98
(Topaz, et al.)	2016	Rule-based	Extraction of wound information	EMR – clinical notes (discharge summaries, outpatient notes)	F-measure =92.7% Wound treatment: F-score = 95.7% Wound size: F-score = 81.9%
[21]	2016	Machine learning	Identify patients with high-risk for heart failure	EMR – Dictated free-text	Sensitivity = 95.3%, specificity = 97.5%, PPV = 97.45%
[73]	2015	Rule-based, machine learning	Risk factors for heart disease	EMR, 2014 i2b2/ UTHealth NLP Challenge, Medical reports	Micro-averaged F-score = 0.915
[70]	2015	Rule-based	Risk factors for heart disease	2014 i2b2 Challenges	F-score = 0.890, precision improved by 10.3% without the use of lexicon

(continued)

Table 23.1 (continued)

Citation	Year	Methodology	Extraction task	Data	Evaluation
[42]	2015	Rule-based	Coronary artery disease screening algorithm	EMR – ICD9 + clinic notes	Including NLP into the CAD algorithm improved the sensitivity of the algorithm in both IBD and DM, with the greatest gains in IBD (14% increase in subjects classified with CAD at 90% PPV)
[71]	2015	Rule-based	Detection of congestive heart failure	Clinical notes	PPV 0.914
[69]	2015	Rule-based, machine learning	Detection of risk factors for heart disease	2014 i2b2/UTHealth Challenge	Overall F1 score = 0.9185, recall = 0.9409, precision = 0.8972
[10]	2014	Rule-based	Identification for heart failure diagnostic criteria	EMR: all clinical notes	Precision = 0.925, recall = 0.896, F-score = 0.910
[52]	2010	Rule-based	Aspirin use among population at risk for cardiovascular events	EMR – clinical notes	Aspirin: sensitivity = 99% (95% CI [97100]), specificity = 91% (95% CI [88 97]). Contraindications: sensitivity = 92% (95% CI [84 97]), specificity = 71% (95% CI [60 80])
[28]	2010	Rule-based	Relations between risk factors and pathologies	Medline repository of research papers	(1) Over 88% of risk factors for coronary heart disease are correct; (2) associated pathologies are correct in about 70% cases
[36]	2010	Rule-based	Genome-wide association for peripheral arterial disease	EMR – clinical notes	Precision = 67% to 100%, recall = 84% to 100%
[48]	2010	Rule-based	Knowledge extraction and representation	Medical literature	Results – ongoing
[18]	2009	Rule-based	Identify QT prolongation	ECG reports – impressions	NLP (UMLS): sensitivity = 0.996, PPV = 1.000 RegEx: sensitivity = 0.999, PPV = 0.982 Baseline (QTc threshold): sensitivity = 0.994–0.046, PPV = 0.07–0.25
[50, 53]	2007	Rule-based, machine learning	Identification of heart failure	EMR – clinical notes	Verified by manual review: NLP: PPV = 38% (95% CI = [36, 40]) ML: PPV = 82% (95% CI = [73, 93])
[50]	2007	Rule-based	Identification of angina/chest pain	EMR – free-text reports	TP rate for unspecified chest pain 62% (95% CI 55–67); exertional chest pain, TP rate was 71% (95% CI 61–80)
[23]	2006	Concept extraction	Concepts relating to congestive heart failure	Radiology reports	CHF (n = 556) sensitivity 0.64 specificity 1.0 Kerley B lines (n = 19) sensitivity 0.21 specificity 1.0; prominent PVa (n = 2337) sensitivity 0.73 specificity 0.99; pulmonary edema (n = 1650) sensitivity 0.73 specificity 1.0; cardiomegaly (n = 5200) sensitivity 0.91 specificity 0.99; pleural effusion (n = 3707) sensitivity 0.78 specificity 1.0
[14]	2005	Rule-based	Concept-value pair extraction	ECG reports	Precision = 99, recall = 78
[58]	2000	Rule-based	Arterial branching relations	Cardiac catheterization reports	Precision = 100, recall = 83
[5]	1998	Rule-based	Anatomical spatial relations	Clinical text	Precision = 0.67, recall = 0.78
[65]	1998	Rule-based	Coronary artery-related terms	Coronary catheterization reports	Precision = 0.88, recall = 0.83

targeted task, methodology, and performance in terms of standard statistical measures. The earlier works in this area were based only on rule-based NLP techniques, and popular applications have been the extraction of cardiac abnormalities from ECG reports, medical literature, clinical notes, etc. [65] and relationships between cardiac anatomical entities [5, 14, 18, 58]. In Pakhomov, Shah, Hanson, Balasubramaniam, and Smith [52], the use of aspirin among cardiac patients was detected by applying rule-based NLP techniques on free-text sections of EMR. Hamon, Graña, Raggio, Grabar, and Naya [28] describe a large-scale study of relation between health condition and over 22,000 risk factors extracted by applying rule-based techniques on published literature in Medline repository. Similarly, genome-wide associations were established using EMR data with factors like medication use, smoking, comorbidities, etc. [36]. Even in 2012, rule-based techniques such as regular expression and string matching were used on ECG reports from the Department of Veteran Affairs (VA) of United States to extract risk factors for heart failure [24]. Authors later published another work on the same data where they used machine learning for tagging sequences of text, in addition to rule-based techniques, to identify quality measure in heart failure procedures from the same data [25]. Extraction of heart failure factors was also performed using rule-based NLP on EMR data by focusing on all mentions of Farmingham's criteria [10].

Recently, a hybrid approach combining rule-based and machine learning techniques was used for risk factor extraction from 1304 medical reports of 296 patients in Yang and Garibaldi [73]. Similar hybrid risk factor extraction and classification model is described in Torii M. F. [69] to extract left ventricular ejection fraction from ECG reports of VA data [35]. Risk factors are extracted from clinical notes using named entity recognition in [70]. A screening algorithm for coronary artery disease (CAD) across cohorts of three different chronic diseases (diabetes, RA, and IBD) is described in [42] where NLP techniques are used to extract information from free-text notes. Cases of congestive heart failure (CHF) were identified using rule-based NLP techniques in clinical notes from healthcare records of the state of Maine in United States [71]. Authors (Afzal et al. [1]) proposed rule-based NLP method to automate the chart review process for identification of peripheral arterial disease (PAD). Dictionary-based keyword extraction has been used for surveillance of the same disease in 1569 clinical reports from Mayo clinic [3]. Similar extraction was performed for wound information in EMR data of cardiac patients (Topaz, et al.). Rule-based NLP extraction techniques have been used to expand vocabulary of terms related to heart disease using ECG reports from VA's data [55].

Recently, more sophisticated rule-based NLP systems and tools have been developed and deployed for information extraction such as Unified Medical Language System (UMLS)[1] and MedTagger [43]. MedTagger was used to extract PAD-related concepts from tens of thousands of clinical notes [2]. cTAKES (Clinical Text Analysis and Knowledge Extraction System) has been used for extraction of relevant concepts to predict CAD using clinical narratives [8]. In 2019, a study was performed to investigate cause of death in UK primary care records focused on myocardial infarction and death [63]. In this study, Foundation Model of Anatomy (FMA) was used which maps diagnosis in free-text EMR to structured format. Another study was performed on EMR of hypertrophic cardiomyopathy (HCM) patients to detect cardiac death risk factors such as family history of HCM, syncopal episode within the last 5 years, etc. [46].

Application of deep learning for the task of information extraction is another modern trend. Popular transformer model, i.e., BERT (Bidirectional Encoder Representations from Transformers), was used for labeling free-text sequences from radiology reports such as chest X-ray, brain MRI, and Babygrams for extraction of spatial relation among biomedical entities [17]. An example of spatial relations is "*Disorder* – extends into – *Anatomical Location.*" Convolutional neural network (CNN) has been used for extraction of predefined radiologic findings from thoracoabdominal radiology reports [54].

State-of-the-Art Classification

Table 23.2 summarizes the publications that targeted classification of the notes/reports using NLP in the cardiovascular medicine domain, and we found eight relevant publications since 2005. Machine learning classifiers like Naïve Bayes and multilayer perceptrons were used on clinical notes to classify patients as suitable or unsuitable candidates for a study regarding congestive heart failure [51]. Chest X-ray reports written in Portuguese were translated to English using machine translation model so that MedLEE can be applied on them for identification of patients with and without support devices [11]. Risk factors for heart failure were identified based on the accuracy of classifier for coronary artery disease detection built using these factors as features [69]. Data from i2b2/UTHealth challenge was used for this system. New York

[1] https://www.nlm.nih.gov/research/umls/index.html.

Table 23.2 Prior publications related to classification applied to the domain of cardiology

Citation	Year	Methodology	Classification Task	Data	Evaluation
[49]	2020	Deep learning	Identify ischemic stroke, acuity, and location	Radiology reports (CT, MRI, CTA, or MRA)	Glove + RNN: AUC = 0.96, 0.98, 0.93 with presence, location, and acuity of ischemic stroke, respectively
[67]	2019	Deep learning	Convert unstructured CTPA reports into structured format	CT pulmonary angiography (CTPA) reports	Accuracy = 91% (with only one label per sentence) Accuracy = 96% (with more than one label per sentence)
[41]	2019	Deep learning	Detection of bleeding events	Expert-annotated clinical notes	Bleeding event annotation: AUC = 0.957, F-score = 0.938
[76]	2018	Machine learning	New York Heart Association classification	EMR – heart failure patient notes	Random forest with n-gram features: F1 = 93.78%.
[75]	2017	Machine learning	New York Heart Association classification	EMR – heart failure patient notes	Rule-based: F-score = 93.37% SVM: F-score = 93.57%
[69]	2015	Machine learning	Identification of risk factors for heart disease	2014 i2b2/UTHealth Challenge	F-score = 0.9185, recall = 0.9409, precision = 0.8972
[11]	2007	Rule-based, machine learning	Thoracic diagnosis for Portuguese reports	Chest X-ray reports	Normal reports: sensitivity =1, specificity = 0.71 Reports with devices (catheter, implants, etc.): sensitivity = 0.97, specificity = 0.97
[51]	2005	Machine learning	Patient selection for congestive heart failure study	Clinical notes	Naïve Bayes: recall on +ve sample = 95%, accuracy = 57% Perceptron: recall on +ve sample = 86%, accuracy = 65% Baseline: recall on +ve sample = 71%, accuracy = 54%

Heart Association (NYHA) functional classification system is used by cardiologists to categorize heart failure patients based on limitation on their physical activity. Patient notes from EMR data have been used to automatically assign this classification to patients. Such classification relies on machine learning-based classifiers such as SVM and random forest classifier [75, 76].

In recent past, deep learning techniques have gained popularity to build sophisticated classification models for cardiology-related text. For example, a sentence-by-sentence bleeding event detector was built using CNN and bidirectional LSTM for notes recorded in EMR [41]. Another sentence-by-sentence deep learning classifier was built to map unstructured CT reports into a template where each sentence is tagged with label (e.g., pulmonary arteries, lungs and airways, pleura, mediastinum and lymph nodes, cardiovascular, soft tissues and bones, upper abdomen, lines/tubes) identifying the type of information it describes [67]. Information regarding ischemic stroke such as its presence, location, and acuity were detected using recurrent neural network (RNN) on the text of radiology reports like CT, MRI, CTA, or MRA [49].

State-of-the-Art Prediction

Table 23.3 presents prediction problems that have been formulated over the years using cardiology-related text. Rule-based prediction model was used to predict quality-of-care measure like reperfusion rate, beta-blockers, and lipid-lowering agent before discharge, and reasonable level of agreement has been found between experts and the rule-based predictors [13]. Decision support system was developed to predict which patients can be weaned off of ventricular assistive device [61]. Modulators for electrocardiographic interval were identified from clinical notes based on their predictive power for the interval value [57]. Simple machine learning classifier was used to predict the risk of readmission of cardiac patient using structured and unstructured information such as clinical notes from EMR data [44]. XGBoost, a machine learning-based classifier, was used to predict suitable patients for cardiac resynchronization therapy using free-text notes from EMR [31]. A large-scale study was conducted to predict mortality and cardiopulmonary arrest among 235,826 patients arriving in Portuguese emergency departments (ED) between 2012 and 2016 using data collected in ED [22].

Meta-Analysis

We performed a multidimensional meta-analysis of the reviewed article (Fig. 23.3) and found that IE from clinical text has been most popular area (53.33%) of NLP research in cardiology domain. Even though the final performance varied based on the targeted tasks, many publications presented >90% accuracy with simple regex rules for detection of abnormalities (Table 23.1). Hybrid models that combine machine learning and rule-based system are also very popular architecture for developing the NLP systems, although sequential deep learning models (12.96%) are adopted recently for extraction of spatial relation among biomedical entities and classification predefined radiologic findings from thoracoabdominal radiology reports (X-ray, CT). Given the difficulties in handling varying free-text clinic narratives due to variations in documentation styles, prediction using NLP is still a challenging area, and limited work has been done. Our analysis also highlights most of the NLP research (43.59%) that has been done of a pre-selected set of clinical narratives where expert opinion has been incorporated for selection. The use of open-source clinical dataset (2014 i2b2/UTHealth Challenge and NIH Chest X-ray dataset) has also generated significant number of interesting publications.

Conclusion

In this chapter, we introduce the basic NLP methodologies from a high level, and we did a systematic review of the published NLP models in the cardiovascular domain starting from the 1990s. We benchmarked 47 NLP publications proposed in the cardiovascular domain in terms of methodology developed, dataset used, and performance. Several NLP systems achieved human-level performance for information extraction and classification, including radiologic findings and cardiovascular outcomes. Even though deep learning models (RNN, CNN, and transformer) became the most popular architectures for NLP tasks for cardiovascular applications recently (starting from 2012), traditional rule-based systems are still widely used. In summary, the field is still advancing by implementing highly efficient algorithm using complex computational methodologies, such as transformer model, CNN, and large open-source de-identified clinical datasets, similar to i2b2, may overcome the training data limitation and serve as a key for the introduction of new advance deep methodologies.

Table 23.3 Prior publications related to prediction applied to the domain of cardiology

Citation	Year	Methodology	Prediction task	Data	Evaluation
[22]	2020	Machine learning	Mortality and cardiopulmonary arrest	EMR patient notes	AUROC = 0.96, AUPRC = 0.31, recall = 0.84, precision = 0.06, F-score = 0.12
[31]	2019	Machine learning	Patient selection for cardiac resynchronization therapy	EMR – free-text reports	Model identified 26% of patients at a PPV of $79\%_{\beta}$ ($\beta = 0.1$) = 77%, recall = 0.26, precision = 0.79, accuracy = 0.65
[44]	2019	Machine learning	Prediction of risk for readmission for heart failure	EMR – clinical notes	AUC 0.6447 [0.6386–0.6508] for combined model and offered 15% Net Benefit over its individual counterparts at a threshold predicted probability of 0.20
[57]	2011	Machine learning	Modulators/factors for electrocardiographic intervals	EMR – clinical notes, billing records	Positive predictive value of 97%
[61]	2010	Machine learning	Decision support model for ventricular assist devise weaning	Expert interviews, patients' clinical data	Hybrid model (expert knowledge + clinical information) performed the best with accuracy = 94.74% (95% confidence interval [75.37– 99.07%])
[13]	2010	Rule-based	Assessment of quality of care for cardiovascular diseases	Hospital discharge notes	Reasonable agreement (k value) with medical experts from 0.65 (early reperfusion rate) to 0.97 for different QC measures in the test set

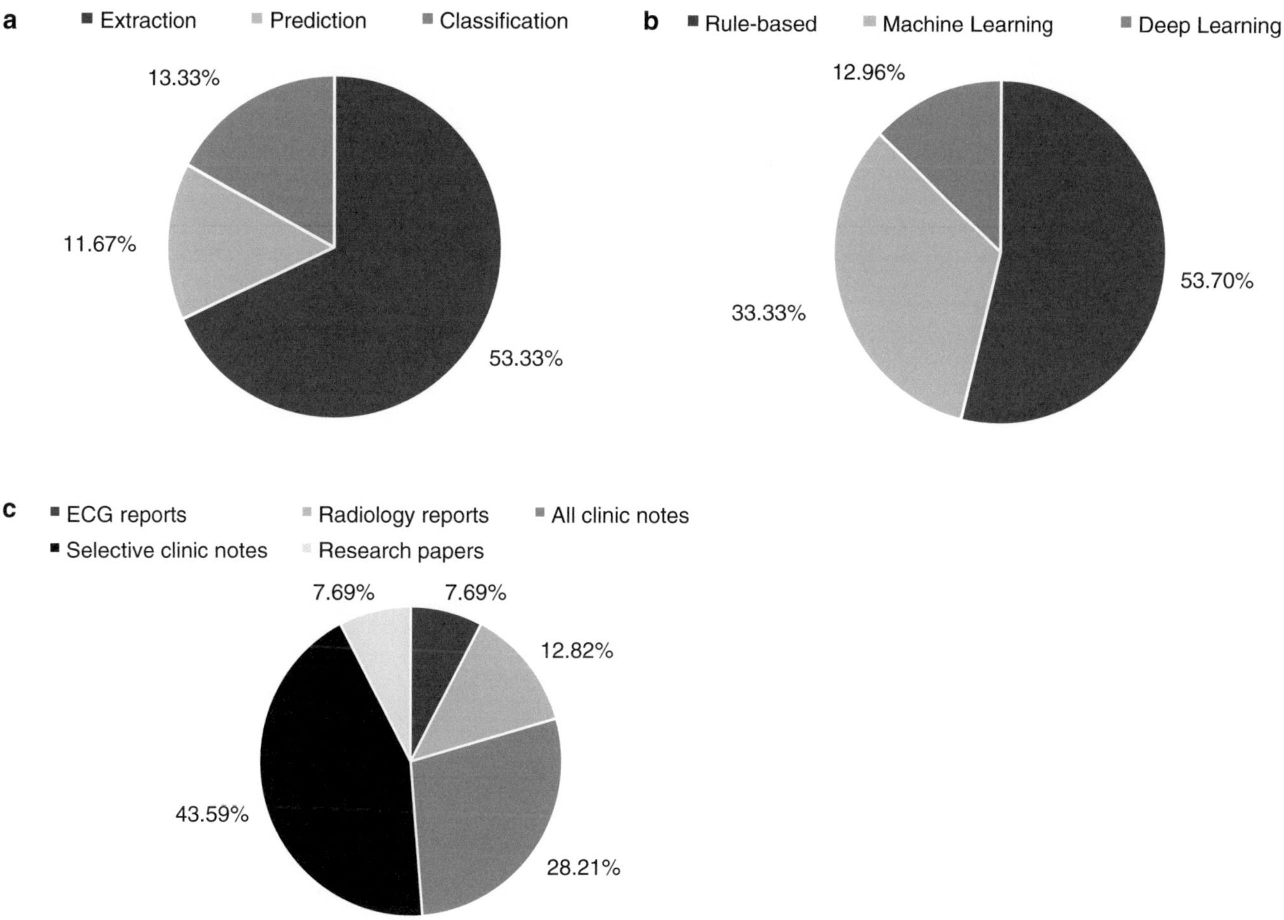

Fig. 23.3 Meta analysis of 47 benchmarked publications shown as pie charts – (**a**) task-wise, (**b**) algorithms, and (**c**) data used

References

1. Afzal N, Sohn S, Abram S, Liu H, Kullo IJ, Arruda-Olson AM. Identifying peripheral arterial disease cases using natural language processing of clinical notes. 2016 IEEE-EMBS International Conference on Biomedical and Health Informatics (BHI). pp. 126–31; 2016.
2. Afzal N, Sohn S, Abram S, Scott CG, Chaudhry R, Liu H, et al. Mining peripheral arterial disease cases from narrative clinical notes using natural language processing. J Vasc Surg. 2017;65:1753–61.
3. Afzal N, Sohn S, Scott CG, Liu H, Kullo IJ, Arruda-Olson AM. Surveillance of peripheral arterial disease cases using natural language processing of clinical notes. AMIA Summits on Translational Science Proceedings; 2017, 28.
4. Banerjee I, Gensheimer MF, Wood DJ, Henry S, Aggarwal S, Chang DT, et al. Probabilistic prognostic estimates of survival in metastatic cancer patients (PPES-Met) utilizing free-text clinical narratives. Sci Rep. 2018;8:1–12.
5. Bean CA, Rindflesch TC, Sneiderman CA. Automatic semantic interpretation of anatomic spatial relationships in clinical text. Proceedings of the AMIA Symposium. p. 897; 1998.
6. Bozkurt S, Alkim E, Banerjee I, Rubin DL. Automated detection of measurements and their descriptors in radiology reports using a hybrid natural language processing algorithm. J Digit Imaging. 2019;32:544–53.
7. Bozkurt S, Lipson JA, Senol U, Rubin DL. Automatic abstraction of imaging observations with their characteristics from mammography reports. J Am Med Inform Assoc. 2015;22:e81–92.
8. Buchan K, Filannino M, Uzuner Ö. Automatic prediction of coronary artery disease from clinical narratives. J Biomed Inform. 2017;72:23–32.
9. Burger G, Abu-Hanna A, de Keizer N, Cornet R. Natural language processing in pathology: a scoping review. J Clin Pathol. 2016;69:949–55.
10. Byrd RJ. Automatic identification of heart failure diagnostic criteria, using text analysis of clinical notes from electronic health records. Int J Med Inform. 2014;83:983–92.
11. Castilla AC, Furuie SS, Mendonça EA. Multilingual information retrieval in thoracic radiology: feasibility study. Stud Health Technol Inform. 2007;129:387.
12. Chen P, Hinote D, Chen G. A rule based solution to co-reference resolution in clinical text. J Am Med Inform Assoc. 2013;20:891–7.
13. Chiang J-H, Lin J-W, Yang C-W. Automated evaluation of electronic discharge notes to assess quality of care for cardiovascular diseases using Medical Language Extraction and Encoding System (MedLEE). J Am Med Inform Assoc. 2010;17:245–52.
14. Chung J, Murphy S. Concept-value pair extraction from semi-structured clinical narrative: a case study using echocardiogram reports. AMIA Ann Symp Proc. 2005;2005:131.
15. Colombet IE. Models to predict cardiovascular risk: comparison of CART, multilayer perceptron and logistic regression. Proceedings. AMIA Symposium, 156–60; 2000.

16. Cury RA. CAD-RADSTM coronary artery disease–reporting and data system. An expert consensus document of the Society of Cardiovascular Computed Tomography (SCCT), the American College of Radiology (ACR) and the North American Society for Cardiovascular Imaging (NASC. J Cardiovasc Comput Tomogr. 2016:269–81.
17. Datta S, Ulinski M, Godfrey-Stovall J, Khanpara S, Riascos-Castaneda RF, Roberts K. Rad-SpatialNet: a frame-based resource for fine-grained spatial relations in radiology reports. LREC... International Conference on Language Resources & Evaluation:[proceedings]. International Conference on Language Resources and Evaluation. p. 2251; 2020.
18. Denny JC, Miller RA, Waitman LR, Arrieta MA, Peterson JF. Identifying QT prolongation from ECG impressions using a general-purpose Natural Language Processor. Int J Med Inform. 2009;78:S34–42.
19. Dublin S, Baldwin E, Walker RL, Christensen LM, Haug PJ, Jackson ML, et al. Natural Language Processing to identify pneumonia from radiology reports. Pharmacoepidemiol Drug Saf. 2013;22:834–41.
20. Edward Choi AS. Using recurrent neuralnetwork models for early detection of heart failure onset. J Am Med Info Assoc. 2016;24:361–70.
21. Evans RS, Benuzillo J, Horne BD, Lloyd JF, Bradshaw A, Budge D, et al. Automated identification and predictive tools to help identify high-risk heart failure patients: pilot evaluation. J Am Med Inform Assoc. 2016;23:872–8.
22. Fernandes M, Mendes R, Vieira SM, Leite F, Palos C, Johnson A, et al. Risk of mortality and cardiopulmonary arrest in critical patients presenting to the emergency department using machine learning and natural language processing. PLoS One. 2020;15:e0230876.
23. Friedlin J, McDonald CJ. A natural language processing system to extract and code concepts relating to congestive heart failure from chest radiology reports. AMIA Ann Symp Proc. 2006;2006:269.
24. Garvin JH, DuVall SL, South BR, Bray BE, Bolton D, Heavirland J, et al. Automated extraction of ejection fraction for quality measurement using regular expressions in Unstructured Information Management Architecture (UIMA) for heart failure. J Am Med Inform Assoc. 2012;19:859–66.
25. Garvin JH, Kim Y, Gobbel GT, Matheny ME, Redd A, Bray BE, et al. Automating quality measures for heart failure using natural language processing: a descriptive study in the department of veterans affairs. JMIR Med Inform. 2018;6:e5.
26. Gridach M. Character-level neural network for biomedical named entity recognition. J Biomed Inform. 2017;70:85–91.
27. Gugerty L. Newell and Simon's logic theorist: historical background and impact on cognitive modeling. Proceedings of the human factors and ergonomics society annual meeting. 2006;50:880–4.
28. Hamon T, Graña M, Raggio V, Grabar N, Naya H. Identification of relations between risk factors and their pathologies or health conditions by mining scientific literature. Medinfo. pp. 964–8; 2010.
29. Hastie T, Tibshirani R, Friedman J. The elements of statistical learning: data mining, inference, and prediction. Springer Science & Business Media; 2009.
30. Hersh WR. Automatic prediction of trauma registry procedure codes from emergency room dictations. MedInfo; 1998.
31. Hu S-Y, Santus E, Forsyth AW, Malhotra D, Haimson J, Chatterjee NA, et al. Can machine learning improve patient selection for cardiac resynchronization therapy? PLoS One. 2019;14:e0222397.
32. Huang Z, Dong W, Ji L, Duan H. Outcome prediction in clinical treatment processes. J Med Syst. 2016;40:8.
33. Hutchins WJ. The Georgetown-IBM experiment demonstrated in January 1954. In: Frederking RE, Taylor KB, editors. Machine translation: from real users to research. Berlin: Springer Berlin Heidelberg; 2004. p. 102–14.
34. Kaur H, Sohn S, Wi C-I, Ryu E, Park MA, Bachman K, et al. Automated chart review utilizing natural language processing algorithm for asthma predictive index. BMC Pulm Med. 2018;18:1–9.
35. Kim Y, Garvin JH, Goldstein MK, Hwang TS, Redd A, Bolton D, et al. Extraction of left ventricular ejection fraction information from various types of clinical reports. J Biomed Inform. 2017;67:42–8.
36. Kullo IJ, Fan J, Pathak J, Savova GK, Ali Z, Chute CG. Leveraging informatics for genetic studies: use of the electronic medical record to enable a genome-wide association study of peripheral arterial disease. J Am Med Inform Assoc. 2010;17:568–74.
37. Lakhani P, Kim W, Langlotz CP. Automated detection of critical results in radiology reports. J Digit Imaging. 2012;25:30–6.
38. LeCun YB. Backpropagation applied to handwritten zip code recognition. Neural Comput. 1989;1:541–51.
39. Ledley RS, Lusted LB. Newell and Simon's logic theorist: historical background and impact on cognitive modeling. Am Assoc Adv Sci. 1959;130:9–31.
40. Leiter RE, Santus E, Jin Z, Lee KC, Yusufov M, Chien I, et al. Deep natural language processing to identify symptom documentation in clinical notes for patients with heart failure undergoing cardiac resynchronization therapy. J Pain Symptom Manage. 2020;60:948–58.
41. Li R, Hu B, Liu F, Liu W, Cunningham F, McManus DD, et al. Detection of bleeding events in electronic health record notes using convolutional neural network models enhanced with recurrent neural network autoencoders: deep learning approach. JMIR Med Inform. 2019;7:e10788.
42. Liao KP, Ananthakrishnan AN, Kumar V, Xia Z, Cagan A, Gainer VS, et al. Methods to develop an electronic medical record phenotype algorithm to compare the risk of coronary artery disease across 3 chronic disease cohorts. PLoS One. 2015;10:e0136651.
43. Liu H, Bielinski SJ, Sohn S, Murphy S, Wagholikar KB, Jonnalagadda SR, et al. An information extraction framework for cohort identification using electronic health records. AMIA Summits on Translational Science Proceedings, American Medical Informatics Association; 2013.
44. Mahajan SM, Ghani R. Combining structured and unstructured data for predicting risk of readmission for heart failure patients. MedInfo. pp. 238–42; 2019.
45. Mohamed A-R, Dahl G, Hinton G. Deep belief networks for phone recognition. In Nips workshop on deep learning for speech recognition and related applications. 2009;1:9.
46. Moon S, Liu S, Scott CG, Samudrala S, Abidian MM, Geske JB, et al. Automated extraction of sudden cardiac death risk factors in hypertrophic cardiomyopathy patients by natural language processing. Int J Med Inform. 2019;128:32–8.
47. Morioka C, Meng F, Taira R, Sayre J, Zimmerman P, Ishimitsu D, et al. Automatic classification of ultrasound screening examinations of the abdominal aorta. J Digit Imaging. 2016;29:742–8.
48. Nuzzo A, Mulas F, Gabetta M, Arbustini E, Zupan B, Larizza C, et al. Text mining approaches for automated literature knowledge extraction and representation. MedInfo. pp. 954–8; 2010.
49. Ong CJ, Orfanoudaki A, Zhang R, Caprasse FP, Hutch M, Ma L, et al. Machine learning and natural language processing methods to identify ischemic stroke, acuity and location from radiology reports. PLoS One. 2020;15:e0234908.
50. Pakhomov SS, Hemingway H, Weston SA, Jacobsen SJ, Rodeheffer R, Roger VL. Epidemiology of angina pectoris: role of natural language processing of the medical record. Am Heart J. 2007a;153:666–73.
51. Pakhomov SV, Buntrock J, Chute CG. Prospective recruitment of patients with congestive heart failure using an ad-hoc binary classifier. J Biomed Inform. 2005;38:145–53.
52. Pakhomov S, Shah N, Hanson P, Balasubramaniam S, Smith S. Automated processing of electronic medical records is a reliable method of determining aspirin use in populations at risk for cardiovascular events. J Innov Health Info. 2010;18:125–33.

53. Pakhomov S, Weston SA, Jacobsen SJ, Chute CG, Meverden R, Roger VL, et al. Electronic medical records for clinical research: application to the identification of heart failure. Am J Manag Care. 2007b;13:281–8.
54. Pandey M, Xu Z, Sholle E, Maliakal G, Singh G, Fatima Z, et al. Extraction of radiographic findings from unstructured thoracoabdominal computed tomography reports using convolutional neural network based natural language processing. PLoS One. 2020;15:e0236827.
55. Patterson OV, Freiberg MS, Skanderson M, Fodeh SJ, Brandt CA, DuVall SL. Unlocking echocardiogram measurements for heart disease research through natural language processing. BMC Cardiovasc Disord. 2017;17:151.
56. Pons E, Braun LM, Hunink MM, Kors JA. Natural language processing in radiology: a systematic review. Radiology. 2016;279:329–43.
57. Ramirez AH, Schildcrout JS, Blakemore DL, Masys DR, Pulley JM, Basford MA, et al. Modulators of normal electrocardiographic intervals identified in a large electronic medical record. Heart Rhythm. 2011;8:271–7.
58. Rindflesch TC, Bean CA, Sneiderman CA. Argument identification for arterial branching predications asserted in cardiac catheterization reports. Proceedings of the AMIA symposium. p. 704; 2000.
59. Rosenblatt F. The perceptron: a probabilistic model for information storage and organization in the brain. Psychol Rev. 1958;65:386–408.
60. Rubin D, Wang D, Chambers DA, Chambers JG, South BR, Goldstein MK. Natural language processing for lines and devices in portable chest x-rays. AMIA Ann Symp Proc. 2010;2010:692.
61. Santelices LC, Wang Y, Severyn D, Druzdzel MJ, Kormos RL, Antaki JF. Development of a hybrid decision support model for optimal ventricular assist device weaning. Ann Thorac Surg. 2010;90:713–20.
62. Schuemie MJ, Sen E, 't Jong GW, van Soest EM, Sturkenboom MC, Kors JA. Automating classification of free-text electronic health records for epidemiological studies. Pharmacoepidemiol Drug Saf. 2012;21:651–8.
63. Shah AD, Bailey E, Williams T, Denaxas S, Dobson R, Hemingway H. Natural language processing for disease phenotyping in UK primary care records for research: a pilot study in myocardial infarction and death. J Biomed Semantics. 2019;10:20.
64. Shickel B, Tighe PJ, Bihorac A, Rashidi P. Deep EHR: a survey of recent advances in deep learning techniques for electronic health record (EHR) analysis. IEEE J Biomed Health Inform. 2018;22:1589–604.
65. Sneiderman CA, Rindflesch TC, Bean CA. Identification of anatomical terminology in medical text. Proceedings of the AMIA symposium. p. 428; 1998.
66. Solti I, Cooke CR, Xia F, Wurfel MM. Automated classification of radiology reports for acute lung injury: comparison of keyword and machine learning based natural language processing approaches. 2009 IEEE international conference on bioinformatics and biomedicine workshop. pp. 314–9; 2009.
67. Spandorfer A, Branch C, Sharma P, Sahbaee P, Schoepf UJ, Ravenel JG, et al. Deep learning to convert unstructured CT pulmonary angiography reports into structured reports. Eur Radiol Exp. 2019;3:37.
68. Tomas Mikolov KC. Efficient estimation of word representations in vector space. Worskhop at ICLR; 2013.
69. Torii MF. Risk factor detection for heart disease by applying text analytics in electronic medical records. J Biomed Inform. 2015;58:S164–70.
70. Urbain J. Mining heart disease risk factors in clinical text with named entity recognition and distributional semantic models. J Biomed Inform. 2015;58:S143–9.
71. Wang Y, Luo J, Hao S, Xu H, Shin AY, Jin B, et al. NLP based congestive heart failure case finding: a prospective analysis on statewide electronic medical records. Int J Med Inform. 2015;84:1039–47.
72. Wong RL, Gaynon P. An automated parsing routine for diagnostic statements of surgical pathology reports. Methods Inf Med. 1971;10:168–75.
73. Yang H, Garibaldi JM. A hybrid model for automatic identification of risk factors for heart disease. J Biomed Inform. 2015;58:S171–82.
74. Liang Z, Zhang G. Deep learning for healthcare decision making with EMRs. International Conference on Bioinformatics and Biomedicine (BIBM); 2014.
75. Zhang R, Ma S, Shanahan L, Munroe J, Horn S, Speedie S. Automatic methods to extract New York heart association classification from clinical notes. 2017 ieee international conference on bioinformatics and biomedicine (bibm). pp. 1296–9; 2017.
76. Zhang R, Ma S, Shanahan L, Munroe J, Horn S, Speedie S. Discovering and identifying New York heart association classification from electronic health records. BMC Med Inform Decis Mak. 2018;18:48.
77. Zou HA. Regularization and variable selection via the elastic net. J R Stat Soc Series B Stat Methodology. 2005;67:301–20.

Artificial Intelligence-Based Evaluation of Coronary Calcium

24

Sanne G. M. van Velzen, Nils Hampe, Bob D. de Vos, and Ivana Išgum

Introduction

Cardiovascular disease (CVD) accounts for approximately one-third of all global deaths [1]. With obesity being a global health concern, worldwide rates of diabetes mellitus on the rise, and an increasing number of smokers in developing countries, the need for early detection of CVD risk is increasingly apparent.

Calcium scoring, a process in which arterial calcifications are detected and quantified in CT, has been shown to be valuable in prediction of cardiovascular events [2]. For instance, calcifications in the aortic arch and carotid arteries have been associated with an elevated risk of stroke [3, 4]. The amount of coronary artery calcification (CAC) is a strong and independent predictor of coronary heart disease (CHD) events [5, 6], and therefore, calcium scoring is most often applied to the coronary arteries.

Calcium scoring is standardly performed in CT scans without contrast enhancement, where lesions are defined as a high-density area of ≥ 130 Hounsfield units (HU) in an artery [7]. Calcifications are standardly quantified into Agatston, volume, and mass scores [8]. The volume score represents the volume of calcified lesions, and it only takes the voxel size into account, while the calcium mass considers both the volume and the density of the lesions. Both scores are used for quantification of calcifications in any artery, while the Agatston score is applied to the coronary arteries only. The Agatston score is a slice-based quantification method that combines the area of a lesion with an ordinal weight term based on the maximum density of the lesion in each slice (<200 HU: 1; <300 HU: 2; <400 HU: 3; ≥400 HU: 4). The total Agatston score is obtained by summing the 2D lesion scores over all slices. Based on the total Agatston score, a patient can be assigned to a risk category that directly relates to a 10-year risk of CVD events [7, 9]. Commonly used risk categories are listed in Table 24.1.

Standard Calcium Scoring

Routinely, only coronary calcium scoring is performed. In clinic, this is done with commercially available software in a semi automatic manner. The interactive software projects an overlay showing all the areas above 130 HU onto a CT slice. Subsequently, the areas in the coronary arteries representing CAC are manually identified by the expert with a mouse click. The software then automatically identifies the whole lesion and labels it according to the artery label provided by the expert. This process is repeated for each CAC lesion and each CT slice. Thereafter, the identified lesions are quantified into Agatston score, volume, and mass. The scores are calculated per artery and over all arteries.

Table 24.1 Commonly used risk categories based on Agatston scores determined in the coronary arteries

Agatston score	Risk
0	Very low
1–10	Low
11–100	Intermediate
100–400	High
>400	Very high

S. G. M. van Velzen, PhD · N. Hampe, PhD · B. D. de Vos, PhD
Department of Biomedical Engineering and Physics, Amsterdam University Medical Centers – location AMC, University of Amsterdam, Amsterdam, the Netherlands

Amsterdam Cardiovascular Sciences, Amsterdam University Medical Centers, Amsterdam, the Netherlands

I. Išgum, PhD (✉)
Department of Biomedical Engineering and Physics, Amsterdam University Medical Centers – location AMC, University of Amsterdam, Amsterdam, the Netherlands

Amsterdam Cardiovascular Sciences, Amsterdam University Medical Centers, Amsterdam, the Netherlands

Department of Radiology and Nuclear Medicine, Amsterdam University Medical Centers – location AMC, University of Amsterdam, Amsterdam, the Netherlands
e-mail: i.isgum@amsterdamumc.nl

AI for Calcium Scoring

Although manual calcium scoring is not considered a difficult task for experts, it can be tedious and time-consuming, especially when large numbers of scans are involved or the image quality is compromised. Therefore, a multitude of artificial intelligence (AI) methods have been developed to automate calcium scoring [10, 11].

Due to large variability in the manifestation of calcified plaque and its look-alikes, designing rule-based algorithms for identifying calcified plaque is far from trivial. Instead, state-of-the art automatic systems utilize machine learning to learn the intuitive rules experts apply when scoring a scan. Calcium scoring is often posed as a classification problem where the machine learning task is to separate arterial calcifications from their look-alikes. In conventional machine learning, classification is performed based on the information describing the potential calcifications (features) that is relevant for the task at hand. In case of calcium scoring, the potential calcifications typically consist of candidate lesions above 130 HU in the scan, which need to be classified into calcifications or other lesions. The features used in automatic calcium scoring typically describe lesion size, shape, texture, and location in the scan. For calcium scoring, it is feasible to obtain labels for the training data, i.e., for each candidate lesion, a label can be obtained that indicates whether the lesion is a true arterial calcification or not. Hence, the training of calcium scoring methods is supervised: the classifier learns to perform the classification based on labeled example data. When training is finished, the free parameters are frozen, and the algorithm can be used to classify previously unseen samples.

While extensive research throughout multiple decades has produced a wide spectrum of machine learning algorithms, hardware and algorithm developments over the last years evoked the creation of an entirely new AI category, termed deep learning. The most distinct difference between deep learning and the conventional machine learning algorithms lies in their ability to learn directly from the data, circumventing the need for designing features. This shifts the focus from carefully designing specific features that incorporate expert knowledge about the task at hand to engineering the network architecture and the optimization process. Furthermore, ability of deep learning approaches to learn optimal features simultaneously with the classification can result in substantially improved performance. Like in calcium scoring using conventional machine learning, deep learning calcium scoring methods predominantly utilize supervised approaches.

We discuss machine learning and deep learning methods for calcium scoring that follow standard identification of calcified lesions in clinic in section "Automatic Coronary Calcium Scoring". Later methods advance coronary calcium scoring to achieve faster and more reproducible measurements. These methods are discussed in section "Advancing the Standard Calcium Scoring Protocol". Finally, section "Future Directions and Conclusions" provides a discussion on the current state of the art and potential future research directions.

Automatic Coronary Calcium Scoring

To date, most automatic coronary calcium scoring methods are closely related to the expert manual calcium scoring procedure using commercial software solutions: Lesion candidates are first extracted based on their image intensity values, and thereafter, the calcifications of interest are identified (Fig. 24.1). Currently, most automatic CAC scoring methods focus on automating the manual lesion identification with a machine learning classifier or deep learning architecture.

In clinical practice, only coronary calcium scoring is routinely performed, and it is done in dedicated calcium scoring CT (CSCT) scans. However, other CT protocols that visualize the heart also allow CAC scoring. Because different CT protocols pose different challenges, we describe automatic CAC scoring per target CT protocol.

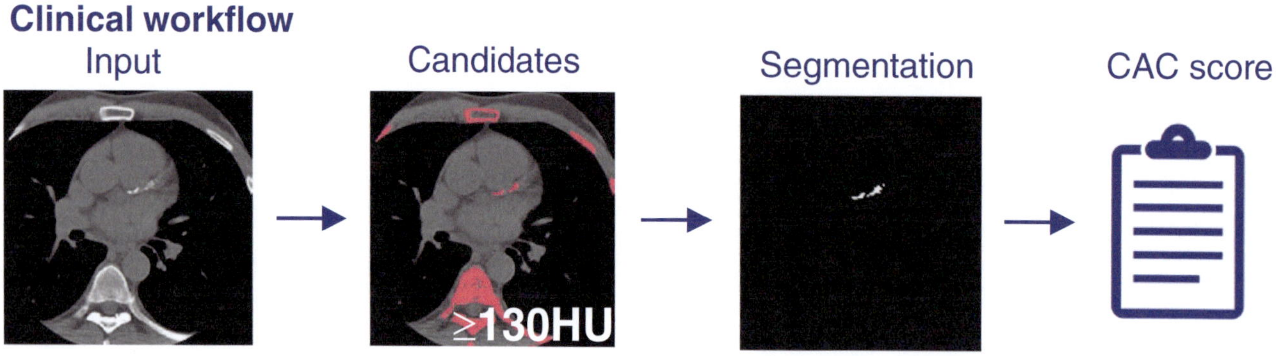

Fig. 24.1 Clinical workflow for CAC quantification: lesion candidates are extracted based on their image intensity values, and thereafter, the arterial calcifications of interest are identified and quantified

Coronary Calcium Scoring in Cardiac CT

For quantification of CAC, a dedicated CSCT is performed without contrast enhancement, with electrocardiography (ECG)-triggering, 120 kVp, and 3 mm slice thickness [12]. The dedicated protocol allows for optimal visualization of coronary calcifications and, hence, accurate quantification of CAC. The absence of contrast agent in the arteries allows for good visualization of the calcified lesions. Moreover, the slice thickness of 3 mm minimizes image noise and therefore allows discrimination between small calcifications and noise voxels. Furthermore, using ECG, image acquisition is triggered to the end-diastolic phase, when the heart is most stable. Minimizing cardiac motion is particularly important for coronary calcium scoring due to its pronounced effect on visualization of the coronary arteries.

Analogous to clinical calcium scoring, earliest AI methods for coronary calcium scoring were generally focused on application in CSCT scans, in which they computed a total CAC score. The typical automation pipeline of these early methods starts with defining the region of interest (ROI). In the defined ROI, the methods identify true calcified lesions among a set of candidates using a supervised machine learning classifier based on handcrafted features [13–18].

Published methods mainly differ in strategies for defining the region of interest (ROI), the choice of machine learning classifier, and the type of computed features. A combination of classifiers typically led to the best performance [13, 14]. Isgum et al. [13] used k-nearest neighbor (kNN) classifiers sequentially, where the result of the first classifier was used as input to the second classifier: In the first stage, obvious positives and obvious negatives were discarded, and subsequently, a new classifier was trained for the remaining, more difficult candidates [13]. Alternative to such a sequential combination, Kurkure et al. [14] proposed to merge the output of an ensemble of multiple support vector machine (SVM) classifiers that were trained separately on different independently sampled subsets of the training data. This way a robust method was trained.

Next to the classifier, the computed features played an essential role in the automation pipeline. Features often describe shape, size, appearance, and location of calcium lesions [13–18]. While shape, size, and appearance features are described directly from the lesions using, for instance, volume, Gaussian filters, and intensity value statistics, their spatial location requires contextual information from the scan. For instance, Išgum et al. [13] described the position of lesions with respect to anatomical structures, i.e., the heart and the aorta. Kurkure et al. [14] defined location features relative to a bounding box around the heart. The features were agnostic to the specific machine learning classifier, and their descriptive power was crucial for algorithm performance.

Besides location information being important for distinguishing true coronary calcifications among candidates, it is useful for computing per artery scores. Therefore, machine learning methods were proposed that, unlike the aforementioned methods, used location information to infer in which coronary artery a lesion may reside in. Brunner et al. [16] used coordinates with respect to manually placed landmarks as features to assign all voxels in a CSCT scan to classes belonging to one of the three main coronary artery branches (LAD, LCX, and RCA) or background with an SVM. By assigning lesion candidates to the predicted coronary artery, artery specific calcium scoring was performed. Other methods utilized an additional set of coronary CT angiography (CCTA) scans, in which an intravenously administered contrast agent enables visualization of the arteries [17, 18]. The CCTA scans were used to define coronary artery atlases, i.e., probabilistic maps of artery locations in typical heart anatomies. Registration of these atlases to CSCT images allowed for obtaining estimates of the coronary artery location and assigning a lesion to an artery. In addition to enabling the computation of artery-specific calcium scores based on the CCTA atlases, Shahzad et al. [17] also exploited artery locations in the form of an additional location feature relative to the arteries. Due to the differences in contrast between CCTA and CSCT, accurate registration is a very challenging task. Therefore, Wolterink et al. [18] proposed to first transfer the CCTA atlases to CSCT atlas scans. The hereby obtained CSCT atlases were subsequently used to estimate artery locations. Moreover, the impact of potential registration errors on classification performance was mitigated by computing location features with respect to all coronary arteries instead of merely the closest one. Furthermore, the authors enabled an additional opportunity for a semi-automatic workflow, in which high uncertainty output of the trained classifier was presented to an expert for potential correction. By referring only lesion candidates with high classifier uncertainty, performance similar to a second observer was achieved, with relatively little manual expert input [18].

Recently, deep learning methods have been proposed for CAC scoring in CSCT. Martin et al. [19] segmented the territories in CSCT that belong to the three main coronary arteries with a segmentation convolutional neural network (CNN). Subsequently, only candidate lesions in the vicinity of the coronary arteries were classified using a neural network that combines spatial coordinate features with features from the segmentation CNN. Van den Oever et al. [20] proposed an approach that employs a CNN to segment CAC by analyzing image slices in three orthogonal directions and, thereafter, combines them to obtain the final segmentation. The evaluation showed that due to the absence of false negative predictions, the method could be used to exclude scans without CAC to relieve the workload of radiologist.

Although direct comparison of attained performances by the presented methods is generally desirable, it is often not possible due to differences in evaluation metrics and used datasets. Therefore, Wolterink et al. [21] organized the orCaScore challenge that provided a set of multi-center and multi-vendor training and test CSCT and CCTA scans and a standardized evaluation of the results. At the workshop that launched the challenge, the performance of five (semi-)automatic calcium scoring methods aimed at CSCT was assessed, including the methods of Shahzad et al. [17] and Wolterink et al. [18]. The authors found that, on a lesion level, some methods can identify CAC in CSCT with a sensitivity and positive predictive value close to that of expert observers. Nevertheless, all evaluated methods made common errors, typically at the coronary ostia, where the exact starting point of the coronary arteries is potentially ambiguous, and in distal segments of the coronary arteries, which are difficult to extract with most coronary artery tracking methods.

Calcium Scoring in Non-contrast CT Showing the Heart

Over 7 million non-contrast chest CT scans are annually acquired for clinical care in the United States alone. This amounts to approximately ten times more acquired chest CT scans than dedicated CSCT scans [22]. Moreover, if lung cancer screening with chest CT would be considered, potentially another 7–10 million low-dose chest CTs per year would be acquired [23]. Furthermore, non-contrast CT scans showing the chest are made for nondiagnostic purposes, e.g., radiotherapy treatment planning CT. All these scans visualize the heart and allow calcium scoring in the coronary arteries and in the aorta (Fig. 24.2). Given the clinical relevance of CAC scoring, the guidelines of the Society of Cardiovascular Computed Tomography and the Society of Thoracic Radiology [12] recommend to quantify and report CAC on *all* such CT scans.

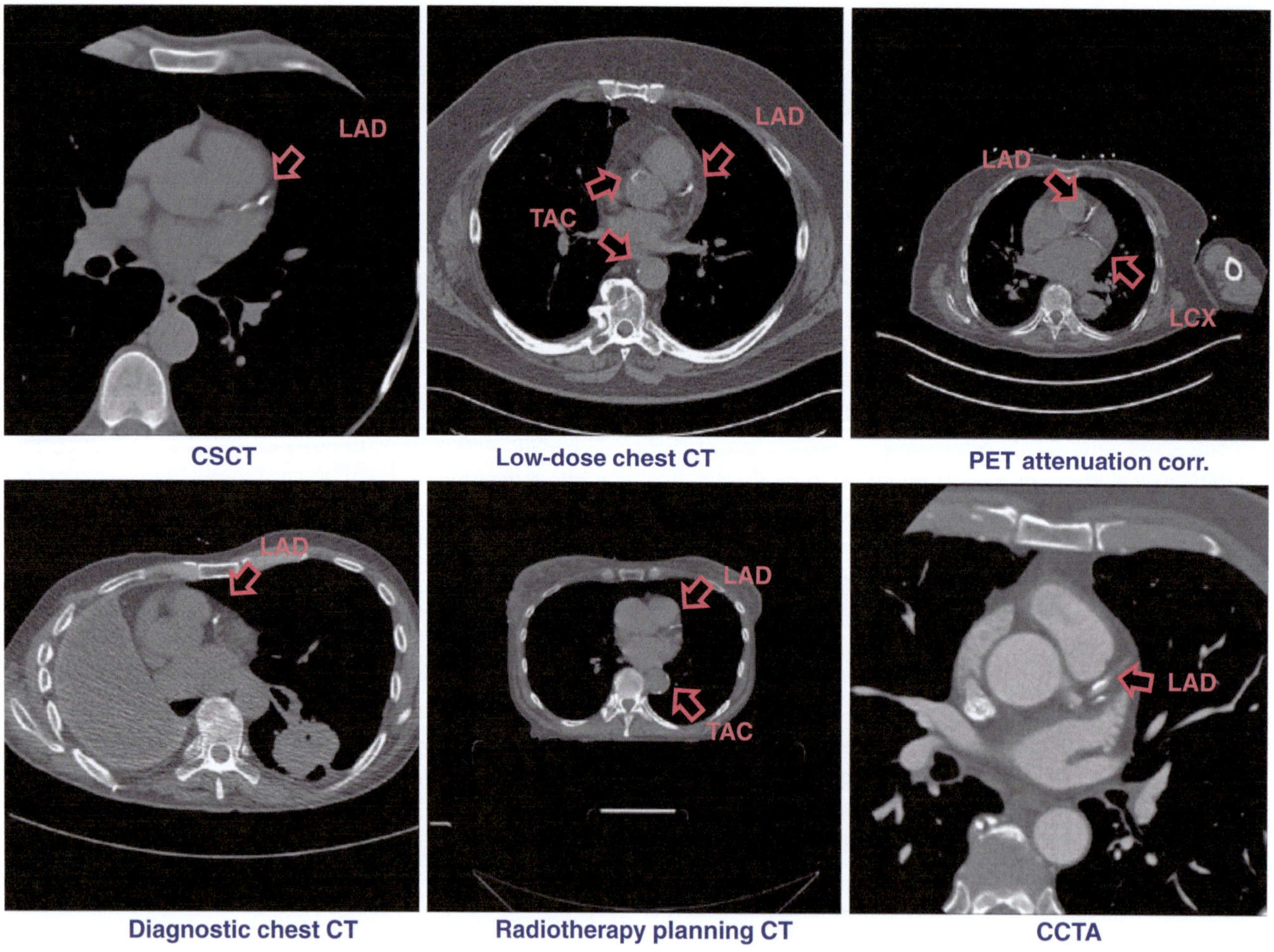

Fig. 24.2 Examples of different CT scan protocols with pronounced differences in field of view, image resolution, cardiac motion, intravenous contrast, and pathology. The arrows indicate calcified lesions in the left anterior descending (LAD) and left circumflex (LCX) artery, and thoracic aorta calcification (TAC)

However, a number of extra challenges arise that are not present in CSCT. Since these scans are made for a wide variety of clinical indications, the field of view is not focused on the heart but contains a larger volume, which necessarily translates to a lower in-plane resolution. Moreover, such CT scans are usually acquired without ECG-triggering, resulting in more pronounced cardiac motion artifacts impacting the appearance of calcifications in the coronary arteries.

Nevertheless, also in these scans, calcium scoring has most frequently been applied to the coronary arteries. Because localization of the coronary arteries is not feasible due to lack of contrast enhancement and cardiac motion artifacts, machine learning methods for CAC scoring often simplify the analysis by defining a ROI or incorporate spatial information. For instance, González et al. [24] defined a bounding box around the heart to determine the ROI using machine learning classifiers that classified the presence of the heart per slice in three orthogonal directions. Thereafter, a rule-based approach was used to classify CAC lesions within the bounding box. Other methods did not specifically restrict the analysis to a certain ROI but incorporated spatial information in a different manner. Išgum et al. [25] explicitly utilized the property that coronary calcifications appear at typical locations in the coronary artery tree. Through image registration of scans with reference segmentations of CAC, a spatial CAC probability map was created that was used to compute spatial features for candidate calcifications. Like in the methods for CAC detection in CSCT, features describing shape, size, appearance, and location of the lesion were computed. These were used to detect CAC lesions with a combination of classifiers. Although the method was developed for low-dose chest CTs, the same method was also applied to attenuation correction CT scans for cardiac perfusion PET scans [26] and radiotherapy planning CT scans of breast cancer patients [27], both with good agreement with reference scores [28].

Owing to the typically large field of view, these scans also allow quantification of extracardiac arterial calcification in, for instance, the thoracic aorta, innominate artery, or carotid arteries. Accordingly, several automatic methods for extracardiac calcium scoring have been developed. For instance, Išgum et al. [29] proposed to quantify calcifications in the thoracic aorta by delineating the aorta using a multi-atlas segmentation approach and classifying candidate lesions within this volume with two sequential kNN classifiers. Similarly, Chellamuthu et al. [30] used two sequential CNNs to detect whether calcified lesions were present in a number of large arteries in the chest and neck. Simultaneously the location of a bounding box around the lesion was regressed, and thereafter a CNN was used to segment the lesion within the bounding box. In both approaches, application of sequential classifiers substantially reduced the amount of false positive lesion detections [29, 30].

Recently, deep learning-based methods were proposed for calcium scoring in low-dose chest CT [31, 32]. Lessmann et al. [31] used two subsequent CNNs to detect calcifications in the coronary arteries, aorta, and cardiac valves. The first CNN exploited dilated convolutions to identify candidate calcification voxels and label them according to their spatial location, and the second CNN identified true calcified voxels among those detected by the first CNN. Note that the voxels were identified instead of the lesions. This was needed to address low-dose CT where high noise levels don't allow region growing of the voxels above the 130 HU extraction threshold.

The aforementioned methods were typically developed and evaluated in a set of scans with uniform image acquisition characteristics. Due to the supervised nature of these methods, they are sensitive to changes in image acquisition parameters and the imaged population. Consequently, a good performance is often suboptimal in CT scans acquired with different acquisition parameters, which limits the clinical applicability. To extend the applicability, in a large-scale multicenter study including CT scans with diverse acquisition protocols, van Velzen et al. [33] evaluated training strategies for the deep learning method proposed by Lessmann et al. [31] for calcium scoring in the coronary arteries and the aorta. The performance was evaluated in CSCT, diagnostic chest CT, radiotherapy planning CT, and attenuation correction CT acquired with cardiac perfusion PET. Training with a combination of all available types of CT scans led to excellent agreement in risk categorization between manual and automatic scoring, i.e., linearly weighted Cohen's kappa > 0.9 [28]. This type of generic method eliminates the need for a specialized network for every type of CT, which is practical for wide application in clinical practice.

Calcium Scoring in Contrast-Enhanced Scans

For CCTA acquisition, an iodine-containing contrast agent is intravenously administered, which enables visualization of blood vessels in the coronary artery tree. Hence, the current diagnostic purpose of CCTA lies in identification of noncalcified plaque, as well as determination of the presence and quantification of the anatomical significance of coronary artery stenosis. Standard calcium scoring is not applicable to CCTA as the contrast agent in the artery typically exceeds the clinical intensity level threshold of 130 HU (Fig. 24.3). This led to application of higher detection thresholds of, for instance, 320 HU [34] or 600 HU [35]. However, due to variations between CCTA scans caused by differences in acquisition protocols, scanners, and contrast agents, using the same detection threshold for all subjects does often not lead to the most optimal results (Fig. 24.3). To address this, the threshold was derived automatically at standardized

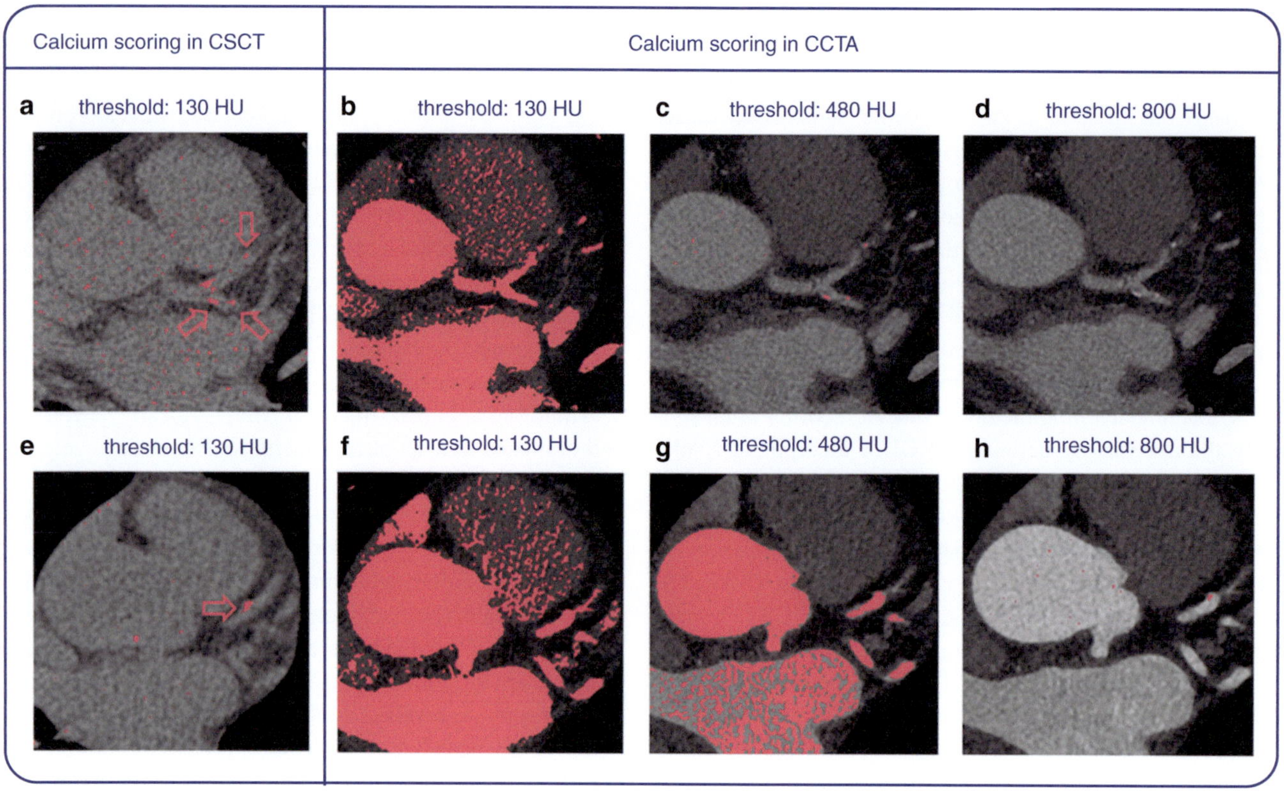

Fig. 24.3 Paired CSCT (**a**; **e**) and CCTA (**b–d**; **f–h**) scans for two different patients (top and bottom). In the CSCT scans, arrows indicate lesions detected by using the clinical intensity level threshold of 130 HU. Different thresholds (130 HU; 480 HU; 800 HU) for calcium scoring in CCTA demonstrate inapplicability of a global threshold and thus the need for adjusted approaches

anatomical locations, e.g., the ascending aorta [36] or the proximal coronary arteries [37].

Automatic methods for CAC scoring in CCTA typically determine the CAC extraction threshold and localize the coronary arteries (and aorta) by finding their centerlines, thereby allowing detection of CAC lesions in the proximity of the detected centerlines. For example, Teßman et al. [38] derived a threshold from the histogram of the localized vessels and applied this threshold to all voxels in the extracted vessel tree. Subsequently, more complex models were developed in which CAC was defined in relation to the local lumen attenuation values [39–41]. Furthermore, Mittal et al. [42] combined machine learning approaches for CAC scoring in CSCT while exploiting the visibility of the coronary arteries in CTA. Namely, the authors trained a random forest classifier based on handcrafted features to identify CAC lesions along an extracted coronary artery centerline.

Later, deep learning approaches were also utilized. Because extraction of the coronary artery centerlines may be challenging especially in the presence of pathology like severe stenosis, Wolterink et al. [43] circumvented this by defining a bounding box around the heart using a deep learning approach [44]. Thereafter, all voxels within the bounding box were classified by an ensemble of four pairs of sequential CNNs, each with either a 2.5D or 3D architecture and varying size of the receptive field. The method showed a high correlation with CSCT reference scores and good agreement of risk categorization [28]. Zreik et al. [45] first extracted coronary artery centerlines and classified the presence of CAC along these centerlines with a combination of a CNN and a recurrent neural network. In this approach, CAC was not segmented, but its presence was detected. A later method by Fischer et al. [46] used a similar approach that combined a CNN and a recurrent neural network for CAC detection. While the method showed a high accuracy for CAC lesion detection, their segmentation was not performed, and hence, quantification of CAC was not evaluated.

Advancing the Standard Calcium Scoring Protocol

While the aforementioned methods employed different methodologies to perform automatic calcium scoring, they all closely followed the clinical workflow using the standard definition of arterial calcification. By adjusting this workflow, several automatic methods have been developed that bring calcium scoring to a new level (Fig. 24.4). For instance, by circumventing the explicit lesion segmentation and directly predicting an Agatston score, methods can be orders

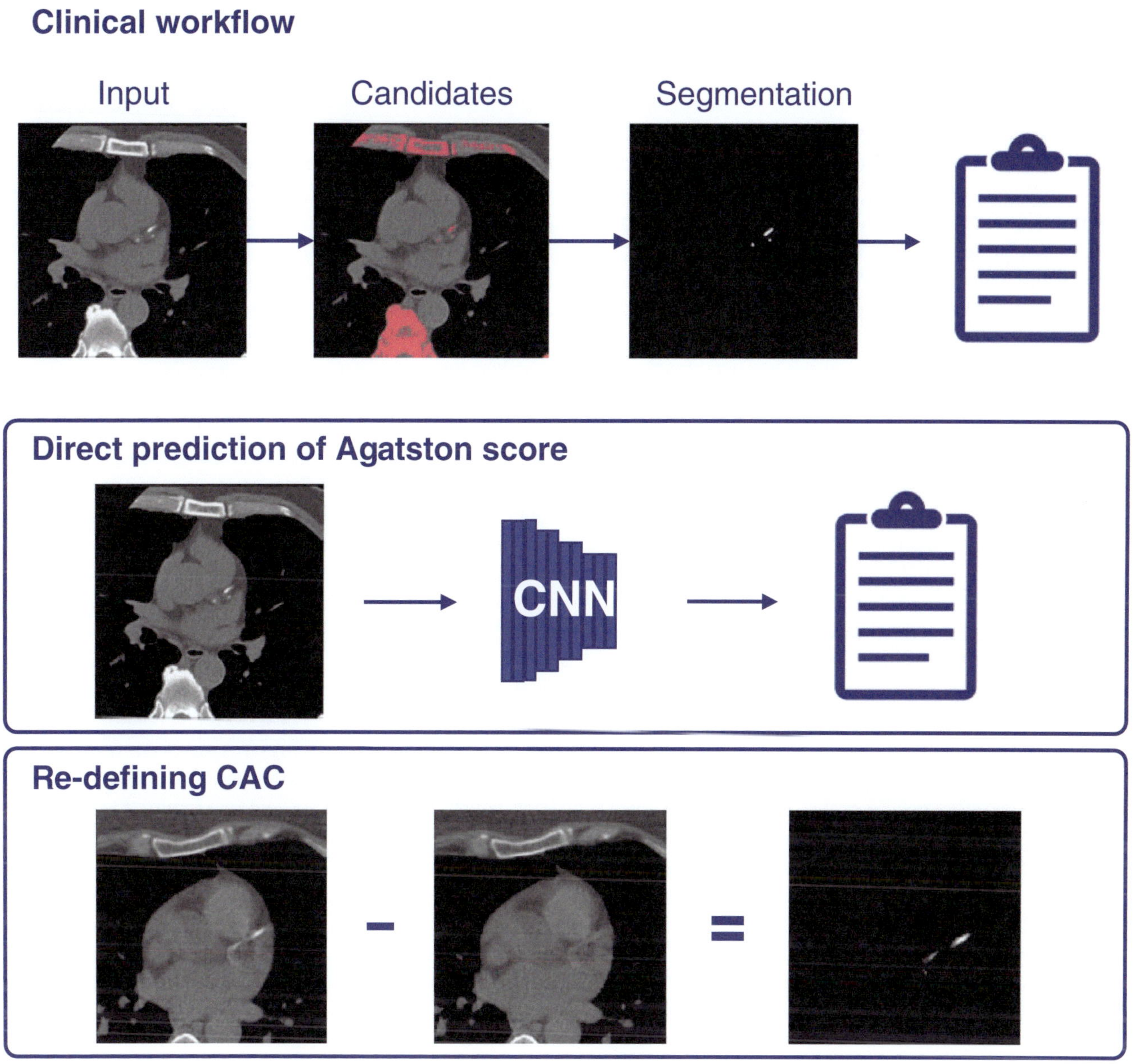

Fig. 24.4 By augmenting the clinical workflow, several automatic methods have been developed that offer new opportunities

of magnitude faster. Furthermore, revisiting the definition of CAC led to a method that provides more reproducible CAC quantification.

Direct Prediction of Coronary Calcium Scores

While the aforementioned methods aimed at calcium scoring in CSCT and other non-contrast CT showing the heart use different approaches, they all follow the manual calcium scoring workflow: Calcified lesions are first identified and thereafter quantified. Although several of the methods show good performance, this comes at a considerable computational cost. Therefore, CAC scoring methods have been proposed that bypass the lesion segmentation step and, instead, directly regress the Agatston score from the CT image [47, 48]. Like other methods, these methods focused the analysis on the heart by first defining a ROI. Cano-Espinoza et al. [48] defined a bounding box around the heart using an object-detection method. After defining the ROI, the Agatston score was regressed by a 3D CNN that analyzed the heart volume. This means that, instead of a categorical label as was used in classification, a continuous calcium score is predicted. However, in 14% of the images, the heart detection failed and the subsequent analysis could not be performed. In contrast to Cano-Espinoza et al., de Vos et al. [47] defined the ROI through registration that aligned the analyzed CT with an atlas image that was constructed from CSCT scans.

Conventional image registration is typically computationally expensive and slow, defying the purpose of a direct calcium scoring method. Therefore, a deep learning image registration framework [49] was used, which is able to register a 3D image volume in less than a second. Thereafter, the method utilized a 2D CNN architecture to predict an Agatston score in the ROI per image slice. This manner of computation mimicked the clinical calculation of the Agatston score, which is performed in 2D axial image slices (Fig. 24.5). Next to an accuracy in risk categorization that was comparable or better than for other state-of-the-art calcium scoring methods in cardiac and chest CT [18, 31], de Vos et al. [47] showed that their direct calcium scoring method was hundreds of times faster.

Improving Reproducibility

Although coronary calcium scoring is an established and effective method for CVD risk categorization, its interscan reproducibility is limited. For example, in dedicated CSCT scans that are optimized for CAC scoring, the interscan difference in Agatston scores was reported to range from 15% to 41% [50–53]. In chest scans, the reproducibility is even more compromised, due to lack of ECG-triggering and the lower image in-plane resolution. In these scans, the reported interscan difference is up to 71%, which led to a difference in risk categorization in 24% of the subjects [54].

Due to the relatively low in-plane resolution especially in non-cardiac CT scans that visualize the heart, the partial volume effect plays a significant role in CAC quantification. The partial volume effect blurs small calcifications so that they remain below the threshold and are missed during segmentation, causing underestimation of the amount of CAC. Another cause of limited scoring reproducibility is the fact that non-cardiac CTs, like chest CTs, are acquired without ECG-triggering. In these scans, extensive cardiac motion can blur lesions or make them invisible.

Increasing the interscan agreement was addressed by many researchers. The earliest approaches adjusted the intensity level threshold for detection of coronary calcifications, instead of using the fixed 130 HU. Groen et al. [55] proposed to use a lesion-specific adaptive threshold that is determined using the maximum intensity of the each CAC lesion in non-ECG-triggered CT [55]. In contrast, Song et al. adapted the threshold in a dedicated CSCT protocol based on the intensity of the background in the vicinity of lesions [56]. Another approach aimed at dedicated CSCT protocols was proposed by Sauer et al. [57], who used a mesh-based algorithm to refine the boundaries of a CAC lesion based on the intensity value profile. However, creating a boundary model for small calcifications or those strongly affected by cardiac motion is very challenging, since typically no intensity plateau is reached because of the partial volume effect, which may hamper performance in CT protocols without ECG-triggering. A different method, aimed at non-ECG-triggered protocols, was proposed by Šprem et al. [58], who built on work by Dehmeshki et al. [59]. The authors based their methods on the fact that, due to the limited spatial resolution and cardiac motion, voxels of lesions can contain a mixture of CAC and other tissues. Using an expectation-maximization algorithm, they determined the partial calcium content in each voxel of a CAC lesion and its vicinity. Subsequently, the volume of the lesion was corrected by the partial calcium content.

Development and evaluation of partial volume correction methods is often hampered by the fact that the true amount of calcium in patients cannot be measured non-invasively, and thus it is not available. Therefore, most partial volume correction methods either used a phantom for development or

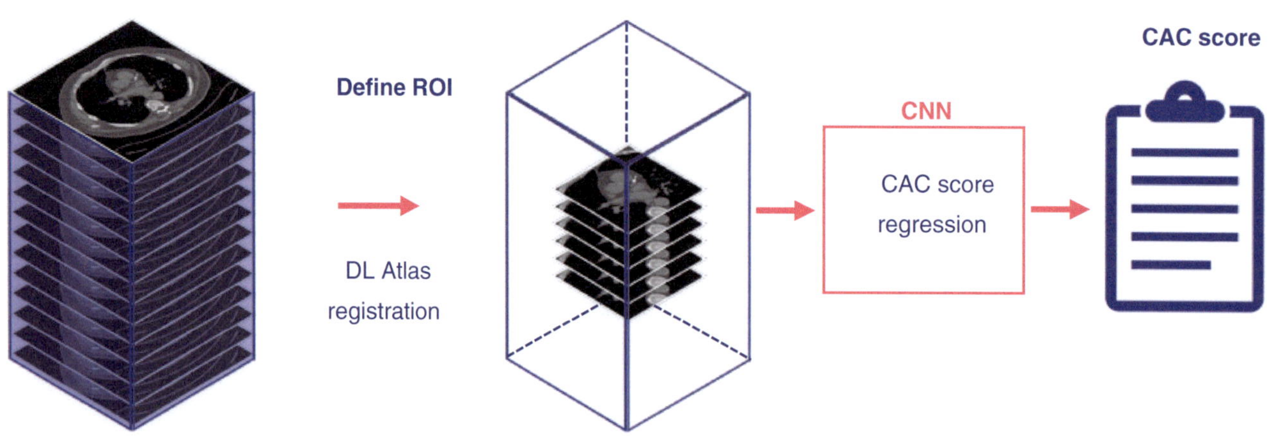

Fig. 24.5 Direct calcium scoring framework by de Vos et al. [47]: First the region of interest (ROI) containing the heart is determined using deep learning (DL) atlas registration. Subsequently, the calcium score is regressed with a CNN

used cadaver data. This is problematic for training AI methods that require large training sets. Unfortunately, thus far, only a few methods have been shown to translate well to patient data [58, 59].

Revisiting the Clinical Definition of Arterial Calcification

As outlined in section "Improving Reproducibility", intensity-level thresholding contributes to the large interscan reproducibility issues of calcium quantification affected by the partial volume effect and cardiac motion artifacts, especially in non-ECG triggered CT scans.

To address this, an automatic CAC scoring method that abandons the clinically used definition of CAC was proposed [60]. Instead of defining lesions using the intensity level threshold, the method defined lesions as the difference between an image visibly containing CAC and a corresponding image without CAC (Fig. 24.6). Because scan pairs of the same patient, where one scan shows CAC and the other one does not, do not exist, image synthesis with a CycleGAN was used to generate images without CAC from images containing CAC. By using labels that indicate whether an image slice contains CAC, image slices can be sorted into two domains: a *containing CAC* domain and a domain *without CAC*. Based on these labels, a CycleGAN was trained to translate images from one domain to the other and vice versa. By defining the task in this manner, the use of a threshold for detection and segmentation was avoided. Instead, the model itself decides which voxels contain CAC from a higher level of abstraction. Thereby, the method allows quantification of lesions that are partially or completely below the threshold and implicitly corrects for partial volume effect and motion artifacts. The method led to substantially lower relative interscan difference than standard manual calcium scoring. This may lead to improved and more reliable CVD risk prediction.

Future Directions and Conclusions

Recent advances in artificial intelligence research have sparked predictions of a future in which no longer radiologists but advanced computer algorithms read medical images. While this future may still seem distant, AI-based automatic image analysis may much sooner become useful as a supportive tool in the clinic, serving as a second pair of eyes or relieving radiologists and image analysts of tedious tasks. Since manual calcium scoring can be tedious and time-consuming, a multitude of AI methods have been developed to automate calcium scoring [10, 11]. Typically, these AI-based image analysis methods are trained and evaluated on single center studies with high risk for selection biases and under exclusion of low-quality scans. For application in clinical routine, software tools need to be robust to variation in image acquisition parameters and variation in the imaged population. Therefore, ideally large, diverse, well-structured and labeled data sets would be available for the development of new methods and validation of existing techniques. In healthcare, legal barriers often hamper data sharing, and therefore, collecting data for large multicenter evaluation studies is often difficult. This underlines the importance of image analysis challenges for benchmarking the performance

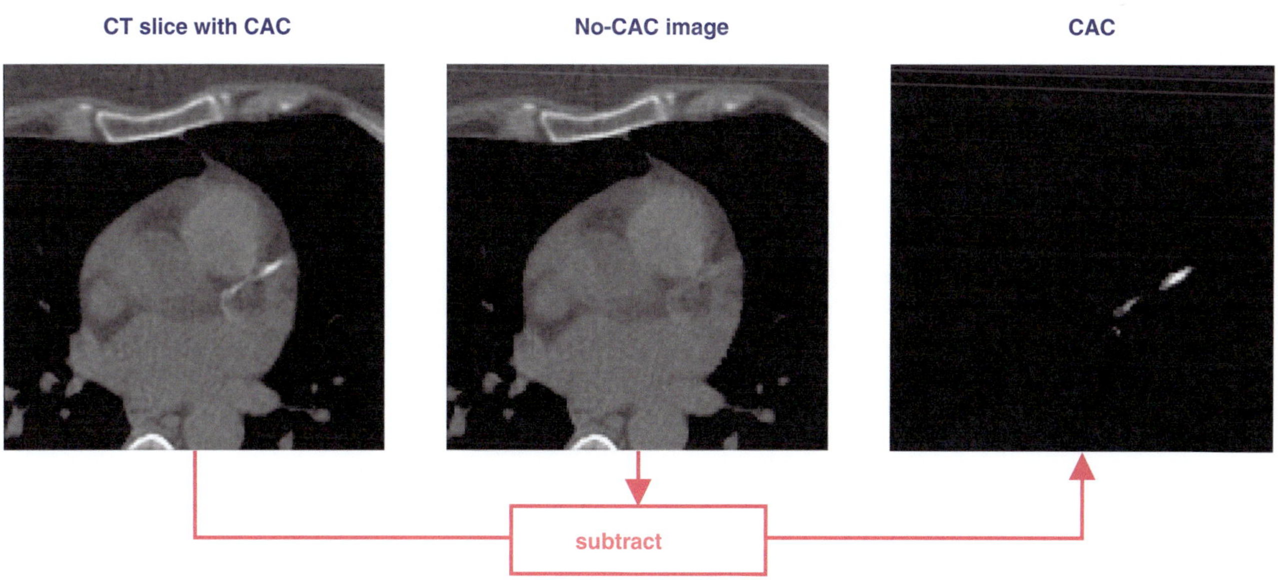

Fig. 24.6 By defining CAC as the difference between an image visibly containing CAC and a corresponding image without CAC, lesions affected by motion and the partial volume effect can be quantified

of methods. The orCaScore challenge [21] provided an evaluation of several automatic methods for calcium scoring in CSCT using multicenter and multi-vendor data. Moreover, a number of methods have proven to be applicable to CTs with different populations or protocols that they were trained on [26, 33, 61]. This versatility and robustness indicate great potential for broad application in clinical practice.

CAC scoring in CSCT is considered a relatively easy task for an expert, and the interobserver agreement is very high in these scans [21]. In non-ECG-synchronized CT, where coronary calcium scoring is more challenging due to, e.g., noise, low resolution, and motion artifacts, the interobserver variability is typically higher. Similar differences over scans are seen in the performance of the automatic methods. While the orCaScore challenge demonstrated excellent performance of automatic methods in CSCT that closely follow expert performance [18, 33, 62], methods applied to other CT scans showing the heart were challenged by image artifacts and low resolution. Nevertheless, also in these cases, the performance of several automatic methods closely followed interobserver agreement [31, 33, 62].

Related to the nature of many AI-driven calcium scoring methods, different approaches were used. Early machine learning methods that were aimed at classifying lesions typically exploit lesion-level labels [13–18, 63]. Later methods were trained to classify candidate voxels with voxel-level labels [31, 33]. Although both approaches require substantial manual labor for obtaining the reference standard, they provide strong supervision, which have been shown to often lead to the best performance compared to other training strategies. Nevertheless, other training strategies also have been successfully used. Methods that directly regress an Agatston score from an image slice use Agatston scores as labels [48, 62]. Because in this approach the labels are defined per image slice instead of per voxel or lesion, the supervision is less strict than with voxel or lesion labels. However, CAC needs to be manually segmented before a reference Agatston score can be derived, which does not alleviate the workload of defining the reference standard. An explicit advantage of this approach is the gain in speed compared to conventional methods that use segmentation. A different approach, which does not use the clinical CAC definition, uses labels that merely indicate whether CAC is present in an image slice [60]. This manner of annotation is less labor-intensive than CAC segmentation. In this approach, the method is trained to derive which voxels contain CAC from information that only indicates whether CAC is present.

For acceptance and application in clinic, the interpretability of a machine learning method is of key importance. Most calcium scoring methods produce a segmentation map, indicating per voxel whether it is part of a calcified lesion, which was used in further quantification. Although the mechanism for prediction of the segmentation map itself is often hidden in the complex algorithm or network, inspection of the calcification segmentation shows the plausibility and accuracy of the calcium scoring result. On the other hand, direct calcium scoring methods only produce an output Agatston score and, as such, act to a greater extent as a black box. De Vos et al. [62] addressed this issue by implementing an optional decision feedback mechanism that shows which parts of the image contributed to the score. Moreover, several types of visualization techniques for CNNs [64–66] have been proposed to visualize CNN decision-making to improve interpretability of CNNs.

Since the ultimate goal of calcium scoring is to derive a risk of CVD, future research could investigate direct prediction of CVD risk from a CT scan. Hard outcome labels like CVD events or CVD mortality provide a powerful and reliable reference. These labels are defined according to strict clinical protocol and definitions [67], which should make them less subject to interobserver variability. Despite the obvious application potential, this area of research is still in its infancy, likely caused by a combination of the challenging problem and difficulties of obtaining sufficient data. Given the data sets of limited size that were available for this research, thus far developed methods used a two-step approach, where first features describing the image [68, 69] were extracted and, thereafter, a classifier was trained to classify patients according to the outcomes. However, much like in conventional machine learning, the first stage was not directly coupled to the final prediction goal. Incorporating clinical patient data for multitask learning [70] or advanced augmentation techniques [71] may make end-to-end training with a limited dataset feasible.

In the era of precision medicine, it has become increasingly important to quantify disease-related parameters to provide a complete overview of the patients' physical state. Because it requires substantial manual effort to quantify all relevant parameters from the plethora of information comprised in a CT scan, automation using AI methods can facilitate and speed up the quantification process. Measuring a broad set of CVD parameters, including calcium scores, may aid medical experts in lifting the practice of personalized medicine to a new level. While the value of careful evaluation should not be forgotten, the incorporation of AI into CVD risk prediction is not a change that clinicians should fear, but rather, one that should be embraced.

References

1. Roth GA, Abate D, Abate KH, Abay SM, Abbafati C, Abbasi N, Abbastabar H, Abd-Allah F, Abdela J, Abdelalim A, et al. Global, regional, and national age-sex-specific mortality for 282 causes of death in 195 countries and territories, 1980–2017: a systematic analysis for the global burden of disease study 2017. Lancet. 2018;392(10159):1736–88.

2. Greenland P, Blaha MJ, Budoff MJ, Erbel R, Watson KE. Coronary calcium score and cardiovascular risk. J Am Coll Cardiol. 2018;72(4):434–47.
3. Iribarren C, Sidney S, Sternfeld B, Browner WS. Calcification of the aortic arch: risk factors and association with coronary heart disease, stroke, and peripheral vascular disease. JAMA. 2000;283(21):2810–5.
4. Nandalur KR, Baskurt E, Hagspiel KD, Finch M, Phillips CD, Bollampally SR, Kramer CM. Carotid artery calcification on CT may independently predict stroke risk. Am J Roentgenol. 2006;186(2):547–52.
5. Hecht HS. Coronary artery calcium scanning: past, present, and future. JACC Cardiovasc Imaging. 2015;8(5):579–96.
6. Budoff MJ, Nasir K, McClelland RL, Detrano R, Wong N, Blumenthal RS, Kondos G, Kronmal RA. Coronary calcium predicts events better with absolute calcium scores than age-sex-race/ethnicity percentiles: MESA (Multi-Ethnic Study of Atherosclerosis). J Am Coll Cardiol. 2009;53(4):345–52.
7. Agatston AS, Janowitz WR, Hildner FJ, Zusmer NR, Viamonte M, Detrano R. Quantification of coronary artery calcium using ultrafast computed tomography. J Am Coll Cardiol. 1990;15(4):827–32.
8. Rumberger JA, Kaufman L. A rosetta stone for coronary calcium risk stratification: Agatston, volume, and mass scores in 11,490 individuals. Am J Roentgenol. 2003;181(3):743–8.
9. Budoff MJ, Young R, Burke G, Jeffrey Carr J, Detrano RC, Folsom AR, Kronmal R, Lima JA, Liu KJ, McClelland RL, et al. Ten-year association of coronary artery calcium with atherosclerotic cardiovascular disease (ASCVD) events: the multi-ethnic study of atherosclerosis (MESA). Eur Heart J. 2018;39(25):2401–8.
10. Hampe N, Wolterink JM, Van Velzen SGM, Leiner T, Išgum I. Machine learning for assessment of coronary artery disease in cardiac CT: a survey. Front Cardiovasc Med. 2019;6:172.
11. Litjens G, Ciompi F, Wolterink JM, de Vos BD, Leiner T, Teuwen J, Išgum I. State-of-the-art deep learning in cardiovascular image analysis. JACC Cardiovasc Imaging. 2019;12(8):1549–65.
12. Hecht HS, Cronin P, Blaha MJ, Budoff MJ, Kazerooni EA, Narula J, Yankelevitz D, Abbara S. 2016 SCCT/STR guidelines for coronary artery calcium scoring of noncontrast noncardiac chest CT scans: a report of the society of cardiovascular computed tomography and society of thoracic radiology. J Cardiovasc Comput Tomogr. 2017;11(1):74–84.
13. I Išgum, A. Rutten, M. Prokop, and B. van Ginneken, "Detection of coronary calcifications from computed tomography scans for automated risk assessment of coronary artery disease," Med Phys, vol. 34. pp. 1450–1461; 2007.
14. Kurkure U, Chittajallu DR, Brunner G, Le YH, Kakadiaris IA. A supervised classification-based method for coronary calcium detection in non-contrast CT. Int J Cardiovasc Imaging. 2010;26(7):817–28.
15. Qian Z, Anderson H, Marvasty I, Akram K, Vazquez G, Rinehart S, Voros S. Lesion-and vessel-specific coronary artery calcium scores are superior to whole-heart Agatston and volume scores in the diagnosis of obstructive coronary artery disease. J Cardiovasc Comput Tomogr. 2010;4(6):391–9.
16. Brunner G, Chittajallu DR, Kurkure U, Kakadiaris IA. Toward the automatic detection of coronary artery calcification in non-contrast computed tomography data. Int J Cardiovasc Imaging. 2010;26(7):829–38.
17. Shahzad R, van Walsum T, Schaap M, Rossi A, Klein S, Weustink AC, de Feyter PJ, van Vliet LJ, Niessen WJ. Vessel specific coronary artery calcium scoring: an automatic system. Acad Radiol. 2013;20(1):1–9.
18. Wolterink JM, Leiner T, Takx RA, Viergever MA, Išgum I. Automatic coronary calcium scoring in non-contrast-enhanced ECG-triggered cardiac CT with ambiguity detection. IEEE Trans Med Imaging. 2015;34(9):1867–78.
19. Martin SS, van Assen M, Rapaka S, Hudson HT, Fischer AM, Varga-Szemes A, Sahbaee P, Schwemmer C, Gulsun MA, Cimen S, Sharma P, Vogl TJ, Schoepf UJ. Evaluation of a deep learning based automated CT coronary artery calcium scoring algorithm. JACC Cardiovasc Imaging. 2020;13(2 Part 1):524–6.
20. van den Oever L, Cornelissen L, Vonder M, Xia C, Bolhuis J, Vliegenthart R, Veldhuis R, Bock G, Oudkerk M, Van Ooijen P. Deep learning for automated exclusion of cardiac CT examinations negative for coronary artery calcium. Eur J Radiol. 2020;129:109114.
21. Wolterink JM, Leiner T, De Vos BD, Coatrieux J-L, Kelm BM, Kondo S, Salgado RA, Shahzad R, Shu H, Snoeren M, et al. An evaluation of automatic coronary artery calcium scoring methods with cardiac CT using the orCaScore framework. Med Phys. 2016;43(5):2361–73.
22. De González AB, Mahesh M, Kim K-P, Bhargavan M, Lewis R, Mettler F, Land C. Projected cancer risks from computed tomographic scans performed in the United States in 2007. Arch Intern Med. 2009;169(22):2071–7.
23. Moyer VA. Screening for lung cancer: US preventive services task force recommendation statement. Ann Intern Med. 2014;160(5):330–8.
24. González G, Washko GR, Estépar RSJ. Automated agatston score computation in a large dataset of non ECG-gated chest computed tomography. In 2016 IEEE 13th International Symposium on Biomedical Imaging (ISBI). pp. 53–57, IEEE; 2016.
25. Isgum I, Prokop M, Niemeijer M, Viergever MA, Van Ginneken B. Automatic coronary calcium scoring in low-dose chest computed tomography. IEEE Trans Med Imaging. 2012;31(12):2322–34.
26. Išgum I, de Vos BD, Wolterink JM, Dey D, Berman DS, Rubeaux M, Leiner T, Slomka PJ. Automatic determination of cardiovascular risk by CT attenuation correction maps in Rb-82 PET/CT. J Nucl Cardiol. 2018;25(6):2133–42.
27. Gernaat SAM, Išgum I, de Vos BD, Takx RAP, Young-Afat DA, Rijnberg N, Grobbee DE, van der Graaf Y, de Jong PA, Leiner T, van den Bongard DHJ, Pignol J-P, Verkooijen HM. Automatic coronary artery calcium scoring on radiotherapy planning CT scans of breast cancer patients: Reproducibility and association with traditional cardiovascular risk factors. PLoS One. 2016;11(12):e0167925.
28. Cohen J. A coefficient of agreement for nominal scales. Educ Psychol Meas. 1960;20(1):37–46.
29. Išgum I, Rutten A, Prokop M, Staring M, Klein S, Pluim JP, Viergever MA, van Ginneken B. Automated aortic calcium scoring on low-dose chest computed tomography. Med Phys. 2010;37(2):714–23.
30. Chellamuthu K, Liu J, Yao J, Bagheri M, Lu L, Sandfort V, Summers RM. Atherosclerotic vascular calcification detection and segmentation on low dose computed tomography scans using convolutional neural networks. In: 2017 IEEE 14th International Symposium on Biomedical Imaging (ISBI 2017). pp. 388–91, IEEE; 2017.
31. Lessmann N, van Ginneken B, Zreik M, de Jong PA, de Vos BD, Viergever MA, Išgum I. Automatic calcium scoring in low-dose chest CT using deep neural networks with dilated convolutions. IEEE Trans Med Imaging. 2018;37:615–25.
32. Lessmann N, Išgum I, Setio AA, de Vos BD, Ciompi F, de Jong PA, Oudkerk M, Willem PTM, Viergever MA, van Ginneken B. Deep convolutional neural networks for automatic coronary calcium scoring in a screening study with low-dose chest CT. In: Medical imaging 2016: computer-aided diagnosis, vol. 9785. p. 978511, International Society for Optics and Photonics; 2016.
33. van Velzen SGM, Lessmann N, Velthuis BK, Bank IE, van den Bongard DH, Leiner T, de Jong PA, Veldhuis WB, Correa A, Terry JG, et al. Deep learning for automatic calcium scoring in CT: validation using multiple cardiac CT and chest CT protocols. Radiology. 2020;295(1):66–79.

34. Otton JM, Lønborg JT, Boshell D, Feneley M, Hayen A, Sammel N, Sesel K, Bester L, McCrohon J. A method for coronary artery calcium scoring using contrast-enhanced computed tomography. J Cardiovasc Comput Tomogr. 2012;6(1):37–44.
35. Glodny B, Helmel B, Trieb T, Schenk C, Taferner B, Unterholzner V, Strasak A, Petersen J. A method for calcium quantification by means of CT coronary angiography using 64-multidetector CT: very high correlation with Agatston and volume scores. Eur Radiol. 2009;19(7):1661–8.
36. Mylonas I, Alam M, Amily N, Small G, Chen L, Yam Y, Hibbert B, Chow BJ. Quantifying coronary artery calcification from a contrast-enhanced cardiac computed tomography angiography study. Eur Heart J Cardiovasc Imaging. 2014;15(2):210–5.
37. Pavitt CW, Harron K, Lindsay AC, Ray R, Zielke S, Gordon D, Rubens MB, Padley SP, Nicol ED. Deriving coronary artery calcium scores from CT coronary angiography: a proposed algorithm for evaluating stable chest pain. Int J Cardiovasc Imaging. 2014;30(6):1135–43.
38. Teßmann M, Vega-Higuera F, Bischoff B, Hausleiter J, Greiner G. Automatic detection and quantification of coronary calcium on 3D CT angiography data. Comput Sci Res Dev. 2011;26(1–2):117–24.
39. Dey D, Cheng VY, Slomka PJ, Nakazato R, Ramesh A, Gurudevan S, Germano G, Berman DS. Automated 3-dimensional quantification of noncalcified and calcified coronary plaque from coronary CT angiography. J Cardiovasc Comput Tomogr. 2009;3(6):372–82.
40. Wesarg S, Khan MF, Firle EA. Localizing calcifications in cardiac CT data sets using a new vessel segmentation approach. J Digit Imaging. 2006;19(3):249–57.
41. Ahmed W, de Graaf MA, Broersen A, Kitslaar PH, Oost E, Dijkstra J, Bax JJ, Reiber JH, Scholte AJ. Automatic detection and quantification of the Agatston coronary artery calcium score on contrast computed tomography angiography. Int J Cardiovasc Imaging. 2015;31(1):151–61.
42. Mittal S, Zheng Y, Georgescu B, Vega-Higuera F, Zhou SK, Meer P, Comaniciu D. Fast automatic detection of calcified coronary lesions in 3D cardiac CT images. In: International Workshop on Machine Learning in Medical Imaging. Springer; 2010. p. 1–9.
43. Wolterink JM, Leiner T, de Vos BD, van Hamersvelt RW, Viergever MA, Išgum I. Automatic coronary artery calcium scoring in cardiac CT angiography using paired convolutional neural networks. Med Image Anal. 2016;34:123–36.
44. de Vos BD, Wolterink JM, de Jong PA, Leiner T, Viergever MA, Išgum I. Convnet-based localization of anatomical structures in 3-D medical images. IEEE Trans Med Imaging. 2017;36(7):1470–81.
45. Zreik M, Van Hamersvelt RW, Wolterink JM, Leiner T, Viergever MA, Išgum I. A recurrent CNN for automatic detection and classification of coronary artery plaque and stenosis in coronary CT angiography. IEEE Trans Med Imaging. 2018;38(7):1588–98.
46. Fischer AM, Eid M, De Cecco CN, Gulsun MA, van Assen M, Nance JW, Sahbaee P, De Santis D, Bauer MJ, Jacobs BE, et al. Accuracy of an artificial intelligence deep learning algorithm implementing a recurrent neural network with long short-term memory for the automated detection of calcified plaques from coronary computed tomography angiography. J Thorac Imaging. 2020;35:S49–57.
47. de Vos BD, Wolterink JM, Leiner T, de Jong PA, Lessmann N, Išgum I. Direct automatic coronary calcium scoring in cardiac and chest CT. In IEEE Transactions on Medical Imaging, vol. 38. pp. 2127–38; 2019.
48. Cano-Espinosa C, González G, Washko GR, Cazorla M, Estépar RSJ. Automated agatston score computation in non-ECG gated CT scans using deep learning. In Proceedings of SPIE–the International Society for Optical Engineering, vol. 10574; 2018.
49. de Vos BD, Berendsen FF, Viergever MA, Sokooti H, Staring M, Išgum I. A deep learning framework for unsupervised affine and deformable image registration. Med Image Anal. 2019;52:128–43.
50. Detrano RC, Anderson M, Nelson J, Wong ND, Carr JJ, McNitt-Gray M, Bild DE. Coronary calcium measurements: effect of CT scanner type and calcium measure on rescan reproducibility: MESA study. Radiology. 2005;236(2):477–84.
51. Mao S, Bakhsheshi H, Lu B, Liu SC, Oudiz RJ, Budoff MJ. Effect of electrocardiogram triggering on reproducibility of coronary artery calcium scoring. Radiology. 2001;220(3):707–11.
52. Hoffmann U, Siebert U, Bull-Stewart A, Achenbach S, Ferencik M, Moselewski F, Brady TJ, Massaro JM, O'Donnell CJ. Evidence for lower variability of coronary artery calcium mineral mass measurements by multi-detector computed tomography in a community-based cohort—consequences for progression studies. Eur J Radiol. 2006;57(3):396–402.
53. Van Hoe LR, De Meerleer KG, Leyman PP, Vanhoenacker PK. Coronary artery calcium scoring using ECG-gated multidetector CT: effect of individually optimized image-reconstruction windows on image quality and measurement reproducibility. Am J Roentgenol. 2003;181(4):1093–100.
54. Jacobs PC, Isgum I, Gondrie MJ, Mali WPTM, van Ginneken B, Prokop M, van der Graaf Y. Coronary artery calcification scoring in low-dose ungated CT screening for lung cancer: interscan agreement. Am J Roentgenol. 2010;194(5):1244–9.
55. Groen J, Dijkstra H, Greuter M, Oudkerk M. Threshold adjusted calcium scoring using CT is less susceptible to cardiac motion and more accurate. Med Phys. 2009;36(2):438–46.
56. Song Y, Eck BL, Levi J, Wilson DL. Improved reproducibility of calcium mass score using deconvolution and partial volume correction. In: Medical Imaging 2019: Biomedical Applications in Molecular, Structural, and Functional Imaging, vol. 10953. p. 109531O, International Society for Optics and Photonics; 2019.
57. Saur SC, Alkadhi H, Desbiolles L, Székely G, Cattin PC. ACCURATUM: improved calcium volume scoring using a mesh-based algorithm—a phantom study. Eur Radiol. 2009;19(3):591–8.
58. Šprem J, De Vos BD, Lessmann N, Van Hamersvelt RW, Greuter MJ, De Jong PA, Leiner T, Viergever MA, Išgum I. Coronary calcium scoring with partial volume correction in anthropomorphic thorax phantom and screening chest CT images. PLoS One. 2018;13(12):e0209318.
59. Dehmeshki J, Ye X, Amin H, Abaei M, Lin X, Qanadli SD. Volumetric quantification of atherosclerotic plaque in CT considering partial volume effect. IEEE Trans Med Imaging. 2007;26(3):273–82.
60. van Velzen SGM, de Vos BD, Verkooijen HM, Leiner T, Viergever MA, Išgum I. Coronary artery calcium scoring: can we do better? In: Medical Imaging 2020: Image Processing, vol. 11313. p. 113130G, International Society for Optics and Photonics; 2020.
61. Gernaat SA, Išgum I, de Vos BD, Takx RA, Young-Afat DA, Rijnberg N, Grobbee DE, van der Graaf Y, de Jong PA, Leiner T, et al. Automatic coronary artery calcium scoring on radiotherapy planning CT scans of breast cancer patients: reproducibility and association with traditional cardiovascular risk factors. PLoS One. 2016;11(12):e0167925.
62. de Vos BD, Wolterink JM, Leiner T, de Jong PA, Lessmann N, Išgum I. Direct automatic coronary calcium scoring in cardiac and chest CT. In: IEEE Transactions on Medical Imaging; 2019.
63. Išgum I, Prokop M, Niemeijer M, Viergever MA, van Ginneken B. Automatic coronary calcium scoring in low-dose chest computed tomography. IEEE Trans Med Imaging. 2012;31(12):2322–34.
64. Zeiler MD, Fergus R. Visualizing and understanding convolutional networks. In: European conference on computer vision. pp. 818–33. Springer; 2014.
65. Selvaraju RR, Cogswell M, Das A, Vedantam R, Parikh D, Batra D. Grad-cam: visual explanations from deep networks via gradient-based localization. In: Proceedings of the IEEE International Conference on Computer Vision. pp. 618–26; 2017.

66. Huo Y, Terry JG, Wang J, Nath V, Bermudez C, Bao S, Parvathaneni P, Carr JJ, Landman BA. Coronary calcium detection using 3d attention identical dual deep network based on weakly supervised learning. In Medical Imaging 2019: Image Processing, vol. 10949. p. 1094917, International Society for Optics and Photonics; 2019.
67. W. H. Organization, et al. The ICD-10 classification of mental and behavioural disorders: diagnostic criteria for research, vol. 2. World Health Organization; 1993.
68. van Velzen SGM, Zreik M, Lessmann N, Viergever MA, de Jong PA, Verkooijen HM, Išgum I. Direct prediction of cardiovascular mortality from low-dose chest CT using deep learning. In: Medical imaging 2019: image processing, vol. 10949. p. 109490X, International Society for Optics and Photonics; 2019.
69. de Vos BD, de Jong PA, Wolterink JM, Vliegenthart R, Wielingen GV, Viergever MA, Išgum I. Automatic machine learning based prediction of cardiovascular events in lung cancer screening data. In: Medical imaging 2015: Computer-Aided Diagnosis, vol. 9414. p. 94140D, International Society for Optics and Photonics; 2015.
70. Guo H, Kruger M, Wang G, Kalra MK, Yan P. Multi-task learning for mortality prediction in LDCT images. In: Medical imaging 2020: computer-aided diagnosis, vol. 11314. p. 113142C, International Society for Optics and Photonics; 2020.
71. Frid-Adar M, Klang E, Amitai M, Goldberger J, Greenspan H. Synthetic data augmentation using GAN for improved liver lesion classification. In: 2018 IEEE 15th International Symposium on Biomedical Imaging (ISBI 2018). pp. 289–293, IEEE; 2018.

Artificial Intelligence-Based Evaluation of Coronary Atherosclerotic Plaques

25

Andrew Lin, Piotr J. Slomka, and Damini Dey

Introduction

Coronary computed tomography angiography (CCTA) is noninvasive first-line modality for the evaluation of coronary artery disease (CAD) [1]. Beyond coronary stenosis, CCTA enables the qualitative and quantitative assessment of atherosclerotic plaque characteristics, providing a wealth of clinically meaningful data [2]. Routine interpretation of CCTA is focused on the visual evaluation of plaque composition and grading of stenosis severity [3], both of which are subject to interobserver variability [4, 5]. Numerous AI algorithms, developed with the aim of automating these tasks, have demonstrated high feasibility and performance. Conventional plaque parameters can also be integrated into ML models for cardiovascular risk prediction. In this chapter, we review state-of-the-art AI applications for the anatomic assessment of coronary atherosclerotic plaques.

Coronary Plaque Detection and Characterization

Coronary artery centerline extraction in CCTA images is a key preprocessing step for AI-based plaque analysis, with conventional automatic extraction methods based on minimum cost paths between proximal and distal artery points [6, 7]. This can be enhanced by the use of random forest [8] or convolutional neural network (CNN) [9] classifiers to verify centerline extraction results. Alternatively, centerlines can be iteratively tracked and extracted using a single seed point, as demonstrated by Wolterink et al. [10] using a 3D CNN. Following centerline extraction, the coronary artery lumen is typically segmented using cross-sectional CCTA images along the centerline, transforming the entire length of the vessel into a single volume [11–13]. Features describing the shape and texture of the vessel wall are then extracted from this volume for the detection and characterization of atherosclerotic plaque.

For the determination of plaque composition, Wei et al. [11] trained a linear classifier combining geometric features of vessels and intensity features of plaque candidates to detect noncalcified plaque (NCP), yielding an area under the receiver operator characteristic curve (AUC) of 0.85. Jawaid et al. [12] utilized a support vector machine (SVM) integrating 80 vessel- and plaque-based features to automatically estimate the position and length of NCP within coronary segments; this model achieved an overall accuracy of 88% compared with expert annotations. Zhao et al. [13] used a multi-class SVM algorithm incorporating intensity, shape, and texture features to detect and classify plaques as calcified, noncalcified, or mixed with an average precision of 92.6%. For the same task, Zreik et al. [14] trained a 3D CNN to automatically extract image features along the coronary artery, which were used as inputs by a recurrent neural network (RNN) for classification.

While many AI algorithms have successfully classified and quantified calcified plaque (Chap. 32), characterization of the individual components of noncalcified plaque is challenging due to the substantial overlap of CT attenuation [15, 16]. Masuda et al. [17] trained a boosted ensemble ML algorithm (XGBoost) using the mean plaque CT attenuation and histogram-based features from intravascular ultrasound (IVUS) to differentiate fibrous from lipid plaque on CCTA. The ML model exhibited a significantly higher AUC than the conventional CT attenuation threshold of 30 Hounsfield units (0.92 vs. 0.83, $p = 0.001$) when referenced against IVUS. Kolossváry et al. [18] used ex vivo coronary plaque specimens as the reference standard and co-registered

A. Lin, MBBS, PhD · D. Dey, PhD (✉)
Biomedical Imaging Research Institute, Cedars-Sinai Medical Center, Los Angeles, CA, USA
e-mail: andrew.lin3@cshs.org; damini.dey@cshs.org

P. J. Slomka, PhD
Artificial Intelligence in Medicine Program, Cedars-Sinai Medical Center, Los Angeles, CA, USA
e-mail: piotr.slomka@cshs.org

C. N. De Cecco et al. (eds.), *Artificial Intelligence in Cardiothoracic Imaging*, Contemporary Medical Imaging,
https://doi.org/10.1007/978-3-030-92087-6_25

histologic slides with CCTA cross-sectional images. A least-angle regression ML model trained with 13 CCTA-derived plaque radiomic features (AUC 0.73) outperformed visual assessment (AUC 0.65) and mean plaque attenuation (AUC 0.53) for distinguishing early from late fibroatheroma. Meanwhile, Yamak et al. [19] utilized additional attenuation data from dual-energy CT as input for supervised ML models (SVM, random forests, and artificial neural networks), which accurately classified noncalcified plaque as fibrous or lipid when trained with organic phantom plaques.

Coronary Stenosis Quantification

Anatomic assessment of coronary artery stenosis severity remains the cornerstone of clinical CCTA reporting. Several AI approaches have been developed to detect and quantify anatomically significant stenosis (≥50% luminal narrowing) from CCTA. Stenosis detection requires a local measurement of the diseased lumen diameter and an estimation of the healthy lumen diameter, measurements which can be derived from automatically extracted coronary centerlines. While numerous centerline extraction techniques assume a circular coronary artery profile [8, 10], diseased vessel segments often have noncircular profiles and thus required more detailed lumen segmentation. Huang et al. used automated coronary centerlines to generate patient-specific 3D masks of coronary segments for the training of a CNN, yielding high performance for lumen segmentation compared with manual annotations (dice similarity coefficient 0.83). Meanwhile, Lee et al. [20] employed an end-to-end CNN to convert a centerline into a 3D tube-shaped shape template, which was then deformed to match the underlying coronary lumen.

Although lumen segmentation is often considered a preprocessing step for AI-based coronary stenosis assessment, the presence and degree of stenosis can also be determined directly from CCTA image data. In an early study, Zuluaga et al. [21] trained a SVM using local intensity-based and second-order metrics to automatically detect coronary artery cross-sections containing lesions, yielding a sensitivity of 81% and specificity of 86% compared with expert readers. Kelm et al. [8] subsequently used random forest regression to compute the lumen cross-sectional area based on local image features along the vessel centerline. Candidate stenosis regions were then identified and graded as significant (≥50%) or nonsignificant (<50%) based on the estimated lumen radius. This method achieved a per-vessel sensitivity of 98% for the detection of significant noncalcified stenosis, with an average processing time of 1.8 seconds.

More recently, Kang et al. [22] utilized a SVM combining quantitative geometric and shape features of coronary lesions to detect the presence of diameter stenosis ≥25%. In this technique, each artery was divided into small volume patches from which nine features were extracted and used by the SVM algorithm to detect the presence of lesions. This was combined with a formula-based analytic method which estimated the degree of stenosis using luminal diameters. This method performed with high sensitivity (93%), specificity (95%), and accuracy (94%) for the detection of stenosis ≥25%, with an AUC of 0.94 when compared to expert visual assessment.

With respect to DL techniques for stenosis detection, Hong et al. [23] trained an end-to-end CNN to automatically quantify percentage diameter stenosis and minimal luminal area using 156 CCTA patient datasets with 716 diseased coronary segments (Fig. 25.1). The resultant DL measurements correlated strongly with expert manual annotations ($r = 0.957$ for stenosis and $r = 0.984$ for minimal luminal area, both $p < 0.001$) (Fig. 25.2). Zreik et al. [14] applied a RNN to multiplanar reformatted CCTA images to classify luminal diameter stenosis as absent, nonsignificant (<50%), or significant (≥50%), achieving an accuracy of 0.80 compared with expert readers. Meanwhile, Freiman et al. [24] used deep sparse autoencoders – a variation on CNNs – combined with denoising of input data to accurately detect coronary cross-sections with intermediate (≥40%) stenosis (AUC 0.84).

Machine Learning Using Plaque Features for Risk Prediction

The prognostic value of anatomical assessment of CAD by CCTA is well established [25]. It follows that CCTA-derived measures of stenosis severity and plaque characteristics have been incorporated into ML models for outcome prediction. In 10,030 patients with suspected CAD, Motwani et al. [26] trained a boosted ensemble ML algorithm (LogitBoost) using 25 clinical variables and 44 visually determined CCTA parameters of coronary atherosclerotic disease extent, severity, and composition for the prediction of 5-year all-cause mortality. The resultant ML score (AUC 0.79) outperformed conventional CCTA segment scores (AUC 0.64 for both segment stenosis score and segment involvement score) and the Framingham risk score (AUC 0.61; all $p < 0.001$) (Fig. 25.3). Among the highest-ranked variables in the ML model were the number of segments with noncalcified plaque and number of vessels with diameter stenosis less than 50%.

CCTA-based quantification of plaque morphology using semi-automated software applications has demonstrated predictive value for future cardiac events, independently of qualitative high-risk plaque features or visual stenosis severity [27, 28]. Quantitative measures of plaque volume and burden have recently been used in ML models for prognostication. In a lesion-level analysis of a patients with incident

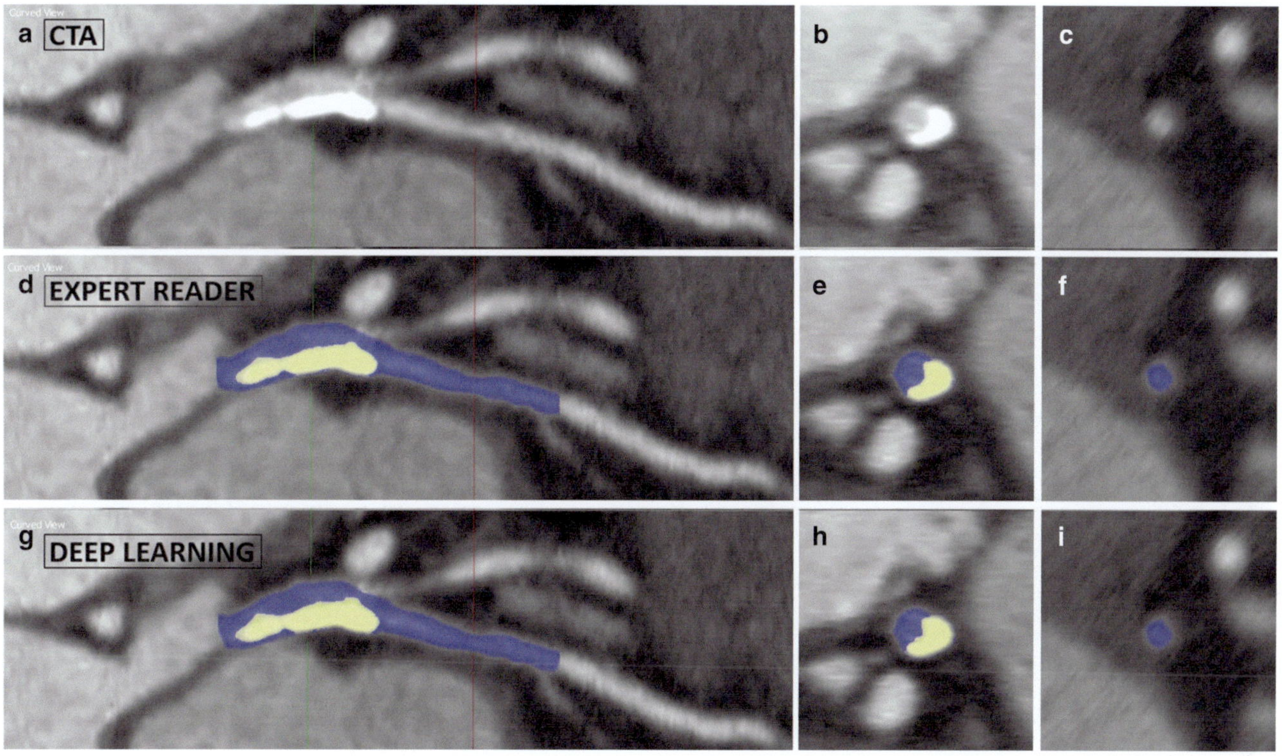

Fig. 25.1 Deep learning-based plaque analysis. Case example of lumen and calcified plaque segmentation on CCTA in a lesion extending from the left main into the left anterior descending artery. Top row: curved planar reformation (**a**) and cross-sections of the lesion (**b**) and healthy lumen (**c**). Middle row: (**d–f**) manual segmentations performed by the expert reader. Bottom row: (**g–i**) automated segmentations performed by the deep learning algorithm

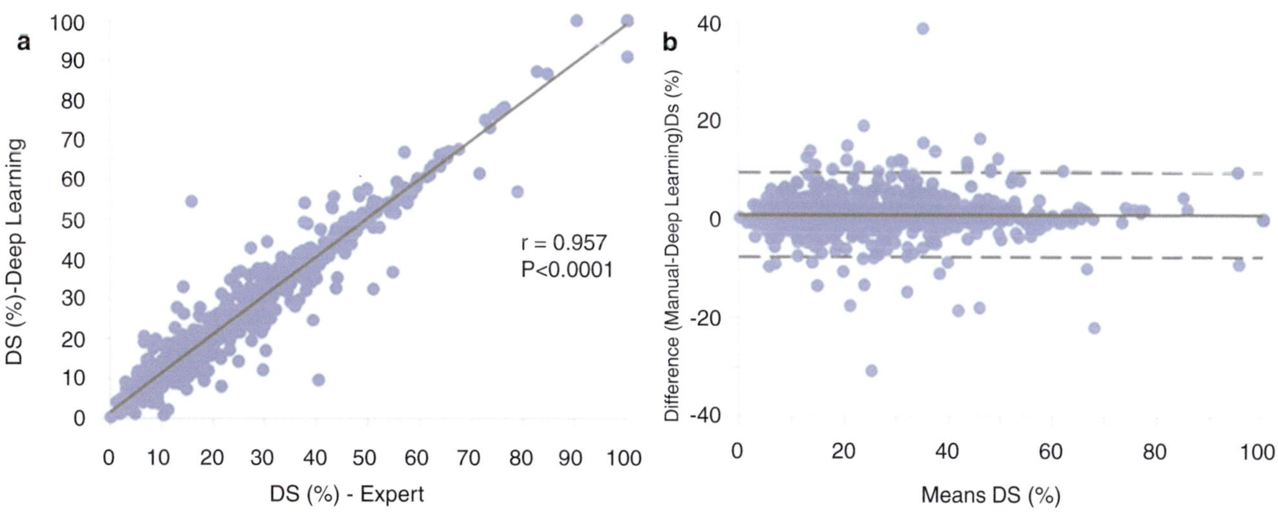

Fig. 25.2 Performance of a deep learning algorithm for stenosis severity quantification. (**a**) Spearman correlation and (**b**) Bland-Altman plots for percentage diameter stenosis between deep learning and manual expert quantification using software. Correlation was excellent ($r = 0.957$), and the 95% limits of agreement were −7.7 to 9.5%

ACS, Al'Aref et al. [29] input qualitative and quantitative plaque features from their baseline CCTA into an XGBoost algorithm for the prediction of culprit lesion precursors. The ML model integrating all features (AUC 0.77) provided superior performance compared with quantitative plaque parameters alone (AUC 0.67), qualitative parameters alone (AUC 0.52), or stenosis severity (AUC 0.60; all $p < 0.01$). Plaque volume per coronary segment and plaque burden at

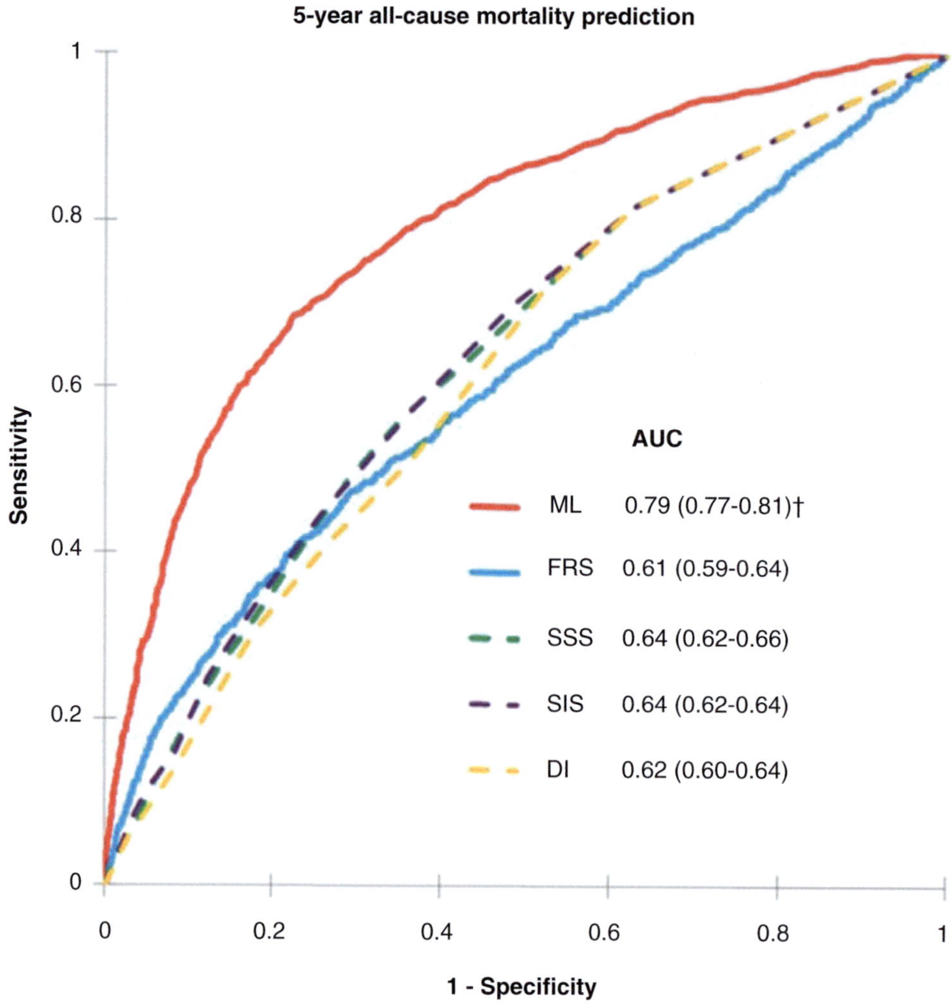

Fig. 25.3 Machine learning model for the prediction of all-cause mortality. Receiver-operating characteristics curves for prediction of 5-year all-cause mortality: a machine learning (ML) risk score integrating clinical and CCTA data exhibited a higher AUC than the Framingham Risk Score (FRS) and CCTA severity scores (segment stenosis score [SSS], segment involvement score [SIS], Duke Index [DI]) ($p < 0.001$†). AUC area under the curve, CCTA coronary computed tomography angiography. (Reproduced with permission from Motwani et al. [26])

the maximally stenotic CCTA cross-section had greatest variable importance in the ML model.

A ML framework has also yielded promising results for the prediction of plaque progression. In patients undergoing serial CCTA over a median of 3.3 years, Han et al. [30] showed a LogitBoost model incorporating baseline clinical variables and qualitative and quantitative plaque parameters to have greater discriminatory value for patients with rapid plaque progression (AUC 0.83) than a ML model with only clinical variables and qualitative plaque parameters (AUC 0.73) or the atherosclerotic cardiovascular disease risk score (AUC 0.60, all $p < 0.001$). Quantitative plaque features provided the highest information gain for ML, followed by qualitative plaque features and clinical variables. Percentage atheroma volume, total plaque volume, and fibrous plaque volume were the highest-ranked quantitative plaque features.

ML integrating plaque measurements can also predict the functional significance of coronary lesions. The current reference standard for lesion-specific ischemia is invasive fractional flow reserve (FFR), which has a well-established association with adverse cardiac events at a threshold of ≤0.80 [31]. In a substudy of the NXT (Analysis of Coronary Blood Flow Using CT Angiography: Next Steps) trial, Dey et al. [32] used ML combining quantitative plaque metrics from CCTA and computed a per-vessel "Ischemia Risk Score," which was the probability of invasive FFR ≤0.80. This ML score (AUC 0.84) exhibited a higher AUC (0.84) compared with stenosis severity (0.76, $p = 0.005$) or clinical pre-test probability of CAD (AUC 0.63, $p < 0.001$). The plaque features with greatest ML information gain (Fig. 25.4) were noncalcified plaque volume and low-attenuation noncalcified plaque volume (noncalcified plaque <30 Hounsfield Units). In a subsequent multicenter study of patients undergoing CCTA for suspected CAD [33], the Ischemia Risk Score predicted early revascularization independently of risk factors and presence of obstructive CAD and provided incremental value beyond a traditional risk model with clinical data and stenosis severity. ML has also been applied to the identification of patients with downstream coronary vascular dysfunction. Dey et al. [34] showed a LogitBoost algorithm trained using quantitative plaque burden, stenosis severity,

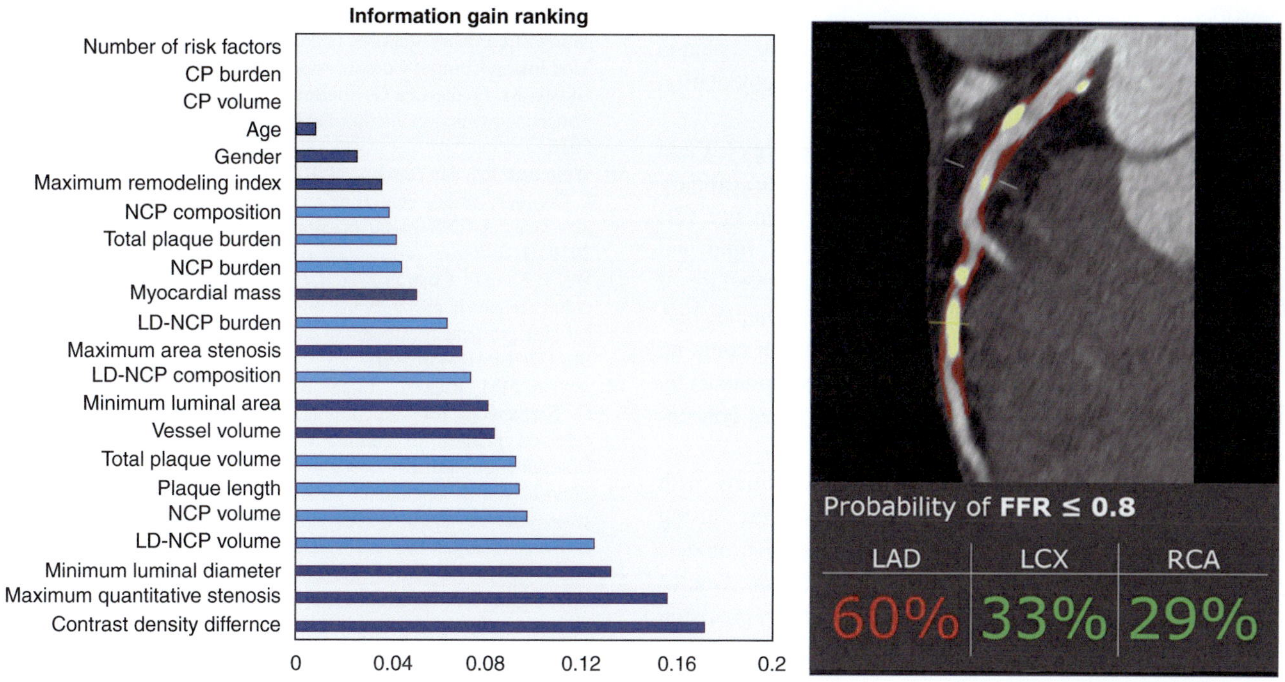

Fig. 25.4 Machine learning prediction of lesion-specific ischemia. The *left panel* shows the information gain ranking of variables in a CCTA-based machine learning Ischemia Risk Score used to predict lesion-specific ischemia by invasive FFR. Quantitative plaque measures are shown in light blue, and other CCTA and clinical variables are shown in dark blue. The *right panel* is a case example of the Ischemia Risk Score applied to a stable patient undergoing CCTA, with noncalcified plaque (NCP) and calcified plaque (CP) shown in red and yellow overlay, respectively. Invasive FFR of LAD was abnormal (0.73). CCTA coronary computed tomography angiography, LAD left anterior descending artery, LD-NCP low-density noncalcified plaque, LCX left circumflex artery, RCA right coronary artery. (Reproduced with permission from Dey et al. [40])

and CT-derived myocardial mass to accurately predict impaired regional myocardial flow reserve on positron emission tomography (AUC 0.83) over and above stenosis severity alone (AUC 0.66, $p = 0.005$).

Coronary Plaque Radiomics

Coronary atherosclerotic plaques are comprised of distinct histological components with different attenuation values on CCTA, enabling the qualitative and quantitative assessment of plaque morphology in vivo [16]. However, visual assessment of high-risk plaque features is subject to inter-reader variability [35], and current plaque quantification derives from absolute voxel attenuation values without considering the complex spatial relationship between voxels. As detailed in Chap. 31, radiomics can provide an objective, mathematical, or AI-based description of plaque incorporating textural and geometric imaging features. Kolossváry et al. [36] showed this approach to outperform conventional quantitative plaque metrics for the identification of "napkin-ring sign" on CCTA. Of 4440 radiomic features analyzed, 418 (9.4%) exhibited high diagnostic accuracy (AUC >0.80), outperforming per-lesion plaque burden (AUC 0.71) and mean plaque attenuation (AUC 0.75; all $p < 0.05$). In another study, the same authors [37] demonstrated that radiomic analysis had superior discriminatory value for IVUS-verified vulnerable plaque beyond current qualitative and quantitative parameters.

Conclusions and Future Perspectives

CCTA is being increasingly adopted in clinical practice and will likely become the dominant first-line test for noninvasive evaluation of CAD in the near future. Here, we demonstrate how AI algorithms can be directly applied to CCTA images for the automated detection and characterization of plaque as well as quantification of anatomic stenosis severity. Conventional plaque parameters can also be incorporated into ML models for cardiovascular risk prediction. Further, the combination of radiomics with AI techniques holds great promise for identifying new imaging biomarkers of the vulnerable plaque. While semi-automated software solutions now enable quantitative assessment of atherosclerotic plaque characteristics, this process is time-consuming and requires considerable input from a human reader. In the near future, fully automated quantification of coronary plaque morphology based on AI methods for image segmentation will likely become available.

Other disruptive technologies such as dual-energy CT and spectral CT will enhance our ability to characterize coronary atherosclerotic plaque. Compared with single-energy CT, dual-energy CT improves the differentiation of lipid and fibrous plaque components with minimum overlap of attenuation ranges [38] and thus could improve plaque characterization. Meanwhile, spectral CT with photon counting can accurately discriminate different plaque components by generating maps of the differences in contrast agent concentration and photon attenuation [39].

Finally, the combination of plaque radiomic features with a patient's genomics, proteomics, or metabolomics using ML will enable the development of comprehensive models for cardiovascular phenotyping and risk prediction. One of the ultimate goals of CCTA will be to provide precision imaging of plaque to facilitate personalized medicine.

Disclosures Outside of the current work, DD and PS received software royalties from Cedars-Sinai Medical Center and hold a patent. AL has no relevant conflicts of interest to disclose.

Funding This work was supported in part by grants from the National Heart, Lung, and Blood Institute [1R01HL133616 and 1R01HL148787-01A1].

References

1. Narula J, Chandrashekhar Y, Ahmadi A, et al. SCCT 2021 Expert consensus document on coronary computed tomographic angiography: a report of the society of Cardiovascular Computed Tomography. J Cardiovasc Comput Tomogr. 15:192–217.
2. Shaw LJ, Blankstein R, Bax JJ, et al. Society of Cardiovascular Computed Tomography / North American Society of Cardiovascular Imaging – Expert Consensus Document on Coronary CT Imaging of Atherosclerotic Plaque. J Cardiovasc Comput Tomogr. 2020;15:93–109.
3. Leipsic J, Abbara S, Achenbach S, et al. SCCT guidelines for the interpretation and reporting of coronary CT angiography: a report of the Society of Cardiovascular Computed Tomography Guidelines Committee. J Cardiovasc Comput Tomogr. 2014;8(5):342–58.
4. Hoffmann H, Frieler K, Hamm B, Dewey M. Intra- and interobserver variability in detection and assessment of calcified and noncalcified coronary artery plaques using 64-slice computed tomography. Int J Cardiovasc Imaging. 2008;24(7):735–42.
5. Arbab-Zadeh A, Hoe J. Quantification of coronary arterial stenoses by multidetector CT angiography in comparison with conventional angiography methods, caveats, and implications. JACC Cardiovasc Imaging. 2011;4(2):191–202.
6. Lesage D, Angelini ED, Bloch I, Funka-Lea G. A review of 3D vessel lumen segmentation techniques: models, features and extraction schemes. Med Image Anal. 2009;13(6):819–45.
7. Schaap M, Metz CT, van Walsum T, et al. Standardized evaluation methodology and reference database for evaluating coronary artery centerline extraction algorithms. Med Image Anal. 2009;13(5):701–14.
8. Kelm BM, Mittal S, Zheng Y, et al. Detection, grading and classification of coronary stenoses in computed tomography angiography. Med Image Comput Comput Assist Interv. 2011;14(Pt 3):25–32.
9. Gülsün M, Funka-Lea G, Sharma P, Rapaka S, Zheng Y. Coronary centerline extraction via optimal flow paths and CNN path pruning; 2016.
10. Wolterink JM, van Hamersvelt RW, Viergever MA, Leiner T, Isgum I. Coronary artery centerline extraction in cardiac CT angiography using a CNN-based orientation classifier. Med Image Anal. 2019;51:46–60.
11. Wei J, Zhou C, Chan H-P, et al. Computerized detection of noncalcified plaques in coronary CT angiography: evaluation of topological soft gradient prescreening method and luminal analysis. Med Phys. 2014;41(8):081901.
12. Jawaid MM, Riaz A, Rajani R, Reyes-Aldasoro CC, Slabaugh G. Framework for detection and localization of coronary noncalcified plaques in cardiac CTA using mean radial profiles. Comput Biol Med. 2017;89:84–95.
13. Zhao F, Wu B, Chen F, et al. An automatic multi-class coronary atherosclerosis plaque detection and classification framework. Med Biol Eng Comput. 2019;57(1):245–57.
14. Zreik M, van Hamersvelt RW, Wolterink JM, Leiner T, Viergever MA, Isgum I. A recurrent CNN for automatic detection and classification of coronary artery plaque and stenosis in coronary CT angiography. IEEE Trans Med Imaging. 2019;38(7):1588–98.
15. Kristanto W, van Ooijen PM, Jansen-van der Weide MC, Vliegenthart R, Oudkerk M. A meta analysis and hierarchical classification of HU-based atherosclerotic plaque characterization criteria. PLoS One. 2013;8(9):e73460.
16. Voros S, Rinehart S, Qian Z, et al. Coronary atherosclerosis imaging by coronary CT angiography: current status, correlation with intravascular interrogation and meta-analysis. JACC Cardiovasc Imaging. 2011;4(5):537–48.
17. Masuda T, Nakaura T, Funama Y, et al. Machine-learning integration of CT histogram analysis to evaluate the composition of atherosclerotic plaques: validation with IB-IVUS. J Cardiovasc Comput Tomogr. 2019;13(2):163–9.
18. Kolossváry M, Karády J, Kikuchi Y, et al. Radiomics versus visual and histogram-based assessment to identify atheromatous lesions at coronary CT angiography: an ex vivo study. Radiology. 2019;293(1):89–96.
19. Yamak D, Panse P, Pavlicek W, Boltz T, Akay M. Non-calcified coronary atherosclerotic plaque characterization by dual energy computed tomography. IEEE J Biomed Health Inform. 2014;18(3):939–45.
20. Lee MCH, Petersen K, Pawlowski N, Glocker B, Schaap M. TeTrIS: template transformer networks for image segmentation with shape priors. IEEE Trans Med Imaging. 2019;38(11):2596–606.
21. Zuluaga MA, Magnin IE, Hernández Hoyos M, Delgado Leyton EJF, Lozano F, Orkisz M. Automatic detection of abnormal vascular cross-sections based on density level detection and support vector machines. Int J Comput Assist Radiol Surg. 2011;6(2):163–74.
22. Kang D, Dey D, Slomka PJ, et al. Structured learning algorithm for detection of nonobstructive and obstructive coronary plaque lesions from computed tomography angiography. J Med Imaging (Bellingham). 2015;2(1):014003.
23. Hong Y, Commandeur F, Cadet S, et al. Deep learning-based stenosis quantification from coronary CT angiography. Proc SPIE Int Soc Opt Eng. 2019;10949:109492I.
24. Freiman M, Manjeshwar R, Goshen L. Unsupervised abnormality detection through mixed structure regularization (MSR) in deep sparse autoencoders. Med Phys. 2019;46(5):2223–31.
25. Min JK, Dunning A, Lin FY, et al. Age- and sex-related differences in all-cause mortality risk based on coronary computed tomography angiography findings results from the International Multicenter CONFIRM (Coronary CT Angiography Evaluation for Clinical Outcomes: An International Multicenter Registry) of 23,854

patients without known coronary artery disease. J Am Coll Cardiol. 2011;58(8):849–60.
26. Motwani M, Dey D, Berman DS, et al. Machine learning for prediction of all-cause mortality in patients with suspected coronary artery disease: a 5-year multicentre prospective registry analysis. Eur Heart J. 2017;38(7):500–7.
27. Williams MC, Kwiecinski J, Doris M, et al. Low-attenuation noncalcified plaque on coronary computed tomography angiography predicts myocardial infarction. Circulation. 2020;141(18):1452–62.
28. Chang HJ, Lin FY, Lee SE, et al. Coronary atherosclerotic precursors of acute coronary syndromes. J Am Coll Cardiol. 2018;71(22):2511–22.
29. Al'Aref SJ, Singh G, Choi JW, et al. A boosted ensemble algorithm for determination of plaque stability in high-risk patients on coronary CTA. JACC Cardiovasc Imaging. 2020:3447.
30. Han D, Kolli KK, Al'Aref SJ, et al. Machine learning framework to identify individuals at risk of rapid progression of coronary atherosclerosis: from the PARADIGM registry. J Am Heart Assoc. 2020;9(5):e013958.
31. Johnson NP, Tóth GG, Lai D, et al. Prognostic value of fractional flow reserve: linking physiologic severity to clinical outcomes. J Am Coll Cardiol. 2014;64(16):1641–54.
32. Dey D, Gaur S, Ovrehus KA, et al. Integrated prediction of lesion-specific ischaemia from quantitative coronary CT angiography using machine learning: a multicentre study. Eur Radiol. 2018;28(6):2655–64.
33. Kwan A, McElhinney P, Tamarappoo B, et al. Prediction of revascularization by coronary CT angiography using a machine learning ischemia risk score. Eur Radiol. 2020 (in press).
34. Dey D, Diaz Zamudio M, Schuhbaeck A, et al. Relationship between quantitative adverse plaque features from coronary computed tomography angiography and downstream impaired myocardial flow reserve by 13N-ammonia positron emission tomography: a pilot study. Circ Cardiovasc Imaging. 2015;8(10):e003255.
35. Puchner SB, Liu T, Mayrhofer T, et al. High-risk plaque detected on coronary CT angiography predicts acute coronary syndromes independent of significant stenosis in acute chest pain: results from the ROMICAT-II trial. J Am Coll Cardiol. 2014;64(7):684–92.
36. Kolossvary M, Karady J, Szilveszter B, et al. Radiomic features are superior to conventional quantitative computed tomographic metrics to identify coronary plaques with napkin-ring sign. Circ Cardiovasc Imaging. 2017;10(12):e006843.
37. Kolossváry M, Park J, Bang J-I, et al. Identification of invasive and radionuclide imaging markers of coronary plaque vulnerability using radiomic analysis of coronary computed tomography angiography. Eur Heart J Cardiovasc Imaging. 2019;20(11):1250–8.
38. Obaid DR, Calvert PA, Gopalan D, et al. Dual-energy computed tomography imaging to determine atherosclerotic plaque composition: a prospective study with tissue validation. J Cardiovasc Comput Tomogr. 2014;8(3):230–7.
39. Boussel L, Coulon P, Thran A, et al. Photon counting spectral CT component analysis of coronary artery atherosclerotic plaque samples. Br J Radiol. 2014;87(1040):20130798.
40. Dey D, Slomka PJ, Leeson P, et al. Artificial intelligence in cardiovascular imaging: JACC state-of-the-art review. J Am Coll Cardiol. 2019;73(11):1317–35.

Artificial Intelligence-Based Coronary Artery Disease Reporting and Data System (CAD-RADS)

26

Giuseppe Muscogiuri, Mattia Chiesa, Claudio Cau, Riccardo Cau, Marco Guglielmo, Andrea Baggiano, Laura Fusini, Andrea I. Guaricci, Luca Saba, Mark G. Rabbat, and Gianluca Pontone

Introduction

In recent years, radiology reporting has been evolving from a free text form to structured reporting [1]. The main advantage of structured reporting over free form reporting is represented by the application of a standardized approach that provides information to clinicians with a progressive hierarchy and focus on clinical query [1]. Although in the early days structured reporting approaches were strictly confined to specific body parts, currently the application of structured reporting involves more or less the whole body [2–8]. In particular, the application of structured reporting in cardiac computed tomography angiography (CCTA) was shown in Coronary Artery Disease Reporting and Data System (CAD-RADS) classification, which has been demonstrated to be useful for the evaluation of coronary artery disease (CAD) [8]. The CAD-RADS classification is an expert consensus document produced by a multi-society, multidisciplinary working group with the goal of improving communication of coronary CT angiography (CTA) results to referring physicians developed in 2016. In particular the development of CAD-RADS classification was performed in order to have a better management of patients with suspicious CAD. This approach, patient-based, is able to stratify the patients allowing a better management of patients standardizing the therapeutic approach [8].

The CAD-RADS classification is composed of the following classes: CAD-RADS 0, no CAD; CAD-RADS 1, minimal non-obstructive CAD; CAD-RADS 2, mild non-obstructive CAD; CAD-RADS 3, moderate stenosis; CAD-RADS 4, severe stenosis; and CAD-RADS 5, total occlusion [8]. An additional class "N" was also identified in the presence of a nondiagnostic study [8] (Table 26.1).

The possibility to provide quick information regarding the CAD burden in a patient-based analysis represents one of the main advantages of CAD-RADS classification, facilitating the management of patients with suspected CAD. The speed of reporting and query is extremely important considering the future widespread use of CCTA in clinical practice following the ESC guidelines; furthermore a standardized approach could be helpful for a correct and objective therapeutic approach [9].

A helpful tool for the evaluation of CAD-RADS in a time-efficient way can be provided from the application of artificial intelligence (AI) [10]. The use of AI in clinical practice, despite primarily confined to research purposes, could represent an important tool in cardiac imaging.

In this chapter, we will highlight the application of AI for CAD-RADS classification.

Application of CAD-RADS in Clinical Practice

In clinical practice, CAD-RADS represents an interesting tool for diagnosis and clinical management [11].

Early literature focused on the evaluation of reliability of CAD-RADS in clinical practice [12, 13]. Abdel Razek et al. evaluated the inter-observer agreement of CAD-RADS score

G. Muscogiuri, MD, PhD · M. Chiesa, PhD · M. Guglielmo, MD
A. Baggiano, MD · L. Fusini, MD · G. Pontone, MD, PhD (✉)
Centro Cardiologico Monzino, IRCCS, Milan, Italy
e-mail: mattia.chiesa@ccfm.it; marco.guglielmo@ccfm.it; andrea.baggiano@ccfm.it; laura.fusini@ccfm.it; gianluca.pontone@ccfm.it

C. Cau, MD · R. Cau, MD · L. Saba, MD
Department of Radiology, Azienda Ospedaliero Universitaria (A.O.U.), di Cagliari - Polo di Monserrato, Cagliari, Italy

A. I. Guaricci, MD
Institute of Cardiovascular Disease, Department of Emergency and Organ Transplantation, University Hospital "Policlinico Consorziale" of Bari, Bari, Italy

M. G. Rabbat, MD
Loyola University of Chicago, Chicago, IL, USA

Edward Hines Jr. VA Hospital, Hines, IL, USA
e-mail: mrabbat@lumc.edu

C. N. De Cecco et al. (eds.), *Artificial Intelligence in Cardiothoracic Imaging*, Contemporary Medical Imaging,
https://doi.org/10.1007/978-3-030-92087-6_26

Table 26.1 CAD-RADS classification

Score	Coronary stenosis	Interpretation	Further investigation	Management
CAD-RADS 0	0%	Absence of CAD	None	Examine other cause of chest pain
CAD-RADS 1	1–24%	Minimal non-obstructive CAD	None	Examine other cause of chest pain Evaluate risk factor modification and preventive therapy
CAD-RADS 2	24–49%	Mild non-obstructive CAD	None	Examine other cause of chest pain Evaluate risk factor modification and preventive therapy
CAD-RADS 3	50–69%	Moderate stenosis	Consider functional evaluation	Evaluate anti-ischemic, preventive therapy and risk factor modification
CAD-RADS 4a	70–99% single or two vessels	Severe stenosis	Functional evaluation or ICA	Evaluate anti-ischemic, preventive therapy and risk factor modification Evaluate other treatments (e.g., revascularization)
CAD-RADS 4b	Left main >50% or 3 vessels ≥70%		ICA	
CAD-RADS 5	100%	Total occlusion	ICA and/or viability evaluation	Evaluate anti-ischemic, preventive therapy and risk factor modification Evaluate other treatments (e.g., revascularization)
CAD-RADS N	Nondiagnostic test	Obstructive CAD cannot be excluded	Additional assessment needed	

in a selected cohort of 96 patients with stable chest pain [13] and demonstrated an overall agreement of $k = 0.862$ [13].

Maroules et al. analyzed the inter-observer agreement for the assessment of CAD-RADS in a setting composed by expert readers and early career readers and compared images with different image quality [12]. The authors found that overall intraclass correlation coefficient (ICC) for categories was excellent (ICC: 0.958). Expert readers demonstrated an ICC of 0.925, while for early career physicians, the ICC was 0.904. Interestingly, in the presence of high image quality, the ICC was 0.944, while in moderate image quality, it was 0.887 [12].

The application of AI will overcome the limitation of reproducibility. Indeed, the AI approach would be independent of reader experience and not prone to fatigue.

Focusing on the impact of CAD-RADS in terms of prognosis, several papers have been published in the literature [14, 15]. According to Xie et al., analyzing the cohort of the CONFIRM study, the 5-year survival in the CAD-RADS score 0–5 ranges from 95.2% to 69.3%, respectively [14]. When compared to the Duke Index and CCTA to predict myocardial infarction, the CAD-RADS approach showed the following results: Duke Index, 0.70; CCTA, 0.70; and CAD-RADS, 0.70 [14]. The increase of CAD-RADS score was positively associated with an increased number of invasive coronary angiography procedures [14]. In a selected cohort of SCOT-HEART trial, Williams et al. analyzed the impact of CAD-RADS in terms of prognosis [15]. The authors found that higher values of CAD-RADS were associated with an increased risk to develop fatal or nonfatal myocardial infarction; in particular, the class with higher risk (represented by the category CAD-RADS 4b) observed a hazard ratio (HR) of 19.4 [15].

In a larger population consisting of 3840 patients, Bittner et al. showed that classification of CAD-RADS can be extremely helpful for accurate risk stratification [16]. Patients with CAD-RADS 4b and 5 showed a HR of 30.80, while in CAD-RADS 1, the HR was 2.66 [16]. This finding was confirmed by adjusting the CAD-RADS score with atherosclerotic cardiovascular disease (ASCVD) risk score showing, for CAD-RADS 1 and CAD-RADS 5, HR values of 2.43 and 21.84, respectively [16].

The application of CAD-RADS in routine clinical practice can be fundamental for correct risk stratification; however as mentioned above, the reporting can differ depending on expertise of readers. Furthermore, the analysis of images can be time-consuming; indeed, the analysis is patient based, and it is mandatory to analyze the burden of CAD in all coronaries. The application of AI could facilitate, improve reproducibility, and speed up the whole CAD-RADS assessment.

Development of CNN for CAD-RADS Analysis

Currently, convolutional neural networks (CNNs) are the most powerful deep learning technique used for diagnosis classification and prediction from medical images [17]. A CNN consists of a series of convolution and pooling operators, followed by a standard fully connected artificial neural network. By an iterative learning phase (called training), a CNN improves itself minimizing the error between the predictions achieved and the ground truth labels [18, 19]. Overall, the first two types of layers, convolution and pooling, perform feature extraction, whereas the fully connected layer maps the extracted features into final output classes. Moreover, the concatenation of consecutive blocks of convolutional and pooling layers allows detecting more and more specific and relevant structures in the image, from single edges to complex objects. Other hyper-parameters allow controlling the complexity and the performance of the CNN. The presence of dropout layers and the regularization limit the overfitting effect [20]. The number of neurons and the number of hidden layers in the full-connected part of the CNN affect the classification performance, and different settings of learning rate, optimizers, epochs, loss function, the number of convolutional filters, and the ratio between training set and test set highly impact the CNN efficacy and efficiency.

Of note, finding the best combination of hyper-parameters is a critical task which should be performed for each specific case. Concerning the CAD-RADS classification, a suitable combination of parameters for implementing a 2-D CNN consisted of a sequence of three blocks of convolutional layer and a max pooling layer. Each convolutional layer should be composed of at least 32 filters (3 × 3 px) and the pooling window size of 2 × 2. A densely connected network with two hidden layers (16 and 8 neurons, respectively) and an output layer is sufficient to predict CAD-RADS classes. To handle the overfitting, a dropout strategy should also be implemented before the first hidden layer (dropout rate, 0.5). The ReLU activation function is the optimal solution for each neuron, except for the output layer (activation function: "softmax"). Moreover, to ensure that the CNN learns highly discriminant patterns, at least 500 iterative epochs and a data augmentation strategy are needed [10].

Finally, many other parameters have to be properly set based on the shape and the format of data. The standard format for storing CT scans is the DICOM standard, usually composed of 256 slices (512 by 512 pixels). On one hand, if a specific frame is selected or a mosaic of frames is generated, the aforementioned architecture is sufficient; on the other hand, if the DICOM is fed into the network as is (3D object: frame by height by width), a 3D CNN configuration has to be implemented.

AI Applications in CAD-RADS

The application of AI in CAD-RADS has mainly focused on the evaluation of CAD-RADS in a short time [10]. To date, only few articles have been published [10, 21, 22].

Our team first described the application of a CNN for CAD-RADS evaluation in 2020 on 288 patients [10]. In particular, we developed a 2D-CNN for identification of correct CAD-RADS, analyzing the diagnostic performance in three different CAD-RADS models. Model A was composed of CAD-RADS 0 vs CAD-RADS 1-2 vs CAD-RADS 3-5, Model 1 was composed of CAD-RADS 0 and CAD-RADS >0, and Model 2 was composed of CAD-RADS 0-2 and CAD-RADS 3-5 [10]. We were successful in developing an algorithm that was able to correctly identify CAD-RADS with a sensitivity, specificity, negative predictive value, positive predictive value, and accuracy in Model A of 47%, 74%, 77%, 46%, and 60%. Model 1 showed a sensitivity, specificity, negative predictive value, positive predictive value, and accuracy of 66%, 91%, 92%, 63%, and 86%, while in Model 2 the sensitivity, specificity, negative predictive value, positive predictive value, and accuracy were 82%, 58%, 74%, 69%, and 71%, respectively [10]. It is important to note that the time of identification of CAD-RADS using the automatic approach was 104.3 ± 1.4 sec vs 530.5 ± 179 sec for human analysis [10].

Similarly, Denzinger et al. developed a CNN algorithm that was able to differentiate the different classes of CAD-RADS in a large cohort of 2867 patients [22]. The authors tested their network using the Model 1 (CAD-RADS 0 vs CAD-RADS 1-5) and Model 2 (CAD-RADS 0-2 vs CAD-RADS 3-5) developed by our team (Muscogiuri et al.) [10]. For Model 1, the authors found an AUC, accuracy, sensitivity, and specificity of 0.860, 0.849, 0.489, and 0.907, respectively, and when combined with a regression of calcification grade, it was able to identify the correct CAD-RADS subgroup with an AUC, accuracy, sensitivity, and specificity of 0.914, 0.888, 0.532, and 0.945, respectively [22]. For Model 2, the AUC, accuracy, sensitivity, and specificity were 0.901, 0.838, 0.879, and 0.759, and when combined with calcification grade, it predicted an AUC, accuracy, sensitivity, and specificity of 0.923, 0.860, 0.891, and 0.802, respectively [22].

Another interesting article published by Huang et al. analyzed the relationship between CAD-RADS analyzed by a deep learning approach and breast arterial calcification (BAC) [21].

In particular, Huang et al. classified CAD-RADS using a deep learning technique in low CAD-RADS (CAD-RADS <3) and high CAD-RADS (CAD-RADS ≥3) [21]. The authors found that high CAD-RADS was associated with higher prevalence of BAC [21].

These papers demonstrate that is possible to develop a successful AI algorithm to automatically provide a CAD-RADS analysis. The algorithms used for the analysis, in the three manuscripts are based on deep learning technique and they showed the possibility to have an accurate evaluation of CAD-RADS using an approach based on AI (Fig. 26.1). Figures 26.2 and 26.3 show two cases of a correct identification of CAD by AI tool. However, it is clearly evident that these investigators were not able to identify the exact category of CAD-RADS, while it was possible to identify some macroareas. It is necessary in the future to develop an algorithm that is able to identify the exact category. In this way, it would be possible to speed up the post-processing of CCTA.

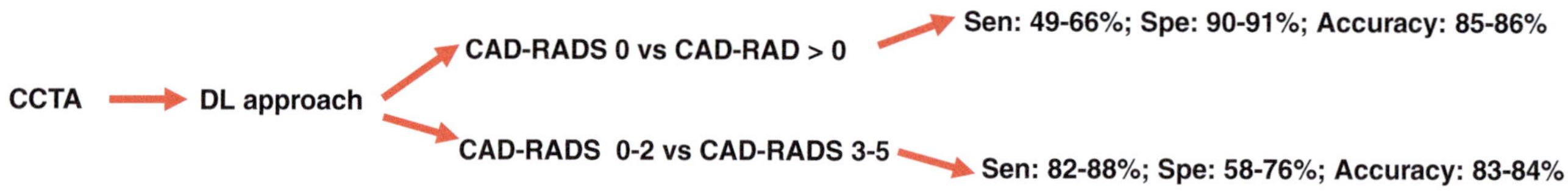

Fig. 26.1 Image showing the current state of the art for CAD-RAD classification using DL algorithms according the manuscript of Muscogiuri et al. [10] and Denziger et al. [22]

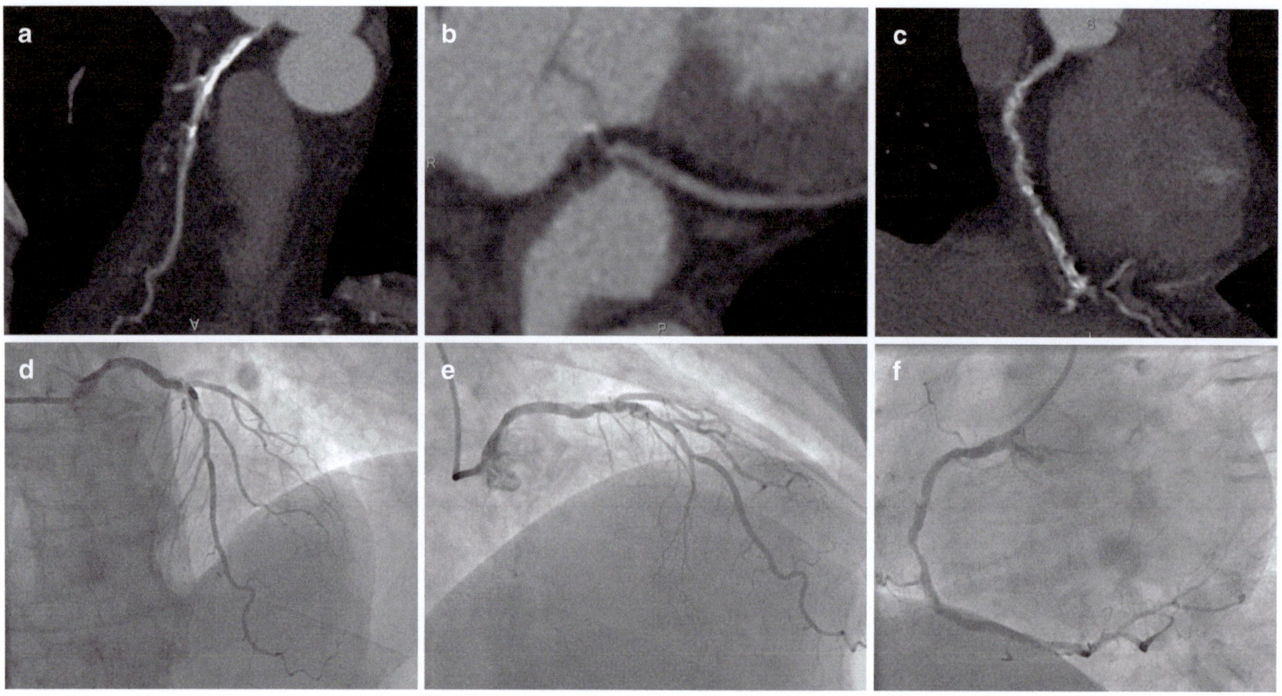

Fig. 26.2 CAD-RADS 4. A 69-year-old patient with typical chest pain demonstrating severe calcified plaques in the left anterior descending artery (**a**), non-calcified moderate stenosis in the left circumflex artery (**b**), and diffuse calcified and non-calcified disease in the right coronary artery with a moderate calcified plaque in the mid-segment (**c**) on coronary computed tomography angiography. These findings were confirmed on invasive coronary angiography of the left anterior descending artery (**d**), left circumflex artery, (**e**) and right coronary artery (**f**)

Conclusion

The application of AI in CAD-RADS assessment should allow the evaluation of CAD-RADS scores in a short time [10]. Development of new AI algorithms will be useful in terms of time reduction and increase of diagnostic accuracy. These developments will be necessary if we consider the increasing number CCTA requests. Although these algorithms may be useful in clinical practice, we need to consider that CAD-RADS assessment should be complemented by the assessment of ischemia and advanced plaque analysis. The development of complex AI algorithms analyzing and combining multiple morphological and functional parameters represents the next step in the AI applied to CAD.

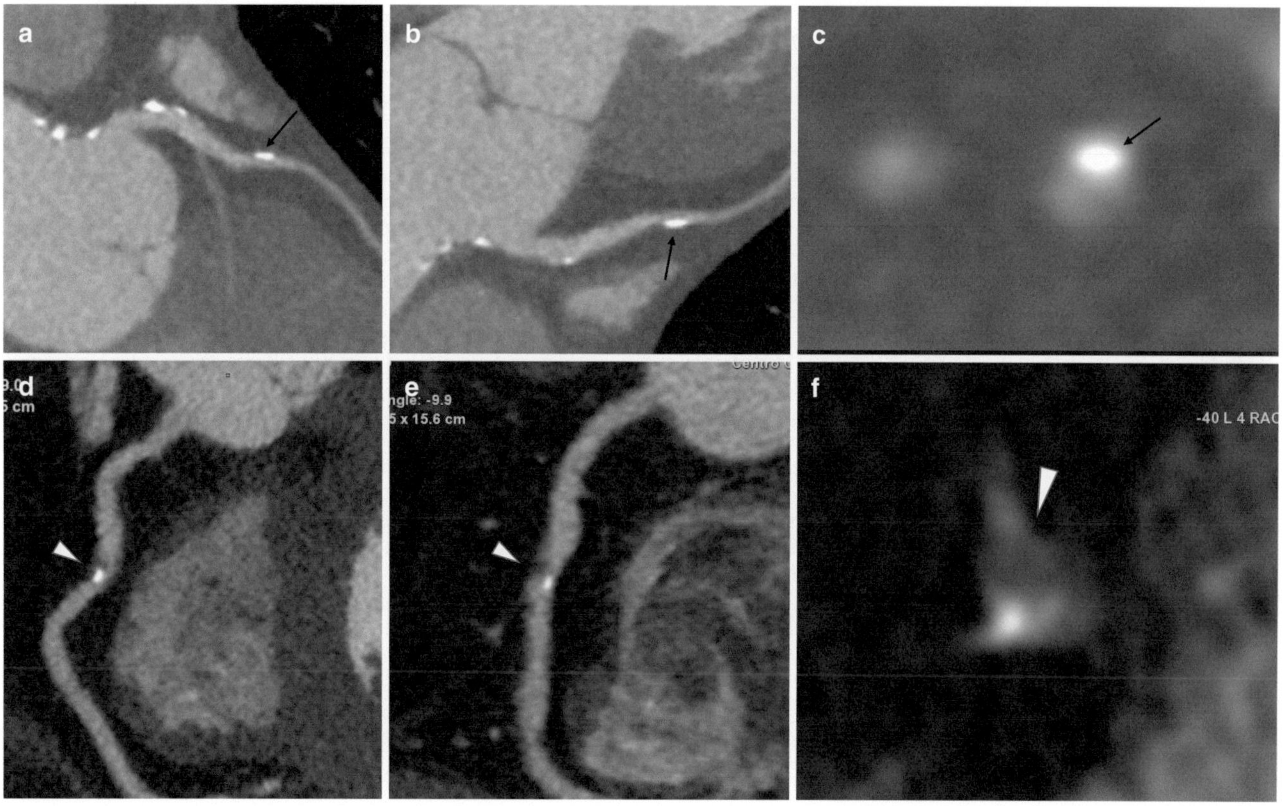

Fig. 26.3 A 76-year-old male patient with atypical chest pain underwent cardiac computed tomography angiography (CCTA) for suspected CAD. CCTA showed on multiplanar reconstructions (arrows A, B) and cross-sectional view (arrow, C) mild calcified plaque in the first diagonal branch of the LAD. A CAD-RADS 2 score was attributed. A 74-year-old patient underwent CCTA for dyspnea during exercise showing severe mixed plaque on multiplanar reconstructions (arrow-heads, D and E) and cross-sectional view (arrow-head, F). The patient was classified as CAD-RADS 4

References

1. Faggioni L, Coppola F, Ferrari R, Neri E, Regge D. Usage of structured reporting in radiological practice: results from an Italian online survey. Eur Radiol. 2017;27:1934–43.
2. Stoian D, Timar B, Derban M, Pantea S, Varcus F, Craina M, Craciunescu M. Thyroid imaging reporting and data system (TI-RADS): the impact of quantitative strain elastography for better stratification of cancer risks. Med Ultrason. 2015;17:327–32.
3. Yee J, Chang KJ, Dachman AH, Kim DH, McFarland EG, Pickhardt PJ, Cash BD, Bruining DH, Zalis ME. The added value of the CT colonography reporting and data system. J Am Coll Radiol. 2016;13:931–5.
4. Mahoney MC, Gatsonis C, Hanna L, DeMartini WB, Lehman C. Positive predictive value of BI-RADS MR imaging. Radiology. 2012;264:51–8.
5. Amor F, Alcazar JL, Vaccaro H, Leon M, Iturra A. GI-RADS reporting system for ultrasound evaluation of adnexal masses in clinical practice: a prospective multicenter study. Ultrasound Obstet Gynecol. 2011;38:450–5.
6. Rothke M, Blondin D, Schlemmer HP, Franiel T. PI-RADS classification: structured reporting for MRI of the prostate. Rofo. 2013;185:253–61.
7. An JY, Unsdorfer KML, Weinreb JC. BI-RADS, C-RADS, CAD-RADS, LI-RADS, lung-RADS, NI-RADS, O-RADS, PI-RADS, TI-RADS: reporting and data systems. Radiographics. 2019;39:1435–6.
8. Cury RC, Abbara S, Achenbach S, Agatston A, Berman DS, Budoff MJ, Dill KE, Jacobs JE, Maroules CD, Rubin GD, Rybicki FJ, Schoepf UJ, Shaw LJ, Stillman AE, White CS, Woodard PK, Leipsic JA. CAD-RADS(TM) Coronary Artery Disease - Reporting and Data System. An expert consensus document of the Society of Cardiovascular Computed Tomography (SCCT), the American College of Radiology (ACR) and the North American Society for Cardiovascular Imaging (NASCI). Endorsed by the American College of Cardiology. J Cardiovasc Comput Tomogr. 2016;10:269–81.
9. Knuuti J, Wijns W, Saraste A, Capodanno D, Barbato E, Funck-Brentano C, Prescott E, Storey RF, Deaton C, Cuisset T, Agewall S, Dickstein K, Edvardsen T, Escaned J, Gersh BJ, Svitil P, Gilard M, Hasdai D, Hatala R, Mahfoud F, Masip J, Muneretto C, Valgimigli M, Achenbach S, Bax JJ, Group ESCSD. ESC guidelines for the diagnosis and management of chronic coronary syndromes. Eur Heart J. 2019;2020(41):407–77.
10. Muscogiuri G, Chiesa M, Trotta M, Gatti M, Palmisano V, Dell'Aversana S, Baessato F, Cavaliere A, Cicala G, Loffreno A, Rizzon G, Guglielmo M, Baggiano A, Fusini L, Saba L, Andreini D, Pepi M, Rabbat MG, Guaricci AI, De Cecco CN, Colombo G, Pontone G. Performance of a deep learning algorithm for the evaluation of CAD-RADS classification with CCTA. Atherosclerosis. 2020;294:25–32.
11. Foldyna B, Szilveszter B, Scholtz JE, Banerji D, Maurovich-Horvat P, Hoffmann U. CAD-RADS - a new clinical decision support tool for coronary computed tomography angiography. Eur Radiol. 2018;28:1365–72.

12. Maroules CD, Hamilton-Craig C, Branch K, Lee J, Cury RC, Maurovich-Horvat P, Rubinshtein R, Thomas D, Williams M, Guo Y, Cury RC. Coronary artery disease reporting and data system (CAD-RADS(TM)): inter-observer agreement for assessment categories and modifiers. J Cardiovasc Comput Tomogr. 2018;12:125–30.
13. Abdel Razek AAK, Elrakhawy MM, Yossof MM, Nageb HM. Inter-observer agreement of the Coronary Artery Disease Reporting and Data System (CAD-RADS(TM)) in patients with stable chest pain. Pol J Radiol. 2018;83:e151–9.
14. Xie JX, Cury RC, Leipsic J, Crim MT, Berman DS, Gransar H, Budoff MJ, Achenbach S, Hartaigh BÓ, Callister TQ, Marques H, Rubinshtein R, Al-Mallah MH, Andreini D, Pontone G, Cademartiri F, Maffei E, Chinnaiyan K, Raff G, Hadamitzky M, Hausleiter J, Feuchtner G, Dunning A, DeLago A, Kim YJ, Kaufmann PA, Villines TC, Chow BJW, Hindoyan N, Gomez M, Lin FY, Jones E, Min JK, Shaw LJ. The Coronary Artery Disease-Reporting and Data System (CAD-RADS): prognostic and clinical implications associated with standardized coronary computed tomography angiography reporting. JACC Cardiovasc Imaging. 2018;11:78–89.
15. Williams MC, Moss A, Dweck M, Hunter A, Pawade T, Adamson PD, Shah ASV, Alam S, Maroules CD, van Beek EJ, Cury R, Nicol ED, Newby DE, Roditi G. Standardized reporting systems for computed tomography coronary angiography and calcium scoring: A real-world validation of CAD-RADS and CAC-DRS in patients with stable chest pain. J Cardiovasc Comput Tomogr. 2020;14:3–11.
16. Bittner DO, Mayrhofer T, Budoff M, Szilveszter B, Foldyna B, Hallett TR, Ivanov A, Janjua S, Meyersohn NM, Staziaki PV, Achenbach S, Ferencik M, Douglas PS, Hoffmann U, Lu MT, Investigators P. Prognostic value of coronary CTA in stable chest pain: CAD-RADS, CAC, and cardiovascular events in PROMISE. JACC Cardiovasc Imaging. 2020;13:1534–45.
17. Litjens G, Kooi T, Bejnordi BE, Setio AAA, Ciompi F, Ghafoorian M, van der Laak J, van Ginneken B, Sanchez CI. A survey on deep learning in medical image analysis. Med Image Anal. 2017;42:60–88.
18. LeCun Y, Bengio Y, Hinton G. Deep learning. Nature. 2015;521:436–44.
19. Bengio Y, Courville A, Vincent P. Representation learning: a review and new perspectives. IEEE Trans Pattern Anal Mach Intell. 2013;35:1798–828.
20. Svristava N, Hinton G, Khrizhevsky A, Sutskever I, Salakhutdinov R. Dropout: a simple way to prevent neural networks from overfitting. J Machine Learning. 2014;15:1929–58.
21. Huang Z, Xiao J, Xie Y, Hu Y, Zhang S, Li X, Wang Z, Li Z, Wang X. The correlation of deep learning-based CAD-RADS evaluated by coronary computed tomography angiography with breast arterial calcification on mammography. Sci Rep. 2020;10:11532.
22. Denzinger F, Wels M, Breininger K, Gülsün MA, Schöbinger M, André F, Buß S, Görich J, Sühling M and Maier A. Automatic CAD-RADS scoring using deep learning. MICCAI 2020; 2020.

Artificial Intelligence-Based CT-Derived Fractional Flow Reserve (CT-FFR)

27

Verena Brandt, Hunter N. Gray, and Christian Tesche

Introduction

Cardiac CT using coronary CT angiography (cCTA) is a clinically proven noninvasive method which has shown excellent evaluation of coronary artery disease (CAD) combining morphological and anatomical assessment of CAD for cardiovascular risk stratification and therapeutic decision-making [1–3], in addition to providing prognostic value for the occurrence of adverse cardiac outcome. In recent decades, cCTA has emerged as a diagnostic tool with high negative predictive value (NPV) and moderate positive predictive value (PPV), comparable to the invasive coronary angiography (ICA) with FFR [4, 5], which is established as the gold standard for the functional and anatomical assessment of CAD [6].

In 2019, the European Society of Cardiology (ESC) classified computed tomography angiography (CTA) as class 1 recommendation for diagnosing stable CAD in symptomatic patients [7]. Considering all aspects, it should be noted that the anatomical assessment by cCTA alone provides poor discriminatory value concerning the prediction of ischemia-specific CAD, which strongly weakens the diagnostic power. Recent advances in CT software applications considerably improved the evaluation of hemodynamically significant stenosis. Coronary computed tomography fractional flow reserve (CT-FFR) has emerged as a new, noninvasive technology that uses CTA images combined with computational fluid dynamic (CFD) techniques to estimate virtual FFR values throughout coronary vessels and offers precise quantification of a specific coronary lesion, regarding hemodynamic consequence [8, 9]. For CT-FFR, several multicenter trials displayed a significantly higher predictive value for functionally obstructive lesions as defined by invasive FFR, which may help direct therapeutic decision-making with the potential to improve efficiency of ICA [10, 11]. However, CFD-based CT-FFR entails potential limitations, such as off-site computation and long process duration. Therefore, new technical approaches for assessment of CT-FFR feature assisting software algorithms, which use artificial intelligence (AI) and machine learning (ML) based on deep neural networks [12, 13].

AI is based on mathematics and computer science using large datasets as well as high performance computational infrastructure with applied algorithms [10]. In medical imaging, most AI systems are based on ML applications, which facilitate improved workflow, superior diagnostic accuracy to identify flow-limiting CAD, better outcome prediction, and more effective decision-making in daily clinical practice [14, 15].

Recent studies demonstrated that ML-based CT-FFR (CT-FFR_{ML}) resolves the abovementioned limitations of CFD-based CT-FFR while also providing higher prognostic value when compared to flow-limiting CAD by cCTA alone. In summary, this grants an option to improve efficiency of ICA and reduce accompanying complications [16–18].

V. Brandt, MD
Division of Cardiovascular Imaging, Department of Radiology and Radiological Science, Medical University of South Carolina, Charleston, SC, USA

Department of Cardiology, Robert-Bosch-Krankenhaus, Stuttgart, Germany

H. N. Gray, BS
Division of Cardiovascular Imaging, Department of Radiology and Radiological Science, Medical University of South Carolina, Charleston, SC, USA
e-mail: grayhu@musc.edu

C. Tesche, MD (✉)
Division of Cardiovascular Imaging, Department of Radiology and Radiological Science, Medical University of South Carolina, Charleston, SC, USA

Department of Cardiology, Robert-Bosch-Krankenhaus, Stuttgart, Germany

Department of Cardiology, Munich University Clinic, Ludwig-Maximilians-University, Munich, Germany

Department of Internal Medicine, St. Johannes-Hospital, Dortmund, Germany

C. N. De Cecco et al. (eds.), *Artificial Intelligence in Cardiothoracic Imaging*, Contemporary Medical Imaging,
https://doi.org/10.1007/978-3-030-92087-6_27

During the further course of this chapter, an overview of the technical background, clinical validation, and implementation of CT-FFR$_{ML}$ as well as a future outlook is given.

Artificial Intelligence Applications in CT-FFR

Principles and Technical Aspects

CT-FFR$_{ML}$ represents an opportunity to detect functional significant CAD through the application of using only noninvasive image post-processing techniques on standard datasets combined with cCTA, previously described in detail [12, 13]. By using a software based on an artificial intelligence algorithm, CT-FFR$_{ML}$ grants a deep learning framework, which inputs the cCTA dataset of the coronary artery tree geometry to compute the functional classification of a coronary lesion. A multilayer neural network is a deep learning model that is trained offline to learn the diverse relationships between the anatomy of the coronary tree and its analogous hemodynamic parameters [12].

By enrolling a large database of certain parameters like artificial coronary anatomies, the ML model can be trained to identify and differentiate anatomical variation and its accompanying hemodynamic conditions from a computational fluid dynamic simulation. An artificial dataset of 12,000 three-dimensional coronary artery models is generated by an algorithm, representing diversified patient characteristics like branch length, degree of tapering, and vessel radius.

Important parameters concerning quantification and analysis of stenosis include total length, maximum degree of radius reduction, location of the stenosis center, length of the stenosis region with minimum radius, and overall degree of tapering along the stenosis. Stenosis is categorized as single or serial, multibranch, or bifurcation [12].

The ML algorithm training phase uses a reduced-order computational blood flow model, which allows calculation of CT-FFR$_{ML}$ values at all locations along the coronary vessels from the given model of the created coronary tree. It is to note that the computational blood flow model has been reevaluated and compared to invasive approaches in recent clinical studies [19, 20].

The artificial deep learning framework consists of 28 different input features, like coronary anatomy, and their interactions in the neural network. Specific features, such as FFR, are represented by a classified scheme from a database of samples with prior analyzed characteristics and outcomes acquired from the computational fluid dynamic approach. Higher diagnostic accuracy is achieved by application of abovementioned ML algorithm against the prior CFD algorithm, as shown by Itu et al. [12]. Technical calculation of CT-FFR$_{ML}$ is shown in Fig. 27.1.

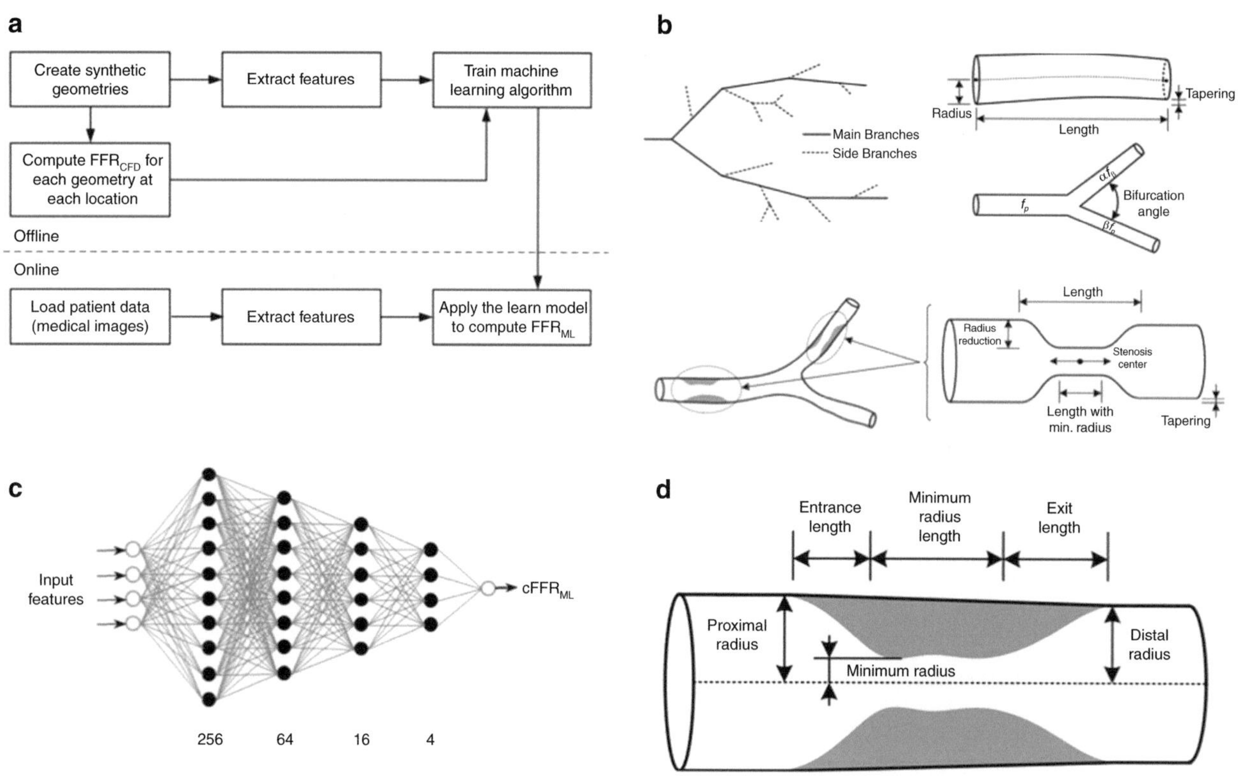

Fig. 27.1 Workflow for the calculation of CT-FFR$_{ML}$. (**a**) Workflow of machine learning-derived CT-FFR (CT-FFR$_{ML}$) calculation. (**b**) Creation of stenotic coronary arteries with modeling of healthy geometry information, stenotic lesions, and radius of the parent branch of the bifurcation. (**c**) Deep learning network architecture to train the CT-FFR$_{ML}$ model. The network consists of four hidden layers and uses a fully connected network model. (**d**) Automatic detection of stenosis-specific features. (Courtesy of Siemens Healthineers)

Current Evidence

Validation and Diagnostic Accuracy

After its introduction in 2016, several studies have confirmed CT-FFR_{ML} as being an equal or superior diagnostic method in comparison to invasive FFR as the standard of reference [12].

So far, the diagnostic performance of CT-FFR_{ML} was evaluated in several single-center studies and one multicenter trial in relation to cCTA. A threshold of ≤0.80 acquired from invasive FFR was established to identify hemodynamically significant stenosis.

Numerous single-center studies have provided insight on CT-FFR_{ML} diagnostic performance: Tesche et al. investigated diagnostic accuracy of CT-FFR compared to CT-FFR_{ML} in a retrospective study [21] which analyzed a cohort of 85 patients (104 vessels). The results showed on a per-lesion and per-patient level a sensitivity of 79% and 90% and a specificity of 94% and 95%, respectively, by CT-FFR_{ML} for detecting lesion-specific ischemia. Additionally, a ROC analysis revealed higher diagnostic performance of CT-FFR_{ML} to cCTA alone, both on a per-lesion and per-patient level (AUCs of 0.89 vs. 0.61, $p < 0.001$ and 0.91 vs. 0.65, $p < 0.001$, respectively).

Another publication demonstrated an analysis regarding the diagnostic performance of CT-FFR_{ML} combined with plaque quantification for detecting lesion-specific ischemia in 84 patients (103 vessels) [22]. CT-FFR_{ML} provided higher discrimination of lesion-specific ischemia in comparison to cCTA (AUC 0.89 vs. AUC 0.61), while a sensitivity and specificity of 82% and 94% for CT-FFR_{ML} were shown. Comparable results regarding sensitivity and specificity (0.91 and 0.96) for CT-FFR_{ML} were shown by Rother et al. in a study with 71 patients (91 vessels), with significantly higher AUC for CT-FFR_{ML} in comparison to visual stenosis grading on cCTA (AUC 0.94 vs. 0.61, $p < 0.05$) [23].

A retrospective multicenter trial was built on the MACHINE registry (named *Diagnostic Accuracy of a Machine-Learning Approach to Coronary Computed Tomographic Angiography-Based Fractional Flow Reserve: Result from the MACHINE Consortium*), including 351 patients (525 vessels) from 5 sites in the United States, Europe, and Asia [16]. The study objective was to evaluate the diagnostic performance of CT-FFR_{ML} in comparison to CT-FFR, using a CFD algorithm (CT-FFR_{CFD}).

First- and second-generation dual-source CT scanners (Somatom Definition or Somatom Definition Flash, Siemens Healthineers, Forchheim, Germany) provided the image source while using a research prototype (cFFR version 2.1, Siemens Healthineers, Forchheim, Germany) for CT-FFR_{ML} analysis.

Significant improvement regarding diagnostic accuracy of CT-FFR_{ML} vs. cCTA (78% vs. 58%) was demonstrated. Additionally, the per-patient accuracy changed from 71% by cCTA to 85% by using machine learning-based CT-FFR, as well as the correction of 73% false-positive cCTA results.

Intermediate Stenosis

In 2018, Kim et al. demonstrated limitations for diagnosis of lesion-specific ischemia in intermediate coronary stenosis by cCTA [24]. CT-FFR_{ML} may have the potential to differentiate between the need of ICA with revascularization and conservative therapy. An investigation by Tang et al. evaluated 101 patients (122 vessels) with intermediate coronary lesion severity (30–69% stenosis grade) in which CT-FFR_{ML} provided high accuracy and specificity (0.89 and 0.94, respectively) for identification of lesion-specific ischemia, compared to cCTA grading alone (AUC: 0.79 vs. 0.53, $p < 0.05$) [25]. Nous et al. presented similar results, when showing a significant reduction of patients requiring additional ICA by availability of on-site CT-FFR on cCTA compared to cCTA alone, which would have changed the initial management strategy significantly [26].

Influence of Coronary Calcification

In a subgroup analysis of the MACHINE registry, authors evaluated the influence of coronary artery calcium (CAC) on the diagnostic performance of CT-FFR_{ML} [27].

A total of 482 vessels in 314 patients (77% male) who underwent cCTA followed by ICA with FFR were investigated by CT-FFR_{ML} with data from the MACHINE registry.

Diagnostic performance of CT-FFR_{ML} to detect lesion-specific ischemia was compared to invasive FFR as the reference standard by using the CAC score quantified by the Agatston method with subsequent CAC categories (CAC 0, > 0 to <100, 100 to <400, and ≥400).

The diagnostic accuracy of CT-FFR_{ML} against invasive FFR was higher than cCTA alone on a per-vessel level (78% vs. 60%) and per-patient level (83% vs. 73%) across all Agatston score categories. High discrimination using CT-FFR_{ML} was shown in vessels with high Agatston scores (CAC ≥400) and high accuracy in low-to-intermediate Agatston scores (CAC > 0 to <400). However, statistically significant CT-derived fractional flow reserve (CT-FFR): differences in the AUCs (AUC, 0.71 [95% CI, 0.57–0.85] vs. 0.85 [95% CI, 0.82–0.89], p = 0.04) were detected. All in all, CT-FFR_{ML} demonstrated higher diagnostic performance over cCTA in vessels with high Agatston scores (p = 0.04) and low-to-intermediate Agatston scores ($p < 0.001$). It is to note that 20 patients (5%) were excluded due to nondiagnostic image quality.

Influence of Gender

The impact of sex on the diagnostic performance of CT-FFR_{ML} was investigated by Baumann and colleagues [28]. A total of 398 vessels in men and 127 vessels in woman were analyzed by machine learning-derived CT-FFR. For men, the sensitivity and specificity were 0.78 and 0.79 compared to 0.75 and 0.81 in women. Summarized CAD diagnostic by CT-FFR_{ML} presented no significant gender difference (p = 0.89). Furthermore, CT-FFR_{ML} showed significantly higher accuracy in men (p = 0.007) to cCTA alone, but none in women (p = 0.12), explained by the authors with limited statistical power by under-representation of women (26.5%).

Influence of Diabetes Mellitus

The prevalence of diabetes mellitus (DM) is growing and has reached epidemic range worldwide [29, 30]. Coronary artery disease (CAD) is the leading cause of death and a major determinant factor of the long-term prognosis in patients with DM. Clinically, there are many reasons for this, including metabolic factors like dyslipidemia, hyperglycemia, and insulin resistance, in addition to hypertension and obesity, which lead to endothelial and microvascular dysfunction with a more diffuse atherosclerosis and abnormal coagulation by impaired platelet function [31–33]. Concerning heart disease, this patient population has a twofold to fourfold increased mortality risk, an increased mortality after myocardial infarction (MI), as well as worse overall prognosis with CAD [34].

CT-FFR is based on the expectation of a normal coronary microvascular response. Nous et al. [35] investigated the diagnostic performance of a machine-learning based application by CT-FFR in patients with and without diabetes mellitus with suspected coronary artery disease.

Overall, 75 diabetic patients with 110 vessels and 276 nondiabetic patients with 415 vessels were evaluated. CT-FFR_{ML} has a diagnostic accuracy of 75% in nondiabetic patients and 83% in diabetic patients (p = 0.088) and demonstrated a higher diagnostic performance over cCTA alone, which was 65% and 58% (p = 0.223), respectively. Nous et al. were able to conclude not only that CT-FFR_{ML} accurately discriminated lesion-specific ischemia in both nondiabetic and diabetic patients but also that CT-FFR_{ML} has an improved diagnostic accuracy compared to cCTA alone.

Clinical Implications

Impact on Patient Management

The insufficient data situation for CT-FFR_{ML} on patient management, outcome, and clinical impact is based primarily on retrospective, single-center studies and needs more scientific evidence in the framework of large, multicenter investigations.

In prior studies, the importance of CT-FFR_{ML} regarding adverse cardiac outcome has been shown in comparison to standard cCTA [17]. Aside from displaying a higher predictive value for MACE (major adverse cardiac events), CT-FFR_{ML} provided stronger discriminatory power over cCTA for stenosis classification alone: after median follow-up of 18.5 months, MACE was identified in 21% (18 of 82 patients), while in multivariable regression analysis, CT-$FFR_{ML} \leq 0.80$ presented the most significant predictor (p = 0.001, odds ratio 7.78). Additional predictive value for future MACE detection by CT-FFR_{ML} in comparison to degree of lumen stenosis on ICA was demonstrated by Duguay et al. [36].

Furthermore, Qiao et al. confirmed these results by showing CT-FFR_{ML} to have higher prognostic value compared to hemodynamic significant coronary stenosis identified with cCTA and argued in view of this for improved therapeutic decision-making with the potential to improve efficiency of ICA by CT-FFR_{ML}.

Another retrospective single-center study investigated therapeutic strategy (optimal medical therapy alone vs. revascularization) and revascularization method (percutaneous coronary intervention vs. coronary artery bypass grafting) by using cCTA/CT-FFR_{ML} versus ICA with invasive FFR as the reference standard [37]. In 49% of the patients (36 of 74), hemodynamically significant CAD was detected by invasive measurement (ICA with FFR). Patients with this diagnosed flow-limiting CAD by ICA/FFR and the cohort with nonsignificant hemodynamically CAD were precisely detected by cCTA/CT-FFR_{ML} with 97% (35 of 36) and 100% (38 of 38), respectively. There was general approval concerning appropriate indication of revascularization therapy by ICA/FFR versus cCTA/CT-FFR_{ML} in 97% (35 of 36). High accuracy (0.99), sensitivity (0.97), and specificity (1.0) underlined correct treatment decision with cCTA/CT-FFR_{ML} in 99% (73 of 74) of the patients. In the light of these results, CT-FFR_{ML} shows promising diagnostic potential for right-guided therapeutic decision-making, especially concerning further reduction of additional ICA procedures and related radiation exposure [28]. Case examples of CT-FFR_{ML}, cCTA, and ICA with corresponding invasive FFR measurements are shown in Figs. 27.2 and 27.3.

Acute chest pain (ACP) is one of the most common reasons for presentation in the emergency department. Because of this, there is a need of improved specificity in identifying patients with significant CAD for further therapeutic strategy. Recent studies showed that the calculation with on-site application of CT-FFR in triple-rule-out CTA (chest-pain CT) improves diagnostic accuracy and was a better predictor concerning MACE and need for coronary revascularization compared to triple-rule-out CTA alone [38, 39]. Therefore, CT-FFR is feasible in the emergency setting and may show improved specificity in identification of patients with ACP and significant CAD.

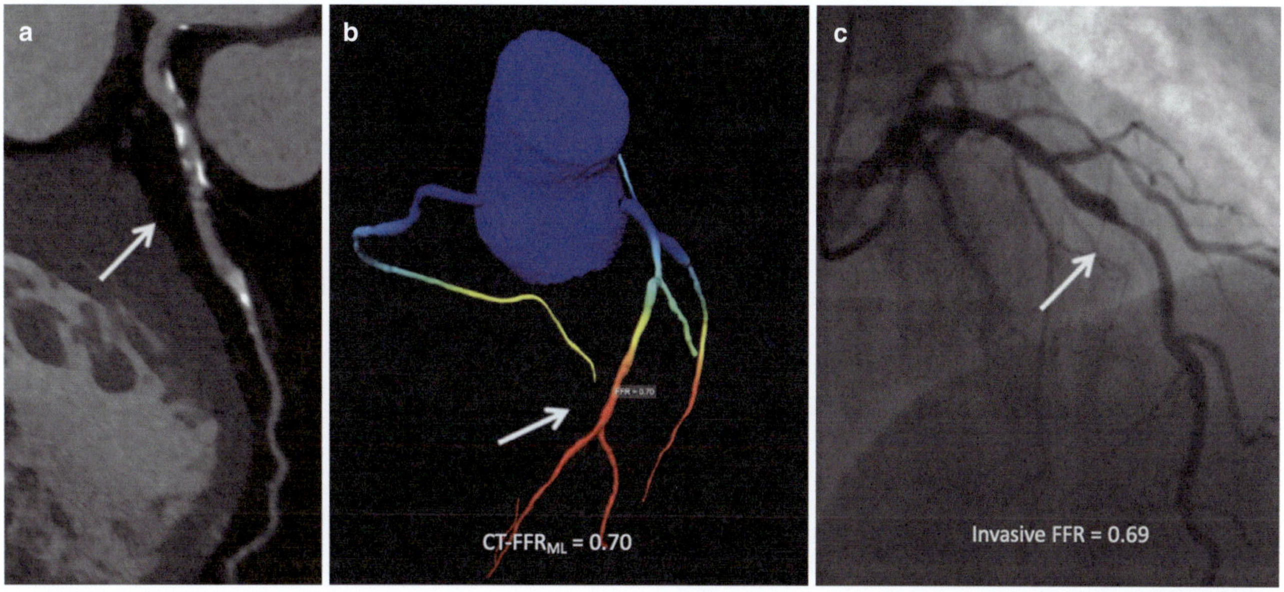

Fig. 27.2 Case example of coronary stenosis on cCTA and ICA with corresponding CT-FFR$_{ML}$ and invasive FFR assessment. Coronary CT angiography is shown in a 61-year-old man presenting to the outpatient service with chest pain. (**a**) Automatically generated curved multiplanar reformations illustrate >70% stenosis of the LAD. (**b**) A three-dimensional color-coded mesh derived from CT-FFR analysis shows a CT-FFR$_{ML}$ value of 0.72, confirming lesion-specific ischemia (arrow). (**c**) Invasive coronary angiography yielded obstructive stenosis of the LAD (arrow) with FFR of 0.72, confirming the hemodynamic significance of the underlying coronary lesion

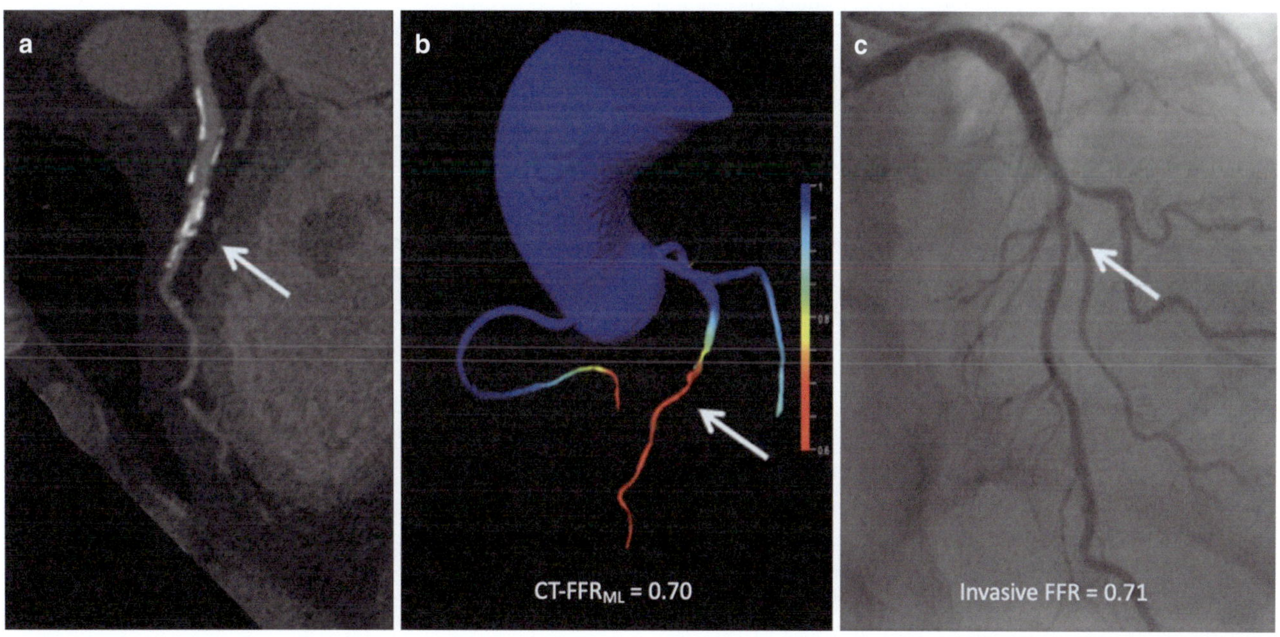

Fig. 27.3 Case example of coronary stenosis on cCTA and ICA with corresponding CT-FFR$_{ML}$ and invasive FFR evaluation. Coronary CT angiography in a 51-year-old woman presenting with chest discomfort. (**a**) Automatically generated curved multiplanar reformations demonstrate >70% stenosis of the LAD. (**b**) Three-dimensional color-coded mesh shows a CT-FFR$_{ML}$ value of 0.72, indicating inducible ischemia (arrow). (**c**) Invasive coronary angiography shows obstructive stenosis of the LAD (arrow) with FFR of 0.72, validating the hemodynamic significance of CAD

Overall, these data need further evaluation in larger cohorts as prospective randomized trials to facilitate an improvement of outcome, resulting in better quality of life, and to achieve cost efficiency for the overall healthcare system.

Limitations and Future Outlook

CT-FFR_{ML} represents an exciting new diagnostic tool in the evaluation of significant CAD and ischemic heart disease. In view of this, the technique is based on a post-processing approach, in which cCTA image data is processed with a CT-FFR_{ML} software and is predisposed by similar factors influencing regular cCTA evaluation.

Major limitations consist of image quality depending on increased image noise, blooming artifacts – due to coronary calcification – as well as patient-related motion artifacts. Aside from technical barriers, it should also be mentioned that CT-FFR_{ML} has neither been commercially available nor approved by the FDA and so far has been used for research purposes only. Any financial reimbursements should be discussed with healthcare providers and patients. Furthermore, additional studies for broader evidence and knowledge regarding application of CT-FFR_{ML} in the clinical setting are necessary.

Future developments regarding precision of CT-FFR_{ML} should further strengthen diagnostic accuracy and therapeutic decision-making, while integration of CT-FFR_{ML} in clinical practice will not only improve functional relevance of CAD but also allow further anatomical knowledge and plaque quantification through cCTA data [8]. Until now CT-FFR_{ML} has been provided by one vendor (Siemens Healthineers, Forchheim, Germany) for research purposes only, while other vendors are beginning to establish similar algorithms, such as Keya Medical's (Beijing, China) DeepVessel FFR application [40].

Additionally, because current FFR-CT algorithms are centering on the noninvasive derivation of flow conditions through a diseased coronary artery, adequate usage of the abovementioned cCTA data in terms of plaque characteristics and vessel remodeling, known as strong predictors for flow obstruction and patient outcome [41–43], is limited and must be expanded in its analysis [44]. Because of this, the application of deep ML facilitates analysis and contemporaneous evaluation of anatomy and function by noninvasive cCTA and allows better characterization of CAD severity, as well as further improvement of risk management, treatment guidelines, and patient outcome prediction [8, 44–46].

Conclusion

In conclusion, CT-FFR_{ML} offers a new, noninvasive diagnostic tool to identify functionally significant coronary lesions with high precision by combination of anatomical and functional analysis by noninvasive cCTA and ML. Recent studies, in which CT-FFR_{ML} analysis software has been validated against invasive FFR, demonstrate high diagnostic accuracy and show that CT-FFR_{ML} could be beneficial when integrated into daily clinical practice, to distinguish between patients who require revascularization and those patients who can safely avoid ICA and therefore reduce interventional complications.

Disclosures C.T. receives honoraria for speaking and consulting from HeartFlow Inc. and Siemens Healthineers. The other authors have no conflict of interest to disclose.

References

1. Chow BJ, Small G, Yam Y, et al. CONFIRM investigators. Incremental prognostic value of cardiac computed tomography in coronary artery disease using CONFIRM: COroNary computed tomography angiography evaluation for clinical outcomes: an International Multicenter registry. Circ Cardiovasc Imaging. 2011;4:463–72.
2. Maroules CD, Rajiah P, Bhasin M, et al. Current evidence in cardiothoracic imaging: growing evidence for coronary computed tomography angiography as a first-line test in stable chest pain. J Thorac Imaging. 2019;34:4–11.
3. Erthal F, Premaratne M, Yam Y, et al. Appropriate use criteria for cardiac computed tomography: does computed tomography have incremental value in all appropriate use criteria categories? J Thorac Imaging. 2018;33:132–7.
4. Meijboom WB, Van Mieghem CA, van Pelt N, et al. Comprehensive assessment of coronary artery stenoses: computed tomography coronary angiography versus conventional coronary angiography and correlation with fractional flow reserve in patients with stable angina. J Am Coll Cardiol. 2008;52:636–43. [PubMed: 18702967].
5. Gonzalez JA, Lipinski MJ, Flors L, Shaw PW, Kramer CM, Salerno M. Meta-analysis of diagnostic performance of coronary computed tomography angiography, computed tomography perfusion, and computed tomography-fractional flow reserve in functional myocardial ischemia assessment versus invasive fractional flow reserve. Am J Cardiol. 2015;116(9):1469–78. [PubMed: 26347004].
6. Neumann FJ, Sousa-Uvu M, Ahlsson A, et al. Group ESCSD. 2018 ESC/EACTS guidelines on myocardial revascularization. Eur Heart J. 2019;40:87–165.
7. Knuuti J, Wijns W, Saraste A, et al. 2019 ESC guidelines for the diagnosis and management of chronic coronary syndromes [published correction appears in Eur Heart J. 2020;41(44):4242]. Eur Heart J. 2020;41(3):407–77. https://doi.org/10.1093/eurheartj/ehz425.
8. Tesche C, Gray HN. Machine learning and deep neural networks applications in coronary flow assessment: the case of computed tomography fractional flow reserve. J Thorac Imaging. 2020;35

Suppl 1:S66–71. https://doi.org/10.1097/RTI.0000000000000483. PMID: 32091446.

9. Zhuang B, Wang S, Zhao S, Lu M. Computed tomography angiography-derived fractional flow reserve (CT-FFR) for the detection of myocardial ischemia with invasive fractional flow reserve as reference: systematic review and meta-analysis. Eur Radiol. 2020;30(2):712–25. https://doi.org/10.1007/s00330-019-06470-8. Epub 2019 Nov 6. PMID: 31696294.
10. Brandt V, Emrich T, Schoepf UJ, Dargis DM, Bayer RR, De Cecco CN, Tesche C. Ischemia and outcome prediction by cardiac CT based machine learning. Int J Cardiovasc Imaging 2020. https://doi.org/10.1007/s10554-020-01929-y. Epub ahead of print. PMID: 32623625.
11. Mathew RC, Gottbrecht M, Salerno M. Computed tomography fractional flow reserve to guide coronary angiography and intervention. Interv Cardiol Clin. 2018;7(3):345–54. https://doi.org/10.1016/j.iccl.2018.03.008.
12. Itu L, Rapaka S, Passerini T, et al. A machine-learning approach for computation of fractional flow reserve from coronary computed tomography. J Appl Physiol (1985). 2016;121:42–52.
13. Taylor CA, Fonte TA, Min JK. Computational fluid dynamics applied to cardiac computed tomography for noninvasive quantification of fractional flow reserve: scientific basis. J Am Coll Cardiol. 2013;61:2233–41.
14. van Assen M, Banerjee I, De Cecco CN. Beyond the artificial intelligence hype: what lies behind the algorithms and what we can achieve. J Thorac Imaging. 2020;35:S3–S10.
15. Dey D, Gaur S, Ovrehus KA, et al. Integrated prediction of lesion-specific ischaemia from quantitative coronary CT angiography using machine learning: a multicentre study. Eur Radiol. 2018;28:2655–64.
16. Coenen A, Kim YH, Kruk M, et al. Diagnostic accuracy of a machine-learning approach to coronary computed tomographic angiography-based fractional flow reserve: result from the MACHINE consortium. Circ Cardiovasc Imaging. 2018;11:e007217.
17. von Knebel Doeberitz PL, De Cecco CN, Schoepf UJ, et al. Impact of coronary computerized tomography angiography- derived plaque quantification and machine learning computerized tomography fractional flow reserve on adverse cardiac outcome. Am J Cardiol. 2019;124:1340–8.
18. Tesche C, De Cecco CN, Albrecht MH, et al. Coronary CT angiography-derived fractional flow reserve. Radiology. 2017;285:17–33.
19. Coenen A, Lubbers MM, Kurata A, et al. Fractional flow reserve computed from noninvasive CT angiography data: diagnostic performance of an on-site clinician-operated computational fluid dynamics algorithm. Radiology. 2015;274:674–83.
20. Renker M, Schoepf UJ, Wang R, et al. Comparison of diagnostic value of a novel noninvasive coronary computed tomography angiography method versus standard coronary angiography for assessing fractional flow reserve. Am J Cardiol. 2014;114:1303–8.
21. Tesche C, De Cecco CN, Baumann S, et al. Coronary CT angiography-derived fractional flow reserve: machine learning algorithm versus computational fluid dynamics modeling. Radiology. 2018;288:64–72.
22. von Knebel Doeberitz PL, De Cecco CN, Schoepf UJ, et al. Coronary CT angiography-derived plaque quantification with artificial intelligence CT fractional flow reserve for the identification of lesion-specific ischemia. Eur Radiol. 2019;29:2378–87.
23. Rother J, Moshage M, Dey D, et al. Comparison of invasively measured FFR with FFR derived from coronary CT angiography for detection of lesion-specific ischemia: results from a PC- based prototype algorithm. J Cardiovasc Comput Tomogr. 2018;12:101–7.
24. Kim C, Hong SJ, Ahn CM, et al. Clinical implications of moderate coronary stenosis on coronary computed tomography angiography in patients with stable angina. Yonsei Med J. 2018;59(8):937–44. https://doi.org/10.3349/ymj.2018.59.8.937.
25. Tang CX, Wang YN, Zhou F, et al. Diagnostic performance of fractional flow reserve derived from coronary CT angiography for detection of lesion-specific ischemia: a multi-center study and meta-analysis. Eur J Radiol. 2019;116:90–7.
26. Nous FMA, Budde RPJ, Lubbers MM, et al. Impact of machine-learning CT-derived fractional flow reserve for the diagnosis and management of coronary artery disease in the randomized CRESCENT trials. Eur Radiol. 2020;30(7):3692–701. https://doi.org/10.1007/s00330-020-06778-w.
27. Tesche C, Otani K, De Cecco CN, Coenen A, De Geer J, Kruk M, Kim YH, Albrecht MH, Baumann S, Renker M, Bayer RR, Duguay TM, Litwin SE, Varga-Szemes A, Steinberg DH, Yang DH, Kepka C, Persson A, Nieman K, Schoepf UJ. Influence of coronary calcium on diagnostic performance of machine learning CT-FFR: results from MACHINE registry. JACC Cardiovasc Imaging. 2020;13(3):760–70. https://doi.org/10.1016/j.jcmg.2019.06.027. Epub 2019 Aug 14. PMID: 31422141.
28. Baumann S, Renker M, Schoepf UJ, et al. Gender differences in the diagnostic performance of machine learning coronary CT angiography-derived fractional flow reserve -results from the MACHINE registry. Eur J Radiol. 2019;119:108657.
29. Danaei G, Finucane MM, Lu Y, et al. National, regional, and global trends in fasting plasma glucose and diabetes prevalence since 1980: systematic analysis of health examination surveys and epidemiological studies with 370 country-years and 2.7 million participants. Lancet. 2011;378:31–40.
30. Go AS, Mozaffarian D, Roger VL, et al. Heart disease and stroke statistics—2014 update: a report from the American Heart Association. Circulation. 2014;129:e28–e292.
31. Suzuki LA, Poot M, Gerrity RG, Bornfeldt KE. Diabetes accelerates smooth muscle accumulation in lesions of atherosclerosis: lack of direct growth-promoting effects of high glucose levels. Diabetes. 2001;50(4):851–60.
32. Williams SB, Cusco JA, Roddy MA, Johnstone MT, Creager MA. Impaired nitric oxide-mediated vasodilation in patients with non-insulin-dependent diabetes mellitus. J Am Coll Cardiol. 1996;27(3):567–74.
33. Vinik AI, Erbas T, Park TS, Nolan R, Pittenger GL. Platelet dysfunction in type 2 diabetes. Diabetes Care. 2001;24(8):1476–85.
34. Aronson D, Edelman ER. Coronary artery disease and diabetes mellitus. Cardiol Clin. 2014;32(3):439–55. https://doi.org/10.1016/j.ccl.2014.04.001.
35. Nous FMA, Coenen A, Boersma E, Kim YH, Kruk MBP, Tesche C, de Geer J, Yang DH, Kepka C, Schoepf UJ, Persson A, Kurata A, Budde RPJ, Nieman K. Comparison of the diagnostic performance of coronary computed tomography angiography-derived fractional flow reserve in patients with versus without diabetes mellitus (from the MACHINE consortium). Am J Cardiol. 2019;123(4):537–43. https://doi.org/10.1016/j.amjcard.2018.11.024. Epub 2018 Nov 24. PMID: 30553510.
36. Duguay TM, Tesche C, Vliegenthart R, et al. Coronary computed tomographic angiography-derived fractional flow reserve based on machine learning for risk stratification of non- culprit coronary narrowings in patients with acute coronary syndrome. Am J Cardiol. 2017;120:1260–6.

37. Tesche C, Vliegenthart R, Duguay TM, et al. Coronary computed tomographic angiography-derived fractional flow reserve for therapeutic decision making. Am J Cardiol. 2017;120:2121–7.
38. Martin S, Mastrodicasa D, van Assen M, et al. Value of machine learning–based coronary CT fractional flow reserve applied to triple-rule-out ct angiography in acute chest pain. Radiol Cardiothorac Imaging. 2020;2:e190137. https://doi.org/10.1148/ryct.2020190137.
39. Eberhard M, Nadarevic T, Cousin A, et al. Machine learning-based CT fractional flow reserve assessment in acute chest pain: first experience. Cardiovasc Diagn Ther. 2020;10(4):820–30. https://doi.org/10.21037/cdt-20-381.
40. Tang CX, Liu CY, Lu MJ, Schoepf UJ, Tesche C, Bayer RR, 2nd, et al. CT FFR for ischemia-specific CAD with a new computational fluid dynamics algorithm: a Chinese multicenter study. JACC Cardiovasc Imaging; 2019.
41. Tesche C, Plank F, De Cecco CN, et al. Prognostic implications of coronary CT angiography-derived quantitative markers for the prediction of major adverse cardiac events. J Cardiovasc Comput Tomogr. 2016;10(6):458–65.
42. Nance JW Jr, Schlett CL, Schoepf UJ, et al. Incremental prognostic value of different components of coronary atherosclerotic plaque at cardiac CT angiography beyond coronary calcification in patients with acute chest pain. Radiology. 2012;264(3):679–90.
43. Motwani M, Dey D, Berman DS, et al. Machine learning for prediction of all- cause mortality in patients with suspected coronary artery disease: a 5-year multicentre prospective registry analysis. Eur Heart J. 2017;38(7):500–7.
44. Tesche C, De Cecco CN, Albrecht MH, Duguay TM, Bayer RR 2nd, Litwin SE, Steinberg DH, Schoepf UJ. Coronary CT angiography-derived fractional flow reserve. Radiology. 2017;285(1):17–33. https://doi.org/10.1148/radiol.2017162641. PMID: 28926310.
45. Lossnitzer D, Chandra L, Rutsch M, Becher T, Overhoff D, Janssen S, Weiss C, Borggrefe M, Akin I, Pfleger S, Baumann S. Additional value of machine-learning computed tomographic angiography-based fractional flow reserve compared to standard computed tomographic angiography. J Clin Med. 2020;9(3):676. https://doi.org/10.3390/jcm9030676. PMID: 32138259; PMCID: PMC7141259.
46. Kumamaru KK, Fujimoto S, Otsuka Y, et al. Diagnostic accuracy of 3D deep-learning-based fully automated estimation of patient-level minimum fractional flow reserve from coronary computed tomography angiography. Eur Heart J Cardiovasc Imaging. 2020;21(4):437–45. https://doi.org/10.1093/ehjci/jez160.

Artificial Intelligence-Based Evaluation of Cardiac Valves

28

Gudrun M. Feuchtner, Vitalijs Zujs, Nikolaos Bonaros, and Fabian Plank

Clinical Use Scenarios

- *3D segmentation of cardiac valves and 3D visualization*

Deep learning (DL) tools provide the unique opportunity to train convolutional neuronal networks (CNNs) for automated segmentation of different cardiac structures. This technique has been successfully translated into clinical practice for cardiac chambers and vessels [1]. However, valvular leaflets, due to their extensive motion during cardiac cycle and their thin layers, are a major challenge for automated contour tracking and leaflet segmentation. Artifacts from leaflet motion are hindering accurate segmentation results easily.

Therefore, CT datasets with high image quality and without cardiac motion are crucial for the development of AI-based quantitative image analysis tools.

In contrast to leaflets, valvular calcification can be segmented much more reliably, due to their high X-ray attenuation (CT density, Hounsfield Units = HU) with values above 350 HU up to 1000 HU, from surrounding soft tissue such as leaflets or the fibrous annulus and valve apparatus. These adjacent fibrous structures are characterized by CT densities ranging from 50 to 160 HU. Advanced post-processing by 3D volume rendering technique (VRT) allows for the application of different color settings, as illustrated for a bicuspid valve (Fig. 28.1). "Black blood" (Fig. 28.1a, b) or inverse "white blood" (Fig. 28.1c) color coding is feasible, allowing for adjusting the CT image visualization to the individual heart team's visual preferences. Valvular calcium is either colored blue (**a**), white (**b**), or black (**c**) and contrasted to aortic valve leaflets and aortic root. 3D visualization of the exact location and estimation of calcium severity (mild, moderate, or severe) are important for the cardiac surgeon to plan a surgical procedure or minimal invasive intervention.

Further, automated segmentation of valvular and mitral annulus annular calcification (Fig. 28.2e) can be performed for planning of valvular interventions such as transcatheter aortic valve implantations (TAVIs) and transcatheter mitral valve repair (TMVR). This technique requires dedicated advanced post-processing software, such as the one provided from *Materialise* (Leuven, Belgium, NL) (Fig. 28.2e). The contours of the different tissue components (leaflets, valvular calcifications, aortic root, or even stent struts from valvular prosthesis) are traced on multiplanar reformations and used to create 3D models with MESH technique.

Another post-processing technique, the quantification of absolute CT attenuation (HU) of valvular masses, has the potential to improve the diagnostic accuracy of differential diagnosis of valvular masses. There is some scientific evidence that [2] pannus after prosthetic heart valve implantation (PHV) can be better differentiated from thrombus by setting a threshold of >145HU (single centric retrospective study). A pannus is a chronic- organized lesion with neovascularization, which is characterized by modest iodine contrast agent uptake and subsequent higher HU. A thrombus, in contrast, has a lower CT attenuation of less than 90 HU, because of its distinct composition consisting of platelets and thrombogenic material, not allowing for an iodine contrast agent update [2]. However, scientific evidence is sparse, and studies with large sample sizes are lacking. Both conditions are mainly observed in patients with smaller (e.g., 19–21 mm for the aortic valve) mechanical valves and in low flow hemodynamic conditions (atrial fibrillation or impaired

G. M. Feuchtner, MD, MBA (✉)
Department of Radiology, Innsbruck Medical University, Innsbruck, Austria
e-mail: gudrun.feuchtner@i-med.ac.at

V. Zujs, MD · N. Bonaros, MD
Department of Cardiac Surgery, Innsbruck Medical University, Innsbruck, Austria
e-mail: Vitalijs.Zujs@tirol-kliniken.at; Nikolaos.Bonaros@tirol-kliniken.at

F. Plank, MD, PhD
Department of Internal Medicine III and Cardiology, Innsbruck Medical University, Innsbruck, Austria
e-mail: Fabian.Plank@tirol-kliniken.at

C. N. De Cecco et al. (eds.), *Artificial Intelligence in Cardiothoracic Imaging*, Contemporary Medical Imaging,
https://doi.org/10.1007/978-3-030-92087-6_28

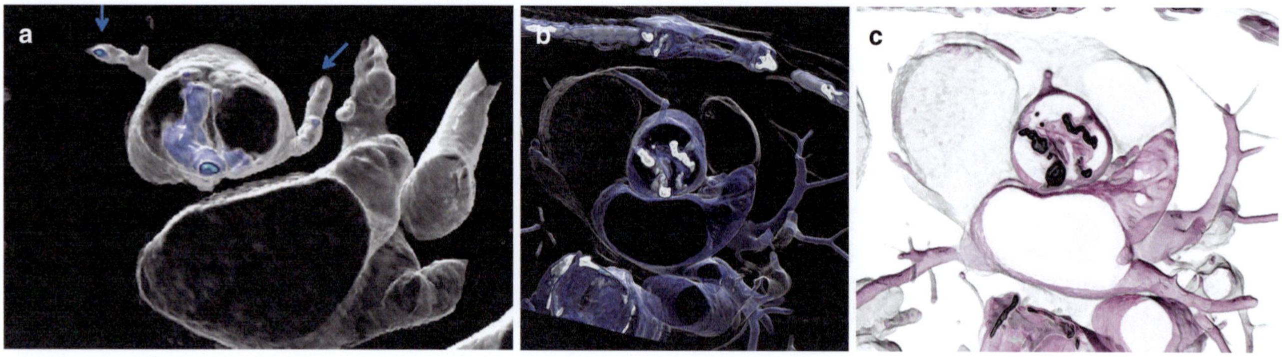

Fig. 28.1 Advanced 3D post-processing of bicuspid aortic valve by 3D volume rendering technique (VRT). (**a**) "Black blood VRT" bicuspid aortic valve (BAV) type 0 (no raphe) with severe calcification of the fused non-coronary and right coronary cusp (blue) (arrow). LCA and RCA ostium (arrows). Calcium is colored blue and, aortic root vessel walls are segmented and colored white. Blood is colored black. (**b**) *Bicuspid aortic valve type I (with raphe between right and left cusp, "fused BAV")* and severe calcifications of all cusps. Mid-systolic phase (25% of RR interval) shows bottom hole narrowing of AVA (0.4 cm^2) correlating with severe aortic stenosis grade III. Different color settings are applied: calcium = white (350 HU–1000 HU). Leaflets and vessel wall are colored blue (50–150 HU). Blood with iodine is colored black (200–350 HU) ("black blood VRT"). (**c**) *Inverse color coding ("white blood VRT").* The same bicuspid valve as show in Panel b is displayed with inversed color settings (calcium = black and leaflets, vessel wall = purple). In clinical practice, adjusting color setting according to interdisciplinary team members' preference is recommended

left ventricular function), or artifacts from prosthesis material are limiting the accuracy of quantification of prosthetic valve masses, depending on the prosthesis model and specific material composition.

Thrombi may be also found attached to native valves, mostly in association with diseases creating a pro-coagulative state, such as autoimmune or hematological such as systemic lupus or antiphospholipid syndrome. Carcinoid disease or other neoplasm may also lead to thrombotic appositions on native valves. Accurate diagnosis is crucial, because the risk of embolization shows a linear increase with growing size and mobility. Early treatment with specific antithrombogenic regimens may improve outcomes and adverse events.

Other valvular masses, such as the most common cardiac valve tumor, the papillary fibroelastoma (PFE), have a very similar appearance on CT: Papillary fibroelastomas are usually small sized masses with lesion size of less than 1 cm, consisting of fibrous elastic tissue with mild iodine contrast agent uptake ranging from 90 to 130 HU. They can often not be accurately differentiated from vegetations developing in patients with infective endocarditis, due to similar HU values, shape, and size. Correlation with the patient's clinical history is necessary for differential diagnosis. In summary to date, AI tools do not play a major role in this setting, due to lack of clinical validation studies.

Another quantitative approach, "radiomics," may have the potential to further improve accuracy of differential diagnosis but is associated with similar inherent limitations. For coronary plaque [3], the sub-analysis of the broad spectrum of "radiomics" (texture based) parameters of the grayscale matrix (up to 4000) of a single image pixel has shown to improve the characterization of "high-risk" vulnerable plaque with signs of plaque inflammation. Whether or not these findings may translate to valvular masses is unknown and has not been investigated yet. However, based on the distinct histological texture of thrombi, tumors, and vegetations, radiomics may allow for a better differential diagnosis. No systematic studies however have been conducted so far, and the reasons are twofold: training DL models requires large data sample sizes with high-quality datasets without motion artifacts and reference standard (e.g., histopathology) for validation. To set up such a database would take a long time period, and motion artifacts are another major great challenge. Most likely, the development and the introduction of novel CT technology such as photon-counting CT, with higher spatial and temporal resolution will have to be awaited to explore this research field.

Dual energy is another specific CT technique allowing for material characterization. The feasibility of improved differential diagnosis of inflammatory cardiac masses in a patient with pulmonary prosthetic valve endocarditis (PVE) after a transcatheter procedure [4] by using dual-energy CT (DECT) and iodine uptake quantification has been demonstrated recently. In clinical practice, ^{18}fluordesoxyglucose-positron emission tomography (^{18}FDG-PET) is the modality of choice for diagnosis of PVE, with a pooled sensitivity of 80.5% and a specificity of 73.1% [5] and slightly lower values for native valve endocarditis (sens. 76.8%, spec. 77.9%). ^{18}FDG-PET provides the advantage of detecting extracardiac foci (17%) [5] and has a higher accuracy as CT; therefore it will certainly remain the clinical reference tool for suspected PVE in practice.

- *3D printing*. Three-dimensional (3D) [6] printing transforms volumetric CT datasets into real 3D objects. Advanced 3D printing allows for segmentation of materials into multiple layers and for creating models of specific cardiac structural pathologies. 3D image segmentation can be performed automatically, for example, for tissue components with different CT attenuation (HU) or manually, by applying manual contour tracing of the target objects. Overall, 3D printing is a relatively time-consuming process which requires advanced post-processing software such as the one developed by Materialise (Leuven, Belgium) (Fig. 28.2e).

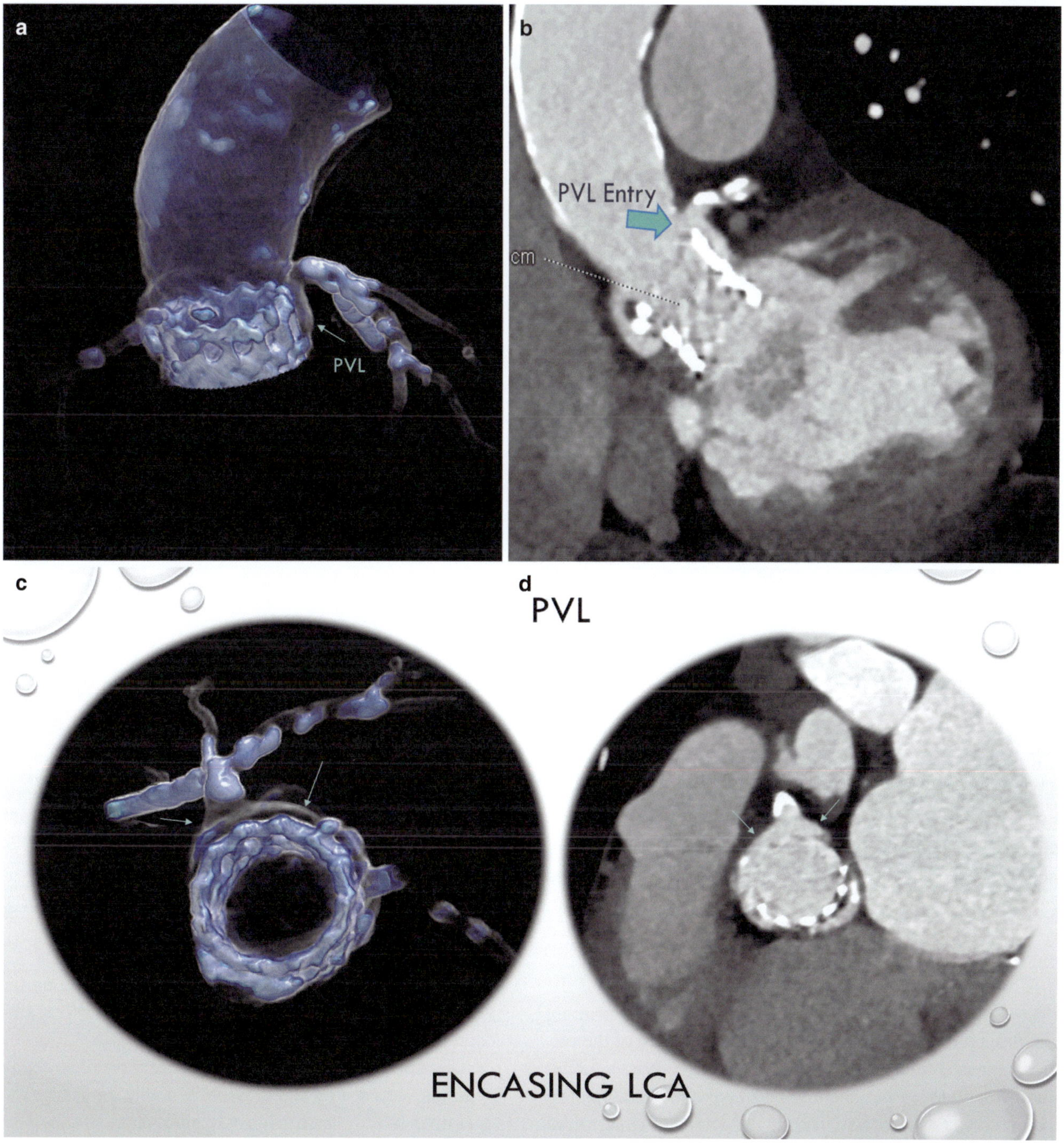

Fig. 28.2 *Paravalvular leak (PVL)* CTA 3D VRT visualization (**a–d**): Left-sided PVL (arrow) after transcatheter aortic valve implantation of a SAPIEN 3 TAVR bioprosthesis. CTA allowed for accurate sizing of the closure device (Amplatz, 14× 3 mm) and the relationship of the LCA ostium to the leak. If the distance between the coronary and the ostium is too short, the LCA is at risk for occlusion and requires protection during the implantation. PVL closure was successful in this patient. *label e* shows 3D segmentation of the aortic root and the prosthesis from the CT dataset using an AI software (*Materialise, Belgium*). These models can be used to create 3D prints. *Panel E.* 3D segmentation of the aortic root and the prosthesis (blue arrow->) and the creation of 3D models (purple arrow->) for 3D printing. PVL paravalvular leak. (Copyright © 2020 Materialise N.V)

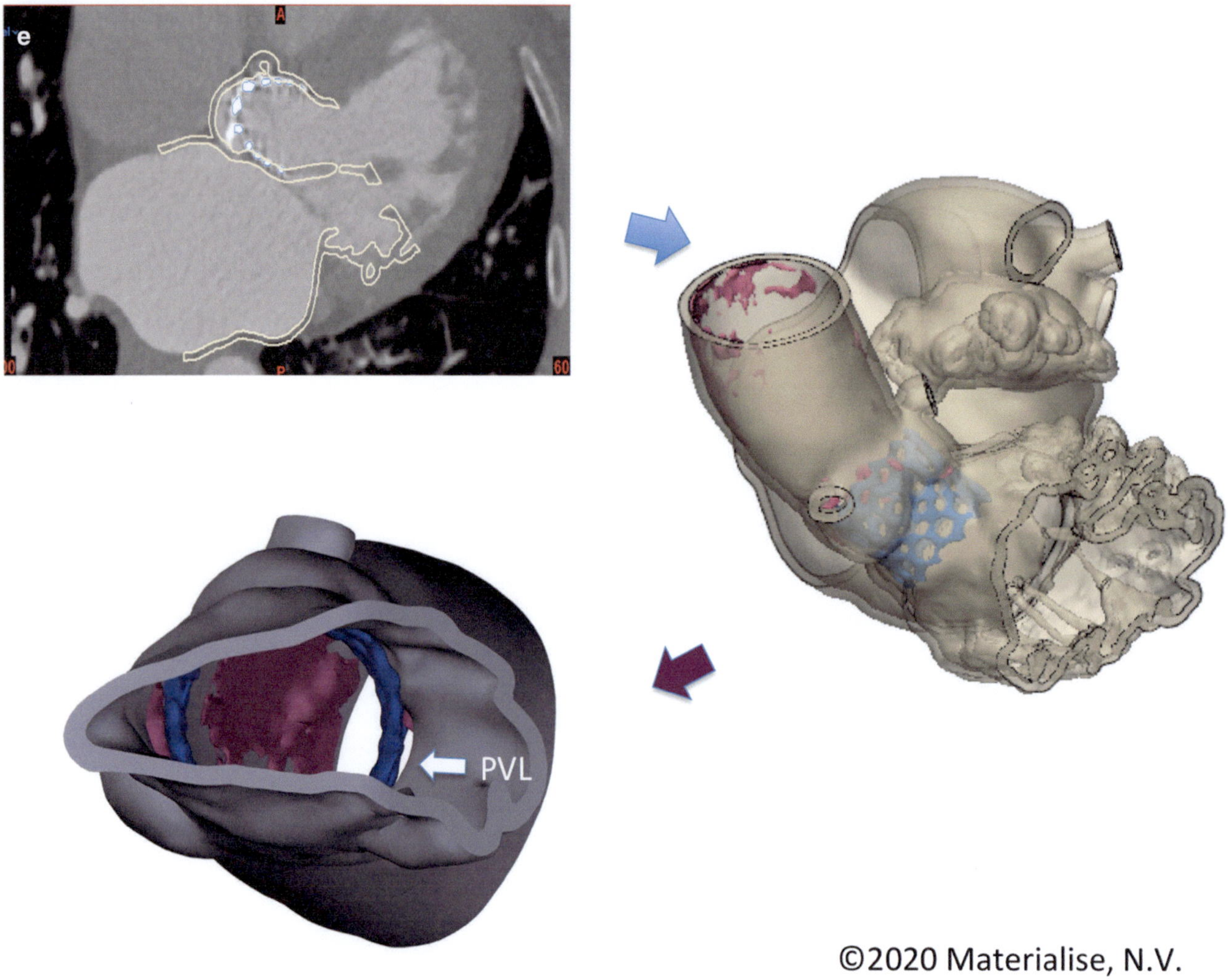

Fig. 28.2 (continued)

3D printing for cardiovascular applications [7, 8] is a relatively new development, with a rapid evolution over the past decade. Especially cardiac surgeons, whose procedure planning is based on the individual patient's pathologies and anatomy, have driven the translation of 3D printing into clinical practice and have proven the usefulness of 3D printed models.

Complex congenital heart disease (CHD) is one of the major applications, in which pre-procedural 3D printing enables a more precise and personalized planning of the surgical interventions ("precision medicine") [9]. Valvular malformations are not uncommon in complex CHD; hence those models usually also include the detailed visualization of rare and unusual valvular anomalies such as quadricuspid valve [10].

3D printing also enables to create models of cardiac devices such as ASD occluders or prosthetic heart valves; hence post-surgical complications – such as an incorrect device position – can be displayed more "real," which facilitates planning of more difficult post-surgical complications (e.g., interventional closure of a paravalvular leak) [11] (Fig. 28.2e).

- *Planning of minimal invasive and transcatheter valve implantations*
  - *Minimal invasive aortic valve replacement*

  Over the last two decades, minimally invasive aortic valve replacement has proven its value and has rapidly decreased the perioperative mortality [12, 13].

  This approach has a comparable safety profile to conventional sternotomy and is associated with reduced post-operative pain, transfusion requirement, respiratory complications, and a shorter hospital stay [14]. The advent of rapid deployment valves has facilitated minimally invasive procedures due to the simplification of valve implantation. Still, the vast majority of the procedures are performed through conventional sternotomy, due to reduced visibility and limitations in surgical access. These difficulties frequently increase cardiopulmonary bypass and aortic cross-clamp time, which have an impact on clinical outcomes. Preoperative computed tomography (CT) scans provide valuable information on anatomical landmarks and reduce the possibility of aortic valve size mismatch or access limitations caused by the smaller surgical incision. The analysis of CT angiographic images has gained major importance in transcatheter valve procedures and can be used to establish an individualized ("personalized") surgical plan. 3D visualization and 3D sizing of thoracic dimensions on CT images in multiple planes are mandatory for planning of minimal invasive approaches. The use of automated software (*3Mensio* ™, *Materialise*, etc.) allows for the creation of 3D volume rendering technique (VRT) images and multiplanar reformations (MPR) in three planes (sagittal, coronal, axial). 3D VRT provides a "realistic" 3D visualization, and MPR allows for accurate sizing of cardiac anatomy and their relationship to mediastinal structures. Measuring these dimensions can improve preoperative cannulation and planning of the myocardial protection strategy [15] . Therefore, CT imaging has become an essential component of the pre-procedural planning by multidisciplinary team. It is important to identify singularities of each patient and analyze numerous individual characteristics. Furthermore, the location of the aortic valve in relation to the outer rib cage and sternal notches can be accurately defined pre-procedural and is helpful to plan the exact location, direction, and length of the incision site. This enables accurate preoperative planning and helps in choosing the best surgical approach for minimally invasive aortic valve replacement procedure [16] such as the selection of the best intercostal space (ICR), which is varying from 3rd up to the 6th ICR.

- *Transcatheter aortic valve implantation (TAVI) planning*. 3D segmentation of aortic valve and annular calcification is very helpful for planning and guiding TAVI procedures. The severity, location, and shape of aortic valve and annular calcification are valuable predictors for intra- and post-procedural complications. Severe protruding annular calcifications increase the risk for paravalvular leaks (PVL), due to inconsistent adaption of the prosthesis stent with the annulus. Furthermore, severe annular and subannular calcifications increase the risk of annulus rupture, another fatal complication during TAVI [17, 18]. 3D printing can further assist TAVI planning by modeling prosthesis fit [19, 20].
- *Valve-in-valve interventions*: 3D segmentation of a failed bioprosthesis allows a thorough examination of the anatomy of the valve and the surrounding structures. Due to the different construction of bioprosthetic valves especially in those with external leaflet positioning (such as the LivaNova *Mitroflow*, Crown, and the Abbott Trifecta), there is a higher risk of malpositioning, high residual gradients, and coronary obstruction. 3D printing provides important information of the aortic root anatomy and the relationship of the valve struts or leaflets to the coronary ostia.
- *Simulation of valve implantation from CT imaging data*: Virtual valve implantation in a specific anatomy can be extremely useful in cases with challenging anatomy, especially mitral valves. The main advantage of the technique is to predict the ideal anatomical position of a valve based on the anatomical features of the fabricate. This is of paramount importance in patients with asymmetric calcifications, low coronary ostia or degenerated bioprosthesis, or mitral valve interventions in order to avoid fatal complications. The exact height of the valve can be simulated to achieve optimal valve expansion and minimize the risk of inflow obstruction. In valve-in-valve (VIV) interventions, a supra-annular positioning of the valve can be achieved using this technique. However, virtual valve implantation is based on software simulations based on the geometrical data from the manufacturer and cannot always predict the position and the degree of expansion of the valve in a calcified native valve or degenerated bioprosthesis. Obviously, there are broad differences in the tissue compliance of different anatomical structures of the aortic root which may lead to different degrees of expansion. For these cases, real 3D printing using different degrees of hardness and valve implantation in a model may increase predictability.
- *Transcatheter mitral valve replacement (TMVR)* represents a greater technical challenge for cardiothoracic surgeons, as compared to aortic valve interventions. In contrast to the aortic valve, the mitral geometry is more complex in shape and morphology. A variety of devices from different vendors have been introduced for TMVR to the market over the past decade, each with distinct shapes and mechanical properties. These novel devices are currently under clinical investigation in several specialized cardiovascular centers worldwide. The first attempts were made using the traditional transcatheter aortic valve prosthesis (*SAPIEN 3, Edwards Lifesciences Inc., Irvine, CA, USA*), with moderate results: The Global Registry of TMVR in patients with significant MAC, Guerrero et al. reported in 64 patients from 32 centers an improvement in New York Heart Association functional class in 84% of patients, while 30-day all-cause mortality was high with almost 30% [21]. Mitral annular calcifications (MACs) [22] are one of the major criteria for planning both minimal invasive mitral valve surgery and TMVR (Fig. 28.3). Mitral

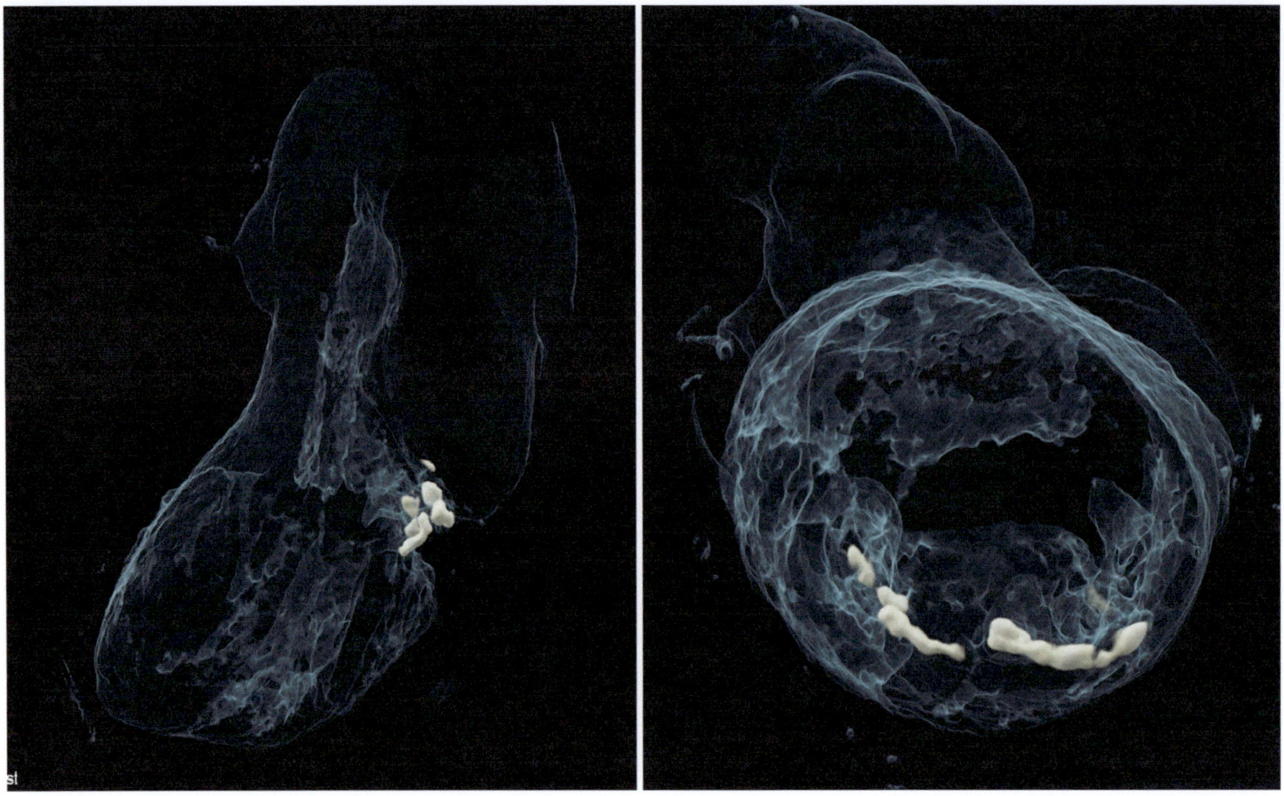

Fig. 28.3 CTA 3D segmentation of mitral annular calcification (MAC) is helpful for planning of minimal invasive mitral valve surgery and transcatheter mitral valve replacement (TMVR): mild posterior basal MAC (left, three-chamber view, and right, short axis view) by 3D volume rendering technique (VRT)

valve annular calcifications are highly varying in shape and size. 3D mapping their position and severity is helpful to select the device model and to define the technical approach.

- During TMVR, the proximity of the mitral valve to the LVOT poses the patient at risk of LVOT obstruction, depending on its individual morphology. It has been shown that the aortomitral angle is a valuable parameter to predict LVOT obstruction [23]. Automated software (*Materialise, Belgium*) with finite element analysis and computed simulation allows for a more accurate procedure planning and patient selection. By modeling shape and size of the predicted LVOT after TMVR implantation ("Neo-LVOT"), a patients' appropriateness for implanting a mitral prosthesis can be defined in advance from CT datasets. The Neo-LVOT has to provide enough space to ensure sufficient LV outflow after the procedure [24, 25] (Fig. 28.4). CT data enable a volumetric calculation of the Neo-LVOT and accurate prediction.
- A variety of different transcatheter mitral valve devices with distinct shapes and material compositions are currently under clinical investigations for transcatheter edge-to-edge repair. One model, the *Tendyne*™, consists of a bioprosthetic valve and an anchoring tether with an apical pad, which is anchored in the LV apex [25]. This device is currently evaluated by an ongoing 1:1 randomized trial (SUMMIT), enrolling patients with severe symptomatic mitral regurgitation (MR) grade III/IV. The preliminary results of SUMMIT trial are promising with 96% technical success, 0% procedure mortality, and 6% mortality at 30 days. The SUMMIT trial consists of two subarms, one head-to-head comparative study with *MitraClip*™ and one subcohort with severe MAC [25]. Severe MAC was defined as >1000 mm^3 calcium volume quantified by CT or visible myocardial invasion on CT scan. So far, in 11 patients with severe MAC, all devices could be placed successfully. For planning of anchoring, 3D models of MAC from CT are segmented, and prosthesis fit is defined (Fig. 28.5).
- For procedure planning, further quantitative measurements from CT (or TEE) are a pre-requisite: i) mitral annular dimensions (two diameters – septal lateral and the intercommissural area), ii) the distance of the mitral annulus from LV apex, and ii) the 3D volume of the predicted Neo-LVOT and aortomitral angle (end-diastolic and end-systolic).

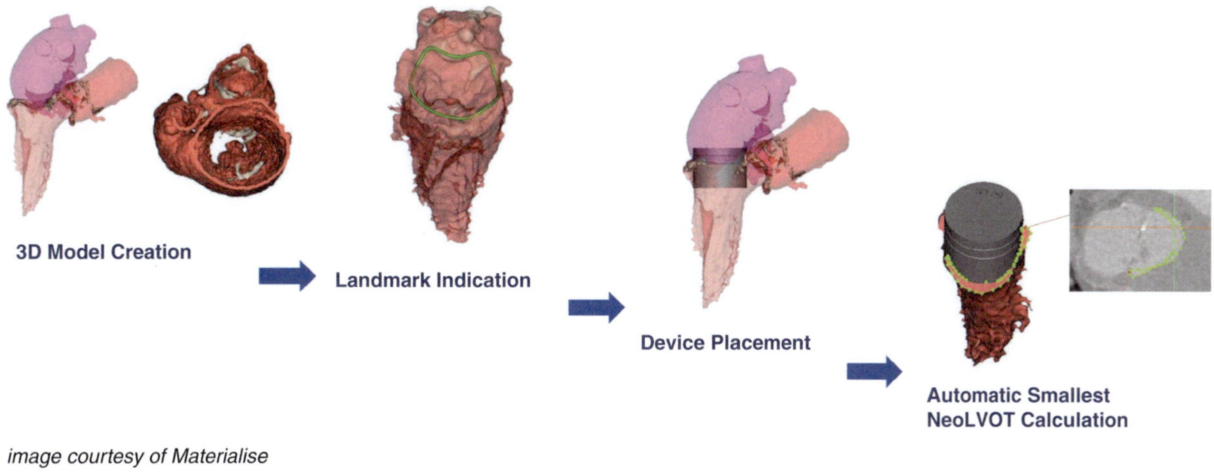

Fig. 28.4 Planning of transcatheter mitral valve replacement (TMVR): Neo-LVOT modeling from CTA, illustrated by four steps: (1) 3D model creation, (2) landmark indication, (3) device placement simulation, and (4) the calculation of the predicted smallest Neo-LVOT. (Copyright © 2020 Materialise N.V)

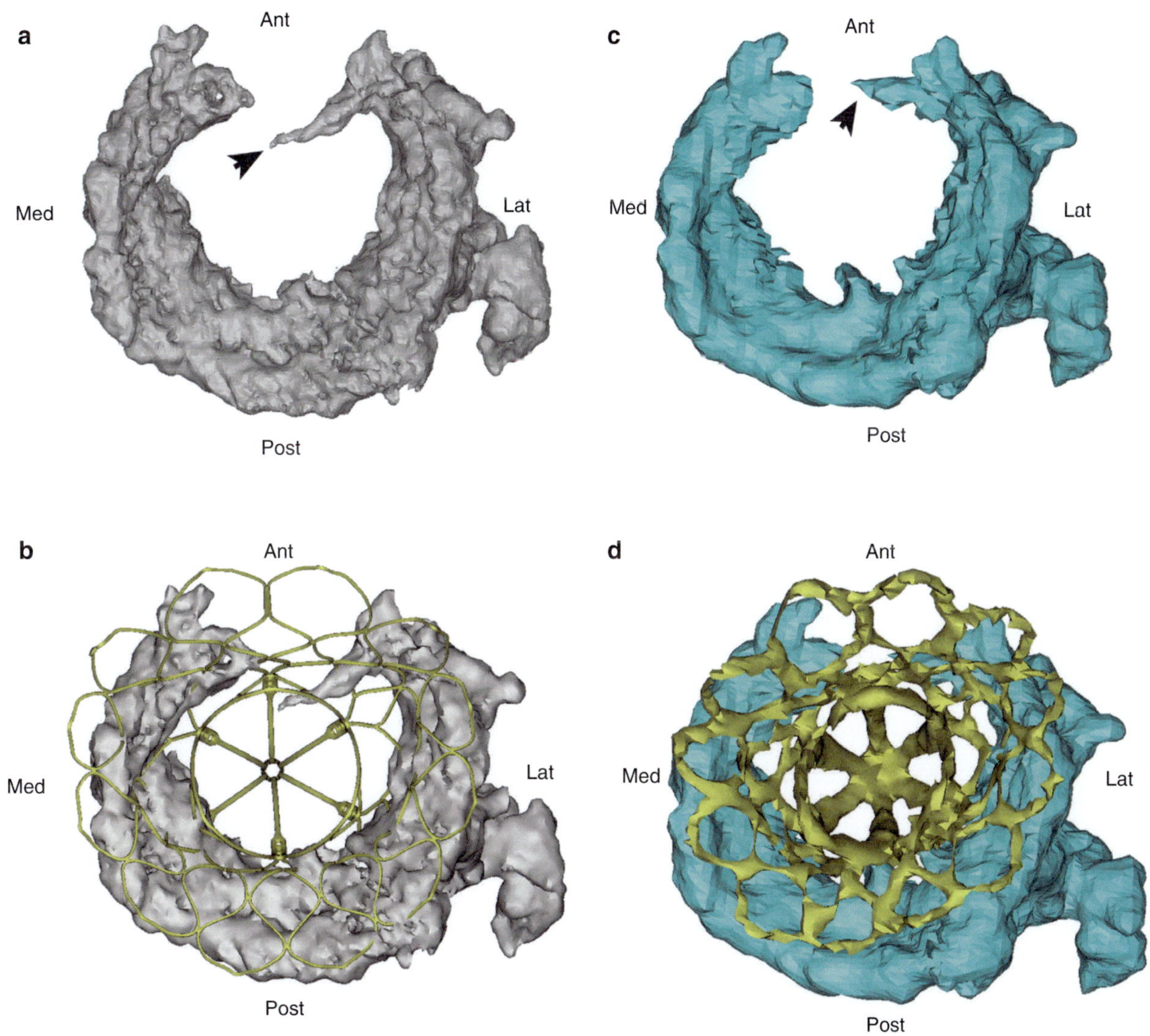

Fig. 28.5 Segmentation of severe circumferential mitral annular calcification (MAC) from CT data (**a**, **c**) and simulation of mitral prosthesis fit (Tendyne™) (**b**, **d**)

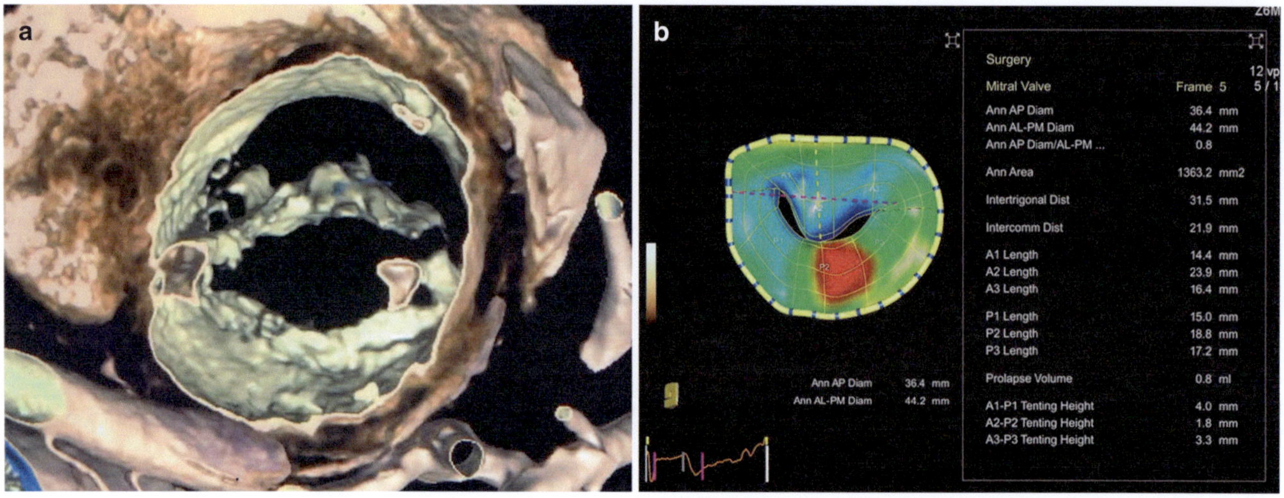

Fig. 28.6 Segmentation of mitral valve and automated 3D measurement of dimensions. (**a**) 3D volume rendering (VR) short axis view of mitral valve from CT (SyngoVia™, Siemens Healthineers). (**b**) Corresponding 3D transesophageal echocardiography (TEE) short axis view using eSie™ Valve Software (Siemens Healthcare, Mountain View, CA, USA). (With the courtesy of Siemens Healthineers). Measurement of the various parameters for surgical planning (AP = anteroposterior diameter (yellow dashed line), Ann = annulus, Dist = distance, A = anterior, P = posterior). Valve dimensions, leaflet length, and tenting height of the different segments of the leaflets (A1-P1, A2-P2, A3-P3), intercommissural distance (purple line), and prolapse volume can be quantified using an AI-based machine learning tool

- *Echocardiographic segmentation of mitral valve using machine learning (ML)* [26–28]: Echocardiographic analysis of mitral valve (MV) is essential for the assessment of MV disease. Current software requires manual input resulting in high interobserver variability. A novel automated software applies artificial intelligence (AI) for MV analysis (eSie™ Valve Software; Siemens Healthcare, Mountain View, CA, USA) which allows for automated contour tracing and segmentation of 3D TEE data. In an explorative study, three examiners analyzed three end-systolic (ES) frames in four patients (total, 36 ES frames). The study found a significant ($p = 0.0083$) correlation for six parameters tested (such as annulus area, perimeter, or non-planarity angle), while the different examiners did not have an effect (Fig. 28.6). These AI algorithms may help to reduce interobserver variability and improve accuracy, since they allow for automated measurements of specific quantitative parameters for MV procedure planning. Both CT and TEE data can be used from modeling [27, 28].

Conclusion

Artificial intelligence (AI)-based cardiac valve evaluation is an emerging field. Cardiac valves, due to their slender leaflets and high level of motion, are a major challenge for AI-based algorithms, beyond general limitations of CNNs [29, 30]. In contrast, calcifications can be more easily 3D mapped and segmented, which plays a pivotal role in surgical procedure planning.

3D segmentation of valvular structures from CT imaging datasets using automated tools has gained clinical application for planning of minimal invasive and transcatheter valve replacement procedures, in order to define a patient's eligibility and to avoid procedure-related complications. 4D real-time navigation and simulation of valvular interventions using virtual reality (VR) based on imaging data could further enhance the field in the future.

AI-assisted image texture-based CT analysis may have the potential to improve the accuracy of differential diagnosis or valvular masses; however this field is currently limited by spatial and temporal resolution, and advancements in CT technology (e.g., photon counting CT) are required.

References

1. Baskaran L, Al'Aref SJ, Maliakal G, Lee BC, Xu Z, Choi JW, Lee SE, Sung JM, Lin FY, Dunham S, Mosadegh B, Kim YJ, Gottlieb I, Lee BK, Chun EJ, Cademartiri F, Maffei E, Marques H, Shin S, Choi JH, Chinnaiyan K, Hadamitzky M, Conte E, Andreini D, Pontone G, Budoff MJ, Leipsic JA, Raff GL, Virmani R, Samady H, Stone PH, Berman DS, Narula J, Bax JJ, Chang HJ, Min JK, Shaw LJ. Automatic segmentation of multiple cardiovascular structures from cardiac computed tomography angiography images using deep learning. PLoS One. 2020;15(5):e0232573.
2. Gündüz S, Özkan M, Kalçik M, Gürsoy OM, Astarcioğlu MA, Karakoyun S, Aykan AÇ, Biteker M, Gökdeniz T, Kaya H, Yesin M, Duran NE, Sevinç D, Güneysu T, Gündüz S, Özkan M, Kalçik M, Gürsoy OM, Astarcioğlu MA, Karakoyun S, Aykan AÇ, Biteker M, Gökdeniz T, Kaya H, Yesin M, Duran NE, Sevinç D, Güneysu T. Sixty-four-section cardiac computed tomography in mechanical prosthetic heart valve dysfunction: thrombus or pannus. Circ Cardiovasc Imaging. 2015;8(12):e003246.

3. Kolossváry M, De Cecco CN, Feuchtner G, Maurovich-Horvat P. Advanced atherosclerosis imaging by CT: radiomics, machine learning and deep learning. J Cardiovasc Comput Tomogr. 2019;13(5):274–80.
4. Priya S, Nagpal P, Vidholia A, Sachdev IS, Ashwath R. Evaluation of transcatheter pulmonary valve endocarditis by dual-energy computed tomography. Cureus. 2020;12(6):e8851.
5. Mahmood M, Kendi AT, Ajmal S, et al. Meta-analysis of 18F-FDG PET/CT in the diagnosis of infective endocarditis. J Nucl Cardiol. 2019;26(3):922–35.
6. Vukicevic M, Mosadegh B, Min JK, Little SH. Cardiac 3D printing and its future directions. JACC Cardiovasc Imaging. 2017;10(2):171–84.
7. Wang DD, Qian Z, Vukicevic M, et al. 3D printing, computational modeling, and artificial intelligence for structural heart disease [published online ahead of print, 2020 Aug 25]. JACC Cardiovasc Imaging. 2020;S1936-878X(20)30515-5.
8. Levin D, Mackensen GB, Reisman M, McCabe JM, Dvir D, Ripley B. 3D printing applications for transcatheter aortic valve replacement. Curr Cardiol Rep. 2020;22(4):23.
9. Shinbane JS, Saxon LA. Virtual medicine: utilization of the advanced cardiac imaging patient avatar for procedural planning and facilitation. J Cardiovasc Comput Tomogr. 2018;12(1):16–27.
10. Feuchtner G. Quadricuspid aortic valve: 3D-visualization by computed tomography. J Cardiovasc Comput Tomogr. 2019:5;S1934-5925(19)30327-2.
11. Motwani M, Burley O, Luckie M, et al. 3D-printing assisted closure of paravalvular leak [published online ahead of print, 2019 Mar 26]. J Cardiovasc Comput Tomogr. 2019;S1934-5925(19)30035-8.
12. Brown JM, O'Brien SM, Wu C, Sikora JAH, Griffith BP, Gammie JS. Isolated aortic valve replacement in North America comprising 108,687 patients in 10 years: changes in risks, valve types, and outcomes in the Society of Thoracic Surgeons national database. J Thorac Cardiovasc Surg. 2008;137:82–90.
13. Bakir I, Casselman FP, Wellens F, et al. Minimally invasive versus standard approach aortic valve replacement: a study in 506 patients. Ann Thorac Surg. 2006;81:1599–604
14. Semsroth S, Matteucci-Gothe R, Heinz A, Dal Capello T, Kilo J, Müller L, Grimm M, Ruttman-Ulmer E. Comparison of anterolateral minithoracotomy versus partial upper hemisternotomy in aortic valve replacement. Ann Thorac Surg. 2015;100:868–73.
15. Johnston DR, Roselli EE. Minimally invasive aortic valve surgery: Cleveland Clinic experience. Ann Cardiothorac Surg. 2015;4:140–7.
16. Ammar R, Porat E, Eisenberg DS, Uretzky G. Utility of spiral CT in minimally invasive approach for aortic valve replacement. Eur J Cardiothorac Surg. 1998;14(Suppl.1):S130–3.
17. Barbanti M, Yang TH, Rodès Cabau J, et al. Anatomical and procedural features associated with aortic root rupture during balloon-expandable transcatheter aortic valve replacement. Circulation. 2013;128(3):244–53.
18. Pollari F, Hitzl W, Vogt F, et al. Aortic valve calcification as a risk factor for major complications and reduced survival after transcatheter replacement. J Cardiovasc Comput Tomogr. 2020;14(4):307–13.
19. Ripley B, Kelil T, Cheezum MK, et al. 3D printing based on cardiac CT assists anatomic visualization prior to transcatheter aortic valve replacement. J Cardiovasc Comput Tomogr. 2016;10(1):28–36.
20. Qian Z, Wang K, Liu S, et al. Quantitative prediction of paravalvular leak in transcatheter aortic valve replacement based on tissue-mimicking 3D printing. JACC Cardiovasc Imaging. 2017;10(7):719–31.
21. Guerrero M, Dvir D, Himbert D, et al. Transcatheter mitral valve replacement in native mitral valve disease with severe mitral annular calcification: results from the first multicenter global Registry. JACC Cardiovasc Interv. 2016;9:1361–71.
22. Karády J, Ntalas I, Prendergast B, et al. Transcatheter mitral valve replacement in mitral annulus calcification – "The art of computer simulation". J Cardiovasc Comput Tomogr. 2018;12(2):153–7.
23. Wang DD, Eng M, Greenbaum A, et al. Predicting LVOT obstruction after TMVR. JACC Cardiovasc Imaging. 2016;9(11):1349–52.
24. Ooms J, Minet M, Daemen J, Van Mieghem N. Pre-procedural planning of transcatheter mitral valve replacement in mitral stenosis with multi-detector tomography-derived 3D modeling and printing: a case report. Eur Heart J Case Rep. 2020;4(3):1–6.
25. Sorajja P, Gössl M, Babaliaros V, Rizik D, Conradi L, Bae R, Burke RF, Schäfer U, Lisko JC, Riley RD, Guyton R, Dumonteil N, Berthoumieu P, Tchetche D, Blanke P, Cavalcante JL, Sun B. Novel transcatheter mitral valve prosthesis for patients with severe mitral annular calcification. J Am Coll Cardiol. 2019;74(11):1431–40.
26. Jeganathan J, Knio Z, Amador Y, Hai T, Khamooshian A, Matyal R, Khabbaz KR, Mahmood F. Artificial intelligence in mitral valve analysis. Ann Card Anaesth. 2017;20(2):129–34.
27. Ionasec R, Voigt I, Georgescu B, Wang Y, Houle H, Vega-Higuera F, Navab N, Comaniciu D. Patient-specific modeling and quantification of the aortic and mitral valves from 4-D cardiac CT and TEE. IEEE Trans Med Imaging. 2010;9:1636–51.
28. Sasa G, Ionasec R, Vitanovski D, Voigt I, Wang Y, Georgescu B, Navab N, Comaniciu D. Complete valvular heart apparatus model from 4D cardiac CT. Med Image Anal. 2012;16(5):1003–14.
29. Nguyen A, Yosinski J, Clune J. Deep neural networks are easily fooled: high confidence predictions for unrecognizable images. Proceedings of the IEEE Computer Society Conference on Computer Vision and Pattern Recognition. 2015:427–436.
30. Al'Aref S, Anchouche K, Singh G, Slomka PJ, Kolli KK, Kumar A, Pandey M, Maliakal G, van Rosendael A, et al. Clinical applications of machine learning in cardiovascular disease and its relevance to cardiac imaging. Eur Heart J. 2019;40(24):1975–86:31.

Artificial Intelligence-Based Diagnosis and Procedural Planning for Aortic Valve Disease

29

Praveen Indraratna and Jonathon Leipsic

Introduction to Aortic Valve Disease

There are two primary pathological manifestations of aortic valve disease – aortic valve stenosis and aortic valve regurgitation. When both conditions become severe, medical therapy is largely ineffective, and valve replacement either by a traditional open surgical or transcatheter approach is considered definitive therapy. Transcatheter approaches are typically heavily reliant on imaging, particularly computed tomography (CT) in order to ensure accurate valve sizing and correct choice of fluoroscopic angles and assessment of the peripheral vasculature (the aorta, iliofemoral system, and/or subclavian arteries) in order to identify individual patient suitability for the procedure.

Aortic Valve Stenosis

In industrialized nations, aortic valve stenosis is the most common valvular abnormality of the heart [1] and has several causes. Generally, aortic stenosis is a disease of the elderly, caused by calcific degeneration of the valve, until leaflet excursion is impaired. Bicuspid aortic valve, the most common congenital cardiac abnormality, is the predominant cause of aortic stenosis in those under the age of 65 [2]. Rheumatic heart disease remains an important cause of aortic stenosis in the developing world. Aortic stenosis is traditionally graded as mild, moderate, or severe. Generally, only severe cases become symptomatic. Symptoms can include dyspnea, chest pain, and, in critical cases, syncope and heart failure. Sudden death is a not infrequent initial presentation. Clinicians may become suspicious of aortic stenosis by the clinical history or by detection of the typical ejection systolic murmur. Other more subtle clinical signs such as an anacrotic (slow-rising), a narrow pulse pressure, and a palpable thrill may become apparent in severe cases. Echocardiography is the mainstay of diagnosis, which is achieved by identifying the typical calcific appearance, leaflet thickening, and poor leaflet excursion. The severity of the lesion is typically defined by a combination of the mean transvalvular gradient, the peak velocity, and the calculated valve area using the continuity equation. Left ventricular hypertrophy may be noted as a consequence of the increased afterload, and in end-stage cases, left ventricular dysfunction develops. CT is often required in equivocal cases, particularly when the cardiac output is low due to cardiac failure. In this setting, the calcium content of the valve (the calcium score) may aid in adjudicating the likelihood of severe aortic stenosis.

Severe, symptomatic cases require valve replacement, as aortic stenosis is an irreversible condition, and will likely be fatal unless treated definitively. Transcatheter valve replacement has emerged as an efficacious and safe alternative to open surgical valve replacement, on the basis of several large randomized controlled trials [2].

Aortic Valve Regurgitation

Aortic valve regurgitation can be caused by damaged or abnormal valve leaflets, such as in the case of bicuspid aortic valve or infective endocarditis. Additionally, disruption of the valve annulus due to conditions causing dilatation of the aortic root or ascending aorta such as hypertension, congenital disorders (Turner syndrome and familial thoracic aortic aneurysm and dissection syndromes), and hereditary connective tissue disorders (Marfan, Ehlers-Danlos, and Loeys-Dietz syndromes) can also cause aortic valve regurgitation.

The diagnosis of aortic valve regurgitation can be challenging, as clinical signs are often subtle, and echocardiography can lead to overestimation or underestimation of the severity of the condition. In many individuals, severe aortic

P. Indraratna, MBBS (✉) · J. Leipsic, MD
Department of Radiology, St. Paul's Hospital, Vancouver, Canada

University of British Columbia, Vancouver, Canada
e-mail: praveen@unsw.edu.au; jleipsic@providencehealth.bc.ca

C. N. De Cecco et al. (eds.), *Artificial Intelligence in Cardiothoracic Imaging*, Contemporary Medical Imaging,
https://doi.org/10.1007/978-3-030-92087-6_29

regurgitation can be tolerated with minimal or no symptoms, but it will inevitably lead to progressive dilatation of the left ventricle and eventually left ventricular dysfunction, both of which can be irreversible if valve replacement does not occur.

The mainstay of treatment is surgical aortic valve replacement, although transcatheter valve replacement is becoming increasingly popular as an option, although the evidence base is not as robust as for aortic valve stenosis [3].

Artificial Intelligence in the Diagnosis of Aortic Stenosis

Where traditional diagnosis of aortic valve stenosis requires clinician referral for echocardiography, several AI-based options may help streamline screening of large populations for the condition. For example, a Korean group developed a deep learning-based algorithm using over 39,000 ECGs 12-lead and single-lead ECGs [4]. The algorithm predominantly used the T-wave axis in leads V1–V4, the QT interval, and the patient's age to detect moderate or severe aortic stenosis. The area under the curve was 0.861, which the authors stated was higher than that of widely used breast cancer and colorectal cancer screening programs. Further study is required to refine the algorithm, but it suggests a promising option for rapidly screening large populations of patients, particularly those in remote communities who may not have access to echocardiography.

Similarly, detection of aortic stenosis by machine learning-based analysis of cardiac murmurs is now offered by several commercial enterprises. One currently available device, which has FDA approval, consists of a digital stethoscope which generates a phonocardiogram and an accompanying smartphone application which uses machine-learning to analyze the recording. An observational study of this technology is currently underway [5]. A similar technique that combined a phonocardiogram obtained from a digital stethoscope with an ECG was used to train a deep learning algorithm that identified bicuspid aortic valves in children. The deep learning model outperformed five trained clinicians, which is not unexpected given that interpretation of cardiac murmurs in children is often more difficult than in adults, owing to their higher baseline heart rates, higher propensity for splitting of heart sounds, and high prevalence of benign "flow" murmurs [6].

Echocardiography remains the mainstay for diagnosis of aortic stenosis and aortic regurgitation. Artificial intelligence has demonstrated several promising roles in the field and theoretically can reduce problems with interobserver variability, as well as increasing efficiency in busy echocardiography laboratories and assisting with echocardiography interpretation in situations and locations where qualified individuals are unavailable. Deep learning algorithms have demonstrated efficacy in identifying left ventricular hypertrophy, which is often observed in aortic stenosis, as well as left ventricular volumes and dysfunction [7], which are particularly relevant to aortic regurgitation (see Fig. 29.1).

As previously described, the use of calcium scoring of the aortic valve can be useful in cases where the echocardiographic results are equivocal or in the context of low-flow, low-gradient aortic stenosis. A deep learning model to automatically segment and score aortic valve calcification has been published [8], although further refinement is required. The authors commented that the model had difficulty distinguishing aortic valve calcification from aortic calcification, which is also a challenge in manual interpretation. While the model was developed from the examination of noncontrast chest CT scans, one would expect that such a model would be more accurate in dedicated scans of the aortic valve which included both contrast and noncontrast acquisition, but further study is required in this field.

Artificial Intelligence in the Diagnosis of Aortic Regurgitation

Similar to the diagnosis of aortic stenosis, AI interpretation of phonocardiograms can be used to diagnose aortic regurgitation. Aortic regurgitation typically causes a characteristic diastolic murmur, which can be difficult for inexperienced clinicians to identify. One system demonstrated an accuracy of over 98% when identifying aortic regurgitation [9].

Cardiac MRI is useful in the diagnosis and grading of aortic regurgitation, particularly in the setting of eccentric regurgitant jets, or suboptimal echocardiographic image quality. Regurgitant volume can be calculated using the phase contrast technique, which identifies the velocity of protons in the blood pool. When this technique is applied to the ascending aorta, both the forward and regurgitant flow can be calculated. Previously, manual segmentation of the ascending aorta was required; however machine learning has been shown to yield comparable results to manual segmentation [10]. Several deep learning models have demonstrated the ability to automatically perform quantification of the left ventricular volume [11, 12], with a high degree of accuracy compared to manual quantification. Left ventricular size is a crucial parameter in determining the need for valve replacement in patients with asymptomatic aortic regurgitation.

Another deep learning model used phase contrast data to identify bicuspid from tricuspid aortic valves [13]. This holds some promise as visual distinction of bicuspid from tricuspid aortic valves can be challenging when there is excess valve calcification and is clinically relevant as, under certain conditions, indications for valve replacement in individuals with bicuspid aortic valve vary from those who have a tricuspid valve.

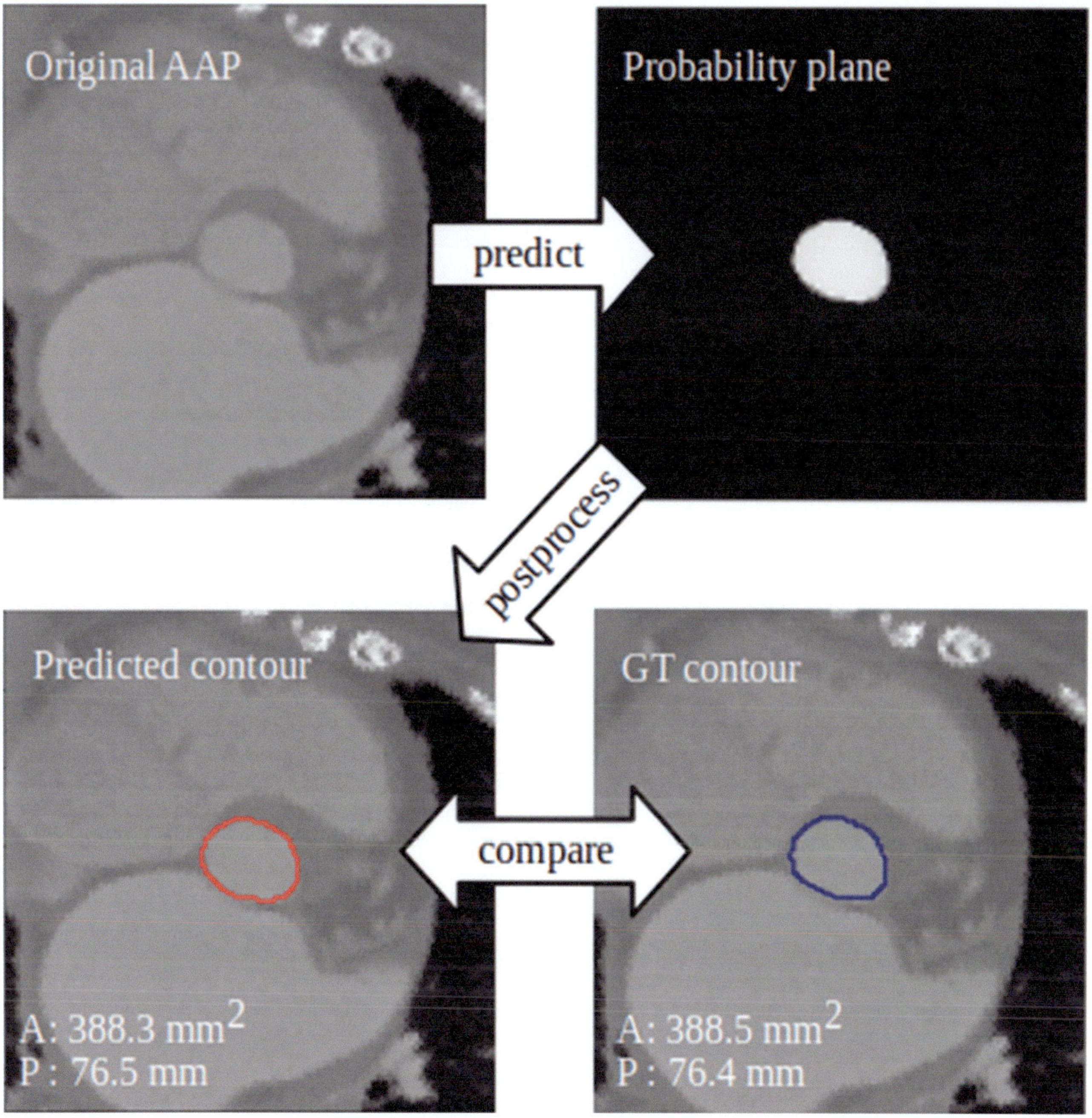

Fig. 29.1 An example of a deep learning algorithm to detect three echocardiographic findings. The shaded areas represent the 95% confidence intervals. (Reproduced from Ghorbani et al. [7] under the terms of the Creative Commons Attribution 4.0 International License)

Artificial Intelligence for Evaluation of the Aorta

A detailed analysis of AI in evaluation of the aorta is covered in Chap. 58. Evaluation of the aorta is particularly important in those with bicuspid aortic valves, as up to 40% of these individuals will have concomitant thoracic aortic dilatation [14], which can predispose to aortic dissection, a frequently fatal condition. In regard to bicuspid aortopathy, a machine learning model has been published, which established the relationship between the morphology of the valve and the pattern of aneurysmal dilatation [15]. Future studies in this area may be useful in determining the timing and nature of aortic surgery in these patients.

Additionally, aortic root dilatation is a cause of aortic valve regurgitation, and thus the aorta should be evaluated in all patients with this condition. Baskaran et al. have published a deep learning method for automatic segmentation of many cardiovascular structures, including the aorta, with excellent accuracy as evidenced by dice scores above 0.95 [16].

The Role of AI in TAVR Planning CT Scans

CT is recommended as a prerequisite investigation in patients undergoing TAVR. CT provides sufficient anatomical detail for both planning of the valve selection and sizing, risk of complications such as annular rupture, as well as an assessment of the peripheral vascular access.

Typically, these scans are analyzed by trained radiologists and may be labor-intensive. The process involves defining the annular plane and making an accurate assessment of the annular size (area and perimeter) in systole using 3D reconstructive software. This method is preferred for valve sizing [17]. Accurate annular sizing is crucial, as underestimation of the annular size can lead to annular rupture and overestimation of annular size can lead to valve embolization, paravalvular regurgitation, and patient-prosthesis mismatch. Apart from annular sizing, further information is gathered by CT, including the height of the coronary arteries from the annular plane, the sizes of the sinuses of Valsalva, and the sinotubular junction, a combination of which can be used to estimate the risk of annular rupture and coronary artery obstruction during the procedure [18].

Annular segmentation can be challenging; however a deep learning method using two models has been studied. Astudillo and colleagues describe a deep learning method that can automatically derive the annulus perimeter and area [19]. After training the models with 355 patients, the method was evaluated on 118 patients. The automatic predictions varied from manual assessment of area and perimeter by a mean of 3.3 mm^2 and 1.3 mm, respectively, which the authors considered to be within the limits of typical interobserver variability (see Fig. 29.2). The processing speed was less than 1 second.

A similar approach based on machine learning was tested in 110 patients [20]. Here, manual measurements were compared to semi-automated and fully automated measurements. The semi-automated method, which allowed readers to accept or modify the annular plane prior to size calculations, required major correction in five patients. Eighty percent of measurements were within an annular area of 0.5 cm^2 which may not be considered an acceptable margin of error. The fully automated method was less accurate.

Thus, AI may be an option to cross-check annular sizing results obtained by manual measurement or may ultimately be a "stand-alone" option.

Image Quality Improvement

Deep learning reconstruction methods have been used widely to improve image quality of CT image across a wide variety of indications [21]. CT scans performed for the purposes of TAVR can be subject to image noise and, as they are performed over the full cardiac cycle, increase radiation exposure to patients compared to other forms of cardiac CT. Image noise can make segmentation of the annulus particularly challenging, especially when there is a high burden of calcification. In a randomized trial, Ippolito et al. subjected 32 patients with aortic stenosis to a low-dose (80 kV vs. 100 kV), low-volume (60 mL of contrast vs. 80 mL) CT, with deep learning iterative reconstruction [22]. This method resulted in a 56% reduction in dose-length product, with no significant difference in image quality, as assessed by two radiologists.

Prediction of Diagnosis and Outcome

Patients undergoing transcatheter valve replacement (TAVR) are at risk of inhospital mortality. This is a result of direct complications of the procedure, as well as comorbidities in a typically frail population. Prediction models of morbidity and mortality are required for judicious patient selection, particularly in resource-limited settings where many patients may not have access to treatment. A machine learning model, NIS-TAVR, was developed and applied to a cohort of over 10,000 TAVR patients with a 3.6% total mortality rate and was found to outperform established risk calculators, with an area under the curve (AUC) of 0.92 [23]. A second machine learning model, tested on 451 patients, was shown to have superior mortality prediction (AUC 0.94–0.97) than the STS risk score (AUC 0.64), although the authors cautioned that procedural complications such as stroke, vascular complications, and bradycardia requiring pacing were not predictable [24]. Abdul Ghaffar and colleagues used a semisupervised automated machine learning approach to classify patients into five phenotypic groups, ordered in regard to estimated mortality, and demonstrated that using this approach in conjunction with the STS risk score improved mortality prediction [25].

Conclusion

Artificial intelligence has been studied in population screening and staging and diagnosis of aortic valve disease, as well as providing options for expediting the planning process for TAVR. Aortic stenosis, in particular, is a common problem in the elderly, and with an aging population in developed countries, there is potential for the demand for diagnosis and treatment that may overwhelm the existing services able to provide them. In this context, AI has promise in streamlining the patient journey and potentially leading to improved outcomes.

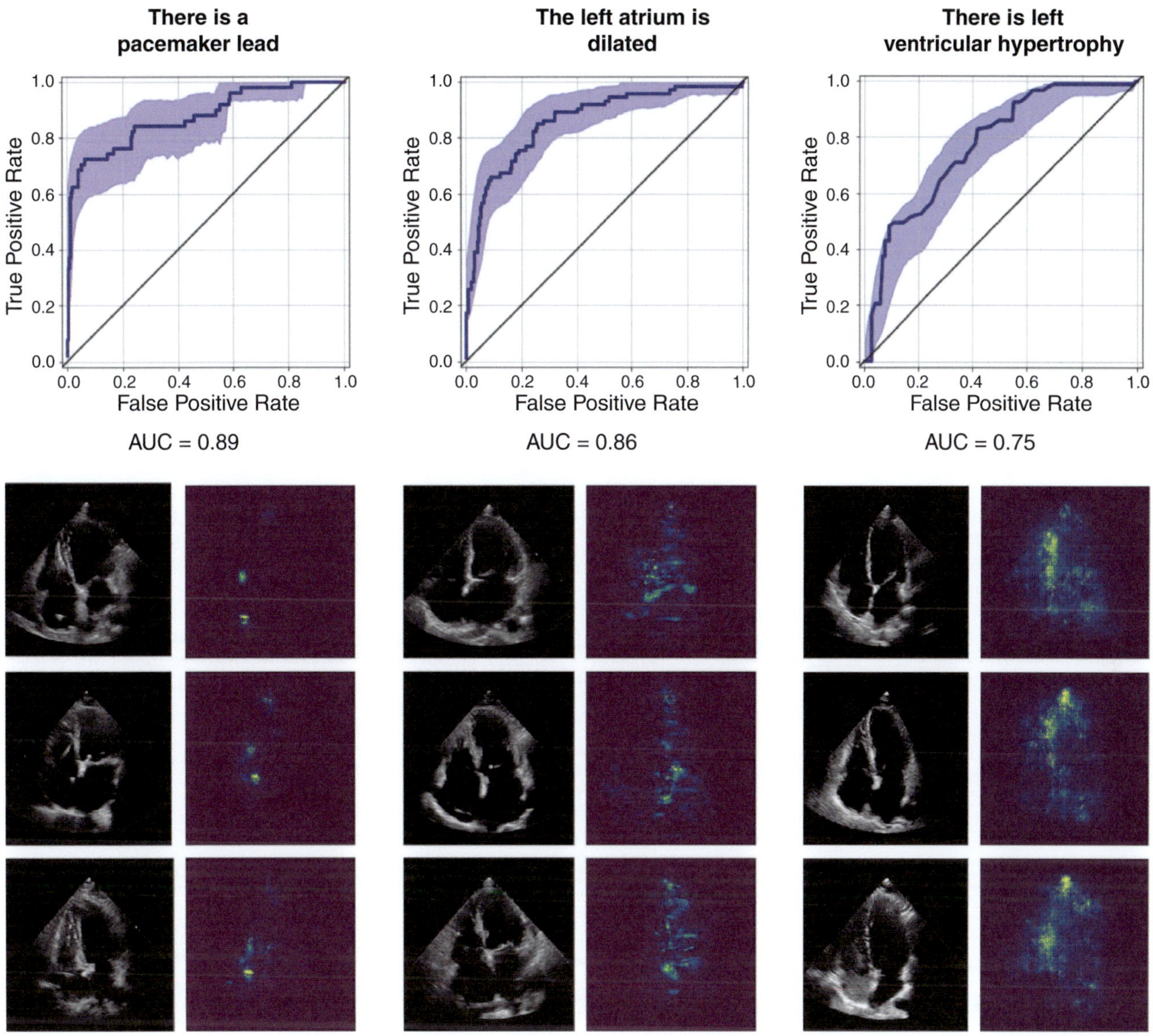

Fig. 29.2 An example of aortic annular plane (AAP) segmentation as derived from a deep convolutional neural network (bottom left) compared to the *ground truth (GT)* derived from manual segmentation (bottom right). (Reproduced from Astudillo et al. [19] under the terms of the Creative Commons Attribution License)

References

1. Nathaniel S, Saligram S, Innasimuthu AL. Aortic stenosis: an update. World J Cardiol. 2010;2(6):135–9.
2. Fedak PW, Verma S, David TE, Leask RL, Weisel RD, Butany J. Clinical and pathophysiological implications of a bicuspid aortic valve. Circulation. 2002;106(8):900–4.
3. Arias EA, Bhan A, Lim ZY, Mullen M. TAVI for pure native aortic regurgitation: are we there yet? Interv Cardiol. 2019;14(1):26–30.
4. Kwon JM, Lee SY, Jeon KH, Lee Y, Kim KH, Park J, et al. Deep learning based algorithm for detecting aortic stenosis using electrocardiography. J Am Heart Assoc. 2020;9(7):e014717.
5. White BE, Shapiro AM, Kanzawa MM, Venkatraman S, Paek J, Pham S, et al. Abstract 13831: handheld wireless digital phonocardiography for machine learning-based detection of mitral regurgitation. Circulation. 2019;140(Suppl_1):A13831-A.
6. Gharehbaghi A, Dutoit T, Sepehri AA, Kocharian A, Lindén M. A novel method for screening children with isolated bicuspid aortic valve. Cardiovasc Eng Technol. 2015;6(4):546–56.
7. Ghorbani A, Ouyang D, Abid A, He B, Chen JH, Harrington RA, et al. Deep learning interpretation of echocardiograms. NPJ Digital Med. 2020;3(1):10.
8. Lessmann N, van Ginneken B, Zreik M, de Jong PA, de Vos BD, Viergever MA, et al. Automatic calcium scoring in low-dose chest CT using deep neural networks with dilated convolutions. IEEE Trans Med Imaging. 2018;37(2):615–25.
9. Sun S. An innovative intelligent system based on automatic diagnostic feature extraction for diagnosing heart diseases. Knowledge-Based Syst. 2015;75:224–38.
10. Bratt A, Kim J, Pollie M, Beecy AN, Tehrani NH, Codella N, et al. Machine learning derived segmentation of phase velocity encoded cardiovascular magnetic resonance for fully automated aortic flow quantification. J Cardiovasc Magn Reson. 2019;21(1):1.

11. Avendi MR, Kheradvar A, Jafarkhani H. A combined deep-learning and deformable-model approach to fully automatic segmentation of the left ventricle in cardiac MRI. Med Image Anal. 2016;30:108–19.
12. Tao Q, Yan W, Wang Y, Paiman EHM, Shamonin DP, Garg P, et al. Deep learning-based method for fully automatic quantification of left ventricle function from cine MR images: a multivendor. Multicenter Study Radiol. 2019;290(1):81–8.
13. Fries JA, Varma P, Chen VS, Xiao K, Tejeda H, Saha P, et al. Weakly supervised classification of aortic valve malformations using unlabeled cardiac MRI sequences. Nat Commun. 2019;10(1):3111.
14. Borger MA, Fedak PWM, Stephens EH, Gleason TG, Girdauskas E, Ikonomidis JS, et al. The American Association for Thoracic Surgery consensus guidelines on bicuspid aortic valve-related aortopathy: full online-only version. J Thorac Cardiovasc Surg. 2018;156(2):e41–74.
15. Wojnarski CM, Roselli EE, Idrees JJ, Zhu Y, Carnes TA, Lowry AM, et al. Machine-learning phenotypic classification of bicuspid aortopathy. J Thorac Cardiovasc Surg. 2018;155(2):461–9.e4.
16. Baskaran L, Al'Aref SJ, Maliakal G, Lee BC, Xu Z, Choi JW, et al. Automatic segmentation of multiple cardiovascular structures from cardiac computed tomography angiography images using deep learning. PLoS One. 2020;15(5):e0232573.
17. Blanke P, Schoepf UJ, Leipsic JA. CT in transcatheter aortic valve replacement. Radiology. 2013;269(3):650–69.
18. Blanke P, Soon J, Dvir D, Park JK, Naoum C, Kueh SH, et al. Computed tomography assessment for transcatheter aortic valve in valve implantation: the Vancouver approach to predict anatomical risk for coronary obstruction and other considerations. J Cardiovasc Comput Tomogr. 2016;10(6):491–9.
19. Astudillo P, Mortier P, Bosmans J, De Backer O, de Jaegere P, De Beule M, et al. Enabling automated device size selection for transcatheter aortic valve implantation. J Interv Cardiol. 2019;2019:3591314.
20. Lou J, Obuchowski NA, Krishnaswamy A, Popovic Z, Flamm SD, Kapadia SR, et al. Manual, semiautomated, and fully automated measurement of the aortic annulus for planning of transcatheter aortic valve replacement (TAVR/TAVI): analysis of interchangeability. J Cardiovasc Comput Tomogr. 2015;9(1):42–9.
21. Zhang H-M, Dong B. A review on deep learning in medical image reconstruction. J Operations Res Soc China. 2020;8(2):311–40.
22. Ippolito D, Riva L, Talei Franzesi C, De Vito A, Cangiotti C, Crespi A, et al. Computed tomography angiography combined with knowledge-based iterative algorithm for transcatheter aortic valve implantation planning: image quality and radiation dose exposure with low-kV and low-contrast-medium protocol. J Comput Assist Tomogr. 2020;44(1):13–9.
23. Hernandez-Suarez DF, Kim Y, Villablanca P, Gupta T, Wiley J, Nieves-Rodriguez BG, et al. Machine learning prediction models for in-hospital mortality after transcatheter aortic valve replacement. JACC Cardiovasc Interv. 2019;12(14):1328–38.
24. Gomes B, Pilz M, Reich C, Leuschner F, Konstandin M, Katus HA, et al. Machine learning-based risk prediction of intrahospital clinical outcomes in patients undergoing TAVI. Clin Res Cardiol. 2021;110:343–56.
25. Abdul Ghffar Y, Osman M, Shrestha S, Shaukat F, Kagiyama N, Alkhouli M, et al. Usefulness of semisupervised machine-learning-based phenogrouping to improve risk assessment for patients undergoing transcatheter aortic valve implantation. Am J Cardiol. 2020;136:122–30.

Artificial Intelligence-Based Quantification of Cardiac Fat

30

Caterina B. Monti, Davide Capra, Francesco Secchi, Marina Codari, and Francesco Sardanelli

Introduction

Epicardial adipose tissue (EAT) is the layer of adipose tissue which is located between the epicardium and the visceral pericardium [1]. The most conspicuous amount of EAT is found in the atrioventricular and interventricular grooves; of note, it is thicker around the right ventricle than the left. EAT represents roughly one fifth of the overall cardiac volume. Another mediastinal adipose tissue, paracardiac adipose tissue (PAT), lies right outside the pericardium, thus surrounding the EAT. Despite their anatomical vicinity, EAT and PAT are two different tissues with different physiological and metabolic profiles.

EAT has been hypothesized to originate from the mesenchymal transformation that can be induced in cells belonging to the epicardium with the expression of the peroxisome proliferator-activated receptor gamma [2]. Thus, EAT is a metabolically active tissue, leaning toward a brown nature during childhood and switching toward a "beige" nature in adulthood [3]. Brown and, to a lesser extent, beige adipose tissues are characterized by the presence of a specific protein, the uncoupling protein 1 also known as thermogenin. While thermogenin is virtually always expressed in brown adipose tissue, its expression in beige adipose tissue is secondary to a process of stimulation and induction called "beiging," which could be mediated by free fatty acids (FFAs) [4]. The action of thermogenin leads to the uncoupling of mitochondrial respiration and the dispersion of energy with a subsequent generation of heat.

Important interactions between EAT and the heart regard the coronary arteries, which are fully enveloped by EAT: it acts like a cushion, protecting them from mechanical strain [5]. Moreover, EAT draws its sustainment from the coronary arteries, which in turn present a direct way of communication between EAT and the heart. In fact, EAT has an important role in the metabolism and turnover of FFAs, which on the one hand provide an energy source for the myocardium, while on the other hand may induce cardiotoxic effects, regulating the level of FFAs to which the heart is exposed (lipotoxicity) [6]. Moreover, EAT can produce and regulate the levels of certain cytokines (adipokines) such as tumor necrosis factor-α, leptin, resistin, and adiponectin. In particular, the last one yields important implications for atherogenesis, as it can stimulate the synthesis of nitric oxide, regulating oxidative stress and inflammation [7].

Given the metabolic relevance of EAT, many studies have aimed to better define its role in cardiac disease. A growing body of evidence plays in favor of a direct positive correlation between EAT thickness or volume and cardiovascular risk: an increase in EAT volume may reflect an overall fat overload and dysmetabolic asset trending toward metabolic syndrome. More recently, EAT radiodensity assessed through computed tomography (CT) has been proposed as a further potential biomarker of cardiovascular risk, more specifically linked to coronary artery disease (CAD) [8].

Epicardial Adipose Tissue Imaging

Noninvasive imaging techniques have been employed for the evaluation of EAT through the years. The first imaging method which has been used with this purpose was

C. B. Monti, MD, PhD (✉) · D. Capra, MD
Department of Biomedical Sciences for Health, Università degli Studi di Milano, Milan, Italy
e-mail: caterina.monti@unimi.it; davide.capra@unimi.it

F. Secchi, MD, PhD · F. Sardanelli, MD
Department of Biomedical Sciences for Health, Università degli Studi di Milano, Milan, Italy

Unit of Radiology, IRCCS Policlinico San Donato, San Donato Milanese, Milan, Italy
e-mail: francesco.secchi@unimi.it; francesco.sardanelli@unimi.it

M. Codari, MSc, PhD
Department of Radiology, School of Medicine, Stanford University, Stanford, CA, USA
e-mail: mcodari@stanford.edu

C. N. De Cecco et al. (eds.), *Artificial Intelligence in Cardiothoracic Imaging*, Contemporary Medical Imaging,
https://doi.org/10.1007/978-3-030-92087-6_30

transthoracic echocardiography (TTE), which was then followed by CT and magnetic resonance imaging (MRI) [9].

Transthoracic Echocardiography

Images acquired with TTE allow the visualization of EAT surrounding the ventricles, showing a different tissue echogenicity as reported by Davidovich et al. [10].

The relative easiness of assessing EAT thickness by TTE made it a possible biomarker of cardiometabolic disease. It can be measured through TTE around the right ventricle and perpendicular to its wall. Given the high operator dependency of this technique, it may be useful to perform more than one measurement of EAT thickness. Cutoff values for EAT thickness indicating a higher potential for cardiovascular pathology are set around 5 mm [11, 12].

Among the main advantages of TTE are its low cost, widespread and ready availability, as well as lack of radiation exposure, which would prove ideal should TTE be proposed as a screening tool. However, TTE also bears some limitations other than reproducibility issues. In fact, pericardial effusion could potentially be mistaken for EAT in some instances where EAT appears especially hypoechoic [13].

Computed Tomography

Chest CT offers a detailed representation of anatomical structures, allowing an accurate volume estimation of EAT. On CT scans, EAT appears as a hypodense tissue, with Hounsfield units (HU) values usually ranging between −190 and −30 HU, located around the heart and inside the pericardium, as depicted in Fig. 30.1. EAT can be visualized similarly on either unenhanced or contrast-enhanced scans, albeit its density might change slightly in the latter case, *i.e.*, after intravenous injection of iodine-based contrast agent [14]. Unenhanced scans may provide an advantage, as, together with calcium score quantification, it would allow a cardiovascular risk assessment also in patients presenting with contraindications to iodine-based contrast agent such as allergic reactions or kidney disease. Of note, even though CT scans acquired with retrospective or prospective electrocardiographic gating show superior quality, EAT can be assessed also by non-gated scans, albeit keeping into consideration that, to obtain reliable measurements, when assessing non-gated scans, acquisition velocity must be high enough as to allow a substantial absence of movement artifacts. Figure 30.2 shows EAT on a slice from a non-gated chest scan.

The entire EAT volume may be quantified from any chest CT examination covering the whole heart, with a higher precision when image slices are thinner. The average volume of EAT in a healthy subject is estimated to be around 15–20% of the overall cardiac volume, which usually means less than 125 mL [15].

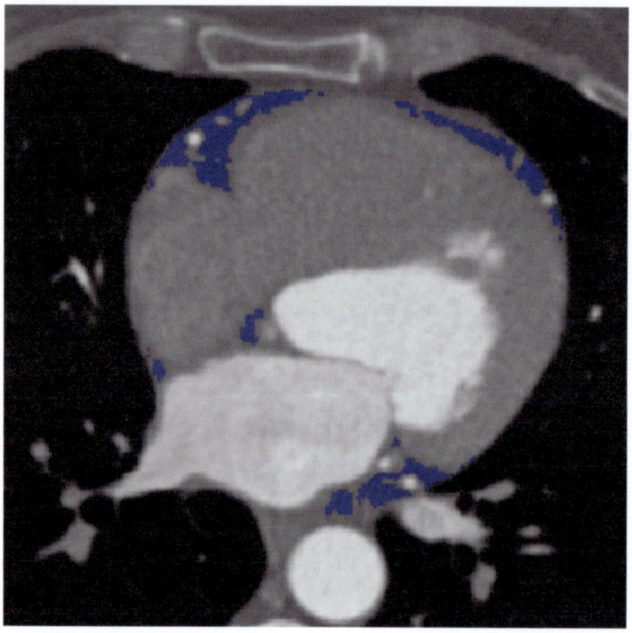

Fig. 30.1 Contrast-enhanced, gated CT scan representing EAT (in blue), segmented with a thresholding for HU values between −190 and −30 HU, directly surrounding the heart

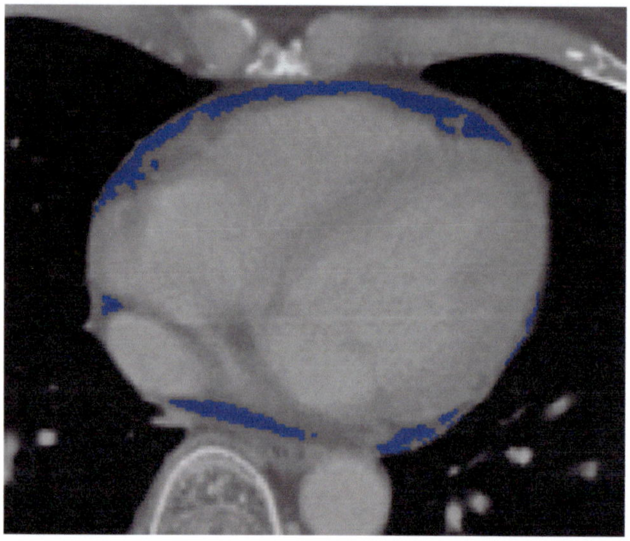

Fig. 30.2 Contrast-enhanced, portal venous phase, non-gated CT scan depicting EAT (in blue), segmented with a thresholding for HU values between −190 and −30 HU, directly surrounding the heart

More recently, a growing number of studies have aimed to review the role of EAT radiodensity as a potential biomarker of cardiovascular risk. While it would seem that radiodensity of the EAT directly surrounding the coronary arteries rises in the presence of CAD, results concerning overall EAT density appear somewhat conflicting so far. In fact, while some works observed an increase in density in patients with CAD, other studies reported density decreasing [16]. These conflicting findings may be due to the fact that EAT density rises in the presence of inflammation, fibrosis, or "beiging," whereas it decreases in case of inactive fat deposition. Therefore, in patients with CAD and likely dyslipidemia or dysregulation of fat metabolism, EAT density in the fat pad right around the coronary arteries, the so-called pericoronary epicardial adipose tissue (pCAT), could increase due to CAD-related inflammation. At the same time, density might decrease at a global level due to the quantitative increase of fat depots, also related to the adipose volumetric increase that is observed in high-risk patients. Other potential explanations for these findings also include the possibility that iodine-based contrast agents further increase the density of EAT in areas presenting with inflammation [17].

While CT yields the advantages of allowing the assessment of EAT volumes at a reasonably high definition, being also widely available, and allowing quick scanning times, its main disadvantages are not negligible such as radiation exposure and potentially very long segmentation times according to spatial resolution, in particular when low slice thickness implies a large number of slices to be segmented.

Magnetic Resonance Imaging

Another noninvasive imaging technique that allows a three-dimensional representation of EAT is MRI. The assessment of EAT with MRI does not require the use of contrast agents However, gated scans are recommended to properly visualize EAT to avoid movement artifacts. Different MRI sequences may be used for evaluating EAT, the most common being bright-blood steady-state free-precession cine acquisitions, as they represent a mainstay in every cardiac MRI examination [18]. On these conventional cine sequences, EAT is visualized as a hyperintense tissue located between the ventricles and the thin (not always well-detectable), hypointense pericardium layer, as shown in Fig. 30.3. Using cine sequences, EAT can be quantified at end-systolic and end-diastolic cardiac phases, which may provide different measurements, as fat around the atria is better visualized during diastole, whereas around the ventricle it may appear more prominent during systole. Other acquisitions that could allow the assessment of EAT include half-Fourier single-shot turbo spin echo (HASTE) [19], but also mapping sequences and all other sequences which allow a clear visualization of the myocardium and pericardium could serve this purpose [20]. Recently, attempts have been made to perform measurements of EAT volumes on scans obtained on open-bore MRI scanners (see Fig. 30.4), which allow imaging of severely obese or claustrophobic patients who would not be able to undergo closed-bore MRI.

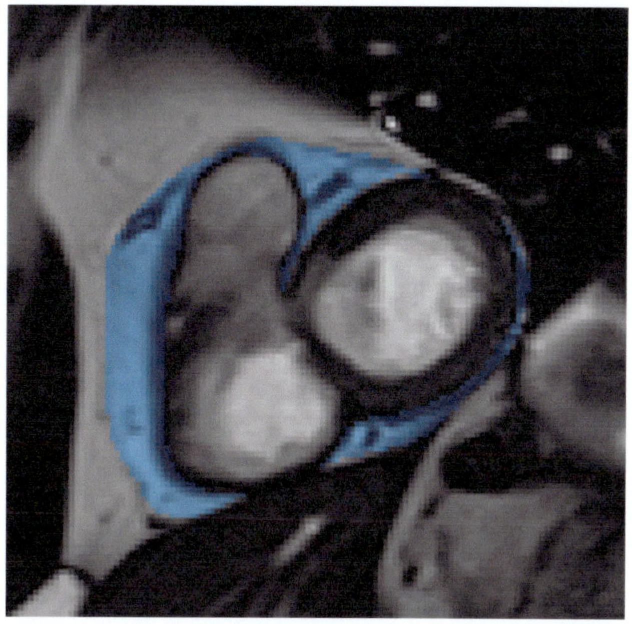

Fig. 30.3 MRI cine bright-blood steady-state free-precession acquisition on a 1.5-T scanner depicting EAT in blue surrounding the heart

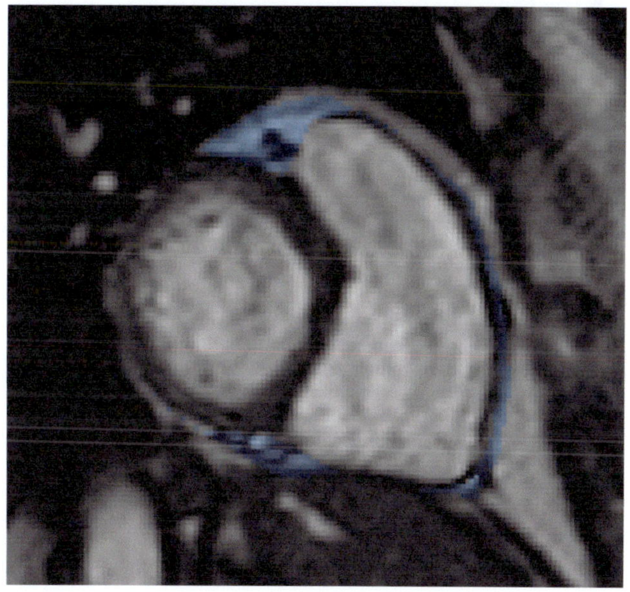

Fig. 30.4 MRI cine bright-blood steady-state free-precession acquisition on an open-bore 1.0-T scanner depicting EAT in blue surrounding the heart

While the volumetric nature of MRI images does allow the evaluation of EAT volumes, although at a lower spatial resolution compared to CT, signal intensity is not standardized as it happens for density on CT scans. Therefore, there has been no widespread interest in ascertaining signal intensity or MRI signal-to-noise ratio in cardiovascular risk assessment.

The main advantage of MRI for EAT evaluation is the lack of radiation exposure, whereas its drawbacks include limited availability, long scanning times, and relatively high costs (if cardiac MRI would be performed for the specific purpose of EAT assessment).

Artificial Intelligence Applications for Epicardial Adipose Tissue Evaluation

Recently, various artificial intelligence (AI) applications have been proposed to solve tasks related to EAT assessment. Their main aims could be classified in two core groups: (i) EAT segmentation and (ii) the development of clinical models including parameters derived from EAT analysis. So far, AI works have been focused on CT imaging.

Epicardial Adipose Tissue Segmentation

Manual segmentation of EAT is cumbersome for several reasons. First, it is extremely time-consuming, especially when working on CT images, as slice thickness (as already stated) may be lower than 1 mm leading to datasets comprising up to a few hundred images. While this issue may be bypassed by only segmenting a smaller number of slices than those available (e.g., one every ten slices), this could potentially lead to a less accurate segmentation and thus less reliable quantitative EAT estimates. Second, reproducibility of EAT parameters may not always be flawless, as the external limit of EAT is represented by the pericardium which may only appear as a thin, tenuous line at imaging, and outside the pericardium lies another fat layer, which could prove a potential confounder. Thus, it may be recommended that segmentation should be performed by readers experienced in cardiovascular imaging [21]. Given the nature of AI methods, their contribution to overcome the presented limitations could prove valuable.

Among the first works to tackle this task with the use of AI, a study by Rodrigues et al. [22] published in 2017 proposed a deep learning framework to automatically segment EAT on unenhanced, gated CT scans. The authors utilized a method which comprised thresholding for adipose tissue between −200 and −30 HU, subsequent image registration, feature extraction, and classification of the adipose tissue voxel based on such features. Their ground truth was represented by images manually segmented by experienced human readers. Working on 878 individual images belonging to 20 patients, the investigators developed different AI models working on a 66% split with tenfold cross-validation. Random forest algorithm showed best performance, with an accuracy of 98.5% for EAT segmentation, with a processing time only slightly longer than a minute.

One subsequent study by Commandeur et al. [23] published in 2018 developed a fully convolutional neural network (CNN) that automatically segments EAT on unenhanced, gated CT scans. In the proposed method, images are used as input for a first fully CNN which extracts image features. Subsequently, dense layers and a subsequent up-sampling allow the classification of intra- and extra-pericardial structures and EAT segmentation. A second fully CNN then inputs the results from the first net and provides an output probability map for the pericardial sac, further adjusting and then thresholding the segmentation. The authors trained their model with tenfold cross-validation on a set of 250 unenhanced, gated CT scans which had been manually segmented by a reader with more than 3 years of experience in cardiovascular imaging for the generation of the ground truth. The AI model obtained a Dice score coefficient (DSC) of 0.823 (interquartile range 0.779–0.860), a bias between 1 and 2 cm^3, and a correlation coefficient of 0.924 ($p < 0.001$), with a segmentation timing on a standard personal computer below 30s.

The same group published a further study in 2020 [24], aiming to retrain and test a slightly different fully CNN on a larger, multicenter database. This approach involved the use of one individual network exploiting residual learning for its deeper layers, which identifies slices containing the heart and segments inside the pericardium with a threshold for adipose tissue between −190 and −30 HU. Ground truth was represented by manual segmentations performed by experienced readers. The authors drew images from four different cohorts scanned at three centers. Training was performed on 614 unenhanced, gated CT scans from 570 subjects comprising three out of the four cohorts, with a tenfold cross-validation and an 80%–10%–10% split for training, validation, and testing, respectively. The model was then perfected and tested on 236 new CT scans from the fourth datasets cohort, achieving a high agreement for EAT volumes with the ground truth ($r = 0.975$, $p < 0.001$) and a bias of around 2 cm^3, with a median processing time of about 2 s when a graphic processing unit was used and around 7 s when only a central processing unit was used.

A further work by He et al. [25] proposed a fully CNN-based method to segment EAT on contrast-enhanced, gated CT scans which employs a three-dimensional U-Net incorporating attention gates. This algorithm was trained on 200 patients who underwent contrast-enhanced cardiac CT with fivefold cross-validation, whereas the ground truth was represented by manual segmentations from two experienced readers. The model achieved a correlation coefficient of 0.949 for cross-validation, with an average volume difference of about 8 cm^3.

The main characteristics and results of the abovementioned studies concerning AI for EAT segmentation are reported in Table 30.1.

Results related to overall EAT volume appear very promising and seem to suggest that AI methods may allow the

Table 30.1 Summary of the main characteristics and results from the reported studies describing the use of AI for EAT segmentation

Author	Year	Image type	Method	Performance	Time
Rodrigues et al. [22]	2017	Noncontrast, gated CT	Random forest	Accuracy: 98.5%	1–2 min
Commandeur et al. [23]	2018	Noncontrast, gated CT	Two CNNs	DSC: 0.823 (0.779–0.860) correlation: $r = 0.924$, $p < 0.001$	<30s
Commandeur et al. [24]	2020	Noncontrast, gated CT	CNN	Correlation: $r = 0.975$, $p < 0.001$	2–7 s
He et al. [25]	2020	Contrast-enhanced, gated CT	CNN	Correlation: $r = 0.949$, $p < 0.001$	N.A.

segmentation of EAT with high accuracy, small volume bias, and within short times. This would indeed pave the way for the inclusion of EAT assessment among the imaging biomarkers that can be readily analyzed on CT scans, such as coronary calcium scoring, which entered clinical practice, being commonly integrated in radiologic reports. Further advancements could include the development of AI methods that also work on other imaging modalities, such as MRI, and the validation of the proposed methods for the assessment of EAT density given its potential role in cardiovascular risk assessment.

Clinical Models Involving Epicardial Adipose Tissue

Another potential application of AI involving the study of EAT is related to the development of models which could help better define the clinical role and scope of EAT parameters. In this regard, AI might, for instance, be of invaluable aid when researchers are faced with the ever-increasing size of available data and the need of generating and perfecting complex models which can integrate multiple variables.

Concerning this purpose, one study by Otaki et al. [26] published in 2015 developed an AI model including EAT volume calculated from unenhanced CT scans to predict the impairment of myocardial flow reserve detected at rest-stress ^{82}Rb positron emission tomography. The authors retrospectively collected data from 85 patients without history of CAD and then used an ensemble-boosting machine learning algorithm, LogitBoost, with tenfold cross-validation to classify patients according to flow reserve impairment (≤ 2.0). Their model included several variables, namely, age, sex, cardiovascular risk factors, calcium scoring, and EAT volume. The authors reported an area under the curve (AUC) of 0.73 for their model, which was significantly greater than those reported for calcium scoring alone (AUC = 0.66, $p = 0.008$) or EAT volume alone (AUC = 0.67, $p = 0.002$).

Subsequent work by Commandeur et al. [27] aimed to use AI to predict patients' long-term risk of myocardial infarction and cardiac death based on clinical variables, calcium scoring, and EAT volume. They used an extreme gradient boosting (XGBoost) model with tenfold cross-validation on a population of 1912 asymptomatic subjects who underwent unenhanced, gated cardiac CT for the calculation of calcium scoring. Their outcome was based on a 14.5-year-long follow-up, during which 76 patients experienced cardiovascular adverse events or death. Their proposed model achieved an AUC of 0.82 (95% confidence interval 0.77–0.87).

While the previously mentioned works focused on EAT volume, which is a well-established biomarker of cardiovascular risk [28], other studies have also aimed to develop AI models including EAT density, especially concerning the pCAT.

One study by Oikonomou et al. [29] proposed an AI model including radiomic analysis of the pCAT to predict cardiovascular risk. The authors performed a radiomic profiling of the pCAT in patients who underwent contrast-enhanced cardiac CT, 101 of whom experienced adverse events in the following 5 years, extracting 1391 individual features from every scan. They proposed a random forest algorithm for a classification task, dividing subjects according to the occurrence of adverse events. They trained the model in 202 patients with an 80%–20% split for training and testing, respectively, a five-fold cross-validation, achieving an AUC of 0.774 (95% confidence interval 0.622–0.926). Afterward, the authors tested their algorithm on a population of 1575 consecutive patients, observing a significant increase in risk prediction accuracy compared to traditional models.

Further work by Lin et al. [30] analyzed the radiomic signature of pCAT in relation to myocardial infarction, in a prospective cohort of 60 patients with acute myocardial infarction, 60 with stable CAD and 60 matched healthy controls without CAD who agreed to undergo a contrast-enhanced cardiac CT. For each patient, the authors extracted 1103 radiomic features, and they subsequently trained an XGBoost classifier with a tenfold cross-validation to identify patients with infarction, achieving an AUC of 0.87 (95% confidence interval 0.82–0.93).

Results from works describing AI approaches to clinical models involving EAT evaluation seem to confirm that EAT features may contribute to cardiovascular risk stratification and that the use of such tools may help better establish their clinical role. Radiomic analyses seem to yield high performances concerning the pCAT, while the overall EAT has not yet been extensively studied so far.

Conclusions

The assessment of EAT is gaining widespread popularity, as it has shown promise in cardiovascular risk stratification related not only to CAD and CAD-associated pathologies such as myocardial infarction but also to structural pathologies such as arrhythmias and to metabolic disease [31]. In this regard, AI may be particularly useful as it could help overcome the difficulties related to EAT segmentation, namely, its being a cumbersome, time-consuming task, requiring experienced readers. Moreover, AI can aid in devising prediction models which include affirmed and potential risk factors, such as EAT volume and density, to achieve higher clinical performances and help in shaping cardiovascular precision medicine.

All AI tasks related to EAT developed so far are performed on CT images. This is due to several reasons. First, EAT volume is a biomarker related to an increased prevalence of CAD and heightened cardiovascular risk, and cardiac CT is a well-established step in the workflow of patients at low risk for CAD, the population for which risk assessment is most useful [32]. Second, EAT density is calculated from CT, obtaining values measured in HU, always standardized to water, while MRI signal intensity is measured in arbitrary units, depending in magnetic field strength and on the sequence type and parameters as well as on the radiofrequency coil. Thus, applications involving the assessment of EAT density need to be based on CT images. Nevertheless, considering that variations in EAT volume may also be correlated with other pathologies involving the myocardium which are usually assessed through MRI, it could be potentially useful to have AI systems able to segment the EAT also on MRI images. More so, while MRI image intensity is not standardized, perhaps AI approach may compensate for this intrinsic limitation, still yielding clinical relevance.

References

1. Talman AH, Psaltis PJ, Cameron JD, Meredith IT, Seneviratne SK, Wong DTL. Epicardial adipose tissue: far more than a fat depot. Cardiovasc Diagn Ther. 2014;4(6):416–29.
2. Yamaguchi Y, Cavallero S, Patterson M, Shen H, Xu J, Kumar SR, et al. Adipogenesis and epicardial adipose tissue: a novel fate of the epicardium induced by mesenchymal transformation and PPARγ activation. Proc Natl Acad Sci [Internet]. 2015;112(7):2070–5. Available from: http://www.pnas.org/lookup/doi/10.1073/pnas.1417232112.
3. Aldiss P, Davies G, Woods R, Budge H, Sacks HS, Symonds ME. 'Browning' the cardiac and peri-vascular adipose tissues to modulate cardiovascular risk. Int J Cardiol [Internet]. 2017;228:265–74. Available from: https://linkinghub.elsevier.com/retrieve/pii/S0167527316335203.
4. Mulya A, Kirwan JP. Brown and Beige adipose tissue. Endocrinol Metab Clin North Am [Internet]. 2016;45(3):605–21. Available from: https://linkinghub.elsevier.com/retrieve/pii/S088985291630041X.
5. Raggi P. Epicardial adipose tissue and progression of coronary artery calcium. JACC Cardiovasc Imaging [Internet]. 2014;7(9):917–9. Available from: https://linkinghub.elsevier.com/retrieve/pii/S1936878X14005385.
6. Iozzo P. Metabolic toxicity of the heart: insights from molecular imaging. Nutr Metab Cardiovasc Dis [Internet]. 2010;20(3):147–56. Available from: https://linkinghub.elsevier.com/retrieve/pii/S0939475309002105.
7. Deng G, Long Y, Yu Y-RR, Li M-RR. Adiponectin directly improves endothelial dysfunction in obese rats through the AMPK–eNOS pathway. Int J Obes [Internet]. 2010;34(1):165–71. Available from: http://www.nature.com/articles/ijo2009205.
8. Alvey NJ, Pedley A, Rosenquist KJ, Massaro JM, O'Donnell CJ, Hoffmann U, et al. Association of fat Density with subclinical atherosclerosis. J Am Heart Assoc [Internet]. 2014;3(4). Available from: https://www.ahajournals.org/doi/10.1161/JAHA.114.000788.
9. Monti CB, Codari M, De Cecco CN, Secchi F, Sardanelli F, Stillman AE. Novel imaging biomarkers: epicardial adipose tissue evaluation. Br J Radiol [Internet]. 2019;20190770. Available from: https://www.birpublications.org/doi/10.1259/bjr.20190770.
10. Davidovich D, Gastaldelli A, Sicari R. Imaging cardiac fat. Eur Hear J Cardiovasc Imaging [Internet]. 2013;14(7):625–30. Available from: https://academic.oup.com/ehjcimaging/article-lookup/doi/10.1093/ehjci/jet045.
11. Lima-Martínez MM, Paoli M, Donis JH, Odreman R, Torres C, Iacobellis G. Punto de corte de espesor de tejido adiposo epicárdico para predecir síndrome metabólico en población venezolana. Endocrinol y Nutr [Internet]. 2013;60(10):570–6. Available from: https://linkinghub.elsevier.com/retrieve/pii/S1575092213001344.
12. Iacobellis G, Assael F, Ribaudo MC, Zappaterreno A, Alessi G, Di Mario U, et al. Epicardial fat from echocardiography: a new method for visceral adipose tissue prediction. Obes Res [Internet]. 2003;11(2):304–310. Available from: https://doi.org/10.1038/oby.2003.45.
13. Cianciulli TF, Saccheri MC, Lax JA, Papantoniou A. Prominent epicardial fat mimicking pericardial effusion on echocardiography. Eur Hear J Case Reports [Internet]. 2018;2(2). Available from: https://academic.oup.com/ehjcr/article/doi/10.1093/ehjcr/yty034/4944673.
14. La Grutta L, Toia P, Farruggia A, Albano D, Grassedonio E, Palmeri A, et al. Quantification of epicardial adipose tissue in coronary calcium score and CT coronary angiography image data sets: comparison of attenuation values, thickness and volumes. Br J Radiol. 2016;89(1062):20150773.
15. Spearman JV, Renker M, Schoepf UJ, Krazinski AW, Herbert TL, De Cecco CN, et al. Prognostic value of epicardial fat volume measurements by computed tomography: a systematic review of the literature. Eur Radiol [Internet]. 2015;25(11):3372–81. Available from: http://link.springer.com/10.1007/s00330-015-3765-5.
16. Liu Z, Wang S, Wang Y, Zhou N, Shu J, Stamm C, et al. Association of epicardial adipose tissue attenuation with coronary atherosclerosis in patients with a high risk of coronary artery disease. Atherosclerosis [Internet]. 2019;284:230–6. Available from: https://linkinghub.elsevier.com/retrieve/pii/S0021915019300577.
17. Goeller M, Achenbach S, Marwan M, Doris MK, Cadet S, Commandeur F, et al. Epicardial adipose tissue density and volume are related to subclinical atherosclerosis, inflammation and major adverse cardiac events in asymptomatic subjects. J Cardiovasc Comput Tomogr [Internet]. 2018;12(1):67–73. Available from: https://linkinghub.elsevier.com/retrieve/pii/S1934592517302460.
18. Petrini M, Alì M, Cannaò PM, Zambelli D, Cozzi A, Codari M, et al. Epicardial adipose tissue volume in patients with coronary artery disease or non-ischaemic dilated cardiomyopathy: evaluation

with cardiac magnetic resonance imaging. Clin Radiol [Internet]. 2019;74(1):81.e1–7. Available from: https://linkinghub.elsevier.com/retrieve/pii/S0009926018305415.
19. Jolly US, Soliman A, McKenzie C, Peters T, Stirrat J, Nevis I, et al. Intra-thoracic fat volume is associated with myocardial infarction in patients with metabolic syndrome. J Cardiovasc Magn Reson [Internet]. 2013;15(1):77. Available from: http://jcmr-online.biomedcentral.com/articles/10.1186/1532-429X-15-77.
20. Nezafat M, Nakamori S, Basha TA, Fahmy AS, Hauser T, Botnar RM. Imaging sequence for joint myocardial T 1 mapping and fat/water separation. Magn Reson Med [Internet]. 2019;81(1):486–94. Available from: https://doi.org/10.1002/mrm.27390.
21. Nerlekar N, Thakur U, Lin A, Koh JQS, Potter E, Liu D, et al. The natural history of Epicardial adipose tissue volume and attenuation: a long-term prospective cohort follow-up study. Sci Rep [Internet]. 2020;10(1):7109. Available from: http://www.nature.com/articles/s41598-020-63135-z.
22. Rodrigues ÉO, Pinheiro VHA, Liatsis P, Conci A. Machine learning in the prediction of cardiac epicardial and mediastinal fat volumes. Comput Biol Med [Internet]. 2017;89:520–9. Available from: https://linkinghub.elsevier.com/retrieve/pii/S0010482517300471.
23. Commandeur F, Goeller M, Betancur J, Cadet S, Doris M, Chen X, et al. Deep learning for quantification of epicardial and thoracic adipose tissue from non-contrast CT. IEEE Trans Med Imaging [Internet]. 2018;37(8):1835–46. Available from: https://ieeexplore.ieee.org/document/8288602/.
24. Commandeur F, Goeller M, Razipour A, Cadet S, Hell MM, Kwiecinski J, et al. Fully automated CT quantification of epicardial adipose tissue by deep learning: a multicenter study. Radiol Artif Intell [Internet]. 2019;1(6):e190045. Available from: https://doi.org/10.1148/ryai.2019190045.
25. He X, Guo BJ, Lei Y, Wang T, Fu Y, Curran WJ, et al. Automatic segmentation and quantification of epicardial adipose tissue from coronary computed tomography angiography. Phys Med Biol [Internet]. 2020;65(9):095012. Available from: https://iopscience.iop.org/article/10.1088/1361-6560/ab8077.
26. Otaki Y, Hell M, Slomka PJ, Schuhbaeck A, Gransar H, Huber B, et al. Relationship of epicardial fat volume from noncontrast CT with impaired myocardial flow reserve by positron emission tomography. J Cardiovasc Comput Tomogr [Internet]. 2015;9(4):303–9. Available from: https://linkinghub.elsevier.com/retrieve/pii/S1934592515000957.
27. Commandeur F, Slomka PJ, Goeller M, Chen X, Cadet S, Razipour A, et al. Machine learning to predict the long-term risk of myocardial infarction and cardiac death based on clinical risk, coronary calcium, and epicardial adipose tissue: a prospective study. Cardiovasc Res [Internet]. 2019. Available from: https://academic.oup.com/cardiovascres/advance-article/doi/10.1093/cvr/cvz321/5680420.
28. Hell MM, Ding X, Rubeaux M, Slomka P, Gransar H, Terzopoulos D, et al. Epicardial adipose tissue volume but not density is an independent predictor for myocardial ischemia. J Cardiovasc Comput Tomogr [Internet]. 2016;10(2):141–9. Available from: https://linkinghub.elsevier.com/retrieve/pii/S1934592516300089.
29. Oikonomou EK, Williams MC, Kotanidis CP, Desai MY, Marwan M, Antonopoulos AS, et al. A novel machine learning-derived radiotranscriptomic signature of perivascular fat improves cardiac risk prediction using coronary CT angiography. Eur Heart J [Internet]. 2019;40(43):3529–43. Available from: https://academic.oup.com/eurheartj/article/40/43/3529/5554432.
30. Lin A, Kolossváry M, Yuvaraj J, Cadet S, McElhinney PA, Jiang C, et al. Myocardial infarction associates with a distinct pericoronary adipose tissue radiomic phenotype. JACC Cardiovasc Imaging [Internet]. 2020;13(11):2371–83. Available from: https://linkinghub.elsevier.com/retrieve/pii/S1936878X2030615X.
31. Le Jemtel TH, Samson R, Ayinapudi K, Singh T, Oparil S. Epicardial adipose tissue and cardiovascular disease. Curr Hypertens Rep. 2019;278:254–60.
32. Schoepf UJ, Becker CR, Ohnesorge BM, Yucel EK. CT of coronary artery disease. Radiology. 2004;232(1):18–37.

Radiomics in Cardiac CT

31

Márton Kolossváry and Pál Maurovich-Horvat

Background

Imaging hardware has undergone remarkable advances in the past decades, which has allowed to access previously unavailable functional (i.e., dynamic perfusion CT) and anatomical data (i.e., compositional assessment of coronary plaque) based on radiological images [1]. These technological developments have increased the use of imaging for clinical diagnostic purpose especially in the past decade [2]. Both the increase in the number of radiological examinations and the available information from these studies have initiated an artificial intelligence (AI) revolution and a change in radiological image interpretation [3].

The key component of all AI applications is the machine learning (ML) algorithms behind them. In brief, ML is grouping term for statistical models which increase their performance in a given task (evaluated by some performance metric) proportional to the amount of experience they possess, without being explicitly programed for the given job (for more details, please see Chap. 6: Machine Learning and Biostatistics) [4].

A key question in ML-based medical image analysis is as follows: what should the input features be to the model? Two main methodologies have developed over the years. One is to use the pixel or voxel intensity values as inputs. This requires a special form of ML, so-called deep learning (DL), which uses neural networks to analyze the images [5, 6]. Each pixel or voxel is fed into a set of perceptrons, the smallest unit of the neural network [7]. These perceptrons are very similar to linear regression equations, where the optimally weighted sum of the inputs is estimated. However, instead of a linear function, the perceptron calculates a nonlinear function of its input values, which allows to model complex nonlinear relationships [8]. These perceptrons can be stacked into multiple layers, hence the term "deep" learning. Here the output of one perceptron serves as the input to another one, mimicking the structure of real-life neuronal networks [9]. DL allows the identification of complex spatial patterns within images, which can be used for classification and regression tasks (for details please refer to Chap. 8: Artificial Intelligence Algorithm Developments for Imaging Purposes).

Radiomics, on the other hand, derives quantitative features from the voxel values prior to statistical modeling [10]. It is based on fundamental work done in texture analysis in the 1970s when researchers were faced with the problem of differentiating urban territories from uninhabited ones on aerial photography [11, 12]. Researchers defined mathematical formulas to quantify spatial heterogeneity using the pixel values of the images. Radiomics builds on these fundamentals and applies these formulas to quantify textural properties of the lesions. Instead of simple volumetric analysis, where all spatial information is discarded, radiomic features use the relative spatial position of the voxels to each other to enumerate lesion morphology. Several hundred different parameters can be calculated, which results in a big data database, where each abnormality is represented by numerous quantitative radiological imaging markers. This in turn can be used to precisely phenotype diseases based on noninvasive radiological imaging. In this chapter, we wish to present the fundamentals of radiomics and its current applications to cardiovascular CT imaging.

Fundamentals of Radiomics

Fundamentally, all objects can be described using three properties: intensity (amount and wavelength of the absorbed or emitted light), texture (spatial pattern of the intensity values), and shape (spatial form of the object). In CT, our intensity values represent the amount of absorbed radiation of a

M. Kolossváry, MD, PhD (✉)
Cardiovascular Imaging Research Center, Massachusetts General Hospital, Boston, MA, USA

P. Maurovich-Horvat, MD, PhD, MPH
MTA-SE Cardiovascular Imaging Research Group, Heart and Vascular Center, Semmelweis University, Budapest, Hungary

C. N. De Cecco et al. (eds.), *Artificial Intelligence in Cardiothoracic Imaging*, Contemporary Medical Imaging,
https://doi.org/10.1007/978-3-030-92087-6_31

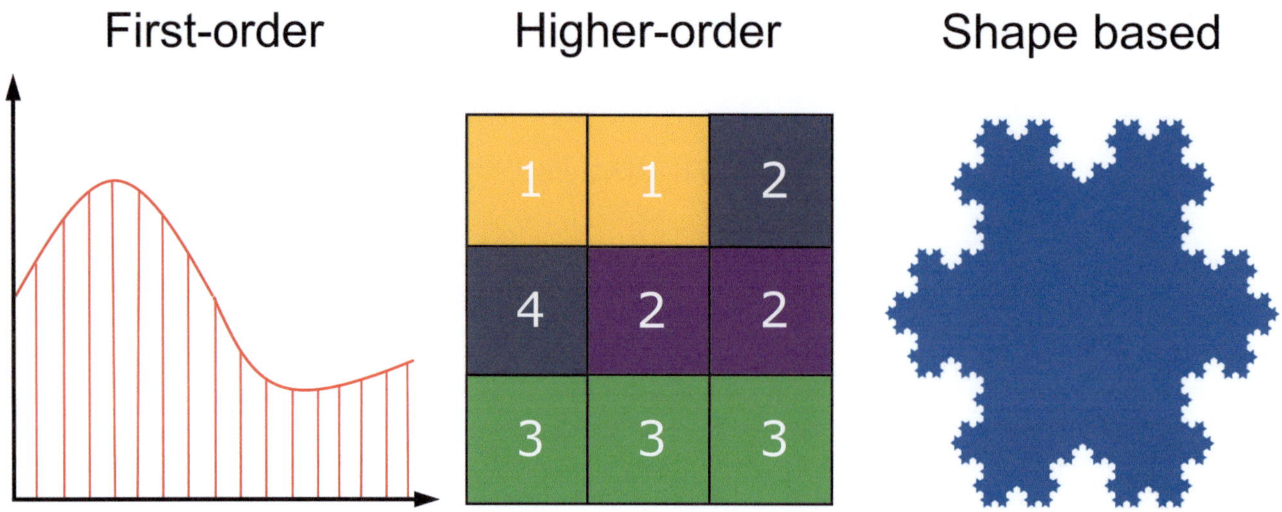

Fig. 31.1 Pictograms of classes of radiomic parameters. First-order parameters calculate statistics based on the intensity distribution of the voxel values and discard all spatial information. Higher-order metrics calculate statistics based on the spatial co-occurrence of specific voxel values. Shape-based statistics quantify the spatial complexity and self-symmetry of the lesion. (Modified based on Kolossváry et al. [6])

given spatial unit, the voxel. The differences in voxel values in close proximity to each other create patterns which are used to differentiate textures on an image which represent different underlying tissues. These voxel groups also outline the shape of the lesion. Radiomics uses mathematical formulas to enumerate these core properties of region or volume of interest [13]. Radiomic features can be grouped into three classes representing these core concepts: first-order features (or intensity-based metrics), higher-order features (or texture-based parameters), and shape-based metrics (Fig. 31.1) [6, 10].

First-order metrics discard all spatial information and only describe the intensity distribution of the voxels. This methodology has also been referred to as histogram analysis, where we describe properties of the intensity histogram, which is basically a mathematical representation of the amount (how many voxels) and wavelength (intensity of the voxels) of the voxel values. Several quantitative parameters can be derived from the histogram, some of which are often used in daily clinical practice, such as the minimum or maximum intensity of the lesion.

Higher-order features quantify the texture of the given area or volume. Instead of observing the individual voxel values, these algorithms quantify how often specific value voxel pairs occur in close proximity to each other. This information is then stored in matrices, from which several different parameters can be extracted. Different methods have evolved to derive these matrices of which the gray-level co-occurrence matrix (GLCM) and gray-level run-length matrix (GLRLM) are the most well-known [11, 12]. The GLCM has as many rows and columns as there are different intensity values in the given region or volume of interest. Each element describes how many times a voxel with intensity value corresponding to the row number co-occurs next to a voxel intensity corresponding to the column number. In case of the GLRLM matrix, the elements of the matrix describe how many times voxel intensities corresponding to the row number are situated next to each other n-times, where n corresponds to the column number.

Shaped-based features describe the spatial form of a given lesion. Volumetric quantification of abnormalities can be considered as a simple form of shape-based feature extraction which has made its way to clinical utility. However, radiomics-based shape parameters provide additional information on the spatial form of the lesion by deriving parameters from the volume and the surface area of the lesion to enumerate, for example, how close the abnormality resembles a sphere. Also, another group of shape-based features uses fractal equations to describe the self-symmetry of the lesion.

These radiomic features can be derived from 2D and 3D medical images using open-source software tools (such as pyradiomics in python or radiomic image analysis [RIA] in R). After feature extraction, the conventional tools of ML can be used to analyze and model the data. For more detailed description of radiomic methodologies, please refer to Chap. 9: Radiomics: Technical Background. In the next section, we wish to present the current applications of radiomics to cardiovascular CT.

Radiomics in Cardiac CT

Several applications of radiomics in cardiac CT have been published in the past years. We wish to present the readers with an overview of topics where radiomics seems to have additive value compared to conventional qualitative and quantitative analyses.

Applications to Quantitatively Identify and Classify Pathologies

One of the core tasks of evaluating radiological images is the identification and classification of lesions into their respective categories. Through the decades, numerous different radiological signs have been described, each a specific marker of a respective pathological processes. However, these signs mostly rely on visual inspection and are dependent on reader experience. Even for such established and commonly used markers, such as the semiquantitative degree of luminal stenosis on coronary CT angiography, there seems to be a considerable variability in reader agreement [14]. Similar discrepancies were also seen when expert readers' opinions were compared regarding the presence of high-risk plaque features [15]. These results show the need for a quantitative approach to identify and classify pathologies in a reproducible manner.

Most radiological signs rely on a specific spatial pattern of the voxels. However, conventional quantitative approaches discard all spatial information and therefore can only achieve limited accuracies to identify these markers. On the other hand, radiomics, through mathematical analysis of texture, has the potential to provide an objective and reproducible method to identify qualitative imaging markers, which can only be identified visually currently.

One of the first applications of radiomics in the cardiovascular domain used these features to quantitatively identify plaque showing the napkin-ring sign [16]. Researchers calculated 4440 radiomic features on 30 plaques with and 30 plaques without the napkin-ring sign, which were matched for degree of calcification, luminal obstruction, localization, and imaging parameters. Since the large number of comparisons between the two groups greatly inflates the false positive rate, Bonferroni corrected p values were used. Overall, 20.6% (916/4440) of the radiomic features while none of the conventional qualitative and quantitative parameters were significantly different between the two types of plaques. Furthermore, the best radiomic features achieved significantly higher cross-validated area under the curve (AUC) values as compared to the conventional markers. Also, the researchers applied cluster analysis to the radiomic features and identified 44 unique clusters in the data potentially implying 44 unique structural components of plaque composition. These results show that radiomics may be able to quantitatively identify high-risk plaque characteristics in an objective manner and that radiomics may be able to extract new plaque phenotypes that remain invisible to the human eye. Similar results were found when researchers used the radiomic features as inputs to a ML model to identify advanced atherosclerotic lesions based on ex vivo imaging [16]. The radiomics-based ML model significantly outperformed the gold standard plaque attenuation pattern classification scheme (AUC = 0.73 vs.0.65, $p = 0.04$) on a validation set consisting of 112 coronary plaque cross sections.

Similar methodologies have been used to identify infarcted myocardium on cardiac CT [17]. Comparing 20 patients with proven acute myocardial infarction with 20 healthy controls with no cardiac abnormalities, they found a significant difference in 2/4 histogram features, 3/4 GLCM features, and 6/11 GLRLM features. A radiomics-based multivariate logistic model was able to achieve an AUC of 0.90 to differentiate patients with or without prior myocardial infarction. These results potentially imply that specific pathologies may be identified using objective numerical methods, as opposed to subjective reader assessment.

Radiomics has also been used to differentiate between the etiologies causing mechanical prosthetic valve obstruction. While possible causes (thrombus, pannus, and vegetation) behind this life-threatening condition do not have specific appearances on CT, they require very different therapeutic solutions. Overall, 52 radiomic features were extracted from the segmentations of 39 periprosthetic masses. Several significant radiomic features were found between pannus and non-pannus lesions. Using a least absolute shrinkage and selection operator logistic regression, a radiomic score was derived. Bootstrapped AUC values showed that a combination of the radiomic score and visual analysis outperformed visual analysis alone to differentiate pannus from other etiologies of mechanical prosthetic valve obstruction. These findings may imply that radiomics may be used as a link between radiology and histology [18].

Radiomics can also help to differentiate between patients presenting with myocardial infarction and patients having stable coronary artery disease [19]. Researchers found that 20.3% of the 1103 radiomic features calculated on pericoronary fat tissue were significant (corrected p value <0.0006) between 60 patients presenting with myocardial infarction and age-sex matched controls. Integrating radiomic features with the best discriminatory power into a ML model resulted in significant improvement (AUC = 0.87) to models containing only pericoronary fat attenuation and clinical factors (AUC: 0.77; $p = 0.001$) or clinical factors alone (AUC: 0.76; $p < 0.001$). Importantly, 6 months after infarction, there was no significant change in the pericoronary fat radiomic profile around the proximal RCA or non-culprit lesions. These results show that radiomic analysis may hold important information above and beyond current clinical and simple quantitative measurements.

Applications to Expand the Capabilities of Imaging Modalities

Previous examples used radiomics to objectively identify pathologies which are currently diagnosed using visual assessment or to increase the diagnostic accuracy of current imaging solutions. However, previous articles found that there seems to be more information in the images that is comprehensible visually. Each imaging modality uses different physical properties to depict the abnormality, while, fundamentally, they are imaging the same thing. Therefore, it may be reasonable to assume that radiomics, which increases the amount of information available to analyze from images, might allow to expand the diagnostic capabilities of current imaging solutions to identify abnormalities currently not possible using a given modality.

Researchers analyzed 44 lesions of 25 individuals who underwent coronary CT angiography, sodium fluoride positron emission tomography (NaF-PET), prior to invasive angiography, where intravascular ultrasound and optical coherence tomography were used [20]. Overall, 935 different radiomic parameters were calculated on the CT images and used to identify high-risk plaque morphologies on the other imaging modalities. Using stratified fivefold cross-validation with 1000 repeats, the results showed that the best radiomic parameter had significantly better discriminatory power (AUC, 0.72 vs. 0.59, $p < 0.001$) to identify attenuated plaques on intravascular ultrasound as compared to the best conventional parameter: noncalcified plaque volume. Similar results were found in case of optical coherence tomography where radiomics outperformed conventional parameters to identify thin-cap fibroatheromas (AUC, 0.80 vs. 0.66, $p < 0.001$). These results indicate that radiomics may have better discriminatory power to identify other imaging modalities' anatomical vulnerability parameters. Interestingly though, radiomics seemed also to outperform conventional parameters to identify plaques showing activity on NaF-PET. The best radiomic parameter achieved good diagnostic accuracy to discriminate between plaques showing NaF-PET positivity, while conventional parameters only had moderate accuracy (AUC, 0.87 vs. 0.65, $p < 0.001$). It seems that radiomics not only provides better discriminatory power to identify anatomical vulnerability, but it seems that it can also extract fine textural information which may be indicative of metabolic vulnerability, therefore allowing identification of PET activity using conventional CT images (Fig. 31.2).

Researchers have also utilized radiomics to identify myocardial infarction from noncontrast low radiation dose examinations [21]. In a retrospective case-control setting of 27 patients with acute myocardial infarction, 30 with chronic myocardial infarction, and 30 controls, 308 radiomic features were extracted from freehand regions of interest of the myocardium and the blood pool. These features were then feed into six different ML models. The results show that the radiomics-based ML models achieved good diagnostic accuracy to differentiate between myocardial infarction patients and healthy controls (AUC = 0.78). However, subjective visual differentiation of controls as well as acute and chronic MI cases on noncontrast CT images was not possible. These results imply that texture analysis is able to identify pathologies from noncontrast low-dose CT images, which is not possible using visual inspection. Therefore, the diagnostic capabilities of imaging modalities might be broader than we currently think.

Applications for Better Cardiovascular Risk Prediction

Previous applications used radiomics to objectively identify diseases potentially even from imaging modalities which previously were not possible. However, the question arises that beyond providing a more accurate disease classification method, does the extracted information have additive value in predicting patient outcomes?

Coronary calcium score is a safe and effective method for screening asymptomatic individuals to predict later cardiovascular outcomes [22]. The Agatston score provides a quantitative methodology to summarize the coronary atherosclerotic disease burden [23]. However, the score only incorporates volumetric information and the density of the lesions and does not incorporate textural or shape-based information. Therefore, researchers extracted 2120 quantitative radiomic features from 318 individuals on whom a radiomic score was developed [24]. This radiomic score was tested on 306 individuals as a validation cohort. Incorporating the radiomic score into a model also including the Agatston score, the discriminatory power was better than Agatston score alone with borderline significance (AUC, 0.79 vs. 0.73; $p = 0.05$) to predict a composite endpoint of clinical events during a median follow-up of 9.1 years. Researchers have also used radiomics on pericoronary fat tissue to extract novel imaging features to increase prognostication in patients undergoing coronary CT angiography [25]. A fat radiomic profile was developed using 1391 coronary perivascular fat radiomic features in 101 patients who experienced major adverse cardiac events within 5 years of having a coronary CT and 101 matched controls without any events. This model was then tested on 1575 consecutive patients to predict adverse outcomes. Individuals with increased radiomic profile score had a 10.8-fold higher risk of adverse outcomes, after adjustment for age, sex, systolic blood pressure, total cholesterol, high-density lipoproteins, diabetes mellitus, smoking, body mass index, obstructive coronary disease, CT scanner type, the presence of high-risk plaque features, and calcium score. Importantly, the fat radiomic profile did not correlate with the presence of high-risk plaque features (Rho = 0.004, $p = 0.87$). These results indicate that radiomics not only provides a better means of disease classification, but it may help outcome prognostication above and beyond currently used methods.

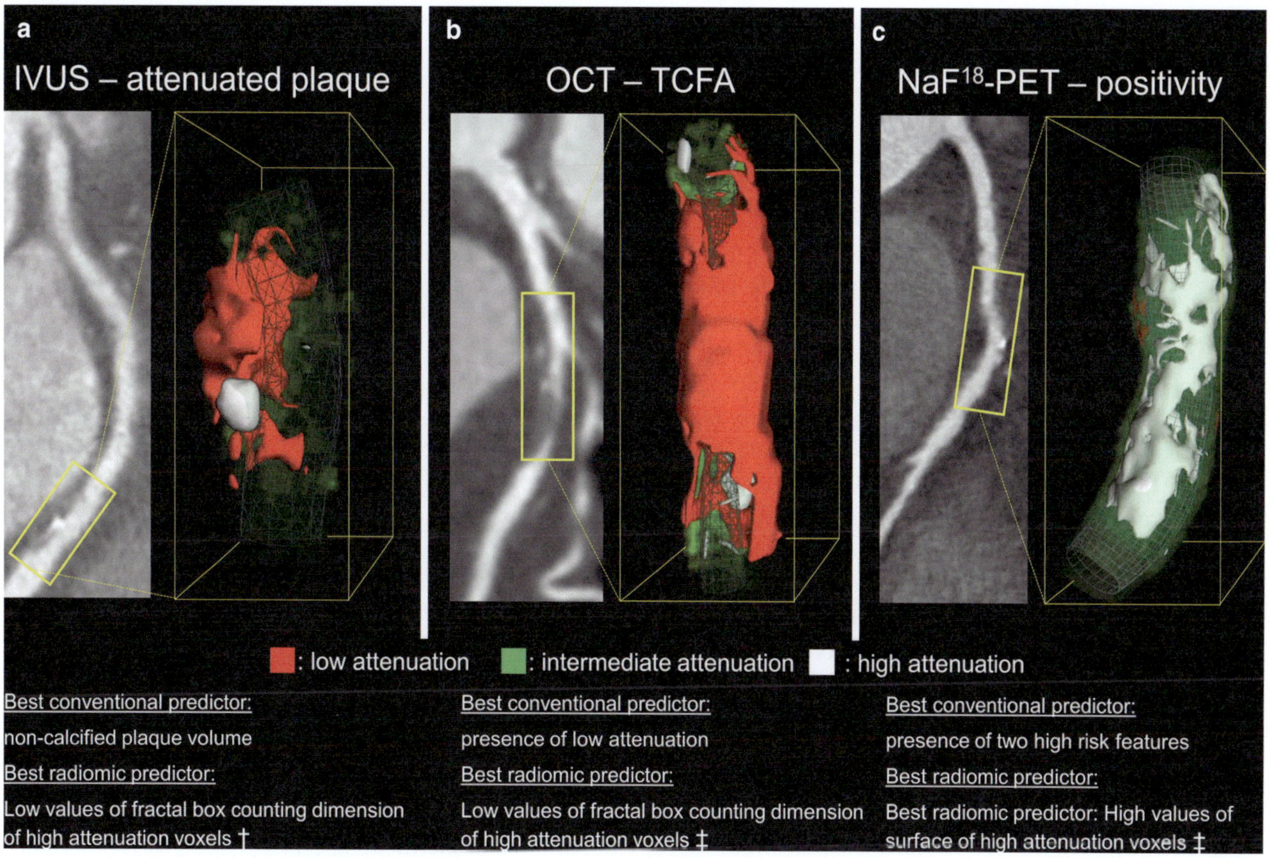

Fig. 31.2 Representative curved multiplanar and volume rendered CT images of three coronary plaques corresponding to specific invasive and radionuclide imaging markers of plaque vulnerability. (**a**) A coronary lesion which scored the lowest on fractal box counting dimension of high attenuation voxels (component 30 when discretizing to 32 equally sized bins) which was indicative of attenuated plaque on IVUS [AUC, 0.72 (0.65–0.78)]. (**b**) Depicts a coronary plaque which scored the lowest on fractal box counting dimension of high attenuation voxels (component 8 when discretizing to eight equally sized bins) which was suggestive of OCT-TCFA [AUC, 0.80 (0.72–0.88)]. (**c**) A coronary lesion which had a high surface of high attenuation voxels (component 8 when discretizing to eight equally sized bins) which was the best parameter to identify NaF-PET positivity [AUC, 0.87 (0.82–0.91)]. AUC, area under the curve; IVUS, intravascular ultrasound; NaF-PET, NaF-positron emission tomography; OCT-TCFA, optical coherence tomography identified thin-cap fibroatheroma. [a]: Component 30 when discretizing to 32 equally sized bins. [b]: Component 8 when discretizing to eight equally sized bins. (Replicated from Kolossváry et al. [20])

Using Radiomics to Precision Phentyping Diseases

Previous radiomic analyses focused on using these technologies to accomplish tasks that humans are also capable of but doing it more efficiently and accurately. Instead of trying to find imaging markers to identify, classify, and prognosticate diseases, *radiogenomics* links radiological images to the most precise information available on diseases, their genetic basis [26, 27]. Genetic phenotyping of tumors is essential for contemporary cancer therapy. The possibility of decoding disease phenotypes from radiological images and linking them to genetic alterations has the potential to revolutionize the diagnostic pathways of not only oncology but also cardiology [28]. Also, these technologies may facilitate connecting the results from the "bench to the bedside," potentially allowing the identification of molecular alterations and pathways based on in vivo radiological imaging [29–31].

Such analyses are scarce in the field of cardiovascular imaging though. However, there are promising results that inflammatory processes can be derived from the attenuation values of perivascular fat [32, 33]. Furthermore, radiomic analysis of the peri-coronary artery tissues has been linked to gene expressions of inflammation (TNFA expression), fibrosis (COL1A1 expression), and vascularity changes (CD31 expression), potentially raising the possibility of differentiating vascular pathology based on radiological images [25]. Researchers have also found that different risk factors have unique contributions to the progression of coronary artery disease [34]. They found that there was no overlap among parameters associated with elevated cardiovascular or cocaine use and HIV infection. The fact that different exposures on coronary atherosclerosis may be distinguishable from each other implies that, rather than having a complex interconnected network of risk factors contributing to the development of atherosclerosis, the effects of individual risk factors may correspond to specific known or unknown pathways of disease progression. Further research is needed to prove that specific pathological processes result in unique radiomic profiles.

Current Limitations of Radiomic Analyses

Despite the promising results, there are major concerns regarding the robustness and generalizability of radiomic techniques in routine clinical practice. Currently we only have small sample size studies which need rigorous validation in the future. Also, differences in image acquisition and quality have been shown to greatly affect model performance [35, 36]. However, there are also results that radiomics may be robust to different scanner settings due to the rigorous downscaling of information done prior to analysis [37, 38]. These limitations may be overcome by increasing the size and variability of the datasets on which the inferences are made and the algorithms are trained. Furthermore, radiological societies have published recommendations on standardization procedures in AI research that may help the generalizability and application of radiomic models in different settings [39, 40]. However, these limitations can only be addressed by conducting randomized controlled clinical trials, assessing the usefulness of radiomics in real-life clinical settings. Furthermore, there still exists the question of legal liability associated with the use of AI for image interpretation. While these algorithms may achieve results on par with clinical experts, there are still a considerable number of misdiagnoses, in which case there is no clear agreement regarding who is responsible in these cases [41].

Conclusions

AI applications such as radiomics have the potential to transform the field of cardiovascular imaging. By providing numerical means of identifying and classifying diseases, they have the potential to improve the quality of healthcare and provide more precise diagnoses and prognoses. While these changes may take place in the next few years as hardware and software technologies are incorporated into commercial solutions, an even more promising application is the use of these techniques for precision phenotyping of diseases. Radiomics has the potential to revolutionize clinical workflows by proving unprecedented detail from radiological images. This new, previously unavailable information may help to further refine our disease taxonomies and provide personalized medical solutions for the masses. However, much work needs to be done regarding the generalizability of these promising results. These methodologies still need to prove their clinical utility as per guidelines of federal regulatory agencies. Nevertheless, if these technologies survive the rigorous assessment and validation ahead of them, they have the potential to transform not only radiology but also the diagnostic and treatment protocols of medicine as we know them today.

References

1. Alexander A, McGill M, Tarasova A, Ferreira C, Zurkiya D. Scanning the future of medical imaging. J Am Coll Radiol. 2019;16:501–7. https://doi.org/10.1016/j.jacr.2018.09.050.
2. Hong AS, et al. Trends in diagnostic imaging utilization among medicare and commercially insured adults from 2003 through 2016. Radiology. 2020;294:342–50. https://doi.org/10.1148/radiol.2019191116.
3. Pesapane F, Codari M, Sardanelli F. Artificial intelligence in medical imaging: threat or opportunity? Radiologists again at the forefront of innovation in medicine. Eur Radiol Exp. 2018;2:35. https://doi.org/10.1186/s41747-018-0061-6.
4. Mitchell TM. Machine learning. McGraw Hill; 1997.
5. Géron A. Hands-on machine learning with scikit-learn, keras, and tensorflow: concepts, tools, and techniques to build intelligent systems. O'Reilly Media, Incorporated; 2019.
6. Kolossvary M, De Cecco CN, Feuchtner G, Maurovich-Horvat P. Advanced atherosclerosis imaging by CT: radiomics, machine learning and deep learning. J Cardiovasc Comput Tomogr. 2019;13:274–80. https://doi.org/10.1016/j.jcct.2019.04.007.
7. McCulloch WS, Pitts W. A logical calculus of the ideas immanent in nervous activity. Bull Math Biophys. 1943;5:115–33. https://doi.org/10.1007/BF02478259.
8. Montavon G, Orr G, Müller KR. Neural networks: tricks of the trade. Berlin Heidelberg: Springer; 2012.
9. Fukushima K. Neocognitron: a self-organizing neural network model for a mechanism of pattern recognition unaffected by shift in position. Biol Cybern. 1980;36:193–202. https://doi.org/10.1007/BF00344251.
10. Kolossvary M, Kellermayer M, Merkely B, Maurovich-Horvat P. Cardiac computed tomography radiomics: a comprehensive review on radiomic techniques. J Thorac Imaging. 2018;33:26–34. https://doi.org/10.1097/RTI.0000000000000268.
11. Haralick RM, Shanmugam K, Dinstein IH. Textural features for image classification. IEEE Transactions on Systems, Man, and Cybernetics SMC-3. 1973:610–21. https://doi.org/10.1109/tsmc.1973.4309314.
12. Galloway MM. Texture analysis using gray level run lengths. Comput Graphics Image Proces. 1975;4:172–9. https://doi.org/10.1016/s0146-664x(75)80008-6.
13. Gillies RJ, Kinahan PE, Hricak H. Radiomics: images are more than pictures, they are data. Radiology. 2016;278:563–77. https://doi.org/10.1148/radiol.2015151169.
14. Lu MT, et al. Central core laboratory versus site interpretation of coronary CT angiography: agreement and association with cardiovascular events in the PROMISE trial. Radiology. 2018;287:87–95. https://doi.org/10.1148/radiol.2017172181.
15. Maroules CD, et al. Coronary artery disease reporting and data system (CAD-RADS(TM)): inter-observer agreement for assessment categories and modifiers. J Cardiovasc Comput Tomogr. 2018;12:125–30. https://doi.org/10.1016/j.jcct.2017.11.014.
16. Kolossvary M, et al. Radiomics versus visual and histogram-based assessment to identify atheromatous lesions at coronary CT angiography: an ex vivo study. Radiology. 2019;293:89–96. https://doi.org/10.1148/radiol.2019190407.

17. Hinzpeter R, et al. Texture analysis of acute myocardial infarction with CT: first experience study. PLoS One. 2017;12:e0186876. https://doi.org/10.1371/journal.pone.0186876.
18. Kolossvary M, Maurovich-Horvat P. Radiomics: the link between radiology and histology? Circ Cardiovasc Imaging. 2019;12:e009990. https://doi.org/10.1161/CIRCIMAGING.119.009990.
19. Lin A, et al. Myocardial infarction associates with a distinct pericoronary adipose tissue radiomic phenotype: a prospective case-control study. JACC Cardiovasc Imaging. 2020;13:2371–83. https://doi.org/10.1016/j.jcmg.2020.06.033.
20. Kolossvary M, et al. Identification of invasive and radionuclide imaging markers of coronary plaque vulnerability using radiomic analysis of coronary computed tomography angiography. Eur Heart J Cardiovasc Imaging. 2019;20:1250–8. https://doi.org/10.1093/ehjci/jez033.
21. Mannil M, von Spiczak J, Manka R, Alkadhi H. Texture analysis and machine learning for detecting myocardial infarction in noncontrast low-dose computed tomography: unveiling the invisible. Invest Radiol. 2018;53:338–43. https://doi.org/10.1097/RLI.0000000000000448.
22. Mitchell JD, Paisley R, Moon P, Novak E, Villines TC. Coronary artery calcium and long-term risk of death, myocardial infarction, and stroke: the Walter reed cohort study. JACC Cardiovasc Imaging. 2018;11:1799–806. https://doi.org/10.1016/j.jcmg.2017.09.003.
23. Agatston AS, et al. Quantification of coronary artery calcium using ultrafast computed tomography. J Am Coll Cardiol. 1990;15:827–32. https://doi.org/10.1016/0735-1097(90)90282-t.
24. Eslami P, et al. Radiomics of coronary artery calcium in the Framingham heart study. Radiol Cardiothorac Imaging. 2020;2:e190119. https://doi.org/10.1148/ryct.2020190119.
25. Oikonomou EK, et al. A novel machine learning-derived radiotranscriptomic signature of perivascular fat improves cardiac risk prediction using coronary CT angiography. Eur Heart J. 2019;40:3529–43. https://doi.org/10.1093/eurheartj/ehz592.
26. Mazurowski MA. Radiogenomics: what it is and why it is important. J Am Coll Radiol. 2015;12:862–6. https://doi.org/10.1016/j.jacr.2015.04.019.
27. Lo Gullo R, Daimiel I, Morris EA, Pinker K. Combining molecular and imaging metrics in cancer: radiogenomics. Insights Imaging. 2020;11:1. https://doi.org/10.1186/s13244-019-0795-6.
28. Aerts HJ, et al. Decoding tumour phenotype by noninvasive imaging using a quantitative radiomics approach. Nat Commun. 2014;5:4006. https://doi.org/10.1038/ncomms5006.
29. Park JE, et al. Prediction of core signaling pathway by using diffusion- and perfusion-based MRI radiomics and next-generation sequencing in isocitrate dehydrogenase wild-type glioblastoma. Radiology. 2020;294:388–97. https://doi.org/10.1148/radiol.2019190913.
30. Bismeijer T, et al. Radiogenomic analysis of breast cancer by linking MRI phenotypes with tumor gene expression. Radiology. 2020;296:277–87. https://doi.org/10.1148/radiol.2020191453.
31. Cho N. Breast cancer radiogenomics: association of enhancement pattern at DCE MRI with deregulation of mTOR pathway. Radiology. 2020;296:288–9. https://doi.org/10.1148/radiol.2020201607.
32. Antonopoulos AS, et al. Detecting human coronary inflammation by imaging perivascular fat. Sci Transl Med. 2017;9. https://doi.org/10.1126/scitranslmed.aal2658.
33. Antoniades C, Antonopoulos AS, Deanfield J. Imaging residual inflammatory cardiovascular risk. Eur Heart J. 2020;41:748–58. https://doi.org/10.1093/eurheartj/ehz474.
34. Kolossváry M, et al. Contribution of risk factors to the development of coronary atherosclerosis as confirmed via coronary CT angiography – a longitudinal radiomics-based study. Radiology in press. 2021. https://doi.org/10.1148/radiol.2020203179.
35. Meyer M, et al. Reproducibility of CT radiomic features within the same patient: influence of radiation dose and CT reconstruction settings. Radiology. 2019;293:583–91. https://doi.org/10.1148/radiol.2019190928.
36. Berenguer R, et al. Radiomics of CT features may be nonreproducible and redundant: influence of CT acquisition parameters. Radiology. 2018;288:407–15. https://doi.org/10.1148/radiol.2018172361.
37. Kolossvary M, et al. Effect of image reconstruction algorithms on volumetric and radiomic parameters of coronary plaques. J Cardiovasc Comput Tomogr. 2019;13:325–30. https://doi.org/10.1016/j.jcct.2018.11.004.
38. Kolossvary M, et al. Effect of vessel wall segmentation on volumetric and radiomic parameters of coronary plaques with adverse characteristics. J Cardiovasc Comput Tomogr. 2020. https://doi.org/10.1016/j.jcct.2020.08.001.
39. Langlotz CP, et al. A roadmap for foundational research on artificial intelligence in medical imaging: from the 2018 NIH/RSNA/ACR/the academy workshop. Radiology. 2019;291:781–91. https://doi.org/10.1148/radiol.2019190613.
40. Zwanenburg A, et al. The image biomarker standardization initiative: standardized quantitative radiomics for high-throughput image-based phenotyping. Radiology. 2020;295:328–38. https://doi.org/10.1148/radiol.2020191145.
41. Liu X, et al. A comparison of deep learning performance against health-care professionals in detecting diseases from medical imaging: a systematic review and meta-analysis. Lancet Digit Health. 2019;1:e271–97. https://doi.org/10.1016/S2589-7500(19)30123-2.

Cardiac MR Guidelines and Clinical Applications: Where Does Artificial Intelligence Fit In?

32

Davide Vignale, Anna Palmisano, and Antonio Esposito

Introduction

Noninvasive cardiovascular imaging with cardiac magnetic resonance (CMR) has become a fundamental tool for the management of patients affected by many cardiovascular conditions, also thanks to the continuous technological advances of recent years. CMR, with its multiparametric capabilities, offers a comprehensive evaluation of cardiac diseases and has an increasingly recognized role in the diagnosis, risk stratification, treatment monitoring, follow-up, and pre-procedural planning, in different clinical settings. This is reflected by the inclusion of CMR in many clinical practice guidelines (CPGs) provided by the most influential European and American cardiological and radiological societies [1–4].

As of 2020, CMR is represented in around 60% of American College of Cardiology/American Heart Association (ACC/AHA) and European Society of Cardiology (ESC) CPGs. Most recommendations (more than 60%) are in class I and IIa, further supporting the high clinical value that CMR can provide for the management of diverse diseases. Interestingly, only a tiny percentage (around 1%) of the recommendations has a level of evidence A, while the majority (more than 50%) is supported by expert opinion (level of evidence C), reflecting the need for large randomized controlled trials (RCTs) to strengthen the current evidence [2] and, for some application, displaying the lack of scanning and post-processing standardization.

The majority of CMR recommendations addresses the diagnostic work-up of patients, followed by risk stratification purposes, and follow-up of patients mainly affected by heart failure or chronic coronary syndromes. No current CPG recommends CMR for disease or treatment monitoring, albeit an increasing body of data shows that CMR is moving from delivering diagnosis and establishing prognosis to guiding patient follow-up and management.

D. Vignale, MD · A. Palmisano, MD, PhD · A. Esposito, MD (✉)
Experimental Imaging Center, IRCCS San Raffaele Scientific Institute, Milan, Italy

School of Medicine, Vita-Salute San Raffaele University, Milan, Italy
e-mail: vignale.davide@hsr.it; palmisano.anna@hsr.it; esposito.antonio@hsr.it

Factors Limiting Broader Application of CMR

Despite the many well-established roles of CMR in multiple clinical settings and the continuous development of new techniques, which are broadening its application, some drawbacks must be noted.

First, the long acquisition time of both the whole CMR examination and of each individual sequence may be intolerable for some patients (e.g., patients suffering from claustrophobia or patients with reduced breath holding capability). This brings to increased incidence of image artifacts and prevents CMR use in the acute setting (for safety concerns or for inability of the patient to collaborate).

Another issue is the time-consuming post-processing that is required for a comprehensive quantitative evaluation of myocardial diseases with CMR. This problem is particularly relevant for more advanced CMR techniques, such as feature tracking, quantitative myocardial perfusion, or 4D flow. In fact, these methods may require lengthy and tedious segmentation, which is limiting their widespread availability in a real-world clinical setting.

Furthermore, despite the major effort to develop standardized protocols for image acquisition, post-processing, and interpretation [5], variability due to different scanner manufacturers, magnetic field strength, and sequence geometry (e.g., the difference in T1 mapping values between 1.5 T and 3 T scanners) still limits the reproducibility of CMR among different centers. Moreover, image quality may depend also on patients' characteristics (e.g., high prevalence of artifacts in arrhythmic patients). Another important source of variability derives from the multiple manual or semiautomatic

C. N. De Cecco et al. (eds.), *Artificial Intelligence in Cardiothoracic Imaging*, Contemporary Medical Imaging,
https://doi.org/10.1007/978-3-030-92087-6_32

segmentations performed for most of the CMR applications, from the segmentation of cine steady-state free precession (SSFP) images for volume and function quantification to advanced analysis of stress CMR perfusion sequences. Artificial intelligence (AI) may offer solutions for most of these limitations.

Artificial Intelligence for Image Acquisition and Reconstruction

The first issue in CMR acquisition is the long examination time. In fact, the speed at which the k-space can be filled is limited by technical factors and physiological properties of the tissues being imaged, and underfilling the k-space in order to shorten scan length leads to violation of the Nyquist theorem and appearance of aliasing artifacts. However, this problem can be overcome with the compressed sensing (CS) reconstruction technique, which is based on the compressibility of MR images (i.e., MR images have a sparse representation in at least a known mathematical transform domain [6]) and allows reconstruction of images from undersampled k-space, without loss of image quality. However, the major drawback of CS is the complexity of the algorithm, which is based on an iterative architecture and requires high computational power and long reconstruction times, especially for dynamic sequences, limiting its application in a real-world clinical setting [7]. Thus, a faster reconstruction technique is needed, and deep learning (DL) shows promising results in speeding up the process, because once a neural network is trained, its processing is not iterative anymore. Initial experiences with DL application to CMR image reconstruction are promising, and several groups are developing different DL approaches to solve this issue. Qin et al. [8] combined a traditional iterative reconstruction algorithm with a convolutional recurrent neural network for the reconstruction of CMR dynamic cine SSFP acquisition that outperformed current reconstruction methods both in terms of accuracy and speed. Schlemper et al. [9] developed a deep cascade of convolutional neural networks that enabled accurate image reconstruction until 11-fold undersampling, together with a reconstruction time of around 10 s for dynamic sequences and 23 ms for 2D images, allowing real-time applications of CMR.

Another issue in CMR acquisition is the prescription of the correct image plane. In fact, differently from other anatomical regions, the heart position and foremost its spatial orientation differ greatly from patient to patient. Thus, the positioning of the correct cardiac planes, a prerequisite for a high-quality examination, is challenging, especially for non-expert technicians. Blansit K. and colleagues [10] have demonstrated the feasibility of using DL to automatically localize the cardiac landmarks necessary for cardiac plane prescription, with an optimal agreement with planes prescribed by an expert physician or technologist, potentially speeding up scan planning and reducing the need for highly qualified personnel.

The last domain of image acquisition in which DL is proving its usefulness is image quality monitoring. In routine clinical practice, the most common artifacts encountered during CMR are related to respiratory motion and arrhythmia, which result in spatial or temporal blurring of the images and consequent reduction of image quality that can lead to inconclusive or erroneous results. Usually, technicians or physicians inspect the image and decide, eventually, to repeat sequences with insufficient quality. However, this approach is time-consuming and poorly reproducible and requires a constant presence of expert personnel during CMR acquisition. Tarroni et al. [11] tackled this issue by developing an AI-based algorithm that performs a real-time fully automated quality control of short-axis CMR images. Their algorithm was able to accurately detect sequences with insufficient longitudinal heart coverage, inter-slice motion, or low image contrast in the cardiac region and consequently to exclude them from the dataset or to trigger a rescan. Küstner et al. [12] went further and developed a DL method capable of performing retrospective motion correction on already acquired images, with optimal results in terms of generation of near-realistic motion-free images. However, this process can potentially hide or modify important features of the original images, leading to wrong or missed diagnosis, and should be validated in the clinical setting.

To sum up, in the setting of image acquisition, DL has many useful potential applications, ranging from scan time reduction to image quality improvement, aimed to increase the number of CMR acquisition slots and to broaden the cohort of patients eligible for a CMR examination.

In the following paragraphs, the use of AI in three clinical scenarios will be described, to exemplify the potential usefulness of this technology when applied to CMR (Fig. 32.1). AI will probably increase reliability and broaden the application of CMR in the next future, with positive impact on CMR indications in the CPGs.

CMR in the Clinical Setting of Heart Failure: Where Does AI Fit In?

One of the clinical settings addressed by the CPGs is heart failure (HF) [13, 14]. In this setting, CMR allows for a comprehensive evaluation of both heart function and myocardial structure that may hint to the underlying etiology [15]. CMR is the gold standard for the evaluation of volumes and

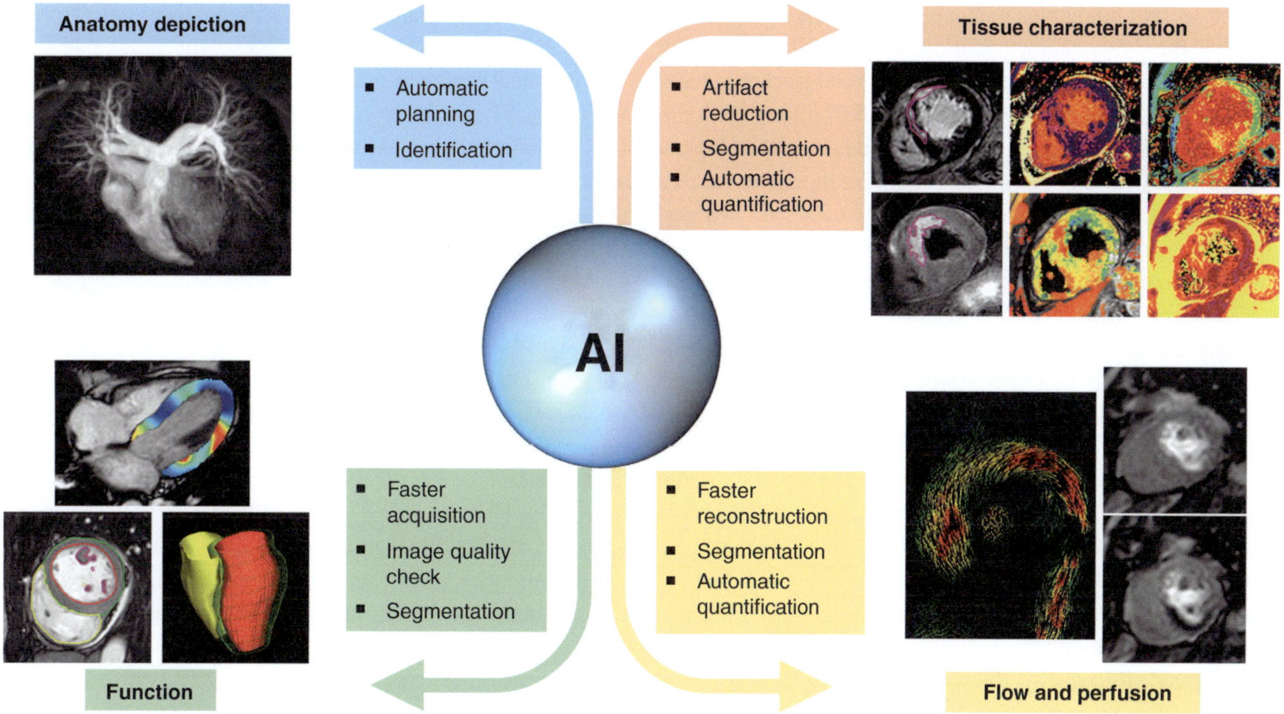

Fig. 32.1 CMR imaging allows a comprehensive evaluation of the cardiovascular structures. Main strengths of CMR include the wonderful capability to depict anatomy, the unique ability to noninvasively characterize myocardial tissue, and the high reliability in the assessment of the heart function, vessels hemodynamics, and myocardial perfusion. CMR presence in the clinical guidelines is progressively increasing thanks to these unique capabilities. Artificial intelligence (AI) tools are being increasingly applied to improve the CMR workflow, with a potential impact on image planning and acquisition, image quality, post-processing, and quantification

ejection fraction (EF) of both ventricles [14], and it is recommended in patients with nondiagnostic echocardiographic studies, especially for the imaging of the right heart. CMR is also useful for detailing anatomy, volumes, and function in patients with complex congenital heart disease, both for planning of the surgical repair and for follow-up, since the complex anatomy of these patients may undermine a correct echocardiographic evaluation. In this setting, CMR is recommended to assess eventual residual hemodynamic lesions after intervention, to identify those patients with structural heart disease at risk of developing arrhythmias, and to diagnose potential acquired heart diseases [14, 16].

The limitation of CMR in calculating chamber volume and function on cine SSFP images is the necessity to perform segmentation of the epicardial and endocardial contours, which is a time-consuming process with accuracy and reproducibility concerns, even when the analysis is performed by experienced readers [17]. Thus, a fully automated segmentation tool is long overdue. A large body of literature has been published about automated CMR segmentation approaches [18]. However, conventional methods are still semiautomated, and manual correction is needed, especially in apical and basal slices, in the right ventricle, and in trabeculated myocardial segments.

The application of AI to the task of segmentation of heart chambers on cine SSFP images for the quantification of volumes and function is showing promising results. In recent years, head-to-head comparisons of different DL-based segmentation algorithms have taken place during international challenges [19], with generally highly accurate results for LV segmentation (Dice similarity coefficients higher than 0.95) while still suboptimal for RV segmentation. However, the main limitation of these results is that the training of the models was performed on a small sample of CMR coming from a single center; thus many doubts remain about the performance of the algorithms in case of patients with more complex anatomy or coming from multiple centers.

Tao et al. [20] overcame issues about accuracy and generalizability by training a CNN on a larger sample of CMR performed on different scanners. The study focused on LV analysis, and the CNN averaged a perpendicular distance between manual and automatic segmentation of about 1 mm, which is comparable to intra- and inter-observer variability.

Thus, the LV segmentation problem seems to be solved. However, more research is needed to develop AI algorithms capable of performing accurate segmentation of the other heart chambers and to maintain their accuracy in the setting of complex congenital heart diseases or anatomical variants.

The second fundamental capability of CMR in the setting of HF is the tissue characterization, which has been recently expanded by the advent of the quantitative relaxometric techniques (i.e., T1, T2, and T2* mapping). CMR allows the identification and quantification of the different pathophysiological mechanism involving the myocardium. STIR sequences, T2 mapping, and native T1 mapping are able to identify myocardial edema due to acute myocardial damage or inflammation; late gadolinium enhancement (LGE) sequences and extracellular volume fraction (ECV) can quantify myocyte necrosis or myocardial fibrosis; hyperemia due inflammation can be assessed using T1 mapping shortening early after contrast administration [21]. However, most of mapping parameters still need further investigation and validation, especially in the chronic setting, despite a relatively large body of literature supporting their application in specific settings. The combined evaluation of CMR biomarkers of tissue characterization may help in defining the etiology of HF, which may be due to many different causes, most importantly ischemic cardiomyopathy, inflammatory cardiomyopathies, toxic cardiomyopathies, infiltrative diseases, storage diseases, and idiopathic dilated cardiomyopathy.

A common feature of most of the pathophysiological processes leading to heart failure is myocardial fibrosis, detected and measured using the late gadolinium enhancement (LGE) sequence. The identification of replacement fibrosis is fundamental since it provides one of the mainstays of differential diagnosis among distinct cardiomyopathies, and its burden is a well-recognized prognostic factor in different clinical settings. However, its quantification in clinical routine requires careful delineation of LV boundaries and manual selection of an area with LGE and/or of a remote area. The segmentation process is subjective and time-consuming and may introduce biases impacting on accuracy and reproducibility among operators and centers [22, 23].

To address these limitations, DL is starting to be applied to the LGE quantification setting. Moccia et al. [24] have developed a fully CNN for automatic quantification of LGE in the setting of ischemic cardiomyopathy, achieving a high performance. However, the limitation of this DL method is that it has been trained and validated only in patients affected by a well-defined disease. Thus, an algorithm capable of quantifying LGE extent independently of the underlying disease, which would make automatic scar burden quantification for each patient available, does not currently exist.

The introduction of the novel quantitative relaxometric sequences, namely, T1, T2, and T2* mapping, has dramatically increased the CMR capabilities of tissue characterization. In fact, their advantage over conventional sequences is that they allow not only the visualization of the disease process but also its quantification. Moreover, differently from usual T1-, T2-, or T2*-weighted images, mapping techniques can identify and quantify also diffuse myocardial diseases, which have historically been a diagnostic challenge [25]. The classical example is the setting of cardiac amyloidosis, in which T1 mapping with extracellular volume fraction (ECV) quantification has significantly higher sensitivity and specificity than conventional late gadolinium enhancement (LGE) sequences [26], and it can also provide a risk stratification of patients [26].

Mapping sequences assume that the acquired signals follow an exponential recovery curve (for T1 mapping) or decay curve (for T2 mapping). Consequently, these exponential curves are built by fitting the signal of each pixel of a series of images that are acquired in different fashions depending on the parameter to be studied. For example, the technique of T1 mapping requires the acquisition of multiple T1-weighted images, prepared with an inversion recovery pulse and each acquired after a different inversion time and on the subsequent estimation of the T1 time at each voxel, which will be used to build the relaxation curve. Since every T1 image is acquired in a different heartbeat, each one is slightly different from the others due to heart rate variability or respiratory motion. Thus, careful segmentation of each T1-weighted image and their alignment by means of image registration are necessary to avoid artifacts.

AI has a role also in this setting, since automatic segmentation could help streamlining this process increasing accuracy and reproducibility. Fahmy et al. have developed a CNN [27] that combines segmentation of all slices and inversion times, their alignment, and T1 quantification, with good agreement in respect to manual segmentation and with interobserver variability comparable to the one between expert readers.

Further into the future of CMR lies the possibility of acquiring multiple tissue properties with a single sequence. The technique of magnetic resonance fingerprinting (MRF) is a step toward this result. Differently from conventional mapping sequences, MRF pulse sequence can sensitize multiple tissue properties at the same time. To reconstruct the correct T1 and T2 relaxation times for each voxel, a dictionary matching technique is used: the process is based on the choice from the dictionary of the signal time course that best fits the measured signal time course. The T1 and T2 values of the best fitting dictionary entry will be assigned to that voxel [28]. MRF has been validated in healthy subjects, and initial clinical experience is promising [28, 29]. However, the process of dictionary creation and of matching the signal to the dictionary may slow down the reconstruction of the images, hampering the clinical availability of the technique. Machine learning (ML) may help overcome these issues. In fact, the process of signal dictionary generation can be significantly accelerated with the use of ML-based algorithms, allowing fast image reconstruction [30].

CMR in the Clinical Setting of Ischemic Cardiomyopathy: Where Does AI Fit In?

The most represented setting in CPGs is ischemic heart disease (IHD) [2]. The 2019 ESC guidelines on chronic coronary syndromes (CCSs) recommend the use of either an anatomical test (computed tomography angiography [CTA]) or a functional test (stress echocardiography, stress CMR, single-photon emission computed tomography, or positron emission tomography) for the diagnosis of coronary artery disease (CAD) in symptomatic patients, depending on pre-test likelihood, patient characteristics, and availability of the test [31]. Stress CMR can assess two different pathophysiological levels along the ischemic cascade (relative and absolute perfusion abnormalities and wall motion abnormalities) [32]. It has been demonstrated that stress-rest CMR perfusion imaging has the highest negative and positive likelihood ratio (0.13 and 7.10, respectively) to rule in or rule out functionally significant CAD across a wide range of pre-test likelihood, using invasive fractional flow reserve (FFR) as the reference standard [33].

CMR also has a role in the CPGs regarding acute coronary syndromes (ACSs). In the setting of ST-segment elevation myocardial infarction (STEMI), the 2017 ESC guidelines established CMR as a valuable risk stratification tool after the acute event [34]. In fact, with its unique capabilities of tissue characterization, it can assess many of the pathophysiological changes induced by myocardial infarction, such as the extent of myocardium at risk, the presence of intramyocardial hemorrhage, the infarct size, and the presence and extent of microvascular obstruction, the latter two having an important impact on long-term mortality and heart failure risk [35, 36]. Furthermore, stress CMR can detect the presence of residual ischemia beyond the infarcted territory, thus allowing targeted revascularization and better long-term outcomes [37].

In the setting of suspected non-ST segment elevation acute coronary syndromes (NSTE-ACS), the 2020 ESC guidelines recommend, in patients without ischemic ECG changes and with normal hs-cTn and no recurring chest pain, an anatomical or functional test for the exclusion of CAD, during hospitalization or shortly after discharge [38]. A negative stress CMR can exclude functional significant CAD with excellent short- and mid-term prognosis [39]. Furthermore, CMR performed in this setting reduces the use of invasive coronary angiography and provides an alternative diagnosis in a non-negligible number of patients [40].

In the current clinical practice, stress CMR perfusion is a qualitative technique based on the comparison of dynamic perfusion images acquired during rest and during pharmacological stress on a basal, mid, and apical LV short axis slice, in order to identify the appearance of areas of relative hypoperfusion due to functionally significant coronary artery stenosis. Besides being one of the most accurate non-invasive imaging modalities for the diagnosis of myocardial ischemia due to epicardial coronary artery disease (CAD) [33], stress CMR also carries important prognostic value, since a negative stress CMR predicts low incidence of cardiac events, including coronary revascularization, and low spending on further testing [41]. A major drawback of this approach is that, in case of balanced three-vessel disease or in case of coronary microvascular dysfunction, both causing a global impairment of myocardial wall perfusion reserve, the absence of normally perfused myocardium to use as a reference may lead to an increase rate of false-negative results [42].

Stress-rest CMR images can be elaborated to measure several semiquantitative analyses of perfusion. One of the most validated is the myocardial perfusion reserve index (MPRI), which is calculated as the ratio between stress and rest maximum upslope of the first-pass myocardial perfusion time-intensity curve divided by the maximum upslope of the first-pass LV cavity time-intensity curve. MPRI has a good diagnostic performance in comparison to invasive evaluation [43].

Furthermore, stress CMR is bound to become a quantitative tool to measure myocardial perfusion in terms of milliliters of blood per minute per gram of myocardium. Quantitative stress-rest CMR perfusion provides an even higher diagnostic accuracy than semiquantitative evaluation in comparison to invasive assessment as reference standard. Furthermore, since quantitative evaluation is based on numerical cutoffs distinguishing between normal and pathological states, it has the advantage of increased reproducibility and easier clinical application [44, 45].

However, segmentation is fundamental also for the quantitative analysis of perfusion, which requires lengthy image post-processing. In fact, it is necessary to delineate both the blood pool (to extract the arterial input function) and the myocardium (to quantify the myocardial blood flow) on each dynamic acquisition and on each slice. Furthermore, the perfusion sequence has peculiar characteristics that challenge the automatic segmentation algorithms, such as the low signal-to-noise ratio and the dynamic contrast enhancement.

AI may help overcome segmentation problems that are impeding the widespread clinical application of quantitative CMR perfusion. Scannell et al. [46] have developed a DL algorithm that automatically performs all the steps necessary for the evaluation of myocardial perfusion, from detection of peak enhancement in the left ventricle cavity and subsequent quantification of the arterial input function to segmentation of the LV wall with automatic quantification of myocardial blood flow. This automatic approach based on DL showed a good agreement with manual segmentation, allowing a dramatic reduction in processing time.

CMR in the Clinical Setting of Hypertrophic Phenotype: Where Does AI Fit In?

Another clinical category in which CMR is recommended by the CPGs is hypertrophic cardiomyopathy (HCM) and, more in general, the hypertrophic phenotype. In patients with suspected left ventricular hypertrophy, CMR is recommended especially when echocardiography is nonconclusive in reaching a diagnosis due to poor acoustic window or when some left ventricle areas are poorly visualized due to anatomical characteristics, for example, the anterolateral wall, the apex, and the right ventricle [47]. CMR is also recommended when the diagnosis of hypertrophic cardiomyopathy is not certain and differential diagnosis with other hypertrophic phenotypes, such as Fabry's disease or amyloidosis, is needed [48]. Interestingly, CMR was already recommended for differential diagnosis even without the novel relaxometric techniques, which have dramatically increased the diagnostic yield of CMR in patients presenting with the hypertrophic phenotype. In fact, both T1 mapping and ECV quantification can provide a reliable diagnosis of amyloidosis, characterized by a significant increase of native T1 and ECV values [49], and of Fabry's disease, characterized by a pathognomonic decrease in native T1 values associated with LGE [50] and increased ECV when scarring fibrosis occurs, mainly in the inferolateral left ventricle wall [51].

Furthermore, CMR is superior to echocardiography in the detection of subtle markers of the disease (e.g., papillary muscle abnormalities or myocardial crypts) which may be due to sarcomeric protein gene mutations [52], enabling an early diagnosis.

In patients with HCM, LGE is present in around 65% of patients [48], typically in the hypertrophic areas, with patchy mid-wall distribution, and at the anterior and posterior right ventricle insertion points on the interventricular septum. LGE etiology in HCM is linked to ischemia due to microvascular impairment in the hypertrophic areas and myocardial metabolic impairment [53]. LGE is associated with adverse left ventricle remodeling, and as in other cardiomyopathies, LGE burden entails a higher risk of heart failure death, cardiovascular mortality, and all-cause death. Furthermore, LGE burden has a significant prognostic value for the prediction of sudden cardiac death; thus its assessment is a valuable risk stratification tool and may aid the patient selection for implantable cardioverter-defibrillator (ICD) therapy. However, no specific recommendation exists for LGE burden quantification, since the most recent CPGs on HCM management date back to 2014 [48] and the speed at which research in the cardiovascular field proceeds constantly outpaces the process of establishing CPGs.

As in the setting of ischemic cardiomyopathy, also in HCM patients, DL is tackling the issue of automatic LGE burden quantification. Fahmy et al. [54] have developed a 3D-CNN for the automatic quantification of LGE in patients with hypertrophic cardiomyopathy, obtaining accurate results in comparison to manual segmentation, thus potentially enabling the exploitation of this important parameter for every examination.

Potential Future Applications of AI in the Clinical Use of CMR: Automatic Diagnosis

When public discussion about AI occurs, the argument of whether AI will ever be able to perform a fully automatic diagnosis is often addressed. However, apart from detection and segmentation tasks, AI has still a very limited role in performing automatic diagnosis based on CMR images. In fact, reaching a diagnosis requires an expert physician to integrate the multiparametric features extracted from the images with clinical information such as age, history, and symptoms. AI is very far from reaching this level of complexity; however initial experience is being gathered in well-defined settings, such as in the classification of myocardial disease phenotypes. In the 2017 "Automatic Cardiac Diagnosis Challenge" [19], different ML algorithms were created for a classification task to identify, on cine SSFP images, healthy patients and patients affected by dilated cardiomyopathy, hypertrophic cardiomyopathy, ischemic cardiomyopathy with depressed ejection fraction, or right ventricle abnormalities. The best algorithm reached a classification accuracy above 92%, even if due to the small sample size of the study further validation is required. Furthermore, the classification of a phenotype is just the first step to reach a diagnosis, since different diseases may share a common phenotype but different etiology and therapeutic strategies.

Potential Future Applications of AI in the Clinical Use of CMR: Prediction

More interestingly than for automatic diagnosis, AI could be applied for CMR-based risk stratification and outcome prediction. Some pilot studies have leveraged the power of ML to build risk prediction algorithms based on image analysis or on a combination of clinical and image data in specific settings. Dawes et al. [55] have built a ML-based tool capable of predicting survival in patients affected by pulmonary hypertension by analyzing 3D contractility patterns of the right ventricle. Interestingly, the algorithm increased the accuracy of conventional imaging and hemodynamic and clinical markers and provided better stratification between high- and low-risk patients. Another study from Diller et al. [56] has demonstrated that, in the setting of patients with repaired Tetralogy of Fallot, a DL-based risk stratification algorithm that automatically segments heart chambers and quantifies myocardial deformation parameters with feature tracking can predict the prognosis.

Conclusions

CMR, thanks to its multiparametric capabilities, is a valuable tool for diagnosis, risk stratification, treatment monitoring, follow-up, and pre-procedural planning in most cardiovascular diseases. Thus, CMR is recommended by radiological and cardiological CPGs in many different clinical settings, such as heart failure, ischemic cardiomyopathy, and cardiac diseases with hypertrophic phenotype.

AI is on the verge of revolutionizing every aspect of the CMR examination, from faster acquisition and reconstruction to automatic segmentation, potential diagnostic aid, and outcome prediction. These advances will give AI-empowered CMR an even more central role in the CPGs. Faster acquisition and reconstruction will increase CMR availability and thus its use in a wider range of clinical settings covered by CPGs. The automatic segmentation and analysis will speed up CMR assessment and reporting, generating at the same time robust results reducing interobserver variability. Ultimately, integrating AI in the CMR workflow will benefit patient management.

References

1. Leiner T, et al. SCMR position paper (2020) on clinical indications for cardiovascular magnetic resonance. J Cardiovasc Magn Reson. 2020;22:76.
2. Esposito A, et al. The current landscape of imaging recommendations in cardiovascular clinical guidelines: toward an imaging-guided precision medicine. Radiol Med. 2020;125:1013–23.
3. Von Knobelsdorff-Brenkenhoff F, Schulz-Menger J. Role of cardiovascular magnetic resonance in the guidelines of the European Society of Cardiology. J Cardiovasc Magn Reson. 2016;18:6.
4. Von Knobelsdorff-Brenkenhoff F, Pilz G, Schulz-Menger J. Representation of cardiovascular magnetic resonance in the AHA/ACC guidelines. J Cardiovasc Magn Reson. 2017;19:70.
5. Schulz-Menger J, et al. Standardized image interpretation and post-processing in cardiovascular magnetic resonance – 2020 update: Society for Cardiovascular Magnetic Resonance (SCMR): Board of Trustees Task Force on standardized post-processing. J Cardiovasc Magn Reson. 2020;22:19.
6. Lustig M, Donoho D, Pauly JM. Sparse MRI: the application of compressed sensing for rapid MR imaging. Magn Reson Med. 2007;58:1182–95.
7. Ye JC. Compressed sensing MRI: a review from signal processing perspective. BMC Biomed Eng. 2019;1:1–17.
8. Qin C, et al. Convolutional recurrent neural networks for dynamic MR image reconstruction. IEEE Trans Med Imaging. 2019;38:280–90.
9. Schlemper J, Caballero J, Hajnal JV, Price AN, Rueckert D. A deep cascade of convolutional neural networks for dynamic MR image reconstruction. IEEE Trans Med Imaging. 2018;37:491–503.
10. Blansit K, Retson T, Masutani E, Bahrami N, Hsiao A. Deep learning–based prescription of cardiac MRI planes. Radiol Artif Intell. 2019;1:e180069.
11. Tarroni G, et al. Learning-based quality control for cardiac MR images. IEEE Trans Med Imaging. 2019;38:1127–38.
12. Küstner T, et al. Retrospective correction of motion-affected MR images using deep learning frameworks. Magn Reson Med. 2019;82:1527–40.
13. Yancy CW, et al. 2013 ACCF/AHA guideline for the management of heart failure: a report of the American college of cardiology foundation/American heart association task force on practice guidelines. Circulation. 2013; https://doi.org/10.1161/CIR.0b013e31829e8776.
14. Ponikowski P, et al. 2016 ESC guidelines for the diagnosis and treatment of acute and chronic heart failure. Eur Heart J. 2016;37:2129–2200m.
15. Di Cesare E, et al. Multimodality imaging in chronic heart failure. Radiol Med. 2020; https://doi.org/10.1007/s11547-020-01245-4.
16. Kilner PJ, et al. Recommendations for cardiovascular magnetic resonance in adults with congenital heart disease from the respective working groups of the European Society of Cardiology. Eur Heart J. 2010; https://doi.org/10.1093/eurheartj/ehp586.
17. Suinesiaputra A, et al. Quantification of LV function and mass by cardiovascular magnetic resonance: multi-center variability and consensus contours. J Cardiovasc Magn Reson. 2015;17:63.
18. Peng P, et al. A review of heart chamber segmentation for structural and functional analysis using cardiac magnetic resonance imaging. MAGMA. 2016;29:155–95.
19. Bernard O, et al. Deep learning techniques for automatic MRI cardiac multi-structures segmentation and diagnosis: is the problem solved? IEEE Trans Med Imaging. 2018;37:2514–25.
20. Tao Q, et al. Deep learning based method for fully automatic quantification of left ventricle function from cine MR images: a multi-vendor, Multicenter Study. Radiology. 2019;290:81–8.
21. Palmisano A, et al. Early T1 myocardial MRI mapping: value in detecting myocardial hyperemia in acute myocarditis. Radiology. 2020;295:316–25.
22. Engblom H, et al. A new automatic algorithm for quantification of myocardial infarction imaged by late gadolinium enhancement cardiovascular magnetic resonance: experimental validation and comparison to expert delineations in multi-center, multi-vendor patient data. J Cardiovasc Magn Reson. 2016;18:27.
23. Palmisano A, et al. Late iodine enhancement cardiac computed tomography for detection of myocardial scars: impact of experience in the clinical practice. Radiol Med. 2020;125:128–36.
24. Moccia S, et al. Development and testing of a deep learning-based strategy for scar segmentation on CMR-LGE images. Magn Reson Mater Phys Biol Med. 2019;32:187–95.
25. Messroghli DR, et al. Clinical recommendations for cardiovascular magnetic resonance mapping of T1, T2, T2 and extracellular volume: a consensus statement by the Society for Cardiovascular Magnetic Resonance (SCMR) endorsed by the European Association for Cardiovascular Imagin. J Cardiovasc Magn Reson. 2017;19:75.
26. Pan JA, Kerwin MJ, Salerno M. Native T1 mapping, extracellular volume mapping, and late gadolinium enhancement in cardiac amyloidosis: a meta-analysis. JACC Cardiovasc Imaging. 2020;13:1299–310.
27. Fahmy AS, El-Rewaidy H, Nezafat M, Nakamori S, Nezafat R. Automated analysis of cardiovascular magnetic resonance myocardial native T1 mapping images using fully convolutional neural networks. J Cardiovasc Magn Reson. 2019;21:7.
28. Liu Y, Hamilton J, Rajagopalan S, Seiberlich N. Cardiac magnetic resonance fingerprinting: technical overview and initial results. JACC Cardiovasc Imaging. 2018;11:1837–53.

29. Cavallo AU, et al. CMR fingerprinting for myocardial T1, T2, and ECV quantification in patients with nonischemic cardiomyopathy. JACC Cardiovasc Imaging. 2019;12:1584–5.
30. Hamilton JI, Seiberlich N. Machine learning for rapid magnetic resonance fingerprinting tissue property quantification. Proc IEEE. 2020;108:69–85.
31. Knuuti J, et al. 2019 ESC guidelines for the diagnosis and management of chronic coronary syndromes. Eur Heart J. 2020;41:407–77.
32. Palmisano A, et al. Feature tracking and mapping analysis of myocardial response to improved perfusion reserve in patients with refractory angina treated by coronary sinus reducer implantation: a CMR study. Int J Cardiovasc Imaging. 2020; https://doi.org/10.1007/s10554-020-01964-9.
33. Knuuti J, et al. The performance of non-invasive tests to rule-in and rule-out significant coronary artery stenosis in patients with stable angina: a meta-analysis focused on post-test disease probability. Eur Heart J. 2018;39:3322–30.
34. Ibanez B, et al. 2017 ESC guidelines for the management of acute myocardial infarction in patients presenting with ST-segment elevation. Eur Heart J. 2018;39:119–77.
35. Stone GW, et al. Relationship between infarct size and outcomes following primary PCI patient-level analysis from 10 randomized trials. J Am Coll Cardiol. 2016; https://doi.org/10.1016/j.jacc.2016.01.069.
36. Eitel I, et al. Comprehensive prognosis assessment by CMR imaging after ST-segment elevation myocardial infarction. J Am Coll Cardiol. 2014; https://doi.org/10.1016/j.jacc.2014.06.1194.
37. Gerber BL, et al. Prognostic value of myocardial viability by delayed-enhanced magnetic resonance in patients with coronary artery disease and low ejection fraction: impact of revascularization therapy. J Am Coll Cardiol. 2012; https://doi.org/10.1016/j.jacc.2011.09.073.
38. Collet J-P, et al. 2020 ESC guidelines for the management of acute coronary syndromes in patients presenting without persistent ST-segment elevation. Eur Heart J. 2020; https://doi.org/10.1093/eurheartj/ehaa575.
39. Ingkanisorn WP, et al. Prognosis of negative adenosine stress magnetic resonance in patients presenting to an emergency department with chest pain. J Am Coll Cardiol. 2006; https://doi.org/10.1016/j.jacc.2005.11.059.
40. Smulders MW, et al. Initial imaging-guided strategy versus routine care in patients with non–ST-segment elevation myocardial infarction. J Am Coll Cardiol. 2019;74:2466–77.
41. Kwong RY, et al. Cardiac magnetic resonance stress perfusion imaging for evaluation of patients with chest pain. J Am Coll Cardiol. 2019;74:1741–55.
42. Knott KD, et al. The prognostic significance of quantitative myocardial perfusion: an artificial intelligence-based approach using perfusion mapping. Circulation. 2020;141:1282–91. https://doi.org/10.1161/CIRCULATIONAHA.119.044666.
43. Thomson LEJ, et al. Cardiac magnetic resonance myocardial perfusion reserve index is reduced in women with coronary microvascular dysfunction: a national heart, lung, and blood institute-sponsored study from the women's ischemia syndrome evaluation. Circ Cardiovasc Imaging. 2015;8:e002481.
44. Mordini FE, et al. Diagnostic accuracy of stress perfusion CMR in comparison with quantitative coronary angiography: fully quantitative, semiquantitative, and qualitative assessment. JACC Cardiovasc Imaging. 2014;7:14–22.
45. Kotecha T, et al. Automated pixel-wise quantitative myocardial perfusion mapping by CMR to detect obstructive coronary artery disease and coronary microvascular dysfunction: validation against invasive coronary physiology. JACC Cardiovasc Imaging. 2019;12:1958–69.
46. Scannell CM, et al. Deep-learning-based preprocessing for quantitative myocardial perfusion MRI. J Magn Reson Imaging. 2020; https://doi.org/10.1002/jmri.26983.
47. Rickers C, et al. Utility of cardiac magnetic resonance imaging in the diagnosis of hypertrophic cardiomyopathy. Circulation. 2005;112:855–61.
48. Zamorano JL, et al. 2014 ESC guidelines on diagnosis and management of hypertrophic cardiomyopathy: the task force for the diagnosis and management of hypertrophic cardiomyopathy of the European Society of Cardiology (ESC). Eur Heart J. 2014; https://doi.org/10.1093/eurheartj/ehu284.
49. Brownrigg J, Lorenzini M, Lumley M, Elliott P. Diagnostic performance of imaging investigations in detecting and differentiating cardiac amyloidosis: a systematic review and meta-analysis. ESC Hear Fail. 2019;6:1041–51.
50. De Cobelli F, et al. Delayed-enhanced cardiac MRI for differentiation of fabry's disease from symmetric hypertrophic cardiomyopathy. Am J Roentgenol. 2009;192:W97.
51. Perry R, et al. The role of cardiac imaging in the diagnosis and management of Anderson-Fabry disease. JACC Cardiovasc Imaging. 2019;12:1230–42.
52. Brouwer WP, et al. Multiple myocardial crypts on modified long-axis view are a specific finding in pre-hypertrophic HCM mutation carriers. Eur Heart J Cardiovasc Imaging. 2012; https://doi.org/10.1093/ehjci/jes005.
53. Esposito A, et al. Impaired left ventricular energy metabolism in patients with hypertrophic cardiomyopathy is related to the extension of fibrosis at delayed gadolinium-enhanced magnetic resonance imaging. Heart. 2009;95:228–33.
54. Fahmy AS, et al. Three-dimensional deep convolutional neural networks for automated myocardial scar quantification in hypertrophic cardiomyopathy: a multicenter multivendor study. Radiology. 2020;294:52–60.
55. Dawes TJW, et al. Machine learning of three-dimensional right ventricular motion enables outcome prediction in pulmonary hypertension: a cardiac MR imaging study. Radiology. 2017;283:381–90.
56. Diller GP, et al. Prediction of prognosis in patients with tetralogy of Fallot based on deep learning imaging analysis. Heart. 2020; https://doi.org/10.1136/heartjnl-2019-315962.

Artificial Intelligence-Based Evaluation of Functional Cardiac Magnetic Resonance Imaging

33

Qian Tao and Rob J. van der Geest

Introduction

With its excellent soft tissue contrast and fine spatial resolution, cardiac magnetic resonance (CMR) is widely considered as the gold standard modality to image the heart [1–3]. Accurate assessment of cardiac function is an important basis for diagnosis and evaluation of a range of cardiovascular diseases [4, 5]. CMR sequences for cardiac functional assessment typically include steady-state free procession (SSFP) cine MRI, which visualizes the heart in motion in a full cardiac cycle, and tagged MRI, which more explicitly tracks the myocardial motion by spatially modulating the longitudinal magnetization in myocardial tissue [6]. In clinical practice, for its relative ease of acquisition and analysis, cine MRI is most frequently used for cardiac function evaluation. The analysis of functional CMR sequences can be performed in a qualitative manner based on the experience of radiologists, as well as quantitatively based on manual or computer-aided image analysis.

Quantification provides more accurate, objective, and in-depth information for individual patient but is not a trivial task either for human or computer. Analysis of a cine MRI sequence, for example, would entail interpretation of more than 300 image frames (number of slices multiplied by the number of cardiac phases), which is extremely tedious and time-consuming if manually performed. Likewise, manual tracking of the tag patterns in a tagged MRI sequence is exhaustive, if not impossible. For this reason, automated and semiautomated analysis of functional CMR has been an active research topic in the medical imaging community over the past three decades [7–10].

In a broad sense, artificial intelligence (AI) is the set of computer methods that imitate human intelligence in accomplishing certain data analysis tasks. While AI has gained enormous popularity in recent years, the history of AI dated back much further, to the 1950s [11, 12]. Along the years, the mainstream AI algorithms for CMR analysis have experienced several paradigm shifts, from image-based methods to model-based methods, now to data-based methods. The latest data-based methods largely rely on "deep learning," the set of machine learning methods that use multilayer neural networks (NNs) [13, 14]. While data-based methods are the state of the art and most popular, this article aims to provide a systematic and historical (albeit not complete) review on a broader range of AI methods that have been developed by generations of researchers for functional CMR analysis.

This chapter is organized as follows: Sect. 2 presents the formulation of the functional CMR analysis problem and its main technical challenges. Sections 3, 4, and 5 review the AI methods in historical order and discuss their rationales. We review the AI methods for three main functional CMR analysis tasks: heart segmentation (Sect. 3), cardiac motion tracking (Sect. 4), and functional parameter estimation (Sect. 5). Finally, Sect. 6 discusses the current limitations and future prospective of AI for functional CMR analysis.

Functional CMR Analysis: Technical Challenges

AI methods for functional CMR aim to automatically or semiautomatically (1) recognize the heart from the field of view and segment the myocardium, (2) track local cardiac motion, and (3) quantify and report clinically relevant functional parameters. Automated detection and segmentation of the heart is a major task for functional CMR analysis, as the basis for quantification of functional parameters including

Q. Tao, PhD (✉)
Department of Imaging Physics, Delft University of Technology, Delft, The Netherlands

Department of Radiology, Leiden University Medical Center, Leiden, The Netherlands
e-mail: q.tao@tudelft.nl

R. J. van der Geest, PhD
Department of Radiology, Leiden University Medical Center, Leiden, The Netherlands

C. N. De Cecco et al. (eds.), *Artificial Intelligence in Cardiothoracic Imaging*, Contemporary Medical Imaging,
https://doi.org/10.1007/978-3-030-92087-6_33

left and right ventricular volume, ejection fraction, myocardial wall thickness, and mass. Tracking of cardiac motion further provides means to assess the myocardial kinetics and allows characterization of wall motion abnormalities. Importantly, it also enables quantification of myocardial strain, which reflects the mechanical properties of heart muscles. Among the four heart chambers, the left ventricle (LV) has been most frequently studied in literature, because of its relatively large size and regular shape. In earlier literature, most AI methods focused on the LV, while in recent work, more AI methods started to tackle right ventricle (RV) and left atrium (LA).

For AI methods, the major technical challenge lies in the high variability of functional CMR images. The variability originates from a wide range of external and internal factors. External factors include the specific MRI scanner, sequence parameter, imaging plane, imaging resolution, contrast, illuminance, bias field, noise pattern, signal-to-noise ratio (SNR), artifact, etc. Internal factors include the large inter-subject variation in cardiac structure, orientation, size, etc., especially for subjects with cardiovascular diseases. As such, the major challenge for a clinically applicable AI tool is to adequately address the substantial variability such that it can handle any arbitrary CMR dataset in clinical practice.

Although the latest deep learning-based methods demonstrate state-of-the-art performance in functional CMR analysis [15, 16], we intend to review a broader range of AI methods developed in the past decades with evolving principles. Along the evolution, we can observe an increasing degree of knowledge integration, which eventually makes it possible to handle the high variability in functional CMR.

AI Methods for Functional Analysis: Cardiac Segmentation

Existing AI methods for functional CMR analysis can be divided into three large categories: image-based, model-based, and data-based, largely in a chronological order.

Image-Based Methods

Early AI methods focused on the image itself at pixel level. From the point of view of a computer algorithm, an image can be seen as a matrix of scalar values. Various image filters can be developed to extract the features that are relevant to the heart object. The myocardial boundary, for example, can be highlighted by applying edge filters such as the Sobel filter or Canny operation [17]. For segmentation, these discrete contour locations need to be connected, which is a nontrivial task for computer. The most intuitive solution is to connect these points using the dynamic programming method in the polar coordinate system for LV segmentation in short axis images [18]. The Snake algorithm, also known as active contours, is another established method to connect edge points around anatomical structures by parametrization and optimization [19]. Compared to dynamic programming, Snake can handle more complex object geometries. The Snake method parametrizes a set of contour points, allowing them to evolve based on minimization of an energy function, which typically contains two terms: one is the internal energy that regulates the shape of the Snake (e.g., smoothness, curvature), and the other is the external energy that enforces the Snake to move close to the boundary of a structure. The Snake is iteratively optimized by the gradient descent method that decreases the energy function step by step. This represents a classical formulation of an image analysis problem by AI: (1) parametrize the variable θ representing the solution space; (2) define a cost function that describes the desired solution when $C(\theta; I)$ is minimized (e.g., smooth contours at the object boundary), where C is the cost function, θ is the variable, and I is the image; and (3) minimize the cost function by iteratively moving down the gradient of the cost function: $\hat{\theta} = \arg\theta \min C(\theta; I)$. In early literature, the Snake method was applied to segmentation of the LV in cine MRI as well as in tagged MRI [20–24].

While Snake is a parametrized curve that iteratively updates itself by energy minimization, its upgraded version, the level set method, represents an unparametrized curve (or surface) [25]. Like the Snake, level set also minimizes an energy function composed of internal and external energy that exert both geometrical and locational constraints. Different from Snakes, however, the curve or surface is implicitly represented as the zero-level set in a higher-dimensional hypersurface, and for this reason, it allows more complex topology and produces more stable results in noise-corrupted situations. The level set method has gained much popularity around 2000, and many variants of the energy function aiming for higher accuracy and robustness were proposed to tackle the challenge of cine MRI segmentation [26–31]. By devising a composite energy function $C(\theta_{\text{endo}}, \theta_{\text{epi}}; I)$ where θ_{endo} parametrizes the endocardial contour and θ_{epi} the epicardial contour, the level set method was also used for simultaneous detection of the endocardial and epicardial contours. The cost function C can meanwhile encode the thickness information of the myocardium [29, 31].

Other popular image-based methods for cine MRI segmentation include morphological operation, graph cut, pixel classification, and clustering [32–36]. It is worth noting that most image-based methods are semiautomated, necessitating a proper initialization, and their results are heavily dependent on the quality of such an initialization. Although many methods worked well on the laboratory dataset, the applicability of such methods to an arbitrary CMR dataset in clinic was questionable. The results can be corrupted due to inappropriate initialization or local minima in optimization. Furthermore, given that the energy function is computed from local image patches, these methods lack a global view of the heart and may easily be trapped by local image artifacts which dominate the energy function. Despite the mathematical soundness of many image-based methods, this category of methods falls short in a real clinical scenario.

Model-Based Methods

With development of AI algorithms and computational power, model-based methods became popular in medical image analysis. Different from the methods that only use information from the image itself, model-based methods introduced the concept of "learning," i.e., they take into consideration not only the information from the given image but also from a priori knowledge of the object. In the active shape model (ASM) method, the shape space, defined as a low-dimensional manifold representing all plausible heart shapes, is learned from a set of aligned heart shapes from manual annotation [37]. This shape space can be derived, for example, by principle component analysis (PCA), a linear dimensionality reduction method that extracts the orthogonal principle components while preserving the largest variance. ASM characterizes the shape of the heart, with the number of principle components far smaller than the original dimensionality, thereby forming a well-constrained shape space. Therefore, when optimizing the cost function, the evolvement of a contour can be confined properly. ASM is therefore sometimes called a "smart Snake," as it can be seen as an active contour model with global shape constraints [37]. The optimization problem can now be expressed as $\hat{\theta} = \arg\theta \min C(\theta;I)$, subject to $\theta \in \Theta$, where Θ is the low-dimensional manifold. Optimization on the low-dimensional manifold largely mitigates the problem of purely image-based methods in which the resulting shape is globally unconstrained, reducing errors caused by local noise or artifact.

An upgraded version of ASM is called active appearance model (AAM), which integrates not only the shape (geometry) of the heart but also the appearance (texture) of the heart. Here "appearance" refers to the signal intensity pattern or distribution in the proximity of the object. AAM gives more constraints to characterize a plausible segmentation: not only the shape of the heart but also the appearance of the myocardium should satisfy a predefined model. In the literature, ASM, AAM, and their variants have been adopted to address the heart segmentation problem for cine MRI [38–41]. In addition, the model was often extended to the time dimension to further encode the variability of shape from cardiac motion [42–44].

With the introduction of prior knowledge on shape and appearance, ASM and AAM methods achieved great improvement compared to purely image-based methods. However, they are still insufficient to handle the extensive variability in functional CMR images. Practical issues further include the difficulty to parametrize the contour for hearts of different size, shape, and orientation, variability of appearance in image from different scanners, as well as the difficulty to properly initialize the segmentation in a fully automated manner. With the development of image registration technique, a more robust model-based method for functional CMR segmentation became popular, named multi-atlas segmentation. "Atlas" refers to a set of CMR images, each paired with its known (manual) segmentation. Atlas extends the information beyond shape and local appearance of the heart, to the content of the entire image (or volume). Given a set of atlases and a new dataset to be segmented, the multi-atlas method works as follows: (1) nonrigid image registration is applied to register the atlas image to the given image, (2) the atlas segmentation is propagated to the given image, and (3) multiple segmentations from Step 2 are synthesized for a final segmentation. Multi-atlas method is fully automated, initialization-free, and noise-insensitive, inheriting multiple advantages from nonrigid image registration techniques. In essence, the multi-atlas method also utilizes an a priori "model" but in a more implicit manner than ASM and AAM. Compared to ASM/AAM, it achieved further improved performance on heart segmentation for functional CMR [45–48].

Data-Based Methods

Data-based methods also rely on prior knowledge but are free of explicit models. They learn directly from much larger datasets than those used in model-based methods. Most data-based methods for CMR analysis are based on neural network, whose success is attributed to (1) the renaissance of convolutional neural network (CNN) that features two-dimensional input and deep architecture [49–51], (2) the development of graphic processing units (GPUs) that enables fast parallel computing, (3) the open-source platforms to realize the complex computation such as TensorFlow [52] and PyTorch [53], and (4) the accumulation of massive datasets in the digital era [54, 55]. For functional CMR, public databases also become available, including the Cardiac Atlas [45], Automated Cardiac Diagnosis Challenge (ACDC) [56], and Multi-Centre, Multi-Vendor & Multi-Disease Cardiac Image Segmentation Challenge (M&Ms) [57].

The rationale of data-based methods appears different from image-based and model-based methods, but it essentially remains an optimization problem with a cost to minimize. Given a set of training data, it optimizes the network parameters through minimization of a cost (more often referred to as "loss" in deep learning) function to map an input to an output [58]. The input of a deep learning CNN is typically an image or an image sequence, while the output can be flexibly defined: depending on the application, it can be a categorical label (classification), a quantitative number (regression), or an output image (segmentation, registration, synthesis). Following this new rationale, the functional CMR analysis problem can be formulated into building CNNs with dedicated loss functions: the input is the cine MRI or tagged MRI, while the output can be heart segmentation, myocardial strain, motion field, or even quantitative measurement (e.g., LVEF).

The main components of a CNN include (1) a well-designed CNN architecture, (2) a dedicated loss function (e.g., cross entropy for segmentation), and (3) an efficient optimizer. Based on the choice of the three components, a variety of CNNs can be built up to tackle the functional CMR analysis problem. Compared to previous methods, the formulation of optimization in data-based methods is simpler, as neither contour parametrization nor prior models are needed.

The simplicity in methodology and superiority in performance make CNN a popular tool for many medical image analysis tasks [15, 16, 59]. In recent years, a large number of CNN-based methods have been developed for functional CMR analysis. Early methods adopted pixel classification CNN, which classifies each pixel in a CMR image by evaluating their context (image patches) [60, 61]. Later work adopted more efficient network architectures such as the fully convolutional neural network (FCN) [62] and U-Net [63], both end-to-end CNNs. By learning from a high number of images with known annotation, the end-to-end CNN is able to perform the complex mapping directly from the original cine image to its segmentation. In [64] a FCN was used to segment both LV and RV from short axis cine MRI and outperformed traditional methods. In [65] the FCN model was applied to cine MRI data of the healthy population of the UK Biobank [66] from the same MRI vendor. In [67] the U-Net model was evaluated on multicenter, multi-vendor, and multi-pathology cine MRI data and demonstrated excellent performance on data of high variability. Representative examples are given in Fig. 33.1, showing the performance of such a well-trained U-Net on multiple-vendor, multicenter cine MRI datasets with substantial variability.

Later work along the line has focused on improvement of network architectures and loss functions. The work includes [20, 21] in which inception modules were introduced to extract features at different scale, [22] in which ResNet replaced the original network module, and [56, 68] in which improved loss functions of weighted Dice and focal loss were proposed. Given that cine MRI is a temporal sequence, and that the radiologists always view it in the cine mode, there are also research works incorporating the time dimension for more temporally coherent segmentation results through a cardiac cycle [69–73].

Despite the technical improvement on CNN architecture and loss function that are pushing further the limits of segmentation accuracy, it is noteworthy that the selection of well-balanced training data and high-quality annotation remains important [74]. In this light, recent development in deep learning research addresses the distribution shift problem by image normalization, transfer learning, and domain adaptation [74–78], and some latest studies adopt adversarial learning techniques to generate artificial training datasets to reduce the effort of extensive data collection and annotation [79, 80].

AI Methods for Functional Analysis: Cardiac Motion Tracking and Strain Analysis

Cardiac motion tracking is another important task for AI in functional CMR analysis. MR tagging technique uses special pulse sequences to spatially modulate the longitudinal magnetization in the myocardial tissue, such that the myocardial tissue is "tagged" hence its motion followed [6, 81–83]. Motion tracking can be performed visually or computationally on the tagged patterns. Recently, motion tracking is also performed directly from cine MRI sequences [84–87], for its ease of acquisition and analysis. With cardiac motion tracking, the myocardial strain and strain rate can be computed from the physical displacement [88]. We review in the following the classical motion tracking methods that dominate the last decades and introduce the latest new trend of data-based CNN methods.

Traditional Methods

There are two established techniques for automatic assessment of cardiac motion and strain [89]: displacement encoding with stimulated echoes (DENSE) [90] and harmonic phase (HARP) [82]. The basic principle of DENSE is a stimulated echo with a bipolar gradient, which directly encodes the motion into the phase of the MRI signal [90]. In comparison, HARP is a post-processing technique proposed for spatial modulation of magnetization (SPAMM) tagged images, and the rationale is that strain can be computed from the local spatial frequency of the tagged lines. HARP computes the spectral peaks in the Fourier domain and extracts motion information by phase demodulation.

In the literature, there is a body of AI methods for cardiac motion tracking. Prior to deep learning, these methods fall roughly into four categories: (1) Snake-based methods and AAM/ASM methods [21, 91–94], which localize the tags with internal and external constraints, (2) optical flow

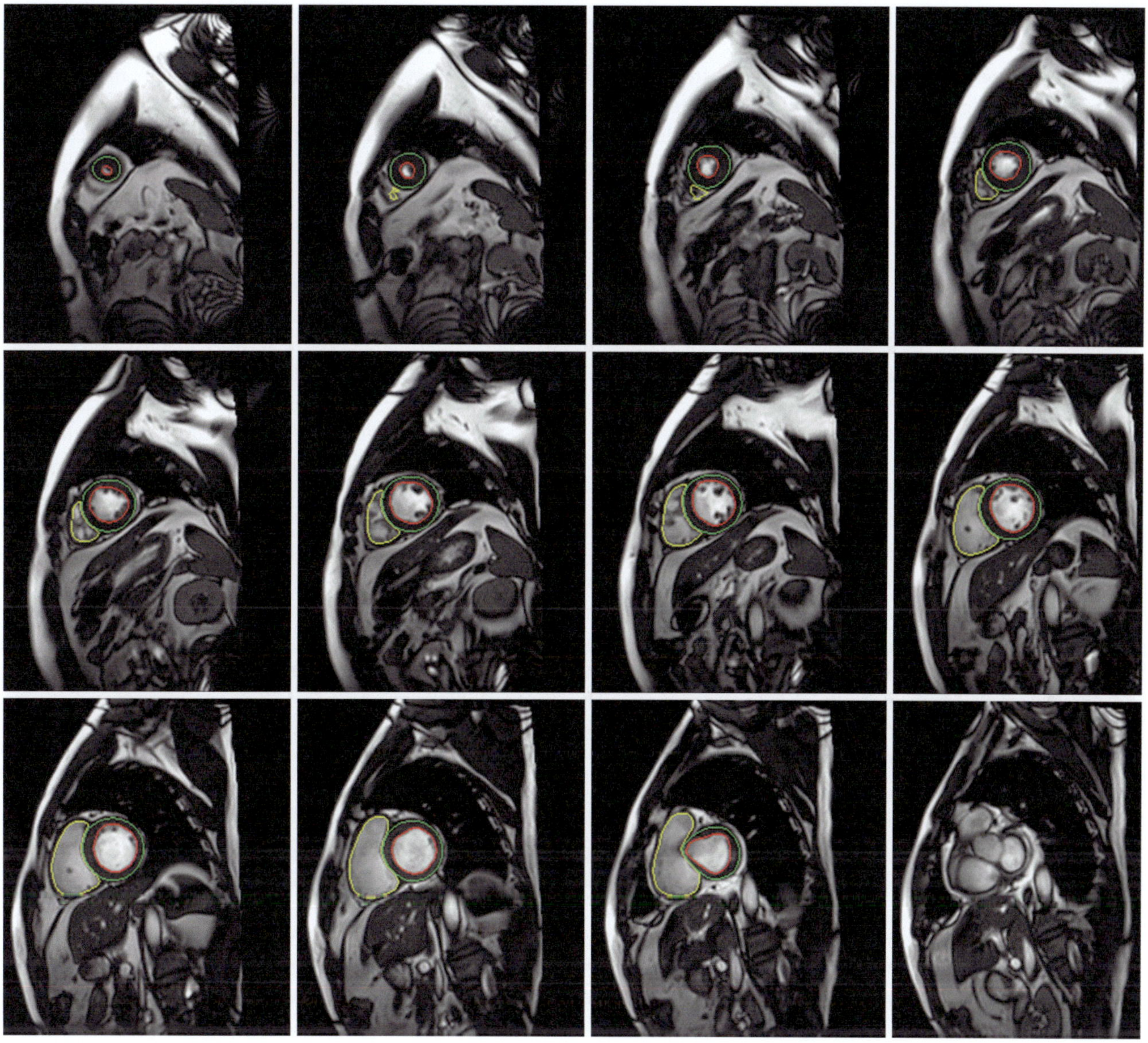

Fig. 33.1 An example of heart segmentation from cine MRI by the data-based method. All contours, including LV endocardial, epicardial, and RV endocardial contours, are fully automatically extracted by a trained U-Net. The method also correctly identifies the range of the heart till the aorta

methods [95, 96], which track the tagged patterns by formulating motion tracking as an optical flow problem [97], including the feature tracking (FT) method that was originally developed for speckle echocardiography and now adopted for cine MRI [84], (3) frequency analysis methods [98, 99], which convert the analysis into the Fourier domain, in a similar spirit as HARP [82], and (4) registration-based methods [100, 101], which matches the tagged pattern by nonrigid image registration [102]. In [101], the authors made a comprehensive comparison among the HARP, Snake, optical flow, and registration methods and concluded that the nonrigid registration method yielded the highest accuracy and robustness.

MR tagging is with limited use in clinical practice, due to restricted availability and lack of standardized analysis tools. Multiple recent studies have validated the use of SSFP cine sequences for motion tracking against the gold standard MR tagging [103, 104]. In the previous section, we have reviewed the mechanisms of AI methods for heart segmentation. Interestingly, many of the methods applied for heart segmentation can also be adapted for cardiac motion tracking. The image-based Snake methods and model-based ASM/AAM methods, for example, can be applied to all image frames in a cardiac cycle, and given that the contour points are parametrized, their correspondence at each cardiac phase can be obtained to track the motion of myocardium at both endocardial and epicardial border. The ASM/AAM can also be extended to an additional time dimension, which further models the shape and appearance variability from cardiac motion. The nonrigid registration method that was used in multi-atlas segmentation can also be applied to find the correspondence of contour location at different cardiac phases and hence track the cardiac motion.

CNN Methods

The latest development of deep learning CNN opens up new possibilities to automatically track cardiac motion. While it is not a common image classification or segmentation task, the flexibility of deep learning allows a "mapping" from a video input to a motion field output. In this framework, cardiac motion tracking can be formulated as identifying the optical flow through frames: to track myocardium edges and anatomical points through a cardiac cycle, using methods such as FlowNetS [105] and FlowNetC [106]. Compared to the original computer vision task to compute optical flow from unconstrained natural scenes, the myocardial motion tracking is a much more constrained problem. Training of the optical flow CNN can therefore be dedicated to cine MRI or tagged MRI. In [85] automated cardiac motion tracking by optical flow CNN was proposed, and its performance was compared to the traditional registration-based methods. The work showed that the CNN is able to track the cardiac motion with higher accuracy and much faster speed than the registration-based method, given that it is trained on a heterogeneous dataset covering a large range of cardiac pathologies. Registration can also be formulated as a regression problem with known motion from synthetic data for supervised training [107] or an amortized version of classical image registration in a fully unsupervised manner [108, 109]. In [110], a CNN framework was proposed to analyze cine MRI data and directly extract motion features to identify chronic myocardial infarction, using late gadolinium-enhanced (LGE) MRI as the gold standard. The study reported a relatively high accuracy in localizing myocardial infarct without the need of contrast agent. In [111], a CNN in combination with a recurrent NN (RNN) was proposed to fully automatically detect and track the tags from tagged MRI, enabling high-throughput image analysis with direct computation of myocardial strain.

AI Methods for Functional Analysis: Functional Parameter Estimation

Clinically relevant functional parameters include myocardial mass, thickness, stroke volume, LVEF, RVEF, longitudinal and circumferential strain, etc. Given that heart segmentation and cardiac motion tracking can be automatically obtained by AI methods, these parameters are readily computable. Studies have reported high accuracy and excellent correlation of AI-derived parameters compared to the manually derived ones [9, 65, 112, 113].

With the superior capability of deep learning CNNs to map any input to any output, there are interesting exploratory studies that directly extract the functional parameters from the original CMR images by regression [114–116]. In [114], a CNN architecture is proposed to directly map the original cine MRI to all structural and functional parameters without intermediate LV segmentation. The CNN architecture consists of an image autoencoder network that extracts the low-dimensional features from the cine MRI and a regression network that makes quantitative predictions from these features. The two networks are jointly optimized by the training data. This type of data-to-parameter mapping demonstrates the strong capability of deep learning methods to perform highly nonlinear and complex mapping and may parallel the way an experienced radiologist views a CMR exam: the radiologist would have an estimation of the stroke volume or LVEF just by looking at the cine CMR without any annotation. However, without intermediate segmentation results, such a method is very difficult to interpret or monitor.

Discussion

Despite decades of development and research, traditional AI methods had difficulties to tackle the high variability in clinical CMR. Today, deep learning has established as the state of the art for functional CMR, showing great promise to enter into clinical practice. The advantages of deep learning-based AI include accuracy, flexibility, and extremely fast computation.

In this chapter, instead of focusing only on data-based deep learning methods, we have reviewed a larger body of AI methods developed in the past decades, namely, image-based methods that only utilize the information from an image and model-based methods that integrate some a priori information. The evolution of AI methods clearly demonstrated the trend of increasing information integration. The manner to integrate a priori information also evolved, from explicit models to implicit models. We argue that the complexity of the CMR images can hardly be fully captured in an explicit model with a limited number of freedom; instead, a more appropriate way is the statistical learning approach covering the data distribution as much as possible from massive dataset.

Despite tremendous improvement of performance by deep learning methods, we note that there is a reduced degree of explainability and controllability, as data-based deep learning methods typically have millions of internal parameters that cannot be intuitively interpreted and conveniently adapted. This differs from the traditional methods such as

Snakes or ASM, in which the parameters are far fewer but have clear physical meanings and can be controlled and fine-tuned accordingly. The lack of explainability and controllability in data-based AI methods poses problems especially in applications related to clinical decisions, when the stakes are high for clinicians and patients. There is a body of research focusing on the explainability of deep CNNs in general [117–119]. In the future, explainability needs to be rigorously investigated specifically for clinical AI analysis tools.

Another weakness of data-based methods is their vulnerability to distribution shift. Deep learning is a statistical method with the underlying assumption that the data should be independent and identically distributed (i.i.d.). When this assumption is violated, i.e., the testing data has a different distribution than the training data, the results become highly unreliable. Sources of distribution shift include different MRI machines and protocols, different centers, and different patient cohorts. This independent and identically distributed assumption also explains the "bias" in data-based methods, as the CNN can only be as good as the data that it is trained on. Another intriguing issue of the deep learning CNN is that they can be susceptible to adversarial attack due to the extremely high freedom in the high-dimensional space [120]. Such weaknesses can negatively influence the practical applicability of CNN and introduce risks in high-stake applications. Recent work has started to focus on distribution shift and adversarial attack issues to address the weakness of deep CNNs from both practical and theoretical angles [74, 80, 118, 119, 121].

Given abovementioned limitations, for data-based AI tools to be deployed for functional CMR analysis in clinical practice, it remains crucial that the tools undergo rigorous validation on a broad and heterogeneous dataset. Furthermore, those AI tools that provide intermediate results (e.g., segmentation) are preferred over a black box, as the intermediate output provides explainability and controllability to an extent and can be easily inspected and manually corrected whenever necessary.

Despite AI's competence to accomplish many labor-intensive, well-defined analysis tasks such as segmentation and tracking, the human qualifications such as higher-level thinking, synthesis, and cognition in the presence of disturbances are still lacking in today's AI. Future developments call for close interdisciplinary collaboration among computer scientists, MRI physicists, radiologists, and cardiologists.

Conclusions

AI methods for functional CMR analysis have been an active research topic in the past three decades. In this chapter, we reviewed a broad range of AI methods developed for functional CMR analysis in a historical order, categorized into (1) image-based methods that only utilize the information from a given image, (2) model-based methods that integrate a priori information from a limited annotated dataset, and (3) data-based methods that learn from massive annotated dataset. For each category of AI methods, we present their high-level working principles and review relevant applications in the literature. The evolution of AI methods demonstrates an increasing trend of information integration and underlies the consistently improving performance. Today, AI for CMR analysis shows great promise to enter into clinical practice, while ongoing research will make AI more explainable, accountable, and controllable.

References

1. La Gerche A, Claessen G, Van de Bruaene A, Pattyn N, Van Cleemput J, Gewillig M, et al. Cardiac MRI: a new gold standard for ventricular volume quantification during high-intensity exercise. Circ Cardiovasc Imaging. 2013;6(2):329–38.
2. de Roos A, Higgins CB. Cardiac radiology: centenary review. Radiology. 2014;273(2 Suppl):S142–59.
3. Puntmann VO, Valbuena S, Hinojar R, Petersen SE, Greenwood JP, Kramer CM, et al. Society for Cardiovascular Magnetic Resonance (SCMR) expert consensus for CMR imaging endpoints in clinical research: part I – analytical validation and clinical qualification. J Cardiovasc Magn Reson [Internet]. 2018 Sep 20 [cited 2020 Nov 24];20. Available from: https://www.ncbi.nlm.nih.gov/pmc/articles/PMC6147157/.
4. Schulz-Menger J, Bluemke DA, Bremerich J, Flamm SD, Fogel MA, Friedrich MG, et al. Standardized image interpretation and post-processing in cardiovascular magnetic resonance - 2020 update. J Cardiovasc Magn Reson. 2020;22(1):19.
5. Kramer CM, Barkhausen J, Bucciarelli-Ducci C, Flamm SD, Kim RJ, Nagel E. Standardized cardiovascular magnetic resonance imaging (CMR) protocols: 2020 update. J Cardiovasc Magn Reson. 2020;22(1):17.
6. Ibrahim E-SH. Myocardial tagging by cardiovascular magnetic resonance: evolution of techniques–pulse sequences, analysis algorithms, and applications. J Cardiovasc Magn Reson. 2011;13(1):36.
7. Kang D, Woo J, Kuo CCJ, Slomka PJ, Dey D, Germano G. Heart chambers and whole heart segmentation techniques: review. JEI. 2012;21(1):010901.
8. Peng P, Lekadir K, Gooya A, Shao L, Petersen SE, Frangi AF. A review of heart chamber segmentation for structural and functional analysis using cardiac magnetic resonance imaging. MAGMA. 2016;29:155–95.
9. Tao Q, Lelieveldt BPF, van der Geest RJ. Deep learning for quantitative cardiac MRI. Am J Roentgenol. 2019;214(3):529–35.
10. Chen C, Qin C, Qiu H, Tarroni G, Duan J, Bai W, et al. Deep learning for cardiac image segmentation: a review. Front Cardiovasc Med [Internet]. 2020 Mar 5 [cited 2020 Nov 18];7. Available from: https://www.ncbi.nlm.nih.gov/pmc/articles/PMC7066212/.
11. Rosenblatt F. The perceptron: a probabilistic model for information storage and organization in the Brain. Psychol Rev. 1958;65:386.
12. Rochester N, Holland J, Haibt L, Duda W. Tests on a cell assembly theory of the action of the brain, using a large digital computer. IRE Trans Inform Theory. 1956;2(3):80–93.
13. LeCun Y, Bengio Y, Hinton G. Deep learning. Nature. 2015;521(7553):436–44.
14. Goodfellow I, Bengio Y, Courville A. Deep learning. Cambridge: The MIT Press; 2016. p. 775.

15. Shen D, Wu G, Suk H-I. Deep learning in medical image analysis. Annu Rev Biomed Eng. 2017;19(1):221–48.
16. Litjens G, Kooi T, Bejnordi BE, Setio AAA, Ciompi F, Ghafoorian M, et al. A survey on deep learning in medical image analysis. Med Image Anal. 2017;1(42):60–88.
17. Canny J. A computational approach to edge detection. IEEE Trans Pattern Anal Mach Intell. 1986;PAMI-8(6):679–98.
18. Geiger D, Gupta A, Costa LA, Vlontzos J. Dynamic programming for detecting, tracking, and matching deformable contours. IEEE Trans Pattern Anal Mach Intell. 1995;17(3):294–302.
19. Kass M, Witkin A, Terzopoulos D. Snakes: active contour models. Int J Comput Vis. 1988;1(4):321–31.
20. Lee H, Codella NCF, Cham MD, Weinsaft JW, Wang Y. Automatic left ventricle segmentation using iterative thresholding and an active contour model with adaptation on short-axis cardiac MRI. IEEE Trans Biomed Eng. 2010 Apr;57(4):905–13.
21. Guttman MA, Zerhouni EA, McVeigh ER. Analysis of cardiac function from MR images. IEEE Comput Graph Appl. 1997;17(1):30–8.
22. Kaushikkar SV, Li D, Haacke EM, Dávila-Román VG. Adaptive blood pool segmentation in three-dimensions: application to MR cardiac evaluation. J Magn Reson Imaging. 1996;6(4):690–7.
23. Hautvast G, Lobregt S, Breeuwer M, Gerritsen F. Automatic contour propagation in cine cardiac magnetic resonance images. IEEE Trans Med Imaging. 2006;25(11):1472–82.
24. Pluempitiwiriyawej C, Moura JMF, Fellow, Wu Y-JL, Ho C. STACS: new active contour scheme for cardiac MR image segmentation. IEEE Trans Med Imaging. 2005;24(5):593–603.
25. Osher S, Fedkiw R. Level set methods and dynamic implicit surfaces [internet]. New York: Springer New York; 2003 [cited 2015 Sep 14]. (Antman SS, Marsden JE, Sirovich L, editors. Applied Mathematical Sciences; vol. 153). Available from: http://link.springer.com/10.1007/b98879.
26. Paragios N. A variational approach for the segmentation of the left ventricle in cardiac image analysis. Int J Comput Vis. 2002;50(3):345–62.
27. Paragios N. A level set approach for shape-driven segmentation and tracking of the left ventricle. IEEE Trans Med Imaging. 2003;22(6):773–6.
28. Lynch M, Ghita O, Whelan PF. Left-ventricle myocardium segmentation using a coupled level-set with a priori knowledge. Comput Med Imaging Graph. 2006;30(4):255–62.
29. Liu Y, Captur G, Moon JC, Guo S, Yang X, Zhang S, et al. Distance regularized two level sets for segmentation of left and right ventricles from cine-MRI. Magn Reson Imaging. 2016;34(5):699–706.
30. Fritscher KD, Pilgram R, Schubert R. Automatic cardiac 4D segmentation using level sets. In: Frangi AF, Radeva PI, Santos A, Hernandez M, editors. Functional imaging and modeling of the heart. Berlin, Heidelberg: Springer; 2005. p. 113–22. (Lecture Notes in Computer Science).
31. Ji Y, Geest RJ van der, Nazarian S, Lelieveldt BPF, Tao Q. Advanced two-layer level set with a soft distance constraint for dual surfaces segmentation in medical images. In: Medical imaging 2018: image processing [Internet]. International Society for Optics and Photonics; 2018 [cited 2020 Nov 19]. p. 105743B. Available from: https://www.spiedigitallibrary.org/conference-proceedings-of-spie/10574/105743B/Advanced-two-layer-level-set-with-a-soft-distance-constraint/10.1117/12.2293246.short.
32. Boudraa A-E-O. Automated detection of the left ventricular region in magnetic resonance images by fuzzy C-means model. Int J Cardiovasc Imaging. 1997;13(4):347–55.
33. Cocosco CA, Niessen WJ, Netsch T, Vonken E-JPA, Lund G, Stork A, et al. Automatic image-driven segmentation of the ventricles in cardiac cine MRI. J Magn Reson Imaging. 2008;28(2):366–74.
34. Kurkure U, Pednekar A, Muthupillai R, Flamm SD, Kakadiaris Ast IA. Localization and segmentation of left ventricle in cardiac cine-MR images. IEEE Trans Biomed Eng. 2009;56(5):1360–70.
35. Albà X, Figueras I, Ventura RM, Lekadir K, Tobon-Gomez C, Hoogendoorn C, Frangi AF. Automatic cardiac LV segmentation in MRI using modified graph cuts with smoothness and interslice constraints. Magn Reson Med. 2013;72:1775.
36. Uzkent B, Hoffman MJ, Cherry E, Cahill N. 3-D MRI cardiac segmentation using graph cuts. In: 2014 IEEE Western New York Image and Signal Processing Workshop (WNYISPW). Rochester, NY, USA; 2014. p. 47–51.
37. Cootes TF, Taylor CJ, Cooper DH, Graham J. Active shape models-their training and application. Comput Vis Image Underst. 1995;61(1):38–59.
38. Mitchell SC, Bosch JG, Lelieveldt BPF, van der Geest RJ, Reiber JHC, Sonka M. 3-D active appearance models: segmentation of cardiac MR and ultrasound images. IEEE Trans Med Imaging. 2002;21(9):1167–78.
39. Mitchell SC, Lelieveldt BP, van der Geest RJ, Bosch HG, Reiber JH, Sonka M. Multistage hybrid active appearance model matching: segmentation of left and right ventricles in cardiac MR images. IEEE Trans Med Imaging. 2001;20(5):415–23.
40. Uzümcü M, van der Geest RJ, Sonka M, Lamb HJ, Reiber JHC, Lelieveldt BPF. Multiview active appearance models for simultaneous segmentation of cardiac 2- and 4-chamber long-axis magnetic resonance images. Investig Radiol. 2005;40(4):195–203.
41. Zhang H, Wahle A, Johnson RK, Scholz TD, Sonka M. 4-D cardiac MR image analysis: left and right ventricular morphology and function. IEEE Trans Med Imaging. 2010 Feb;29(2):350–64.
42. Lelieveldt BPF, van der Geest RJ, Reiber JHC, Bosch JG, Mitchell SC, Sonka M. Time-continuous segmentation of cardiac image sequences using active appearance motion models. In: Insana MF, Leahy RM, editors. Information processing in medical imaging. Berlin, Heidelberg: Springer; 2001. p. 446–52. (Lecture Notes in Computer Science).
43. Mitchell SC, Lelieveldt BPF, Geest RJ van der, Bosch HG, Reiber JHC, Sonka M. Time-continuous segmentation of cardiac MR image sequences using active appearance motion models. In: Medical imaging 2001: image processing [Internet]. International Society for Optics and Photonics; 2001 [cited 2020 Nov 21]. p. 249–56. Available from: https://www.spiedigitallibrary.org/conference-proceedings-of-spie/4322/0000/Time-continuous-segmentation-of-cardiac-MR-image-sequences-using-active/10.1117/12.431094.short.
44. Stegmann MB, Pedersen D. Bi-temporal 3D active appearance models with applications to unsupervised ejection fraction estimation. In: Medical imaging 2005: image processing [Internet]. International Society for Optics and Photonics; 2005 [cited 2020 Nov 21]. p. 336–50. Available from: https://www.spiedigitallibrary.org/conference-proceedings-of-spie/5747/0000/Bi-temporal-3D-active-appearance-models-with-applications-to-unsupervised/10.1117/12.594930.short.
45. Lorenzo-Valdés M, Sanchez-Ortiz GI, Mohiaddin R, Rueckert D. Atlas-based segmentation and tracking of 3D cardiac MR images using non-rigid registration. In: Dohi T, Kikinis R, editors. Medical Image Computing and Computer-Assisted Intervention — MICCAI 2002. Berlin, Heidelberg: Springer; 2002. p. 642–50. (Lecture Notes in Computer Science).
46. Zhuang X, Hawkes DJ, Crum WR, Boubertakh R, Uribe S, Atkinson D, et al. Robust registration between cardiac MRI images and atlas for segmentation propagation. In: Medical imaging 2008: image processing [Internet]. International Society for Optics and Photonics; 2008 [cited 2020 Nov 21]. p. 691408. Available from: https://www.spiedigitallibrary.

org/conference-proceedings-of-spie/6914/691408/Robust-registration-between-cardiac-MRI-images-and-atlas-for-segmentation/10.1117/12.769445.short.

47. Zhuang X, Rhode KS, Razavi RS, Hawkes DJ, Ourselin S. A registration-based propagation framework for automatic whole heart segmentation of cardiac MRI. IEEE Trans Med Imaging. 2010;29(9):1612–25.
48. Shahzad R, Tao Q, Dzyubachyk O, Staring M, Lelieveldt BPF, van der Geest RJ. Fully-automatic left ventricular segmentation from long-axis cardiac cine MR scans. Med Image Anal. 2017;39:44–55.
49. LeCun Y, Boser B, Denker JS, Henderson D, Howard RE, Hubbard W, et al. Backpropagation applied to handwritten zip code recognition. Neural Comput. 1989;1(4):541–51.
50. He K, Zhang X, Ren S, Sun J. Deep residual learning for image recognition. In: 2016 IEEE Conference on Computer Vision and Pattern Recognition (CVPR). Las Vegas, NV, USA; 2016. p. 770–8.
51. Huang G, Liu Z, Maaten LVD, Weinberger KQ. Densely connected convolutional networks. In: 2017 IEEE Conference on Computer Vision and Pattern Recognition (CVPR). Honolulu, HI, USA; 2017. p. 2261–9.
52. Abadi M, Agarwal A, Barham P, Brevdo E, Chen Z, Citro C, et al. TensorFlow: large-scale machine learning on heterogeneous distributed systems. 2015 [cited 2018 Feb 14]; Available from: https://research.google.com/pubs/pub45166.html.
53. Introduction to PyTorch — PyTorch Tutorials 1.7.0 documentation [Internet]. [cited 2020 Nov 28]. Available from: https://pytorch.org/tutorials/beginner/nlp/pytorch_tutorial.html.
54. Deng J, Dong W, Socher R, Li L, Kai Li, Li Fei-Fei. ImageNet: a large-scale hierarchical image database. In: 2009 IEEE conference on computer vision and pattern recognition. Miami, FL, USA; 2009. p. 248–255.
55. Russakovsky O, Deng J, Su H, Krause J, Satheesh S, Ma S, et al. ImageNet large scale visual recognition challenge. Int J Comput Vis. 2015;115(3):211–52.
56. Bernard O, Lalande A, Zotti C, Cervenansky F, Yang X, Heng P-A, et al. Deep learning techniques for automatic MRI cardiac multi-structures segmentation and diagnosis: is the problem solved? IEEE Trans Med Imaging. 2018;37(11):2514–25.
57. Scannell CM, Chiribiri A, Veta M. Domain-adversarial learning for multi-centre, multi-vendor, and multi-disease cardiac mr image segmentation. arXiv:200811776 [cs, eess] [Internet]. 2020 Aug 26 [cited 2020 Nov 24]; Available from: http://arxiv.org/abs/2008.11776.
58. Rumelhart DE, Hinton GE, Williams RJ. Learning representations by back-propagating errors. Nature. 1986;323(6088):533.
59. Zhou SK, Greenspan H, Davatzikos C, Duncan JS, van Ginneken B, Madabhushi A, et al. A review of deep learning in medical imaging: Image traits, technology trends, case studies with progress highlights, and future promises. arXiv:200809104 [cs, eess] [Internet]. 2020 Aug 2 [cited 2020 Nov 26]; Available from: http://arxiv.org/abs/2008.09104.
60. Avendi MR, Kheradvar A, Jafarkhani H. A combined deep-learning and deformable-model approach to fully automatic segmentation of the left ventricle in cardiac MRI. Med Image Anal. 2016;30:108–19.
61. Kamnitsas K, Ledig C, Newcombe VFJ, Simpson JP, Kane AD, Menon DK, et al. Efficient multi-scale 3D CNN with fully connected CRF for accurate brain lesion segmentation. Med Image Anal. 2017;36:61–78.
62. Long J, Shelhamer E, Darrell T. Fully convolutional networks for semantic segmentation. arXiv:14114038 [cs] [Internet]. 2015 Mar 8 [cited 2020 Nov 17]; Available from: http://arxiv.org/abs/1411.4038.
63. Ronneberger O, Fischer P, Brox T. U-Net: convolutional networks for biomedical image segmentation. In: Navab N, Hornegger J, Wells WM, Frangi AF, editors. Medical Image Computing and Computer-Assisted Intervention – MICCAI 2015. Springer International Publishing; 2015. p. 234–41. (Lecture Notes in Computer Science).
64. Tran PV. A fully convolutional neural network for cardiac segmentation in short-axis MRI. arXiv:160400494 [cs] [Internet]. 2017 Apr 26 [cited 2020 Nov 17]; Available from: http://arxiv.org/abs/1604.00494.
65. Bai W, Sinclair M, Tarroni G, Oktay O, Rajchl M, Vaillant G, et al. Automated cardiovascular magnetic resonance image analysis with fully convolutional networks. J Cardiovasc Magn Reson. 2018;20(1):65.
66. Sudlow C, Gallacher J, Allen N, Beral V, Burton P, Danesh J, et al. UK biobank: an open access resource for identifying the causes of a wide range of complex diseases of middle and old age. PLoS Med. 2015;12(3):e1001779.
67. Tao Q, Yan W, Wang Y, Paiman EHM, Shamonin DP, Garg P, et al. Deep learning-based method for fully automatic quantification of left ventricle function from cine MR images: a multivendor, multicenter study. Radiology. 2019;290(1):81–8.
68. Yang X, Bian C, Yu L, Ni D, Heng P-A. Class-balanced deep neural network for automatic ventricular structure segmentation. In: Pop M, Sermesant M, Jodoin P-M, Lalande A, Zhuang X, Yang G, et al., editors. Statistical atlases and computational models of the heart ACDC and MMWHS challenges. Cham: Springer International Publishing; 2018. p. 152–60. (Lecture Notes in Computer Science).
69. Poudel RPK, Lamata P, Montana G. Recurrent fully convolutional neural networks for multi-slice MRI cardiac segmentation. arXiv:160803974 [cs, stat] [Internet]. 2016 Aug 13; Available from: http://arxiv.org/abs/1608.03974.
70. Yan W, Wang Y, Li Z, van der Geest RJ, Tao Q. Left ventricle segmentation via optical-flow-net from short-axis cine MRI: preserving the temporal coherence of cardiac motion. Medical Image Computing and Computer-Assisted Intervention – MICCAI 2018. p. 613–321.
71. Savioli N, Vieira MS, Lamata P, Montana G. Automated segmentation on the entire cardiac cycle using a deep learning work-flow. In: 2018 Fifth International Conference on Social Networks Analysis, Management and Security (SNAMS). Valencia, Spain; 2018. p. 153–158.
72. Yan W, Wang Y, van der Geest RJ, Tao Q. Cine MRI analysis by deep learning of optical flow: adding the temporal dimension. Comput Biol Med. 2019;1(111):103356.
73. Luo C, Shi C, Li X, Gao D. Cardiac MR segmentation based on sequence propagation by deep learning. PLoS One. 2020;15(4):e0230415.
74. Yan W, Huang L, Xia L, Gu S, Yan F, Wang Y, et al. MRI manufacturer shift and adaptation: increasing the generalizability of deep learning segmentation for MR images acquired with different scanners. Radiology Artif Intell. 2020;2(4):e190195.
75. Vesal S, Ravikumar N, Maier A. Automated multi-sequence cardiac MRI segmentation using supervised domain adaptation. arXiv:190807726 [cs, eess]. 2020;12009:300–308.
76. Yan W, Wang Y, Xia M, Tao Q. Edge-guided output adaptor: highly efficient adaptation module for cross-vendor medical image segmentation. IEEE Signal Proc Lett. 2019;26(11):1593–7.
77. Chen C, Bai W, Davies RH, Bhuva AN, Manisty CH, Augusto JB, et al. Improving the generalizability of convolutional neural network-based segmentation on CMR images. Front Cardiovasc Med [Internet] 2020 [cited 2020 Nov 22];7. Available from: https://www.frontiersin.org/articles/10.3389/fcvm.2020.00105/full.
78. Wang J, Huang H, Chen C, Ma W, Huang Y, Ding X. Multi-sequence cardiac MR segmentation with adversarial domain adaptation network. arXiv:191012514 [cs, eess] [Internet]. 2019

Oct 28 [cited 2020 Nov 22]; Available from: http://arxiv.org/abs/1910.12514.
79. Chaitanya K, Karani N, Baumgartner C, Donati O, Becker A, Konukoglu E. Semi-supervised and task-driven data augmentation. arXiv:190205396 [cs, stat] [Internet] 2019 Feb 28 [cited 2020 Nov 22]; Available from: http://arxiv.org/abs/1902.05396.
80. Chen C, Qin C, Qiu H, Ouyang C, Wang S, Chen L, et al. Realistic Adversarial Data Augmentation for MR Image Segmentation. In: Martel AL, Abolmaesumi P, Stoyanov D, Mateus D, Zuluaga MA, Zhou SK, et al., editors. Medical Image Computing and Computer Assisted Intervention – MICCAI 2020. Cham: Springer International Publishing; 2020. p. 667–77. (Lecture Notes in Computer Science).
81. Zerhouni EA, Parish DM, Rogers WJ, Yang A, Shapiro EP. Human heart: tagging with MR imaging–a method for noninvasive assessment of myocardial motion. Radiology 1988 169(1):59–63.
82. Osman NF, Kerwin WS, McVeigh ER, Prince JL. Cardiac motion tracking using CINE harmonic phase (HARP) magnetic resonance imaging. Magn Reson Med. 1999;42(6):1048–60.
83. Moore CC, McVeigh ER, Zerhouni EA. Quantitative tagged magnetic resonance imaging of the normal human left ventricle. Top Magn Reson Imaging. 2000;11(6):359–71.
84. Pedrizzetti G, Claus P, Kilner PJ, Nagel E. Principles of cardiovascular magnetic resonance feature tracking and echocardiographic speckle tracking for informed clinical use. J Cardiovasc Mag Res [Internet] 2016 Dec [cited 2017 Aug 21];18(1). Available from: http://jcmr-online.biomedcentral.com/articles/10.1186/s12968-016-0269-7.
85. Qiao M, Wang Y, Guo Y, Huang L, Xia L, Tao Q. Temporally coherent cardiac motion tracking from cine MRI: traditional registration method and modern CNN method. Med Phys. 2020;47:4189.
86. Obokata M, Nagata Y, Wu VC-C, Kado Y, Kurabayashi M, Otsuji Y, et al. Direct comparison of cardiac magnetic resonance feature tracking and 2D/3D echocardiography speckle tracking for evaluation of global left ventricular strain. Eur Heart J Cardiovasc Imaging. 2016;17(5):525–32.
87. Wu L, Germans T, Güçlü A, Heymans MW, Allaart CP, van Rossum AC. Feature tracking compared with tissue tagging measurements of segmental strain by cardiovascular magnetic resonance. J Cardiovasc Magn Reson. 2014;16(1):10.
88. Amzulescu MS, De Craene M, Langet H, Pasquet A, Vancraeynest D, Pouleur AC, et al. Myocardial strain imaging: review of general principles, validation, and sources of discrepancies. Eur Heart J Cardiovasc Imaging. 2019;20(6):605–19.
89. Kuijer JPA, Hofman MBM, Zwanenburg JJM, Marcus JT, van Rossum AC, Heethaar RM. DENSE and HARP: two views on the same technique of phase-based strain imaging. J Magn Reson Imaging. 2006;24(6):1432–8.
90. Aletras AH, Ding S, Balaban RS, Wen H. DENSE: displacement encoding with stimulated echoes in cardiac functional MRI. J Magn Reson. 1999;137(1):247–52.
91. Amini AA, Chen Y, Curwen RW, Mani V, Sun J. Coupled B-snake grids and constrained thin-plate splines for analysis of 2-D tissue deformations from tagged MRI. IEEE Trans Med Imaging. 1998;17(3):344–56.
92. Guttman MA, Prince JL, McVeigh ER. Tag and contour detection in tagged MR images of the left ventricle. IEEE Trans Med Imaging. 1994;13(1):74–88.
93. Suinesiaputra A, Frangi AF, Kaandorp TAM, Lamb HJ, Bax JJ, Reiber JHC, et al. Automated detection of regional wall motion abnormalities based on a statistical model applied to multislice short-axis cardiac MR images. IEEE Trans Med Imaging. 2009;28(4):595–607.
94. Suinesiaputra A, McCulloch AD, Nash MP, Pontre B, Young AA. Cardiac image modelling: breadth and depth in heart disease. Med Image Anal. 2016;33:38–43.
95. Prince JL, Gupta SN, Osman NF. Bandpass optical flow for tagged MRI. Med Phys. 2000;27(1):108–18.
96. Carranza-Herrezuelo N, Bajo A, Sroubek F, Santamarta C, Cristobal G, Santos A, et al. Motion estimation of tagged cardiac magnetic resonance images using variational techniques. Comput Med Imaging Graph. 2010;34(6):514–22.
97. Beauchemin SS, Barron JL. The computation of optical flow. ACM Comput Surv. 1995;27(3):433–66.
98. Zhang S, Douglas MA, Yaroslavsky L, Summers RM, Dilsizian V, Fananapazir L, et al. A Fourier based algorithm for tracking SPAMM tags in gated magnetic resonance cardiac images. Med Phys. 1996;23(8):1359–69.
99. Clarysse P, Basset C, Khouas L, Croisille P, Friboulet D, Odet C, et al. Two-dimensional spatial and temporal displacement and deformation field fitting from cardiac magnetic resonance tagging. Med Image Anal. 2000;4(3):253–68.
100. Rougon N, Petitjean C, Prêteux F, Cluzel P, Grenier P. A non-rigid registration approach for quantifying myocardial contraction in tagged MRI using generalized information measures. Med Image Anal. 2005;9(4):353–75.
101. Smal I, Carranza-Herrezuelo N, Klein S, Niessen W, Meijering E. Quantitative comparison of tracking methods for motion analysis in tagged MRI. In: 2011 IEEE international symposium on biomedical imaging: from nano to macro. Chicago, IL, USA; 2011. p. 345–348.
102. Viergever MA, Maintz JBA, Klein S, Murphy K, Staring M, Pluim JPW. A survey of medical image registration – under review. Med Image Anal. 2016;1(33):140–4.
103. Hor KN, Gottliebson WM, Carson C, Wash E, Cnota J, Fleck R, et al. Comparison of magnetic resonance feature tracking for strain calculation with harmonic phase imaging analysis. JACC Cardiovasc Imaging. 2010;3(2):144–51.
104. Cao JJ, Ngai N, Duncanson L, Cheng J, Gliganic K, Chen Q. A comparison of both DENSE and feature tracking techniques with tagging for the cardiovascular magnetic resonance assessment of myocardial strain. J Cardiovasc Magn Reson [Internet]. 2018 Apr 19 [cited 2020 Nov 24];20. Available from: https://www.ncbi.nlm.nih.gov/pmc/articles/PMC5907464/.
105. Fischer P, Dosovitskiy A, Ilg E, Häusser P, Hazırbaş C, Golkov V, et al. FlowNet: learning optical flow with convolutional networks. arXiv:150406852 [cs] [Internet]. 2015 May 4 [cited 2020 Nov 24]; Available from: http://arxiv.org/abs/1504.06852.
106. Ilg E, Mayer N, Saikia T, Keuper M, Dosovitskiy A, Brox T. FlowNet 2.0: evolution of optical flow estimation with deep networks. arXiv:161201925 [cs] [Internet]. 2016 Dec 6 [cited 2020 Nov 24]; Available from: http://arxiv.org/abs/1612.01925.
107. Morales MA, Izquierdo-Garcia D, Aganj I, Kalpathy-Cramer J, Rosen BR, Catana C. Implementation and validation of a three-dimensional cardiac motion estimation network. Radiology Artif Intell. 2019;1(4):e180080.
108. Balakrishnan G, Zhao A, Sabuncu MR, Dalca AV, Guttag J. An unsupervised learning model for deformable medical image registration. In: 2018 IEEE/CVF conference on computer vision and pattern recognition. 2018. p. 9252–9260.
109. de Vos BD, Berendsen FF, Viergever MA, Staring M, Išgum I. End-to-end unsupervised deformable image registration with a convolutional neural network. arXiv:170406065 [cs]. 2017;10553:204–212.
110. Zhang N, Yang G, Gao Z, Xu C, Zhang Y, Shi R, et al. Deep learning for diagnosis of chronic myocardial infarction on nonenhanced cardiac cine MRI. Radiology. 2019;291(3):606–17.
111. Ferdian E, Suinesiaputra A, Fung K, Aung N, Lukaschuk E, Barutcu A, et al. Fully automated myocardial strain estimation from cardiovascular MRI–tagged images using a deep learning framework in the UK biobank. Radiology: Cardiothoracic Imaging. 2020;2(1):e190032.

112. Leiner T, Rueckert D, Suinesiaputra A, Baeßler B, Nezafat R, Išgum I, et al. Machine learning in cardiovascular magnetic resonance: basic concepts and applications. J Cardiovasc Magn Reson. 2019;21(1):61.
113. Colletti PM. Deep learning for cardiac MRI: the time has come. Radiology. 2018;290(1):89.
114. Xue W, Lum A, Mercado A, Landis M, Warringto J, Li S. Full quantification of left ventricle via deep multitask learning network respecting intra- and inter-task relatedness. arXiv:170601912 [cs] [Internet]. 2017 Jun 6; Available from: http://arxiv.org/abs/1706.01912.
115. Wang W, Wang Y, Wu Y, Lin T, Li S, Chen B. Quantification of full left ventricular metrics via deep regression learning with contour-guidance. IEEE Access. 2019;7:47918–28.
116. Du X, Zhang W, Zhang H, Chen J, Zhang Y, Warrington JC, et al. Deep regression segmentation for cardiac bi-ventricle MR images. IEEE Access. 2018;6:3828–38.
117. Zhang Q, Zhu S-C. Visual interpretability for deep learning: a survey. arXiv:180200614 [cs] [Internet]. 2018 Feb 7 [cited 2020 Nov 28]; Available from: http://arxiv.org/abs/1802.00614.
118. Singh A, Sengupta S, Lakshminarayanan V. Explainable deep learning models in medical image analysis. arXiv:200513799 [cs, eess] [Internet]. 2020 May 28 [cited 2020 Nov 24]; Available from: http://arxiv.org/abs/2005.13799.
119. Zheng Q, Delingette H, Ayache N. Explainable cardiac pathology classification on cine MRI with motion characterization by semi-supervised learning of apparent flow. Med Image Anal. 2019;1(56):80–95.
120. Goodfellow I, Pouget-Abadie J, Mirza M, Xu B, Warde-Farley D, Ozair S, et al. Generative adversarial nets. In: Ghahramani Z, Welling M, Cortes C, Lawrence ND, Weinberger KQ, editors. Advances in neural information processing systems 27 [Internet]. Curran Associates, Inc.; 2014 [cited 2019 Oct 10]. p. 2672–80. Available from: http://papers.nips.cc/paper/5423-generative-adversarial-nets.pdf.
121. Liu X, Thermos S, Chartsias A, O'Neil A, Tsaftaris SA. Disentangled representations for domain-generalized cardiac segmentation. arXiv:200811514 [cs, eess] [Internet]. 2020 Aug 26 [citeed 2020 Nov 24]; Available from: http://arxiv.org/abs/2008.11514.

Magnetic Resonance Imaging-Based 4D Flow: The Role of Artificial Intelligence

34

Eva S. Peper, Sebastian Kozerke, and Pim van Ooij

Introduction

Since its advent in the mid-1990s [1], 4D flow MRI has developed into an attractive tool for the multidimensional assessment of hemodynamics (dynamics of blood flow) in a wide variety of cardiovascular diseases. In 4D flow MRI, motion-sensitive MRI gradients and ECG gating are employed to measure the time-resolved velocity vector fields of blood flow in a volume of interest.

The sequence provides three series of 3D and time-resolved (=4D) anatomical images (consisting of the MRI signal magnitude) and velocity images (consisting of the difference between multiple MRI signal phases) for each principal directions [2]. From the velocity images, three-dimensional velocity vectors can be reconstructed for each voxel (3D pixel). Air (lungs and body surroundings) encoded as noise in the phase images and static tissue should have a velocity of zero, while the magnitude and direction of the velocity of moving tissue can be quantified and visualized by the reconstructed vector. By displaying the volumetric velocity vectors over time, the behavior of blood flow over the cardiac cycle can be visualized, and the differences between healthy and diseased flow and velocity can be studied. Furthermore, the fully quantitative nature of 4D flow MRI allows derivation of other parameters that are relevant for insights in pathological hemodynamic alterations such as wall shear stress (WSS), pulse wave velocity, (turbulent) kinetic energy, viscous energy loss, and pressure difference.

4D flow MRI has proven useful in several cardiothoracic diseases. For example, 4D flow MRI is suited for the quantification of regurgitant flow over the heart valves [3, 4] and has been used to describe abnormal left ventricular hemodynamics in hypertrophic [5, 6] and dilated cardiomyopathy [7]. In patients with atrial fibrillation, it was found that lower blood flow velocities in the left atrium correlated with an increased risk for stroke [8]. In patients with chronic obstructive pulmonary disease (COPD), retrograde flow in the superior vena cava was associated with emphysema [9]. Patients with pulmonary hypertension had higher right ventricular 4D flow MRI-derived kinetic energy and higher viscous energy loss in the pulmonary arteries than healthy subjects [10]. Furthermore, aortic WSS, the shear force of blood flow on the vessel wall, was higher than normal in patients with bicuspid aortic valves and aortic valve stenosis [11], which was associated with elastic fiber thinning in the aortic wall [12, 13]. Lastly, in patients with Marfan syndrome, 4D flow MRI-derived pulse wave velocity and thus aortic stiffness were high [14], and subtle abnormal hemodynamic properties are present at a young age in the proximal descending aorta which is a known location for vessel wall rupture [15, 16].

The comprehensive but complex acquisition and data processing methods for 4D flow MRI come with several drawbacks that hinder an efficient clinical workflow: (1) acquisition times are long on the order of 15–30 minutes, (2) image reconstruction times are long on the order of 15 minutes, (3) vessel segmentation processes are manual or semi-automatic at best and therefore time-consuming, and (4) measurement noise and artifacts compromise 4D flow MRI data consistency. Many research groups worldwide are investigating methods to overcome these drawbacks, many of which are based on artificial intelligence, e.g., machine learning, the study of computer algorithms to, in this case, automate workflows and improve image reconstruction and

E. S. Peper, PhD · S. Kozerke, PhD
Institute for Biomedical Engineering, ETH Zurich and University Zurich, Zurich, Switzerland
e-mail: peper@biomed.ee.ethz.ch; kozerke@biomed.ee.ethz.ch

P. van Ooij, PhD (✉)
Department of Radiology & Nuclear Medicine, Amsterdam University Medical Centers, Location AMC, Amsterdam, The Netherlands

Department of Pediatric Cardiology, Wilhelmina Children's Hospital, University Medical Center Utrecht, Utrecht, The Netherlands
e-mail: p.vanooij@amsterdamumc.nl

C. N. De Cecco et al. (eds.), *Artificial Intelligence in Cardiothoracic Imaging*, Contemporary Medical Imaging,
https://doi.org/10.1007/978-3-030-92087-6_34

data inference in the presence of random and systematic measurement errors.

In this chapter, we (1) review the MRI physics and techniques behind 4D flow MRI and recent improvements, (2) discuss reconstruction and segmentation algorithms and how machine learning can improve these, (3) discuss machine learning algorithms to improve image quality, (4) discuss basic visualization and hemodynamic quantification methods, and (5) give an overview of the current clinical relevance of 4D flow MRI-derived parameters.

4D Flow MRI Acquisition

Encoding Strategies

4D flow MRI encodes motion of magnetization along three spatial directions in a 3D and time-resolved domain. This is done by applying additional, motion-sensitive gradients of a bipolar shape to the regular sequence Scheme [17, 18]. Bipolar gradients, shown in Fig. 34.1a, will lead to a phase accumulation for moving spins proportional to the velocity with which they travel along the gradients' direction. Stationary spins in contrast will accumulate a phase during the first gradient lobe, which is compensated for in the second lobe, leading to a net phase accumulation of zero if field inhomogeneity is ignored. The phase accumulation ϕ over time t after applying the gradient G along direction x can be written as $\phi(t)=\gamma\int G_x(\tau)x(\tau)d\tau$, where γ denotes the gyromagnetic ratio. Approximating the particle position $x(\tau)$ using Taylor expansion, this equation can be rewritten as

$$\phi(t)=\gamma x_0\int_0^t G_x(\tau)d\tau+\gamma v_0\int_0^t G_x(\tau)\tau d\tau + \frac{\gamma}{2}a_0\int_0^t G_x(\tau)\tau^2 d\tau+\ldots$$

with x_0, v_0, and a_0 being position, velocity, and acceleration along the applied gradient direction at the expansion point. Constant acceleration can be disregarded if the expansion point is set to be at the center of gravity of the bipolar gradient. The gradient moments, defined as $m_{n,x}=\int G_x(\tau)\tau^n d\tau$, describe the accumulated phase for stationary and moving spins. For stationary spins, the accumulated phase is 0, with m_0 and v_0 being zero too. For moving spins, the accumulated phase is, under the aforementioned assumptions, proportional to v_0 and the first moment m_1, $\phi(t)=\gamma v_0 m_{1,x}=\gamma v_0\int_0 G_x(\tau)\tau d\tau=\gamma v_0 At$ with gradient area A, as shown in Fig. 34.1b. Flow encoding strategies can also be combined with flow compensation to minimize flow artifacts.

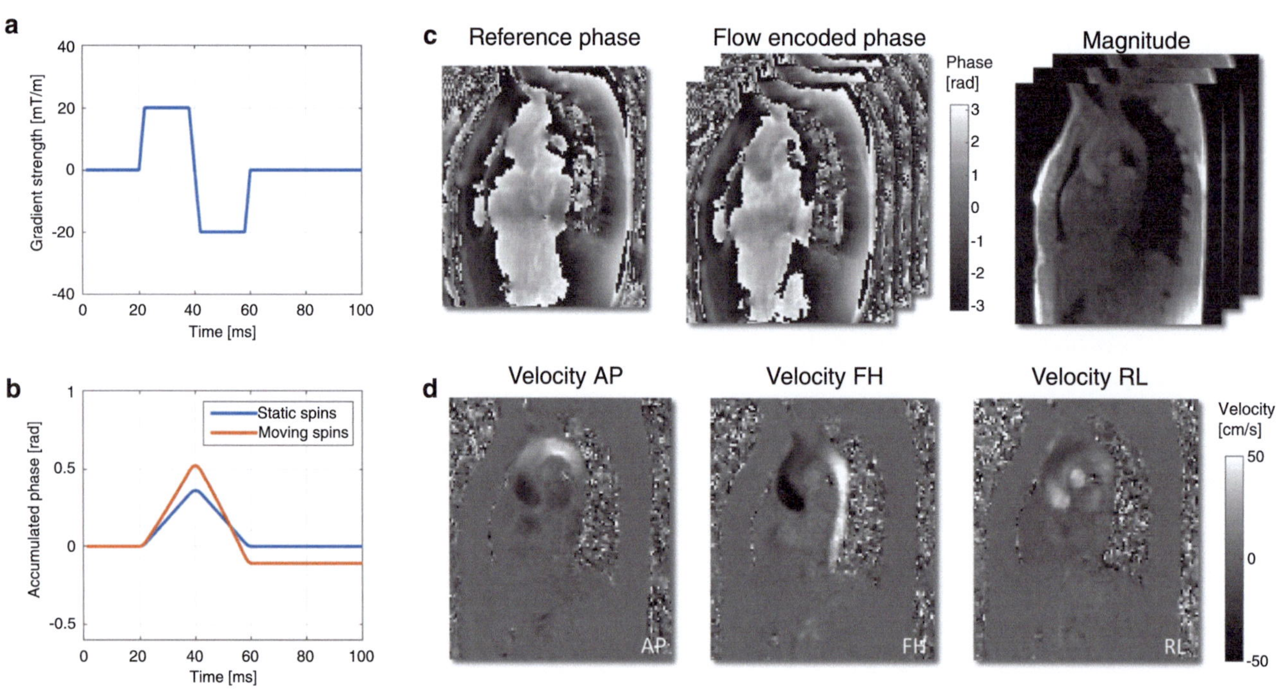

Fig. 34.1 (**a**) Bipolar gradients applied along one direction. (**b**) Phase accumulation for static spins and for spins moving along the gradients' direction. (**c**) Phase images (including phase wraps due to additional background phase) of a reference and the flow-encoded scans as well as corresponding magnitude images. (**d**) Phase difference images or – after scaling with the VENC – velocity maps, resulting from subtracting the flow-encoded phase from the reference phase. This is done for each flow encoding gradient directions separately

As the accumulated phase includes contributions from the background phase, typically, in so-called referenced (or non-balanced) flow encoding schemes, a separate measurement is done, which does not include any motion-encoding gradients (Fig. 34.1c). The phase difference image between a flow-encoded and non-flow-encoded scan is expressed as a velocity map as shown in Fig. 34.1d. It can be obtained by complex division of the signals S_1 (non-flow-encoded) and S_2 (flow-encoded): $\Delta\phi = \arg S_2 - \arg S_1 = \arg\left(\frac{S_2}{S_1}\right) = \gamma v \Delta m_{1,x}$. The encoding strategy, so far demonstrated for the x direction, can be repeated for all three principal directions. 4D flow encoding can then be acquired with a common "four-point encoding" scheme in which phase accumulations for v_x, v_y, v_z are acquired separately with one non-flow-encoded reference scan.

An important parameter to characterize the relation between applied gradients and resulting phase accumulation is the VENC (velocity encoding): $\mathrm{VENC} = \frac{\pi}{\gamma \left|\Delta m_{1,x}\right|}$. The range of + and – VENC corresponds to a phase accumulation of + and – π. It is favorable that the VENC is set slightly larger than the encoded velocity, as a low VENC would result in wrapping of the phase, called aliasing. A VENC much larger than the maximum encoded velocity, however, would result in a low velocity-to-noise ratio.

Gating and Duration of 4D Flow MRI Sequences

The repetitive, pulsatile blood flow in the healthy aorta reaches maximum velocities of up to 160 cm/s during systole and minimum velocities of 10 cm/s during diastole (maximum net flow 400–500 ml/s; see Fig. 34.2). As not only average velocities and flow rates are of clinical interest, one would like to know the time-resolved behavior of velocities in the heart and aorta. This means that the flow encoding

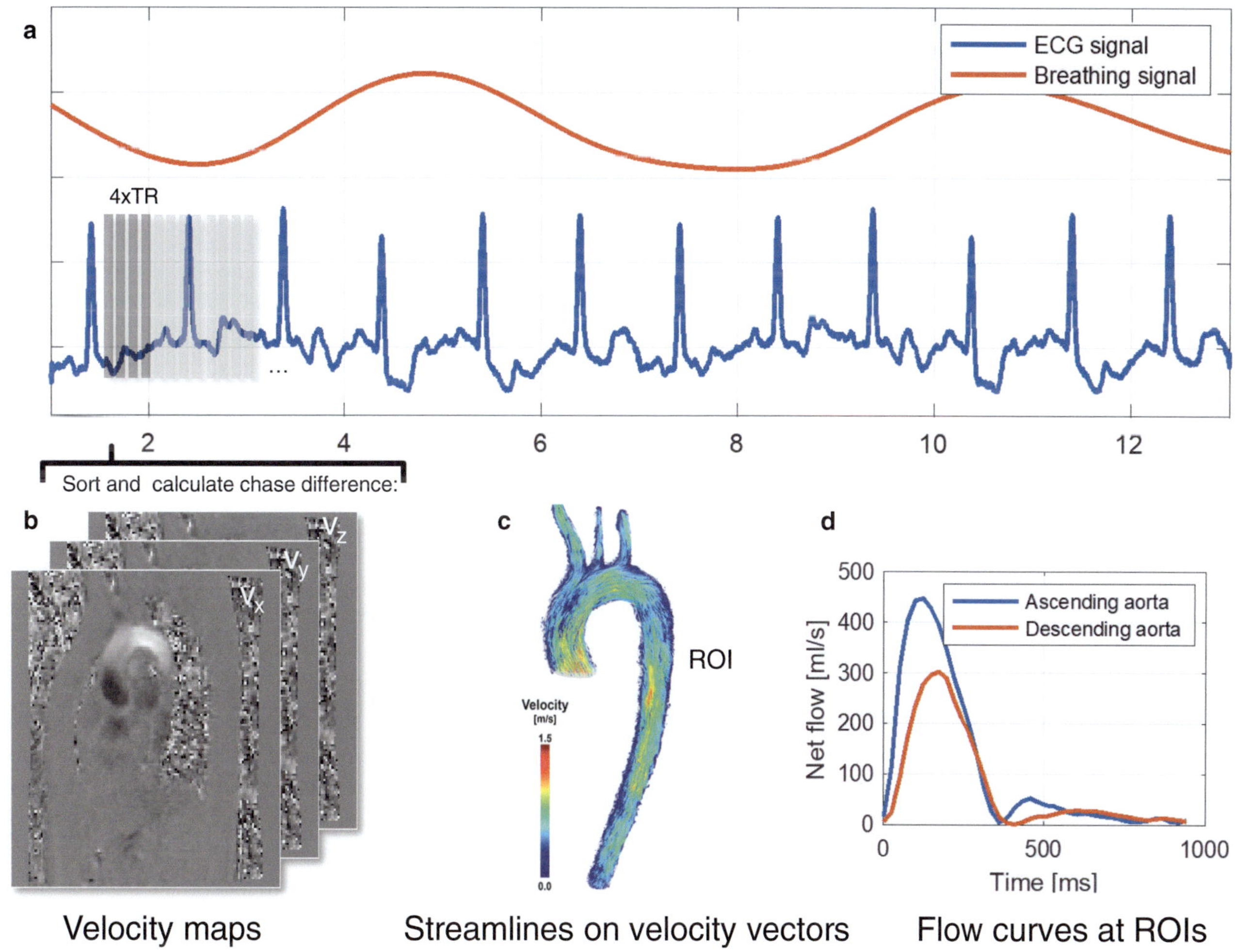

Fig. 34.2 (**a**) The 4D flow MRI acquisition needs to be synchronized with cardiac and respiratory motion. The acquisition of each k-space line (of duration TR) is repeated and assigned to a certain time point with respect to the R peak of the ECG. Like that, k-space can be filled over multiple heartbeats and sorted in one average heartbeat retrospectively. The four flow encoding gradients are played out after each other. (**b**) The four phase images are combined into three phase difference or velocity maps, all assigned to one time point of the cardiac cycle. At the end of the acquisition, a 3D dataset at each time point of the cardiac cycle is acquired. (**c**) The time-resolved velocity vector can then be calculated and streamlines can be derived. (**d**) Net flow can be determined through an ROI perpendicular to the aorta

strategy has to be repeated for a multitude of time points of the cardiac cycle. To this end, the acquisition is split up into measurement data subsections, which are sampled during different heartbeats. Like this, an acquisition can last up to half an hour. The time point within the cardiac cycle is assigned using the ECG signal which is either sampled alongside with the MRI data (called retrospective triggering) or which is controlling the MRI acquisition (called prospective triggering or gating). In both cases, the reconstructed and sorted data will provide a 3D volume for each time point of an averaged cardiac cycle (Fig. 34.2b).

As breathing introduces motion artifacts, 4D flow sequences can be gated using a navigator signal, a pencil beam MRI acquisition detecting diaphragmatic motion, which, however, can disrupt the magnetization steady state of the sequence. Alternative techniques are tracking the breathing motion with self-gating techniques [19] or, on newer MRI systems, with in-bore cameras [20].

Speeding Up 4D Flow MRI Acquisitions

Long scan times are problematic in terms of patient comfort, costs, and image quality, which can be corrupted by motion and physiological variation. In order to speed up the multidimensional and therefore lengthy 4D flow MRI sequences, simply less data can be acquired. This so-called (sub-Nyquist) undersampling allows for faster scan times but does not provide the full information content necessary for sharp and artifact-free images. Yet, there are several techniques that use prior information, for example, on the spatial distribution of the coil sensitivities (SENSE [21]) to recover the full image information from an undersampled dataset.

Another approach is to exploit the inherent sparsity of 4D flow MRI data. Sparsity, a condition entailing a substantial number of zero components in the data, can, for instance, be found in angiograms, in which all voxels except for the blood vessel are zero or below a certain threshold. Similarly, time-resolved data can be sparse in a certain transform domain, such as the finite differences or total variation (TV) transform over time [22]. The TV transform assumes that the sum of the absolute variation between time frames is mostly zero. 4D flow MRI is highly correlated in time, which has been exploited in acceleration techniques such as k-t BLAST [23], k-t GRAPPA [24], k-t PCA [25], and compressed sensing (CS) [26] reconstruction techniques of undersampled data. Iterative CS reconstructions have shown to achieve high acceleration rates in 4D flow MRI [27]. It requires incoherent sampling [22], creating noise-like undersampling artifacts. The iterative reconstruction

$$\text{Minimize}\left\|\psi \text{m}\right\|_1, \text{ s.t. } \left\|\text{F}_\text{U}\text{m}-\text{y}\right\|_2 < \varepsilon$$

enforces sparsity of the reconstructed image m under transform ψ (e.g., TV) and data consistency with the sampled data y. In this equation, F_u represents the undersampled Fourier operator, and ε is chosen approximately equal to the noise level. CS sampling schemes and advanced reconstruction algorithms for 4D flow MRI data have been implemented for Cartesian [27–29] and non-Cartesian [30] sampling strategies, enabling 10–30 times faster scans. The bottleneck of these applications and their clinical feasibility are typically the long reconstruction time of 15–30 min, depending on matrix size, number of coil elements, and temporal resolution. A solution next to the usage of GPUs and parallel reconstructions might be the implementation of neural networks for the image recovery from undersampled data, as discussed in the next section.

4D Flow MRI Reconstruction and Processing Using Machine Learning

Image Reconstruction and Machine Learning

As described in the previous chapter, data acquisition can be accelerated by acquiring a subset of the necessary data. The goal of image reconstruction techniques, such as partial Fourier, parallel imaging, k-t PCA, or CS, is to recover the missing data by exploiting redundancies and prior information. However, iterative reconstructions are computationally expensive and take very long (up to several hours). Additionally, standard k-t PCA and CS reconstructions need tuning of hyperparameters, which diminishes image accuracy if tuned badly, is operator dependent, and costs additional reconstruction time. Machine learning could have a major impact on clinical feasibility of 4D flow MRI if image reconstructions could be learned and images would be available within seconds.

One approach of using machine learning for undersampled image reconstruction would be mapping directly from k-space to image space by approximating the inverse sensor function, as is done by Zhu et al. [31]. In that case, the reconstruction transform is learned from MR images in a data-driven supervised task, however, requiring fully connected network layers to map the reciprocal data-image domain relation. Accordingly, these networks may not generalize sufficiently. Another approach would be to train on zero-filled undersampled images using a fully sampled ground truth using a similarity measure as a reconstruction error. Hammernik et al. [32] trained a variational network (VN) on retrospectively undersampled Cartesian data, to which regular and pseudo-random undersampling was applied. The VN used measured k-space, zero-filled image space data, and corresponding coil sensitivity maps as inputs. The error of the output images was compared against the fully sampled datasets and back-propagated to the VN. An image reconstruction framework for undersampled 4D flow MRI as presented in Vishnevskiy et al. (FlowVN) [33] interlaces data consistency step with convolutional layers similar to Hammernik et al. The model-based neural network used retrospectively undersampled k-space data for training, activating the network with the zero-filled image space data (Fig. 34.3). In contrast to Hammernik et al., the FlowVN was adapted by additional 3D filter banks. 4D convolutions were avoided, and instead 3D convolution was performed for real and imaginary parts of the data. After training, the application of the FlowVN took 21 s for a 3D acquisition with four flow encoding directions (in contrast to a 10-min CS local low rank reconstruction for data of the same size). The FlowVN was tested on reconstructing prospectively undersampled clinical 4D flow data in aortic stenosis patients. It could be shown that in (10 times retrospectively undersampled) patient data with abnormal flow, the FlowVN led to a lower nRMSE (1.5%) in comparison with a CS local low rank reconstruction (2.6%) for magnitude images. More importantly, the relative error in the velocity magnitude during peak systole was lower in the FlowVN (19.7%) than in the CS reconstruction (22.1%). Prospectively undersampled data (13 times accelerated) led to a deviation from the gold standard of −1.59% for peak velocities and of −0.05% for peak flow for the FlowVN. The deviation for the corresponding CS reconstruction was −1.18% for peak velocities and 0.36% for peak flow.

Overall, networks which solely learn to create artifact-free images from zero-filled data are closer to image post-processing than image reconstruction techniques and can show insufficient generalization. Using neural networks which are not enforcing closeness to the measured data will lead to inaccuracies, even at lower undersampling factors [34].

Segmentation and Machine Learning

Cardiothoracic 4D flow MRI allows for quantification of many hemodynamic parameters in the heart, aorta, and pulmonary arteries [35]. Quantification of velocity and velocity-derived energy parameters in the heart on the great vessels requires accurate 3D delineation of the heart chambers and aortic wall. Especially for techniques sensi-

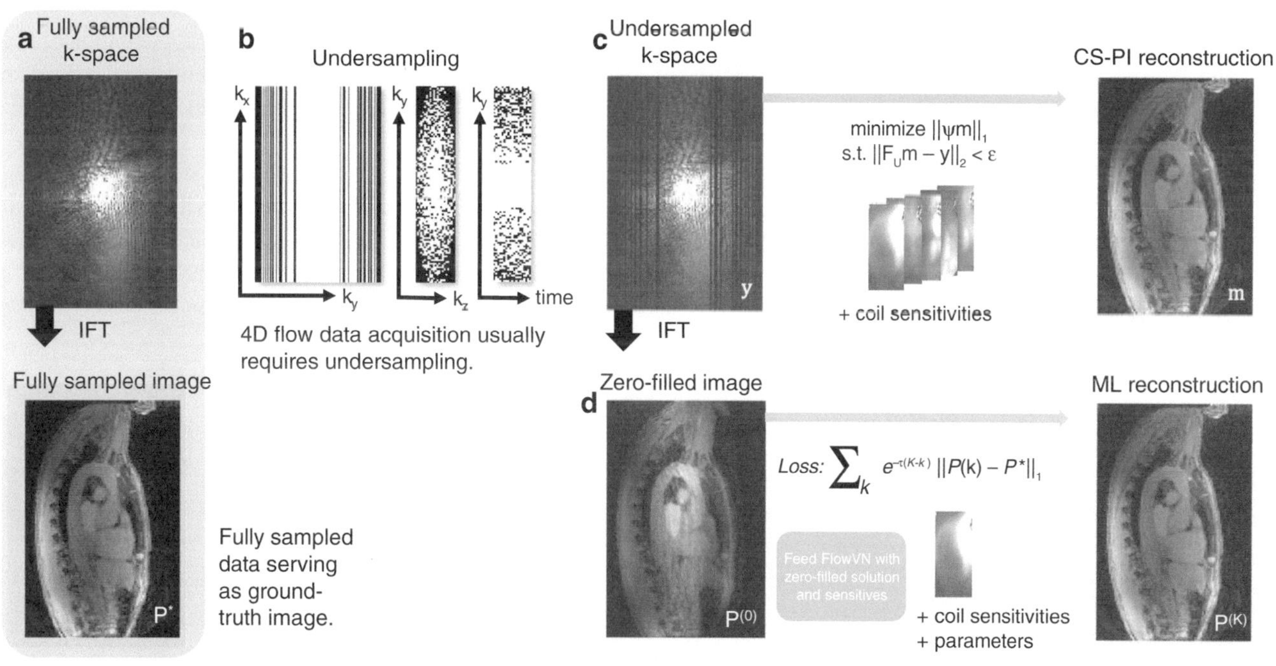

Fig. 34.3 (**a**) Fully sampled k-space and corresponding image space. (**b**) For image acquisition, undersampling is usually necessary to speed up the scan time. Undersampling can be applied in all dimensions of *k*-space k_x, k_y, k_z and in time. The readout direction k_x is usually fully sampled, as frequency encoding is very fast and would not shorten scan time substantially. Irregular sampling as shown here is used for compressed sensing (CS) types of image reconstruction. (**c**) Undersampled *k*-space can be used in an iterative CS reconstruction, together with the coil information and a sparse transform domain, to achieve high-quality images. The reconstruction time can take between 10 and 50 min. (**d**) Undersampled *k*-space can be zero-filled and transformed into image space using an inverse Fourier transform (IFT). In this case, undersampling artifacts will distort the image. The zero-filled image can serve as an initialization of, for example, the FlowVN training [33]. Training loss is calculated in comparison to a fully sampled image. After training, the FlowVN can be applied to recover undersampled images, which takes around 20 s for a three-dimensional image and four flow encoding directions

tive to wall location, such as WSS estimation, time-resolved segmentations are preferred, which are able to capture the motion of the aorta, which is up to 8 mm in the aortic root along the cardiac cycle [36, 37]. Assessment of aortic wall movement is also a measure of distensibility and desirable to achieve within a 4D flow measurement, as a reduced vessel elasticity is highly correlated with cardiovascular disease [38]. 4D flow data provides phase-contrast magnitude images and velocity information, constraining the regions of vessel lumen. Static PC magnetic resonance angiograms (PC-MRAs), representing the PC magnitude-weighted absolute value of the velocity vector averaged over all time frames, help in delineation of the vessel lumen. Therefore, areas of slow flow, such as regions close to the vessel wall or in aneurysms, are problematic for accurate delineation. Also, diastolic time frames provide very little flow contrast, which is why high contrast magnitude images or additionally acquired balanced SSFP datasets are needed for time-resolved segmentations. Usually PC-MRA images are segmented using manual or semiautomatic threshold, watershed, and drawing/erasing algorithms which have shown to be reproducible for peak systolic aortic velocity and WSS quantification [39]. However, segmentation of static PC-MRA images does not take aortic or cardiac motion into account, which necessitates removal of all diastolic time frames. Recent methods have shown improvement of these drawbacks but require high-quality images, preferably acquired with contrast administration, which is not always desirable [40].

Machine learning methods have proven essential for segmentation methods in other sequences and imaging modalities. For segmentation, not only classification but also a voxel-based localization of the tissue is necessary to achieve a segmentation map with dimensions as the input image. Convolutional neural networks (CNN) for segmentation like the U-net [41, 42] therefore consist not only of pooling (down-sampling of spatial information or encoding) but also of up-sampling operators (decoding) allowing for localization and accurate spatial information (Fig. 34.4). A voxel-based classification task to differentiate between vessel lumen and wall can be trained on time-averaged 4D flow MRI datasets by using manual segmentations on the PC-MRA images as a ground truth [43, 44].

In Berhane et al. [44], a CNN (3D U-net [42] with DenseNET [45] layers replacing the convolutional layers) was trained to achieve 3D time-averaged segmentations of 4D flow MRI data. Manual segmentations from PC-MRA data of 669 subjects at different scanners (1.5 T and 3 T) and including BAV (354) and ascending aortic aneurysm (219) patients were used to train and validate the network. With this approach, they achieved 3D segmentations with Dice scores of 0.953 (first observer) and 0.958 (second observer). The performance was similar to other automatic segmentation methods for 2D flow MRI [46, 47]. Berhane et al. also developed a CNN for aortic and pulmonary segmentation using a relatively low number of 4D flow MRI data acquired at two sites and at two vendor systems ($n = 42$ and $n = 25$), which showed good correspondence (Dice scores ~0.90) between machine learning and manual segmentations [48]. This result is in line with findings of Froeling et al. who also used a U-net and found good correspondence (Dice scores ~0.90) in a relatively small cohort ($n = 73$) [43].

It would be of interest to achieve time-resolved segmentation likewise, which is still difficult due to the lack of ground-truth annotations and missing velocity contrast. For 4D flow MRI, it has been tested in Scott et al. [49] to use a slightly

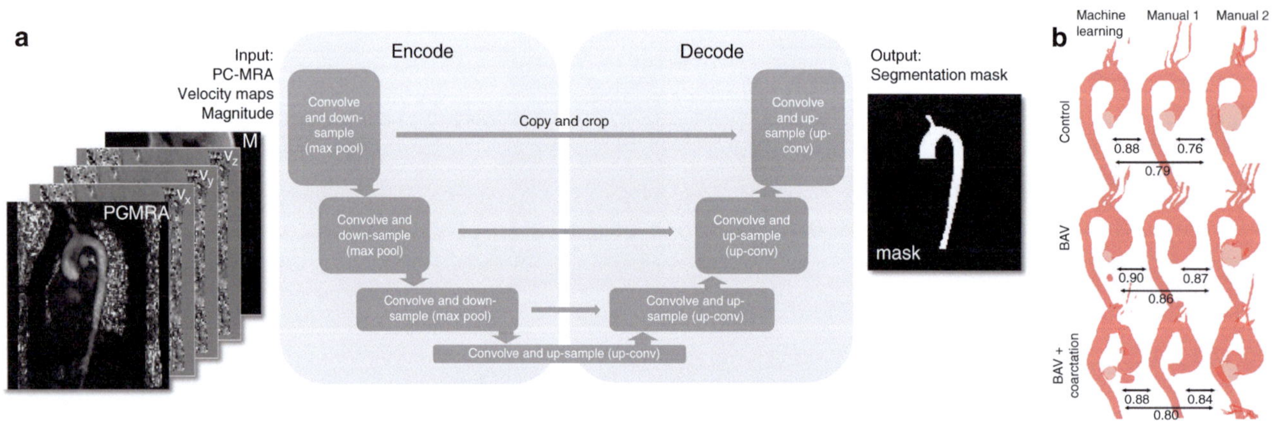

Fig. 34.4 (**a**) Schematic visualization of the U-net [42]. As input for the 4D flow MRI segmentation pipeline, velocity maps and magnitude images are used. Phase-contrast magnetic resonance angiograms (PC-MRAs) can subsequently be calculated as the velocity vectors' absolute value. The U-net is able to classify and localize tissue. Dice values can be calculated in comparison to 3D manual segmentations or even with 2D annotations in MR images with a better time-resolved tissue contrast. (**b**) The performance of the U-net has been shown previously on comparisons between ML results and manual segmentations for healthy controls and patients with a bicuspid aortic valve (BAV) without and with repaired coarctation

unsupervised approach [50], by retraining a network on time-resolved magnitude images, which was originally trained on time-averaged PC-MRA images. As no manual time-resolved segmentations were available, a substitute ground truth was used (ancillary model containing a bounding box encoder), and the CNN was retrained and validated on time-averaged magnitude data to then perform segmentations of time-resolved magnitude images. It remained challenging to provide ground-truth time-resolved segmentations of 4D flow MRI data, which is why 2D cine acquisitions were necessary to determine accuracy of time-resolved vessel wall delineation. The Dice values of this approach were at 0.87 for the static candy cane aorta view.

ML segmentations using voxel-wise classification allow for fast computation times and Dice values. To be accurate, they should be constrained by additional information on shape or hemodynamics. Future applications might include physics-informed segmentation networks that are trained on simulated data and applied to measured 4D flow MRI data to define a clear boundary between moving blood and tissue. Segmentations can also be designed as a regression problem, with segmentations defined as a smooth vector mesh, for example, by smooth circles along an aortic centerline, partially accounting for partial volume effects.

Image Quality Improvement and Derivation of Hemodynamics Using Machine Learning

By solving the Navier-Stokes equations, blood flow simulations that employ computational fluid dynamics (CFD) provide high-resolution cardiovascular velocity fields without noise. The accuracy of these models, however, depends on their input data, such as inflow conditions and patient specific vessel geometries.

CFD simulations can be combined with 4D flow MRI data, and uncertainties in CFD parameters can be fitted to 4D flow MRI measurements of the vessel lumen, which are, however, lower in resolution and have higher noise levels [51]. Another approach would be to use high-resolution, patient-specific CFD data to train a neural network and to enhance 4D flow MRI-derived velocity fields. This would improve the resolution of 4D flow MRI which is limited by scan time restrictions and by inherent flow encoding properties that lead to imperfections of the flow field. Ferdian et al. showed with their 4DFlowNet [52] that – using CFD simulations and synthetic 4D flow MRI data – a neural network can be trained to create noise-free super-resolution 4D flow MR images. The challenge was to apply existing super-resolution frameworks to 4D flow MRI data, consisting of phase and magnitude images. Using a voxel-wise mean squared error for each velocity component, which usually tends to blur images, and a weighted velocity gradient loss term to correct for that, the network was trained on synthetic 4D flow MRI data. The 4DFlowNet was tested on in vivo data. High-resolution aortic 4D flow MRI data (2 mm) predicted from a low-resolution 4D flow MRI scan (4 mm) was compared against an additional 2 mm 4D flow MRI ground-truth dataset. Additionally, in order to demonstrate performance, the low-resolution scans were interpolated to 2 mm resolution. Results show that the high-resolution 4DFlowNet had smaller relative errors at inlet (−0.6%) and outlet (5.8%) than interpolated data at inlet (7%) and outlet (5.8%) with respect to ground truth. Similarly, Rutkowski et al. [53] successfully augmented 4D flow MRI data by using a CFD-informed convolutional neural network for the application in intracranial aneurysms (Fig. 34.5).

Machine learning applications can also enable derivation of hemodynamic parameters, which 4D flow MRI cannot measure. For instance, it remains challenging to retrieve absolute pressure from 4D flow MRI data, although it is one of the most important clinical parameters. Up to now, invasive catheter-based pressure measurements are done. Physics-informed neural networks encode the physics of a given dataset following the principles of mass and momentum conservation and allow for the prediction of pulse wave propagation. In Kissas et al., partial differential equations were solved (similar to Raissi et al. [54]) using a trained neural network, matching the measurements of the system and the underlying physical principles [55]. The network provided mathematically correct predictions of flow and pressure from noisy 4D flow MRI data. The network was trained on simulations in a carotid bifurcation using one-dimensional Navier-Stokes equations. However, the simulated models require an accurate setting of the boundary conditions and the inclusion of downstream flow. Similarly, Fathi et al. trained a deep neural network using data fidelity for 4D flow MRI data and a regularization term enforcing fluid flow physics to achieve super-resolution reconstructions [56]. Once properly trained, a physics-informed neural network, however, could be directly applied to the 4D flow measurement points of individual scans, from which velocity, pressure, and cross-sectional area over time could be determined on noisy clinical data. Future models of this kind will include vessel curvature and other three-dimensional features.

Complex nonlinear functions used for numerical flow simulations are computationally expensive. Learning networks to approximate the solution of partial differential equations [54], such as the Navier-Stokes equations, in a data-driven way will enable faster simulations. For special cases such as turbulence modeling, iterative approximations of the Navier-Stokes equations are particularly slow or even unfeasible [57]. Learning laminar or turbulent flow models from large simulations will provide a solution to this problem.

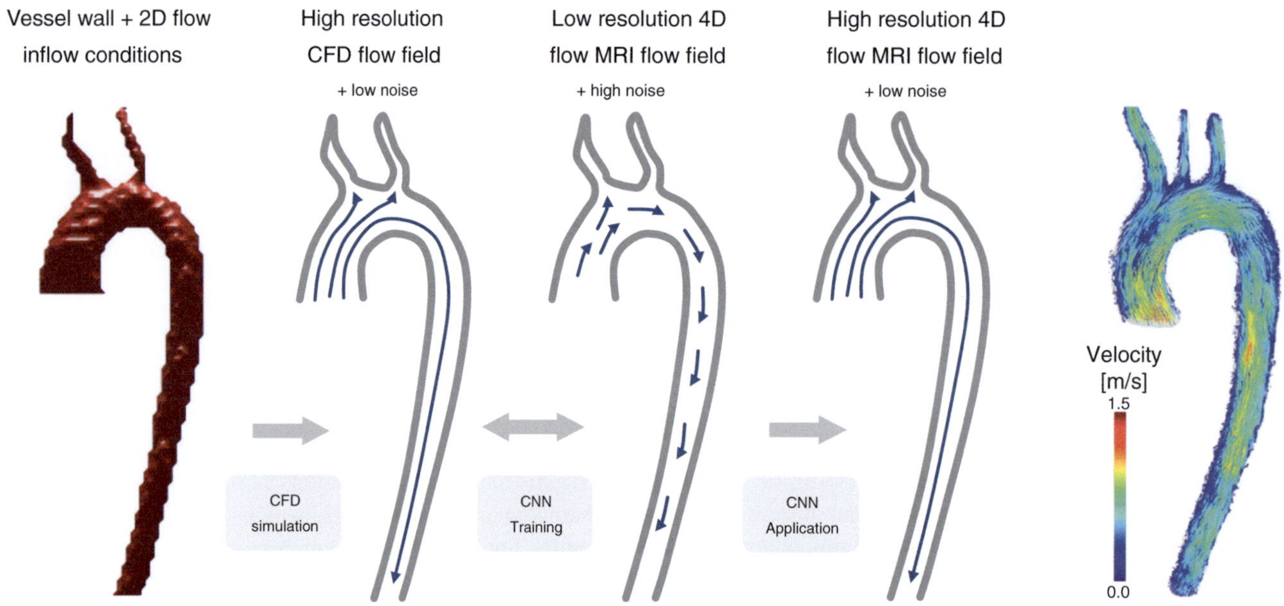

Fig. 34.5 CFD simulations based on 4D flow MRI-derived vessel geometries provide high-resolution streamlines without noise. A ML application as presented in [53] learns how to improve low-resolution, noisy 4D flow MRI data based on the CFD model. (Figure schematically adapted from [53])

The general problem of flow simulations with ML techniques, however, is that 4D flow MRI data is heterogeneous and non-stationary. Advances in physics-informed machine learning provide the connecting link for integrating theoretical models and real-world data.

Learning Clinical Outcomes from 4D Flow MRI

4D flow MRI provides comprehensive visualization and quantification of abnormal blood flow, such as, for example, helical flow in the aorta. Classification of characteristic features of diseased and healthy flow using ML techniques has huge potential to support diagnosis and prediction. Dinh et al. [58] predicted diabetes and cardiovascular disease from a cohort study and identified features exacerbating disease such as weight and age. Wojnarski et al. [59] investigated morphological CT data of patients with BAV, using unsupervised ML clustering methods to then be able to identify three different types of aortopathies. Niemann et al. [60] studied feature-based classification of 4D flow MRI data of patients with bicuspid aortic valve (BAV) ($N = 22$) and healthy volunteers ($N = 90$). Within their study, they extracted qualitative features such as vortices and quantitative features such as heart rate, vessel diameter, and hemodynamic parameters, calculated from multiple planes along an aortic centerline. These features (197 in total) were used for a classification task using five algorithms (CART decision tree, random forest, gradient boosted trees, support vector machines, and least absolute shrinkage and selection operator). For classification of healthy volunteers and BAV patients, the best model found the following features: time-to-peak-vorticity, time-to-peak-in-plane-velocity, and peak-systolic-in-plane-mean-velocity. An interesting future aspect of high-dimensional 4D flow MRI data is to learn and predict clinical outcomes from real or simulated data.

4D Flow MRI Hemodynamic Parameters and Clinical Relevance

Vectors, Streamlines, and Pathlines

Combining the three phase difference images allows reconstruction and visualization of the direction and magnitude of the velocity vector [61, 62]. The vector is usually color-coded according to its velocity magnitude. By connecting the velocity vectors in one time frame, streamlines are created, which represent the instantaneous velocity field tangent to the vectors. Streamlines do thus not take the time dimension into account and do not represent the time-varying trajectory a particle would travel through the blood flow. Pathlines are particle traces that are tangent to the velocity vectors for all points in time and display the trajectories of particles over the entire cardiac cycle [63]. Examples of cardiothoracic 4D flow MRI-derived velocity vectors, streamlines, and pathlines in a healthy volunteer are displayed in Fig. 34.6.

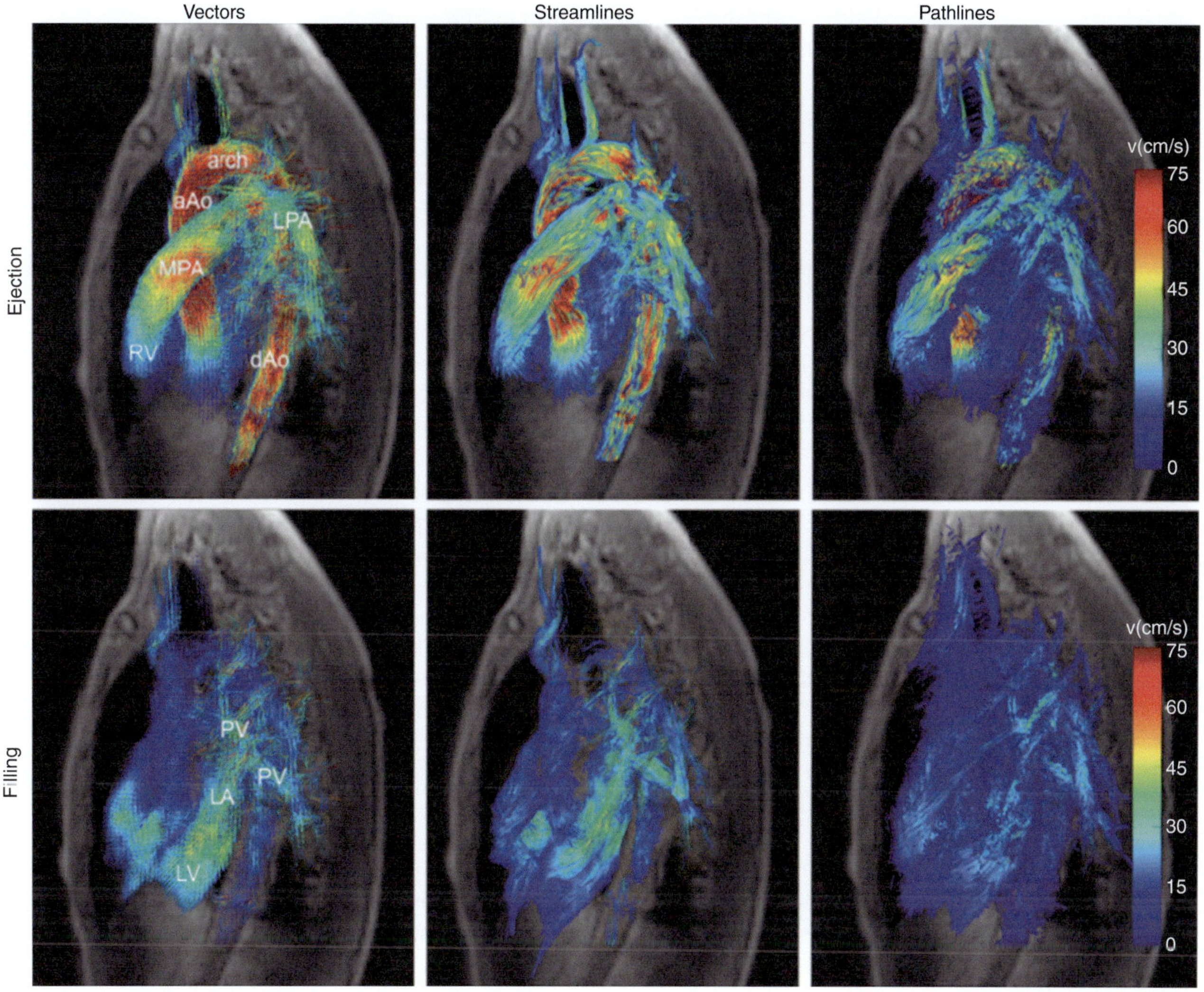

Fig. 34.6 Velocity vectors, streamlines, and pathlines for the ejection and the filling cardiac phases. Blood flow in the right ventricle (RV), main pulmonary artery (MPA), left pulmonary artery (LPA), pulmonary veins (PV), left atrium (LA), left ventricle (LV), ascending aorta (aAo), aortic arch (arch), and descending aorta (dAo) is visualized

Component Flow and Kinetic Energy

Pathlines calculated forward and backward in time can be used to separate time-resolved cardiac blood flow into four different components. After particle emission from a plane placed in the left atrium, *direct flow* is defined as the volume of pathlines relative to the end-diastolic left ventricular (LV) volume that cross planes placed in the mitral vena contracta and the left ventricular outflow tract (LVOT). *Retained flow* is defined as the volume of pathlines that do not cross the plane in the LVOT. *Delayed ejection flow* is the volume of pathlines emitted from the plane in the LVOT that did not cross the plane in the mitral vena contracta. *Residual volume* is the volume of blood that remains in the left ventricle between two cardiac phases and defined of the difference between the end-diastolic volume and the other flow components [64–66]. The flow component methodology was used to calculate the kinetic energy of a pathline defined as $KE = 0.5 * \rho * V * v^2$ where ρ is the density of blood, V the volume of a pathline, and v the velocity.

Turbulent Kinetic Energy

Kinetic energy as described in the previous paragraph can also be regarded as the mean KE (MKE), i.e., the energy based on the average of all velocity values in a voxel. A second energy term can be derived from the intravoxel velocity standard deviation (IVSD), which represents small-scale changes of the flow within the fluctuating velocity field i.e., the irregularity and randomness of turbulence, and is therefore called turbulent kinetic energy (TKE) [67]. IVSD can be calculated by the natural log of phase-contrast magnitude signals acquired with unequal gradients, ideally one with a zero first gradient moment. A combination of MKE and TKE provides a comprehensive assessment of kinetic energy in blood flow.

Viscous Energy Loss

Viscous energy loss (EL) is thermal energy irreversibly lost to the system due to friction between non-turbulent viscous fluid layers and between the fluid and its boundaries. It can be calculated from the velocity fields using a reformulation of the viscous portion of the Navier-Stokes equation [68, 69]. Quantification of EL does depend heavily on spatial resolution [70, 71].

Wall Shear Stress

Wall shear stress (WSS) is the tangential shear force of blood flow on the surface of the endothelial cell layer on the blood vessel wall. It is calculated by extracting the velocity gradient at the wall surface in the direction of the inward normal vector [72–74]. By deriving TKE close to the vessel wall, turbulent WSS can be calculated as well [75]. The limited spatial resolution of 4D flow MRI limits the accurate assessment of velocity profiles close to wall resulting in WSS underestimation. However, relative WSS quantification and cohort comparisons are possible and provide valuable information on the effects of flow on the vessel wall [12, 72, 76].

Pulse Wave Velocity

Pulse wave velocity (PWV) is the velocity with which the pulse pressure wave travels along the vascular system. PWV is a proxy for vessel stiffness, i.e., the higher the PWV, the higher the vessel stiffness. It can be calculated from 4D flow MRI by placing orthogonal planes to the aorta and calculating the difference in time between the upslope of flow [77]. The temporal resolution of 4D flow MRI needs to be sufficient for accurate PWV measurements.

Pressure Difference

The pressure difference can be derived from 4D flow MRI data by using the Navier-Stokes equation $\nabla p = -\rho \frac{DV}{Dt} + \mu \nabla^2 \mathbf{V} + \mathbf{F}$ where ∇p is the pressure gradient, ρ is the density of blood, V is the velocity vector field, DV/Dt is the time derivative of the velocity field, μ is viscosity of blood, and $\mathbf{F}$ represents the body force components such as gravity [78, 79].

Clinical Relevance

In Table 34.1, an overview is given of the most important recent findings of 4D flow MRI in cardiothoracic pathology.

Conclusion

In this chapter, we described the basics of 4D flow MRI in terms of acquisition, image processing, hemodynamic quantification, and clinical relevance in cardiothoracic disease. In particular, we reviewed the current literature in which the progress of using machine learning-based techniques for the application in cardiothoracic 4D flow MRI is presented.

Despite the demonstrated clinical relevance of 4D flow MRI in the assessment of biomarkers for cardiothoracic disease, the technique is employed by approximately a dozen expert centers worldwide. The main reasons for the limited use of 4D flow MRI are the long image acquisition and reconstruction time and the complex and semiautomatic and thus potentially cumbersome processing of the data. Machine learning techniques can have a tremendous impact on accelerating the 4D flow MRI workflow, especially when combined with methods to accelerate the acquisition by undersampling the data.

Many methods to accelerate the acquisition are based on undersampling of the data in a sparse and random manner. With advanced mathematics, e.g., iterative compressed sensing algorithms, the image can be reconstructed without much loss of quality and information. However, due to the iterative nature of these algorithms, reconstruction times can be lengthy which limits clinical applicability. Image reconstruction by machine learning algorithms can drastically shorten reconstruction times [33]. Furthermore, machine learning reconstruction algorithms allow implementation of equations that describe the laws of physics for the behavior of flow. As a result, measurement noise in the images can be reduced, and the images portrayed more detail [52]. Another important application of machine learning is that, for extraction of hemodynamic parameters from the data, segmentation can be automatically performed in a fraction of the semiautomatic segmentation time [44]. Finally, machine learning can be used for the extraction of flow features and use those for classification of healthy or diseased patients. By combining these machine learning applications in the clinical 4D flow MRI workflow, the assessment of hemodynamic biomarkers in cardiothoracic disease can be greatly facilitated.

At this point in time, however, the discussed machine learning algorithms are not yet extensively tested on varieties of data acquired on different vendor systems and field strengths. Furthermore, the knowledge and availability of the discussed machine learning possibilities are still limited to

Table 34.1 Important findings of 4D flow MRI in cardiothoracic pathology

Pathology	What is it?	What are the consequences?	What are important 4D flow MRI findings?
Heart			
Atrial fibrillation	Irregular motion of the atria	Thrombosis, stroke, and heart failure	Left and right mean and peak atrial velocities are lower, and stasis is higher in patients compared to young and age-matched healthy volunteers [80, 81] Left atrial velocity decreased and stasis increased with increasing CHA_2SD_2-VASc (risk for stroke) score [82], and left atrial vortex size correlated with CHA_2SD_2-VASc [83]
Dilated cardiomyopathy	Dilation of the heart chambers	Weakening of the heart's pump function may lead to heart failure	The proportion of LV inflow that passes directly to ejection and the diastolic kinetic energy is lower in patients compared to healthy subjects [7] Systolic and diastolic LV kinetic energy in patients with heart failure (dilated cardiomyopathy and ischemic heart disease) are higher than controls [84]
Hypertrophic cardiomyopathy	Genetic thickening of the myocardial wall	Heart failure or sudden cardiac death	Viscous EL in the LV outflow tract is higher in patients compared to healthy controls and correlated with fibrosis (extracellular volume from T1 mapping) [5]
Tetralogy of Fallot	Congenital heart disease including pulmonary stenosis, a ventricular septal defect, right ventricular hypertrophy, and an overriding aorta	Oxygen deficiency in blood (cyanosis)	Patients with repaired tetralogy of Fallot have decreased LV systolic peak KE compared to controls [85] Patients with repaired tetralogy of Fallot had regurgitation in the pulmonary arteries and higher peak velocities in the pulmonary trunk. There's a tendency for higher blood flow in the right pulmonary artery compared to the left [86]
Univentricular hearts/ Fontan	A genetic disorder where one ventricle is not developed. The other ventricle pumps oxygen-deprived blood to the body	Oxygen deficiency in blood (cyanosis)	Intraventricular kinetic energy is elevated compared to controls [87] Intraventricular viscous EL is elevated compared to controls [88] Intraventricular KE and viscous EL increased significantly after dobutamine stress which correlated with VO_2max [89]
Aorta			
Aortic atherosclerosis	Plaque buildup (fatty deposits) in the aortic wall	Plaque rupture may cause stroke	Aortic PWV in patients correlates with aortic wall thickness [90, 91] Aortic PWV in patients is significantly higher than younger controls but not in age-matched controls [77, 91]
Aortic coarctation	A congenital narrowing of the proximal descending aorta	High blood pressure causing heart thickening and failure	Coarctation alters blood flow patterns in the descending aorta [92] even after surgical repair [93] WSS is significantly increased in the aorta [93] but mainly distal from the coarctation region [94] compared to volunteers 4D flow MRI-based pressure difference mapping is feasible and an alternative for invasive pressure measurements [95]
Aortic valve stenosis	Hardening and subsequent narrowing of the aortic valve	Chronic higher left ventricular pressure may lead to heart failure	TKE in patients is significantly higher than normal volunteers and correlates with echocardiography [96, 97] Viscous EL and WSS are elevated in patients compared to healthy volunteers [11, 68] Differences between 4D flow MRI and echocardiography are related to flow eccentricity [98]

(continued)

Table 34.1 (continued)

Pathology	What is it?	What are the consequences?	What are important 4D flow MRI findings?
Bicuspid aortic valve disease	A congenital fusion of two aortic valve leaflets	Aortic valve stenosis, aortic regurgitation, and dilation of the ascending aorta	Viscous EL, WSS, and pressure drop in the aorta are higher in BAV patients with stenosis compared to patients without and higher for both compared to healthy volunteers [11, 99, 100] Aortic PWV does not differ between non-dilated BAV patients compared to healthy controls and decreases with aortic diameter [14] Peak velocity and WSS correlated with LV mass [101]
Marfan syndrome	A genetic disorder that affects connective tissue	Aortic aneurysms and dissection	WSS is reduced in Marfan patients compared to healthy volunteers in the proximal ascending aorta and proximal descending aorta [15] Aortic PWV is higher for Marfan patients compared to non-dilated BAV patients and healthy controls [14]
Pulmonary			
Pulmonary hypertension	Increased blood pressure in the lung circulation	Right heart failure	Normalized KE over the tricuspid and pulmonary valve is lower, whereas viscous EL in the main pulmonary artery is higher in patients than healthy subjects [10] Flow parameters and WSS in the main, right, and left pulmonary artery are lower in patients than controls [102] The duration of the presence of a vortex strongly correlates with blood pressure in the mean pulmonary artery [103]
Chronic obstructive pulmonary disease (COPD)	A group of lung conditions that cause breathing difficulties including damage to air sacs in the lungs (emphysema) and inflammation of airways (bronchitis)	Shortness of breath, coughing, exercise limitation	Greater percent emphysema (CT) is associated with retrograde flow in the superior and inferior venae cavae and the tricuspid valve [9] Reduced vortex formation in the LV which correlated with CT and echocardiography metrics and with 6-minute walk test [104]
Others			
Fontan conduit (TCPC, total cavopulmonary connection)	A surgically placed connection that, in the absence of a right ventricle, routes the venous return directly to the pulmonary circulation	Cyanosis, exercise limitation, liver dysfunction	The superior and inferior venae cavae have a preferential distribution to the right and left pulmonary artery, respectively [105]. Pulmonary arterial cross-sectional artery correlated with flow distribution [106] Flow distributions varied significantly between respiratory phases [87]

expert groups. Future efforts should thus focus on distributing knowledge, data, and algorithms and on multicenter collaborations to develop algorithms based on combined data.

With widely applicable and validated machine learning algorithms for 4D flow MRI, the impact of 4D flow MRI in the clinic can only increase, thereby providing invaluable clinical support in the management of thoracic cardiovascular disease.

References

1. Wigstrom L, Sjoqvist L, Wranne B. Temporally resolved 3D phase-contrast imaging. Magn Reson Med. 1996;36:800–3.
2. Markl M, Frydrychowicz A, Kozerke S, Hope M, Wieben O. 4D flow MRI. J Magn Reson Imaging. 2012;36:1015–36.
3. Roes SD, Hammer S, van der Geest RJ, Marsan NA, Bax JJ, Lamb HJ, Reiber JHC, de Roos A, Westenberg JJM. Flow assessment through four heart valves simultaneously using 3-dimensional 3-directional velocity-encoded magnetic resonance imaging with retrospective valve tracking in healthy volunteers and patients with valvular regurgitation. Investig Radiol. 2009;44:669–75.
4. Blanken CPS, Westenberg JJM, Aben J-P, Bijvoet GP, Chamuleau SAJ, Boekholdt SM, Nederveen AJ, Leiner T, van Ooij P, Planken RN. Quantification of mitral valve regurgitation from 4D flow MRI using semiautomated flow tracking. Radiol Cardiothorac Imaging. 2020;2:e200004.
5. van Ooij P, Allen BD, Contaldi C, Garcia J, Collins J, Carr J, Choudhury L, Bonow RO, Barker AJ, Markl M. 4D flow MRI and T1-mapping: assessment of altered cardiac hemodynamics and extracellular volume fraction in hypertrophic cardiomyopathy. J Magn Reson Imaging. 2016;43:107–14.
6. Pruijssen JT, Allen BD, Barker AJ, Bonow RO, Choudhury L, Carr JC, Markl M, van Ooij P. Hypertrophic cardiomyopathy is

associated with altered left ventricular 3D blood flow dynamics. Radiol Cardiothorac Imaging. 2020;2:e190038.
7. Eriksson J, Bolger AF, Ebbers T, Carlhäll C-J. Four-dimensional blood flow-specific markers of LV dysfunction in dilated cardiomyopathy. Eur Heart J Cardiovasc Imaging. 2013;14:417–24.
8. Lee DC, Markl M, Ng J, Carr M, Benefield B, Carr JC, Goldberger JJ. Three-dimensional left atrial blood flow characteristics in patients with atrial fibrillation assessed by 4D flow CMR. Eur Heart J Cardiovasc Imaging. 2016;17:1259–68.
9. Rahman O, Markl M, Balte P, Berhane H, Blanken C, Suwa K, Dashnaw S, Wieben O, Bluemke DA, Prince MR, Lima J, Michos E, Ambale-Venkatesh B, Hoffman EA, Gomes AS, Watson K, Sun Y, Carr J, Barr RG. Reproducibility and changes in vena caval blood flow by using 4D flow MRI in pulmonary emphysema and Chronic Obstructive Pulmonary Disease (COPD): the Multi-Ethnic Study of Atherosclerosis (MESA) COPD substudy. Radiology. 2019;292:585–94.
10. Han QJ, Witschey WRT, Fang-Yen CM, Arkles JS, Barker AJ, Forfia PR, Han Y. Altered right ventricular kinetic energy work density and viscous energy dissipation in patients with pulmonary arterial hypertension: a pilot study using 4D flow MRI. PLoS One. 2015;10:e0138365.
11. van Ooij P, Markl M, Collins JD, Carr JC, Rigsby C, Bonow RO, Chris Malaisrie S, McCarthy PM, Fedak PWM, Barker AJ. Aortic valve stenosis alters expression of regional aortic wall shear stress: new insights from a 4-dimensional flow magnetic resonance imaging study of 571 subjects. J Am Heart Assoc. 2017;6:1–14.
12. Guzzardi DG, Barker AJ, van Ooij P, Malaisrie SC, Puthumana JJ, Belke DD, Mewhort HEM, Svystonyuk DA, Kang S, Verma S, Collins J, Carr J, Bonow RO, Markl M, Thomas JD, Mccarthy PM, Fedak PWM. Valve-related hemodynamics mediate human bicuspid aortopathy: insights from wall shear stress mapping. J Am Coll Cardiol. 2015;66:892–900.
13. Bollache E, Guzzardi DG, Sattari S, Olsen KE, Di Martino ES, Malaisrie SC, van Ooij P, Collins J, Carr J, McCarthy PM, Markl M, Barker AJ, Fedak PWM. Aortic valve-mediated wall shear stress is heterogeneous and predicts regional aortic elastic fiber thinning in bicuspid aortic valve-associated aortopathy. J Thorac Cardiovasc Surg. 2018;156:2112–2120.e2.
14. Guala A, Rodriguez-Palomares J, Dux-Santoy L, Teixido-Tura G, Maldonado G, Galian L, Huguet M, Valente F, Gutiérrez L, González-Alujas T, Johnson KM, Wieben O, Sao Avilés A, Garcia-Dorado D, Evangelista A. Influence of aortic dilation on the regional aortic stiffness of bicuspid aortic valve assessed by 4-dimensional flow cardiac magnetic resonance: comparison with Marfan syndrome and degenerative aortic aneurysm. JACC Cardiovasc Imaging. 2019;12:1020–9.
15. van der Palen RLF, Barker AJ, Bollache E, Garcia J, Rose MJ, van Ooij P, Young LT, Roest AAW, Markl M, Robinson JD, Rigsby CK. Altered aortic 3D hemodynamics and geometry in pediatric Marfan syndrome patients. J Cardiovasc Magn Reson. 2017;19:30.
16. Geiger J, Hirtler D, Gottfried K, Rahman O, Bollache E, Barker AJ, Markl M, Stiller B. Longitudinal evaluation of aortic hemodynamics in Marfan syndrome: new insights from a 4D flow cardiovascular magnetic resonance multi-year follow-up study. J Cardiovasc Magn Reson. 2017;19:33.
17. Pelc NJ, Bernstein matt A, Shimakawa A, Glover GH. Encoding strategies for three-direction phase-contrast MR imaging of flow. J Magn Reson Imaging. 1991;1:405–13.
18. Bernstein MA, King KF, Zhou XJ. Handbook of MRI pulse sequences. Amsterdam: Elsevier Academic Press; 2004.
19. Uribe S, Beerbaum P, Sorensen TS, Rasmusson A, Razavi R, Schaeffter T. Four-dimensional (4D) flow of the whole heart and great vessels using real-time respiratory self-gating. Magn Reson Med. 2009;62:984–92.
20. Gottwald LM, Blanken CPS, Tourais JL, Smink J, Planken RN, Boekholdt SM, Coolen BF, Strijkers GJ, Nederveen AJ, van Ooij P. Retrospective camera-based respiratory gating in clinical whole-heart 4D flow MRI. J Magn Reson Imaging. 2021;54(2):440–51.
21. Pruessmann KP, Weiger M, Scheidegger MB, Boesiger P. SENSE: sensitivity encoding for fast MRI. Magn Reson Med. 1999;42:952–62.
22. Lustig M, Donoho D, Pauly JM. Sparse MRI: the application of compressed sensing for rapid MR imaging. Magn Reson Med. 2007;58:1182–95.
23. Carlsson M, Toger J, Kanski M, Bloch KM, Stahlberg F, Heiberg E, Arheden H. Quantification and visualization of cardiovascular 4D velocity mapping accelerated with parallel imaging or k-t BLAST: head to head comparison and validation at 1.5 T and 3 T. J Cardiovasc Magn Reson. 2011;13:55.
24. Schnell S, Markl M, Entezari P, Mahadewia R, Semaan E, Stankovic Z, Collins J, Carr JBJ. k-t GRAPPA. Magn Reson Med. 2015;344:1173–8.
25. Knobloch V, Boesiger P, Kozerke S. Sparsity transform k-t principal component analysis for accelerating cine three-dimensional flow measurements. Magn Reson Med. 2013;70:53–63.
26. Lustig M, Donoho DL, Santos JM, Pauly JM. Compressed sensing MRI. Signal Process Mag IEEE. 2008;25:72–82.
27. Cheng JY, Hanneman K, Zhang T, Alley MT, Lai P, Tamir JI, Uecker M, Pauly JM, Lustig M, Vasanawala SS. Comprehensive motion-compensated highly accelerated 4D flow MRI with ferumoxytol enhancement for pediatric congenital heart disease. J Magn Reson Imaging. 2016;43:1355–68.
28. Walheim J, Dillinger H, Kozerke S. Multipoint 5D flow cardiovascular magnetic resonance - accelerated cardiac- and respiratory-motion resolved mapping of mean and turbulent velocities. J Cardiovasc Magn Reson. 2019;21:1 13.
29. Peper ES, Gottwald LM, Zhang Q, Coolen BF, van Ooij P, Nederveen AJ, Strijkers GJ. Highly accelerated 4D flow cardiovascular magnetic resonance using a pseudo-spiral Cartesian acquisition and compressed sensing reconstruction for carotid flow and wall shear stress. J Cardiovasc Magn Reson. 2020;22:7.
30. Dyvorne H, Knight Greenfield A, Jajamovich G, Besa C, Cui Y, Stalder A, Markl M, Taouli B. Abdominal 4D flow MR imaging in a breath hold: combination of spiral sampling and dynamic compressed sensing for highly accelerated acquisition. Radiology. 2015;275:245–54.
31. Zhu B, Liu JZ, Cauley SF, Rosen BR, Rosen MS. Image reconstruction by domain-transform manifold learning. Nature. 2018;555:487–92.
32. Hammernik K, Klatzer T, Kobler E, Recht MP, Pock T, Knoll F, States U, States U. HHS Public Access. 2019;79:3055–71.
33. Vishnevskiy V, Walheim J, Kozerke S. Deep variational network for rapid 4D flow MRI reconstruction. Nat Mach Intell. 2020;2:228–35.
34. Antun V, Renna F, Poon C, Adcock B, Hansen AC. On instabilities of deep learning in image reconstruction and the potential costs of AI. Proc Natl Acad Sci U S A. 2020;117:30088.
35. Markl M, Kilner PJ, Ebbers T. Comprehensive 4D velocity mapping of the heart and great vessels by cardiovascular magnetic resonance. J Cardiovasc Magn Reson. 2011;13:7.
36. Beller CJ, Labrosse MR, Thubrikar MJ, Robicsek F. Role of aortic root motion in the pathogenesis of aortic dissection. Circulation. 2004;109:763–9.
37. Kozerke S, Scheidegger MB, Pedersen EM, Boesiger P. Heart motion adapted cine phase-contrast flow measurements through the aortic valve. Magn Reson Med. 1999;42:970–8.
38. van Popele NM, Grobbee DE, Bots ML, Asmar R, Topouchian J, Reneman RS, Hoeks AP, van der Kuip DA, Hofman A, Witteman JC. Association between arterial stiffness and atherosclerosis: the Rotterdam study. Stroke. 2001;32:454–60.

39. van Ooij P, Powell AL, Potters WV, Carr JC, Markl M, Barker AJ. Reproducibility and interobserver variability of systolic blood flow velocity and 3D wall shear stress derived from 4D flow MRI in the healthy aorta. J Magn Reson Imaging. 2016;43:236–48.
40. Bustamante M, Gupta V, Forsberg D, Carlhäll C-J, Engvall J, Ebbers T. Automated multi-atlas segmentation of cardiac 4D flow MRI. Med Image Anal. 2018;49:128–40.
41. Ronneberger O, Fischer P, Brox T. U-net: convolutional networks for biomedical image segmentation. In: Navab N, Hornegger J, Wells WM, Frangi AF, editors. Med. Image Comput. Comput. Interv. – MICCAI, vol. 2015. Cham: Springer International Publishing; 2015. p. 234–41.
42. Çiçek Ö, Abdulkadir A, Lienkamp SS, Brox T, Ronneberger O. 3D U-net: learning dense volumetric segmentation from sparse annotation. In: Ourselin S, Joskowicz L, Sabuncu MR, Unal G, Wells W, editors. Med. Image Comput. Comput. Interv. – MICCAI, vol. 2016. Cham: Springer International Publishing; 2016. p. 424–32.
43. Froeling M, Farag ES, Planken RN, Leiner T, van Ooij P. Machine learning for automatic three-dimensional segmentation of the aorta in 4D flow MRI. Proc Intl Soc Mag Reson. 2019;27:0088.
44. Berhane H, Scott M, Elbaz M, Jarvis K, McCarthy P, Carr J, Malaisrie C, Avery R, Barker AJ, Robinson JD, Rigsby CK, Markl M. Fully automated 3D aortic segmentation of 4D flow MRI for hemodynamic analysis using deep learning. Magn Reson Med. 2020;84:2204–18.
45. Huang G, Liu Z, Van Der Maaten L, Weinberger KQ. Densely connected convolutional networks. Proc – 30th IEEE Conf Comput Vis Pattern Recognition, CVPR 2017 2017-Janua:2261–2269.
46. Herment A, Kachenoura N, Lefort M, Bensalah M, Dogui A, Frouin F, Mousseaux E, De Cesare A. Automated segmentation of the aorta from phase contrast MR images: validation against expert tracing in healthy volunteers and in patients with a dilated aorta. J Magn Reson Imaging. 2010;31:881–8.
47. Bratt A, Kim J, Pollie M, Beecy AN, Tehrani NH, Codella N, Perez-Johnston R, Palumbo MC, Alakbarli J, Colizza W, Drexler IR, Azevedo CF, Kim RJ, Devereux RB, Weinsaft JW. Machine learning derived segmentation of phase velocity encoded cardiovascular magnetic resonance for fully automated aortic flow quantification. J Cardiovasc Magn Reson. 2019;21:1.
48. Berhane HB, Scott MB, Fujiwara T, Browne L, Robinson JD, Rigsby CK, Markl M, Barker AJ. Fully automated multivendor and multisite artificial intelligence-based 3D segmentation of the proximal arteries from 4D flow MRI. Proc Intl Soc Mag Reson. 2020;28:0776.
49. Scott MB, Berhane HB, Kalisz KR, Trabzonlu TA, Lee J, Messina M, Malaisrie C, Mccarthy P, Carr J, Barker AJ, Avery R. Verification of fully automated deep learning-based 4D segmentation of the thoracic aorta from 4D flow MRI. Proc Intl Soc Mag Res Med. 2020;28:2229.
50. Ibrahim MS, Vahdat A, Ranjbar M, Macready WG. Semi-supervised semantic image segmentation with self-correcting networks. Proc. IEEE/CVF Conf. Comput. Vis. Pattern Recognit. 2018. p. 12715–25.
51. Töger J, Zahr MJ, Aristokleous N, Markenroth Bloch K, Carlsson M, Persson PO. Blood flow imaging by optimal matching of computational fluid dynamics to 4D-flow data. Magn Reson Med. 2020;84:2231–45.
52. Ferdian E, Suinesiaputra A, Dubowitz DJ, Zhao D, Wang A, Cowan B, Young AA. 4DFlowNet: super-resolution 4D flow MRI using deep learning and computational fluid dynamics. Front Phys. 2020;8:138.
53. Rutkowski DR, Roldán-alzate A, Johnson KM. In-vivo application of a trained neural network using a fusion of computational fluid dynamic and 4D flow MRI data. Proc Intl Soc Mag Res Med. 2020;28:0774.
54. Raissi M, Perdikaris P, Karniadakis GE. Physics-informed neural networks: a deep learning framework for solving forward and inverse problems involving nonlinear partial differential equations. J Comput Phys. 2019;378:686–707.
55. Kissas G, Yang Y, Hwuang E, Witschey WR, Detre JA, Perdikaris P. Machine learning in cardiovascular flows modeling: predicting arterial blood pressure from non-invasive 4D flow MRI data using physics-informed neural networks. Comput Methods Appl Mech Eng. 2020;358:112623.
56. Fathi MF, Perez-Raya I, Baghaie A, Berg P, Janiga G, Arzani A, D'Souza RM. Super-resolution and denoising of 4D-flow MRI using physics-informed deep neural nets. Comput Methods Prog Biomed. 2020;197:105729.
57. Brunton SL, Noack BR, Koumoutsakos P. Machine learning for fluid mechanics. Annu Rev Fluid Mech. 2020;52:477–508.
58. Dinh A, Miertschin S, Young A, Mohanty SD. A data-driven approach to predicting diabetes and cardiovascular disease with machine learning. BMC Med Inform Decis Mak. 2019;19:1–15.
59. Wojnarski CM, Roselli EE, Idrees JJ, Zhu Y, Carnes TA, Lowry AM, Collier PH, Griffin B, Ehrlinger J, Blackstone EH, Svensson LG, Lytle BW. Machine-learning phenotypic classification of bicuspid aortopathy. J Thorac Cardiovasc Surg. 2018;155:461–469.e4.
60. Niemann U, Neog A, Behrendt B, Lawonn K, Gutberlet M, Spiliopoulou M, Preim B, Meuschke M. Cardiac cohort classification based on morphologic and hemodynamic parameters extracted from 4D PC-MRI data. arXiv preprint arXiv:2010.05612. 2020.
61. Kilner PJ, Yang GZ, Mohiaddin RH, Firmin DN, Longmore DB. Helical and retrograde secondary flow patterns in the aortic arch studied by three-directional magnetic resonance velocity mapping. Circulation. 1993;88:2235–47.
62. Mohiaddin RH, Yang GZ, Kilner PJ. Visualization of flow by vector analysis of multidirectional cine MR velocity mapping. J Comput Assist Tomogr. 1994;18:383–92.
63. Buonocore MH. Visualizing blood flow patterns using streamlines, arrows, and particle paths. Magn Reson Med. 1998;40:210–26.
64. Bolger AF, Heiberg E, Karlsson M, Wigström L, Engvall J, Sigfridsson A, Ebbers T, Kvitting J-PE, Carlhäll CJ, Wranne B. Transit of blood flow through the human left ventricle mapped by cardiovascular magnetic resonance. J Cardiovasc Magn Reson. 2007;9:741–7.
65. Eriksson J, Carlhäll CJ, Dyverfeldt P, Engvall J, Bolger AF, Ebbers T. Semi-automatic quantification of 4D left ventricular blood flow. J Cardiovasc Magn Reson. 2010;12:9.
66. Stoll VM, Loudon M, Eriksson J, Bissell MM, Dyverfeldt P, Ebbers T, Myerson SG, Neubauer S, Carlhäll C-J, Hess AT. Test-retest variability of left ventricular 4D flow cardiovascular magnetic resonance measurements in healthy subjects. J Cardiovasc Magn Reson. 2018;20:15.
67. Dyverfeldt P, Kvitting JP, Sigfridsson A, Engvall J, Bolger AF, Ebbers T. Assessment of fluctuating velocities in disturbed cardiovascular blood flow: in vivo feasibility of generalized phase-contrast MRI. J Magn Reson Imaging. 2008;28:655–63.
68. Barker AJ, van Ooij P, Bandi K, Garcia J, Albaghdadi M, McCarthy P, Bonow RO, Carr J, Collins J, Malaisrie SC, Markl M. Viscous energy loss in the presence of abnormal aortic flow. Magn Reson Med. 2014;72:620–8.
69. Elbaz MSM, van der Geest RJ, Calkoen EE, de Roos A, Lelieveldt BPF, Roest AAW, Westenberg JJM. Assessment of viscous energy loss and the association with three-dimensional vortex ring formation in left ventricular inflow: in vivo evaluation using four-dimensional flow MRI. Magn Reson Med. 2017;77:794–805.
70. Casas B, Lantz J, Dyverfeldt P, Ebbers T. 4D flow MRI-based pressure loss estimation in stenotic flows: evaluation using numerical simulations. Magn Reson Med. 2016;75:1808–21.

71. Binter C, Gülan U, Holzner M, Kozerke S. On the accuracy of viscous and turbulent loss quantification in stenotic aortic flow using phase-contrast MRI. Magn Reson Med. 2016;76:191–6.
72. Stalder A, Russe M, Frydrychowicz A, Bock J, Hennig J, Markl M. Quantitative 2D and 3D phase contrast MRI: optimized analysis of blood flow and vessel wall parameters. Magn Reson Med. 2008;60:1218–31.
73. Bieging ET, Frydrychowicz A, Wentland A, Landgraf BR, Johnson KM, Wieben O, Francois CJ. In vivo three-dimensional MR wall shear stress estimation in ascending aortic dilatation. J Magn Reson Imaging. 2011;33:589–97.
74. Potters WV, van Ooij P, Marquering HA, VanBavel E, Nederveen AJ. Volumetric arterial wall shear stress calculation based on cine phase contrast MRI. J Magn Reson Imaging. 2015;41:505–16.
75. Ziegler M, Lantz J, Ebbers T, Dyverfeldt P. Assessment of turbulent flow effects on the vessel wall using four-dimensional flow MRI. Magn Reson Med. 2017;77:2310–9.
76. van Kesteren F, Wollersheim LW, Baan J, Nederveen AJ, Kaya A, Boekholdt SM, de Mol BA, van Ooij P, Planken RN. Four-dimensional flow MRI of stented versus stentless aortic valve bioprostheses. Eur Radiol. 2018;28:257–64.
77. Markl M, Wallis W, Brendecke S, Simon J, Frydrychowicz A, Harloff A. Estimation of global aortic pulse wave velocity by flow-sensitive 4D MRI. Magn Reson Med. 2010;63:1575–82.
78. Tyszka JM, Laidlaw DH, Asa JW, Silverman JM. Three-dimensional, time-resolved (4D) relative pressure mapping using magnetic resonance imaging. J Magn Reson Imaging. 2000;12:321–9.
79. Ebbers T, Wigström L, Bolger AF, Engvall J, Karlsson M. Estimation of relative cardiovascular pressures using time-resolved three-dimensional phase contrast MRI. Magn Reson Med. 2001;45:872–9.
80. Markl M, Lee DC, Ng J, Carr M, Carr J, Goldberger JJ. Left atrial 4-dimensional flow magnetic resonance imaging: stasis and velocity mapping in patients with atrial fibrillation. Investig Radiol. 2016;51:147–54.
81. Markl M, Carr M, Ng J, Lee DC, Jarvis K, Carr J, Goldberger JJ. Assessment of left and right atrial 3D hemodynamics in patients with atrial fibrillation: a 4D flow MRI study. Int J Cardiovasc Imaging. 2016;32:807–15.
82. Markl M, Lee DC, Furiasse N, Carr M, Foucar C, Ng J, Carr J, Goldberger JJ. Left atrial and left atrial appendage 4D blood flow dynamics in atrial fibrillation. Circ Cardiovasc Imaging. 2016;9:e004984.
83. Garcia J, Sheitt H, Bristow MS, Lydell C, Howarth AG, Heydari B, Prato FS, Drangova M, Thornhill RE, Nery P, Wilton SB, Skanes A, White JA. Left atrial vortex size and velocity distributions by 4D flow MRI in patients with paroxysmal atrial fibrillation: associations with age and CHA2 DS2-VASc risk score. J Magn Reson Imaging. 2020;51:871–84.
84. Kanski M, Arvidsson PM, Töger J, Borgquist R, Heiberg E, Carlsson M, Arheden H. Left ventricular fluid kinetic energy time curves in heart failure from cardiovascular magnetic resonance 4D flow data. J Cardiovasc Magn Reson. 2015;17:111.
85. Sjöberg P, Bidhult S, Bock J, Heiberg E, Arheden H, Gustafsson R, Nozohoor S, Carlsson M. Disturbed left and right ventricular kinetic energy in patients with repaired tetralogy of Fallot: pathophysiological insights using 4D-flow MRI. Eur Radiol. 2018;28:4066–76.
86. Geiger J, Markl M, Jung B, Grohmann J, Stiller B, Langer M, Arnold R. 4D-MR flow analysis in patients after repair for tetralogy of Fallot. Eur Radiol. 2011;21:1651–7.
87. Rutkowski DR, Barton G, François CJ, Bartlett HL, Anagnostopoulos PV, Roldán-Alzate A. Analysis of cavopulmonary and cardiac flow characteristics in fontan patients: comparison with healthy volunteers. J Magn Reson Imaging. 2019;49:1786–99.
88. Kamphuis VP, Elbaz MSM, van den Boogaard PJ, Kroft LJM, van der Geest RJ, de Roos A, Helbing WA, Blom NA, Westenberg JJM, Roest AAW. Disproportionate intraventricular viscous energy loss in Fontan patients: analysis by 4D flow MRI. Eur Heart J Cardiovasc Imaging. 2019;20:323–33.
89. Kamphuis VP, Elbaz MSM, van den Boogaard PJ, Kroft LJM, Lamb HJ, Hazekamp MG, Jongbloed MRM, Blom NA, Helbing WA, Roest AAW, Westenberg JJM. Stress increases intracardiac 4D flow cardiovascular magnetic resonance -derived energetics and vorticity and relates to VO2max in Fontan patients. J Cardiovasc Magn Reson. 2019;21:43.
90. Wehrum T, Günther F, Kams M, Wendel S, Strecker C, Mirzaee H, Harloff A. Quantification of aortic stiffness in stroke patients using 4D flow MRI in comparison with transesophageal echocardiography. Int J Cardiovasc Imaging. 2018;34:1629–36.
91. Jarvis K, Soulat G, Scott M, Vali A, Pathrose A, Syed AA, Kinno M, Prabhakaran S, Collins JD, Markl M. Investigation of aortic wall thickness, stiffness and flow reversal in patients with cryptogenic stroke: a 4D flow MRI study. J Magn Reson Imaging. 2021;53(3):942–52.
92. Hope MD, Meadows AK, Hope TA, Ordovas KG, Saloner D, Reddy GP, Alley MT, Higgins CB. Clinical evaluation of aortic coarctation with 4D flow MR imaging. J Magn Reson Imaging. 2010;31:711–8.
93. Frydrychowicz A, Markl M, Hirtler D, Harloff A, Schlensak C, Geiger J, Stiller B, Arnold R. Aortic hemodynamics in patients with and without repair of aortic coarctation: in vivo analysis by 4D flow-sensitive magnetic resonance imaging. Investig Radiol. 2011;46:317–25.
94. Farag ES, van Ooij P, Boekholdt SM, Planken RN, Dukker KC, Bouma BJ, Groenink M, Koolbergen DR, Sojak V, Nederveen AJ, Hazekamp MG, de Mol BA, Kluin J. Abnormal blood flow and wall shear stress are present in corrected aortic coarctation despite successful surgical repair. J Cardiovasc Surg. 2019;60:152–4.
95. Riesenkampff E, Fernandes JF, Meier S, Goubergrits L, Kropf S, Schubert S, Berger F, Hennemuth A, Henneumuth A, Kuehne T. Pressure fields by flow-sensitive, 4D, velocity-encoded CMR in patients with aortic coarctation. JACC Cardiovasc Imaging. 2014;7:920–6.
96. Dyverfeldt P, Hope MD, Tseng EE, Saloner D. Magnetic resonance measurement of turbulent kinetic energy for the estimation of irreversible pressure loss in aortic stenosis. JACC Cardiovasc Imaging. 2013;6:64–71.
97. Binter C, Gotschy A, Sündermann SH, Frank M, Tanner FC, Lüscher TF, Manka R, Kozerke S. Turbulent kinetic energy assessed by multipoint 4-dimensional flow magnetic resonance imaging provides additional information relative to echocardiography for the determination of aortic stenosis severity. Circ Cardiovasc Imaging. 2017;10:e005486.
98. Adriaans BP, Westenberg JJM, van Cauteren YJM, Gerretsen S, Elbaz MSM, Bekkers SCAM, Veenstra LF, Crijns HJGM, Wildberger JE, Schalla S. Clinical assessment of aortic valve stenosis: comparison between 4D flow MRI and transthoracic echocardiography. J Magn Reson Imaging. 2020;51:472–80.
99. Elbaz MSM, Scott MB, Barker AJ, McCarthy P, Malaisrie C, Collins JD, Bonow RO, Carr J, Markl M. Four-dimensional virtual catheter: noninvasive assessment of intra-aortic hemodynamics in bicuspid aortic valve disease. Radiology. 2019;293:541–50.
100. Fatehi Hassanabad A, Burns F, Bristow MS, Lydell C, Howarth AG, Heydari B, Gao X, Fedak PWM, White JA, Garcia J. Pressure drop mapping using 4D flow MRI in patients with bicuspid aortic

valve disease: a novel marker of valvular obstruction. Magn Reson Imaging. 2020;65:175–82.

101. Geiger J, Rahsepar AA, Suwa K, Powell A, Ghasemiesfe A, Barker AJ, Collins JD, Carr JC, Markl M. 4D flow MRI, cardiac function, and T1 -mapping: association of valve-mediated changes in aortic hemodynamics with left ventricular remodeling. J Magn Reson Imaging. 2018;48:121–31.
102. Barker AJ, Roldán-Alzate A, Entezari P, Shah SJ, Chesler NC, Wieben O, Markl M, François CJ. Four-dimensional flow assessment of pulmonary artery flow and wall shear stress in adult pulmonary arterial hypertension: results from two institutions. Magn Reson Med. 2015;73:1904–13.
103. Reiter G, Reiter U, Kovacs G, Olschewski H, Fuchsjäger M. Blood flow vortices along the main pulmonary artery measured with MR imaging for diagnosis of pulmonary hypertension. Radiology. 2015;275:71–9.
104. Schäfer M, Humphries S, Stenmark KR, Kheyfets VO, Buckner JK, Hunter KS, Fenster BE. 4D-flow cardiac magnetic resonance-derived vorticity is sensitive marker of left ventricular diastolic dysfunction in patients with mild-to-moderate chronic obstructive pulmonary disease. Eur Heart J Cardiovasc Imaging. 2018;19:415–24.
105. Bächler P, Valverde I, Pinochet N, Nordmeyer S, Kuehne T, Crelier G, Tejos C, Irarrazaval P, Beerbaum P, Uribe S. Caval blood flow distribution in patients with Fontan circulation: quantification by using particle traces from 4D flow MR imaging. Radiology. 2013;267:67–75.
106. Jarvis K, Schnell S, Barker AJ, Garcia J, Lorenz R, Rose M, Chowdhary V, Carr J, Robinson JD, Rigsby CK, Markl M. Evaluation of blood flow distribution asymmetry and vascular geometry in patients with Fontan circulation using 4-D flow MRI. Pediatr Radiol. 2016;46:1507–19.

Magnetic Resonance Imaging-Based Coronary Flow: The Role of Artificial Intelligence

35

Tiziano Passerini, Yitong Yang, Teodora Chitiboi, and John N. Oshinski

Introduction

Cardiovascular disease remains the major cause of morbidity and mortality in the western world, and coronary artery disease (CAD) is the underlying etiology in the majority of cardiovascular disease cases [1]. Therefore, it is only natural that artificial intelligence (AI) and especially machine learning (ML) and deep learning (DL) techniques would be applied to help diagnose and improve management of patients with CAD. Recently, several studies using large clinical databases have examined how AI can improve patient management by correlating a range of diagnostic data to clinical endpoints. These studies can help guide treatment plans in patients with ischemic (CAD-based) or non-ischemic heart failure [2–5]. Importantly, many of these studies employ large databases with all-cause mortality or major adverse cardiac events (MACE) as endpoints, ensuring that these studies will have an impact on system-wide patient management [2, 5]. Imaging is playing an increasingly large role in these AI studies. Although most of the larger studies using clinical databases have predominately included echocardiography data because of its widespread use in patient management, computed tomography (CT) and cardiovascular magnetic resonance (CMR) imaging have begun to be used in studies applying AI to CAD patient management [6, 7]. The richness and complexity of CMR image data make it an attractive modality to use in ML studies that include image analysis to inform patient management. Many studies that have used CMR data have concentrated on segmentation of the left ventricle (LV) from cine images, but many other applications such as tissue characterization through late gadolinium enhancement and assessment of metabolism through blood oxygenation level-dependent (BOLD) contrast imaging have also been pursued [8–10].

In this review, we concentrate on the use of AI in the major methods used by CMR imaging for diagnosis of CAD. Therefore, the goal of this chapter is to review the role of AI in direct imaging of the coronary arteries, imaging to determine coronary flow-based metrics, and myocardial perfusion imaging. A review of the imaging methodology, a survey of work accomplished to date, and future directions for work in each of the three applications will be covered.

T. Passerini, PhD
Siemens Healthineers, Princeton, NJ, USA
e-mail: tiziano.passerini@siemens-healthineers.com

Y. Yang, BS
Wallace Coulter Department of Biomedical Engineering, Georgia Institute of Technology and Emory University, Emory University School of Medicine, Atlanta, GA, USA
e-mail: yitong.yang@emory.edu

T. Chitiboi, PhD
Wallace Coulter Department of Biomedical Engineering, Georgia Institute of Technology and Emory University, Emory University School of Medicine, Atlanta, GA, USA

EMEA Scientific Partnerships, Siemens Healthcare GmbH, Hamburg, Deutschland
e-mail: teodora.chitiboi@siemens-healthineers.com

J. N. Oshinski, PhD (✉)
Wallace Coulter Department of Biomedical Engineering, Georgia Institute of Technology and Emory University, Emory University School of Medicine, Atlanta, GA, USA

Department of Radiology and Imaging Sciences, Emory University School of Medicine, Atlanta, GA, USA
e-mail: jnoshin@emory.edu

Imaging of the Coronary Arteries

Overview

The goal of direct imaging of the coronary arteries is to evaluate the 3D geometry of the coronary arteries and evaluate the epicardial vessels for the presence of coronary stenosis. Currently, coronary artery imaging is done with X-ray-based angiography in the catheterization lab or with CT coronary angiography (CTCA). X-ray angiography is the reference standard for determining the anatomical severity of stenoses, but it is invasive and expensive. CTCA enables a less invasive

C. N. De Cecco et al. (eds.), *Artificial Intelligence in Cardiothoracic Imaging*, Contemporary Medical Imaging,
https://doi.org/10.1007/978-3-030-92087-6_35

assessment of coronary geometry, with high sensitivity but low specificity for the diagnosis of CAD, resulting in the classification of non-hemodynamically significant lesions as severe in up to 50% of the cases. Challenges associated with the use of CTCA for CAD assessment include the achievable spatial resolution of the acquired images and the use of ionizing radiation. Moreover, the CT exam provides limited functional information which would be instead available by CMR. With the promise of a noninvasive and comprehensive solution for CAD assessment, development of coronary magnetic resonance angiography (MRA) has remained a topic of extensive research. The challenges with imaging the coronary arteries include their small size, tortuous 3D geometry, and cardiac and respiratory motion. The first studies of coronary MRA used multiple, single-slice breath-hold techniques [11]. Further developments extended imaging to 2D and 3D navigator echo gated techniques often with the addition of contrast agents [12–14]. The navigator echo allowed for imaging to be done at higher resolution as imaging time was not limited to a breath-hold duration. More recently, 4D techniques have been developed using either image- or k-space-based navigators to provide respiratory motion correction or motion binning [15, 16]. These methods have been extended to 5D where data is acquired continuously and retrospectively binned into sets of 3D data at various cardiac and respiratory phases [17, 18]. The 4D and 5D techniques allow for more efficient use of imaging time. Compressed sensing is used to reconstruct these highly under-sampled 3D datasets.

Use of AI in Coronary Artery Imaging

The development of novel MR image reconstruction methods over the past decade has enabled shorter acquisition times and enabled reconstruction of large image volumes with high spatial and temporal resolution from under-sampled k-space data [19]. These iterative reconstruction methods remove the aliasing artifacts and noise and fill in the unacquired k-space data. The methods include sensitivity encoding (SENSE), generalized auto-calibrating partially parallel acquisition (GRAPPA), compressed sensing (CS), dictionary-based methods, and low-rank patch-based methods. SENSE utilizes coil sensitivity maps to restore the full field of view in the reconstructed image [20]. GRAPPA reconstructs under-sampled acquisition by generating the missing data in k-space from weighted sum of several blocks of acquired data [20]. The methods which use CS to accelerate MR imaging rely on two underlying assumptions: 1) there is sparsity of the unknown image in some transform domain due to either spatial, temporal, or coil domain redundancies and 2) an incoherent sampling pattern was used to acquire k-space [21]. While CS utilizes known transforms such as total variation and wavelet transforms to enforce sparsity, dictionary-based methods (sometimes referred to as blind compressed sensing, BCS) utilize sparse transforms learned from under-sampled k-space data [22]. Low-rank matrix modeling of k-space exploits spatial or temporal redundancies, and patch-based methods learn a sparse transform from reconstructed images of under-sampled data by splitting the reconstructed image into patches and determining similarities across different patches [23–25]. Even though these methods have shown the ability to reconstruct cardiac volumes with image quality that is often comparable to the fully sampled data, they suffer from long reconstruction times due to the non-linear nature of the optimization problem, high computational costs required to find the regularization parameters, and difficulty of finding the sparse transform space that corresponds to a specific geometry [19]. For high acceleration factors, CS-based methods can also be affected by residual aliasing artifacts [26]. Also, since analytical reconstruction methods often assume a priori information about the image, such as piecewise constant total variation, their accuracy can be insufficient for images with finer details such as coronary arteries [25, 27]. Therefore, there is a need to accelerate the reconstruction pipeline in dynamic cardiac imaging to enable higher temporal resolution and in magnetic resonance angiography (MRA) to enable higher spatial resolution, reduce image artifacts, and reduce noise. In recent years, AI-based methods have been implemented to achieve these goals.

AI- and specifically ML- and DL-based reconstruction methods have been mainly used in two applications of cardiac magnetic resonance (CMR): dynamic cine imaging and whole-heart coronary MRA. The goal of AI-based reconstruction is to automatically learn optimal reconstruction and regularization parameters that find the underlying complete images from the under-sampled k-space data. If a ground-truth (i.e., fully sampled) image serves as a reference to train the reconstruction network, and one computes an image difference measure to this ground truth, then such methods are by definition "supervised." "Unsupervised" methods on the other hand do not have one-to-one corresponding ground truth. The input data can be either the under-sampled k-space, or blurred/corrupted images reconstructed from the under-sampled k-space, or both. The AI-based networks that have been used for CMR image reconstruction can be organized into four groups: *image domain denoiser*, *image domain denoiser with data consistency*, *end-to-end cascaded learning*, and *k-space learning* (Fig. 35.1).

The first type of network, the *image domain denoiser* reconstruction model, takes images directly reconstructed from under-sampled k-space as input and finds the network parameters that map these to the ground-truth images reconstructed from fully sampled k-space data. Wang et al. utilized a convolutional neural network (CNN) to map the corrupted images created from zero-filled retrospectively under-sampled k-space data to ground-truth images created from

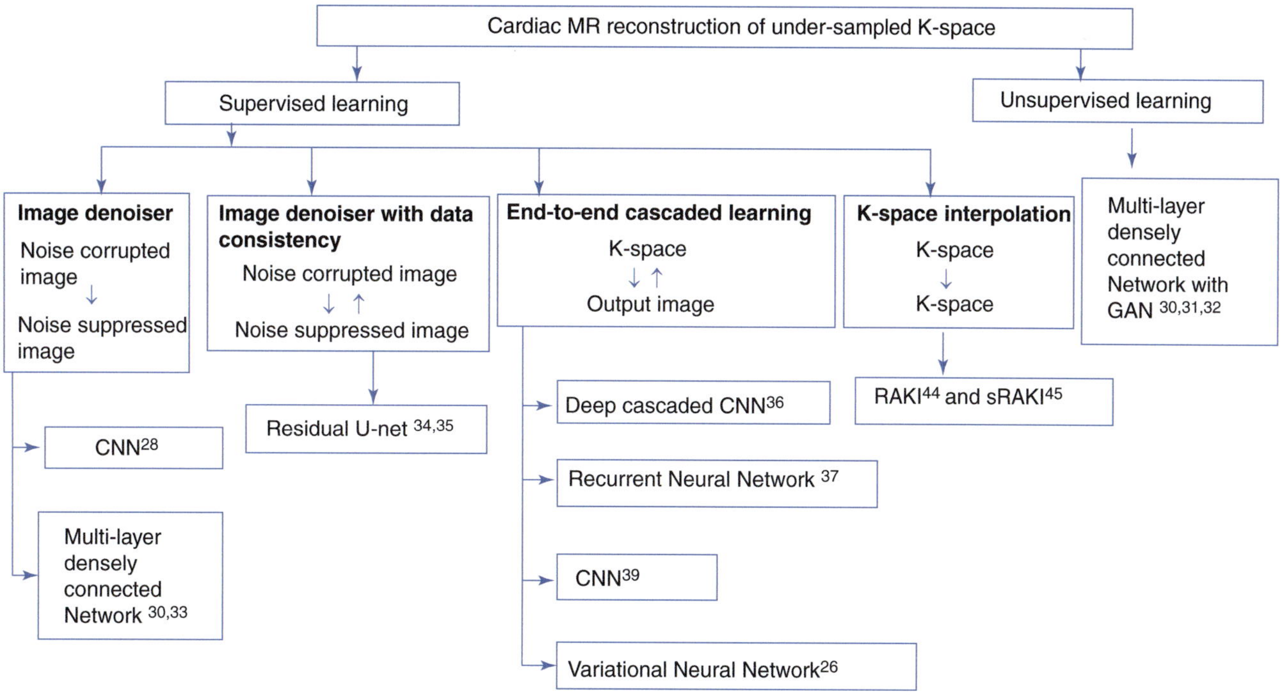

Fig. 35.1 Overview of AI-based CMR reconstruction techniques. Supervised and unsupervised methods for deep learning-based reconstruction techniques have different requirements for use of ground-truth images in training. In supervised learning, there are four main types of reconstruction: the image domain denoiser uses CNNs to map a noise-corrupted images to a ground-truth images; the image domain denoiser with data consistency enforces data consistency through residual connection in an encoder-and-decoder design; end-to-end cascaded learning uses DL to model the iterative reconstruction by enforcing data consistency in learning the regularization parameters; and k-space interpolation is a DL method for parallel imaging that learns the unacquired k-space lines from under-sampled k-space

fully sampled k-space data to restore the fine details of MR brain images [28]. They also demonstrated that the proposed network can be incorporated in an online constrained reconstruction pipeline after training to achieve the "noise-free" images in less than 1 second. Deeper convolutional networks with denser connections (i.e., DenseNet) have been developed to elevate a network's ability to extract characteristic input image features and enhance information flow [29, 30]. However, memory consumption limits the number of layers that can be practically implemented. Chen et al. proposed a multilevel densely connected network (mDCN) which reserves concatenation and direct connection to the reconstruction layer as is done in DenseNet but decomposes a single DenseBlock (DB) in DenseNet into several shallower blocks. An added 1 × 1 × 1 convolutional layer before DB reduces memory consumption and equally weighs each DenseBlock outputs to achieve the final prediction [27]. The developed mDCN can be further optimized by incorporating an unsupervised generative adversarial network (GAN)-based loss function [31] to output high-resolution images from low-resolution input in brain MR images [30]. A further extension to mDCN has been applied on 5D dynamic cardiac images to reconstruct highly under-sampled dynamic cardiac images with more than 40,000 frames by using partially separable low-rank modeling of the underlying complete images and using mDCN deep learning network to recover spatial feature spaces within the low-rank model [32, 33].The proposed approach recovers the feature space from low-rank tensor in 0.39 seconds compared to 20 minutes using conventional iterative methods.

The second type of DL-based reconstruction method is an *image denoiser with data consistency*. It is also based on image domain mapping but differs from the image domain denoiser by the addition of data consistency enforcement through a residual connection encoder-decoder network structure [26]. A modified multi-scale CNN architecture has been utilized on real-time CMR to suppress the spatiotemporal artifacts [34, 35]. The trained network has shown the ability to reconstruct congenital heart disease patients' real-time scans ~5.6 times faster compared to compressed sensing, and the image quality was superior using the deep artifact suppression network [34].

The third type of deep learning-based reconstruction network is called *end-to-end cascaded learning*. In cascaded learning, the input data is under-sampled k-space, and the target images are reconstructed by iteratively updating the output images and k-space data and employing an extra data consistency layer. Schlemper et al. proposed a cascaded CNN that concatenates two CNN structures that work together to predict the unknown k-space values from under-sampled k-space [36]. In this cascaded CNN, one CNN structure consists only of data consistency layers, while the other one consists only of denoising layers. This approach has been shown to preserve anatomical structures from real-time MRI that is under-sampled up to 11-fold and reconstructs each slice in 23 milliseconds for 2D cine and 8.2 seconds for 3D case. Qin et al. proposed a novel convolutional recurrent neural network (CRNN) which uses a recurrent neural network (RNN) to reconstruct under-sampled dynamic cardiac images [37]. The recurrent backward and forward connections in the RNN not only mimic the conventional iterative reconstruction structure but also exploit global spatial and temporal correlations between slices. This CRNN was shown to accurately reconstruct dynamic cardiac images and reduce background noise compared to a 3D CNN. Besides the application to real-time MRI, a CNN with an additional data consistency layer has been used to reconstruct under-sampled, 3D, non-Cartesian, variable density image-based navigator (iNAV) coronary MRA [38, 39]. The 3D iNAV DL model reconstructs CMRA data in 0.83 seconds compared to 1.68 seconds in iterative reconstruction techniques and improves right and left coronary artery sharpness [39, 40]. Fuin et al. developed a multi-scale variational neural network (MS-VNN) that accelerates the reconstruction of prospectively under-sampled 3D whole-heart coronary MR angiography motion-compensated using image-based 2D translational navigator [41, 42]. The MS-VNN enforces data consistency between input and output in each layer and learns the regularization parameters for both magnitude and phase images. Compared to wavelet-based CS reconstruction and other variational neural networks, it was shown that the MS-VNN achieved lower mean square error when results from these methods were evaluated against the fully sampled images [26]. The reconstruction time for MS-VNN is only 14 seconds after training compared to a 5-minute reconstruction time for wavelet-based compressed sensing reconstruction.

The fourth type of AI-based reconstruction pipeline is *k-space learning*. Conventional k-space interpolation methods such as GRAPPA use linear convolution to estimate missing k-space lines, and this approach is known to be sensitive to noise [43]. Therefore, the aim of k-space learning methods is to learn the entire k-space from the under-sampled k-space data with improved noise resilience. A robust artificial-neural-network for k-space interpolation (RAKI) reconstruction method demonstrated improved noise resilience at high acceleration rates compared to GRAPPA [44]. RAKI estimates the k-space lines from the acquired under-sampled k-space data using nonlinear convolution. Self-consistent RAKI (sRAKI) uses the RAKI framework but combines the iterative self-consistent parallel imaging reconstruction (SPIRiT), which iteratively interpolates local k-space data and enforces data consistency with nonlinear interpolation using a CNN. sRAKI reconstructed coronary MRI with an acceleration factor of 2–5 with reduced noise and blurring artifacts and an 11% improvement in vessel sharpness over SPIRiT [45].

Besides improving reconstruction speed and improving image quality of under-sampled k-space data, AI has also been used to assess image quality. A deep learning convolutional neural network for image quality assessment algorithm (IQ-DCNN) [46] was developed based on a very deep convolutional neural network (VGG 16 model) previously developed [47]. The DL network results lie within the range of inter- and intra-observer variance when compared to grading by human experts [48]. The IQ-DCNN can be used to track image quality improvements gained with increasing iterations for a compressed sensing reconstruction pipeline [49].

Future Directions

One of the most critical factors in deriving an accurate and generalized image domain noise suppression method is the quality and quantity of fully sampled k-space data for training. Since the fully sampled dataset for training usually comes from a single center and has been acquired on a specific cardiac imaging sequence, it is hard to train a denoising model that is able to reconstruct the full image from any specific imaging sequence. This data availability issue can be potentially resolved in the following ways. First, one can choose to implement DL-based scan-specific k-space interpolation methods as in RAKI and sRAKI [44] which do not require a training database. Second, a multicenter study could potentially collect many fully sampled datasets from a variety of imaging sequences to train a generalized network that could robustly adapt to input sequences. Third, using a physics-inspired reconstruction method inherently requires less training data. The mDCN model with unsupervised GAN is able to generate realistic features with high resolution and SNR from limited training data and to discriminate the artificial features [27]. Yaman et al. developed a self-supervised learning via data under-sampling (SSDU) for physics-guided deep learning reconstruction of highly accelerated acquisition without using fully sampled data for training and were able to achieve results comparable to supervised training with fully sampled data [50]. Finally, directly integrating the reconstruction pipeline on the scanner console opens the door for clinical use.

Coronary Flow and Flow Metrics

Overview

Measurement of coronary flow has the goal of determining the absolute flow through coronary vessels that perfuse the myocardium. These flow values can be used to determine and localize perfusion defects caused by either epicardial lesions or microvascular coronary artery disease. Coronary flow measurement techniques are used primarily to determine coronary flow reserve (CFR), which is the ratio of baseline coronary vascular flow to hyperemic flow [51, 52], or myocardial flow reserve (MFR), the ratio of tissue level flow at baseline to hyperemic flow. Although there are some important differences, CFR and MFR are generally taken as equivalent measures made with different modalities, and they reflect a combination of epicardial disease (stenoses) and microvascular disease [53–55]. The measurement has traditionally been accomplished in two different ways: the direct measurement of blood velocity and vessel area in the coronary arteries (in units of *cm/sec* or *ml/min* for the derived flow rate) and the measurement of flow delivered to the myocardial tissue (in units of *ml/min/gram*). The former (direct measurement) is used primarily in the catheterization laboratory where Doppler ultrasound catheter can measure blood velocity and estimate vessel cross-sectional area. The latter (tissue flow) is used primarily by nuclear medicine techniques (SPECT and PET).

CMR can measure CFR/MFR by using first-pass perfusion with or without quantitative modeling [56, 57]. CMR can also measure CFR by measuring flow in the coronary sinus using phase-contrast magnetic resonance (PCMR) at rest and hyperemia (stress) [58–60]. The CFR measurement in the coronary sinus is a quantitative global measure, whereas the measurement using myocardial perfusion is a regional semiquantitative measurement.

Coronary flow measurements can also be used to determine fractional flow reserve (FFR). FFR is the ratio of flow through a vessel to the hypothetical flow with no stenosis present [61]. Since flow without the stenosis is not possible to measure, FFR is estimated by the ratio of pressures measured distal to and upstream of a stenosis under maximal hyperemia in the catheterization lab. The maximal hyperemia reduces downstream resistance and ensures pressure is proportional to flow. FFR reflects only the resistance across the epicardial stenosis and therefore has shown value in guiding the use of percutaneous coronary intervention (PCI) and stent placement [48, 62]. Computed tomography (CT) has been used to determine FFR using a combination of CT coronary angiography (CTCA) and computational fluid dynamics (CFD) [63]. Although a number of assumptions are required to determine FFR based on CT, it has shown good correlation with invasive FFR [63–65]. AI has been used extensively in training CT-based FFR algorithms [66–68]. Recent studies demonstrated that FFR could be simulated with CMR by using a combination of PCMR measurements and anatomical imaging of the coronary arteries as shown in Fig. 35.2 [69, 70, 71].

Use of AI in Coronary Flow

CMR has demonstrated great potential for the application to noninvasive blood flow measurement. Phase-contrast magnetic resonance (PCMR) allows for quantitative local estimation of blood velocity on a pixel-by-pixel basis [72]. Coronary and systemic vascular flow can be measured with a rapid 2D measurement [73] or a 4D flow measurement technique (three spatial dimensions plus time) [74]. PCMR offers greater detail on the flow structures compared to what is possible with other noninvasive techniques, such as Doppler ultrasound velocimetry. However, accurate measurement of local velocity is dependent on image quality as determined by image parameter settings, spatial and temporal resolution, as well as the size of the anatomical structures of interest. While important technical advances also based on AI have significantly expanded the capability of PCMR to provide accurate velocity estimation for a wide range of applications (*see* Chap. 44), some open challenges still remain. Flow estimation in the coronary tree is one such challenge, since the anatomical structures of interest are small and they are moving during the cardiac cycle. In this case, measurements of

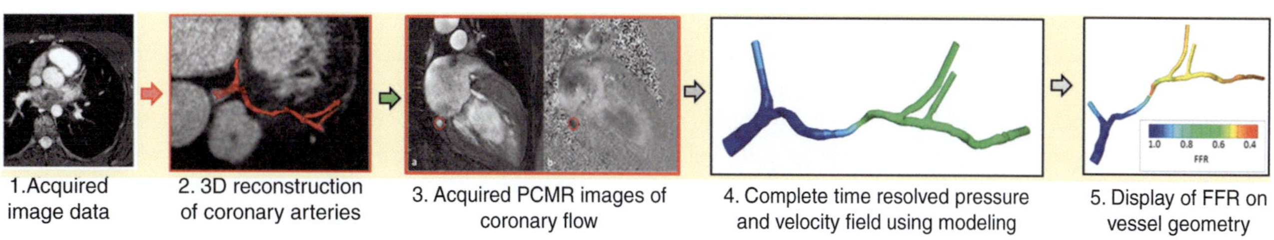

Fig. 35.2 Illustration of a workflow for determining FFR using MRA and flow data and modeling: 1) Images of the coronary vessels are acquired with a 3D coronary MRA technique as described in the chapter section entitled "Imaging of the Coronary Arteries", 2) 3D reconstruction of the coronary vasculature is done from the MR image, 3) PCMR data is acquired in the coronary arteries and/or coronary sinus at rest and stress conditions to use as flow boundary conditions for data assimilation in the modeling step (note the sparsity of data on the coronary flow images due to the small size of the coronary vessels), 4) Modeling solves the governing equations of fluid flow (Navier-Stokes equation) over the 3D geometry to determine time-varying flow, 5) Parameters calculated from the flow/pressure field such as the fractional flow reserve (FFR) can be directly displayed on the vessels

flow as well as anatomy tend to be corrupted by noise, and the achievable spatial and temporal resolution may hinder the possibility of directly resolving the temporal and spatial flow dynamics.

The traditional approach to blood flow estimation from noisy data (both for the purpose of anatomy reconstruction and velocity estimation) is formulating the problem as a data assimilation (DA) problem. In this formulation, data is combined with the governing principles of the phenomenon that is observed, in order to obtain a model that is consistent with the data while satisfying the constraints of the physical laws. Typically, available data is sparse, is irregularly distributed in space and in time, and is subject to noise. The DA model allows estimates of the physical quantities of interest in the entire region of interest with a measurable discrepancy from the direct measurements. Several examples of DA applied to the estimation of blood flow have been documented in the literature, focusing mostly on medium-to-large vessels or in regions of interest that are not significantly affected by motion, such as cerebral vasculature. Toger et al. [75] recently demonstrated that a DA approach to 4D flow measurements significantly improves the accuracy of blood flow rate estimates in cerebrovascular geometries compared to standard 4D flow imaging; 2D PCMR measurements of flow rate on a vascular cross section were taken as reference. Gaidzik et al. [76] considered the problem of flow measurement by 4D flow in complex vascular networks, in which some vessels may be too small to be properly resolved by PCMR. Using a model of blood flow in the entire circle of Willis, DA enabled a significant reduction in the estimated uncertainty of the PCMR measurements compared to traditional image-based flow modeling approaches. This is of particular interest in regions of the vascular network that cannot be resolved given the image resolution.

A limitation of traditional approaches to data assimilation frameworks is that they rely on the definition of an anatomical model of the region of interest for blood flow modeling. Most traditional approaches assume the geometry of the vasculature to be known or at least that uncertainty on the position of the vascular wall is less significant than uncertainty on the blood velocity values. The dynamics of blood velocity is characterized by significant variability during the cardiac cycle, both in time and space. Peak velocity values can vary by 40–50% from diastole to systole, and the spatial profile of blood velocity in vascular cross sections can be complex in curved or tortuous vessels, potentially requiring higher spatial resolution than what is needed to delineate the vessel wall. In the case of coronary vasculature, the aforementioned assumptions cannot be directly applied, both because coronary branches that can be affected by significant coronary artery disease may be small and because the time dynamics of the vessel wall has the same complexity as the time dynamics of coronary blood velocity. Explicitly incorporating the uncertainty on the anatomical model in traditional DA frameworks typically increases the complexity of the problem often making it intractable.

AI-based approaches to the DA problem have been recently proposed. These approaches significantly reduce the complexity of the problem in cases in which the uncertainty on the anatomical geometry cannot be neglected. In such scenarios, the choice of the underlying physics model to be used to assimilate the data can have a significant impact on the estimation of the quantities of interest. In particular, the geometry of the vessels imposes hard constraints on the expected physical phenomena, causing agreement with the data to be potentially more difficult to achieve. Raissi et al. [77–79] in a series of recent works described a data-driven approach to defining models of fluid dynamics, which is using the governing principles as a method to regularize the process of training neural networks. The resulting model represents flow in the sense that it associates relevant physical quantities (e.g., velocity, pressure) to a tuple of point coordinates and time frames provided as an input; this is similar to what a traditional computational model would do. A neural network can be trained to represent such model, when enough samples of input tuples associated with output physical quantities are provided: however, traditional learning approaches would fall short of enabling the final model to generalize to configurations not seen during the training phase (e.g., variations in the geometry or flow regime).

Physics-informed neural networks (PINN) add the laws of motion as expressed by the fluid dynamics equations to the training procedure. They aim at learning a relationship between the output variables and their derivatives, defined according to the governing equations and computed using automatic differentiation. Thus, during training, the neural network achieves the joint objective to minimize the discrepancy between predicted physical quantities and ground-truth values as well as minimize additional quantities expressing, for instance, the conservation of mass in an incompressible fluid or the conservation of momentum in the predicted output variables. Applications of this approach to the study of cardiovascular flow have been recently explored by Kissas et al. [80]. The authors showed that the estimation of physical quantities in networks of blood vessels can be achieved using a physics-informed neural network, when the input information consists of the topology of the network and measurements of blood velocity, plus area on a few vessel cross sections. Knowledge of the topology of the network allows to separate the problem into multiple components. A dedicated neural network is trained to predict flow quantities in each vessel, and interface conditions are prescribed following a standard flow modeling procedure. The system of neural networks is trained using ground-truth physical values produced by a computational model of blood flow, as well as time series of measurements acquired at specified vascular locations. In simple vascular configurations, the authors show increased accuracy in predicting blood velocity values compared to traditional computational approaches. These results suggest that the proposed approach would be suitable for estimating flow in a network of arteries, when reliable data was only available on a limited number of vascular cross sections. Therefore, a combination of high-resolution 2D PCMR measurements and relatively lower-resolution 3D imaging (for defining the network topology) could be sufficient to achieve competitive accuracy in flow estimation while moving away from hard constraints on the governing principles of flow as adopted in traditional DA approaches. This approach shows potential, but there are a number of limitations. The use of reduced order models as underlying physics models for the training of the neural network limits by design the network to only predict averaged flow quantities (e.g., the average pressure on a vascular cross section). Setting up the training database and training the network is complex and time-consuming. Most importantly, the analysis of uncertainty in the network predictions, as determined by uncertainty in the acquired data, is still lacking and remains an active topic of research.

Uncertainty quantification of blood flow estimations in the coronary tree has been recently explored by several groups, with specific focus on quantities of interest for assessing CAD. Sankaran et al. [81] considered in particular the problem of accurate estimation of blood pressure in epicardial coronary vessels, as relevant to the estimation of FFR. They analyzed the impact of uncertainty in the input data, including the definition of the geometry of the blood vessels, measurements of blood velocity, as well as assumptions on the physical properties of blood. They also focused the study on the potential impact of uncertainty from model-derived FFR values on the accuracy of a classification system for severe versus non-severe coronary lesions. They identified a significant dependency of the model-derived FFR on the estimated geometrical properties of the stenosis area, suggesting that in cases in which anatomical information cannot be obtained accurately from the images, the model prediction would have to be presented as interval estimates rather than point estimates and with a confidence level. Similar findings and conclusions were echoed by Yin et al. [82] who also reported the stenosis geometry being the most significant determinant of FFR in computational models of coronary blood flow. Among model parameters, the estimated peripheral resistance was also identified as a critical determinant of model predictions, suggesting a crucial role of the parameter identification method.

Traditional approaches to uncertainty quantification for physics systems rely on mathematical models describing the governing principles. They are based on the analysis of the behavior of the system under controlled conditions or when the model inputs and parameters are assumed to follow certain probability distributions. A principled approach such as this is valuable for the evaluation of the intrinsic uncertainty in clinically relevant quantities estimated by image-based flow models. This approach enables understanding the source of uncertainty and explains the impact of data noise or modeling assumptions on measures that could be directly involved in the clinical decision-making process. On the other hand, a large body of literature has developed in recent years, providing innovative solutions to the problem of uncertainty quantification in multiple scenarios such as computer vision, in which typically large quantities of data are available, but strong prior information on the data structure or distribution is not assumed. These approaches demonstrated great promise in scalability and ability to capture complex probability distributions of the model outputs, which are typically not well modeled by traditional uncertainty quantification methods [83]. New paradigms for model development, such as physics-informed neural networks, have the potential to offer competitive modeling solutions for contexts in which data is limited or affected by noise, in which models purely based on governing principles could implicitly enforce too strong prior information, while purely data-driven models would tend to lack robustness. This in turn can unlock novel approaches to uncertainty quantification in physics systems, leveraging state-of-the-art AI-based techniques. Zhu et al. [84] explored the use of physics-constrained deep learning models for the construction of emulators to be used in traditional uncertainty quantification approaches. They demonstrated the definition of surrogate models of physics phenomena requiring no labeled data (thus, no numerical solution of the original physics equations) while achieving better generalization to out-of-distribution test inputs compared to alternative data-driven surrogates. Yang et al. [85] developed a deep learning framework to estimate uncertainty associated with the outputs of physics-informed neural networks, based on a probabilistic representation of their states. This approach enables performing probabilistic computations for uncertain systems, as well as performing uncertainty propagation studies without the need to evaluate forward models based on computational solution of partial differential equations – which is an important source of complexity in traditional uncertainty quantification approaches for physical systems. These promising advantages come at the cost of requiring tailored training techniques, making practical application still challenging in this early stage.

Future Directions

The combination of AI-based data assimilation techniques with AI-based uncertainty quantification techniques has the potential to drive optimized imaging protocols focusing on acquiring the amount of data required to ensure estimation of quantities relevant to clinical practice, with a controlled level of accuracy.

The recent research trend on physics-informed or physics-constrained neural networks is particularly relevant in the context of noninvasive coronary flow quantification. The task of defining a flow model of the coronary circulation based on anatomical information derived from imaging and knowledge of the underlying governing principle implies strict requirements on the accuracy of the anatomical model as well as the model parameters and boundary conditions. The quantities of interest (blood velocity, blood pressure) produced by the model will depend in a predictable way on the estimated uncertainty of the input data. On the other hand, the correlation of image content with the quantities of interest (blood velocity, vessel wall position) is very difficult to model explicitly especially in scenarios in which spatial resolution is limited – such as in small or stenotic coronary arteries. Data-driven approaches have proven superior performance compared to principled modeling in discovering the correlation between input and output in similar context for various computer vision applications. Physics-informed approaches to developing data-driven models hold the promise to finding an optimal balance between explaining the correlation of input data with output quantities of interest while maximizing the consistency of the output data with expected behavior of the physical system. Additionally, the intrinsic challenges in acquiring imaging data of the coronary tree, with complex topology and vascular anatomy as well as complex motion patterns, make it crucial that data uncertainty can be properly accounted for. Further development of AI techniques for the efficient quantification of uncertainty propagation in models of physics systems is expected to be a crucial component of automated noninvasive quantification of coronary flow with impact on the clinical workflow.

Myocardial Perfusion Imaging

Overview

The goal of CMR-based myocardial perfusion imaging is to determine the extent and location of regional myocardial ischemia. Myocardial perfusion imaging utilizes an intravenous injection of a gadolinium-based T1 shortening agent followed by rapid acquisition of multiple magnetization-prepared slices in the left ventricle (LV) in each cardiac cycle. Acquisition is performed during the first pass of the contrast agent and during vasodilator-induced hyperemia. Signal intensity as a function of time over a number of cardiac cycles gives a qualitative measure of regional perfusion and perfusion reserve [56]. Areas with delayed or reduced signal intensity on the perfusion images are areas where blood flow is reduced or delayed and represent ischemia. A literature review of the T1-weighted first-pass perfusion imaging sequences is available [86], although there is no consensus on the best imaging method to use.

Quantitative perfusion imaging is based on the assumption that the concentration of contrast agent is proportional to the signal intensity. However, in perfusion MRI, there is a nonlinear relationship between the two at high contrast agent concentrations, which causes an underestimation of the arterial input function (AIF). In order to obtain a more accurate AIF for myocardial blood flow (MBF) quantification, dual bolus or dual sequence approaches can be employed for quantification [87]. These methods use a high concentration of contrast agent for analysis of the myocardium but a lower concentration to maintain a linear signal in the LV blood pool [88].

In clinical practice, CMR perfusion images have for the most part been assessed subjectively. Visual interpretation of the images is a complex time-consuming task that depends on the level of training and experience of the operator [89, 90]. Quantifying the MBF from MR perfusion images has the potential to be less operator-dependent and to enable the detection of balanced ischemia in three-vessel disease compared to semi-quantitative methods [90]. MBF also enables the quantification of myocardial perfusion reserve (MPR), defined as the ratio of stress to rest MBF, which is another biomarker for CAD and potential predictor for the outcome of CAD patients. A pixel-by-pixel MBF quantification can be achieved by solving partial differential equations from blood tissue exchange models [88].

Recent studies have shown that myocardial perfusion imaging with MRI employing a gadolinium-based contrast agent and a vasodilator stress agent is superior to single-photon emission computed tomography (SPECT) using 18FDG for detection of CAD. In the CE-MARC study, the sensitivity of CMR perfusion and SPECT was 86.5% and 66.5%, respectively. The sensitivity and negative predictive value of CMR and SPECT differed significantly, and specificity and positive predictive value were equivalent [91–96]. Similar results have been seen in other trials [93, 94]. Therefore, the use of CMR-based myocardial perfusion imaging has increased, playing a role as gatekeeper to identify subjects who should be examined in the catheterization lab due to the high probability of needing to undergo PCI to relieve ischemia.

Use of AI in Myocardial Perfusion Imaging

Machine learning has helped with the important tasks required to develop automatic quantification of MBF from first-pass perfusion MRI. Figure 35.3 shows the image analysis steps involved in the automatic quantification of perfusion MRI [97]. First, a heart bounding box is determined. The next required step is the registration of the cardiac images that may be acquired during different cardiac or respiratory phases. Many rigid and non-rigid registration solutions have been proposed in the literature to tackle this problem [98–100].

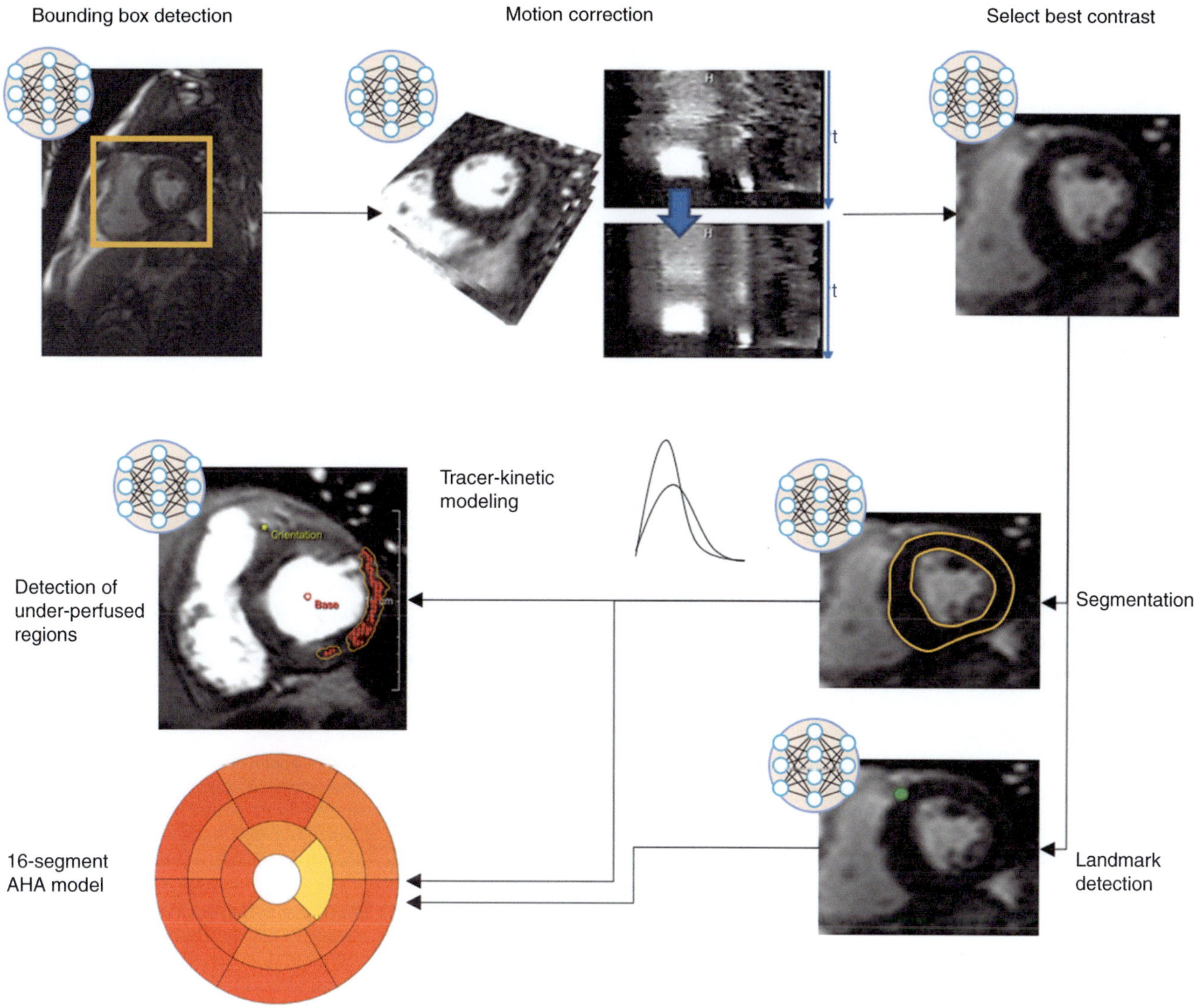

Fig. 35.3 AI-enabled image analysis steps that contribute to fully automatic quantification of myocardial perfusion MRI: heart bounding box detection, motion correction, creating/identifying a representative image with optimal contrast from the series, landmark detection, myocardial segmentation, applying a tracer kinetic model to compute a parameter map (e.g., represented using the 16-segment AHA model), and automatic detection of under-perfused myocardial regions

Myocardium segmentation is the next requisite in automatic quantification. An image frame with optimal contrast between the myocardium and blood pool is typically chosen for segmentation, or alternatively, the image series is combined into one single-frame representation using maximum intensity projection. Deep learning has great potential for accurate and robust automatic segmentation for perfusion MRI [101, 102]. A recent study by Xue et al. [103, 104] trained a convolutional neural network (CNN) on imaging data from more than 1000 patients to produce segmentation results with a low average error within the intersubject variability range.

Next, MBF is computed using a tracer kinetic model for the registered myocardium pixels. In order to automatically generate a 16-segment AHA model report for the perfusion parameters, a reference point, such as the right ventricular insertion point, is necessary to define the individual segments and provide the plot's orientation. This landmark can be automatically detected using DL methods such as image partitioning [105, 106] and deep reinforcement learning [105, 106].

Physics-informed neural networks can also be trained to fit the observed perfusion MR measured data while respecting the underlying physical laws as described by a multi-compartment exchange model [107]. Preliminary work also showed the potential of machine learning to automatically segment under-perfused regions in the myocardium using object-based image analysis [108]. The automatic quantification pipeline has been recently integrated on the MRI scanner console, allowing results to be available immediately following acquisition [103]. These techniques were combined in recent studies aiming to validate the automatic quantification of myocardial perfusion with the goal of using these methods to automatically detect CAD [89, 90, 109–111]. A recent multicenter study by Knott et al., the largest to date, including more than 1000 patients shows a significant association of reduced MBF and MPR with major adverse cardiovascular events (MACE), indicating that quantitative perfusion has prognostic value beyond detecting local ischemia.

Future Directions

One of the main reasons why first-pass myocardial perfusion MRI has not been more widely adopted in clinical practice is the challenging visual interpretation of the results and the laborious manual contouring required for quantitative analysis. In recent years, deep learning has been applied to this problem and has shown there is potential for completely automated analysis, which could contribute to a wider use of CMR perfusion in the detection of CAD. Recent findings such as the strong predictive power of reduced MPR for cardiovascular mortality, as measured both with PET (CFR) and first-pass perfusion MRI, provide the basis for more routine use of the method, but randomized controlled trials are still needed to further validate these findings.

Conclusion

AI techniques, and in particular ML and DL, have begun to play a role in diagnosis and management of patients with CAD. The use of ML and DL techniques in MRI is widespread, and studies have now begun where AI is used in cardiovascular applications of MRI to aid in image interpretation and to speed up image reconstruction and processing. These AI techniques have enabled improved reconstruction of coronary anatomy from sparsely sampled data, improved measurement and modeling of coronary flow, and automated the process of quantitative myocardial perfusion analysis. The concepts and information presented in this chapter are based on research results that are not commercially available. Future availability cannot be guaranteed.

References

1. Virani SS, Alonso A, Aparicio HJ, Benjamin EJ, Bittencourt MS, Callaway CW, Carson AP, Chamberlain AM, Cheng S, Delling FN, Elkind MSV, Evenson KR, Ferguson JF, Gupta DK, Khan SS, Kissela BM, Knutson KL, Lee CD, Lewis TT, Liu J, Loop MS, Lutsey PL, Ma J, Mackey J, Martin SS, Matchar DB, Mussolino ME, Navaneethan SD, Perak AM, Roth GA, Samad Z, Satou GM, Schroeder EB, Shah SH, Shay CM, Stokes A, VanWagner LB, Wang NY, Tsao CW, American Heart Association Council on E, Prevention Statistics C, Stroke Statistics S. Heart disease and stroke statistics-2021 update: a report from the american heart association. Circulation. 2021;143(8):e254-e743 . Epub 2021/01/28. https://doi.org/10.1161/CIR.0000000000000950. PubMed PMID: 33501848.
2. Jing L, Ulloa Cerna AE, Good CW, Sauers NM, Schneider G, Hartzel DN, Leader JB, Kirchner HL, Hu Y, Riviello DM, Stough JV, Gazes S, Haggerty A, Raghunath S, Carry BJ, Haggerty CM, Fornwalt BK. A machine learning approach to management of heart failure populations. JACC Heart Fail 2020;8(7):578–587. Epub 2020/05/11. https://doi.org/10.1016/j.jchf.2020.01.012. PubMed PMID: 32387064.
3. Shah SJ, Katz DH, Selvaraj S, Burke MA, Yancy CW, Gheorghiade M, Bonow RO, Huang CC, Deo RC. Phenomapping for novel classification of heart failure with preserved ejection fraction. Circulation. 2015;131(3):269–79. Epub 2014/11/16. https://doi.org/10.1161/CIRCULATIONAHA.114.010637. PubMed PMID: 25398313; PMCID: PMC4302027.
4. Mortazavi BJ, Downing NS, Bucholz EM, Dharmarajan K, Manhapra A, Li SX, Negahban SN, Krumholz HM. Analysis of machine learning techniques for heart failure readmissions. Circ Cardiovasc Qual Outcomes. 2016;9(6):629–40. Epub 2017/03/07. https://doi.org/10.1161/CIRCOUTCOMES.116.003039. PubMed PMID: 28263938; PMCID: PMC5459389.
5. Ahmad T, Lund LH, Rao P, Ghosh R, Warier P, Vaccaro B, Dahlstrom U, O'Connor CM, Felker GM, Desai NR. Machine learning methods improve prognostication, identify clinically distinct phenotypes, and detect heterogeneity in response to therapy in a large cohort of heart failure patients. J Am Heart Assoc. 2018;7(8). Epub 2018/04/14. https://doi.org/10.1161/JAHA.117.008081. PubMed PMID: 29650709; PMCID: PMC6015420.
6. Henglin M, Stein G, Hushcha PV, Snoek J, Wiltschko AB, Cheng S. Machine learning approaches in cardiovascular imaging. Circ Cardiovasc Imaging. 2017;10(10). Epub 2017/09/29. https://doi.org/10.1161/CIRCIMAGING.117.005614. PubMed PMID: 28956772; PMCID: PMC5718356.
7. Martin-Isla C, Campello VM, Izquierdo C, Raisi-Estabragh Z, Baessler B, Petersen SE, Lekadir K. Image-based cardiac diagnosis with machine learning: a review. Front Cardiovasc Med. 2020;7:1. Epub 2020/02/11. https://doi.org/10.3389/fcvm.2020.00001. PubMed PMID: 32039241; PMCID: PMC6992607.
8. Graves CV, Moreno RA, Rebelo MS, Nomura CH, Gutierrez MA. Improving the generalization of deep learning methods to segment the left ventricle in short axis MR images. Annu Int Conf IEEE Eng Med Biol Soc 2020;2020:1203–1206. Epub 2020/10/07. https://doi.org/10.1109/embc44109.2020.9175256. PubMed PMID: 33018203.
9. Karimi-Bidhendi A, Malekzadeh-Arasteh O, Lee MC, McCrimmon CM, Wang PT, Mahajan A, Liu CY, Nenadic Z, Do AH, Heydari P. CMOS ultralow power brain signal acquisition front-ends: design and human testing. IEEE Trans Biomed Circuits Syst. 2017;11(5):1111–22. Epub 2017/08/08. https://doi.org/10.1109/TBCAS.2017.2723607. PubMed PMID: 28783638; PMCID: PMC6508959.
10. Leiner T, Rueckert D, Suinesiaputra A, Baessler B, Nezafat R, Isgum I, Young AA. Machine learning in cardiovascular magnetic resonance: basic concepts and applications. J Cardiovasc Magn Reson. 2019;21(1):61. Epub 2019/10/09. https://doi.org/10.1186/s12968-019-0575-y. PubMed PMID: 31590664; PMCID: PMC6778980.

11. Manning WJ, Li W, Edelman RR. A preliminary report comparing magnetic resonance coronary angiography with conventional angiography. N Engl J Med 1993;328(12):828–832. Epub 1993/03/25. https://doi.org/10.1056/NEJM199303253281202. PubMed PMID: 8285929.
12. Oshinski JN, Hofland L, Mukundan S, Jr., Dixon WT, Parks WJ, Pettigrew RI. Two-dimensional coronary MR angiography without breath holding. Radiology 1996;201(3):737–743. Epub 1996/12/01. https://doi.org/10.1148/radiology.201.3.8939224. PubMed PMID: 8939224.
13. Lam A, Mora-Vieira LF, Hoskins M, Lloyd M, Oshinski JN. Performance of 3D, navigator echo-gated, contrast-enhanced, magnetic resonance coronary vein imaging in patients undergoing CRT. J Interv Card Electrophysiol. 2014;41(2):155–60. Epub 2014/09/18. https://doi.org/10.1007/s10840-014-9934-7. PubMed PMID: 25227865; PMCID: PMC4192024.
14. Ma H, Tang Q, Yang Q, Bi X, Li H, Ge L, Lin K, Xu D, Du X, Lu J, An J, Jin L, Jerecic R, Li K, Li D. Contrast-enhanced whole-heart coronary MRA at 3.0T for the evaluation of cardiac venous anatomy. Int J Cardiovasc Imaging. 2011;27(7):1003–9. Epub 2010/12/02. https://doi.org/10.1007/s10554-010-9757-2. PubMed PMID: 21120611; PMCID: PMC3182318.
15. Pang J, Bhat H, Sharif B, Fan Z, Thomson LE, LaBounty T, Friedman JD, Min J, Berman DS, Li D. Whole-heart coronary MRA with 100% respiratory gating efficiency: self-navigated three-dimensional retrospective image-based motion correction (TRIM). Magn Reson Med. 2014;71(1):67–74. Epub 2013/02/13. https://doi.org/10.1002/mrm.24628. PubMed PMID: 23401157; PMCID: PMC3655135.
16. Ginami G, Bonanno G, Schwitter J, Stuber M, Piccini D. An iterative approach to respiratory self-navigated whole-heart coronary MRA significantly improves image quality in a preliminary patient study. Magn Reson Med. 2016;75(4):1594–604. Epub 2015/05/12. https://doi.org/10.1002/mrm.25761. PubMed PMID: 25960337.
17. Masala N, Bastiaansen JAM, Di Sopra L, Roy CW, Piccini D, Yerly J, Colotti R, Stuber M. Free running 5D coronary MR angiography at 1.5T using LIBRE water excitation pulses. Magn Reson Med. 2020;84(3):1470–485. Epub 2020/03/08. https://doi.org/10.1002/mrm.28221. PubMed PMID: 32144824.
18. Feng L, Coppo S, Piccini D, Yerly J, Lim RP, Masci PG, Stuber M, Sodickson DK, Otazo R. 5D whole-heart sparse MRI. Magn Reson Med. 2018;79(2):826–38. Epub 2017/05/13. https://doi.org/10.1002/mrm.26745. PubMed PMID: 28497486; PMCID: PMC5681898.
19. Bustin A, Fuin N, Botnar RM, Prieto C. From compressed-sensing to artificial intelligence-based cardiac MRI reconstruction. Front Cardiovasc Med. 2020;7(17) https://doi.org/10.3389/fcvm.2020.00017.
20. Lin F-H, Kwong KK, Belliveau JW, Wald LL. Parallel imaging reconstruction using automatic regularization. Magn Reson Med. 2004;51:559–67. https://doi.org/10.1002/mrm.10718.
21. Ye JC. Compressed sensing MRI: a review from signal processing perspective. BMC Biomedi Eng. 2019;1(1):8. https://doi.org/10.1186/s42490-019-0006-z.
22. Ravishankar S, Bresler Y. MR image reconstruction from highly undersampled k-space data by dictionary learning. IEEE Trans Med Imaging. 2011;30(5):1028–41. https://doi.org/10.1109/TMI.2010.2090538.
23. Haldar JP. Low-rank modeling of local k-space neighborhoods (LORAKS) for constrained MRI. IEEE Trans Med Imaging. 2014;33(3):668–81. https://doi.org/10.1109/TMI.2013.2293974.
24. Bustin A, Rashid I, Cruz G, Hajhosseiny R, Correia T, Neji R, Rajani R, Ismail TF, Botnar RM, Prieto C. 3D whole-heart isotropic sub-millimeter resolution coronary magnetic resonance angiography with non-rigid motion-compensated PROST. J Cardiovasc Magn Reson. 2020;22(1):24. https://doi.org/10.1186/s12968-020-00611-5.
25. Qu X, Hou Y, Lam F, Guo D, Zhong J, Chen Z. Magnetic resonance image reconstruction from undersampled measurements using a patch-based nonlocal operator. Med Image Anal. 2014;18(6):843–56. https://doi.org/10.1016/j.media.2013.09.007.
26. Fuin N, Bustin A, Küstner T, Oksuz I, Clough J, King AP, Schnabel JA, Botnar RM, Prieto C. A multi-scale variational neural network for accelerating motion-compensated whole-heart 3D coronary MR angiography. Magn Reson Imaging. 2020;70:155–67. https://doi.org/10.1016/j.mri.2020.04.007.
27. Chen Y, Shi F, Christodoulou A, Zhou Z, Xie Y, Li D. Efficient and accurate MRI super-resolution using a generative adversarial network and 3D multi-level densely connected network. ArXiv. 2018;abs/1803.01417.
28. Wang S, Su Z, Ying L, Peng X, Zhu S, Liang F, Feng D, Liang D. Accelerating magnetic resonance imaging via deep learning. Proc IEEE Int Symp Biomed Imaging 2016;2016:514–517. Epub 2016/06/16. https://doi.org/10.1109/ISBI.2016.7493320. PubMed PMID: 31709031.
29. Huang G, Liu Z, Weinberger KQ. Densely connected convolutional networks. 2017 IEEE Conference on Computer Vision and Pattern Recognition (CVPR). 2017:2261–2269.
30. Chen Y, Xie Y, Zhou Z, Shi F, Christodoulou A, Li D. Brain MRI super resolution using 3D deep densely connected neural networks. 2018 IEEE 15th International Symposium on Biomedical Imaging (ISBI 2018). 2018:739–42.
31. Ledig C, Theis L, Husz r F, Caballero J, Aitken AP, Tejani A, Totz J, Wang Z, Shi W. Photo-realistic single image super-resolution using a generative adversarial network. 2017 IEEE Conference on Computer Vision and Pattern Recognition (CVPR). 2017:105–114.
32. Chen Y, Shaw JL, Xie Y, Li D, Christodoulou AG. Deep learning within a priori temporal feature spaces for large-scale dynamic MR image reconstruction: application to 5-D cardiac MR multitasking. Med Image Comput Comput Assist Interv 2019;11765:495–504. Epub 2019/10/10. https://doi.org/10.1007/978-3-030-32245-8_55. PubMed PMID: 31723946.
33. Zhao B, Haldar JP, Christodoulou AG, Liang Z-P. Image reconstruction from highly undersampled (k, t)-space data with joint partial separability and sparsity constraints. IEEE Trans Med Imaging 2012;31(9):1809–1820. Epub 2012/06/08. https://doi.org/10.1109/TMI.2012.2203921. PubMed PMID: 22695345.
34. Hauptmann A, Arridge S, Lucka F, Muthurangu V, Steeden JA. Real-time cardiovascular MR with spatio-temporal artifact suppression using deep learning–proof of concept in congenital heart disease. Magn Reson Med. 2019;81(2):1143–56. https://doi.org/10.1002/mrm.27480.
35. Kofler A, Dewey M, Schaeffter T, Wald C, Kolbitsch C. Spatio-temporal deep learning-based undersampling artefact reduction for 2D radial cine MRI with limited training data. IEEE Trans Med Imaging 2020;39(3):703–717. Epub 2019/08/14. https://doi.org/10.1109/tmi.2019.2930318. PubMed PMID: 31403407.
36. Schlemper J, Caballero J, Hajnal JV, Price AN, Rueckert D. A deep cascade of convolutional neural networks for dynamic MR image reconstruction. IEEE Trans Med Imaging. 2018;37(2):491–503. https://doi.org/10.1109/TMI.2017.2760978.
37. Qin C, Schlemper J, Caballero J, Price AN, Hajnal JV, Rueckert D. Convolutional recurrent neural networks for dynamic MR image reconstruction. IEEE Trans Med Imaging. 2019;38(1):280–90. https://doi.org/10.1109/TMI.2018.2863670.
38. Luo J, Addy NO, Ingle RR, Baron CA, Cheng JY, Hu BS, Nishimura DG. Nonrigid motion correction with 3D image-based navigators for coronary MR angiography. Magn Reson Med. 2017;77(5):1884–93. Epub 2016/05/14. https://doi.org/10.1002/mrm.26273. PubMed PMID: 27174673; PMCID: PMC5107365.

39. MalavÈ MO, Baron C, Koundinyan SP, Sandino CM, Ong F, Cheng JY, Nishimura D. Reconstruction of undersampled 3D non-Cartesian image based navigators for coronary MRA using an unrolled deep learning model. Magn Reson Med. 2020;84:800–12.
40. Uecker M, Lai P, Murphy MJ, Virtue P, Elad M, Pauly JM, Vasanawala SS, Lustig M. ESPIRiT—an eigenvalue approach to autocalibrating parallel MRI: where SENSE meets GRAPPA. Magn Reson Med. 2014;71(3):990–1001. https://doi.org/10.1002/mrm.24751.
41. Ma LE, Yerly J, Piccini D, Di Sopra L, Roy CW, Carr JC, Rigsby CK, Kim D, Stuber M, Markl M. 5D flow MRI: a fully self-gated, free-running framework for cardiac and respiratory motion-resolved 3D hemodynamics. Radiol Cardiothorac Imaging. 2020;2(6):e200219. Epub 2021/01/02. https://doi.org/10.1148/ryct.2020200219. PubMed PMID: 33385164; PMCID: PMC7755133 J.Y. disclosed no relevant relationships. D.P. Activities related to the present article: disclosed no relevant relationships. Activities not related to the present article: employment with and stock/stock options for Siemens Healthineers. Other relationships: disclosed no relevant relationships. L.D.S. disclosed no relevant relationships. C.W.R. disclosed no relevant relationships. J.C.C. Activities related to the present article: disclosed no relevant relationships. Activities not related to the present article: consultancy for Bracco; consultancy, grants/grants pending, and payment for lectures from Bayer and Siemens Healthineers; grants/grants pending from Guerbet. Other relationships: disclosed no relevant relationships. C.K.R. disclosed no relevant relationships. D.K. disclosed no relevant relationships. M.S. disclosed no relevant relationships. M.M. Activities related to the present article: disclosed no relevant relationships. Activities not related to the present article: consultancy and grants/grants pending for Circle Cardiovascular Imaging, grants/grants pending from Cryolife and Siemens Healthineers. Other relationships: disclosed no relevant relationships.
42. Henningsson M, Smink J, Razavi R, Botnar RM. Prospective respiratory motion correction for coronary MR angiography using a 2D image navigator. Magn Reson Med. 2013;69(2):486–94. https://doi.org/10.1002/mrm.24280.
43. Huang F, Akao J, Vijayakumar S, Duensing GR, Limkeman M. k-t GRAPPA: a k-space implementation for dynamic MRI with high reduction factor. Magn Reson Med 2005;54(5):1172–1184. Epub 2005/09/30. https://doi.org/10.1002/mrm.20641. PubMed PMID: 16193468.
44. Akçakaya M, Moeller S, Weingärtner S, Uğurbil K. Scan-specific robust artificial-neural-networks for k-space interpolation (RAKI) reconstruction: database-free deep learning for fast imaging. Magn Reson Med. 2019;81(1):439–53. https://doi.org/10.1002/mrm.27420.
45. Hosseini SAH, Zhang C, Weingärtner S, Moeller S, Stuber M, Ugurbil K, Akçakaya M. Accelerated coronary MRI with sRAKI: a database-free self-consistent neural network k-space reconstruction for arbitrary undersampling. PLoS One 2020;15(2):e0229418-e. https://doi.org/10.1371/journal.pone.0229418. PubMed PMID: 32084235.
46. Piccini D, Demesmaeker R, Heerfordt J, Yerly J, Sopra LD, Masci PG, Schwitter J, Ville DVD, Richiardi J, Kober T, Stuber M. Deep learning to automate reference-free image quality assessment of whole-heart MR images. Radiology Artif Intell. 2020;2(3):e190123. https://doi.org/10.1148/ryai.2020190123.
47. Simonyan K, Zisserman A. Very deep convolutional networks for large-scale image recognition. CoRR. 2015;abs/1409.1556.
48. De Bruyne B, Fearon WF, Pijls NH, Barbato E, Tonino P, Piroth Z, Jagic N, Mobius-Winckler S, Rioufol G, Witt N, Kala P, MacCarthy P, Engstrom T, Oldroyd K, Mavromatis K, Manoharan G, Verlee P, Frobert O, Curzen N, Johnson JB, Limacher A, Nuesch E, Juni P, Investigators FT. Fractional flow reserve-guided PCI for stable coronary artery disease. N Engl J Med 2014;371(13):1208–1217. Epub 2014/09/02. https://doi.org/10.1056/NEJMoa1408758. PubMed PMID: 25176289.
49. Piccini D, Feng L, Bonanno G, Coppo S, Yerly J, Lim RP, Schwitter J, Sodickson DK, Otazo R, Stuber M. Four-dimensional respiratory motion-resolved whole heart coronary MR angiography. Magn Reson Med. 2017;77(4):1473–84. https://doi.org/10.1002/mrm.26221.
50. Yaman B, Hosseini SAH, Moeller S, Ellermann J, Uğurbil K, Akçakaya M. Self-supervised learning of physics-guided reconstruction neural networks without fully sampled reference data. Magn Reson Med. 2020;84(6):3172–91. Epub 2020/07/03. https://doi.org/10.1002/mrm.28378. PubMed PMID: 32614100; PMCID: PMC7811359.
51. Lee JM, Jung JH, Hwang D, Park J, Fan Y, Na SH, Doh JH, Nam CW, Shin ES, Koo BK. Coronary flow reserve and microcirculatory resistance in patients with intermediate coronary stenosis. J Am Coll Cardiol 2016;67(10):1158–1169. Epub 2016/03/12. https://doi.org/10.1016/j.jacc.2015.12.053. PubMed PMID: 26965536.
52. Pepine CJ, Anderson RD, Sharaf BL, Reis SE, Smith KM, Handberg EM, Johnson BD, Sopko G, Bairey Merz CN. Coronary microvascular reactivity to adenosine predicts adverse outcome in women evaluated for suspected ischemia results from the National Heart, Lung and Blood Institute WISE (Women's Ischemia Syndrome Evaluation) study. J Am Coll Cardiol. 2010;55(25):2825–32. Epub 2010/06/29. https://doi.org/10.1016/j.jacc.2010.01.054. PubMed PMID: 20579539; PMCID: PMC2898523.
53. Ahn SG, Suh J, Hung OY, Lee HS, Bouchi YH, Zeng W, Gandhi R, Eshtehardi P, Gogas BD, Samady H. Discordance between fractional flow reserve and coronary flow reserve: insights from intracoronary imaging and physiological assessment. JACC Cardiovasc Interv 2017;10(10):999–1007. Epub 2017/05/20. https://doi.org/10.1016/j.jcin.2017.03.006. PubMed PMID: 28521932.
54. Johnson NP, Gould KL. How do PET myocardial blood flow reserve and FFR differ? Curr Cardiol Rep. 2020;22(4):20. Epub 2020/02/14. https://doi.org/10.1007/s11886-020-1274-x. PubMed PMID: 32052198; PMCID: PMC7015869.
55. Leucker TM, Valenta I, Schindler TH. Positron emission tomography-determined hyperemic flow, myocardial flow reserve, and flow gradient-Quo Vadis? Front Cardiovasc Med. 2017;4:46. Epub 2017/08/05. https://doi.org/10.3389/fcvm.2017.00046. PubMed PMID: 28770213; PMCID: PMC5511843.
56. Quinaglia T, Jerosch-Herold M, Coelho-Filho OR. State-of-the-art quantitative assessment of myocardial ischemia by stress perfusion cardiac magnetic resonance. Magn Reson Imaging Clin N Am 2019;27(3):491–505. Epub 2019/07/08. https://doi.org/10.1016/j.mric.2019.04.002. PubMed PMID: 31279452.
57. Hamirani YS, Kramer CM. Cardiac MRI assessment of myocardial perfusion. Future Cardiol. 2014;10(3):349–58. Epub 2014/07/01. https://doi.org/10.2217/fca.14.18. PubMed PMID: 24976472; PMCID: PMC4152773.
58. Dandekar VK, Bauml MA, Ertel AW, Dickens C, Gonzalez RC, Farzaneh-Far A. Assessment of global myocardial perfusion reserve using cardiovascular magnetic resonance of coronary sinus flow at 3 Tesla. J Cardiovasc Magn Reson. 2014;16:24. Epub 2014/03/29. https://doi.org/10.1186/1532-429X-16-24. PubMed PMID: 24674383; PMCID: PMC3977939.
59. Nakamori S, Sakuma H, Dohi K, Ishida M, Tanigawa T, Yamada A, Takase S, Nakajima H, Sawai T, Masuda J, Nagata M, Ichikawa Y, Kitagawa K, Fujii E, Yamada N, Ito M. Combined assessment of stress myocardial perfusion cardiovascular magnetic resonance and flow measurement in the coronary sinus improves prediction of functionally significant coronary stenosis determined by fractional flow reserve in multivessel disease. J Am Heart Assoc. 2018;7(3).

Epub 2018/02/13. https://doi.org/10.1161/JAHA.117.007736. PubMed PMID: 29432130; PMCID: PMC5850257.

60. Shomanova Z, Florian A, Bietenbeck M, Waltenberger J, Sechtem U, Yilmaz A. Diagnostic value of global myocardial perfusion reserve assessment based on coronary sinus flow measurements using cardiovascular magnetic resonance in addition to myocardial stress perfusion imaging. Eur Heart J Cardiovasc Imaging 2017;18(8):851–859. Epub 2017/04/04. https://doi.org/10.1093/ehjci/jew315. PubMed PMID: 28369259.
61. Pijls NH, van Son JA, Kirkeeide RL, De Bruyne B, Gould KL. Experimental basis of determining maximum coronary, myocardial, and collateral blood flow by pressure measurements for assessing functional stenosis severity before and after percutaneous transluminal coronary angioplasty. Circulation 1993;87(4):1354–1367. Epub 1993/04/01. https://doi.org/10.1161/01.cir.87.4.1354. PubMed PMID: 8462157.
62. Fearon WF, Nishi T, De Bruyne B, Boothroyd DB, Barbato E, Tonino P, Juni P, Pijls NHJ, Hlatky MA, Investigators FT. Clinical outcomes and cost-effectiveness of fractional flow reserve-guided percutaneous coronary intervention in patients with stable coronary artery disease: three-year follow-up of the FAME 2 trial (fractional flow reserve versus angiography for multivessel evaluation). Circulation 2018;137(5):480–487. Epub 2017/11/04. https://doi.org/10.1161/CIRCULATIONAHA.117.031907. PubMed PMID: 29097450.
63. Zarins CK, Taylor CA, Min JK. Computed fractional flow reserve (FFTCT) derived from coronary CT angiography. J Cardiovasc Transl Res. 2013;6(5):708–14. Epub 2013/08/13. https://doi.org/10.1007/s12265-013-9498-4. PubMed PMID: 23934536; PMCID: PMC3790916.
64. Min JK, Koo BK, Erglis A, Doh JH, Daniels DV, Jegere S, Kim HS, Dunning AM, Defrance T, Lansky A, Leipsic J. Usefulness of noninvasive fractional flow reserve computed from coronary computed tomographic angiograms for intermediate stenoses confirmed by quantitative coronary angiography. Am J Cardiol 2012;110(7):971–976. Epub 2012/07/04. https://doi.org/10.1016/j.amjcard.2012.05.033. PubMed PMID: 22749390.
65. Douglas PS, Pontone G, Hlatky MA, Patel MR, Norgaard BL, Byrne RA, Curzen N, Purcell I, Gutberlet M, Rioufol G, Hink U, Schuchlenz HW, Feuchtner G, Gilard M, Andreini D, Jensen JM, Hadamitzky M, Chiswell K, Cyr D, Wilk A, Wang F, Rogers C, De Bruyne B, Investigators P. Clinical outcomes of fractional flow reserve by computed tomographic angiography-guided diagnostic strategies vs. usual care in patients with suspected coronary artery disease: the prospective longitudinal trial of FFR(CT): outcome and resource impacts study. Eur Heart J. 2015;36(47):3359–67. Epub 2015/09/04. https://doi.org/10.1093/eurheartj/ehv444. PubMed PMID: 26330417; PMCID: PMC4677273.
66. Mastrodicasa D, Albrecht MH, Schoepf UJ, Varga-Szemes A, Jacobs BE, Gassenmaier S, De Santis D, Eid MH, van Assen M, Tesche C, Mantini C, De Cecco CN. Artificial intelligence machine learning-based coronary CT fractional flow reserve (CT-FFRML): impact of iterative and filtered back projection reconstruction techniques. J Cardiovasc Comput Tomogr 2019;13(6):331–335. Epub 2018/11/06. https://doi.org/10.1016/j.jcct.2018.10.026. PubMed PMID: 30391256.
67. Coenen VA, Schlaepfer TE, Reinacher PC, Mast H, Urbach H, Reisert M. Machine learning-aided personalized DTI tractographic planning for deep brain stimulation of the superolateral medial forebrain bundle using HAMLET. Acta Neurochir (Wien). 2019;161(8):1559–69. Epub 2019/05/31. https://doi.org/10.1007/s00701-019-03947-9. PubMed PMID: 31144167; PMCID: PMC6616222.
68. Tesche C, De Cecco CN, Baumann S, Renker M, McLaurin TW, Duguay TM, Bayer RR, 2nd, Steinberg DH, Grant KL, Canstein C, Schwemmer C, Schoebinger M, Itu LM, Rapaka S, Sharma P, Schoepf UJ. Coronary CT angiography-derived fractional flow reserve: machine learning algorithm versus computational fluid dynamics modeling. Radiology 2018;288(1):64–72. Epub 2018/04/11. https://doi.org/10.1148/radiol.2018171291. PubMed PMID: 29634438.
69. Deng Z, Fan Z, Lee SE, Nguyen C, Xie Y, Pang J, Bi X, Yang Q, Choi BW, Kim JS, Berman D, Chang HJ, Li D. Noninvasive measurement of pressure gradient across a coronary stenosis using phase contrast (PC)-MRI: a feasibility study. Magn Reson Med. 2017;77(2):529–37. Epub 2016/12/27. https://doi.org/10.1002/mrm.26579. PubMed PMID: 28019028; PMCID: PMC5556934.
70. Hair JM SR, Samady, HS, Oshinski JN, editor. Effect of coronary flow reserve values on the accuracy of virtual fractional flow reserve values: implications for MRI-based FFR calculations. Society for Cardiovascular Magnetic Resonance (SCMR) scientific sessions; 2021 February 18-20, 2021; Virtual.
71. Hair J, Timmins, El Sayed R, Samady H, Oshinski J. Effect of patient-specific coronary flow reserve values on the accuracy of mri-based virtual fractional flow reserve. Front. Cardiovasc. Med. 2021. https://doi.org/10.3389/fcvm.2021.663767.
72. Nayak KS, Nielsen JF, Bernstein MA, Markl M, Peter DG, R MB, Saloner D, Lorenz C, Wen H, B SH, Epstein FH, J NO, Raman SV. Cardiovascular magnetic resonance phase contrast imaging. J Cardiovasc Magn Reson. 2015;17:71. Epub 2015/08/10. https://doi.org/10.1186/s12968-015-0172-7. PubMed PMID: 26254979; PMCID: PMC4529988.
73. Johnson K, Sharma P, Oshinski J. Coronary artery flow measurement using navigator echo gated phase contrast magnetic resonance velocity mapping at 3.0 T. J Biomech. 2008;41(3):595–602. Epub 2007/11/27. https://doi.org/10.1016/j.jbiomech.2007.10.010. PubMed PMID: 18036532; PMCID: PMC2759278.
74. Markl M, Frydrychowicz A, Kozerke S, Hope M, Wieben O. 4D flow MRI. J Magn Reson Imaging 2012;36(5):1015–1036. Epub 2012/10/24. https://doi.org/10.1002/jmri.23632. PubMed PMID: 23090914.
75. Töger J, Zahr MJ, Aristokleous N, Markenroth Bloch K, Carlsson M, Persson P-O. Blood flow imaging by optimal matching of computational fluid dynamics to 4D-flow data. Magn Reson Med. 2020;84(4):2231–45. https://doi.org/10.1002/mrm.28269.
76. Gaidzik F, Pathiraja S, Saalfeld S, Stucht D, Speck O, Thévenin D, Janiga G. Hemodynamic data assimilation in a subject-specific circle of Willis geometry. Clin Neuroradiol. 2020; https://doi.org/10.1007/s00062-020-00959-2.
77. Raissi M, Yazdani A, Karniadakis G. Hidden fluid mechanics: a Navier-stokes informed deep learning framework for assimilating flow visualization data. ArXiv. 2018;abs/1808.04327.
78. Raissi M, Perdikaris P, Karniadakis G. Physics informed deep learning (part I): data-driven solutions of nonlinear partial differential equations. ArXiv. 2017;abs/1711.10561.
79. Raissi M, Perdikaris P, Karniadakis G. Physics informed deep learning (part II): data-driven discovery of nonlinear partial differential equations. ArXiv. 2017;abs/1711.10566.
80. Kissas G, Yang Y, Hwuang E, Witschey WR, Detre JA, Perdikaris P. Machine learning in cardiovascular flows modeling: predicting arterial blood pressure from non-invasive 4D flow MRI data using physics-informed neural networks. Comput Methods Appl Mech Eng. 2020;358:112623. https://doi.org/10.1016/j.cma.2019.112623.
81. Sankaran S, Kim HJ, Choi G, Taylor CA. Uncertainty quantification in coronary blood flow simulations: impact of geometry, boundary conditions and blood viscosity. J Biomech. 2016;49(12):2540–7. https://doi.org/10.1016/j.jbiomech.2016.01.002.
82. Yin M, Yazdani A, Karniadakis GE. One-dimensional modeling of fractional flow reserve in coronary artery disease: uncertainty quantification and Bayesian optimization. Comput Methods Appl Mech Eng. 2019;353:66–85. https://doi.org/10.1016/j.cma.2019.05.005.

83. Abdar M, Pourpanah F, Hussain S, Rezazadegan D, Liu L, Ghavamzadeh M, Fieguth P, Cao X, Khosravi A, Acharya U, Makarenkov V, Nahavandi S. A review of uncertainty quantification in deep learning: techniques, applications and challenges. ArXiv. 2020;abs/2011.06225.
84. Zhu Y, Zabaras N, Koutsourelakis P, Perdikaris P. Physics-constrained deep learning for high-dimensional surrogate modeling and uncertainty quantification without labeled data. ArXiv. 2019;abs/1901.06314.
85. Yang Y, Perdikaris P. Adversarial uncertainty quantification in physics-informed neural networks. J Comput Phys. 2019;394:136–52. https://doi.org/10.1016/j.jcp.2019.05.027.
86. Kellman P, Arai AE. Imaging sequences for first pass perfusion – a review. J Cardiovasc Magn Reson 2007;9(3):525–537. Epub 2007/03/17. https://doi.org/10.1080/10976640601187604. PubMed PMID: 17365232.
87. Christian TF, Rettmann DW, Aletras AH, Liao SL, Taylor JL, Balaban RS, Arai AE. Absolute myocardial perfusion in canines measured by using dual-bolus first-pass MR imaging. Radiology 2004;232(3):677–684. Epub 2004/07/31. https://doi.org/10.1148/radiol.2323030573. PubMed PMID: 15284436.
88. Hsu L-Y, Groves DW, Aletras AH, Kellman P, Arai AE. A quantitative pixel-wise measurement of myocardial blood flow by contrast-enhanced first-pass CMR perfusion imaging: microsphere validation in dogs and feasibility study in humans. JACC Cardiovasc Imaging. 2012;5(2):154–66. https://doi.org/10.1016/j.jcmg.2011.07.013.
89. Scannell CM, Veta M, Villa ADM, Sammut EC, Lee J, Breeuwer M, Chiribiri A. Deep-learning-based preprocessing for quantitative myocardial perfusion MRI. J Magn Reson Imaging. 2020;51(6):1689–96. Epub 2019/11/12. https://doi.org/10.1002/jmri.26983. PubMed PMID: 31710769; PMCID: PMC7317373.
90. Knott KD, Camaioni C, Ramasamy A, Augusto JA, Bhuva AN, Xue H, Manisty C, Hughes RK, Brown LAE, Amersey R, Bourantas C, Kellman P, Plein S, Moon JC. Quantitative myocardial perfusion in coronary artery disease: a perfusion mapping study. J Magn Reson Imaging. 2019;50(3):756–62. https://doi.org/10.1002/jmri.26668.
91. Greenwood JP, Motwani M, Maredia N, Brown JM, Everett CC, Nixon J, Bijsterveld P, Dickinson CJ, Ball SG, Plein S. Comparison of cardiovascular magnetic resonance and single-photon emission computed tomography in women with suspected coronary artery disease from the Clinical Evaluation of Magnetic Resonance Imaging in Coronary Heart Disease (CE-MARC) trial. Circulation 2014;129(10):1129–1138. Epub 2013/12/21. https://doi.org/10.1161/CIRCULATIONAHA.112.000071. PubMed PMID: 24357404.
92. Greenwood JP, Maredia N, Younger JF, Brown JM, Nixon J, Everett CC, Bijsterveld P, Ridgway JP, Radjenovic A, Dickinson CJ, Ball SG, Plein S. Cardiovascular magnetic resonance and single-photon emission computed tomography for diagnosis of coronary heart disease (CE-MARC): a prospective trial. Lancet. 2012;379(9814):453–60. Epub 2011/12/27. https://doi.org/10.1016/S0140-6736(11)61335-4. PubMed PMID: 22196944; PMCID: PMC3273722.
93. Schwitter J, Wacker CM, Wilke N, Al-Saadi N, Sauer E, Huettle K, Schonberg SO, Debl K, Strohm O, Ahlstrom H, Dill T, Hoebel N, Simor T, investigators M-I. Superior diagnostic performance of perfusion-cardiovascular magnetic resonance versus SPECT to detect coronary artery disease: The secondary endpoints of the multicenter multivendor MR-IMPACT II (Magnetic Resonance Imaging for Myocardial Perfusion Assessment in Coronary Artery Disease Trial). J Cardiovasc Magn Reson. 2012;14:61. Epub 2012/09/04. https://doi.org/10.1186/1532-429X-14-61. PubMed PMID: 22938651; PMCID: PMC3443449.
94. Schwitter J, Wacker CM, Wilke N, Al-Saadi N, Sauer E, Huettle K, Schonberg SO, Luchner A, Strohm O, Ahlstrom H, Dill T, Hoebel N, Simor T, Investigators M-I. MR-IMPACT II: Magnetic Resonance Imaging for Myocardial Perfusion Assessment in Coronary artery disease Trial: perfusion-cardiac magnetic resonance vs. single-photon emission computed tomography for the detection of coronary artery disease: a comparative multicentre, multivendor trial. Eur Heart J. 2013;34(10):775–81. Epub 2012/03/07. https://doi.org/10.1093/eurheartj/ehs022. PubMed PMID: 22390914.
95. Jaarsma C, Leiner T, Bekkers SC, Crijns HJ, Wildberger JE, Nagel E, Nelemans PJ, Schalla S. Diagnostic performance of noninvasive myocardial perfusion imaging using single-photon emission computed tomography, cardiac magnetic resonance, and positron emission tomography imaging for the detection of obstructive coronary artery disease: a meta-analysis. J Am Coll Cardiol 2012;59(19):1719–1728. Epub 2012/05/05. https://doi.org/10.1016/j.jacc.2011.12.040. PubMed PMID: 22554604.
96. Kamiya K, Sakakibara M, Asakawa N, Yamada S, Yoshitani T, Iwano H, Komatsu H, Naya M, Chiba S, Yamada S, Manabe O, Kikuchi Y, Oyama-Manabe N, Oba K, Tsutsui H. Cardiac magnetic resonance performs better in the detection of functionally significant coronary artery stenosis compared to single-photon emission computed tomography and dobutamine stress echocardiography. Circ J 2014;78(10):2468–2476. Epub 2014/08/12. https://doi.org/10.1253/circj.cj-13-1454. PubMed PMID: 25109426.
97. Gupta V, Kirişli HA, Hendriks EA, van der Geest RJ, van de Giessen M, Niessen W, Reiber JH, Lelieveldt BP. Cardiac MR perfusion image processing techniques: a survey. Med Image Anal 2012;16(4):767–785. Epub 2012/02/03. https://doi.org/10.1016/j.media.2011.12.005. PubMed PMID: 22297264.
98. Lennart T, Hennemuth A, Andersson M, Seeger A, Knutsson H, Friman O. "Phase-based non-rigid registration of myocardial perfusion mri image sequences." In 2010 IEEE international symposium on biomedical imaging: from nano to macro. Rotterdam, Netherlands: IEEE, 2010:516–19. https://doi.org/10.1109/ISBI.2010.5490297.
99. Chefd'hotel C, Hermosillo G, Faugeras O. "Flows of diffeomorphisms for multimodal image registration." In proceedings IEEE international symposium on biomedical imaging. Washington, DC, USA: IEEE, 2002;753–56. https://doi.org/10.1109/ISBI.2002.1029367.
100. Scannell CM, Villa ADM, Lee J, Breeuwer M, Chiribiri A. Robust non-rigid motion compensation of free-breathing myocardial perfusion MRI data. IEEE Trans Med Imaging. 2019;38(8):1812–20. https://doi.org/10.1109/tmi.2019.2897044. Epub 2019/02/05. . PubMed PMID: 30716032; PMCID: PMC6699991.
101. Emad O, Yassine IA, Fahmy AS. Automatic localization of the left ventricle in cardiac MRI images using deep learning Annu Int Conf IEEE Eng Med Biol Soc 2015;2015:683–686. Epub 2016/01/07. https://doi.org/10.1109/embc.2015.7318454. PubMed PMID: 26736354.
102. Kim YC, Kim KR, Choe YH. Automatic myocardial segmentation in dynamic contrast enhanced perfusion MRI using Monte Carlo dropout in an encoder-decoder convolutional neural network. Comput Methods Prog Biomed 2020;185:105150. Epub 2019/11/02. https://doi.org/10.1016/j.cmpb.2019.105150. PubMed PMID: 31671341.
103. Xue H, Davies RH, Brown LAE, Knott KD, Kotecha T, Fontana M, Plein S, Moon JC, Kellman P. Automated inline analysis of myocardial perfusion MRI with deep learning. Radiology. Artif Intell. 2020;2(6):e200009. https://doi.org/10.1148/ryai.2020200009.
104. Xue H, Tseng E, Knott KD, Kotecha T, Brown L, Plein S, Fontana M, Moon JC, Kellman P. Automated detection of left ventricle in arterial input function images for inline perfusion mapping

using deep learning: a study of 15,000 patients. Magn Reson Med. 2020;84(5):2788–800. https://doi.org/10.1002/mrm.28291.

105. Xu Z, Huang Q, Park J, Chen M, Xu D, Yang D, Liu D, Zhou SK, editors. Supervised action classifier: approaching landmark detection as image partitioning. Cham: Springer International Publishing; 2017.

106. Ghesu FC, Georgescu B, Zheng Y, Grbic S, Maier A, Hornegger J, Comaniciu D. Multi-scale deep reinforcement learning for real-time 3D-landmark detection in CT scans. IEEE Trans Pattern Anal Mach Intell 2019;41(1):176–189. Epub 2018/07/11. https://doi.org/10.1109/tpami.2017.2782687. PubMed PMID: 29990011.

107. Herten R, Chiribiri A, Breeuwer M, Veta M, Scannell C. Physics-informed neural networks for myocardial perfusion MRI quantification. 2020. arxiv.org.

108. Chitiboi T, Hennemuth A, Tautz L, Stolzmann P, Donati OF, Linsen L, Hahn HK, editors. Automatic detection of myocardial perfusion defects using object-based myocardium segmentation. Computing in cardiology. Publisher IEEE, conference location Zaragoza, Spain. 2013;2013.

109. Hsu LY, Jacobs M, Benovoy M, Ta AD, Conn HM, Winkler S, Greve AM, Chen MY, Shanbhag SM, Bandettini WP, Arai AE. Diagnostic performance of fully automated pixel-wise quantitative myocardial perfusion imaging by cardiovascular magnetic resonance. JACC Cardiovasc Imaging 2018;11(5):697–707. Epub 2018/02/20. https://doi.org/10.1016/j.jcmg.2018.01.005. PubMed PMID: 29454767.

110. Lockie T, Ishida M, Perera D, Chiribiri A, De Silva K, Kozerke S, Marber M, Nagel E, Rezavi R, Redwood S, Plein S. High-resolution magnetic resonance myocardial perfusion imaging at 3.0-tesla to detect hemodynamically significant coronary stenoses as determined by fractional flow reserve. J Am Coll Cardiol 2011;57(1):70–75. Epub 2010/12/28. https://doi.org/10.1016/j.jacc.2010.09.019. PubMed PMID: 21185504.

111. Sandfort V, Jacobs M, Arai AE, Hsu LY. Reliable segmentation of 2D cardiac magnetic resonance perfusion image sequences using time as the 3rd dimension. Eur Radiol 2020 . Epub 2020/11/29. https://doi.org/10.1007/s00330-020-07474-5. PubMed PMID: 33247342.

Artificial Intelligence-Based Evaluation of Congenital Heart Disease

36

Jennifer A. Steeden, Vivek Muthurangu, and Aurelio Secinaro

Introduction

Congenital heart disease (CHD) affects approximately 1 in every 100 children, and many of these children will require significant interventions throughout their lives. Imaging plays an important role in clinical decision-making in CHD and has become a vital part of follow-up. The main non-invasive techniques are echocardiography, magnetic resonance imaging and computed tomography. Although these modalities are now routinely used in clinical practice, there are some limitations in terms of acquisition, post-processing, interpretation and prediction of outcomes.

Over the past few years, artificial intelligence has shown great potential across the field of medical imaging. Machine learning (ML) has been used to overcome some of the challenges associated with acquisition and reconstruction of imaging data, and it has been used to automate the post-processing and analysis of images, as well as improving diagnosis and outcome predictions. Machine learning has potential benefits in CHD, including discovery of new clinical markers, more precise classification of CHD phenotypes as well as predicting disease progression and optimizing treatment plans and interventions.

However, there is currently limited demonstration of the use of machine learning techniques in CHD. This is in part due to the significant anatomical heterogeneity found in CHD and the limited amount of data available for training. In this chapter, we review the use of machine learning within medical imaging applied to patients with CHD and discuss unmet clinical needs, current barriers to translation and future directions.

Artificial Intelligence for Image Reconstruction

Biomedical imaging relies on accurate reconstruction of data for correct diagnosis and monitoring of CHD. The reconstruction algorithm transforms the collected signals into images. However, this problem is often computationally intensive and difficult to translate to the clinical environment. However, machine learning has shown promise in image reconstruction with lower residual artefacts and faster reconstruction speeds, compared to state-of-the-art technologies. There have been a number of recent review articles in the use of artificial intelligence (AI) for image reconstruction, which cover the technical aspects as well as application beyond CHD [1–3].

Despite a huge explosion in the number of proof-of-principle studies in ML for biomedical image reconstruction, there have been relatively few demonstrating their effectiveness in the CHD population.

Echocardiography

Echocardiography is the most commonly used imaging technique in CHD, as it is widely available and easy to use. However, it is highly operator dependent and often hampered by poor image quality. Machine learning has shown great potential in improving image quality from ultrasound imaging [4], as well as enabling miniaturized low-cost devices [5]. However, demonstration in CHD is limited.

J. A. Steeden, PhD · V. Muthurangu, MD
UCL Centre for Cardiovascular Imaging, University College London, London, UK
e-mail: jennifer.steeden@ucl.ac.uk; v.muthurangu@ucl.ac.uk

A. Secinaro, MD (✉)
Advanced Cardiothoracic Imaging Unit, Department of Imaging, Bambino Gesù Children's Hospital, IRCCS, Rome, Italy
e-mail: aurelio.secinaro@opbg.net

C. N. De Cecco et al. (eds.), *Artificial Intelligence in Cardiothoracic Imaging*, Contemporary Medical Imaging,
https://doi.org/10.1007/978-3-030-92087-6_36

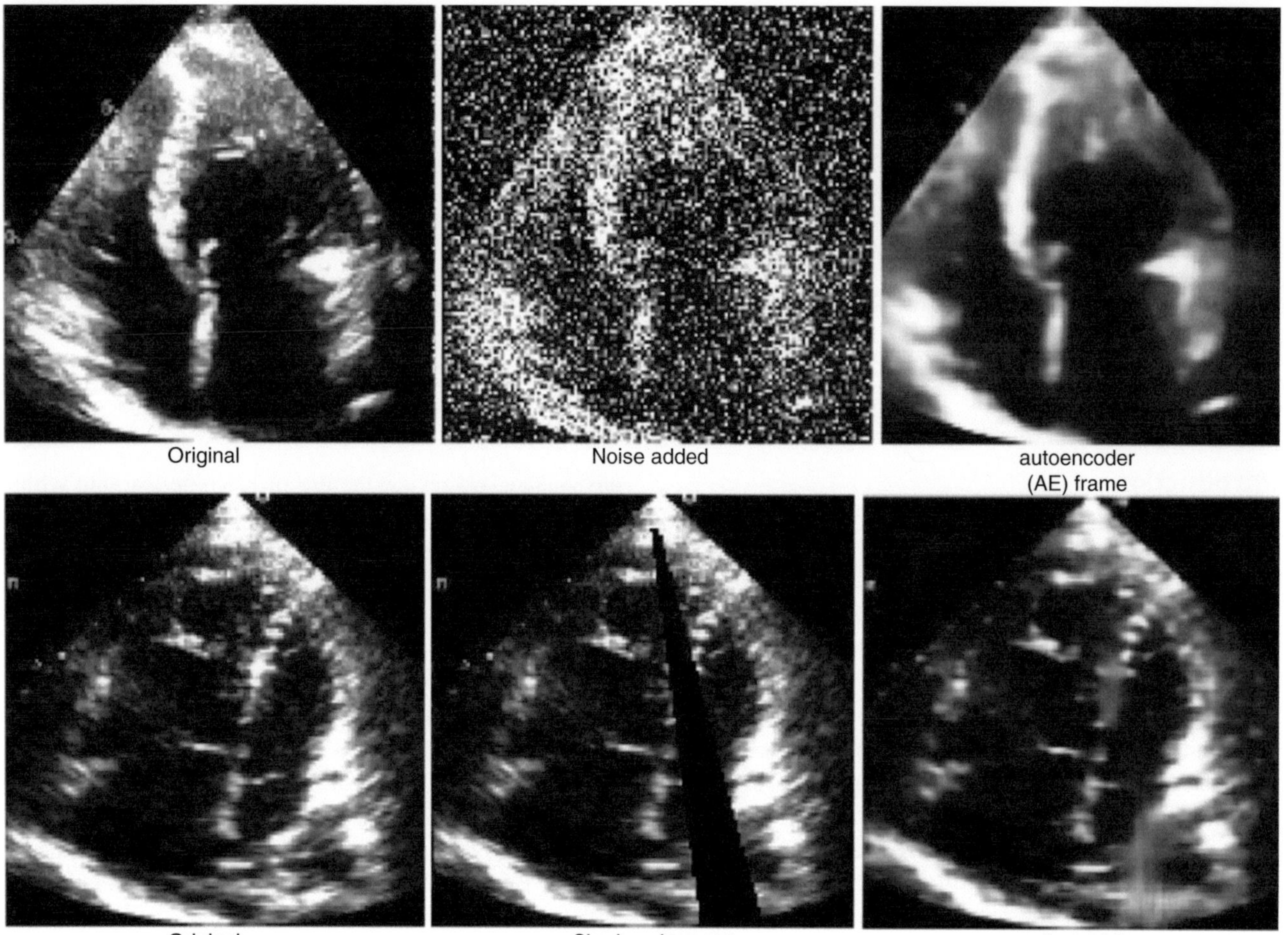

Fig. 36.1 Representative results of the auto-encoders trained for removing random noise (top row) and removing shadowing artefacts (bottom row). Sample images are from a patient with corrected transposition of the great arteries. Results shown are from auto-encoder trained jointly on normal and congenital samples. (Adapted from [6]. Permission obtained for reproduction)

Machine learning has been used to enhance transthoracic echocardiographic images in patients with CHD [6]. Auto-encoder networks were trained to perform noise removal and removal of acoustic shadowing artefacts on echocardiographic apical four-chamber views. Synthetic training data was created from a large database of retrospective 2D echocardiograms, by adding random noise to the images or zeroing sectors of the image (see Fig. 36.1). They showed that automatic denoising and removal of segmental acoustic artefacts were feasible using auto-encoder networks, with reasonable resulting image quality (see Fig. 36.1). They also demonstrated that models exposed to CHD hearts during the training process performed significantly better to models entirely trained on normal hearts, even for structurally normal hearts. However, no tests were performed on prospective data, so it is unclear how the network would perform on real images. Future work is required on real-world examples, as well as extension to 3D echocardiography.

Magnetic Resonance Imaging

Magnetic resonance imaging (MRI) is increasingly used in evaluation of congenital heart disease. In fact, several studies have demonstrated its superiority over echocardiography for evaluation of ventricular function and blood flow [7, 8]. However, conventional images are acquired over multiple heartbeats, and breath-holding is required to remove respiratory motion artefacts. Unfortunately, this can be challenging in children and is one of the main impediments to broader use of CMR in the paediatric population. There has been a huge focus on speeding up MR imaging over the last 20 years, including parallel imaging and compressed sensing. Although these may enable high acceleration factors, the reconstruction times can be prohibitive in the clinical environment, and image quality is often degraded. There have been many approaches to machine learning MRI reconstruction; a number of review articles summarizing these techniques can be found [1, 9–11].

Despite the large number of publications showing technical advances in machine learning for MRI reconstruction, many do not demonstrate clinical utility, and very few have been shown in CHD. Those that have shown demonstration in the CHD population apply AI in image space as an image enhancement problem.

One study aimed to enable quantification of ventricular volumes in real time, in patients with CHD. This enabled total scan times for a complete short-axis stack (SAX) to be reduced from ~280 s (for a conventional acquisition, where each 2D slice is acquired in a separate breath-hold) to ~18 s (during free-breathing). They used a radial sequence, with 13-fold undersampling [12]. A simple gridding reconstruction of this data results in streaking artefacts in the images (as can be seen in Fig. 36.2). In this study, a 3D (2D + time) residual U-net network was used to suppress artefacts (similar to denoising). Synthetic training data was created from a large database of conventional breath-hold, cardiac gated Cartesian SAX data. For prospective data, a compressed sensing (CS) reconstruction (GRASP, golden-angle radial sparse parallel MRI [13]) was also performed on the same raw data to compare image quality and computational time. They found that the overall reconstruction time with the machine learning network was five times faster than CS. The ML reconstructed images had superior image quality and more accurate left and right volumetric measurements than the compressive sensing reconstruction (see Fig. 36.2).

Another important area of CMR in CHD is vascular imaging. There are not any papers showing speedups in the acquisition of vascular imaging using data undersampling with machine learning reconstructions, as described for ventricular imaging. However, several studies have shown demonstration in CHD using other image enhancement techniques.

One study aimed to reduce the scan times (by threefold) for 3D whole-heart images acquired in patients with CHD,

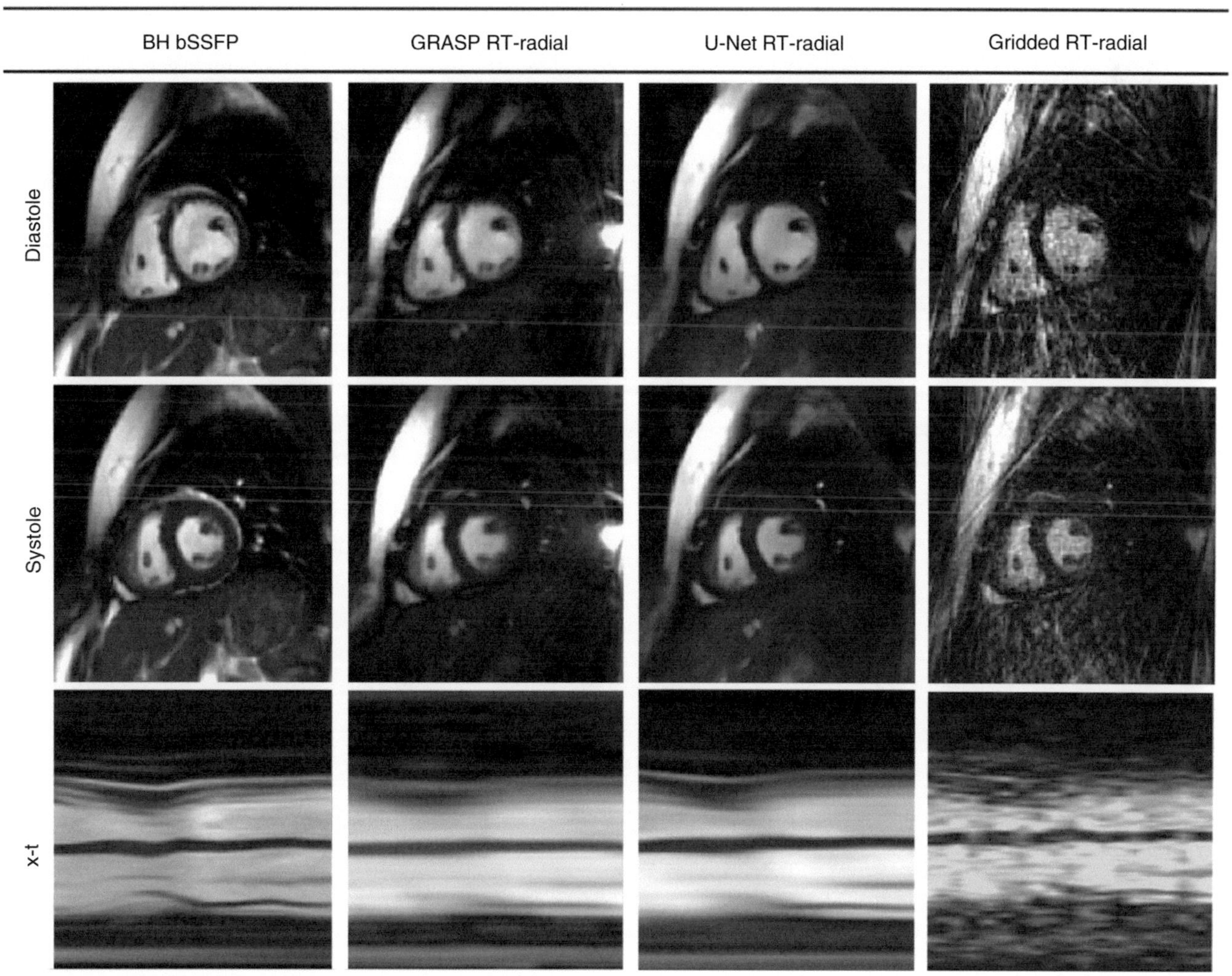

Fig. 36.2 Example of image quality in one prospective patient, shown in peak systole and peak diastole, as well as an x-t plot, from the reference Cartesian breath-hold (BH) bSSFP sequence and the real-time radial sequence reconstructed with GRASP and the residual U-net. (Adapted from [12].)

by acquiring lower-resolution data. A machine learning network was used to recover the high-resolution features from these rapidly acquired low-resolution whole-heart images [14]. Synthetic training data was created from a large database of conventional high-resolution 3D whole-heart images. They demonstrated that the network was able to provide good recovery of the features lost in the low-resolution data, which was particularly evident in small vessels (see Fig. 36.3). Additionally, vessel diameter measurements found that the low-resolution data significantly overestimated diameters in several of the great vessels; however, no significant differences were found with the super-resolution data. The authors also evaluated diagnostic accuracy and confidence, demonstrating that the super-resolution images enabled improved diagnostic confidence compared to low-resolution images. Importantly this technique does not require the use of any specialized sequences, as super-resolution reconstruction is applied as a simple post-processing step, taking ~0.7 s per volume.

Another study aimed to reduce the dose of gadolinium-based contrast agent (to 20%) used in contrast-enhanced magnetic resonance angiography (CE-MRA) in patients with CHD [15]. A machine learning network was trained to recover high-dose CE-MRA characteristics from low-dose images. Similar to the other studies described in this section, they created a large synthetic training data set from

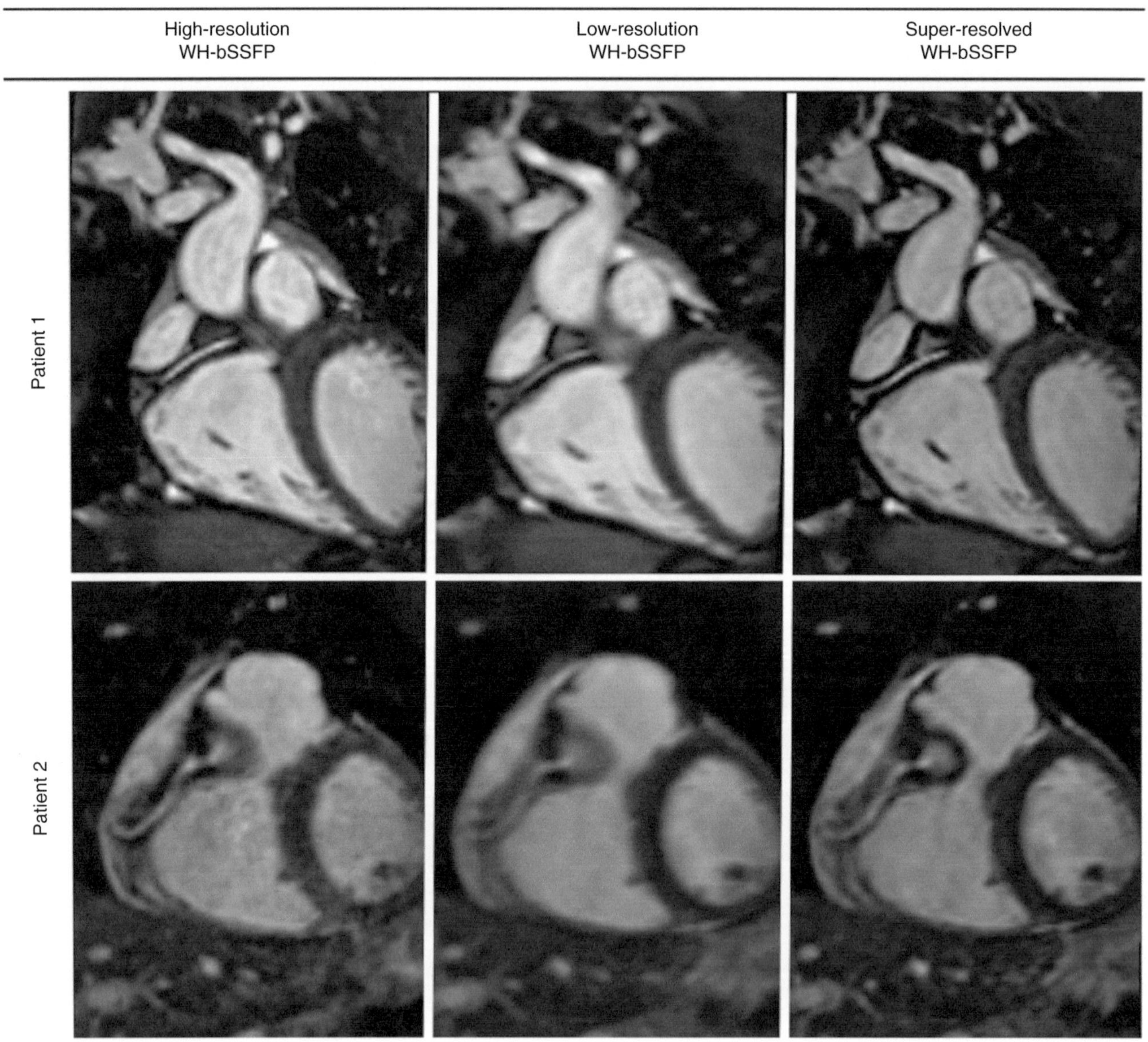

Fig. 36.3 Sample images of the coronaries from the prospective study. Multiplanar reformats of the coronary artery from the high-resolution and low-resolution acquisitions, as well as the super-resolved result. (Adapted from [14])

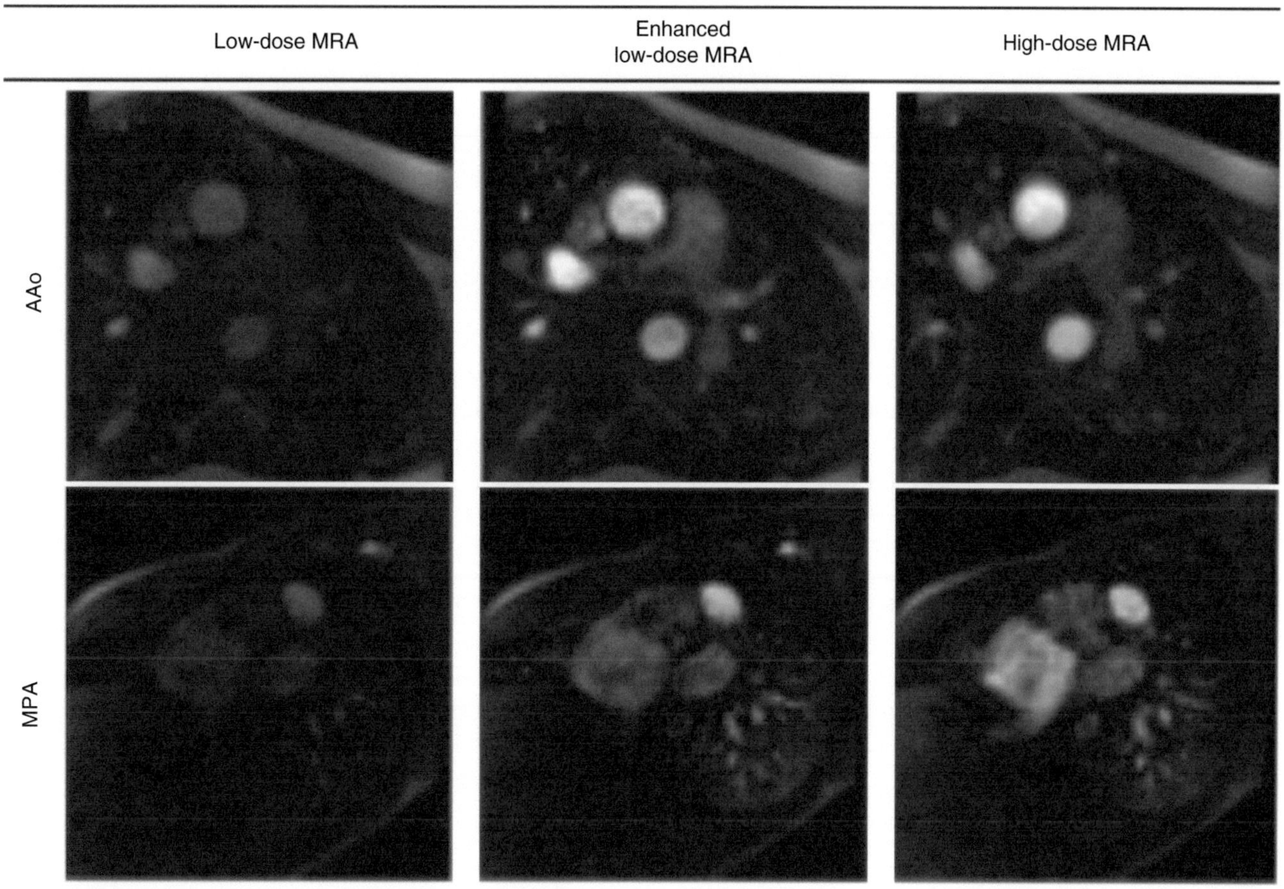

Fig. 36.4 Representative images of vessels from the prospective study. Multiplanar reformats of the ascending aorta (AAO) and main pulmonary artery (MPA) from the low-dose and high-dose MR angiographies, as well as the low-dose images which were enhanced using the trained neural network. (Adapted from CHD [15]. Permission not required as it is an open access article)

retrospective full-dose CE-MRAs. The resulting network was tested on a synthetic test data, as well as a large prospective population with CHD (where both a low-dose MRA and a high-dose MRA were acquired). They demonstrated that image quality from the ML-enhanced low-dose MRA images was comparable to the reference standard high-dose MRA data and significantly better than the low-dose MRA data (see Fig. 36.4). The method improved diagnostic confidence over low-dose MRA data, and vessel diameter measurements were found to agree well with ground-truth high-dose measurements. This method has the potential to reduce both the cost and the associated risk (including nephrogenic systemic fibrosis in patients with renal disease and deposition of gadolinium) of using contrast agents.

ML has an important role in image reconstruction, particularly in MRI. It offers the possibility of fast reconstructions without the requirement for high-end hardware. However, a significant amount of validation is still required before such techniques can be used routinely in congenital heart disease.

Post-processing Techniques Using AI for CHD

One of the major bottlenecks in CHD imaging is post-processing of images. This is particularly true for cross-sectional techniques such as MRI and CT (computed tomography). Both modalities require laborious manual segmentation of vessels and cardiac chambers in three dimensions. This is time-consuming and subject to intra- and inter-observer variability [16–19]. Despite the number of automated tools for segmentation of adult cardiac disease, currently these are not robust in congenital heart disease. This is because the segmentation problem in congenital heart disease is more complicated than other cardiac diagnoses, as both vascular and cardiac structures require segmentation, often in three dimensions.

Segmentation is a very general image processing problem with diverse applications from self-driving cars to light microscopy. Consequently, this is a highly researched area in which AI is becoming increasingly important. The difficulty in developing AI algorithms for segmentation in CHD is further compounded by significant anatomical heterogeneity and a limited amount of labelled data for training. Thus, segmentation of CHD data requires a more sophisticated approach to be successful.

Magnetic Resonance Imaging

The challenges of segmenting CHD data are recognized within the community, and a public competition for segmentation of CHD 3D vascular MRI data was set up by MICCAI (Medical Image Computing and Computer-Assisted Interventions) in 2016 [20]. They provided 20 3D whole-heart images in patients with CHD, along with manual segmentation of the blood pool and ventricular myocardium (HVSMR – Whole-Heart and Great Vessel Segmentation from 3D Cardiovascular MRI in Congenital Heart Disease). In the challenge, ten data sets were used for training and ten for testing. Although the challenge was not restricted to the use of machine learning, the winners (both first [21] and second [22] places) used ML approaches. This challenge has yielded several interesting approaches that have been subsequently built on to develop robust 3D vascular segmentation in CHD.

These top two submissions both used 3D convolutional neural networks (CNNs) as the basis for their segmentation algorithms [21, 22]. Thus, they inherently attempted to segment data in three dimensions. However, several modifications had to be implemented to overcome the complexity of the problem and the small training data set. Both studies used data augmentation to enlarge the training data set (including rotation and image flipping) along with a multiscale network to achieve good results.

The winning submission, 3D FractalNet [21], consists of multiple paths with different receptive fields, which are organized in a self-similar fractal scheme to capture the hierarchical features of the myocardium and vessels. The algorithm demonstrated high levels of agreement compared to manual segmentation (see Fig. 36.5a), with dice scores of ~0.75 for the myocardium and ~ 0.93 for the blood pool in the test data set.

The second place submission also leveraged multiscale features but used stacks of dilated convolutions to achieve this attribute [22]. This method used a patch-based segmentation, based on a classifier (myocardium, blood pool and background classes). The algorithm demonstrated high levels of agreement compared to manual segmentation (see Fig. 36.5b), with dice scores of ~0.80 for the myocardium and ~ 0.93 for the blood pool in the test data set.

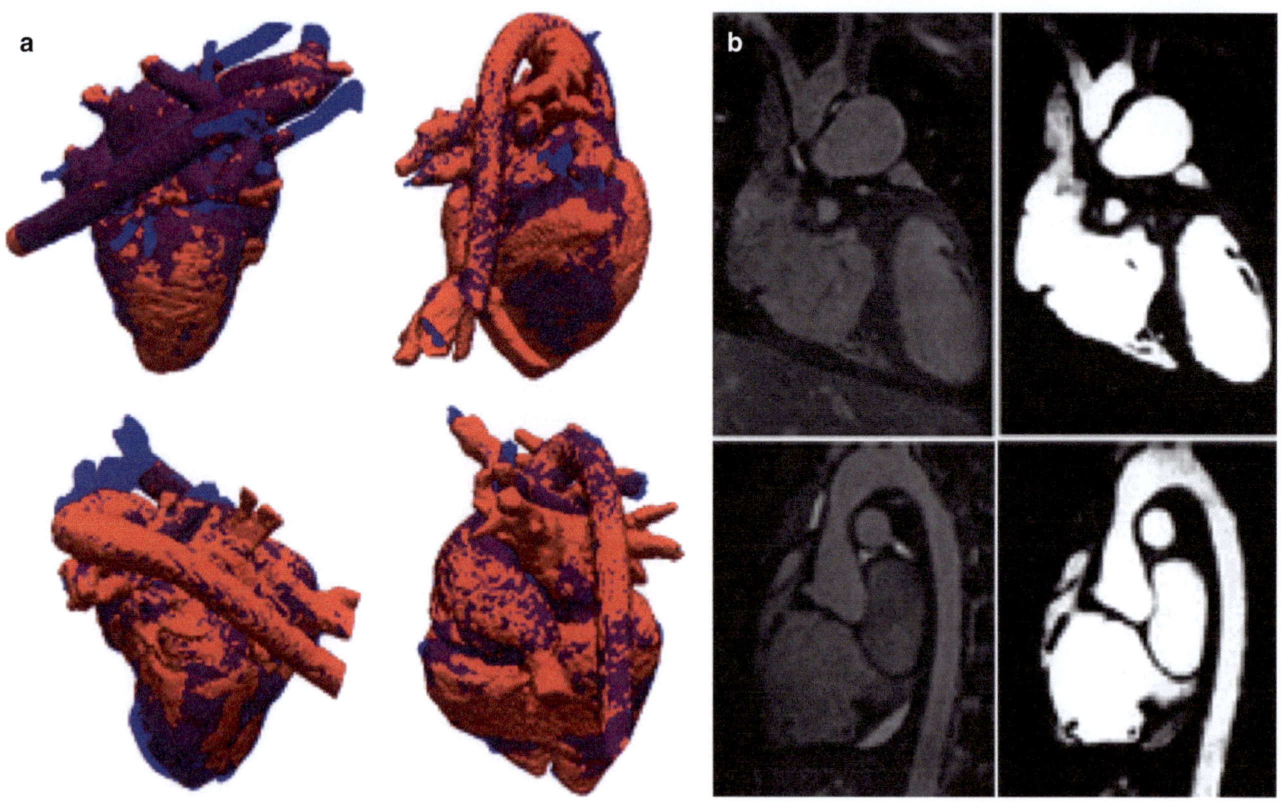

Fig. 36.5 (**a**) Surface-to-surface comparison of the 3D FractalNet segmentation results (blue) with ground truth (red) in four subjects. (Adapted from [21] with permission). (**b**) Left: CMR image slice. Right: Probabilistic blood pool maps from the CNN. (Adapted from [22] with permission)

More recently these approaches have been improved using densely connected CNNs. *DenseVoxNet* [23] uses a densely connected volumetric CNN, which is easier to train and reduces overfitting. This was demonstrated to achieve marginally better results than 3D FractalNet on the same HVSMR data set.

The three-dimensional approach is not the only method of segmenting cross-sectional data. Recurrent convolutional neural networks were created to leverage a series of data. Although classically used for time series, recurrent networks can also be used for 3D data in the form of a series of 2D images [24] (which also demonstrated the use of this network on the HVSMR data set). Recurrent networks have also been combined with generative adversarial networks that use an additional discriminator network (which tries to distinguish a segmentation image coming from the ground truth or from the generator network) to improve segmentation accuracy [25] (also demonstrated on the HVSMR data set).

CNNs are not the only approach to the segmentation problem. Another approach, demonstrated on the HVSMR data set, is to classify individual pixels based on some feature sets that include local pixel intensities. In this study, a random forest is used for multi-label appearance-based fully automatic segmentation [26]. However, this method can be sensitive to noise, and therefore, pre-processing is necessary to remove inhomogeneities/noise (here they used total variation). Nevertheless, excellent results are seen (see Fig. 36.6).

Another important area of CHD is assessment of ventricular volumes, for which CMR is the reference standard method. This data is typically acquired as a stack of 2D cine images. To calculate the volumes, it is necessary to segment the left and right ventricles at both end-diastole and end-systole. A fully convolutional network has been demonstrated to perform reasonably well for this task [27]. However, due to the challenges in obtaining large training data sets, the study additionally augmented a small training data set (of 26 patients) using a generative adversarial network (GAN) to artificially synthesize CMR images and their corresponding segmentation [27]. The resulting GAN was used to create a much larger paired data set, which was used to train the final fully convolutional network to perform the segmentation task (see Fig. 36.7). The study demonstrated superior results when trained with the additional synthetic data.

An alternative approach to reduce the need for large training data sets is to use transfer learning. Transfer learning has been used to enhance the accuracy of a U-net to perform segmentation of 2D phase-contrast (PCMR) data in CHD [28]. The U-net was previously trained on a large atherosclerosis data set, and transfer learning was used to subsequently train the network to segment PCMR data in patients with TOF. An improvement in segmentation accuracy was seen when using transfer learning.

An important real-world test of ventricular segmentation is to ascertain if functional data acquired through ML segmentation is prognostic. Diller et al. [29] developed a risk prediction algorithm using ML ventricular segmentation of single slices across all cardiac phases. In their cohort of patients with repaired tetralogy of Fallot, median follow-up time was 10 years, and 23 patients experienced an event (7 deaths/aborted cardiac arrest and 16 documented non-sustained ventricular tachycardias). They were able to show that ML-based ventricular parameters correlated significantly with patient outcome.

This pioneering work represents a proof of principle; however, there are some clinical and technical limitations that must be considered. Among others, the event rate was low with only 7 patients experiencing aborted cardiac arrest or death, while the remaining 16 (70%) experienced non-sustained ventricular tachycardia (NSVT). However, the paper is an encouraging early demonstration that a machine learning segmentation algorithm can be used to provide clinically useful data. However, significant further work is required before ML segmentation becomes routinely used in the clinical environment.

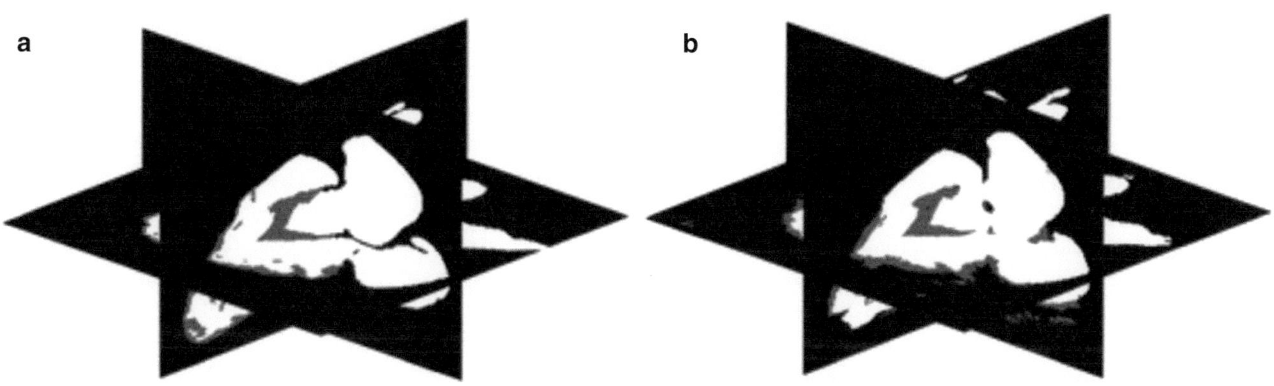

Fig. 36.6 Example of whole-heart segmentation. (**a**) Manual segmentation. (**b**) Total variation random forest method. (Reproduced with permission from [26]. Reproduced with permission)

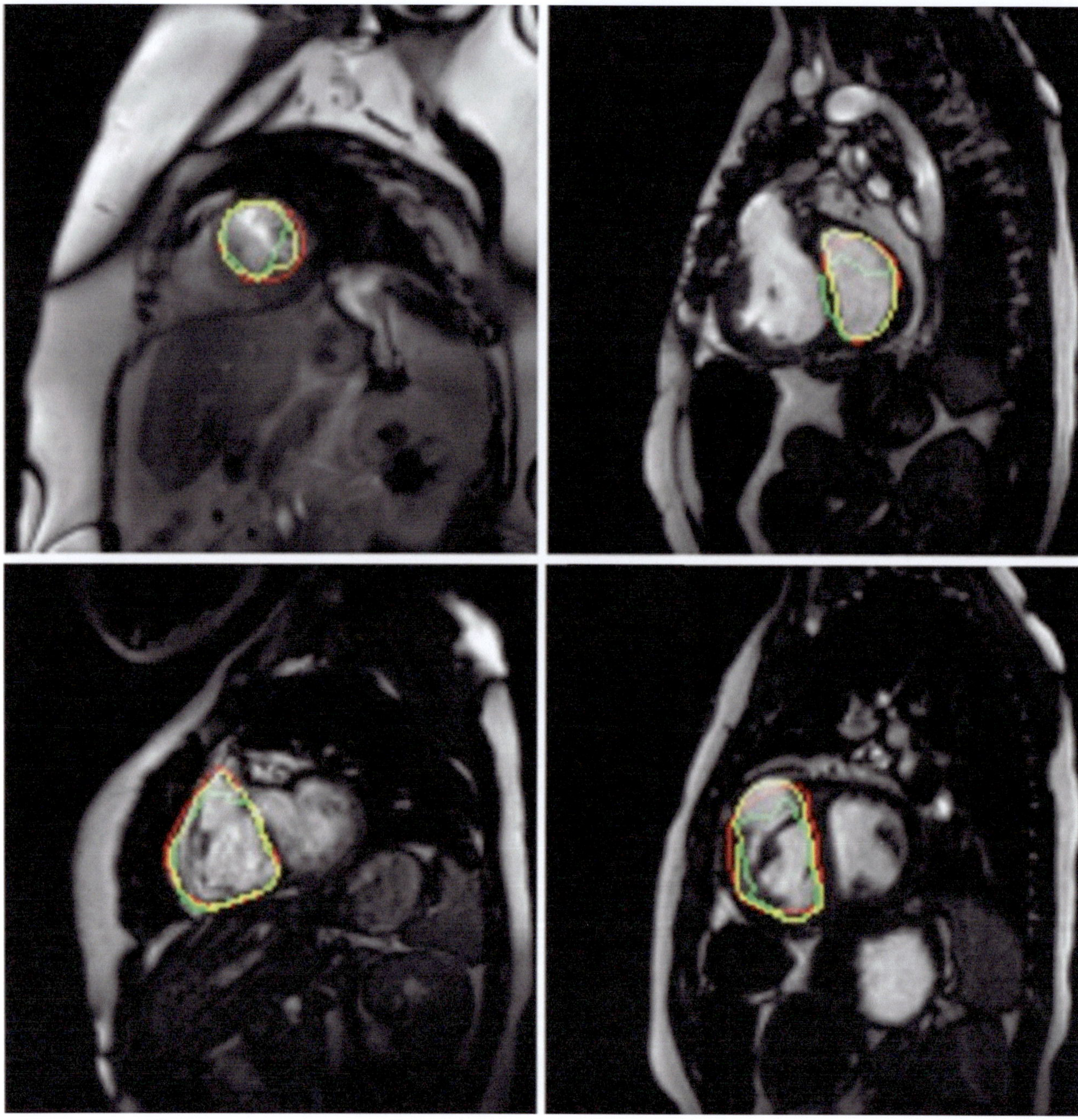

Fig. 36.7 Sample segmentation; red contours correspond to the ground truth, green is result from fully convolutional network trained without the additional synthetic data, and yellow is result from fully convolutional network trained with the additional synthetic data created by a GAN. (From [27].)

Computed Tomography

Segmentation and classification of cardiac structures in 3D CT are also challenging in CHD, and fully automated methods are currently very limited. Xu et al. [30] have demonstrated a fully automated segmentation tool, which uses deep learning and shape similarity analysis method. They use a deep learning network to segment the four chambers and myocardium and a separate deep learning network to segment the blood pool. A refinement step takes the results from these two segmentation networks, to further improve the boundaries. From these segmentation results, the connection features are extracted between the great arteries (aorta and pulmonary artery), the ventricles (left and right ventricle), and the ventricles and atrium (left ventricle and left atrium, as well as right ventricle and right atrium). The final data is then used to determine the classification of all the vessels. This technique was demonstrated on the publicly available data set: ImageCHD [31].

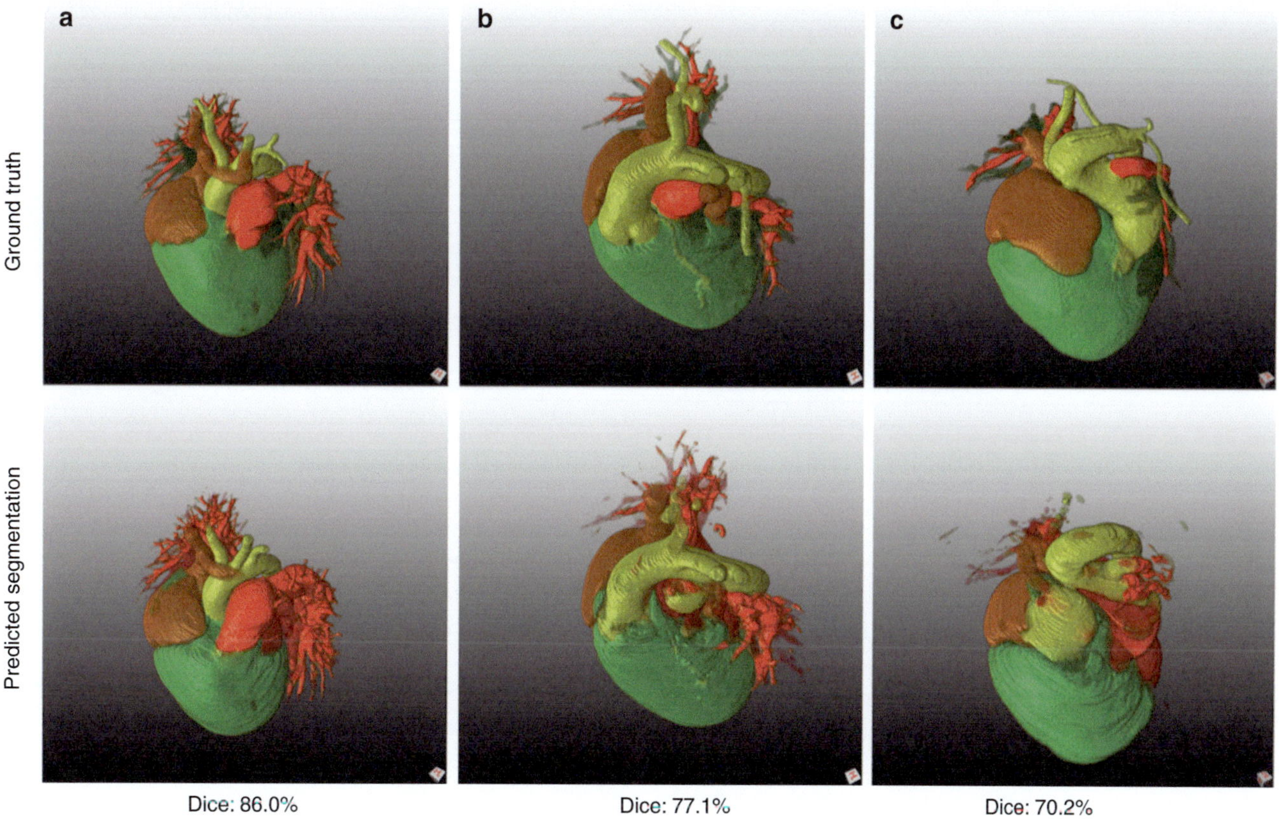

Fig. 36.8 Visualization of the ML segmentation results and the ground truth. (Adapted from [32] with permission)

A similar technique was shown to have slight improvements, through the use of graph reasoning and shape constraints [32]. In this work, graph reasoning is used through projecting a set of features into the interaction space for relation reasoning. From this, shape information can be calculated and added to the loss function as prior knowledge, to improve the prediction accuracy (see Fig. 36.8).

Echocardiography

Similarly, in echocardiography, machine learning has been demonstrated for segmentation and disease classification in CHD. A convolutional neural network has been trained to classify patients by diagnosis [33]: transposition of the great arteries after atrial switch procedure (TGA), congenitally corrected TGA (ccTGA) or normal anatomy. The network was trained using apical four-chamber or parasternal short-axis views from routine transthoracic echocardiograms. The resulting network was able to correctly identify >95% of frames. In the same study, an independent U-net was trained to segment the ventricles in the apical four-chamber view, with separate networks for ccTGA, TGA and normal hearts. The resulting networks were able to correctly identify the systemic ventricle and achieved a high performance in segmenting the systemic right or left ventricle (as seen in Fig. 36.9).

Diagnosis and Outcome Using AI for CHD

Diagnosis, outcome and prediction of events in CHD patients are extremely challenging because of the complex interactions mediating physiologic processes. This often results in traditional regression techniques failing. However, ML has emerged with the necessary tools for both identifying complex patterns within data sets and using those patterns to make better predictions.

Development of AI systems in predictive models requires training data that are generated from clinical activities, including screening, diagnosis and treatment. Monitoring of CHD requires frequent imaging tests, which, combined with ML, has the potential to enable early disease recognition, risk prediction and accurate diagnosis. In order to do this, the data sets need to be queried to explore what is known, perform trend analysis and predict what is about to happen. Probing models that can decrypt the data and pick features that can lead to disease prediction will play a pivotal role in inching closer to personalized medicine [34].

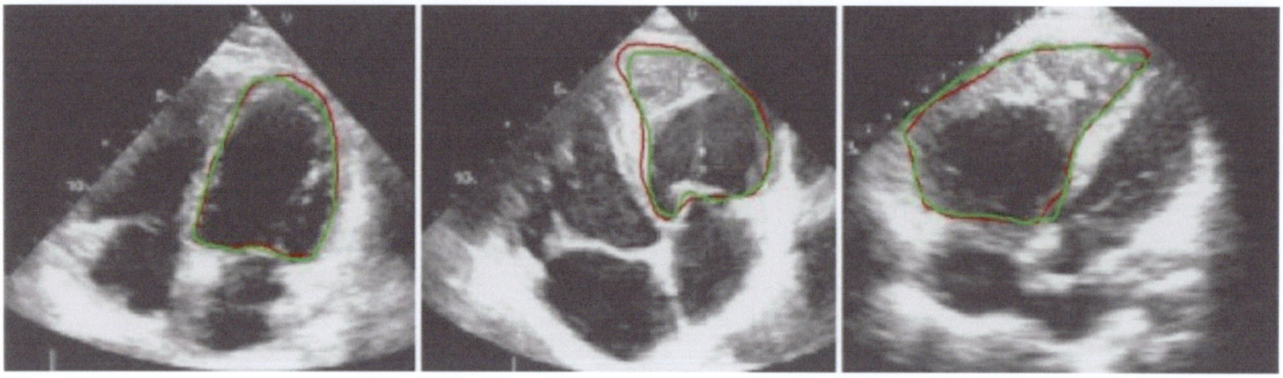

Fig. 36.9 Examples of systemic ventricular ML segmentation. The red line represents the manually provided ground-truth, and the green line is the automatically generated segmentation by the deep learning algorithm. (Adapted from [33] with permission)

X-Ray-Based Prediction Model

Chest radiography can be useful in evaluating pulmonary blood flow status in patients with CHD. However, the predictive value of chest radiography is limited by the subjective and qualitative nature of the interpretation. In a retrospective observational study using cardiac catheterizations and chest radiographs, a deep learning model was used to predict the pulmonary to systemic flow ratio [35]. It was shown that the model significantly correlated with the values calculated using the Fick method, with significantly higher diagnostic concordance than that of experts (64 of 100 cases vs 49 of 100 cases). This may allow clinicians to quantify otherwise qualitative and subjective findings of pulmonary vascularity from chest radiographs.

Echo-Based Interpretation

In echocardiography, the main role of AI in interpretation is in foetal diagnosis. Foetal survey ultrasound is recommended worldwide for prenatal diagnosis of CHD; however, it has poor sensitivity (as low as 30% [36]). Recently, the prenatal ultrasound nine-segment sequential analysis method has been shown to increase accuracy in the diagnosis of foetal CHD [37]. Nevertheless, fully automated methods are desirable.

One study [36] used a large database of retrospective echocardiograms to develop three separate ML models to (i) perform view classification, (ii) distinguish between normal hearts and complex CHD and (iii) perform segmentation to calculate standard foetal cardiothoracic measurements. They showed that the view classification network was able to correctly identify standard views with high sensitivity and specificity (90% and 78%, respectively). Based on the results from the view classification networks, a composite disease classification network was also able to achieve high sensitivity and specificity (95% and 96%, respectively). These deep learning results represent a doubling of sensitivity and specificity, compared to community-level results, on a population-based test set.

A similar ML framework, based on a random forest pipeline, has been presented [38] for detection prediction of congenital heart disease using foetal echocardiography and more recently a large study.

MRI-Based Prediction Algorithm

Prediction of clinical outcomes and prognosis from cardiac MR images have mostly been applied to repaired tetralogy of Fallot patients. Tetralogy of Fallot (TOF) represents the most common cyanotic congenital heart defect at birth, and these patients have an increased risk of ventricular arrhythmias and sudden cardiac death.

In their study, Samad et al. sought to predict the deterioration of right ventricular performance in patients with repaired TOF using ML [39]. The increasing mortality risk generally coincides with progressive dilation and dysfunction of both the left and right ventricles (LV and RV, respectively) [40, 41], and there is growing evidence of a link between dysfunction and poor outcomes, such as death or sustained ventricular tachycardia. The study used both baseline clinical variables and cardiac mechanics from MRI scans to predict repaired TOF patient's deterioration. They showed baseline left LV ejection fraction, LV circumferential strain and pulmonary regurgitation were most useful for achieving accurate predictions. Overall, the network was able to predict deterioration with mean area under the curve (AUC) >0.77. In the future, larger registry-based studies are required to determine if more sophisticated methods can be used to determine events and timing.

CT-Based Prediction Algorithm

There is a growing interest in alternative methods to evaluate pulmonary arterial pressure, using non-invasive image-based metrics. One study [42] demonstrated the use of machine learning classifiers for predicting high-risk mean pulmonary arterial pressure (mPAP >15 mmHg) based on preoperative cardiac CT in staged single-ventricle palliative surgery (post-Glenn shunt). Based on univariate analysis, seven morphologic parameters were manually extracted from CT images. These were used to train a random forest model, which was able to predict post-Glenn shunt patients with a high risk of mPAP >15 mmHg, with mean AUC of 0.79, sensitivity of 78%, specificity of 75% and accuracy of 76%.

Conclusion

In this chapter, we have set out the three main areas where AI can aid in imaging for CHD. These are image reconstruction, post-processing and development of prediction models. AI is particularly relevant to MRI and CT reconstruction and post-processing due to their time-consuming nature. However, there are also important uses of AI in echocardiography, such as image quality enhancement.

Machine learning techniques have also emerged as highly effective computer algorithms for the stratification of patterns in medical data sets with a multitude of variables, facilitating the build-up of models for data-driven prediction or classification. Both supervised and unsupervised ML can be applied to clinical data for developing robust risk models and redefining patient classes. ML promises to revolutionize cardiac imaging with more accurate and more reproducible interpretation delivered almost instantaneously. But transferring promise into clinical delivery is a considerable task, and we fall behind other fields [43].

All of the studies cited in this chapter fall into the category of proof of concept. Thus, large-scale validation studies are required in all areas, prior to routine clinical translation. Nevertheless, AI does have the potential to significantly improve imaging in CHD.

References

1. Wang G, Ye JC, Mueller K, Fessler JA. Image reconstruction is a new frontier of machine learning. IEEE Trans Med Imaging. 2018;37:1289–96.
2. Ben Yedder H, Cardoen B, Hamarneh G. Deep learning for biomedical image reconstruction: a survey. Artif Intell Rev. 2020; https://doi.org/10.1007/s10462-020-09861-2.
3. Zhang H-M, Dong B. A review on deep learning in medical image reconstruction. J Oper Res Soc China. 2020;8:311–40. https://doi.org/10.1007/s40305-019-00287-4.
4. Huijben IAM, Veeling BS, Janse K, Mischi M, Sloun RJG, v. Learning sub-sampling and signal recovery with applications in ultrasound imaging. IEEE Trans Med Imaging. 2020;39:3955–66. https://doi.org/10.1109/TMI.2020.3008501.
5. van Sloun RJG, Cohen R, Eldar YC. Deep learning in ultrasound imaging. Proc IEEE. 2020;108:11–29. https://doi.org/10.1109/JPROC.2019.2932116.
6. Diller G-P, et al. Denoising and artefact removal for transthoracic echocardiographic imaging in congenital heart disease: utility of diagnosis specific deep learning algorithms. Int J Cardiovasc Imaging. 2019;35:2189–96. https://doi.org/10.1007/s10554-019-01671-0.
7. Krupickova S, et al. Echocardiographic arterial measurements in complex congenital diseases before bidirectional Glenn: comparison with cardiovascular magnetic resonance imaging. Eur Heart J Cardiovasc Imaging. 2016;18:332–41. https://doi.org/10.1093/ehjci/jew069.
8. Moledina S, et al. Prognostic significance of cardiac magnetic resonance imaging in children with pulmonary hypertension. Circulation Cardiovasc Imaging. 2013;6:407–14. https://doi.org/10.1161/CIRCIMAGING.112.000082.
9. Montalt-Tordera J, Muthurangu V, Hauptmann A, Steeden JA. Machine learning in Magnetic Resonance Imaging: Image reconstruction. Physica Medica. 2021;83:79–87. https://doi.org/10.1016/j.ejmp.2021.02.020.
10. Knoll F, et al. Deep-learning methods for parallel magnetic resonance imaging reconstruction: a survey of the current approaches, trends, and issues. IEEE Signal Process Mag. 2020;37:128–40. https://doi.org/10.1109/MSP.2019.2950640.
11. Liang D, Cheng J, Ke Z, Ying L. Deep magnetic resonance image reconstruction: inverse problems meet neural networks. IEEE Signal Process Mag. 2020;37:141–51. https://doi.org/10.1109/MSP.2019.2950557.
12. Hauptmann A, Arridge S, Lucka F, Muthurangu V, Steeden JA. Real-time cardiovascular MR with spatio-temporal artifact suppression using deep learning–proof of concept in congenital heart disease. Magn Reson Med. 2019;81:1143–56. https://doi.org/10.1002/mrm.27480.
13. Feng L, et al. Golden-angle radial sparse parallel MRI: combination of compressed sensing, parallel imaging, and golden-angle radial sampling for fast and flexible dynamic volumetric MRI. MRM. 2014;72:707–17. https://doi.org/10.1002/mrm.24980.
14. Steeden JA, et al. Rapid whole-heart CMR with single volume super-resolution. J Cardiovasc Magn Reson. 2020;22:56. https://doi.org/10.1186/s12968-020-00651-x.
15. Montalt-Tordera J, Quail M, Steeden JA, Muthurangu V. Reducing contrast agent dose in cardiovascular MR angiography with deep learning. JMRI. 2021;54:795.
16. Petitjean C, Dacher J-N. A review of segmentation methods in short axis cardiac MR images. Med Image Anal. 2011;15:169–84. https://doi.org/10.1016/j.media.2010.12.004.
17. Tavakoli V, Amini AA. A survey of shaped-based registration and segmentation techniques for cardiac images. Comput Vis Image Underst. 2013;117:966–89. https://doi.org/10.1016/j.cviu.2012.11.017.
18. Heimann T, Meinzer H-P. Statistical shape models for 3D medical image segmentation: a review. Med Image Anal. 2009;13:543–63. https://doi.org/10.1016/j.media.2009.05.004.
19. Suinesiaputra A, et al. A collaborative resource to build consensus for automated left ventricular segmentation of cardiac MR images. Med Image Anal. 2014;18:50–62. https://doi.org/10.1016/j.media.2013.09.001.
20. Zuluaga MA, Bhatia K, Kainz B, Moghari MH, Pace DF. Reconstruction, segmentation, and analysis of medical images: first international workshops, RAMBO 2016 and HVSMR 2016,

held in conjunction with MICCAI 2016, Athens, Greece, October 17, 2016, revised selected papers. Vol. 10129 (Springer, 2017).

21. Yu L, Yang X, Qin J, Heng PA. 3D FractalNet: Dense Volumetric Segmentation for Cardiovascular MRI Volumes. In: Zuluaga M, Bhatia K, Kainz B, Moghari M, Pace D. (eds) Reconstruction, Segmentation, and Analysis of Medical Images. RAMBO 2016, HVSMR 2016. Lecture Notes in Computer Science, vol 10129. Springer, Cham. 2017. https://doi.org/10.1007/978-3-319-52280-7_10.
22. Wolterink JM, Leiner T, Viergever MA, Išgum I. Dilated Convolutional Neural Networks for Cardiovascular MR Segmentation in Congenital Heart Disease. In: Zuluaga M., Bhatia K., Kainz B., Moghari M., Pace D. (eds) Reconstruction, Segmentation, and Analysis of Medical Images. RAMBO 2016, HVSMR 2016. Lecture Notes in Computer Science, vol 10129. Springer, Cham. 2017. https://doi.org/10.1007/978-3-319-52280-7_9.
23. Yu L. et al. Automatic 3D Cardiovascular MR Segmentation with Densely-Connected Volumetric ConvNets. In: Descoteaux M, Maier-Hein L, Franz A, Jannin P, Collins D, Duchesne S. (eds) Medical Image Computing and Computer-Assisted Intervention – MICCAI 2017. MICCAI 2017. Lecture Notes in Computer Science, vol 10434. Springer, Cham. 2017. https://doi.org/10.1007/978-3-319-66185-8_33.
24. Poudel R.P.K., Lamata P., Montana G. Recurrent Fully Convolutional Neural Networks for Multi-slice MRI Cardiac Segmentation. In: Zuluaga M., Bhatia K., Kainz B., Moghari M., Pace D. (eds) Reconstruction, Segmentation, and Analysis of Medical Images. RAMBO 2016, HVSMR 2016. Lecture Notes in Computer Science, vol 10129. Springer, Cham. 2017. https://doi.org/10.1007/978-3-319-52280-7_8.
25. Rezaei M, Yang H, Meinel C. Recurrent generative adversarial network for learning imbalanced medical image semantic segmentation. Multimed Tools Appl. 2020;79:15329–48. https://doi.org/10.1007/s11042-019-7305-1.
26. Mukhopadhyay A. Total Variation Random Forest: Fully Automatic MRI Segmentation in Congenital Heart Diseases. In: Zuluaga M., Bhatia K., Kainz B., Moghari M., Pace D. (eds) Reconstruction, Segmentation, and Analysis of Medical Images. RAMBO 2016, HVSMR 2016. Lecture Notes in Computer Science, vol 10129. Springer, Cham. 2017. https://doi.org/10.1007/978-3-319-52280-7_17.
27. Karimi-Bidhendi S, et al. Fully-automated deep-learning segmentation of pediatric cardiovascular magnetic resonance of patients with complex congenital heart diseases. J Cardiovasc Magn Reson. 2020;22:80. https://doi.org/10.1186/s12968-020-00678-0.
28. Jani VP, et al. Transfer learning for automated aortic segmentation and assessment of aortic mechanics in tetralogy of fallot: multi-ethnic study of atherosclerosis and the German Competence Network for congenital heart defects. Circulation. 2019;140:–A16044. https://doi.org/10.1161/circ.140.suppl_1.16044.
29. Diller GP, et al. Prediction of prognosis in patients with tetralogy of Fallot based on deep learning imaging analysis. Heart. 2020;106:1007–14.
30. Xu X. et al. Whole Heart and Great Vessel Segmentation in Congenital Heart Disease Using Deep Neural Networks and Graph Matching. In: Shen D. et al. (eds) Medical Image Computing and Computer Assisted Intervention – MICCAI 2019. MICCAI 2019. Lecture Notes in Computer Science, vol 11765. Springer, Cham. 2019. https://doi.org/10.1007/978-3-030-32245-8_53.
31. Xu X. et al. ImageCHD: A 3D Computed Tomography Image Dataset for Classification of Congenital Heart Disease. In: Martel AL. et al. (eds) Medical Image Computing and Computer Assisted Intervention – MICCAI 2020. MICCAI 2020. Lecture Notes in Computer Science, vol 12264. Springer, Cham. 2020. https://doi.org/10.1007/978-3-030-59719-1_8.
32. Liu T, Tian Y, Zhao S, Huang X. Graph Reasoning and Shape Constraints for Cardiac Segmentation in Congenital Heart Defect. In: Martel A.L. et al. (eds) Medical Image Computing and Computer Assisted Intervention – MICCAI 2020. MICCAI 2020. Lecture Notes in Computer Science, vol 12264. Springer, Cham. 2020. https://doi.org/10.1007/978-3-030-59719-1_59.
33. Diller G-P, et al. Utility of machine learning algorithms in assessing patients with a systemic right ventricle. Eur Heart J Cardiovasc Imaging. 2019;20:925–31. https://doi.org/10.1093/ehjci/jey211.
34. Thomford NE, et al. Implementing artificial intelligence and digital health in resource-limited settings? Top 10 lessons we learned in congenital heart defects and cardiology. OMICS J Integr Biol. 2020;24:264–77.
35. Toba S, et al. Prediction of pulmonary to systemic flow ratio in patients with congenital heart disease using deep learning–based analysis of chest radiographs. JAMA Cardiol. 2020;5:449–57. https://doi.org/10.1001/jamacardio.2019.5620.
36. Arnaout R, et al. Expert-level prenatal detection of complex congenital heart disease from screening ultrasound using deep learning. medRxiv, 2020.2006.2022.20137786. https://doi.org/10.1101/2020.06.22.20137786.
37. Qiu X, et al. Prenatal diagnosis and pregnancy outcomes of 1492 fetuses with congenital heart disease: role of multidisciplinary-joint consultation in prenatal diagnosis. Sci Rep. 2020;10:7564. https://doi.org/10.1038/s41598-020-64591-3.
38. Le TK, et al. Application of machine learning in screening of congenital heart diseases using fetal echocardiography. J Am Coll Cardiol. 2020;75:648.
39. Samad MD, et al. Predicting deterioration of ventricular function in patients with repaired tetralogy of Fallot using machine learning. Eur Heart J Cardiovasc Imaging. 2018;19:730–8.
40. Valente AM, Powell AJ. Clinical applications of cardiovascular magnetic resonance in congenital heart disease. Magn Reson Imaging Clin N Am. 2007;15:565–77.
41. Geva T, Sandweiss BM, Gauvreau K, Lock JE, Powell AJ. Factors associated with impaired clinical status in long-term survivors of tetralogy of Fallot repair evaluated by magnetic resonance imaging. J Am Coll Cardiol. 2004;43:1068–74.
42. Huang L, et al. Prediction of pulmonary pressure after Glenn shunts by computed tomography–based machine learning models. Eur Radiol. 2020;30:1369–77.
43. Davies R, Babu-Narayan SV. Deep learning in congenital heart disease imaging: hope but not haste. Heart. 2020;106:960. https://doi.org/10.1136/heartjnl-2019-316496.

Cardiac Nuclear Medicine: The Role of Artificial Intelligence

37

Marina Piccinelli and Ernest V. Garcia

Introduction

Over the past 50 years, the nuclear cardiology imaging field has evolved and developed enormously, becoming an integral part of current clinical practice and playing crucial roles in detection, risk stratification, and treatment selection for patients with known or suspected cardiovascular disease [1, 2]. Single-photon emission computed tomography (SPECT) myocardial perfusion imaging (MPI) is the most widely performed noninvasive technique to detect coronary artery disease (CAD) – the single most common cause of death in the developed world – with several million procedures performed worldwide annually [3, 4]. More recently, the introduction of cardiac positron emission tomography (PET) to clinical environments with its ability to quantify absolute myocardial blood flow has exhibited improved image quality, reduction in radiation dose, and greater diagnostic and prognostic value [5, 6]. While nuclear imaging modalities are certainly powerful tools to study cardiovascular pathophysiology, a key aspect for their widespread clinical usage over other modalities has been the continuous development of algorithms and techniques for automated processing, quantification, and display [7–9]. A number of software packages have been developed, validated, and commercialized since as early as 1985 by investigators at Cedars-Sinai Medical Center [10], Emory University [11], University of Michigan [12], and Yale University [13], and currently, 3D SPECT and PET images are automatically analyzed with minimal user input or supervision. Current software can identify the left ventricle and extract a wealth of indexes to depict myocardial perfusion, left ventricular (LV) function, synchrony of contraction, myocardial metabolism, innervation, and inflammation. Decades of investigations and extensive evidence have proven the reproducibility of these measurements and the improved accuracy when compared to qualitative visual assessment by expert readers. The flip side of the coin is that in some regards, diagnostic imaging has become more complicated. Physicians are now required to provide a precise diagnosis or foresee an outcome by integrating dozens of variables from growing amount of heterogeneous data, not just image-derived data and often not even from a single modality, but also from clinical information and by mastering an ever-expanding knowledge in a steadily shrinking time.

As, in recent years, artificial intelligence (AI)-based techniques and methods have crossed over from applications such as search engines, natural language processing, and self-driving cars to healthcare and medicine, they have found in nuclear cardiology imaging a particularly rich and adapt field, already inherently quantitative due to a wealth of parameters and indexes with essential diagnostic and prognostic value routinely extracted [7–9]. For instance, from static to gated to dynamic images acquired for CAD assessment, the following index and variables are routinely provided: perfusion polar maps, total perfusion deficit (TPD), segmental perfusion scores (SSS, SRS, SDS), ischemic burden, LV extraction fraction (EF), end-diastolic (EDV) and end-systolic volumes (ESV), cardiac output, myocardial mass, transient ischemic dilatation, wall thickening, LV systolic dyssynchrony, rest and stress absolute myocardial blood flow (MBF), and flow reserve (MFR). It should come as no surprise that nuclear cardiology turned early on to computer-aided diagnosis methods and expert systems [14], which can be described as early expressions of AI-based techniques. Of note, an expert system developed at Emory University used AI to automatically generate a structured natural language report with a diagnostic performance comparable to those of experts [15]. It is one

M. Piccinelli, PhD (✉) · E. V. Garcia, PhD
Department of Radiology and Imaging Sciences, Emory University School of Medicine, Atlanta, GA, USA
e-mail: mpiccin@emory.edu; ernest.garcia@emory.edu

C. N. De Cecco et al. (eds.), *Artificial Intelligence in Cardiothoracic Imaging*, Contemporary Medical Imaging,
https://doi.org/10.1007/978-3-030-92087-6_37

of the few AI-driven diagnostic systems that have been FDA cleared and commercially available. But the field is bound to further benefit from the introduction of highly efficient AI tools such as machine learning (ML), deep learning (DL), and particularly convolutional neural networks (CNNs), which have been shown to be very effective in many imaging applications. These techniques can be applied to a variety of tasks including enhancing image quality, image segmentation, diagnosis, and especially risk stratification and outcome prediction. The ability of these techniques to consume large amounts of heterogeneous data, directly learning from it, and extrapolate patterns often invisible to the human eye moves clinicians and scientists a little closer to the holy grail of *precise medicine*, a tailored clinical and therapeutical approach to each patient based on his/her characteristics. ML- and DL-based methods have not entered clinical routine yet, and important limitations need to be addressed and emphasized, but in the last few years, a number of investigations have demonstrated not only the feasibility of AI techniques in nuclear cardiology but also its usefulness.

Artificial Intelligence, Machine Learning, and Deep Learning: Basic Principles and Nomenclature

Artificial intelligence was introduced in the 1950 as a field in computer science. Alan Turing, one of its founders, developed the *Turing Test* [16] – originally named the *imitation game* – as a way to determine if a computer could exhibit intelligence similar to that of human beings. As such, AI can be comprehensively described as computational techniques created to complete tasks that would normally require human intelligence to accomplish, such as problem-solving and decision-making [17]. In cardiovascular medicine, AI applications translate into the creation of software and algorithms that analyze images, identify diseases, and predict outcomes based on image-derived information, electronic health records (EHR), outcome results, biometrics from wearable devices, and, possibly, data from the recently introduced "omics" technologies (genomics, metabolomics, proteomics). The *big data* [18] generated by cardiovascular imaging is heterogeneous, ever-increasing, and constantly changing. Their integration and analysis have the potential to discover new patterns within datasets as well as improve current diagnostic and prognostic algorithms, but since medical applications contain too many variables with complex interactions that cannot be interpreted and analyzed with traditional processing techniques, it wasn't until recently that scientists have been able to address crucial clinical questions. In recent years, developments in computer hardware and sophisticated methods to stratify and weight data [19, 20] as well as the accessibility to user-friendly software packages (such as TensorFlow, Scikit-learn, Microsoft Cognitive Toolkit, Theano, and Keras) have created the perfect environment for medical applications of AI techniques to flourish at an unprecedented rate [21]. While an in-depth technical description of AI-based techniques for cardiovascular imaging is beyond the scope of this writing and we point the readers to recent reviews on the matter [22–28], we here wish to introduce the basic terminology and methodologies as they will be often recalled in the following sections.

Machine learning is a subset of AI that broadly indicates algorithms with the ability to autonomously acquire knowledge by extracting patterns and learning rules from the analysis of large amount of data without being specifically programmed in decision-making, such as with expert systems. The development of ML techniques starts from a "training" phase, for the creation of the model and the adjustment of its parameters, followed by a "testing" one to validate the model predictions when new data are supplied. The original datasets are often enriched by additional information about the data commonly called *features*, which are individual measurable image property or data characteristic to be used by the computational method. In imaging, examples of features could be specific pixel brightness or the presence of an edge or the value of an image-derived parameter. ML approaches can be classified into supervised and unsupervised learning. In *supervised learning*, algorithms use labeled datasets to predict a desired outcome; *feature selection*, which is the identification of relevant variables, is a crucial step of these approaches. Learning occurs as the algorithm makes a prediction of a known outcome and adjusts the model parameters in order to refine its performance. Supervised learning is commonly used in classification and regression problems, and examples of algorithms include linear and logistic regression [29], artificial neural network [24, 28] (ANN), support vector machine [30] (SVM), and decision trees [31]. *Unsupervised learning*, on the other hand, utilizes unlabeled data to predict an unknown result, and the algorithms themselves try autonomously to derive a conclusion by identifying unknown patters in the data provided. Examples of unsupervised learning techniques include principal component analysis and clustering analysis. Lastly, *deep learning* [32] is a subset of ML that further aims at simulating brain functioning and human cognition using multiple layers of interconnected ANNs. In Fig. 37.1, the typical ANN structure is depicted. Originally inspired by the structure of the human neurons, ANNs are formed by layers of connected nodes. Each node can have multiple inputs that are multiplied by a weight and combined into a single output through a nonlinear function. The information moves across nodes and layers, and the final output is compared to the known outcome. Errors in classification or prediction are moved backward to adjust the weights between

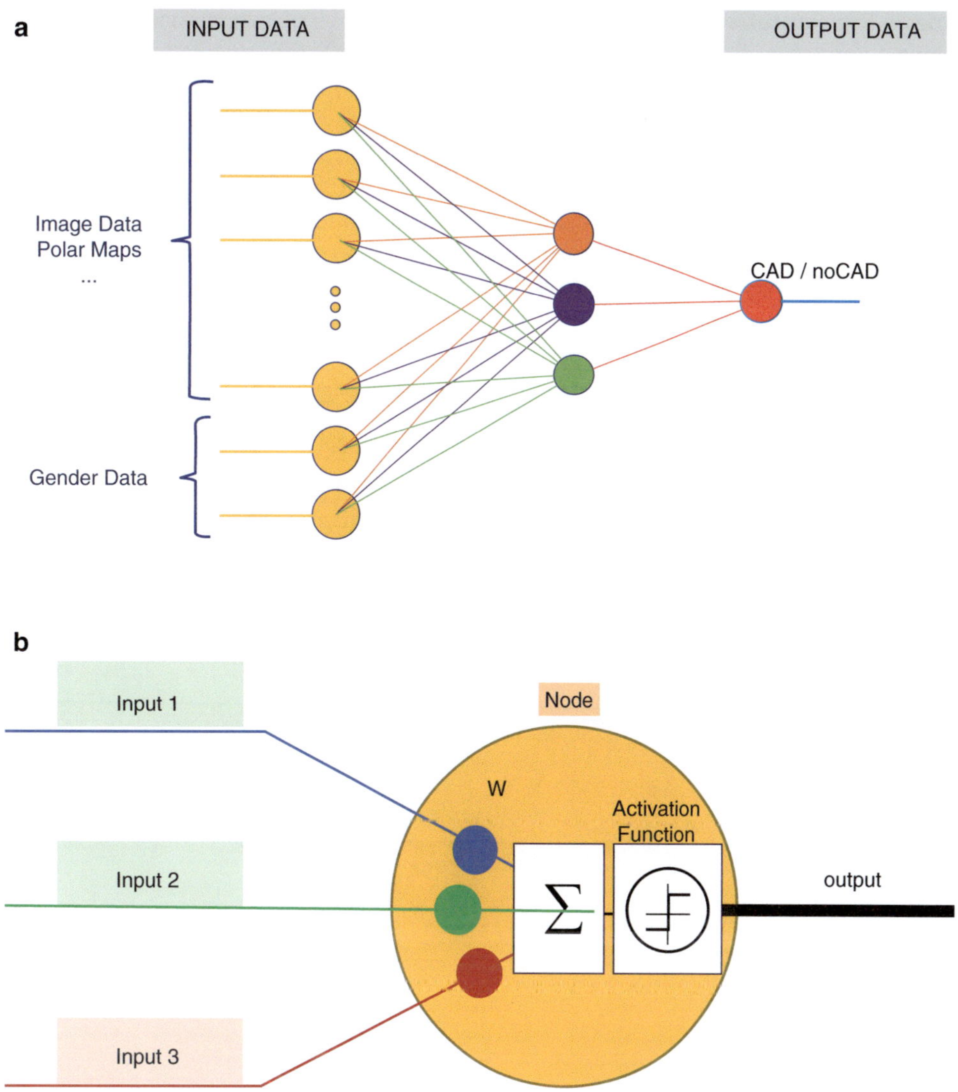

Fig. 37.1 (**a**) Diagram for artificial neural network. (**b**) Individual neural network node. The diagram shows how values from three inputs are weighted (W) and summed (∑). If the sum exceeds a preset threshold, the neuron will fire

the various nodes and improve model performance. The strength of ANNs resides in the fact that highly complex and nonlinear relationships can be modeled improving accuracy while also overcoming the need for the definition of input features if trained in unsupervised mode. ANNs have been around since 1950 and have witnessed some successful applications to medical imaging during the 1990s, but given their complexity, only recently have scientists been able to deploy their full potential thanks to the availability of affordable computational power. Convolution neural networks (CNNs) are presently the most commonly used DL architecture for image analysis and the ones that have shown preeminent results [33]. They can have multiple layers stacked on top of each other usually between 10 and 50, but the use of convolutional operations, hence their name, allows the efficient detection of image features while saving memory.

Image Processing and Quantification

The widespread clinical acceptance of nuclear cardiac studies for the assessment of a variety of cardiovascular diseases is largely due to the highly quantitative nature of these imaging tests. For at least three decades now, nuclear cardiology has witnessed the development and clinical deployment of numerous automated algorithms for image processing and quantification [7–9, 34]. In Fig. 37.2, the main results from the automated processing of a PET MPI study are displayed. While these techniques were not necessarily “styled” as AI-based techniques, they have brought about the ability to perform completely automatic motion correction, image reorientation, image segmentation, and high-level analysis of the results, all tasks that would otherwise require human intervention.

Image Reorientation and Reslicing

The majority of nuclear image processing and visualization occurs in cardiac standard orientation, i.e., short axis (SA) and horizontal and vertical long axes (Fig. 37.2a). Reorientation of transaxial images into standard view has been the focus of many investigations in the 1990 [35–37], and all clinical software presently include automated algorithms for reorienting images. The approach by Germano et al. [35] starts by identifying the LV with thresholding operations and ruled-based location/shape/size criteria. A refinement of this initial region is then performed by extracting mid-myocardial profiles and fitting them to a quadratic surface. The final LV long axis corresponds to the long axis of the resulting 3D ellipsoid which is ultimately used for reslicing. The method was tested in 400 cases, resulting in correct LV reorientation in 394 instances (98.5% success). Mullick et al. [36] also start their algorithm with a threshold based on image intensity histogram followed by a complex

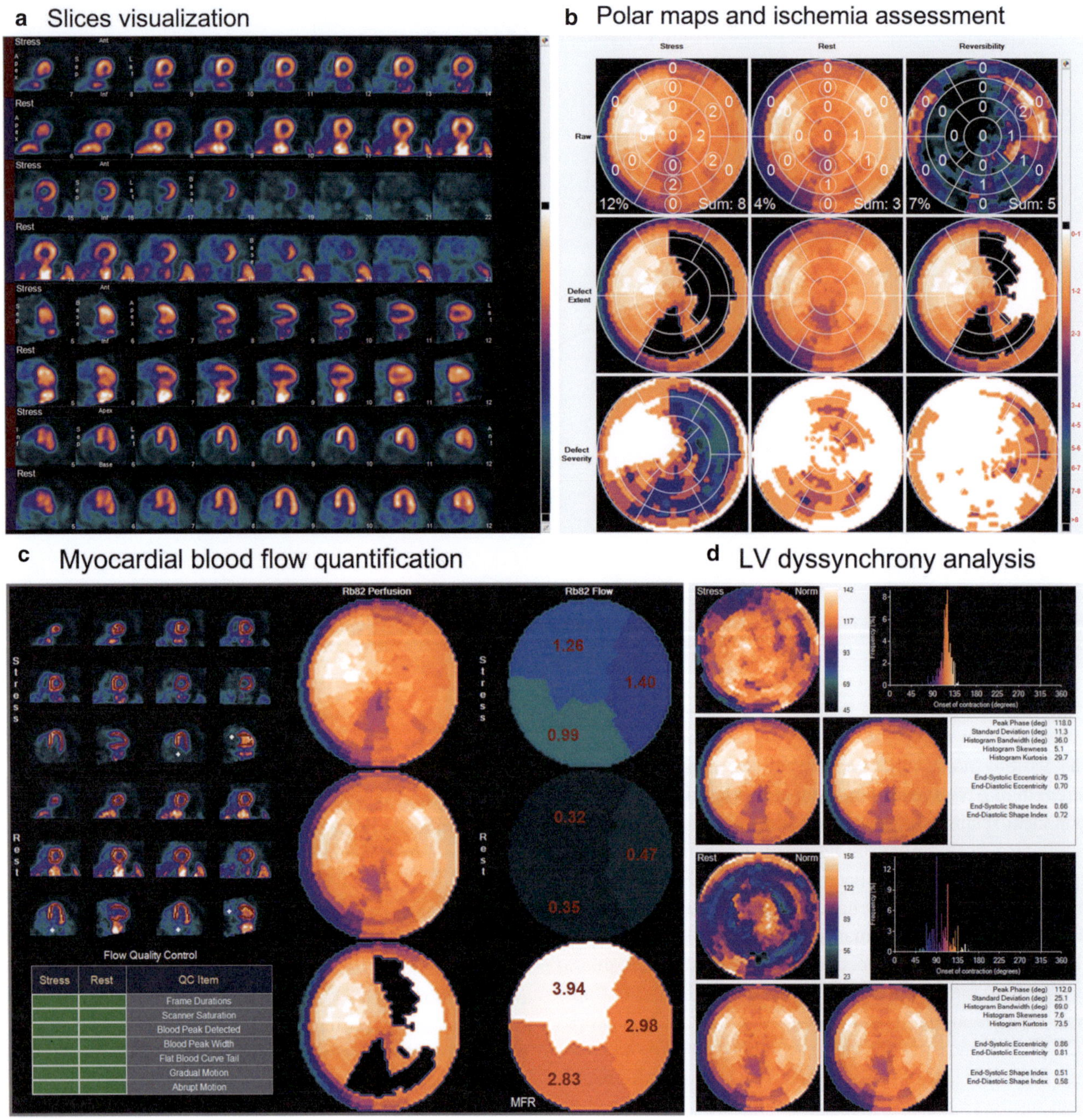

Fig. 37.2 Major processing modules from a rest/stress ^{82}Rb PET MPI study analyzed with ECTb software [11]. (**a**) Original images in SA orientation. (**b**) Polar map representation and myocardial ischemia quantification. (**c**) Stress, rest myocardial absolute blood flow and flow reserve quantification. (**d**) LV dyssynchrony analysis. (**e**) LV function analysis

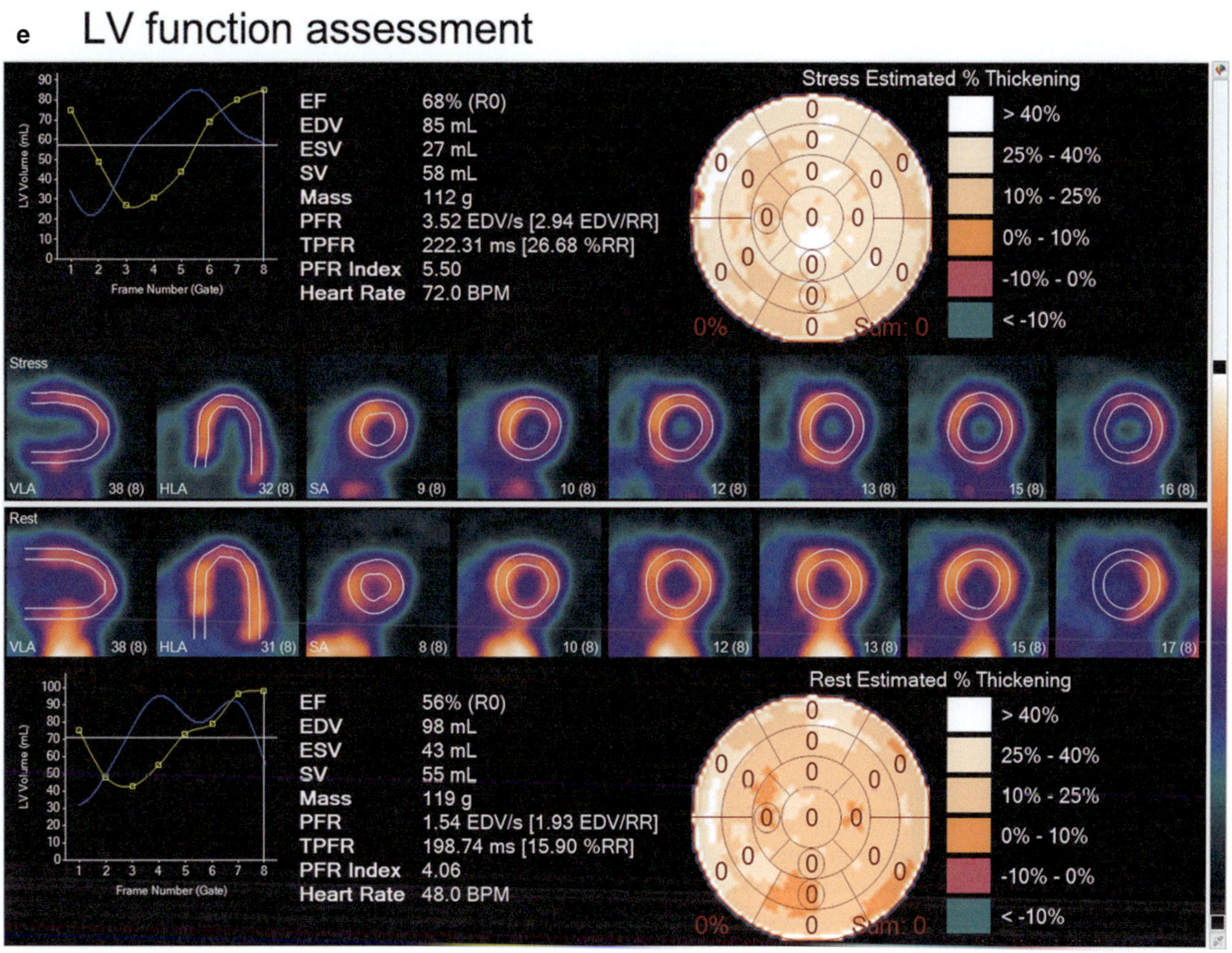

Fig. 37.2 (continued)

series of heuristic rules to refine the selection. A binary mask of the LV region is created and a 3D surface model extracted. Three-dimensional normal vectors to the surface are used to point inward to the LV long axis, which is extracted as the 3D straight line that fits the intersections of the vector directions. The method was tested in 124 normal and abnormal (i.e., exhibiting perfusion defects) subjects, succeeding in 116 (93.5%). Slomka et al. [37] approached the reorientation problem differently, by creating male and female template images with known LV orientation. Each new dataset is registered and scaled to the template minimizing the sum of absolute differences between the two images being registered. The method was tested in 48 subjects and by visual evaluation never failed.

Image Segmentation

Following image reslicing, accurate LV segmentation is crucial for a reliable assessment of myocardial perfusion. Nuclear imaging cardiology can also detail a long record of studies dated back to the 1990 for the automation of this particular image processing task [7–9, 34]. Once the center of the LV chamber and the basal and apical slices have been identified, an automated 3D sampling procedure is performed to extract maximum count profiles from each SA slice. Depending on the approach, the sampling scheme may be ellipsoidal [10, 13] or with a hybrid design [11]. These 3D perfusion distributions are ultimately mapped to a standard template, a 2D polar map that maps count profiles into concentric rings [7]. A countless number of papers have tested and successfully validated these approaches.

Yet, recent technological advancements have further increased the LV segmentation robustness. A quality control algorithm was developed to evaluate the automatically obtained contours and detect segmentation failure [38]. Two error flags were implemented to check the LV shape and the location of the mitral valve. The software was validated against expert readers in the identification of segmentation errors and significantly reduced human supervision. Further, ML techniques were recently used in the implementation of an algorithm for the automated identification of the valve

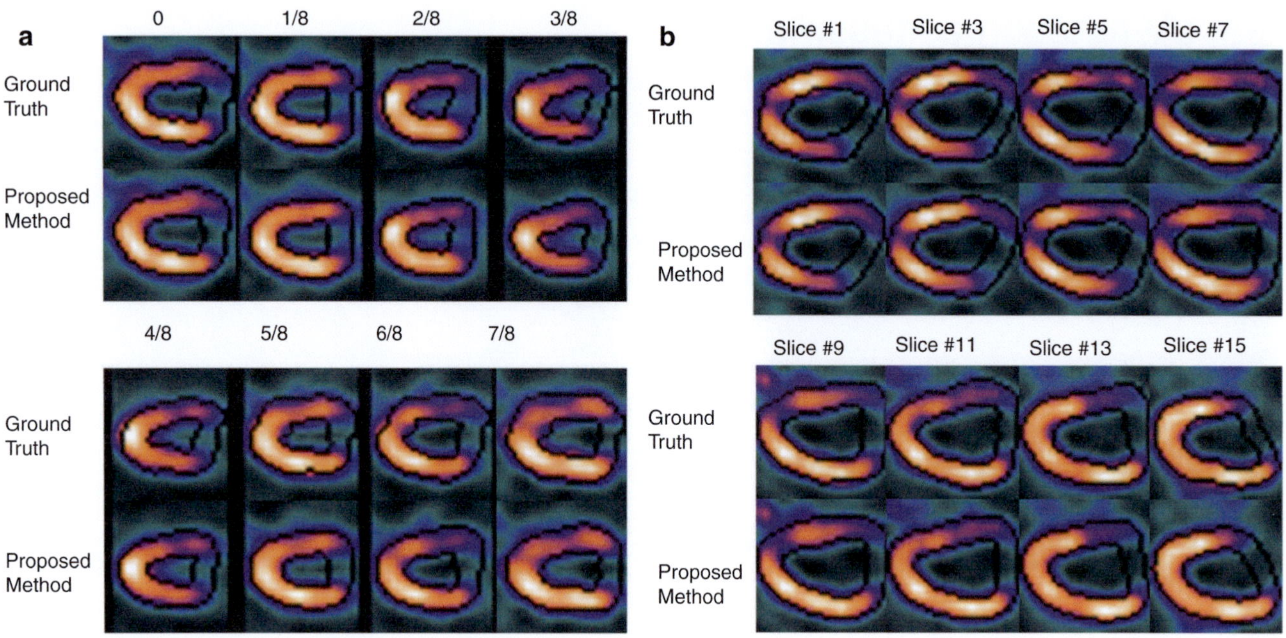

Fig. 37.3 Epicardial and endocardial borders identified with a DL-based technique compared to manual delineation as ground truth. (**a**) Segmentation of the same slice over the eight-frame cardiac cycle (normal case); (**b**) segmentation of phase 0 for an abnormal case. (Reprinted with permissions from Wang et al. [40])

plane (VP) from SPECT images [39]. The quantitative assessment of ischemia greatly relies on correct rest and stress relative perfusion maps, which in turn depend on the proper VP identification during segmentation. The authors created high-level image features – 22 features related to VP location, shape, and intensity as well as from gated acquisitions – as input into an algorithm based on SVM techniques that efficiently include expert knowledge and the anatomical variations of VP location. Coronary CT angiography was used to validate the VP location, and TPD was employed to assess diagnostic accuracy of the model. This fully automated method exhibited a diagnostic performance equivalent to that obtained after correction by experienced readers. Another team leveraged the potential of DL techniques to develop a model for the delineation of LV epicardial and endocardial profiles from gated SPECT images [40]. The method was implemented as an end-to-end fully CNN trained with LV contours delineated by clinicians. Preliminary results on 56 subjects demonstrated excellent precision in assessing LV myocardium volumes with an error of 1.09 ± 3.66%. In Fig. 37.3, the results of this methodology are reported for a normal and abnormal case.

Image Interpretation and Outcome Prediction

The field of image-based diagnosis and outcome prediction is possibly the sector of nuclear cardiology that has experienced the largest progress since the latest technological and methodological developments brought about by ML and DL techniques. In early approaches to CAD investigations with AI methods [41–47], ANNs have been employed to determine if ischemia was present, to what extent, and which coronary was likely to have a stenotic lesion by using sample of myocardial perfusion data as input and corresponding invasive coronary angiography (ICA) results as output. But the works presented in this section provide evidence of the ability of more sophisticated approaches to integrate a substantial number of heterogeneous variables from a large number of subjects and deliver powerful diagnostic tools and prediction models. In Arsanjani et al. [48], the authors presented a fully automated algorithm to compute TPD, compared it to visual assessment by expert readers – currently the recommended standard clinical practice – and validated with angiographic findings on 665 patients who underwent SPECT MPI. The overall accuracy of the automated analysis proved equivalent to the expert reading on a per-patient basis, while it was in cases superior to visual assessment in identifying lesions ≥70% on a per-vessel analysis. The authors then proceeded to apply a fully ML-based approach using SVM techniques [49] to combine several quantitative variables to detect CAD from a cohort of 957 SPECT studies. The algorithm integrated perfusion and functional indexes, namely, TPD, ischemic changes and EF changes between rest and stress, and regional LV wall motion and thickening scores. The diagnostic accuracy was compared to visual interpretation by two expert readers and validated with ICA results. Each individual quantitative measure had been extensively used to assess CAD, but their integration has remained challenging to perform. The study showed an improved diagnostic accuracy for the SVM technique with an ROC AUC of 0.92 vs 0.88 and 0.87 for the two readers. Furthermore, in a follow-up investigation [50] which included 1181 rest/stress SPECT studies, the authors demonstrated additional improvements achieved with ML when quantitative perfusion measures and clinical variables were combined. The ML results were once again tested against an expert reader with an AUC of 0.94 vs 0.89 ($p < 0.001$). As integration of numerous heterogeneous variables can prove challenging and given that MPI interpretation largely depends on readers' experience, the inclusion of such automated assessment could provide fundamental assistance to radiologists in the future, particularly in less experienced centers. The search for improved diagnostic accuracy has as its ultimate goal outcome prediction and, particularly, in the case of CAD, the identification of subjects that would benefit from earlier intervention. In Arsanjani et al. [51], the authors aimed at investigating if early revascularization could be effectively predicted by combining clinical data with quantitative SPECT MPI-derived features. A database of 713 rest/stress studies with a total of 372 revascularization events was analyzed, and an automated feature selection algorithm was used to extract the relevant parameters from a collection of 33 indexes and variables. The performance of the ML model was compared to that of two readers. The results were mixed: in predicting revascularization, the ML algorithm exhibited a sensitivity comparable to that of one experienced reader, higher than the second one, but similar to stand-alone perfusion measures; its specificity was better than both readers but similar to TPD. In a multicenter study, Hu et al. [52] also used a ML algorithm to predict per-vessel early revascularization within 90 days from SPECT MPI. The model used 18 clinical variables, 9 from stress testing plus additional 28 imaging features from a database of 1980 patients for a total of 5590 vessel observations. The AUC of the ML method was compared to expert analysis and quantitative assessment; it outperformed current quantitative methods per patient and per vessel and also expert interpretation. The urge to predict revascularization is an important clinical need in CAD assessment, as a significant number of patients that are scheduled for invasive angiography ultimately do not have obstructive disease.

DL-based techniques have also been extensively used in CAD diagnosis and prognosis studies, with the algorithms identifying patterns independently. Its first use is described in Betancur et al. [53] with a deep CNN modeled to directly interpret perfusion polar maps and identify obstructive disease. In Fig. 37.4, the algorithm schematic is displayed. A database of 1638 patients was used to implement the model and was compared to quantitative assessment by TPD: per-vessel sensitivity improved from 64.4% (TPD) to 69.8% (CNN) by only using as input imaging data. The technique was further developed to include upright and supine data [54], an acquisition approach routinely used to mitigate attenuation artifacts with some solid-state cameras. The DL algorithm was trained on polar maps, hypoperfusion defects, and hypoperfusion severity and similarly evaluated to detect obstructive CAD. Compared to combined quantitative assessment, the DL model showed improved AUC in predicting disease both per patient and vessel, as well as enhanced sensitivity and specificity. The same team also developed a ML model for risk stratification and prediction of major

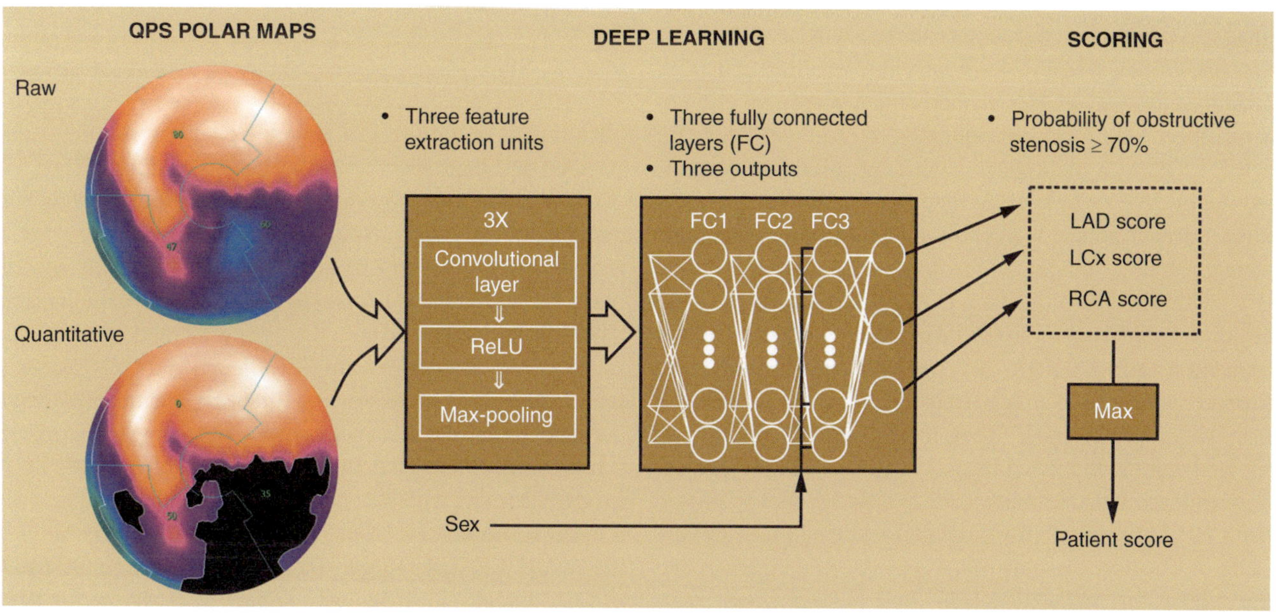

Fig. 37.4 Schematic for DL-based algorithm for the direct detection of obstructive coronary artery disease from polar maps in left anterior descending artery (LAD), left circumflex artery (LCX), and right coronary artery (RCA) territories. (Reprinted with permission from Betancur et al. [53])

adverse cardiovascular events (MACE) by combining clinical data and imaging features from 2619 SPECT [55]. When ML was compared to expert visual interpretation, automated stress TPD, and automated ischemic TPD, the AUCs were 0.81 vs 0.65 vs 0.73 vs 0.71, respectively ($p < 0.01$).

While these models and investigations may strike for their complexity, particularly in terms of input data and feature selection, in a recent work by Juarez-Orozco et al. [56], a ML algorithm was developed from easily accessible clinical and functional variables for the detection of myocardial ischemia as determined through quantitative PET perfusion, namely, PET-derived MFR < 2.0. A database of 1234 patients was used for the model implementation and testing, and its performance was evaluated against a simple logistic regression model with the same variables. ML achieved an AUC of 0.72 compared to 0.67 obtained with traditional regression techniques. In another effort to provide simper methods, Alonso et al. [57] estimated patient's risk of cardiac death based on SPECT MPI and clinical data with multiple ML models by selecting subsets of variables from a group of 122 potential features. Models were trained and tested on 8321 patients and compared to standard regression techniques. The authors identified a model with 6 features and an AUC of 0.77 that outperformed more complex regression models that used up to 14 features.

Image Accuracy and Efficiency

As AI-based techniques have entered cardiac medical imaging, they have been primarily used in image processing, diagnosis, and risk stratification. But other equally important fields of nuclear imaging, such as dose reduction and image reconstruction techniques, are expected to experience new and clinically useful developments [58]. Shiri et al. [59] recently proposed a CNN method aimed at the reduction of acquisition time, and consequently of radiation dose, for SPECT MPI by either reducing the acquisition time per projection by 50% or by halving the number of angular projections. For each patient in a cohort of 363, 4 sets of projections were generated from the acquisition list mode data: full time (FT) with 20 s per projection, half time (HT) with 10 s per projection, full projection (FP) with 32 projections, and half projection (HP) with 16. The convolutional network performed an image-to-image transformation to predict FT from HT and FP from HP. Their results, though preliminary, showed that the predicted images obtained with HT projection achieved a better image quality than the ones predicted from HP. Other feasibility studies investigated the applicability of low-dose imaging [60, 61] by developing DL-based techniques for image denoising that outperformed traditional image processing techniques. Particularly, Ramon et al. [60] used a supervised DL approach to remove the high image noise typical of low-dose acquisitions by using pairs of full-dose and low-dose images. The study included 1052 SPECT MPI datasets and tested 2 common reconstruction techniques (FBP and OSEM). The results indicate that DL methods can significantly improve noise reduction while enhancing diagnostic accuracy. Figure 37.5 depicts the results of the technique in the presence of a perfusion defect with progressive decreases of injected dose.

Interestingly for decades as a means to reduce effective radiation exposure by up to 60% and cancel unnecessary tests, stress-only protocols have been proposed. Yet, these protocols remain severely underutilized. A ML-based algorithm was recently proposed [62] for risk prediction based on stress-only MPI and clinical data to select the low-risk patients that could benefit from rest test cancellation. The study included 20,414 subjects with 98 features trained and tested to provide risk of MACE as a continuous probability of future events indicated as ML score. Three different thresholds of ML score were derived by matching the cancellation rates achieved by a physician interpretation and two clinical guidelines, and the annual MACE rates for patients selected for rest test cancellation were compared between the different approaches. Patients selected for rest cancellation with ML-guided cancellation recommendations exhibited a lower MACE rates than those chosen based on physician's interpretation or clinical guidelines. In Fig. 37.6, two examples of ML-guided recommendation are displayed with ranked contribution of individual features to ML score.

Another important area of nuclear cardiology imaging that based on preliminary investigations will potentially greatly benefit from AI-based techniques is that of attenuation correction (AC) with low-dose CT. Decades of investigations on SPECT MPI have shown that AC reduces ambiguity and increases diagnostic accuracy. But since SPECT/CT devices are expensive and not always available, non-AC SPECT images are commonly used for diagnosis. DL methods have recently presented clinicians with a possible solution in the form of generative adversarial networks (GANs) and their specific application in creating images of one modality from those of another. A feasibility study for generating AC maps from nuclear SPECT images was recently published. Shi et al. [63] developed a 3D model based on GANs that was trained to estimate attenuation maps solely from SPECT images. The study included 65 patients (normal and abnormal) with SPECT and AC CT. The synthetic attenuation maps were qualitatively and quantitatively consistent with the true maps with a mean absolute error of 3.6%. Analogously, the two sets of AC-corrected SPECT images (true and with synthetic AC) were highly similar with a mean absolute error of 0.26%. Noteworthy, after training, the model was able to generate a synthetic AC map from SPECT images in 1 second. Figure 37.7 shows for two patients the true vs synthetic AC maps, as well as the final perfusion polar maps obtained with true and synthetic AC vs without AC.

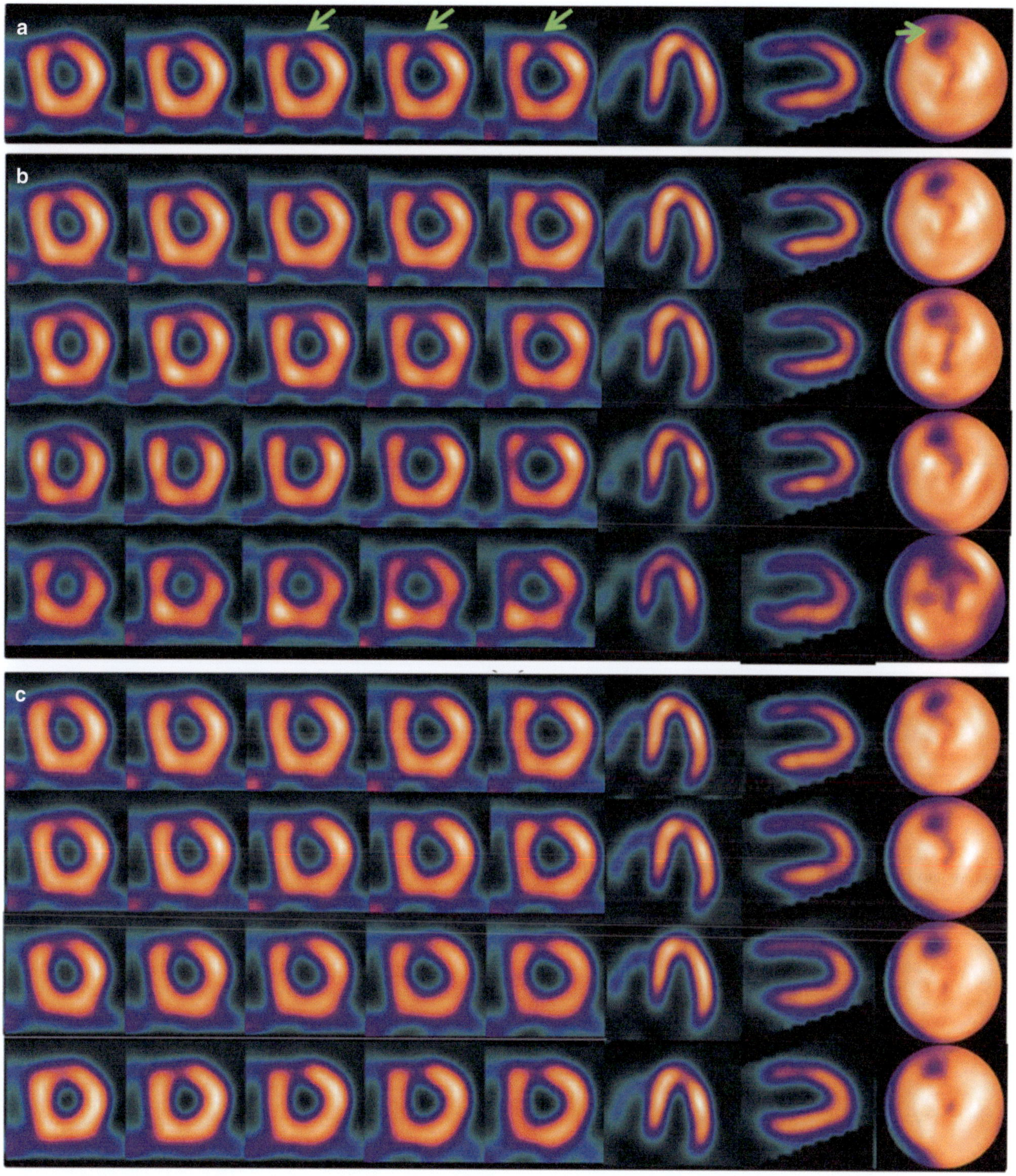

Fig. 37.5 Results from DL-based denoising technique for low-dose SPECT MPI. Images for male subject (age 65, BMI = 37.4) with (**a**) OSEM from full-dose data, (**b**) OSEM from reduced dose data, and (**c**) DL processing. A perfusion defect in the LAD territory is indicated with green arrow. In (**b**) and (**c**), the rows from top to bottom correspond to 1/2, 1/4, 1/8, and 1/16 dose, respectively. In the DL processing, the extent of the defect is better preserved than in OSEM even at much lowered dose levels. The normal region of the LV wall is also more uniform after DL procedure. LAD left anterior descending artery, DL deep learning, OSEM ordered subset expectation maximization. (Reprinted with permission from Ramon et al. [60])

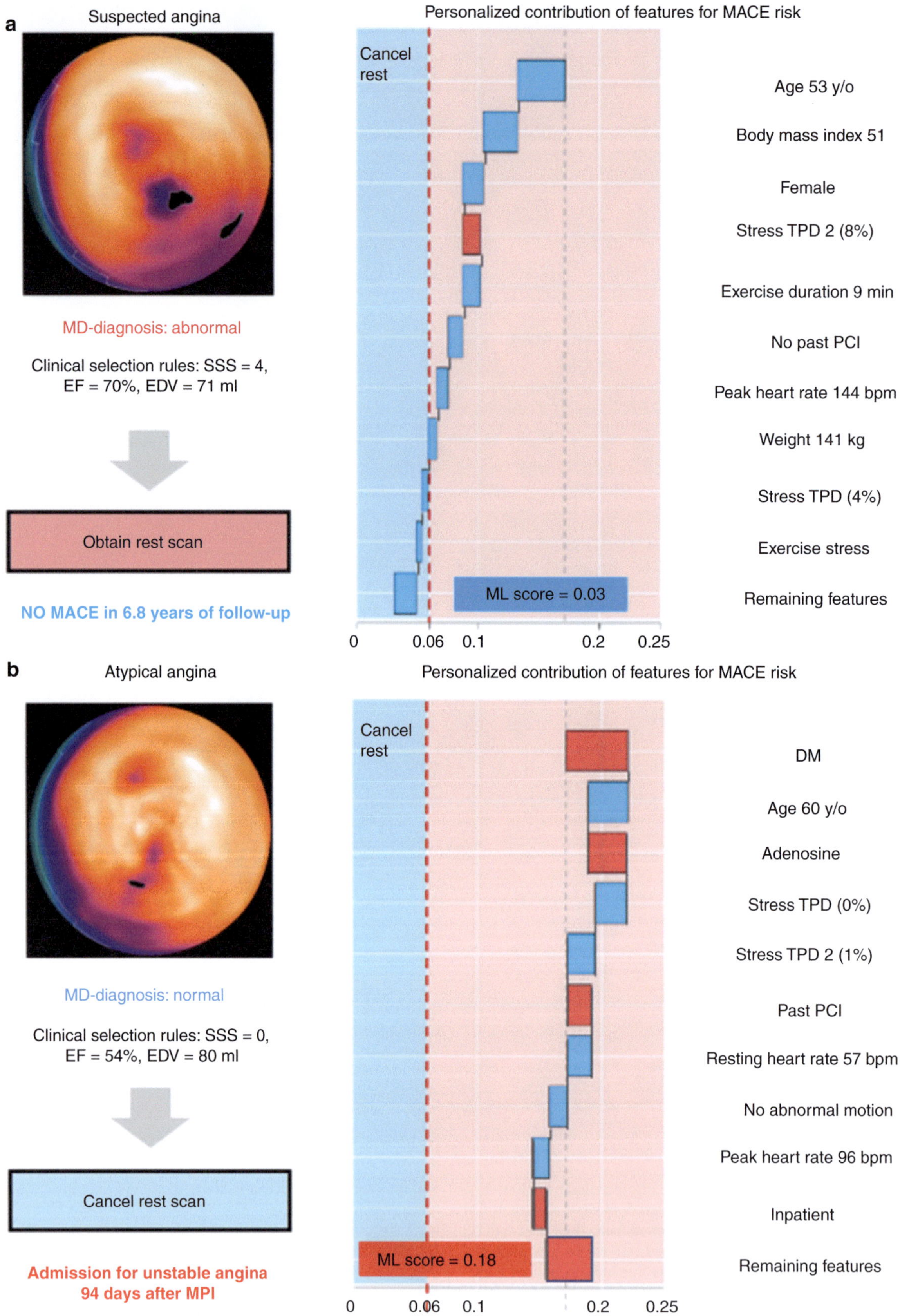

Fig. 37.6 Examples of ML-guided decision for rest test cancellation for stress-only protocols. Polar maps with clinical recommendation (left) and personalized explanations of the ML recommendation (right) are shown in (**a**) a case with a ML score below the ML score threshold and final ML-guided recommendation to cancel the rest scan and (**b**) a case with a ML score higher than the threshold and therefore ML recommendation to proceed with the rest scan. The individual contributions of the top 10 features to the overall risk for each patient are shown (blue bars = decreasing risk, red bars = increasing risk). (Reprinted with permission from Hu et al. [62])

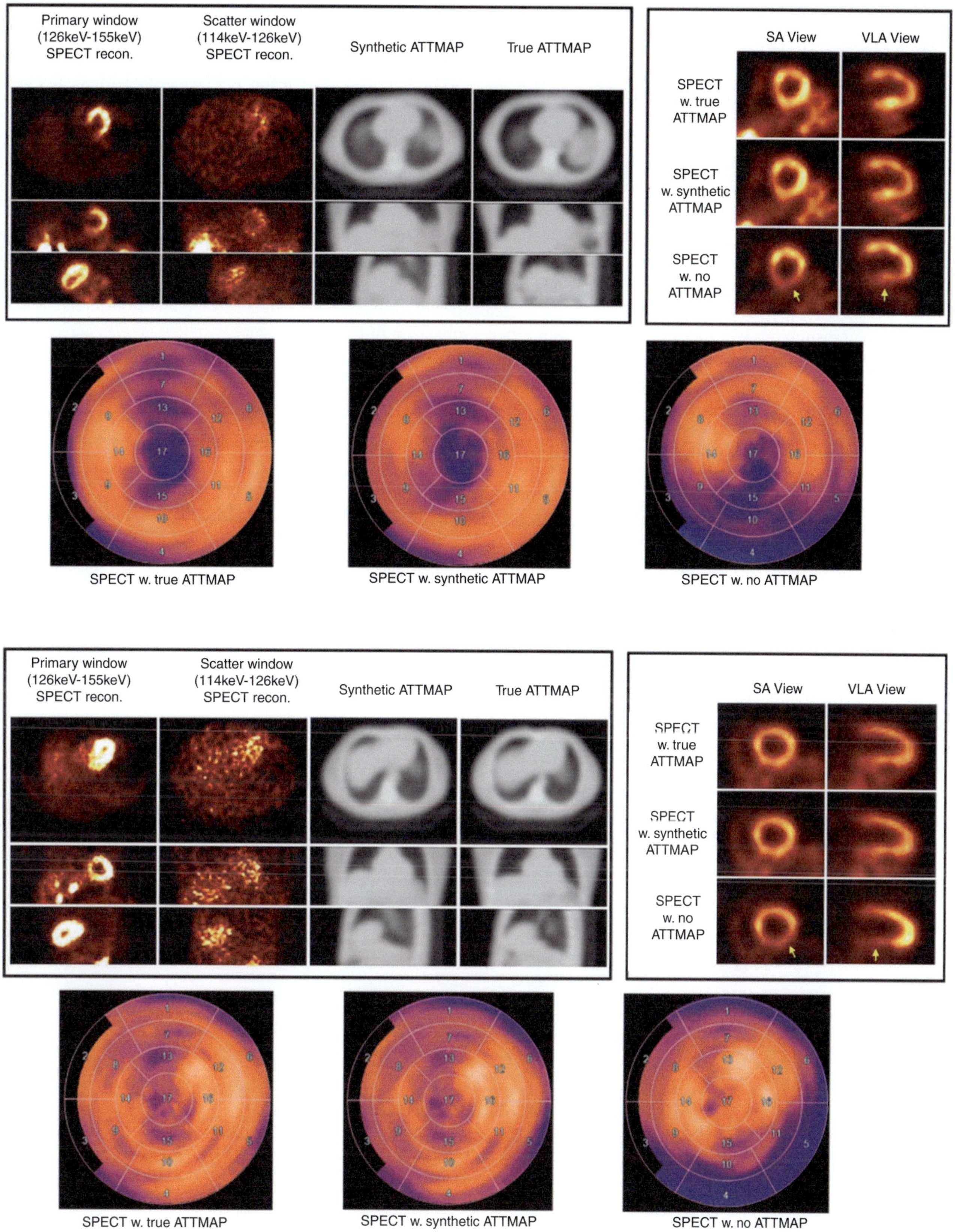

Fig. 37.7 Results from DL-based generation of attenuation correction maps from SPECT MPI images. Upper left: the primary/scatter window SPECT reconstructions, the synthetic attenuation maps, and the CT-based attenuation (true) maps in the axial, coronal, and sagittal views. Upper right: SPECT reconstructed images corrected using CT-based (true) attenuation maps and synthetic attenuation maps generated by the GAN and without attenuation correction in short-axis (SA) and vertical long-axis (VLA) views. Bottom: the polar map comparisons. ATTMAP attenuation map, w with, w.no without. (Reprinted with permission from Shi et al. [63])

Nuclear Imaging Databases for AI

A major prerequisite for AI-based techniques and methodologies to be scrupulously trained, validated, and tested is the availability of large amount of data, commonly referred to as "big data." In principle, the larger the amount of data available, the better the model performance, be it for a segmentation task that has to take into account high anatomical variability or an outcome prediction model that has to integrate and explore all possible interactions between several variables. In the context of medicine and medical imaging, another significant challenge is related to data standardization, particularly when data are collected from different centers. Imaging datasets pooled from different institutions will likely be obtained with different imaging devices and protocols, quantitative variables may be computed with different software, and different nomenclature may be in use. The quality and consistency of the data will impact the accuracy and applicability of the algorithm, independently from the AI approach utilized. Control over these aspects of data collection is crucial to generalize new models and algorithms. The team at Cedars-Sinai Medical Center have recently established a large multicenter registry [64] – *re*gistry of *f*ast myocardial perfusion *i*maging with *ne*xt generation SPECT (REFINE) – of imaging and clinical data with diagnostic and prognostic endpoints from nine international centers. At the time of this writing, 24,025 complete SPECT MPI datasets had been collected [26], with over 290 perfusion and function variables automatically quantified from each study and integrated with clinical data. In terms of diagnosis, results from ICA performed <6 months from imaging were obtained. In terms of prognosis, follow-up was performed to record MACE. In Fig. 37.8, an overview of the REFINE registry is depicted. Various collaborative projects have been developed as a result of this notable effort [52, 62, 65].

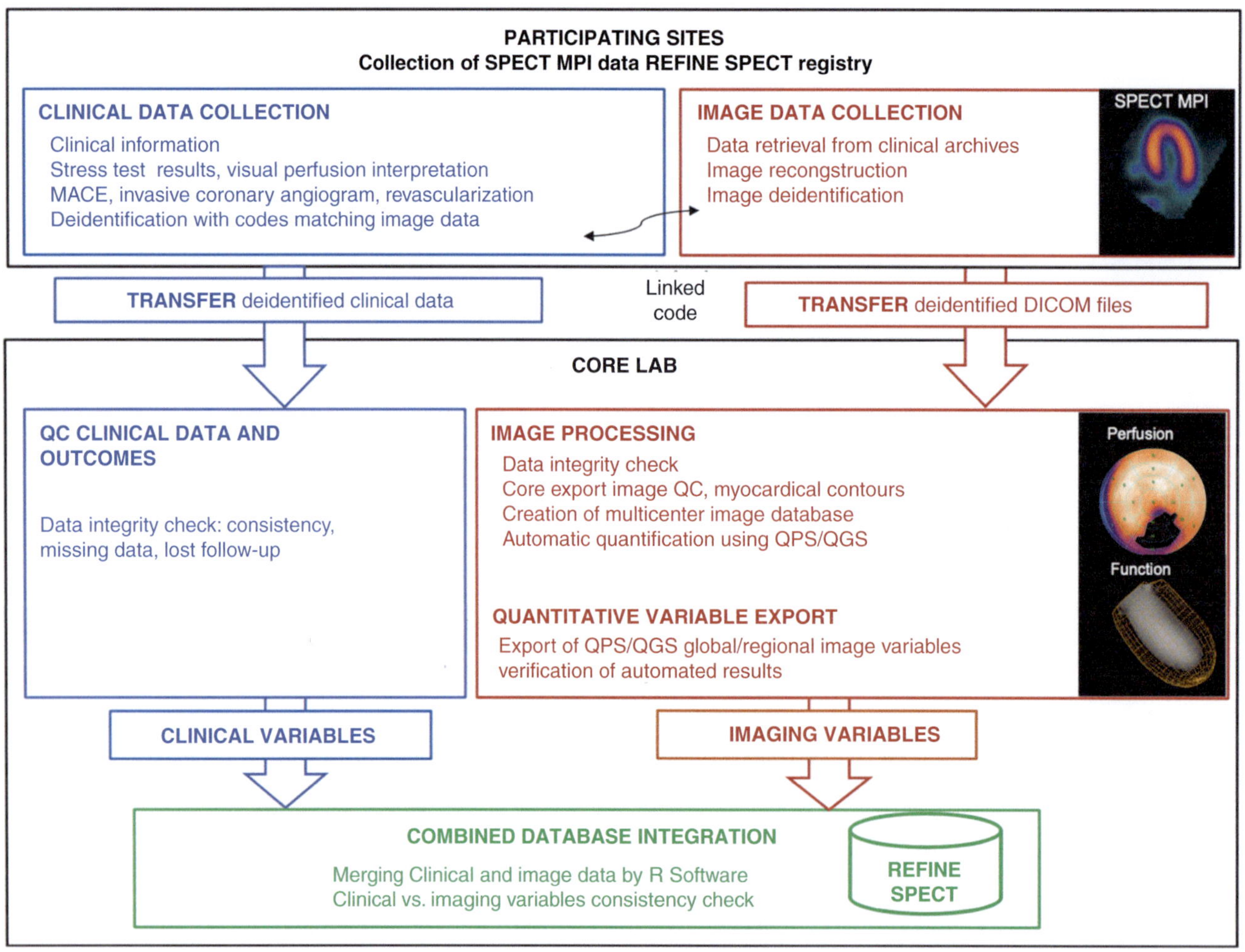

Fig. 37.8 Overview of the data acquisition and processing scheme for REFINE SPECT registry. The activities include clinical data (blue) and image (red) collection and de-identification at participating sites, data transfer to core laboratory for further data processing (quality control, quantification in QPS/QGS software), and combined database integration (green) DICOM Digital Imaging and Communications in Medicine, MACE major adverse cardiovascular event, QC quality control, QPS/QGS quantitative perfusion SPECT/quantitative gated SPECT software. (Reprinted with permission from Slomka et al. [64])

Explainable Artificial Intelligence

The "black box" nature of AI has always been the Achilles heel of these methodologies and a deterrent for its adoption or support from the clinical community. To overcome this hurdle, techniques have recently emerged in computer science that provide "explainable AI," that is, they explicitly present the "reasons" for a specific determination or a recommendation by the algorithm. For instance, CNN methods can identify the specific region in the image that has triggered a certain event and highlight them in the form of *heat maps* as an explanatory tool to users [66, 67]. Originally developed for natural images, these visual explanations can be applied in nuclear cardiology to generate heat map on perfusion polar maps (see Fig. 37.6 in [26]). ML-based prediction or risk stratification models – as those introduced in previous sections – also allow more transparent translation of their inner workings by providing a ranking of the used clinical and image-based features in terms of their individual contribution to the final risk score or outcome prediction (Fig. 37.6). Practical examples of these explanatory tools can be found in Hu et al. [52, 62], Betancur et al. [55], and Alonso et al. [57] and constitute a crucial step to remove the general suspicion that these methodologies have to overcome in the medical community.

Conclusions

AI-based methodologies have the potential to revolutionize the way we approach patient's care and medical imaging, including nuclear cardiology imaging. The research detailed in the previous sections already illustrate the vast applicability of these techniques at least to myocardial perfusion imaging. The feasibility of complex integrations of clinical and imaging variables by ML-based methods has permitted a wide range of studies on image interpretation, outcome prediction, and risk stratification. But other fields of nuclear imaging directed to improve image quality and acquisition efficiency have started to explore the capabilities of these techniques to improve otherwise difficult tasks (such as generation of AC maps, image denoising, and low-dose protocols), which, in addition to appearing less controversial than image interpretation and patients' management, can greatly benefit nuclear cardiology imaging as a whole and consequently patient's care.

The medical community is understandably suspicious of these techniques which they perceive as black boxes with obscure inner workings and possibly even threats to their work and integrity. Yet, the value of some of these methods is difficult to dismiss, especially in the context of AI entering clinical environments and practice not to supplant physicians' decision-making but to support it almost as a second opinion. This is particularly true when methods for explainable AI are also deployed as a means to make models and predictions more transparent to clinicians. On the other hand, in the context of certain applications such as genomics or radiomics – which is the search for patterns in texture from raw imaging data – the human eye or traditional statistical methods will not suffice, and AI ability to learn independently could prove advantageous.

Nevertheless, significant challenges and hurdles remain, hampering AI adoption into clinical settings for the near future. The most important one is certainly the fact that these techniques require large training datasets often manually labeled to provide accurate results. Additionally, validation of the models needs to be performed with a different cohort to assure that a proper generalization has been achieved. Efforts are already ongoing to create large international multicenter registries to be shared among physicians and scientists, but legal barriers exist within our healthcare systems about sharing this type of medical data. A fundamental aspect of this endeavor in data collection is also quality control and data standardization as the reliability of the algorithms will largely depend on the quality of the input data, as well as a seamless integration of HER to the images.

In conclusions, cardiac nuclear imaging already benefits from a wealth of techniques for reliable image acquisition, image processing, diagnosis, and prognosis. AI has recently appeared on the stage as a novel collection of tools that could be embraced or rejected. Continued progress resides in our commitment as scientists to thoughtfully and critically invest in new technologies with patients' care in mind.

References

1. Salerno M, Beller GA. Noninvasive assessment of myocardial perfusion. Circ Cardiovasc Imaging. 2009;2:412–24.
2. Einstein AJ, Pascual TNB, Mercuri M, et al. Current worldwide nuclear cardiology practices and radiation exposure: results from the 65 country IAEA Nuclear Cardiology Protocols Cross-Sectional Study (INCAPS). Eur Heart J. 2015;36:1689–96.
3. Slomka P, Xu Y, Berman D, et al. Quantitative analysis of perfusion studies: strengths and pitfalls. J Nucl Cardiol. 2012;19:338–46.
4. Nuclear Medicine Market Outlook Report 2018. Available from: https://imvinfo.com/product/nuclear-medicine-market-outlook-report-2018/ Accessed on 12/30/2020.
5. Schindler T, Schelbert HR, Quercioli A, et al. Cardiac PET for the detection and monitoring of coronary artery disease and microvascular health. JACC Cardiovasc Imaging. 2010;3:623–40.
6. Al Badarin FJ, Malhotra S. Diagnosis and prognosis of coronary artery disease with SPECT and PET. Curr Cardiol Rep. 2019;21:57.
7. Garcia E, Slomka P, Moody JB, et al. Quantitative clinical nuclear cardiology, part 1: established applications. J Nucl Med. 2019;60:1507–16.
8. Slomka PJ, Moody JB, Miller RJ, et al. Quantitative clinical nuclear cardiology, part 2: evolving/emerging applications. J Nucl Med. 2020. https://doi.org/10.2967/jnumed.120.242537.

9. Motwani M, Berman DS, Germano G, et al. Automated quantitative nuclear cardiology methods. Cardiol Clin. 2016;34:47–57.
10. Germano G, Kavanagh PB, Slomka PJ, et al. Quantitation in gated perfusion SPECT imaging: the Cedars-Sinai approach. J Nucl Cardiol. 2007;14:433–54.
11. Garcia EV, Faber TL, Cooke CD, et al. The increasing role of quantification in clinical nuclear cardiology: the Emory approach. J Nucl Cardiol. 2007;14:420–32.
12. Ficaro EP, Lee BC, Kritzman JN, et al. Corridor4DM: the Michigan method for quantitative nuclear cardiology. J Nucl Cardiol. 2007;14:455–65.
13. Liu Y-H. Quantification of nuclear cardiac images: the Yale approach. J Nucl Cardiol. 2007;14:483–91.
14. Garcia EV, Klein JL, Taylor AT. Clinical decision support systems in myocardial perfusion imaging. J Nucl Cardiol. 2014;21:427–39.
15. Garcia EV, Klein JL, Moncayo V, et al. Diagnostic performance of an artificial intelligence-driven cardiac-structured reporting system for myocardial perfusion SPECT imaging. J Nucl Cardiol. 2020;27:1652–64.
16. Turing AM. Computing machinery and intelligence. Mind. 1950;LIX:433–60.
17. Russel S, Norvel P. Artificial intelligence: A modern approach. 2nd ed. Upper Saddle River: Prentice Hall; 2003.
18. De Mauro A, Greco M, Grimaldi M. A formal definition of big data based on its essential features. Libr Rev. 2016;65:122–35.
19. Nilsson N. The quest for artificial intelligence: a history of ideas and achievements. New York: Cambridge University Press; 2009.
20. Szolovits P, Patil RS, Schwartz WB. Artificial intelligence in medical diagnosis. Ann Inter Med. 1988;108:80–7.
21. CB Insights Research. Healthcare remains the hottest AI category for deals. 2017. Available from: https://www.cbinsights.com/research/artificial-intelligence-healthcare-startups-investors/ Accessed 21 Jan 2021.
22. Dey D, Slomka PJ, Leeson P, et al. Artificial intelligence in cardiovascular imaging. J Am Coll Cardiol. 2019;73:1317–35.
23. Al'Aref SJ, Anchouche K, Singh G, et al. Clinical applications of machine learning in cardiovascular disease and its relevance to cardiac imaging. Eur Heart J. 2019;40:1975–86.
24. Dilsizian ME, Siegel EL. Machine meets biology: a primer of artificial intelligence in cardiology and cardiac imaging. Curr Cardiol Rep. 2018;20:139.
25. Litjens G, Ciompi F, Wolterink JM, et al. State-of-the-art deep learning in cardiovascular image analysis. J Am Coll Cardiol Img. 2018;12:1549–65.
26. Slomka PJ, Miller RJH, Isgum I, et al. Applications and translation of artificial intelligence to cardiovascular imaging in nuclear medicine and non-contrast CT. Semin Nucl Med. 2020;50:357–66.
27. Henglin M, Stein G, Pavel V, et al. Machine learning approaches in cardiovascular imaging. Circ Cardiovasc Imaging. 2017. https://doi.org/10.1161/CIRCIMAGING.117.005614.
28. Juarez-Orozco LE, Martinez-Manzanera O, Nesterov SV, et al. The machine learning horizon in cardiac hybrid imaging. Eur J Hybrid Imaging. 2018;2:15.
29. Mayr A, Binder H, Gefeller O, et al. The evolution of boosting algorithms. From machine learning to statistical modeling. Methods Inf Med. 2014;53:419–27.
30. Smola AJ, Schölkopf B. A tutorial on support vector regression. Stat Comput. 2004;14:199–222.
31. Breiman L. Random forests. Mach Learn. 2001;45:5–32.
32. LeCun Y, Bengio Y, Hinton G. Deep learning. Nature. 2005;521:436–44.
33. Krizhevsky A, Sutskever I, Hinton GE. Imagenet classification with deep convolutional neural networks. Proc Adv Neural Inf Process Sys. 2012;25:1097–105.
34. Gomez J, Doukky R, Germano G, et al. New trends in quantitative nuclear cardiology methods. Curr Cardiovasc Imaging Rep. 2018;11:1. https://doi.org/10.1007/s12410-018-9443-7.
35. Germano G, Kavanaugh PB, Su HT, et al. Automatic reorientation of 3-dimensional transaxial myocardial perfusion SPECT images. J Nucl Med. 1995;36:1107–14.
36. Mullick R, Ezquerra NF. Automatic determination of left ventricular orientation from SPECT data. IEEE Trans Med Imaging. 1995;14:88–99.
37. Slomka PJ, Hurwitz GA, Stephenson J, et al. Automated alignment and sizing of myocardial stress and rest scans to three-dimensional normal templates using an image registration algorithm. J Nucl Med. 1995;36:1115–22.
38. Xu Y, Kavanaugh PB, Fish MB, et al. Automated quality control for segmentation of myocardial perfusion. J Nucl Med. 2009;50:1418–26.
39. Betancur J, Rubeaux M, Fuchs TA, et al. Automatic valve plane localization in myocardial perfusion SPECT/CT by machine learning: anatomic and clinical validations. J Nucl Med. 2017;58:961–7.
40. Wang T, Lei Y, Tang H, et al. A learning-based automatic segmentation and quantification method of left ventricle in gated myocardial perfusion SPECT imaging: a feasibility study. J Nucl Cardiol. 2020;27:976–87.
41. Fujita H, Katafuchi T, Uehara T, et al. Application of neural network to computer-aided diagnosis of coronary artery disease in myocardial SPECT bull's eye images. J Nucl Med. 1992;33:272–6.
42. Porenta G, Dorffner G, Kundrat S, et al. Automated interpretation of planar thallium-201-dipyridamole stress-redistribution scintigrams using artificial neural networks. J Nucl Med. 1994;35:2041–7.
43. Hamilton D, Riley PJ, Miola UJ, et al. A feed-forward neural network for classification of bull's eye myocardial perfusion images. Eur J Nucl Med. 1995;22:108–15.
44. Lindhal D, Palmer J, Ohlsson M, et al. Automated interpretation of myocardial SPECT perfusion images using artificial neural networks. J Nucl Med. 1997;38:1870–5.
45. Lindhal D, Palmer J, Edenbrandt L. Myocardial SPECT: artificial neural networks describe extent and severity of perfusion defects. Clin Physiol. 1999;19:497–503.
46. Lindhal D, Toft J, Hesse B, et al. Scandinavian test of artificial neural network for classification of myocardial perfusion images. Clin Physiol. 2000;20:253–61.
47. Allison JS, Heo J, Iskandrian AE. Artificial neural network modeling of stress single-photon emission computed tomographic imaging for detecting extensive coronary artery disease. Am J Cardiol. 2005;95:178–81.
48. Arsanjani R, Xu Y, Hayes SW, et al. Comparison of fully automated computer analysis and visual scoring for detection of coronary artery disease from myocardial perfusion SPECT in a large population. J Nucl Med. 2013;54:221–8.
49. Arsanjani R, Xu Y, Dey D, et al. Improved accuracy of myocardial perfusion SPECT for the detection of coronary artery disease using a support vector machine algorithm. J Nucl Med. 2013;54:549–55.
50. Arsanjani R, Xu Y, Dey D, et al. Improved accuracy of myocardial perfusion SPECT for detection of coronary artery disease by machine learning in a large population. J Nucl Cardiol. 2013;20:553–62.
51. Arsanjani R, Dey D, Khachatryan T, et al. Prediction of revascularization after myocardial perfusion SPECT by machine learning in a large population. J Nucl Cardiol. 2015;22:877–84.
52. Hu LH, Betancur J, Sharir T, et al. Machine learning predicts per-vessel early coronary revascularization after fast myocardial perfusion SPECT: results from multicenter REFINE SPECT registry. Eur Heart J Cardiovasc Imaging. 2020;12:549–59.

53. Betancur J, Commandeur F, Motlagh M, et al. Deep learning for prediction of obstructive disease from fast myocardial perfusion SPECT: a multicenter study. JACC Cardiovasc Imaging. 2018;11:1654–63.
54. Betancur J, Hu LH, Commandeur F, et al. Deep learning analysis of upright-supine high-efficiency SPECT myocardial perfusion imaging for prediction of coronary artery disease: a multicenter study. J Nucl Med. 2019;60:664–70.
55. Betancur J, Otaki Y, Motwani M, et al. Prognostic value of combined clinical and myocardial perfusion imaging data using machine learning. JACC Cardiovasc Imaging. 2018;11:1000–9.
56. Juarez-Orozco LE, Knol RJJ, Sanches-Catasus CA, et al. Machine learning in the integration of simple variables for identifying patients with myocardial ischemia. J Nucl Cardiol. 2020;27:147–55.
57. Alonso DH, Wernick MN, Yang Y, et al. Prediction of cardiac death after adenosine myocardial perfusion SPECT based on machine learning. J Nucl Cardiol. 2019;26:1746–54.
58. Garcia EV. Deep learning, another important tool for improving acquisition efficiency in SPETC MPI imaging. J Nucl Cardiol. 2020. https://doi.org/10.1007/s12350-020-02188-z.
59. Shiri I, Sabet KA, Arabi H, et al. Standard SPECT myocardial perfusion estimation from half-time acquisitions using deep convolutional residual neural networks. J Nucl Cardiol. 2020. https://doi.org/10.1007/s12350-020-02119-y.
60. Ramon AJ, Yang Y, Pretorius PH, et al. Improving diagnostic accuracy in low-dose SPECT myocardial perfusion imaging with convolution denoising networks. IEEE Trans Med Imaging. 2020;39:2893–903.
61. Song C, Yang Y, Wernick MN, et al. Low-dose cardiac-gated SPECT studies using a residual convolutional neural network. 2019 IEEE 16th International Symposium on Biomedical Imaging (ISBI 2019). 2019; pp. 653–656.
62. Hu LH, Miller RJH, Sharir T, et al. Prognostically safe stress-only single-photon emission computed tomography myocardial perfusion imaging guided by machine learning: report from REFINE SPECT. Eur Heart J Cardiovasc Imaging. 2021;22:705–14.
63. Shi L, Onofrey JA, Liu H, et al. Deep learning-based attenuation map generation for myocardial perfusion SPECT. Eur J Nucl Med Mol Imaging. 2020;47:2383–95.
64. Slomka PJ, Betancur J, Liang JX, et al. Rationale and design of the registry of fast myocardial perfusion imagining with next generation SPECT (REFINE). J Nucl Cardiol. 2020;27:1010–21.
65. Otaki Y, Betancur J, Sharir T, et al. 5-year prognostic value of quantitative vs visual myocardial perfusion imaging in subtle perfusion defects: results from the REFINE SPECT registry. JACC Cardiovasc Imaging. 2020;13:774–85.
66. Zeiler MD, Fergus R. Visualizing and understanding convolutional networks. European Conference on Computer Vision. Springer. 2014; 818–833.
67. Selvaraju RR, Cogswell M, Das A. Grad-cam: Visual explanations from deep networks via gradient-based localization. Proceedings of the IEEE International Conference on Computer Vision, 2017; 618–626.

Cardiac Ultrasound Imaging: The Role of Artificial Intelligence

38

Karthik Seetharam and Partho P. Sengupta

Introduction

Cardiovascular imaging is at the cusp of a significant transformation which will drastically alter the landscape of medicine, and echocardiography is at the forefront of this revolution [1, 2]. Tremendous progress in computer processing capabilities and cloud networks has vastly expanded the frontiers of echocardiography [3, 4]. As we move toward this supposed golden age in echocardiography, we are approaching a precipice [5]. Technological advances have led to the addition of parameters in imaging modalities which can overwhelm providers with abundant information [6, 7]. A number of complexities arise if data arises from multiple sources of information which can include electronic records, smartphone applications, and handheld devices [1]. The inflow of information imposes a significant burden in medical management [8].

As the integration of technology with healthcare is becoming evident, newer approaches are necessary to fully utilize the information present in the vast repositories of echocardiography [9]. Artificial intelligence (AI) can overcome the widening divide between healthcare and technology [10]. Machine learning (ML), a branch of AI, can explore information in a variety of manners. It can automate a number of tasks and find patterns hidden within information, leading to data-driven discoveries [11]. In this chapter, we explore the role of AI in echocardiography.

K. Seetharam, MD
West Virginia University Medicine Heart & Vascular Institute, Morgantown, WV, USA

P. P. Sengupta, MD, DM (✉)
West Virginia University Medicine Heart & Vascular Institute, Morgantown, WV, USA

Rutgers Robert Wood Johnson Medical School, Rutgers University, New Jersey, NJ, USA
e-mail: Partho.Sengupta@wvumedicine.org

Expansion of Data

Echocardiography is the most common diagnostic modality used in cardiovascular imaging [12]. A single scan can produce petabytes of information [10]. As data continues to become larger and complex, conventional statistics will reach the limits of their capabilities [10]. Prediction is not a particular strong attribute of conventional statistics [13]. In contrary, ML algorithms become increasingly effective with bigger datasets, and the predictive accuracy also correspondingly increases [7]. Conventional statistics are quite rigid in nature, but ML is quite dynamic in nature [14]. ML approaches information in a multi-linear manner and can branch off in a number of alternative possibilities. It provides rich insight and can extrapolate information present deep within data matrices.

Nexus Between AI and Echocardiography

In recent times, cardiologists and imaging technicians have a vast array of imaging modalities at the tip of their palms [15]. For practical purposes, very few of these modalities can truly match the versatility and efficiency of echocardiography. It permits assessment of cardiac volumes and can evaluate cardiac function. It can detect and identify a vast number of pathological entities with minimal difficulty. The emergence of speckle tracking echocardiography can enable superior evaluation of cardiac function beyond the ejection fraction seen in echocardiography [9]. Unfortunately, the burdensome nature and time restraints of speckle tracking echocardiography have hindered the advancement of this approach in clinical practice. The integration of AI and ML algorithms will be absolutely quintessential for further advancement of echocardiography. It can introduce new pipelines which can streamline a multitude of processes in clinical practice. In the near future, AI can facilitate incorporation of speckle tracking echocardiography in day-to-day medical care which

C. N. De Cecco et al. (eds.), *Artificial Intelligence in Cardiothoracic Imaging*, Contemporary Medical Imaging,
https://doi.org/10.1007/978-3-030-92087-6_38

Table 38.1 Recent examples of machine learning in echocardiography

Study	Type of machine learning	Description
Improved clinical interpretation		
Narula et al. [16]	Supervised learning	To differentiate between hypertrophic cardiomyopathy and athlete's heart
Sengupta et al. [17]	Supervised learning	To distinguish between restrictive cardiomyopathy and constrictive pericarditis
Increased accuracy		
Zhang et al. [22]	Deep learning	To evaluate automated assessment in echocardiography
Madani et al. [20]	Deep learning	To assess view classification between board-certified physicians and ML
Madani et al. [21]	Deep learning	To assess automatic interpretation of echocardiograms
Enhanced evaluation of cardiac function		
Asch et al. [18]	ML algorithm	To assess automated assessment of ejection fraction
Kusonose et al. [20]	Deep learning	To assess automated ejection fraction
Kusonose et al. [21]	Deep learning	To identify regional wall motion abnormalities
Knackstedt et al. [19]	AI	To assess automated ejection fraction
Identification of unique phenotypes in echocardiography		
Casaclang-Verzosa et al. [26]	Topological data analysis	Phenotypic recognition of left ventricular responses during the course of aortic stenosis
Kwak et al. [27]	Unsupervised learning	To detect clusters associated with cardiovascular complications in aortic stenosis
Todoki et al. [28]	Unsupervised learning	To predict major adverse cardiac events and complications
Phenotypic clustering in congestive heart failure		
Lancaster et al. [29]	Unsupervised learning	To identify high-risk phenotypes in heart failure with diastolic dysfunction
Omar et al. [30]	Unsupervised learning	To assess the magnitude of diastolic dysfunction
Omar et al. [31]	Supervised learning	To evaluate left ventricular filling pressure in diastolic dysfunction patients
Tabassian et al. [32]	Supervised learning	To detect patients with heart failure with preserved ejection fraction during exercise and rest during left ventricular strain
Mishra et al. [33]	Unsupervised learning	To identify heart failure hospitalization in various clusters
Przewlocka-Kosmala et al. [34]	Unsupervised learning	To detect clusters in heart failure with preserved ejection fraction
Cho et al. [35]	Unsupervised learning	To predict complications in various clusters of heart failure patients

can open new pathways for a number of cardiac conditions. Many academic centers have explored the potential of ML in echocardiography and have experienced promising results (Table 38.1).

Advanced Clinical Interpretation

A number of clinical conditions may mimic one another which can lead to erroneous medical management. This can be especially more daunting for younger cardiologists and technicians. ML algorithms can find pattern beyond human perception which can enhance diagnostic accuracy [15]. Narula et al. utilized an ensemble algorithm for deciphering hypertrophic cardiomyopathy from an athlete's heart [16]. Volume (IG = 0.24) and mid-left ventricular segment (IG = 0.134) were the best predictors for separating the two entities. Sengupta et al. used an associate memory classifier ML algorithm in speckle tracking echocardiography for differentiating constrictive pericarditis from restrictive cardiomyopathy [17]. The diagnostic area under the curve was 89.2% and 96.2% with echocardiographic parameters.

Enhanced Evaluation of Cardiac Function

Automated approaches can vastly improve the accuracy of various processes in echocardiography. Asch assessed ML automated echocardiographic quantification of left ventricular ejection fraction in 99 patients with 3 reference experts [18]. There was excellent agreement with reference values ($r = 0.95$) between automated and average manual approaches and an excellent consistency (mean absolute deviation = 2.9%). Knackstedt et al. examined an ML algorithm for differentiating automated and manual ejection fraction measurements in 255 patients [19]. The interclass correlation coefficients and Bland-Altman analysis exhibited good agreements with automated ejection fraction (IC = 0.78 to 0.86) for local or reference center manual tracking. Similarly, Kusonose used deep learning to demonstrate comparable ML-derived ejection fraction with a validation group ($r = 0.82 \pm 0.02$, $p < 0.001$) [20]. Kusonose et al. showed deep learning was superior than medical residents in identifying wall motion abnormalities (AUC 0.99 vs 0.90, $p = 0.002$) and surrounding territories (AUC = 0.97 vs 0.83, $p = 0.003$) in 300 patients with history of myocardial infarction [21]. The ML architecture performed similarly to experienced cardiologists.

Increased Accuracy

The interpretation of clinical images is heavily dependent on the experience and expertise of the imager. Another important aspect is the quality of images obtained from each patient. ML algorithms can extract features and rapidly identify various conditions. Zhang et al. evaluated the role of a CNN for automated image interpretation in 14,035 echocardiograms [22]. It was trained for identifying 23 viewpoints and segmentation of cardiac chamber across 5 common views. The CNN was successful in identifying views (96% for parasternal long axis) and enabled segmentation of cardiac chambers. Madani et al. used deep learning in 267 transthoracic echocardiograms [23]. They showed a 91.7% accuracy for the ML algorithm in comparison to 70.2 to 84.0% for board-certified physicians. In addition, Madani et al. assessed deep learning for automatic interpretation in echocardiography [24]. They demonstrated an accuracy of 94.4% for echocardiographic classification and 91.2% accuracy for binary left ventricular hypertrophy grouping.

Identification of New Phenotypes

ML algorithms, especially unsupervised learning, can identify new clusters or subset of patients [25]. Identification of these clusters can enhance our understanding of a number of pathological conditions. Casaclang-Verzosa et al. explored the role of TDA to characterize the phenotypic left ventricular responses during the evolution of aortic stenosis [26] (Fig. 38.1). A loop was created which separated mild and severe aortic stenosis (AS) ($p < 0.001$) on two different sides. The two groups are connected through moderate AS on the top and bottom aspects with reduced and preserved ejection fraction ($p < 0.001$). It was further shown in mice ($p < 0.001$). Similarly, Kwak et al. utilized unsupervised learning for AS phenotypic clustering; there was a significant difference between complications between the three clusters (mortality rate, 13.3% vs 19.8% vs 6.0%, $p < 0.001$) [27]. Todoki et al. evaluated unsupervised learning approaches by incorporating echocardiographic characteristics from the left ventricle to predict major adverse cardiac events (MACE) in 866 individuals [28]. A loop sectioned patient into four unique groups. The Kaplan-Meier curves clearly showed substantial differences in MACE-related events and mortality (both $p < 0.001$).

Phenotypic Clustering in Congestive Heart Failure

A number of studies have used clustering algorithms to further characterize congestive heart failure with unique findings. Lancaster et al. explored the role of a clustering ML model which detected diastolic dysfunction in 559 of 866 patients with 2 distinct groups [29] (Fig. 38.2). Furthermore, it revealed moderate agreement with conventional classification (kappa = 0.41, $p < 0.001$). Omar et al. utilized cluster analysis of LA and LV strain parameters in diastolic dysfunction patients [30]. The speckle tracking features isolated patients into three groups with elevating levels of dysfunction and left ventricular filling pressure. In a subsequent study, further analysis utilized 14 speckle tracking attributes to distinguish left ventricular filling pressure [31]. The ML algorithm detected 80% of patients with pulmonary capillary wedge pressure > 18 mm Hg. Tabassian et al. obtained velocity, strain, and strain rate curves from all 18 segments of the left ventricle in 100 patients [32]. The strain rate parameters provided the highest accuracy for segregating subjects into four groups (overall 57%, HFpEF patients 81%) and two classes (asymptomatic vs symptomatic; AUC = 0.89; accuracy = 85%; sensitivity = 86%; specificity = 82%). Mishra et al. also utilized unsupervised learning to identify clusters with varying levels of HF hospitalization risk [33]. In another similar study in HFpEF clustering, Przewlocka-Kosmala et al. suggested that reduced LV systolic reserve is associated with exercise intolerance in these patients [34]. Cho et al. applied an ML framework with multidimensional LV parameters in 297 patients for automated phenotyping. It identified four clusters; cluster IV had a higher prevalence of stage C or D heart failure (78%, $p < 0.001$) and higher incidence of MACE ($p < 0.001$) [35].

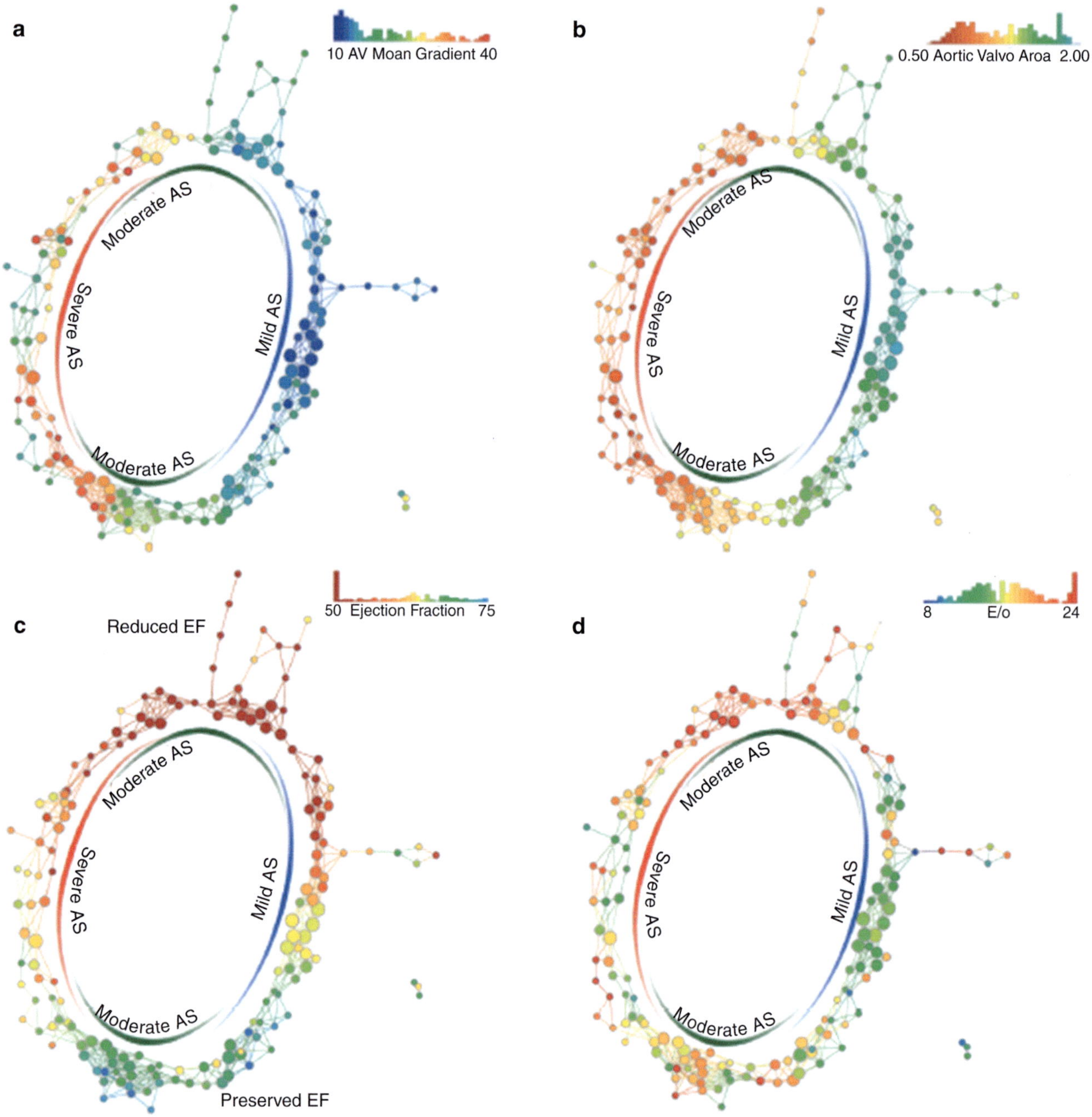

Fig. 38.1 The similarity network draws aggregation of patients with severe and mild AS in two opposite ends and moderate AS in the top and bottom arms of the loop. The red color represents the abnormal values, whereas blue represents the normal or minor malady in the disease space. (**a**) Spectrum of mean gradient in humans identified in the network of disease space. High gradients aggregated on the left side, whereas the low gradients were on the right side with moderate gradients in the middle. (**b**) Distribution of valve area on the network. (**c**) Patient similarity network revealing preserved and reduced ejection fractions (EFs) in patients with aortic stenosis (AS). The top arm clustered patients with the reduced EF, whereas the bottom arm described the patients with preserved EF. The red nodes consist of patients with EFs of ≤50%, whereas the blue nodes consist of patients with EFs of ≥65%. (**d**) Distribution of E/e' as a feature of diastolic dysfunction revealing the pattern of E/e' around moderate and severe AS. TDA topological data analysis

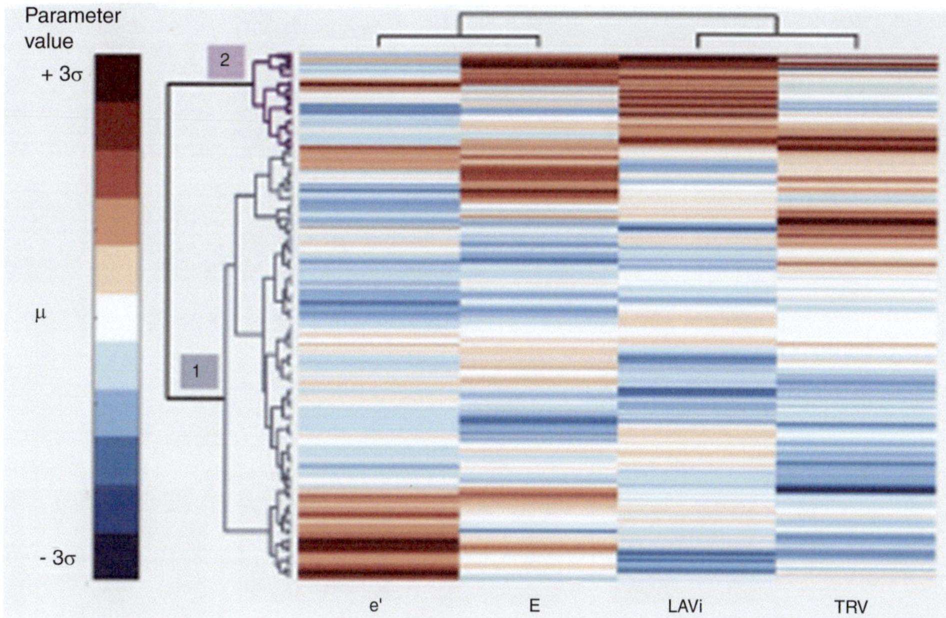

Fig. 38.2 Hierarchical clustering used the Ward method. μ parameter mean, Ó parameter standard deviation, E Doppler-derived early diastolic mitral flow, e' early diastolic tissue Doppler-derived mitral annular velocity, LAVi left atrial volume index; TRV tricuspid regurgitation velocity

Contemporary Beliefs of Machine Learning

As we move forward in this data-driven era in healthcare, existing ideologies must evolve to accept new paradigms in cardiovascular imaging and clinical care. ML algorithms can analyze information in a variety of manners which can vastly expand our understanding [3]. The ability of ML algorithms to adapt and evolve must be incorporated in our current research dogmas. All of research moves in a linear fashion from a hypothesis to a conclusion [14]. We should allow preliminary data analysis to modify our initial hypothesis to enable the investigator to reach more effective conclusions [14]. Furthermore, data-driven analytics can evaluate the logistics of a project and determine feasibility and resource allocation. It could be very useful in randomized clinical trials [36]. This versatility and multi-linear thinking will allow our research to be more dynamic.

Many of the aforementioned studies emphasize a very important concept regarding ML algorithms and cardiology. Cardiovascular diseases are heterogeneous in nature [6]. Many of the existing classifications do not truly embrace the diverse aspects of these conditions. There is a constant interplay among varuous genetic, biologival and environmental factors which can modify the manifestations of these conditions [37]. By further delineating subtypes in various conditions such as aortic stenosis or congestive heart failure, it provides additional insight. This can lead to novel innovative approaches which can appropriately treat the underlying condition [10]. This can lead to tailored regimens which meet the need of each individual and facilitate the growth of precision medicine [38].

The growth of smartphone apps and miniaturized devices will have profound effects in the field of cardiology [9]. In our earlier experiences, we have experienced the first-hand benefits of handheld echocardiography in underserved regions of the world [39]. The incorporation of cloud technology with these devices can allow information to be sent to providers and dictate management. Integration of AI with mHealth can allow tremendous growth in this aspect. The information can be analyzed in real time and automate a number of aspects (Fig. 38.3). Advances in deep learning can allow these algorithms to provide rapid medical diagnosis [40]. AI can help bridge the gap in healthcare and underserved regions of the world [9].

Though ML opens a world of countless possibilities, we must thread with caution at each and every step. ML lacks a moral compass [41]. A number of unintentional biases may creep into the algorithm. This could affect the performance of the algorithm and lead to inaccurate results. False discovery is another important aspect [13]. This can occur with small datasets. The clinical investigator must work with the engineer at each and every step of the algorithm [13] (Fig. 38.4). The medical team must play a vigilant role. The investigator must clearly know the purpose of the project beforehand. It will facilitate effective execution of any given project.

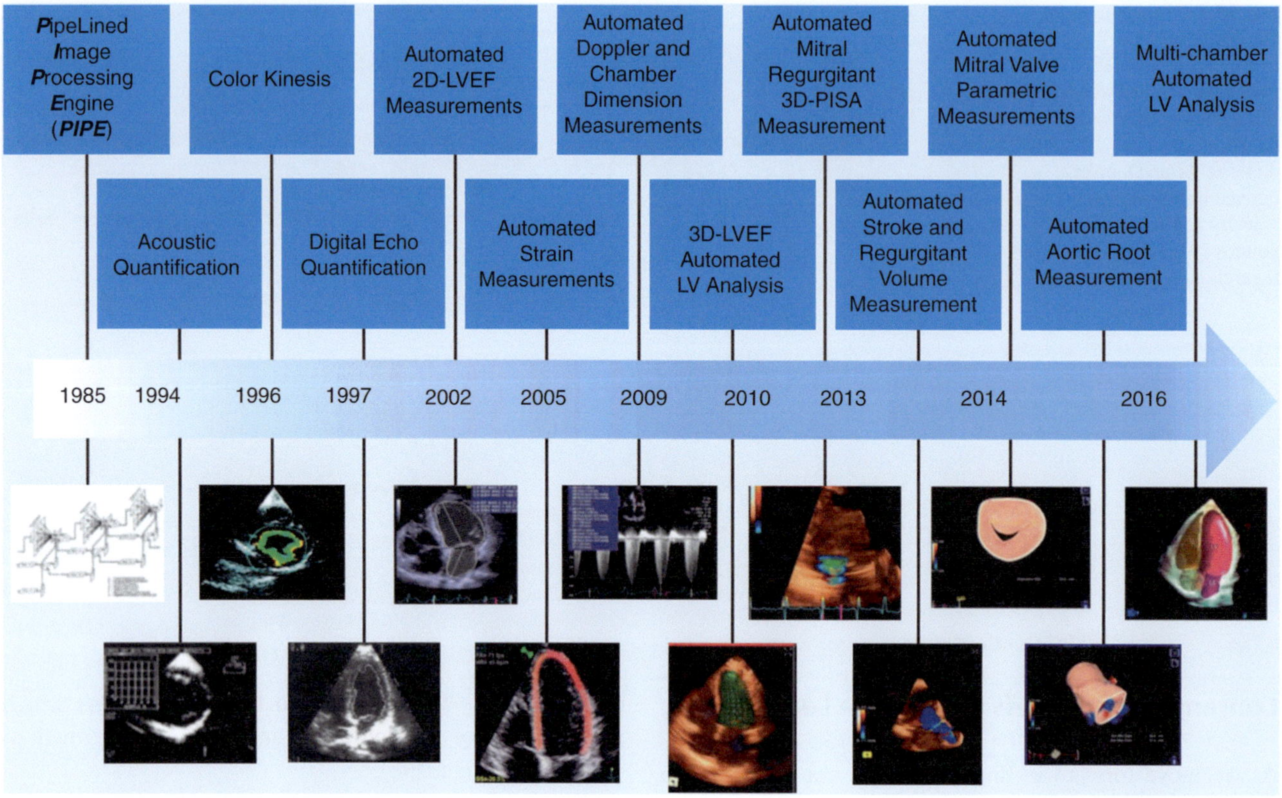

Fig. 38.3 Temporal progression in automated quantification in echocardiography. (Adapted from Nolan et al. [42]. Permission obtained from publisher)

Conclusion

ML is ushering a new era in healthcare which will have a tremendous impact in echocardiography. It can automate a series of tasks and enable data-driven discoveries. Physicians will have more time for patient interactions and divert their mental faculties toward medical management. As the worlds of information technology and echocardiography are coming closer and closer, precision medicine is going to become an inevitable reality.

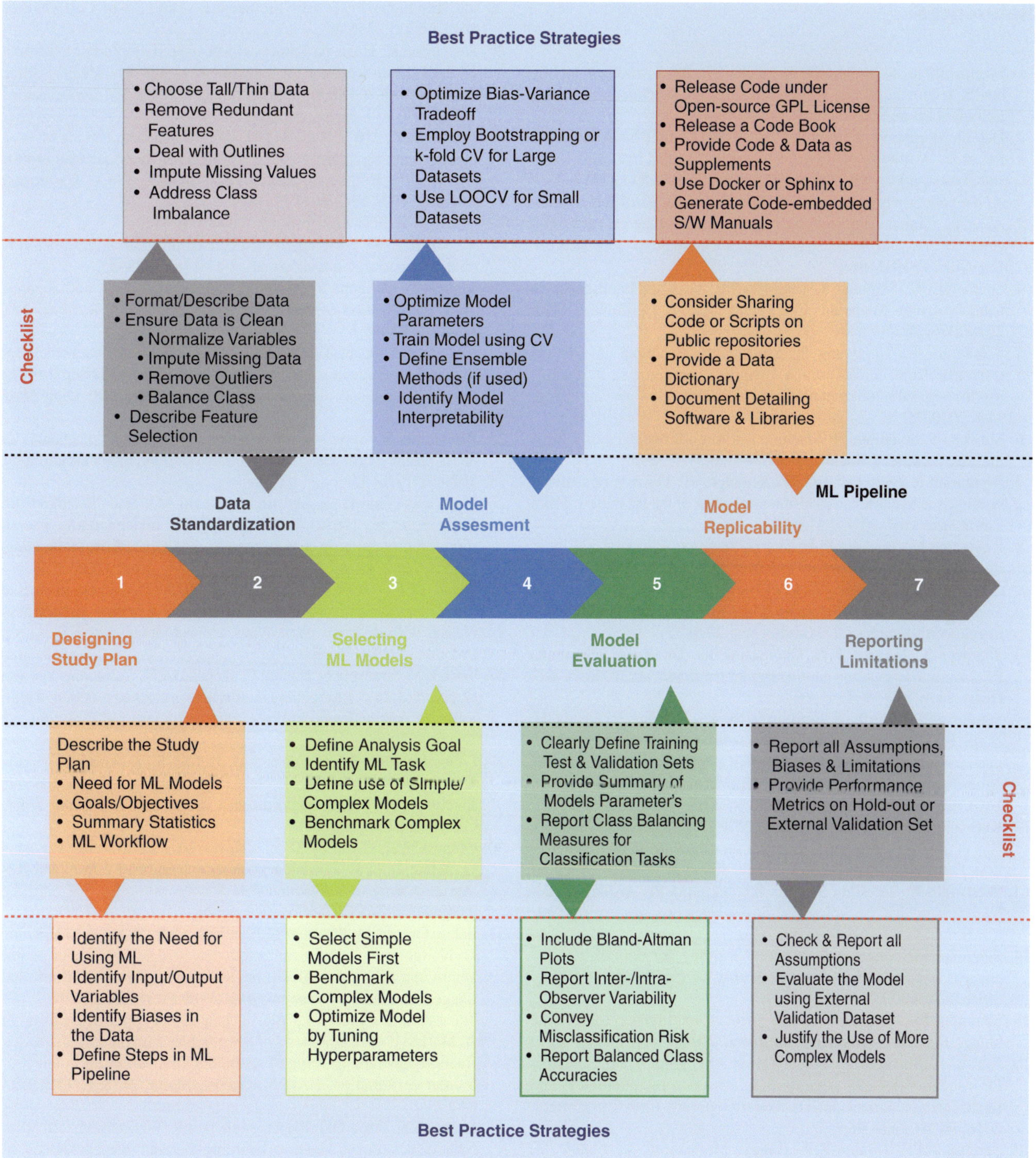

Fig. 38.4 Steps for building a machine learning pipeline and the reporting items in a checklist. (Adapted from Sengupta et al. [11]. Permission obtained from the publisher)

References

1. Seetharam K, Kagiyama N, Sengupta PP. Application of mobile health, telemedicine and artificial intelligence to echocardiography. Echo Res Pract. 2019;6(2):R41–r52.
2. Dey D, Slomka PJ, Leeson P, Comaniciu D, Shrestha S, Sengupta PP, et al. Artificial intelligence in cardiovascular imaging: JACC state-of-the-art review. J Am Coll Cardiol. 2019;73(11):1317–35.
3. Al'Aref SJ, Anchouche K, Singh G, Slomka PJ, Kolli KK, Kumar A, et al. Clinical applications of machine learning in cardiovascular disease and its relevance to cardiac imaging. Eur Heart J. 2019;40(24):1975–86.
4. Seetharam K, Shrestha S, Sengupta PP. Artificial Intelligence in Cardiovascular Medicine. Curr Treat Options Cardiovasc Med. 2019;21(6):25.
5. Seetharam K, Kagiyama N, Shrestha S, Sengupta P. Clinical inference from cardiovascular imaging: paradigm shift towards machine-based intelligent platform. Curr Treat Options Cardiovasc Med 2020;22.
6. Shrestha S, Sengupta PP. Machine learning for nuclear cardiology: the way forward. J Nucl Cardiol. 2019;26(5):1755–8.
7. Seetharam K, Brito D, Farjo PD, Sengupta PP. The role of artificial intelligence in cardiovascular imaging: state of the art review. Front Cardiovasc Med. 2020;7:618849.
8. Kagiyama N, Shrestha S, Farjo PD, Sengupta PP. Artificial intelligence: practical primer for clinical research in cardiovascular disease. J Am Heart Assoc. 2019;8(17):e012788.
9. Seetharam K, Raina S, Sengupta P. The role of artificial intelligence in echocardiography. Curr Cardiol Rep 2020;22.
10. Shameer K, Johnson KW, Glicksberg BS, Dudley JT, Sengupta PP. Machine learning in cardiovascular medicine: are we there yet? Heart. 2018;104(14):1156–64.
11. Sengupta PP, Shrestha S, Berthon B, Messas E, Donal E, Tison GH, et al. Proposed requirements for cardiovascular imaging-related machine learning evaluation (PRIME): a checklist: reviewed by the American College of Cardiology Healthcare Innovation Council. JACC Cardiovasc Imaging. 2020;13(9):2017–35.
12. Kulina R, Seetharam K, Agarwal S, Wiley BM, Narula J, Chaudhry FA, et al. Beamforming algorithms for endocardial border detection. Echocardiography. 2018;35(10):1499–506.
13. Seetharam K, Shresthra S, Mills JD, Sengupta PP. Artificial intelligence in nuclear cardiology: adding value to prognostication. Curr Cardiovasc Imaging Rep 2019;12(5).
14. Sengupta PP, Shrestha S. Machine learning for data-driven discovery: the rise and relevance. JACC Cardiovasc Imaging. 2019;12(4):690–2.
15. Sengupta PP, Adjeroh DA. Will artificial intelligence replace the human Echocardiographer? Circulation. 2018;138(16):1639–42.
16. Narula S, Shameer K, Salem Omar AM, Dudley JT, Sengupta PP. Machine-learning algorithms to automate morphological and functional assessments in 2D echocardiography. J Am Coll Cardiol. 2016;68(21):2287–95.
17. Sengupta PP, Huang YM, Bansal M, Ashrafi A, Fisher M, Shameer K, et al. Cognitive machine-learning algorithm for cardiac imaging: a pilot study for differentiating constrictive pericarditis from restrictive cardiomyopathy. Circ Cardiovasc Imaging 2016;9(6).
18. Asch FM, Poilvert N, Abraham T, Jankowski M, Cleve J, Adams M, et al. Automated echocardiographic quantification of left ventricular ejection fraction without volume measurements using a machine learning algorithm mimicking a human expert. Circ Cardiovasc Imaging. 2019;12(9):e009303.
19. Knackstedt C, Bekkers SC, Schummers G, Schreckenberg M, Muraru D, Badano LP, et al. Fully automated versus standard tracking of left ventricular ejection fraction and longitudinal strain: the FAST-EFs multicenter study. J Am Coll Cardiol. 2015;66(13):1456–66.
20. Kusunose K, Haga A, Yamaguchi N, Abe T, Fukuda D, Yamada H, et al. Deep learning for assessment of left ventricular ejection fraction from echocardiographic images. J Am Soc Echocardiogr. 2020;33(5):632–5.e1.
21. Kusunose K, Abe T, Haga A, Fukuda D, Yamada H, Harada M, et al. A deep learning approach for assessment of Regional Wall motion abnormality from echocardiographic images. JACC Cardiovasc Imaging. 2020;13(2 Pt 1):374–81.
22. Zhang J, Gajjala S, Agrawal P, Tison GH, Hallock LA, Beussink-Nelson L, et al. Fully automated echocardiogram interpretation in clinical practice. Circulation. 2018;138(16):1623–35.
23. Madani A, Arnaout R, Mofrad M, Arnaout R. Fast and accurate view classification of echocardiograms using deep learning. NPJ Digit Med 2018;1.
24. Madani A, Ong JR, Tibrewal A, Mofrad MRK. Deep echocardiography: data-efficient supervised and semi-supervised deep learning towards automated diagnosis of cardiac disease. NPJ Digit Med. 2018;1:59.
25. Seetharam K, Sengupta PP, Bianco CM. Cardiac mechanics in heart failure with preserved ejection fraction. Echocardiography. 2020;37:1936–43.
26. Casaclang-Verzosa G, Shrestha S, Khalil MJ, Cho JS, Tokodi M, Balla S, et al. Network tomography for understanding phenotypic presentations in aortic stenosis. JACC Cardiovasc Imaging. 2019;12(2):236–48.
27. Kwak S, Lee Y, Ko T, Yang S, Hwang IC, Park JB, et al. Unsupervised cluster analysis of patients with aortic stenosis reveals distinct population with different phenotypes and outcomes. Circ Cardiovasc Imaging. 2020;13(5):e009707.
28. Tokodi M, Shrestha S, Bianco C, Kagiyama N, Casaclang-Verzosa G, Narula J, et al. Interpatient similarities in cardiac function: a platform for personalized cardiovascular medicine. JACC Cardiovasc Imaging. 2020.
29. Lancaster MC, Salem Omar AM, Narula S, Kulkarni H, Narula J, Sengupta PP. Phenotypic clustering of left ventricular diastolic function parameters: patterns and prognostic relevance. JACC Cardiovasc Imaging. 2018.
30. Omar AMS, Narula S, Abdel Rahman MA, Pedrizzetti G, Raslan H, Rifaie O, et al. Precision phenotyping in heart failure and pattern clustering of ultrasound data for the assessment of diastolic dysfunction. JACC Cardiovasc Imaging. 2017;10(11):1291–303.
31. Salem Omar AM, Shameer K, Narula S, Abdel Rahman MA, Rifaie O, Narula J, et al. Artificial intelligence-based assessment of left ventricular filling pressures from 2-dimensional cardiac ultrasound images. JACC Cardiovasc Imaging. 2018;11(3):509–10.
32. Tabassian M, Sunderji I, Erdei T, Sanchez-Martinez S, Degiovanni A, Marino P, et al. Diagnosis of heart failure with preserved ejection fraction: machine learning of spatiotemporal variations in left ventricular deformation. J Am Soc Echocardiogr. 2018;31(12):1272–84 e9.
33. Mishra RK, Tison GH, Fang Q, Scherzer R, Whooley MA, Schiller NB. Association of Machine Learning-Derived Phenogroupings of echocardiographic variables with heart failure in stable coronary artery disease: the heart and soul study. J Am Soc Echocardiogr. 2020;33(3):322–31.e1.
34. Przewlocka-Kosmala M, Marwick TH, Dabrowski A, Kosmala W. Contribution of cardiovascular reserve to prognostic categories of heart failure with preserved ejection fraction: a classification based on machine learning. J Am Soc Echocardiogr. 2019;32(5):604–15.e6.
35. Cho J, Shrestha S, Kagiyama N, Hu L, Abdul Ghaffar Y, Casaclang-Verzosa G, et al. A network-based 'Phenomics' approach for discovering patient subtypes from high-throughput cardiac imaging data. JACC Cardiovasc Imaging. 2020.

36. Krittanawong C, Johnson KW, Tang WW. How artificial intelligence could redefine clinical trials in cardiovascular medicine: lessons learned from oncology. Per Med. 2019;16(2):83–8.
37. Leopold JA, Maron BA. Precision medicine in pulmonary arterial hypertension. Circ Res. 2019;124(6):832–3.
38. Johnson KW, Torres Soto J, Glicksberg BS, Shameer K, Miotto R, Ali M, et al. Artificial Intelligence in Cardiology. J Am Coll Cardiol. 2018;71(23):2668–79.
39. Bhavnani SP, Sola S, Adams D, Venkateshvaran A, Dash PK, Sengupta PP. A randomized trial of pocket-echocardiography integrated Mobile health device assessments in modern structural heart disease clinics. JACC Cardiovasc Imaging. 2018;11(4):546–57.
40. Krittanawong C, Johnson KW, Rosenson RS, Wang Z, Aydar M, Baber U, et al. Deep learning for cardiovascular medicine: a practical primer. Eur Heart J. 2019;40(25):2058–73.
41. Seetharam K, Shrestha S, Sengupta P. Artificial Intelligence in Cardiac Imaging. US Cardiol Rev. 2020;13:110–6.
42. Nolan MT, et al. Automated quantification in echocardiography. JACC Cardiol Imaging. 2019;12(6):1073–92.

Artificial Intelligence-Based Cardiovascular Risk Stratification

39

Abdallah Malkawi, Zaid Almarzooq, Mouaz H. Al-Mallah, and Subhi J. Al'Aref

Introduction

Throughout the years, accurate estimation of incident cardiovascular (CV) risk has been a cornerstone of clinical practice. It has important implications on the expected net benefit of any therapeutic strategy a patient is offered, and as such, risk assessment has been incorporated and emphasized across numerous societal guidelines [1]. Traditional CV risk assessment methods, such as the Framingham risk score or the more recently developed American Heart Association/American College of Cardiology (AHA/ACC) atherosclerotic cardiovascular risk estimator, have relied on the use of patient-level characteristics. Recent studies have highlighted the role of novel aspects of risk stratification that include imaging, such as coronary computed tomography angiography (CCTA), coronary artery calcium (CAC) scoring, as well as polygenic risk scores [2]. These factors have since been used as complementary tools to classic CV risk scores. Yet, despite the ease of implementation, classic risk scores have important limitations. CV disease is multifaceted and complex with many interactions between different internal and external variables, some of which have nonlinear and nonhomogeneous relationships. Including all these in a regression model can be very challenging and impractical. In addition, there are many assumptions with using these regression models that may not be met (e.g., collinearity between variables, homogeneous effect of each variable on the outcome). They are also limited in their generalizability to non-studied populations. Finally, they do not incorporate the additional data that is readily available in electronic health records (EHRs) including imaging results. Recent advances in data storage and computational power have led the way in implementing more sophisticated methods in data processing for healthcare solutions. These automated techniques, which include machine learning (ML), can analyze complex multidimensional data in large datasets, taking into account these heterogeneous nonlinear interactions between variables. Ultimately, this can translate into better predictive performance that can help prognosticate and direct clinical management in a more precise manner than traditional risk scores. In this chapter, we discuss the various applications of machine learning in CV risk stratification (Table 39.1, Figs. 39.1 and 39.2).

A. Malkawi, MD · S. J. Al'Aref, MD (✉)
Division of Cardiology, Department of Medicine, University of Arkansas for Medical Sciences (UAMS), Little Rock, AR, USA
e-mail: sjalaref@UAMS.edu

Z. Almarzooq, MBBCh
Brigham and Women's Hospital Heart and Vascular Center, Boston, MA, USA

M. H. Al-Mallah, MD
Department of Cardiology, Houston Methodist DeBakey Heart & Vascular Center, Houston, TX, USA

Main Domains of Machine Learning Use in Cardiovascular Risk Stratification

Machine Learning Use in Cardiovascular Care

Approaches to Utilizing Electronic Health Record-Based Data

EHRs constitute a rich source of clinical data and variables, from which meaningful information and patterns could be extracted and utilized to perform complex tasks. The majority of clinical data in EHRs is inherently in a non-image format, which makes it challenging to utilize powerful classification algorithms (e.g., neural networks), since these algorithms have been mostly developed for image analysis.

In general, data derived from EHRs can be divided into two types: structured and unstructured. Structured data refers to variables that can be extracted from pre-existing fields within EHRs, such as laboratory values, vital signs, and demographic information. Unstructured data mainly refers

C. N. De Cecco et al. (eds.), *Artificial Intelligence in Cardiothoracic Imaging*, Contemporary Medical Imaging,
https://doi.org/10.1007/978-3-030-92087-6_39

Table 39.1 Key studies evaluating the application of machine learning algorithms in cardiovascular risk prediction

Authors	Date	Data/study type	Population	Data science	Key findings
Byrd et al. [4]	2014	EHR	6355 incident heart failure in primary care clinic	NLP	NLP can help extract Framingham diagnostic criteria for heart failure from unstructured EHR data (precision score 0.925, F-score 0.910)
Mayampurath et al. [8]	2019	EHR	115,825 hospital admissions	CNN	Converting EHR data to two-dimensional visual data and then using conventional DL image classification algorithms can help predict in-hospital mortality (AUC 0.91)
Alaa et al. [10]	2019	EHR	423,604 participants in the UK Biobank	Multiple algorithmic framework (AutoPrognosis)	ML predicted 5-year CVD risk better than Framingham risk score (AUC 0.774). The improved prediction in ML was more driven by information gain than modeling gain
Ambale-Venkatesh et al. [11]	2017	Cohort study	6,184 participants from the MESA cohort	Random forest	ML improved prediction of mortality and CVD events better than Framingham risk score and ASCVD (higher C-index and lower Brier index by 10–25%)
Quesada et al. [12]	2019	Cohort study	38,527 asymptomatic patients with increased CVD risk	Quadratic discriminant analysis	ML had a better 5-year risk prediction of mortality and CVD hospitalizations than the SCORE and REGICORE risk scores (AUC 0.708)
Zhao et al. [13]	2019	EHR, genomic	109,490 patients in a single center (10,162 with genomic data)	Gradient boosting and CNN	ML models incorporating temporal information predicted 10-year CVD risk better than traditional score (AUC 0.782), and adding genomic data when available improved risk prediction over EHR-only data by 2.1%
Hernesniemi et al. [15]	2019	EHR	9077 patients with ACS from a single center	XGBoost	ML predicted 6-month mortality post ACS better than GRACE score (AUC 0.890)
Ahmad et al. [16]	2018	EHR	44,886 patients from the Swedish Heart Failure Registry	Random forest and K-means clustering	Random forest can predict mortality better than LVEF in heart failure patients (C-statistic 0.82) Cluster analysis can help identify groups with differential response to different heart failure therapies (C-statistic 0.67)
Cikes et al. [18]	2018	Cohort study	1106 patients from the MADIT-CRT trial	Dimensionality reduction, K-means clustering	Some phenotypic clusters identified by ML showed a significantly differential response to CRT-D versus ICD (i.e., better response)
Mortazavi et al. [20]	2019	Registry	3,316,465 PCI procedures from NCDR registry	XGBoost	XGBoost algorithm was able to identify patients at risk of major bleed post PCI with a better performance than existing models (C-statistic 0.81)
Raghunath et al. [26]	2020	EHR (ECG)	1,169,662 ECGs from 253,397 patients at a single center	DNN	DNN model was able to predict 1-year mortality using ECG data only with a better performance than traditional risk scores (FRS, CCI) (AUC 0.855)
Myers et al. [27]	2017	ECG data from Holter monitors	4395 NSTEMI patients	ANN	ANN model improved risk prediction for 1-year mortality after NSTEMI when compared to TIMI risk score, by incorporating temporal dynamic changes of ST segments from ECG monitors (AUC 0.743)

(continued)

Kwon et al. [28]	2020	EHR (ECG)	22,875 patients from the KorMI registry	ANN	The deep learning model improved mortality risk prediction after MI when compared to GRACE and TIMI scores (AUC 0.905)
Samad et al. [30]	2019	EHR (TTE)	171,510 patients who underwent 331,317 TTE in a single large regional health system	Random forest	ML could predict 5-year all-cause mortality with a high performance by using a variety of EHR and TTE measurements (AUC 0.893)
Omar et al. [33]	2020	EHR (stress TTE)	455 patients with negative stress TTE	Clustering	Cluster techniques were able to better risk stratify patients with a negative stress echocardiogram
Van Rosendael et al. [45]	2018	CCTA	8844 patients from the CONFIRM registry without prior CVD	XGBoost	ML-based CCTA risk score improved prediction of major outcomes when compared to traditional risk scores (AUC 0.771)
Betancur et al. [65]	2019	MPI-SPECT	1160 patients from the REFINE SPECT registry	DNN	ML model significantly outperformed the standard methods in predicting CAD on both per-patient (AUC of 0.81 vs. 0.78) and per-vessel basis (AUC of 0.77 vs. 0.73); $P < 0.001$ for both
Chen et al. [68]	2019	cMRI	98 patients with dilated cardiomyopathy	Naive Bayes classifier	ML model significantly outperformed both MAGGIC score and LVEF (AUC 0.877 vs. 0.599 vs. 0.504, respectively); $P < 0.01$ for both
Motwani et al. [46]	2017	Registry	10,030 patients from the CONFIRM registry	LogitBoost	ML-based CCTA risk score improved prediction of 5-year all-cause mortality in patients compared to traditional scores (AUC 0.79)
Al'Aref et al. [51]	2020	Registry	13,054 patients from the CONFIRM registry	XGBoost	ML model improved prediction of obstructive CAD on CCTA compared to traditional scores (AUC 0.773)
Dogan et al. [74]	2018	Genomic	1545 patients with CHD from the Framingham heart study	Random forest	ML model improved classification of CHD in a test dataset (sensitivity 0.75, specificity 0.80)

Abbreviations: *ML* machine learning, *EHR* electronic medical records, *NLP* natural language processing, *CNN* convolutional neural network, *DL* deep learning, *AUC* area under the curve, *UK* United Kingdom, *CVD* cardiovascular disease, *MESA* Multi-Ethnic Study of Atherosclerosis, *ASCVD* atherosclerotic cardiovascular disease, *LVEF* left ventricular ejection fraction, *CRT-D* cardiac resynchronization therapy-defibrillator, *ICD* implantable cardioverter defibrillator, *PCI* percutaneous coronary intervention, *ECG* electrocardiogram, *DNN* deep learning neural networks, *FRS* Framingham risk score, *CCI* Charlson Comorbidity Index, *NSTEMI* non-ST elevation MI, *ANN* artificial neural networks, *MI* myocardial infarction, *TTE* transthoracic echocardiography, *CCTA* coronary computed tomography angiography, *MPI-SPECT* myocardial perfusion imaging with single-photon emission computed tomography, *cMRI* cardiac MRI, *CHD* coronary heart disease to medical notes written by healthcare providers, which need some kind of processing to extract meaningful variables that can be used by ML algorithms [3]. Natural language processing (NLP) is a growing field in artificial intelligence (AI) research. It has the potential to extract prognostically meaningful variables from unstructured EHR data. In a study by Byrd et al., NLP was used to extract and label affirmations or denials of Framingham heart failure diagnostic criteria from primary care notes, with a precision of 0.925, a recall of 0.896, and an F-score of 0.910 [4]. Implementing such algorithms could potentially aid in more readily identifying these patients using unstructured data for both clinical and research purposes. In a study by Wang et al., an ML algorithm utilized structured and unstructured EHR data to predict stroke and bleeding risk in atrial fibrillation patients, with a comparable performance to the commonly used risk scores in this context (CHA2DS2-VASc and HAS-BLED scores) [5]. In another example, Daghistani et al. built multiple ML models to predict in-hospital length of stay for cardiac patients based on structured EHR data from admission. Choosing predictor variables for the models was also done using an ML concept called "information gain," a commonly used method to describe the importance "weight" of a specific variable in a prediction model. The best performing model used a random forest algorithm and achieved an AUROC of 0.94 on internal validation [6]. Another study by Sakr et al. demonstrated the potential use of ML models to predict the risk of developing hypertension based on stress test data and other demographic and clinical variables [7]. These are just some of the many examples of how ML can be applied to build powerful decision-making tools that are readily available for clinicians within EHR systems and maximize the utilization of the rich information contained within the exponentially growing EHR data.

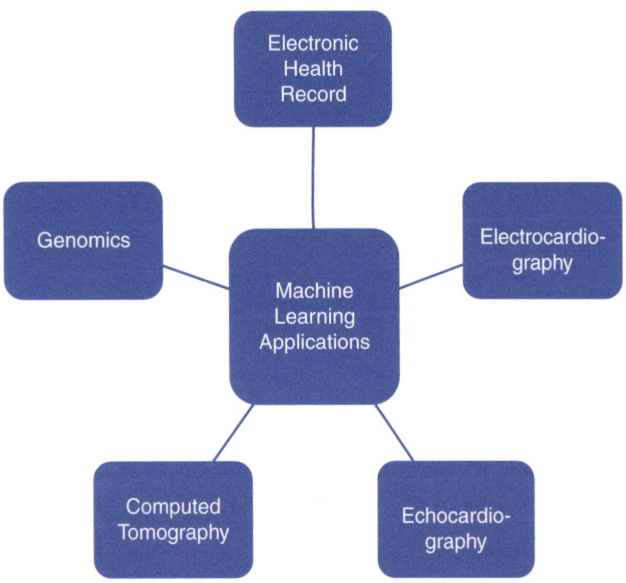

Fig. 39.1 Applications of machine learning within the various cardiovascular domains

Other approaches to using ML for EHR data have been studied. One such method is converting EHR data into an image format that enables the use of ML algorithms that were originally developed for image processing, like convolutional neural networks. Mayampurath et al. created a framework whereby longitudinal structured EHR data was transformed into a two-dimensional visual representation that was then processed as a simple image (Fig. 39.3) [8]. The image created for each patient plotted 156 clinical variables (laboratory tests, vital signs, medications, interventions, diagnostic tests, as well as nursing examinations) on the Y-axis and time (the first 48 hours) on the X-axis. EHR data from 115,825 hospital admissions were converted into their image formats, and the dataset was split into 70% derivation and 30% validation sets, with the outcome of interest being the prediction of in-hospital mortality. The results were promising with the best performing convolutional neural networks achieving an area under the curve (AUC) of 0.91 on the validation set. This outperformed some currently used standard clinical models like the Modified Early Warning Score (MEWS) (AUC of 0.76) and the Sequential Organ Failure Assessment (SOFA) score (AUC of 0.57). Class activation heatmaps were also utilized to highlight areas of the images that were most important in making the prediction, thus providing some insight to clinicians on the factors that contributed to an individual's predicted outcome. This emphasizes an important point about tackling the "black box" issue that is commonly faced when using deep learning (DL) algorithms in clinical practice, which we will discuss later in this chapter [8].

Fig. 39.2 Workflow for the development of machine learning models within the realm of cardiovascular risk assessment

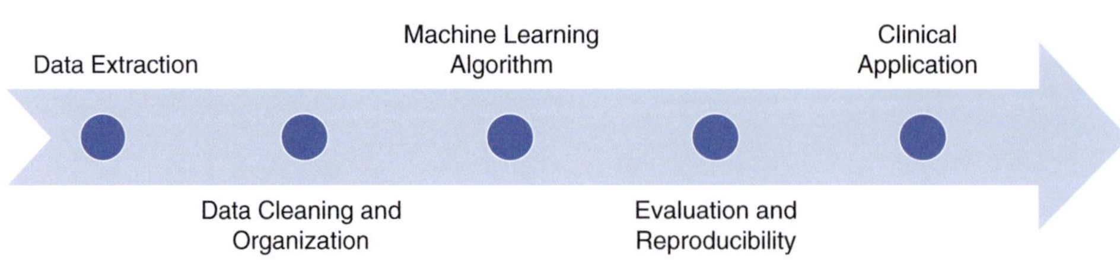

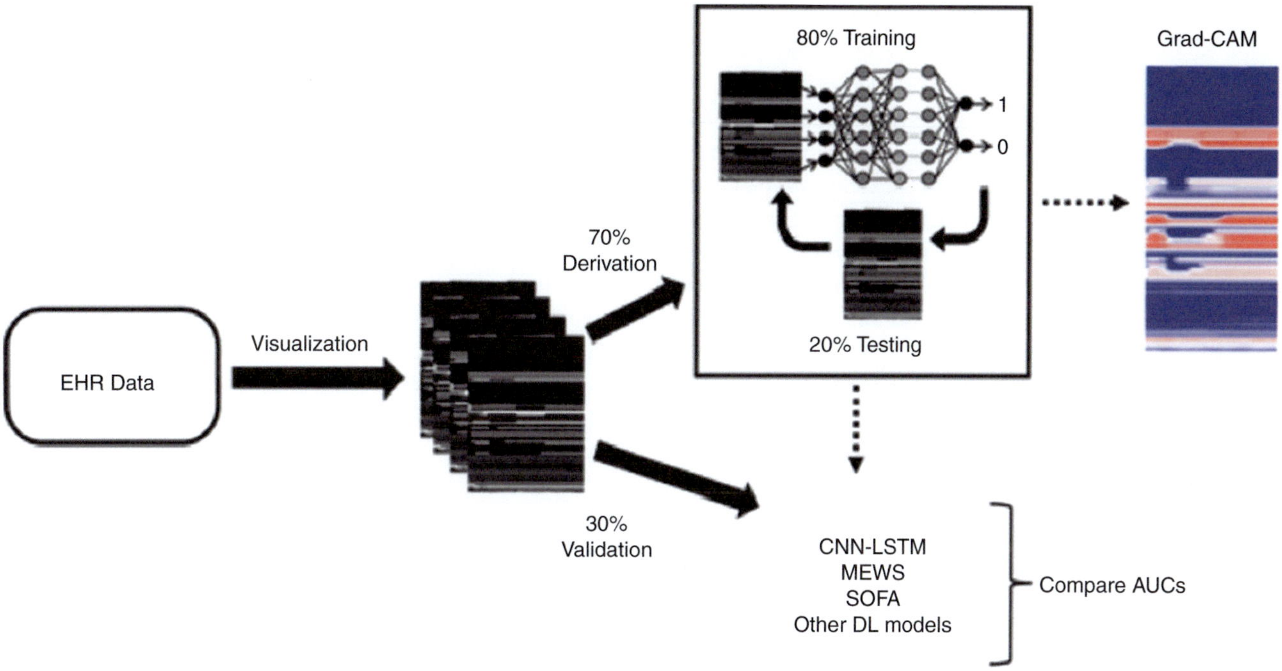

Mayampurath A, Sanchez-Pinto LN, Carey, KA, Venable LR, Churpek M (2019) Combining patient visual timelines with deep learning to predict mortality, PLOS ONE 14(7): e0220640. http://doi.org/10.1371/journal.pone.0220640
https://journals.plos.org/plosone/article?id=10.1371/journal.pone.0220640

Fig. 39.3 Process of visual conversion of EHR data for machine learning application

Primary Coronary Artery Disease Prevention

ML-based risk prediction models will soon be an essential pillar of primary care. Building a unifying cardiovascular risk stratification algorithm that would automatically extract demographic variables and lab results in addition to other available data in the EHR of an individual and process them immediately to come up with an accurate risk assessment score when an individual presents for a preventive visit can help practitioners focus on the appropriate management and risk factor modification strategy in a more precise manner. This approach is commonly referred to as "precision medicine." Such models need to have a balance between predictive performance on one hand and simplicity, applicability, and transparency on the other hand. A lot of the complex ML and DL models can achieve high classification performance but have a "black box" nature that can hinder their application. Weng et al. used a large database from UK family practices, which included 378,526 patients without known CV disease and a 10-year follow-up period. They compared different ML techniques to the traditional ACC/AHA pooled cohort risk equation for CV disease risk prediction. In this study, the various ML models were associated with improved predictive accuracy compared to the established ACC/AHA equation [9].

In another study, Alaa et al. utilized the UK Biobank database, which included 423,604 patients and 473 available variables, to build multiple CV disease risk prediction models using both ML-based and traditional statistical modeling. One of the questions they were trying to answer is whether the predictive performance is more data-driven (information gain) or model-driven (model gain), i.e., whether the amount of variables matters more than the complexity of the model. They built multiple standard ML models and then created a complex ensemble model made out of the standard models by applying an algorithmic framework (AutoPrognosis) that uses a Bayesian optimization technique. They compared these different models against the Framingham risk score for predicting 5-year risk of CV disease events. The AutoPrognosis model that used all 473 variables (AUC 0.774 ± 0.005) outperformed all the other models including the Framingham risk score (AUC 0.724 ± 0.004) and the Cox proportional hazard model that used all variables (AUC 0.758 ± 0.005). In addition, by comparing the different models that used different sets of variables and techniques, they concluded that "information gain" achieved by including more risk factors was significantly higher than "modeling gain" achieved by implementing more complex models. Another important point illustrated in this study was the superior performance of the ML model in patients with diabetes mellitus as opposed to the Framingham risk score (AUC 0.713 ± 0.010 vs. 0.578 ± 0.018; $p < 0.001$). This could be attributed to the "co-linearity" assumed in traditional statistical models that does not take into consideration the nonlinear complex interactions between variables [10].

Few studies are described in the literature where ML-based models are built and trained on cohorts from previous CV disease studies to predict risk. Ambale-Venkatesh et al. built a random forest model to predict mortality and CV disease events. The model was trained using the Multi-Ethnic Study of Atherosclerosis (MESA) cohort of 6184 participants and 735 clinical variables (including imaging). They built a random forest model with all available variables and another random forest model using only the top 20 variables. Both random forest models had a comparable performance and outperformed the Framingham and atherosclerotic cardiovascular disease (ASCVD) risk scores in predictive function (higher C-index and lower Brier index by 10–25%) [11]. In another study, Quesada et al. designed 15 different ML models and trained them on a population derived from the ESCARVAL RISK cohort from Spain to predict 5-year all-cause mortality and cardiovascular-related hospitalizations. The study included 38,527 asymptomatic patients with cardiac risk factors and a follow-up interval of 5 years. For comparison, they used two popular risk scores in Europe: SCORE and REGICORE. The ML models were built using only five variables (age, sex, cholesterol, systolic blood pressure, tobacco use) which are the same variables used in SCORE. For REGICORE, they included these five variables in addition to three additional variables. The ML models significantly outperformed the traditional risk scores. The ML model with the highest predictive function used a quadratic discriminant analysis (AUC 0.708; CI 0.6885–0.7288). The REGICORE (AUC 0.6342; CI 0.6142–0.6542) and SCORE (AUC 0.6333; CI 0.6131–0.6536) scales ranked 11th and 12th in predictive function out of all the models tested. The use of five variables only in the ML models was to prove the concept that more advanced ML methods can help improve discriminatory function and solve higher-dimensional problems by taking into consideration the nonlinear relationships between variables and outcomes and the interactions between variables [12].

The recent advances in data-driven sciences like genomics and radiomics have inspired researchers to utilize the large amount of information contained in different databases (images, genetics, EKG, etc.) in an attempt to increase the accuracy of risk prediction models. Zhao et al. utilized the EHR of Vanderbilt University Medical Center to extract data on 109,490 patients who had follow-up for over 17 years between 2000 and 2016. They divided this period into a 7-year learning "observation" window (2000–2006) during which there was no diagnosis of CV disease. This window was used to train the algorithms to learn the properties of participants before any events. Thereafter, they used a 10-year prediction window (2007–2016) during which 9842 individuals developed CV events. They trained multiple ML models to predict the 10-year CV disease risk in a supervised manner and compared it to the ACC/AHA pooled risk cohort equation as a benchmark. They included different sets of variables in each model, in an attempt to see if the type of variables would have an incremental effect on the performance of a model. When they only used the same variables included in ACC/AHA equation, the ML models (gradient boosting, random forest, logistic regression) achieved a slightly better performance with an AUC of 0.751 for the highest performing ML model (gradient boosting) vs. 0.732 for the ACC/AHA equation. They later added some aggregate values for EHR variables (e.g., blood pressure, lab values) over the 7-year "learning" period, and this improved the ML model performance, with the best model (gradient boosting) achieving an AUC of 0.782. They later incorporated temporal (year-to-year) changes in the EHR variables and added to the comparison a convolutional neural network model. The addition of temporal information further improved the performance of both the gradient boosting and convolutional neural network models. The next experiment was to incorporate the genotype information that was available on a subset of patients (genotyped cohort of 10,162 individuals with 2452 cases and 7710 controls). They used a "two-stage late fusion" approach for this experiment, and this resulted in an improved AUC by 2.1% indicating the potential utility of merging EHR data with other available databases to improve risk prediction [13].

Secondary Coronary Artery Disease Prevention

EHRs could also be turned into a powerful tool for predicting the risk of adverse events after an acute coronary syndrome (ACS) event by applying different ML techniques. Multiple studies have compared the performance of ML models in risk prediction after ACS with the commonly used tools for this purpose like the thrombolysis in myocardial infarction (TIMI) score and the Global Registry of Acute Coronary Events (GRACE) score. Some studies failed to show a significant improvement in prediction compared to these well-validated scores. For example, Shouval et al. built six different ML models to predict 30-day mortality post-STEMI and compared their performance to the TIMI and GRACE scores. They included 2782 patients in the study and utilized structured EHR data to extract 54 predictor variables. The random forest model was the best performing ML model, with an AUC of 0.91 +/− 0.04. This outperformed the TIMI score that had an AUC of 0.82 +/− 0.06 ($p < 0.005$); however, it was not significantly different from GRACE score that had an AUC of 0.87 +/− 0.06 [14]. In a different study, Hernesniemi et al. used a single-center patient cohort from Finland that included 9077 patients with ACS. After a 6-month follow-up, 7.3% of patients had died. Two ML models, using logistic regression and XGBoost, were developed using the cohort. These were compared with the GRACE score for predicting all-cause mortality. Only the XGBoost model outperformed the GRACE score (AUC 0.890 versus 0.822; P-value <0.001), as the logistic regression model did not (AUC 0.867 vs. 0.822; p-value 0.012) [15].

Heart Failure

Significant effort has been spent over the years in order to understand and classify heart failure. Current classification is based on left ventricular ejection fraction (LVEF). However, given the heterogeneity in patients with similar LVEF, this classification can seem too simplistic for such a complex syndrome with a wide range of pathology and outcomes. Using this classification has limited our ability to truly personalize risk assessment and treatment options for patients with various phenotypic manifestations of heart failure. This is an important area of investigation and a gap that ML has been proposed to fill. For example, Ahmad et al. used the Swedish Heart Failure Registry to analyze the records of 44,886 patients. They used 86 clinical variables to train a random forest model to predict 1-year survival after a hospital discharge or an outpatient clinic visit. After ranking variables based on their predictive value, they used the eight strongest predictors and applied an unsupervised ML technique (K-means clustering) to classify the patients into four clusters. To compare the results, patients were also classified into four strata based on LVEF (preserved, mild, moderate, and severe reduction in LVEF). As expected, the random forest model showed a superior discriminatory function to predict 1-year mortality (C-statistic of 0.82 for random forest model versus 0.52 for LVEF). The four clusters created by the unsupervised ML model were able to predict mortality with a C-statistic of 0.67. More importantly, the clusters, which were propensity matched for age, gender, and LVEF, were able to show interactions with some guideline-directed medical therapies (e.g., diuretics, angiotensin-converting enzyme inhibitors, beta-blockers) revealing the significant heterogeneity in response to these medications even after correcting for LVEF [16]. This analysis demonstrates the role that ML can play in risk stratifying heart failure patients and informs clinicians on the utility of guideline-directed medical therapies in a more accurate manner. The phenotypic heterogeneity in patients with heart failure with preserved ejection fraction (HFpEF) is far more than that of patients with heart failure with reduced ejection fraction (HFrEF). This has been deemed one of the key reasons behind the generally disappointing results of clinical trials trying to find effective therapy in HFpEF. Cluster analysis is an unsupervised ML technique that has the ability to find naturally occurring invisible subclasses within data. This technique has the potential to improve our understanding of syndromes like HFpEF, where a better diagnostic detection and classification of patients into more homogeneous groups can help improve risk stratification and prediction of response to treatment. Shah et al. applied cluster analysis on 397 patients with HFpEF using a large set of variables including clinical, laboratory, ECG, echocardiographic, and hemodynamic data. Cluster analysis was blinded to clinical outcomes and managed to classify patients into three distinct phenotypes with significant differences in clinical characteristics and outcomes. Cox regression analysis demonstrated differential outcomes in heart failure mortality and hospitalizations even after adjustment for common risk predictors (e.g., B-type natriuretic peptide [BNP] and the Meta-Analysis Global Group in Chronic Heart Failure [MAGGIC] risk score). For example, group 3 had an increased risk of heart failure hospitalization compared to group 1 after adjustment for traditional risk factors (adjusted HR 4.2 [95% CI 2.0–9.1]) [17]. Cikes et al. also demonstrated the potential applications of unsupervised machine learning in detecting the heterogeneity of therapy response of heart failure patients. In this example, they specifically attempted to identify patient groups with a beneficial response to cardiac resynchronization therapy (CRT). They included 1106 patients from the MADIT-CRT trial that compared CRT-defibrillator (CRT-D) to implantable cardioverter defibrillator (ICD) only. The initial input data included 1682 variables, encompassing 50 clinical and ECG parameters, in addition to 1632 echocardiographic variables on LV volume and strain traces. In order to make it possible to find the clinically relevant patterns given the large number of variables per patient, they applied dimensionality reduction technique using multiple kernel learning algorithms. Dimensionality reduction simply transforms high-dimensional data into lower-dimensional more compact data while retaining the meaningful properties that are relevant for classification, which can potentially provide a new insight on the pathophysiological factors and the clinical predictors that affect response to therapy and general outcomes. After reducing dimensionality, they applied another unsupervised technique using a K-means algorithm to divide patients into four clinically relevant clusters. Regression analysis was then applied on each cluster to compare the effect of therapy (CRT-D vs. ICD) on the primary endpoint (all-cause mortality or heart failure event). Two of the four clusters showed a significantly better response to CRT-D compared to ICD (hazard ratio (HR) 0.35, $p = 0.0005$, and HR 0.36, $p = 0.0001$), while the other two groups did not have a significant difference between CRT-D and ICD ($p = 0.77$ and $p = 0.344$, respectively) [18]. Feeny et al. implemented a similar approach (dimensionality reduction followed by K-means clustering) on a database of 12-lead ECG for a group of CRT patients (n = 946). The unsupervised ML technique was again able to identify two natural clusters within the dataset (based on subtle 12-lead QRS characteristics) that had differential outcomes in terms of mortality and LVEF improvement, even among patients with left bundle branch block and QRS >150 ms, which could potentially enhance the selection criteria for CRT patients in the future beyond the traditional electrocardiogram (ECG) criteria [19].

Procedure Risk Prediction

ML-based risk prediction models can also utilize EHR-derived variables to predict risk from procedures. Mortazavi et al. built a model using XGBoost to predict major bleeding events post percutaneous coronary intervention (PCI) using data from the National Cardiovascular Data Registry (NCDR). The XGBoost model outperformed the existing logistic regression-based NCDR model in predicting major bleeding events post PCI while using the same ten variables, with a C-statistic of 0.81 (95% CI 0.80–0.81) for XGBoost versus 0.77 (95% CI 0.77–0.77) for the logistic regression-based model [20]. Similarly, Huang et al. evaluated an ML model using XGBoost to predict acute kidney injury post PCI. This model also outperformed the existing NCDR acute kidney injury model [21].

Machine Learning and Electrocardiography

ECG is a low-cost readily available diagnostic test that is widely available and constitutes an essential part of work-up for a spectrum of cardiovascular conditions. Despite its widespread use, ECG assessment has not been found to be useful for risk stratification, especially in asymptomatic individuals [22, 23]. As a result, recent ML research has focused on leveraging ECG data for prognostication of outcomes. ECG-based risk prediction models have mostly been based on conventional ML techniques like logistic regression and Bayesian classification rather than neural networks because of the latter's complexity [24, 25]. In addition, conventional models can provide insight into the importance of included features and their influence on the pre-specified outcome by comparing the weights of these features, while the black box nature of neural networks can deem them less desirable when the goal is to stratify patients into different risk groups. However, neural networks are still powerful tools that can perform sophisticated functions and detect subtle patterns in multidimensional complex datasets, which ultimately translates into a high performance in outcome prediction. They also do not typically require the feature selection step that is usually required by conventional ML techniques. Neural networks also have the advantage of exploiting aspects of complex data that cannot be approached by conventional techniques. In a recent study, Raghunath et al. evaluated the use of neural networks in resting ECG to predict 1-year mortality. They trained a deep neural network algorithm on a single-center ECG database, which included 1,169,662 ECGs from 253,397 patients, to learn the spatial and temporal features of the voltage-time signals in a standard 12-lead ECG to predict mortality. The model was then tested on a separate holdout test set of 168,914 patients with 14,207 events, where a single random ECG was chosen for each patient. The deep neural network achieved an AUC of 0.855 for predicting 1-year all-cause mortality when using ECG signals alone and 0.876 when age and sex were added as additional input variables. To compare the deep neural network performance to conventional ML techniques, they trained an XGBoost model on the same dataset using ECG variables (40 clinical ECG features including both numerical measurements and diagnostic patterns). The AUC of the XGBoost model with ECG measures was 0.817, which improved to 0.860 with the addition of age and sex. This was comparable to the deep neural network performance. Both models significantly outperformed traditional risk scores that were used for comparison, namely, Framingham risk score (AUC of 0.648) and the Charlson Comorbidity Index (AUC of 0.816) [26].

Neural networks have the advantage of incorporating temporal ECG patterns on continuous monitors (e.g., temporal evolution of ST changes), while conventional ML methods are usually limited to simple summary statistics of these ECG features that might lead to potential loss of valuable information contained within these patterns. Myers et al. used a non-ST elevation MI (NSTEMI) cohort of 4395 patients to evaluate an artificial neural network model that integrated temporal data of ST segment features from Holter monitors and combined it with a logistic regression model based on demographic and historical data. They trained the artificial neural network model to predict 1-year cardiovascular mortality. The model outperformed the TIMI-NSTE ACS risk score (AUC 0.743 versus 0.670; $p < 0.001$) and was able to retain its predictive power in subgroups of patients who were misclassified as low-moderate risk based on TIMI-NSTE ACS risk score. For instance, only 20% of the patients in that cohort were classified as high risk by the TIMI-NSTE ACS risk score, while 54% of deaths occurred in patients classified as low-moderate risk [27]. In another study, Kwon et al. built a DL model utilizing ECG and EHR variables to stratify mortality risk in patients presenting with an acute myocardial infarction (AMI). They utilized the Korean MI registry, KorMI, of 22,875 patients from 59 hospitals presenting with AMI. The dataset was split into two: training (12,152 patients) and validation (10,723 patients) based on the hospitals rather than individuals to avoid "overlearning" of specific hospital characteristics. The model was built using readily available variables from an initial presentation (demographic information, initial laboratory values, initial vitals, and the presence of ST segment elevation). The outcomes were in-hospital and 12-month mortality. They also built traditional ML models, using random forest and logistic regression, for comparison. The validation group was separated into ST elevation MI (STEMI) and NSTEMI groups since both TIMI and GRACE risk scores have different formulas based on the presence of ST elevation. In both the STEMI and NSTEMI validation groups, the DL model outperformed all other models with an AUC of 0.905 and 0.870, respectively [28].

Machine Learning and Echocardiography

Echocardiography is a simple, low-cost, noninvasive procedure that has always been an essential part of cardiovascular evaluation [29]. Despite the multiple technological advances in this field (e.g., speckle tracking, 3D echocardiography, semiautomated analysis), it remains largely operator dependent. For these reasons, ML algorithms have been developed to improve the diagnostic capabilities and reproducibility of echocardiography. The applications of ML in echocardiography for risk stratification are an area of great interest. Samad et al. suggested the use of echocardiography to predict all cause mortality. They utilized a large database of 171,510 patients who underwent 331,317 echocardiograms in a large regional health system. They trained multiple ML models to predict mortality at different points of time (from 6 months to 60 months). One hundred and fifty-eight predictor variables were used in the models, 100 of which are EHR variables, in addition to 58 non-redundant echocardiographic measurements including LVEF. The best performing ML model was the random forest model with an AUC of 0.893 (0.892–0.895) for predicting 5-year all-cause mortality, while the AUC for Framingham risk score was 0.62, 0.74 for the ACC/AHA guideline score, and 0.79 for the Charlson Comorbidity Index. The logistic regression model also achieved a better AUC than traditional scores of 0.864 (0.862–0.866) but was inferior to the nonlinear random forest. On variable rank importance analysis, they found that the top 10 variables were needed to achieve 95.5% of the maximum predicted accuracy, with six of the ten being echocardiographic variables. Interestingly, the tricuspid regurgitation jet maximum velocity ranked higher than LVEF in importance in predicting mortality [30]. In another study, Kwon et al. suggested predicting in-hospital mortality in cardiac patients utilizing echocardiographic reports. They evaluated 25,776 patients hospitalized with coronary heart disease (CHD) and/or HF, all of which underwent echocardiography during hospitalization. There were 1026 deaths in the cohort. The predictor variables included 54 categorical and 11 continuous variables that were solely extracted from echocardiographic reports. However, they also included non-echocardiographic data that are usually part of the report, such as age and biometric information (weight, height, heart rate). A DL model was built using the derivation data and was tested on an external validation set of 604 patients with CHD. This model significantly outperformed the GRACE and TIMI risk scores (AUC 0.958 [95% CI 0.950–0.987] vs. 0.881 [95% CI 0.794–0.942] vs. 0.806 [95% CI 0.715–0.886], respectively), with the caveat that the cohort was not predominantly an ACS cohort. The DL model was also tested on another external validation set of 760 patients with heart failure and also outperformed traditional risk scores such as the MAGGIC and Get With The Guidelines (GWTG) heart failure risk scores (AUC of 0.913 [95% CI 0.872–0.947] vs. 0.806 [95% CI 0.756–0.852] vs. 0.783 [95% CI 0.716–0.848], respectively) [31].

Stress echocardiography is a valuable tool that has been well established for risk stratification of coronary artery disease. However, like any other test, it can misclassify patients [32]. Patients with a negative exercise stress echocardiography are generally considered low risk; however, such an aggregate measure does not reflect patient-to-patient risk as some are still prone to developing short- and/or long-term cardiovascular events. Clustering, an unsupervised ML method that can detect invisible heterogeneity within data, has been proposed to further improve risk stratification and CV event prediction in conventionally classified low-risk patients. Omar et al. studied a group of 455 patients who had a negative stress echocardiography. They used clinical and stress test variables to build a cluster model that stratified patients into low-, intermediate-, and high-risk categories, with significant differences in outcomes between the clusters in major adverse cardiovascular events (all-cause mortality, MI, stroke) and hospitalizations [33]. As mentioned earlier in the Heart Failure section, clustering techniques have been applied on echocardiographic data in stress echocardiography to better detect HFpEF, utilizing the ability of ML techniques to analyze the large amount of spatiotemporal data contained in stress echocardiography [34, 35].

Machine Learning and Computed Tomography

Noninvasive imaging has played a central role in patient care since its inception. For example, CCTA is now recognized by numerous societies as the first-line imaging modality in the work-up of patients suspected of having coronary artery disease (CAD) [36, 37]. This has been driven by recent large trials demonstrating the diagnostic and prognostic utility of CCTA within the CV realm, with emphasis on the PROMISE and SCOT-HEART trials [38, 39]. This has naturally led to an exponential increase in CCTA utilization in clinical practice, combined with the rapid developments in data storage technologies, which has facilitated the creation of large CCTA datasets and registries [40]. These datasets comprise a perfect substrate for the rapidly developing ML and DL algorithms that can perform complex computational tasks to analyze hidden patterns and features on a radiomic level [41]. Multiple CCTA-based risk scores have been developed to better estimate risk, akin to traditional CAD classification (e.g., CAD-RADS) [42, 43]. Such scores incorporate plaque features, most commonly as a measure of diameter stenosis, which get incorporated into traditional regression models that assume linearity between patient-level characteristics and CAD extent. However, CV outcomes often depend on a complex interaction between anatomy, physiology, and other patient vulnerability [44]. Therefore, ML algorithms have been proposed to account for this complexity. Van Rosendael et al. proposed a CCTA risk score by utilizing a nonlinear ML algorithm that would maximize the information gain from commonly used CCTA variables. They included 8844 patients from the CONFIRM registry without prior CAD who later died or had an MI (609 events) during a ~5-year follow-up period. They built an XGBoost model incorporating 35 CCTA-only variables (encompassing measures of stenosis severity and plaque composition) to predict the composite outcome of death or nonfatal MI. The variables were selected using the XGBoost feature selection with no prior assumptions on causative factors. The model was evaluated in a test set ($N = 1769$) that showed improved performance compared to traditional CCTA scores (AUC 0.771 versus AUC ranging between 0.685 and 0.701 for the Duke prognostic index, the CCTA Leaman score, the segment stenosis score, the segment involvement score, and the traditional CAD classification; P-value <0.001 for ML model compared with all) [45]. Motwani et al. evaluated the use of ML to predict 5-year all-cause mortality in patients with suspected CAD who underwent CCTA. They used an ensemble method (LogitBoost) to build a model using 19 clinical and 35 CCTA variables derived from 10,030 patients from the CONFIRM registry. There were 745 deaths during the 5-year follow-up. The ML model had improved performance compared to clinical or CCTA parameters alone for prediction of 5-year all-cause mortality (AUC 0.79 for ML model versus 0.61 for Framingham risk score versus 0.64 for segment stenosis score versus 0.64 for segment involvement score versus 0.62 for modified Duke index; $P < 0.001$ for all) [46]. Another important ML application demonstrated in this study was the automated feature selection using the "information gain attribute ranking" method. Out of the initial 66 clinical and CCTA variables extracted from patients, 54 variables were selected by this method. This is a distinguishing feature of ML from traditional prognostic methods, since it makes no assumptions about causative factors and allows an unbiased exploration of all available data rather than the traditional hypothesis-driven methods for risk prediction. This helps avoid overlooking important but unexpected predictor variables or interactions, as well as enabling the identification of clinically important risk among patients with several marginal risk factors [46].

With the expanding use of CCTA in clinical practice, a significant number of patients undergoing CCTA end up having minimal or no CAD [47]. This has led to a growing interest in determining the pretest likelihood of having CAD in order to minimize unnecessary testing. Multiple risk scores have been proposed for this purpose, such as the updated Diamond Forrester and the CAD consortium risk score [48–50]. Al'Aref et al. proposed an ML-based risk scoring system for this purpose using a tree-based ensemble algorithm (XGBoost) utilizing clinical and demographic variables (e.g., age, sex, high-density lipoprotein level, diabetes status, etc.) for a binary classification task: the presence or absence of obstructive CAD (defined as the detection of > = 50% coronary stenosis on CCTA). They compared the ML model against the CAD consortium and updated Diamond Forrester risk scores. They included 13,054 patients from the CONFIRM registry. The ML model outperformed these risk scores (AUC 0.773 for ML model versus 0.734 for CAD consortium score versus 0.682 for updated Diamond Forrester score; P-value <0.05 for all comparisons). They also added coronary artery calcium score to both the ML model and CAD consortium score, with significant improvement in the discriminative function for both (AUC 0.881, 95% CI 0.869–0.895, for ML model and 0.866, 95% CI 0.852–0.879, for CAD consortium score) [51].

Another use of ML has involved the discrimination between stable and rapid plaque progression, which has been found to correlate with a higher risk of future cardiovascular events [52, 53]. Han et al. used a cohort of 1038 patients from the PARADIGM registry who underwent serial CCTAs and extracted multiple qualitative and quantitative plaque measurements using conventional methods for CCTA interpretation. Again, feature selection was done using information gain attribute ranking and model building using LogitBoost technique; the best performing model was the one using clinical and lab data, in addition to qualitative and quantitative plaque features. The AUROC was 0.83 for prediction of rapid plaque progression (defined as annual progression of percent atheroma volume > 1.0%). Due to the lack of conventional models for prediction of rapid plaque progression, they used the ASCVD risk score (AUC of 0.60) and Duke CAD risk scores (AUC of 0.74) as benchmark. They also built a logistic regression model using the same selected features which showed a performance comparable to that of the LogitBoost model, highlighting the benefit of advanced feature selection approaches in identifying new disease risk factors that were not previously elucidated [54].

Physiologic testing during invasive angiography such as fractional flow reserve (FFR) has been shown to improve outcomes by guiding revascularization strategies for lesion-specific ischemia [55]. Noninvasive functional measures during anatomical evaluation, such as CT-derived FFR (FFR_{CT}), have been evaluated in DISCOVER-FLOW, DEFACTO, and NXT (among other trials) [56–58]. FFR_{CT} utilizes computational fluid dynamics, which is computationally expensive and time-consuming. However, newer ML algorithms have been used to make CT-based FFR estimation simpler and more available. Itu et al. evaluated a DL neural network algorithm for CT-FFR calculation. The algorithm was trained by creating 12,000 synthetic 3D coronary models of various anatomies. It was then validated against computational fluid dynamics using invasive FFR as a reference standard. The DL algorithm significantly reduced average execution time by a factor of 80 leading to near real-time assessment of FFR while maintaining a very comparable performance [59, 60]. In another study, Dey et al. proposed an ML-based risk score to predict the presence of lesion-specific ischemia by utilizing CCTA-derived quantitative variables combined with demographic variables. They included 254 patients from the NXT trial, 80 of which had lesion-specific ischemia by invasive FFR among a total of 100 vessels. The variables included were selected using the "information gain attribute ranking" method, and then a LogitBoost algorithm was used to predict the presence of lesion-specific ischemia (as defined by invasive FFR <0.80). The model had improved performance compared to individual CCTA quantitative measures, LD-NCP volume, total plaque volume, and pretest likelihood of CAD (AUC 0.84 vs. 0.76 vs. 0.77 vs. 0.74 vs. 0.63, respectively; p-value <0.006) [61]. In a more recent study, Kwan et al. proposed another ML-based risk score for lesion-specific ischemia based on CCTA quantitative variables to predict the need for revascularization. They conducted a post hoc analysis on a prospective cohort of 352 patients with 1052 analyzable vessels who underwent CCTA followed by coronary angiography within 3 months. The primary outcome, revascularization, occurred in 26% of the vessels. The ML risk score ranged between 0 and 81% and was significantly higher in vessels that received revascularization (33.6% (21.1–55.0) vs. 13.0% (4.5–29.1), $p < 0.0001$) [62].

Lastly, Shah et al. proposed using non-cardiac CT to better stratify patients based on their risk of death. They included 2924 patients from the Framingham Heart Study who underwent chest and abdomen CT scans. The median follow-up for all-cause mortality was 9.6 years. They extracted CT-derived variables quantifying valvular and vascular calcification, adiposity, and liver and muscular fat attenuation. They then utilized unsupervised ML techniques to cluster patients into two phenotypically different clusters. These were also found to be prognostically significant on Cox regression analysis. After adjusting for Framingham 10-year risk of CHD, CAC score, and visceral fat, the unfavorable cluster had a HR of 2.61 (95% CI 1.74–3.92, $P < 00.001$) for all-cause mortality compared to the favorable one [63].

Machine Learning and Nuclear Medicine

Myocardial perfusion imaging with single-photon emission computed tomography (MPI-SPECT) is a well-established tool in the diagnosis and prognostication of cardiovascular diseases. ML techniques can further enhance the prognostic value of this tool by maximizing the utilization of data collected within these studies. Alonso et al. built multiple ML models to predict cardiovascular death utilizing a wide range of variables (122 variables) including MPI-SPECT, ECG, and clinical variables. They utilized a dataset of 8321 patients who underwent MPI-SPECT with adenosine stress ± walking stress, of which 551 had a cardiac death event during the follow-up period of 3.15 ± 1.99 years. For comparison, they built a baseline LR model utilizing 14 predictor variables (AUC of 0.76 for predicting CV death). All the ML models significantly outperformed the baseline LR model in predicting CV death, with the highest performing algorithm being a linear SVM with sequential forward selection procedure, which achieved an AUC of 0.83 (49 features, $p < 0.0001$) [64]. In a different study, Betancur et al. built a model using deep convolutional neural networks to predict obstructive CAD by using polar maps of SPECT-MPI. They included 1160 patients from the REFINE SPECT registry who underwent upright and supine SPECT-MPI from 4 different centers and underwent subsequent invasive coronary angiography within 6 months, with 718 patients (62%) found to have obstructive CAD (defined as >70% diameter stenosis in any of the 3 major coronary vessels or > 50% in the left main artery, without the use of FFR). Four DL models were trained on three centers and externally validated on a fourth center left aside each time, and then the performance of these four models was merged for comparison with standard methods. The model's performance was assessed on a per-vessel and per-patient level. The standard methods used for comparison were combined stress total perfusion defect (cTPD) and clinical reads by experts. The DL model significantly outperformed the cTPD in predicting CAD on both per-patient (AUC of 0.81 vs. 0.78) and per-vessel basis (AUC of 0.77 vs. 0.73) with $P < 0.001$ for both. When the model's specificity threshold was matched to the specificity of a normal clinical read, the DL had a sensitivity comparable to that of an on-site clinical read (84.8% vs. 82.6%, $P = 0.3$). Furthermore, the model execution time was <1 s, which could provide a powerful real-time risk assessment tool in the clinical setting for appropriate decision-making [65]. The same group also proposed using ML to predict early vessel revascularization within 90 days after a rest/stress SPECT/MPI, by utilizing clinical, stress, and imaging variables for outcome prediction. Their model achieved an AUC of 0.81 with 95% CI of 0.79–0.83 for predicting early vessel revascularization on a per-patient level and an AUC of 0.79 with 95% CI of 0.77–0.80 for "per-vessel" risk prediction, which significantly outperformed automated MPI quantification by TPD (stress TPD, combined-view TPD, and ischemic TPD), all having $P < 0.001$ [66].

Machine Learning and Cardiac MRI

Cardiac MRI (cMRI) provides invaluable information on cardiac structure and function, which could ultimately be translated into better risk stratification. ML research has focused on automated data extraction and quantification from cMRI; examples include extracellular volume quantification, myocardial strain quantification, myocardial scar mapping, and intracardiac blood flow hemodynamic measurements. Few studies so far have attempted to directly apply ML techniques on cMRI data for risk prediction [67]. Chen et al. studied 98 dilated cardiomyopathy patients who underwent cMRI. Clinical and demographic variables were extracted in addition to cMRI data, and information gain ranking method was used to choose the highest ranking features that were strong predictors of the outcome (18 variables). They trained a naive Bayes classifier to predict the primary endpoint of any cardiovascular event, including cardiac death, hospitalization, or cardiac transplant. All of the included patients had an LVEF <35 and no significant coronary artery disease at baseline, and over a median follow-up period of 18 months, 22 patients developed the primary endpoint. MAGGIC score and LVEF were used as benchmark models. The ML model achieved an AUC of 0.877, which significantly outperformed both MAGGIC score (AUC of 0.599) and LVEF (AUC of 0.504), with $P < 0.01$ for both [68]. Dawes et al. demonstrated another example of how ML can be used to improve risk prediction in the context of cMRI. They evaluated the potential role of three-dimensional cardiac motion pattern data derived from cMRI in improving survival prediction in pulmonary hypertension patients. They included 256 patients with newly diagnosed pulmonary hypertension who had cMRI available at the time of diagnosis, with a median follow-up of 4 years. To extract cardiac motion data from CMRIs, semiautomated segmentation was applied on short-axis cine cMR images, followed by construction of 3D models for the motion patterns of the endocardial surface of the right ventricle and septum during systole. In order to summarize this large amount of complex input data, a supervised principal component analysis approach was used to identify the patterns "markers" that were most strongly associated with survival. In addition, they extracted basic demographic variables, RV volumetric measurements from cine images, hemodynamic data from right heart catheterization, and functional data from the 6-minute walk test. The authors reported that adding 3D cardiac motion data to other clinical and hemodynamic variables resulted in improved survival risk prediction (AUC improved from 0.60 to 0.73, $P < 0.001$) and greater differentiation in median survival time difference between high- and low-risk groups (13.8 years vs. 10.7 years, $P < 0.001$) [69].

Application on Genomics and Other "-omics" for Cardiac Risk Stratification

Data-driven sciences like genomics and other "-omics" operate by discovering properties and patterns from large-scale databases rather than testing preconceived models and hypotheses [70]. As with other risk models in medicine, logistic regression has been the most commonly used method for analysis of microarray data, disease classification, and polygenic risk scoring [71, 72]. Recent advances in data storage and availability along with computational capacity have made it possible to develop and utilize more sophisticated ML techniques like neural networks that have the ability to detect high-dimensional features and nonlinear relationships which are not usually detected by traditional regression techniques. Deep learning has successfully been deployed in multiple areas of genomic research [73]. Single nucleotide polymorphisms (SNPs) have been one of the main targets in genomic research where complex ML techniques can improve individualized disease risk prediction and precision medicine [71]. Many recent studies have focused on utilizing ML and genomics to build cardiovascular risk prediction models. Dogan et al. proposed using ML to predict the risk of developing symptomatic CHD in patients who are previously asymptomatic using integrated genetic-epigenetic data. They used a cohort of 1545 patients with CHD from the Framingham Heart Study. Genome-wide array chips were used to obtain epigenetic (DNA methylation loci) and genetic (SNP) profiles for the cohort. The initial large number of variables (403,192 SNPs and 472,822 DNA methylation (CpG) loci) had to be reduced using multiple techniques in order to fit into ML models. After multiple technical steps for variable reduction, four CpG loci, two SNPs along with age, and gender were retained for prediction and were used to train eight random forest models. An ensemble of the eight models was then built and predicted symptomatic CHD with an accuracy, sensitivity, and specificity of 78%, 0.75, and 0.80, respectively. To compare the performance of genetic-epigenetic variables with the commonly used CHD predictors, they trained a similar random forest-based ensemble model using common CHD risk factors as predictor variables, namely, age, gender, systolic blood pressure, hemoglobin A1c, total cholesterol, self-reported smoking, and high-density lipoprotein, with an accuracy, sensitivity, and specificity of 0.65, 0.42, and 0.89, respectively (in the test set). Despite the multiple limitations and the lack of generalizability in this study, it demonstrates some important lessons. For example, there are a large number of possible combinations of SNPs, methylation loci, and phenotype variables that could be used in future studies to build more powerful predictive models. In addition, further analyses of the methylation signatures could potentially map these signatures to known CV risk factors and medication use, which in turn could be useful in guiding therapeutic interventions, management of risk factors, and monitoring the efficacy of treatment and lifestyle modification [74].

Oguz et al. suggested the use of ML techniques on SNPs to predict advanced CAC score (calculated by the Agatson method), which is an established surrogate marker for major adverse cardiovascular outcomes. They identified a set of 30 SNPs that correlated with advanced CAC score (defined as 89th–99th percentile in the derivation and replication cohorts), and trained different RF models to binarily classify patients into advanced and non-advanced CAC score based on clinical and SNP variables. The random forest models that used the 30 SNPs as predictor variables achieved an AUC of 0.80–0.85 in the testing set, while the random forest model that used only clinical variables achieved an AUC of 0.61 [75].

Biomarkers have always been an essential part of cardiovascular risk stratification. The search for biomarkers that could reliably predict future CV events and improve risk stratification to help direct interventions is a continuously growing field. The advent of big data is shifting this search from a single biomarker approach to proteome-wide testing with the goal of identifying biomarker patterns and signatures that could predict CV disease with a high accuracy. ML models are naturally an essential part of this search process, given their ability to recognize patterns and classify data in higher dimensions. Urinary proteomic analysis has been previously explored and showed the potential to predict CAD and improve risk prediction [76, 77]. Htun et al. used a support vector machine (SVM) classifier, an ML algorithm commonly used to classify data in high-dimensional data space. They analyzed the urinary proteome of 84 patients who later developed ACS in a 5-year follow-up period. This was compared with proteomic data of another 84 matched controls. They identified a set of urinary biomarkers with specific patterns related to ACS and incorporated that into a predictive model to predict 5-year ACS events. The model achieved a reasonable discriminatory function (C-statistic of 0.644) which was similar to that of Framingham risk score when applied on a separate testing set of 42 cases and 42 controls. This demonstrates the potential of such noninvasive approaches to improve risk prediction when used alone or in combination with other traditional methods [78].

Current Use and Limitations of ML

One of the most commonly described limitations of ML implementation in clinical practice is the "black box" problem, which results from the mathematical complexity of some algorithms hindering the ability to interpret the factors behind the final outcome [79]. As seen in the many examples in this chapter, the performance of prediction models is usually assessed by prediction accuracy, with less emphasis on model interpretability. The typical algorithms that have a black box nature are DL algorithms (neural networks), in addition to some nonlinear complex techniques like random forest, SVM, and k-NN. "Black box" can be particularly problematic when building a risk prediction model, since knowing the factors behind an increased risk is important for targeting therapy and modifying the treatment plan. For instance, it would be hard for a clinician to justify extensive testing or surveillance in a seemingly healthy person if the algorithm classified them as a "high risk" with no clear insight of the factors leading to that classification. The interest in ML interpretability is rapidly growing, with multiple techniques and algorithms being developed for this purpose. Examples of such techniques include saliency maps used in neural networks, feature importance, LIME interpretability technique, MofN algorithm, and FERNN algorithm. Elshawi et al. demonstrated the utility of such techniques in understanding the logic behind a complex model. They applied different interpretability algorithms on a random forest model previously developed by the same group to predict hypertension. The authors suggested that such techniques can help improve our understanding of the risk factors for multifactorial diseases such as hypertension in this example [80].

Another important challenge when building an ML risk prediction model is choosing the training dataset. Regardless of the complexity of the algorithm being used, the quality and the quantity of the raw data being fed into the model are detrimental to the model's performance and generalizability. For example, ML algorithms can sometimes learn subtle patterns in data and assume their clinical relevance for risk prediction, while these patterns could simply be present due to systematic errors in data collection or biased datasets. Another example is the variations in CT acquisition parameters (slice thickness, scanner type, tube voltage, and pitch), which can affect the validity of a "radiomic marker" detected by an algorithm on one dataset when applied to external data [81]. ML algorithms can also function poorly in smaller datasets where validated traditional risk scores, based on simpler regression algorithms, maintain their integrity. For example, Dimopoulos et al. built three different ML models (DT, random forest, and k-NN) and trained them to predict 10-year CV risk using a small database (n = 2020 patients) from the Greek ATTICA study. They compared these ML models with a validated risk score (HellenicSCORE) which is a modified model of the ESC SCORE based on prevalence of CV risk factors in Greece and is commonly used in practice there. The ML models performed very comparably to the HellenicSCORE but were more computationally demanding. The k-NN model had the poorest performance due to overfitting [82].

In addition, there is the ethical component of the story, with the need for more adaptive ethical regulations for ML use in healthcare [83]. For instance, when training an algorithm using an ethnically homogeneous dataset to predict risk, it can lead to underestimation or overestimation biases when applied on patients of different ethnicities. This was demonstrated by Gijsberts et al. when they used data from Framingham Risk Study which was based mostly on white population; to predict the risk in non-white patients, they used simple linear regression models and found significant biases in risk prediction associated with ethnicities (both overestimation and underestimation) [84]. This can be even more challenging when using "black box" algorithms when there is no clear insight of whether such factors play a role in risk prediction. Furthermore, the legal regulations need to adapt with the rapidly changing way of utilizing AI in healthcare from simple diagnostic tasks to more complex decision-making tools. The US FDA considers diagnostic software tools as Class 2 (medium-risk) devices. However, with the growing application in risk prediction and automating treatment, this might need a revision of classification into Class 3 (high-risk) devices [41].

Conclusion

ML research in cardiovascular care, as in other fields of medicine, is generally moving from simple diagnostic tasks to more complex decision-making tasks. This is mainly facilitated by the exponential growth in datasets due to improved data extraction and storage technologies, along with the rapid improvements in computational power. This chapter highlights the growing application of ML and DL for improved cardiovascular risk assessment, within the context of the ever-expanding clinical, imaging, and genomic data.

Disclosures S.J.A. is supported by NIH 2R01 HL127661–05 and receives royalty fees from Elsevier. All other authors have reported that they have no conflicts relevant to the contents of this paper to disclose.

References

1. Arnett DK, Blumenthal RS, Albert MA, Buroker AB, Goldberger ZD, Hahn EJ, et al. 2019 ACC/AHA guideline on the primary prevention of cardiovascular disease: A report of the american college of cardiology/american heart association task force on clinical practice guidelines. J Am Coll Cardiol. 2019;74(10):e177–232.
2. Aragam KG, Natarajan P. Polygenic scores to assess atherosclerotic cardiovascular disease risk: clinical perspectives and basic implications. Circ Res. 2020;126(9):1159–77.
3. Schlesinger DE, Stultz CM. Deep learning for cardiovascular risk stratification. Curr Treat Options Cardiovasc Med. 2020;22(8):15.
4. Byrd RJ, Steinhubl SR, Sun J, Ebadollahi S, Stewart WF. Automatic identification of heart failure diagnostic criteria, using text analysis of clinical notes from electronic health records. Int J Med Inform. 2014;83(12):983–92.
5. Wang SV, Rogers JR, Jin Y, Bates DW, Fischer MA. Use of electronic healthcare records to identify complex patients with atrial fibrillation for targeted intervention. J Am Med Inform Assoc. 2017;24(2):339–44.
6. Daghistani TA, Elshawi R, Sakr S, Ahmed AM, Al-Thwayee A, Al-Mallah MH. Predictors of in-hospital length of stay among cardiac patients: A machine learning approach. Int J Cardiol. 2019;288:140–7.
7. Sakr S, Elshawi R, Ahmed A, Qureshi WT, Brawner C, Keteyian S, et al. Using machine learning on cardiorespiratory fitness data for predicting hypertension: The Henry Ford ExercIse Testing (FIT) Project. PLoS One. 2018;13(4):e0195344.
8. Mayampurath A, Sanchez-Pinto LN, Carey KA, Venable L-R, Churpek M. Combining patient visual timelines with deep learning to predict mortality. PLoS One. 2019;14(7):e0220640.
9. Weng SF, Reps J, Kai J, Garibaldi JM, Qureshi N. Can machine-learning improve cardiovascular risk prediction using routine clinical data? PLoS One. 2017;12(4):e0174944.
10. Alaa AM, Bolton T, Di Angelantonio E, Rudd JHF, van der Schaar M. Cardiovascular disease risk prediction using automated machine learning: A prospective study of 423,604 UK Biobank participants. PLoS One. 2019;14(5):e0213653.
11. Ambale-Venkatesh B, Yang X, Wu CO, Liu K, Hundley WG, McClelland R, et al. Cardiovascular event prediction by machine learning: the multi-ethnic study of atherosclerosis. Circ Res. 2017;121(9):1092–101.
12. Quesada JA, Lopez-Pineda A, Gil-Guillén VF, Durazo-Arvizu R, Orozco-Beltrán D, López-Domenech A, et al. Machine learning to predict cardiovascular risk. Int J Clin Pract. 2019;73(10):e13389.
13. Zhao J, Feng Q, Wu P, Lupu RA, Wilke RA, Wells QS, et al. Learning from longitudinal data in electronic health record and genetic data to improve cardiovascular event prediction. Sci Rep. 2019;9(1):717.
14. Shouval R, Hadanny A, Shlomo N, Iakobishvili Z, Unger R, Zahger D, et al. Machine learning for prediction of 30-day mortality after ST elevation myocardial infraction: An Acute Coronary Syndrome Israeli Survey data mining study. Int J Cardiol. 2017;246:7–13.

15. Hernesniemi JA, Mahdiani S, Tynkkynen JA, Lyytikäinen L-P, Mishra PP, Lehtimäki T, et al. Extensive phenotype data and machine learning in prediction of mortality in acute coronary syndrome - the MADDEC study. Ann Med. 2019;51(2):156–63.
16. Ahmad T, Lund LH, Rao P, Ghosh R, Warier P, Vaccaro B, et al. Machine learning methods improve prognostication, identify clinically distinct phenotypes, and detect heterogeneity in response to therapy in a large cohort of heart failure patients. J Am Heart Assoc. 2018;7(8):e008081.
17. Shah SJ, Katz DH, Selvaraj S, Burke MA, Yancy CW, Gheorghiade M, et al. Phenomapping for novel classification of heart failure with preserved ejection fraction. Circulation. 2015;131(3):269–79.
18. Cikes M, Sanchez-Martinez S, Claggett B, Duchateau N, Piella G, Butakoff C, et al. Machine learning-based phenogrouping in heart failure to identify responders to cardiac resynchronization therapy. Eur J Heart Fail. 2019;21(1):74–85.
19. Feeny AK, Rickard J, Trulock KM, Patel D, Toro S, Moennich LA, et al. Machine learning of 12-Lead QRS waveforms to identify cardiac resynchronization therapy patients with differential outcomes. Circ Arrhythm Electrophysiol. 2020;13(7):e008210.
20. Mortazavi BJ, Bucholz EM, Desai NR, Huang C, Curtis JP, Masoudi FA, et al. Comparison of machine learning methods with national cardiovascular data registry models for prediction of risk of bleeding after percutaneous coronary intervention. JAMA Netw Open. 2019;2(7):e196835.
21. Huang C, Murugiah K, Mahajan S, Li S-X, Dhruva SS, Haimovich JS, et al. Enhancing the prediction of acute kidney injury risk after percutaneous coronary intervention using machine learning techniques: A retrospective cohort study. PLoS Med. 2018;15(11):e1002703.
22. Lanza GA. The electrocardiogram as a prognostic tool for predicting major cardiac events. Prog Cardiovasc Dis. 2007;50(2):87–111.
23. US Preventive Services Task Force, Curry SJ, Krist AH, Owens DK, Barry MJ, Caughey AB, et al. Screening for cardiovascular disease risk with electrocardiography: US preventive services task force recommendation statement. JAMA. 2018;319(22):2308–14.
24. Bigi R, Gregori D, Cortigiani L, Desideri A, Chiarotto FA, Toffolo GM. Artificial neural networks and robust Bayesian classifiers for risk stratification following uncomplicated myocardial infarction. Int J Cardiol. 2005;101(3):481–7.
25. Harrison RF, Kennedy RL. Artificial neural network models for prediction of acute coronary syndromes using clinical data from the time of presentation. Ann Emerg Med. 2005;46(5):431–9.
26. Raghunath S, Ulloa Cerna AE, Jing L, vanMaanen DP, Stough J, Hartzel DN, et al. Prediction of mortality from 12-lead electrocardiogram voltage data using a deep neural network. Nat Med. 2020;26(6):886–91.
27. Myers PD, Scirica BM, Stultz CM. Machine learning improves risk stratification after acute coronary syndrome. Sci Rep. 2017;7(1):12692.
28. Kwon J-M, Jeon K-H, Kim HM, Kim MJ, Lim S, Kim K-H, et al. Deep-learning-based risk stratification for mortality of patients with acute myocardial infarction. PLoS One. 2019;14(10):e0224502.
29. Mitchell C, Rahko PS, Blauwet LA, Canaday B, Finstuen JA, Foster MC, et al. Guidelines for performing a comprehensive transthoracic echocardiographic examination in adults: recommendations from the American society of echocardiography. J Am Soc Echocardiogr. 2019;32(1):1–64.
30. Samad MD, Ulloa A, Wehner GJ, Jing L, Hartzel D, Good CW, et al. Predicting survival from large echocardiography and electronic health record datasets: optimization with machine learning. JACC Cardiovasc Imaging. 2019;12(4):681–9.
31. Kwon J-M, Kim K-H, Jeon K-H, Park J. Deep learning for predicting in-hospital mortality among heart disease patients based on echocardiography. Echocardiography. 2019;36(2):213–8.
32. Sicari R, Cortigiani L. The clinical use of stress echocardiography in ischemic heart disease. Cardiovasc Ultrasound. 2017;15(1):7.
33. Omar AMS, Ramirez R, Haddadin F, Sabharwal B, Khandaker M, Patel Y, et al. Unsupervised clustering for phenotypic stratification of clinical, demographic, and stress attributes of cardiac risk in patients with nonischemic exercise stress echocardiography. Echocardiography. 2020;37(4):505–19.
34. Sanchez-Martinez S, Duchateau N, Erdei T, Kunszt G, Aakhus S, Degiovanni A, et al. Machine learning analysis of left ventricular function to characterize heart failure with preserved ejection fraction. Circ Cardiovasc Imaging. 2018;11(4):e007138.
35. Tabassian M, Sunderji I, Erdei T, Sanchez-Martinez S, Degiovanni A, Marino P, et al. Diagnosis of heart failure with preserved ejection fraction: machine learning of spatiotemporal variations in left ventricular deformation. J Am Soc Echocardiogr. 2018;31(12):1272–1284.e9.
36. Smeeth L, Skinner JS, Ashcroft J, Hemingway H, Timmis A, Chest Pain Guideline Development Group. NICE clinical guideline: chest pain of recent onset. Br J Gen Pract. 2010;60(577):607–10.
37. Knuuti J, Wijns W, Saraste A, Capodanno D, Barbato E, Funck-Brentano C, et al. 2019 ESC Guidelines for the diagnosis and management of chronic coronary syndromes. Eur Heart J. 2020;41(3):407–77.
38. Douglas PS, Hoffmann U, Patel MR, Mark DB, Al-Khalidi HR, Cavanaugh B, et al. Outcomes of anatomical versus functional testing for coronary artery disease. N Engl J Med. 2015;372(14):1291–300.
39. SCOT-HEART investigators. CT coronary angiography in patients with suspected angina due to coronary heart disease (SCOT-HEART): an open-label, parallel-group, multicentre trial. Lancet. 2015;385(9985):2383–91.
40. Min JK, Dunning A, Lin FY, Achenbach S, Al-Mallah MH, Berman DS, et al. Rationale and design of the CONFIRM (Coronary CT Angiography Evaluation For Clinical Outcomes: An International Multicenter) Registry. J Cardiovasc Comput Tomogr. 2011;5(2):84–92.
41. Oikonomou EK, Siddique M, Antoniades C. Artificial intelligence in medical imaging: A radiomic guide to precision phenotyping of cardiovascular disease. Cardiovasc Res. 2020;116(13):2040–54.
42. Cury RC, Abbara S, Achenbach S, Agatston A, Berman DS, Budoff MJ, et al. CAD-RADS(TM) Coronary Artery Disease - Reporting and Data System. An expert consensus document of the Society of Cardiovascular Computed Tomography (SCCT), the American College of Radiology (ACR) and the North American Society for Cardiovascular Imaging (NASCI). Endorsed by the American College of Cardiology. J Cardiovasc Comput Tomogr. 2016 Aug;10(4):269–81.
43. Xie JX, Cury RC, Leipsic J, Crim MT, Berman DS, Gransar H, et al. The Coronary Artery Disease-Reporting and Data System (CAD-RADS): prognostic and clinical implications associated with standardized coronary computed tomography angiography reporting. JACC Cardiovasc Imaging. 2018;11(1):78–89.
44. Ahmadi A, Stone GW, Leipsic J, Shaw LJ, Villines TC, Kern MJ, et al. Prognostic determinants of coronary atherosclerosis in stable ischemic heart disease: anatomy, physiology, or morphology? Circ Res. 2016;119(2):317–29.
45. van Rosendael AR, Maliakal G, Kolli KK, Beecy A, Al'Aref SJ, Dwivedi A, et al. Maximization of the usage of coronary CTA derived plaque information using a machine learning based algorithm to improve risk stratification; insights from the CONFIRM registry. J Cardiovasc Comput Tomogr. 2018;12(3):204–9.
46. Motwani M, Dey D, Berman DS, Germano G, Achenbach S, Al-Mallah MH, et al. Machine learning for prediction of all-cause mortality in patients with suspected coronary artery disease: a 5-year multicentre prospective registry analysis. Eur Heart J. 2017;38(7):500–7.

47. Meinel FG, Schoepf UJ, Townsend JC, Flowers BA, Geyer LL, Ebersberger U, et al. Diagnostic yield and accuracy of coronary CT angiography after abnormal nuclear myocardial perfusion imaging. Sci Rep. 2018;8(1):9228.
48. Bittencourt MS, Hulten E, Polonsky TS, Hoffman U, Nasir K, Abbara S, et al. European society of cardiology-recommended coronary artery disease consortium pretest probability scores more accurately predict obstructive coronary disease and cardiovascular events than the diamond and forrester score: the partners registry. Circulation. 2016;134(3):201–11.
49. Genders TSS, Steyerberg EW, Hunink MGM, Nieman K, Galema TW, Mollet NR, et al. Prediction model to estimate presence of coronary artery disease: retrospective pooled analysis of existing cohorts. BMJ. 2012;344:e3485.
50. Genders TSS, Steyerberg EW, Alkadhi H, Leschka S, Desbiolles L, Nieman K, et al. A clinical prediction rule for the diagnosis of coronary artery disease: validation, updating, and extension. Eur Heart J. 2011;32(11):1316–30.
51. Al'Aref SJ, Maliakal G, Singh G, van Rosendael AR, Ma X, Xu Z, et al. Machine learning of clinical variables and coronary artery calcium scoring for the prediction of obstructive coronary artery disease on coronary computed tomography angiography: analysis from the CONFIRM registry. Eur Heart J. 2020;41(3):359–67.
52. Ahmadi A, Leipsic J, Blankstein R, Taylor C, Hecht H, Stone GW, et al. Do plaques rapidly progress prior to myocardial infarction? The interplay between plaque vulnerability and progression. Circ Res. 2015;117(1):99–104.
53. Yokoya K, Takatsu H, Suzuki T, Hosokawa H, Ojio S, Matsubara T, et al. Process of progression of coronary artery lesions from mild or moderate stenosis to moderate or severe stenosis: A study based on four serial coronary arteriograms per year. Circulation. 1999;100(9):903–9.
54. Han D, Kolli KK, Al'Aref SJ, Baskaran L, van Rosendael AR, Gransar H, et al. Machine learning framework to identify individuals at risk of rapid progression of coronary atherosclerosis: from the PARADIGM registry. J Am Heart Assoc. 2020;9(5):e013958.
55. Pijls NHJ, Fearon WF, Tonino PAL, Siebert U, Ikeno F, Bornschein B, et al. Fractional flow reserve versus angiography for guiding percutaneous coronary intervention in patients with multivessel coronary artery disease: 2-year follow-up of the FAME (Fractional Flow Reserve Versus Angiography for Multivessel Evaluation) study. J Am Coll Cardiol. 2010;56(3):177–84.
56. Koo B-K, Erglis A, Doh J-H, Daniels DV, Jegere S, Kim H-S, et al. Diagnosis of ischemia-causing coronary stenoses by noninvasive fractional flow reserve computed from coronary computed tomographic angiograms. Results from the prospective multicenter DISCOVER-FLOW (Diagnosis of Ischemia-Causing Stenoses Obtained Via Noninvasive Fractional Flow Reserve) study. J Am Coll Cardiol. 2011;58(19):1989–97.
57. Nakazato R, Park H-B, Berman DS, Gransar H, Koo B-K, Erglis A, et al. Noninvasive fractional flow reserve derived from computed tomography angiography for coronary lesions of intermediate stenosis severity: results from the DeFACTO study. Circ Cardiovasc Imaging. 2013;6(6):881–9.
58. Nørgaard BL, Leipsic J, Gaur S, Seneviratne S, Ko BS, Ito H, et al. Diagnostic performance of noninvasive fractional flow reserve derived from coronary computed tomography angiography in suspected coronary artery disease: the NXT trial (Analysis of Coronary Blood Flow Using CT Angiography: Next Steps). J Am Coll Cardiol. 2014;63(12):1145–55.
59. Itu L, Rapaka S, Passerini T, Georgescu B, Schwemmer C, Schoebinger M, et al. A machine-learning approach for computation of fractional flow reserve from coronary computed tomography. J Appl Physiol. 2016;121(1):42–52.
60. Tesche C, De Cecco CN, Baumann S, Renker M, McLaurin TW, Duguay TM, et al. Coronary CT angiography-derived fractional flow reserve: machine learning algorithm versus computational fluid dynamics modeling. Radiology. 2018;288(1):64–72.
61. Dey D, Gaur S, Ovrehus KA, Slomka PJ, Betancur J, Goeller M, et al. Integrated prediction of lesion-specific ischaemia from quantitative coronary CT angiography using machine learning: a multicentre study. Eur Radiol. 2018;28(6):2655–64.
62. Kwan AC, McElhinney PA, Tamarappoo BK, Cadet S, Hurtado C, Miller RJH, et al. Prediction of revascularization by coronary CT angiography using a machine learning ischemia risk score. Eur Radiol. 2020;
63. Shah RV, Yeri AS, Murthy VL, Massaro JM, D'Agostino R, Freedman JE, et al. Association of multiorgan computed tomographic phenomap with adverse cardiovascular health outcomes: the framingham heart study. JAMA Cardiol. 2017;2(11):1236–46.
64. Haro Alonso D, Wernick MN, Yang Y, Germano G, Berman DS, Slomka P. Prediction of cardiac death after adenosine myocardial perfusion SPECT based on machine learning. J Nucl Cardiol. 2019;26(5):1746–54.
65. Betancur J, Hu L-H, Commandeur F, Sharir T, Einstein AJ, Fish MB, et al. Deep learning analysis of upright-supine high-efficiency SPECT myocardial perfusion imaging for prediction of obstructive coronary artery disease: a multicenter study. J Nucl Med. 2019;60(5):664–70.
66. Hu L-H, Betancur J, Sharir T, Einstein AJ, Bokhari S, Fish MB, et al. Machine learning predicts per-vessel early coronary revascularization after fast myocardial perfusion SPECT: results from multicentre REFINE SPECT registry. Eur Heart J Cardiovasc Imaging. 2020;21(5):549–59.
67. Tao Q, Lelieveldt BPF, van der Geest RJ. Deep learning for quantitative cardiac MRI. AJR Am J Roentgenol. 2020;214(3):529–35.
68. Chen R, Lu A, Wang J, Ma X, Zhao L, Wu W, et al. Using machine learning to predict one-year cardiovascular events in patients with severe dilated cardiomyopathy. Eur J Radiol. 2019;117:178–83.
69. Dawes TJW, de Marvao A, Shi W, Fletcher T, Watson GMJ, Wharton J, et al. Machine learning of three-dimensional right ventricular motion enables outcome prediction in pulmonary hypertension: a cardiac MR imaging study. Radiology. 2017;283(2):381–90.
70. Brown PO, Botstein D. Exploring the new world of the genome with DNA microarrays. Nat Genet. 1999;21(1 Suppl):33–7.
71. Ho DSW, Schierding W, Wake M, Saffery R, O'Sullivan J. Machine learning SNP based prediction for precision medicine. Front Genet. 2019;10:267.
72. Liao JG, Chin K-V. Logistic regression for disease classification using microarray data: model selection in a large p and small n case. Bioinformatics. 2007;23(15):1945–51.
73. Eraslan G, Avsec Ž, Gagneur J, Theis FJ. Deep learning: new computational modelling techniques for genomics. Nat Rev Genet. 2019;20(7):389–403.
74. Dogan MV, Grumbach IM, Michaelson JJ, Philibert RA. Integrated genetic and epigenetic prediction of coronary heart disease in the Framingham Heart Study. PLoS One. 2018;13(1):e0190549.
75. Oguz C, Sen SK, Davis AR, Fu Y-P, O'Donnell CJ, Gibbons GH. Genotype-driven identification of a molecular network predictive of advanced coronary calcium in ClinSeq® and Framingham Heart Study cohorts. BMC Syst Biol. 2017;11(1):99.
76. Brown CE, McCarthy NS, Hughes AD, Sever P, Stalmach A, Mullen W, et al. Urinary proteomic biomarkers to predict cardiovascular events. Proteomics Clin Appl. 2015;9(5–6):610–7.
77. Delles C, Schiffer E, von Zur MC, Peter K, Rossing P, Parving H-H, et al. Urinary proteomic diagnosis of coronary artery disease: identification and clinical validation in 623 individuals. J Hypertens. 2010;28(11):2316–22.

78. Htun NM, Magliano DJ, Zhang Z-Y, Lyons J, Petit T, Nkuipou-Kenfack E, et al. Prediction of acute coronary syndromes by urinary proteome analysis. PLoS One. 2017;12(3):e0172036.
79. Castelvecchi D. Can we open the black box of AI? Nature. 2016;538(7623):20–3.
80. Elshawi R, Al-Mallah MH, Sakr S. On the interpretability of machine learning-based model for predicting hypertension. BMC Med Inform Decis Mak. 2019;19(1):146.
81. Berenguer R, Pastor-Juan MDR, Canales-Vázquez J, Castro-García M, Villas MV, Mansilla Legorburo F, et al. Radiomics of CT features may be nonreproducible and redundant: influence of CT acquisition parameters. Radiology. 2018;288(2):407–15.
82. Dimopoulos AC, Nikolaidou M, Caballero FF, Engchuan W, Sanchez-Niubo A, Arndt H, et al. Machine learning methodologies versus cardiovascular risk scores, in predicting disease risk. BMC Med Res Methodol. 2018;18(1):179.
83. Char DS, Shah NH, Magnus D. Implementing machine learning in health care - addressing ethical challenges. N Engl J Med. 2018;378(11):981–3.
84. Gijsberts CM, Groenewegen KA, Hoefer IE, Eijkemans MJC, Asselbergs FW, Anderson TJ, et al. Race/ethnic differences in the associations of the framingham risk factors with carotid IMT and cardiovascular events. PLoS One. 2015;10(7):e0132321.

Part IV

Artificial Intelligence: Thoracic Applications

Artificial Intelligence-Based Evaluation of Patients with Chronic Obstructive Pulmonary Disease (COPD)

40

Josua A. Decker, Tilman Emrich, U. Joseph Schoepf, Dhiraj Baruah, Jeremy R. Burt, and Akos Varga-Szemes

Epidemiology

Chronic obstructive pulmonary disease (COPD) is the third leading cause of death due to noncommunicable diseases worldwide and resulted in 3.2 million deaths in 2017 [1–3]. The worldwide prevalence is estimated to be 2.3% [4] and is higher in Western countries such as the United States with 6.3% [5]. With 81.6 million disability-adjusted life years worldwide, COPD ranks sixth for all diseases [1]. It is accompanied by a high socioeconomic burden resulting in increasing yearly projected health expenses in the United States from $32.1 billion in 2010 to $49 billion in 2020 [6, 7]. For a long time, COPD was considered a disease of men, but with changes in social factors, this pattern of distribution also changed over the last decade and is now affecting men and women in a similar fashion, and in some countries, women even show higher prevalence and mortality than men [8–10]. Patients with COPD are at increased risk for squamous cell lung carcinoma and other comorbidities such as type 2 diabetes mellitus and at increased risk for overall mortality [11–14].

Pathophysiology and Clinical Aspects

COPD is a chronic, progressive, airway-narrowing lung disease that limits the ability to adequately exhale and may be complicated by episodes of acute worsening. It is characterized by lung function impairment and more specifically a limitation of airflow due to disease of the airways, pulmonary emphysema, or a combination of both. The "syndrome" COPD comprises different clinical entities that ultimately lead to an irreversible destruction of lung parenchyma with consecutive overinflation and remodeling of airway walls, leading to increased airway resistance [15, 16]. More specifically, the entities chronic bronchitis, chronic respiratory failure, and pulmonary emphysema are under the umbrella of COPD [17]. Dyspnea, cough, and sputum production represent classical symptoms of COPD and may show intermittent periods of acute exacerbations. The disease itself is incurable and gradually progressive over time, which is why the treatment focuses on maintaining quality of life and reduction of breathlessness [17, 18]. As the pathological changes progress over many years, COPD is considered a disease of the elderly, which leads to an underdiagnosis in patients younger than 50 years of age, in which therapeutic steps like smoking cessation can have a much more significant impact on progression of the disease [10, 19, 20].

J. A. Decker, MD
Division of Cardiovascular Imaging, Department of Radiology and Radiological Science, Medical University of South Carolina, Charleston, SC, USA

Department of Diagnostic and Interventional Radiology, University Hospital Augsburg, Augsburg, Germany
e-mail: Josua.decker@uk-augsburg.de

T. Emrich, MD
Division of Cardiovascular Imaging, Department of Radiology and Radiological Science, Medical University of South Carolina, Charleston, SC, USA

Department of Diagnostic and Interventional Radiology, University Medical Center of the Johannes Gutenberg University Mainz, Mainz, Germany

German Centre for Cardiovascular Research (DZHK), Partner Site Rhine-Main, Mainz, Germany
e-mail: emrich@musc.edu

U. J. Schoepf, MD · A. Varga-Szemes, MD, PhD (✉)
Division of Cardiovascular Imaging, Department of Radiology and Radiological Science, Medical University of South Carolina, Charleston, SC, USA
e-mail: schoepf@musc.edu; vargaasz@musc.edu

D. Baruah, MD · J. R. Burt, MD
Division of Cardiovascular Imaging, Department of Radiology and Radiological Science, Medical University of South Carolina, Charleston, SC, USA

Division of Thoracic Imaging, Department of Radiology and Radiological Science, Medical University of South Carolina, Charleston, SC, USA
e-mail: baruah@musc.edu; burtje@musc.edu

C. N. De Cecco et al. (eds.), *Artificial Intelligence in Cardiothoracic Imaging*, Contemporary Medical Imaging,
https://doi.org/10.1007/978-3-030-92087-6_40

Known risk factors for COPD are lung exposure to inhaled noxious agents such as tobacco smoke or air pollution or exposure to biomass fuel [21, 22]. It has to be noted that an estimated 24% of patients with COPD in the United States have no history of smoking [23–25]. The pathological mechanisms behind the consecutive pulmonary changes are likely related to a chronic inflammatory response to inhaled noxious particles that leads to remodeling and destruction of the affected tissue [26].

Diagnosis

The diagnosis of COPD is made on the basis of clinical symptoms and is traditionally supported by spirometry, which represents the most reproducible and objective measurement of airflow limitation [18, 27]. During spirometry, the volume of the first second of forced expiration (FEV1) and the full forced vital capacity (FVC) at maximum inspiration are measured. A FEV1/FVC ratio, also called the Tiffeneau index (TI), of less than 0.7 indicates the presence of an obstructive lung disease, and the diagnosis of COPD can be made. Using the classification of the Global Initiative for Chronic Obstructive Lung Disease (GOLD), the disease is categorized into four grades (grades A–D). These grades have formerly been differentiated only by FEV1 with percentages of ≥80, 50–79, 30–49, and < 30 for GOLD A to D, respectively. Following multiple recommendations, GOLD has recently updated the ABCD assessment tool in which the evaluation of clinical criteria, such as exacerbations, is also considered, rather than solely spirometry measurements [18, 28]. With these recent changes, other diagnostic methods, such as computed tomography (CT), are gaining influence in the diagnosis and evaluation of COPD patients.

Computed Tomography (CT) in COPD

Current guidelines consider CT as an additional diagnostic modality to rule out concomitant lung diseases including bronchiectasis, lung cancer, or interstitial lung abnormalities [18, 28, 29]. However, with advancements in CT technology over the last two decades, the target-oriented use of CT in COPD patients has provided a variety of new applications for diagnosis, risk assessment, and quantitative evaluation. For example, Coxson et al. found that a decline in lung density is related to smoking and gender, and it is also associated with pulmonary blood parameters such as surfactant protein D (SP-D) or soluble receptor for advanced glycation end product (sRAGE) [30]. Furthermore, Wells et al. showed that enlargement of the pulmonary artery is associated with severe exacerbations of COPD [31]. Many other studies that will be described in more detail below report additional significant correlations between CT findings and clinical parameters. Experts are now suggesting inclusion of chest CT in the diagnostic workflow of COPD [10].

Application of CT is especially useful in structural, qualitative, and quantitative assessment of emphysema, which is defined as an irreversible overinflation of the alveolar airspace with accompanying alveolar wall destruction [32, 33]. While spirometry only allows for the evaluation of global lung function, CT can visualize small structural changes and the anatomical distribution pattern of emphysema [32]. COPD patients within the same GOLD stage may show differing CT morphological patterns [34]. Some patients may present predominantly with emphysema, which can be further divided into paraseptal, panlobular, and centrilobular emphysema, whereas others may present with a more airway-predominant type [33, 35]. The visual differentiation between those types, known as phenotyping, has been shown to correlate with different clinical findings and outcomes [34]. For example, patients with emphysema-predominant disease may have more severe dyspnea and lower body mass index (BMI) [36, 37], whereas patients with predominant airway involvement may show more frequent exacerbations and chronic chough [38, 39].

To diagnose emphysema on CT, the radiologist traditionally looks for abnormal lung parenchyma with lower attenuation in comparison to adjacent normal lung parenchyma. These changes are then subjectively interpreted with regard to extent and emphysema pattern. However, this approach has limitations in detecting minor changes and monitoring follow-up, especially if different radiologists interpret the results. The quantitative assessment of emphysema and the evaluation of morphologic changes can help in characterizing COPD patients which may lead to better individualized treatment.

Quantitative CT (QCT) Based on Lung Densitometry

Using attenuation of the lung parenchyma, measured in Hounsfield units (HU), the extent of emphysema can be assessed quantitatively providing a comparable result that is less susceptible to interobserver variability than subjective interpretation. As emphysema is defined as overinflation, the proportion of air is increased in the affected parts of the lung parenchyma. Thresholds of low-attenuating parenchyma with −910 HU and − 950 HU have been established and histopathologically validated to identify mild and severe emphysematous changes of the lung tissue [40–43]. Such changes can be quantified by the volume or percentage of pathological parenchyma in relation to the total lung parenchyma by performing quantitative CT (QCT) analysis. QCT using lung densitometry provides objective measurements and comparable results as advantages over qualitative emphysema assessment [44–46]. To analyze the proportion of emphysema in the lungs, first, anatomical segmentation of the whole lung parenchyma is performed in three-dimensional CT datasets. Second, subsequent segmentation and quantitative analysis of the low-attenuating parenchyma are performed, mostly by using the thresholds mentioned above. In the past, this process was done manually; however, the availability of different novel AI-assisted software methods has the potential to facilitate certain parts of this process, such as image preparation/normalization or segmentation, using region-growing algorithms and/or measurements. Currently, many open-source software tools, including ITK-SNAP (www.itksnap.org) or 3D Slicer (www.slicer.org), and also multiple vendor-specific commercial solutions are available for CT segmentation and quantitative analysis.

QCT based on lung densitometry may help in early detection of spirometrically silent COPD cases. Previous research has shown that a substantial proportion of smokers without abnormalities in spirometry show changes in CT, potentially leading to an underestimation of the disease and a delay in adequate treatment [47, 48]. Especially in emphysema cases with apical predominance, spirometry results may show inappropriately low TI that may lead to misinterpretation of the results [49]. As early diagnosis of COPD with resulting adequate treatment has a significant impact on the prognostic course of the disease [50] and emphysema extent shows strong correlation with survival [51], the role of CT imaging in suspected cases might be even more impactful.

The Role of AI in QCT of COPD Patients

In contrast to manual segmentation or the use of fixed thresholds over the whole lung volume, different AI-assisted semi-automatic approaches have been developed including edge-based segmentation, region-based techniques, or region-growing algorithms that may assist in preparation of the parenchyma that is to be examined [52]. Quantification of the pathological parenchyma can then be used to describe the current state of disease such as the overall extent of emphysema. However, using greater cohorts in COPD research, further AI-assisted methods can be applied to evaluate CT findings with regard to clinical parameters, e.g., spirometric results, episodes of exacerbation, or mortality. At this stage, machine learning algorithms come into play, as methods such as regression, random forest, support vector machine, k-means, or k-nearest neighbor can be used to build models that may predict a clinical parameter using the information assessed in QCT. These methods have been extended even further in the use of radiomics, which represents a comprehensive use of the imaging data (data mining) where a wide variety of imaging parameters are used to build models that may predict clinical parameters or outcome [53, 54]. A more detailed description about the technical aspects of radiomics is presented in Part I, Chap. 9.

AI-Assisted Evaluation of CT in COPD Patients

Using quantification methods in CT, many research teams have addressed the significance of densitometric lung parenchymal changes in patients with COPD. Schroeder et al. showed that the percentage of low-attenuating lung volume (LAV) in QCT correlates with FEV1 and TI in spirometry [55]. Akira et al. described that percentages of LAV differ significantly between GOLD stages with notable higher percentages in higher GOLD stages [56]. There are also a large number of studies showing that findings in CT densitometry positively correlate with stages of COPD and mortality [57–60]. Adding to this, Sorensen et al. provided machine learning-assisted assessments of CT densitometry and a comparison to lung texture analysis to evaluate emphysema patterns in COPD patients. This additional texture-based information achieved superior results compared with a densitometric approach [61–63].

Machine Learning Approaches in the Evaluation of COPD

With even more integration of AI, machine learning approaches in the evaluation of COPD patients have been performed in different ways. A texture-based framework (similar to radiomics) was performed by Ginsburg et al. and could discriminate among normal lung tissue, centrilobular nodularity, and centrilobular emphysema [64]. An exploratory radiomics-based approach by Lafata et al. showed potential to assess changes in lung function with routine CT imaging [65]. Castaldi et al. trained an algorithm for detection of different emphysema patterns (mild, moderate, and severe centrilobular emphysema and pleural-based and panlobular emphysema) that could differentiate between GOLD stages and provide information toward clinical measures [66]. Also addressing different emphysema patterns, Binder et al. trained an unsupervised framework that showed associations between emphysema subtypes and clinical parameters [67]. Using manifold learning, Zulueta-Coarasa et al. classified emphysema types showing good agreement with visual assessment [68]. A different approach of emphysema classification by using a multi-scale deep convolutional neural network has been performed by Peng and colleagues, which showed a 92.7% accuracy to radiologists' annotations [69]. Westcott et al. used a quadratic support vector machine to train a model that could generate ventilation maps by using CT textures and their correlation to hyperpolarized helium 3 MRI ventilation maps [70].

Limitations of AI-Assisted QCT

To measure LAV in lung densitometry, first a segmentation of the whole lung parenchyma has to be performed. Over the last few years, different software were developed to aid in segmentation, but manual input or control is still needed in many cases. Studies mentioned in the paragraph above used different methods including manual segmentation, HU-based segmentation, region-growing algorithms, or neural networks to assess the lung volume. Most of the time, manual input in the form of corrections was required when using these methods. These steps can make quantitative evaluation a tedious and time-consuming process that is almost exclusively used in research studies without practical application in everyday clinical practice [71]. In spite of many technical advantages as well as commercially available software solutions, lung densitometry does not represent a "stand-alone" procedure and should only be performed after traditional visual analysis [45]. AI-assisted quantitative CT methods also require strict adherence to uniform acquisition parameters in addition to manual input, which are subject to increased inter-patient and interobserver variability [72]. Also, the previously mentioned studies that used machine learning approaches were trained on different and often smaller cohorts with different diagnostic goals. This leads to only limited generalizability of the results due to variances in patients, CT scanners, and protocols. With strengths in pattern recognition and segmentation, further evolved AI-based algorithms that have been trained on larger and more diverse cohorts can significantly improve quantification of parenchymal changes and have great potential in the analysis of chest CT [73–76]. In addition, they save time and may reduce interobserver and inter-patient variability, presenting an advantage over semiquantitative methods [71].

Deep Learning in the Evaluation of COPD Patients

In contrast to the machine learning approaches above, deep learning enables the possibility that an algorithm may choose features to differentiate between imaging biomarkers such as emphysema patterns by itself without the need of prior human input. However, this independency in bypassing the identification of features of interest can only be achieved using much larger datasets to train the algorithm. This training requires high computational power and may take a long time which, however, may be a valuable investment since the successive analyses are much faster in the long run.

One of the first applications of deep learning in COPD patients was performed by Gonzales et al. and published in 2018 [77]. The research group used 7983 CT scans from participants of the Genetic Epidemiology of COPD (COPDGene) study [78] to train a convolutional neural network (CNN) that was afterward evaluated using 1000 non-overlapping COPDGene participants and 1672 subjects of the ECLIPSE study (Evaluation of COPD Longitudinally to Identify Predictive Surrogate End-points [79]). For detection of COPD, the accuracy for the exact COPD stage was 51.1% and 29.4% and detection within one stage 75% and 74.6% for COPDGene and ECLIPSE evaluations, respectively, resulting in an area under the receiver operating characteristic curve (AUC) of 0.856. Also, CNN was able to fairly predict smokers who are most likely to have acute respiratory events and those with the highest mortality [77].

Another deep learning algorithm combining a CNN with a long short-term memory layer (recurrent neural network) was established by Humphries and colleagues in 2019 to classify emphysema according to the Fleischner criteria [80]. For training, they also used participants of the COPDGene study (2407 for training and 100 for validation and parameter tuning). Evaluation was performed using 7143 participants of the COPDGene and 1962 subjects of the ECLIPSE studies. For comparison, they used visual scores and clinical parameters including lung function tests. The algorithm was able to differentiate between emphysema classifications and showed correlation to clinical parameters as well as risk of mortality [80].

More recently, Tang et al. examined three deep residual networks for the automated detection of COPD using random subsets of CT scans. The algorithms were independently trained using participants of the Pan-Canadian Early Detection of Lung Cancer (PanCan) study [81], which enrolled former smokers and active smokers at high risk for lung cancer. Validation was performed using 2153 CT scans from the ECLIPSE study, which included spirometric data to evaluate the degree of COPD. The research group found all three models to achieve similar performance with the best performing model reaching an AUC of 0.889. What is special about this study is that they used an external dataset to test and verify the generalizability of the model, which represents a major issue in selectively trained algorithms [82].

With increasing attention of researchers and clinicians, AI-based evaluation of COPD patients also moved into the focus of software developers for commercial applications. A prototype of AI-Rad Companion Chest CT (Siemens Healthineers, Erlangen, Germany) was used by Fischer et al. for fully automated emphysema quantification, and the results were correlated to clinical parameters. The automated segmentation algorithm used by this application is a deep image-to-image network (DI2IN), which represents a multilayer convolutional network (convolution image-to-image network, CIN) and has already been described and applied in liver segmentation [83]. The algorithm has been trained and tested on over 10,000 CT datasets, of which about 5500 were used for training [72]. CIN uses three-dimensional volumes of CT scans as input to create probability maps in which each voxel is labeled as how likely it belongs to a certain region of the lung. In these studies, the process was not yet fully end-to-end capable because the research team checked the segmentation manually for each patient. Different reconstruction methods of chest CT were used but yielded nearly identical results. The research group showed that AI-based, fully automated lung segmentation and emphysema quantification has a high test-retest reliability (ICC 1.0) and shows good correlation with clinical parameters like the GOLD stages or TI [72, 84, 85]. Examples of automated segmentation and emphysema quantification using AI-Rad Companion Chest CT and Imbio LDA (Imbio, LLC, Minneapolis, MN, USA) are shown in Figs. 40.1 and 40.2, respectively.

Limitations

Of course, many of the studies presented above are very recent and were performed using novel applications of AI methods like deep learning in the analysis of chest CT with regard to COPD. This represents a relatively new and constantly evolving field in radiology which is why all results have to be taken with a grain of salt. Many of the algorithms that the different research groups used have been built and tested on pertinently diseased patients. In those patients, other clinical diagnostics like spirometry have been performed, which already indicates that a pulmonary disease was suspected which leads to a limited comparability to the general population. The underlying structures of these algorithms are different from each other, and it is not yet known what exactly the individual strengths and limitations of the different approaches are. There is no standard algorithm, which means that many further investigations have to be performed in order to achieve reliable and generalizable results.

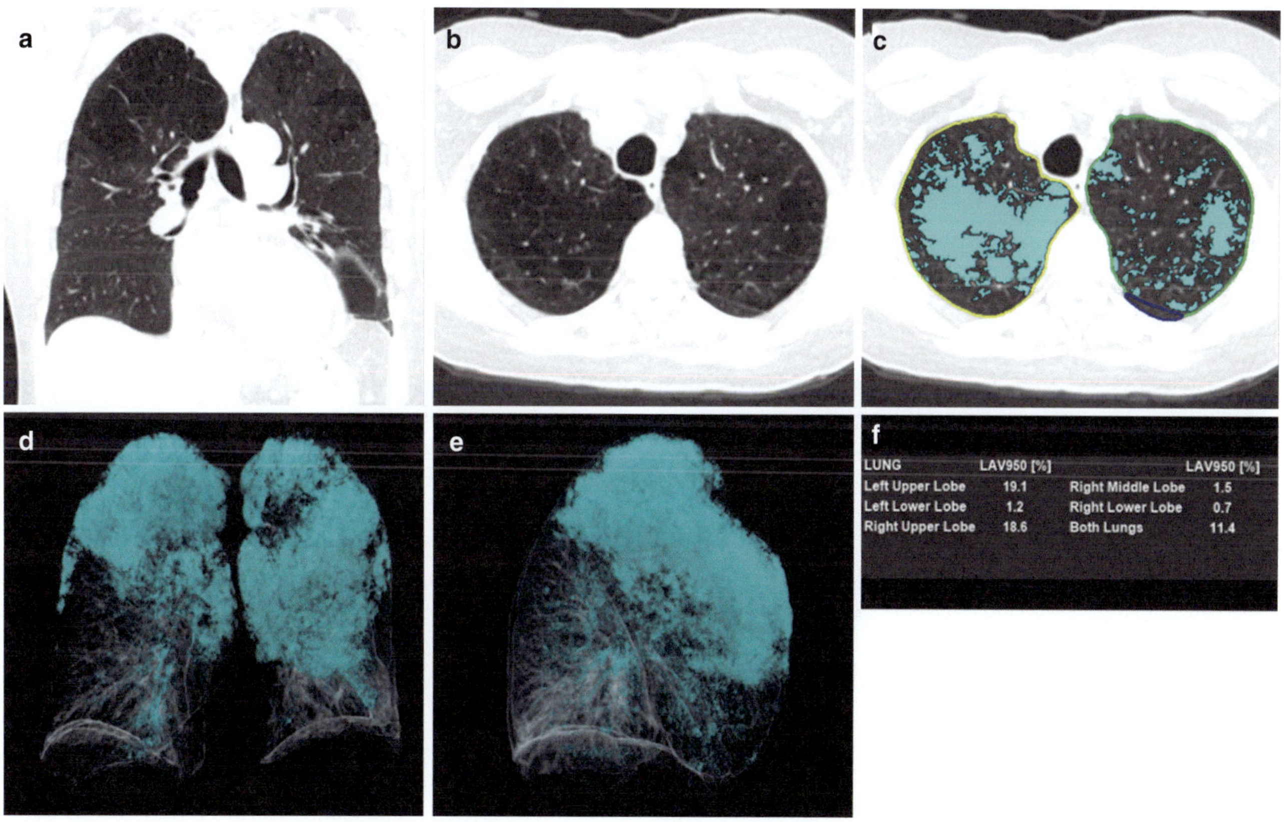

Fig. 40.1 Patient with COPD and upper lobe emphysema analyzed with AI-Rad Companion Chest CT (Siemens Healthineers, Erlangen, Germany). (**a**) Coronal reformation and (**b**) axial image of native chest CT in lung window. (**c**) Axial image after automated lung segmentation (yellow line, right upper lobe; green line, left upper lobe; dark-blue line, left lower lobe; light-blue areas, lung parenchyma with radiodensity below 950 HU). (**d**, **e**) Three-dimensional reconstructions of emphysematous parenchyma. (**f**) Report showing percentages of emphysema in each lobe and in the whole lung. LAV950 low-attenuating volume with a threshold of 950 Hounsfield units

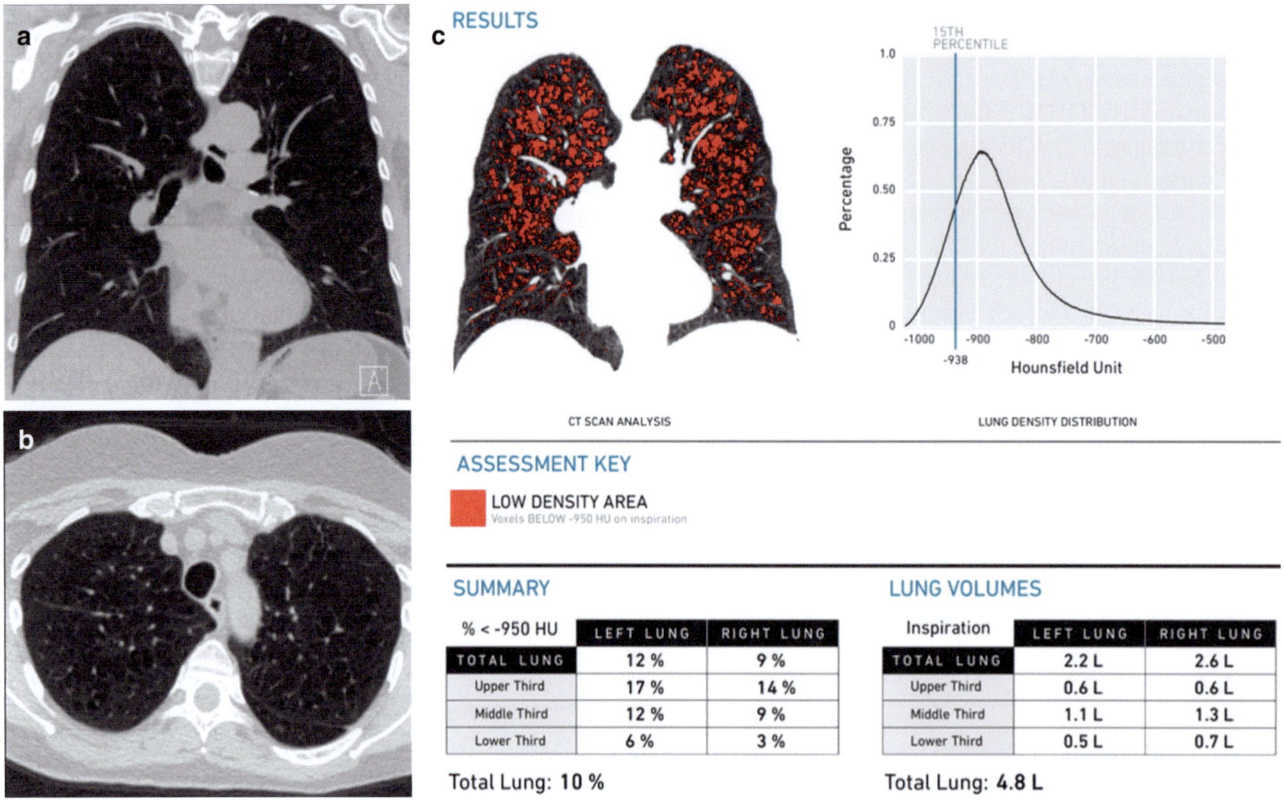

Fig. 40.2 Lung cancer screening patient with centrilobular emphysema. Lung density analysis was performed using Imbio LDA (Imbio, LLC, Minneapolis, MN, USA). (**a**) Coronal reformation and (**b**) axial image of native chest CT in lung window. (**c**) Imbio LDA report showing low-density areas in red color and summaries of emphysema distribution and lung volumes

Conclusion

AI applications in image analysis are a rapidly growing sector in radiology research and already have some clinical applications. The number of performed CT scans is rising steadily overall [86–89]. With the presented growing evidence of use and benefits in COPD patients and also growing voices for implementing CT in the diagnosis of COPD patients, the number of chest CT studies may rise as well. As the number of radiologists does not grow as fast [90], this development may lead to manpower shortages that lead to more studies to be evaluated by a single radiologist and potential for an increased rate of errors or discrepancies [91–93]. Adding to this, the creation of radiological reports is getting more complicated with the application of more detailed imaging criteria, classifications, and guidelines.

As their development evolves and manual input is reduced or no longer needed, AI-based software applications may be able to facilitate this workflow. In the evaluation of COPD patients, AI may aid in different ways in the future. It may add a reliable quantitative assessment of the disease in the form of emphysema extent and its distribution or patterns that can lead to a better comparability between exams and over the course of the disease. It also has the potential to be used in CT scans performed for other reasons, e.g., in lung cancer screening or for cardiac diagnostics. Here, patients in earlier stages of the disease may be identified, which would improve the underdiagnosis of COPD [20]. However, further controlled studies are needed to optimize management of incidentally detected COPD and decide whether spirometry is needed to confirm the diagnosis [82]. An assisted standardized evaluation of patients may also be combined with applications such as structured reporting, which can ease the workflow and provide structured data for future research studies [94–96]. While residents could benefit from a support in their learning process, senior radiologists may be able to shorten the time required for each study.

An AI-based, independent, objective, and comparable interpretation in correlation with a radiologist's experience may help patients suspected of having COPD receive an earlier diagnosis, with the potential to decrease morbidity and increase survival.

References

1. Vos T, Lim SS, Abbafati C, et al. Global burden of 369 diseases and injuries in 204 countries and territories, 1990–2019: a systematic analysis for the Global Burden of Disease Study 2019. Lancet. 2020;396(10258):1204–22. https://doi.org/10.1016/S0140-6736(20)30925-9.
2. James SL, Abate D, Abate KH, et al. Global, regional, and national incidence, prevalence, and years lived with disability for 354 diseases and injuries for 195 countries and territories, 1990–2017: a systematic analysis for the Global Burden of Disease Study 2017. Lancet. 2018;392(10159):1789–858. https://doi.org/10.1016/S0140-6736(18)32279-7.
3. Rabe KF, Watz H. Chronic obstructive pulmonary disease. Lancet. 2017;389(10082):1931–40. https://doi.org/10.1016/S0140-6736(17)31222-9.
4. Soriano JB, Abajobir AA, Abate KH, et al. Global, regional, and national deaths, prevalence, disability-adjusted life years, and years lived with disability for chronic obstructive pulmonary disease and asthma, 1990–2015: a systematic analysis for the Global Burden of Disease Study 2015. Lancet Respir Med. 2017;5(9):691–706. https://doi.org/10.1016/S2213-2600(17)30293-X.
5. Zhang X, Holt JB, Lu H, et al. Multilevel regression and poststratification for small-area estimation of population health outcomes: a case study of chronic obstructive pulmonary disease prevalence using the behavioral risk factor surveillance system. Am J Epidemiol. 2014;179(8):1025–33. https://doi.org/10.1093/aje/kwu018.
6. Ford ES, Murphy LB, Khavjou O, Giles WH, Holt JB, Croft JB. Total and state-specific medical and absenteeism costs of COPD among adults aged 18 years in the United States for 2010 and projections through 2020. Chest. 2015;147(1):31–45. https://doi.org/10.1378/chest.14-0972.
7. COPD Costs. Published July 5, 2019. Accessed 28 Jan 2021. https://www.cdc.gov/copd/infographics/copd-costs.html
8. Adeloye D, Chua S, Lee C, et al. Global and regional estimates of COPD prevalence: systematic review and meta-analysis. J Glob Health. 2015;5(2):020415. https://doi.org/10.7189/jogh.05-020415.
9. Landis SH, Muellerova H, Mannino DM, et al. Continuing to confront COPD international patient survey: methods, COPD prevalence, and disease burden in 2012-2013. Int J Chron Obstruct Pulmon Dis. 2014;9:597–611. https://doi.org/10.2147/COPD.S61854.
10. Celli BR, Wedzicha JA. Update on clinical aspects of chronic obstructive pulmonary disease. N Engl J Med. 2019;381(13):1257–66. https://doi.org/10.1056/NEJMra1900500.
11. Mannino DM, Thorn D, Swensen A, Holguin F. Prevalence and outcomes of diabetes, hypertension and cardiovascular disease in COPD. Eur Respir J. 2008;32(4):962–9. https://doi.org/10.1183/09031936.00012408.
12. Divo MJ, Celli BR, Poblador-Plou B, et al. Chronic obstructive pulmonary disease (COPD) as a disease of early aging: evidence from the EpiChron Cohort. PLoS One. 2018;13(2):e0193143. https://doi.org/10.1371/journal.pone.0193143.
13. Durham AL, Adcock IM. The relationship between COPD and lung cancer. Lung Cancer. 2015;90(2):121–7. https://doi.org/10.1016/j.lungcan.2015.08.017.
14. Raviv S, Hawkins KA, DeCamp MM, Kalhan R. Lung cancer in chronic obstructive pulmonary disease: enhancing surgical options and outcomes. Am J Respir Crit Care Med. 2011;183(9):1138–46. https://doi.org/10.1164/rccm.201008-1274CI.
15. Agustí A, Hogg JC. Update on the pathogenesis of chronic obstructive pulmonary disease. N Engl J Med. 2019;381(13):1248–56. https://doi.org/10.1056/NEJMra1900475.
16. Coxson HO, Rogers RM. Quantitative computed tomography of chronic obstructive pulmonary Disease1. Acad Radiol. 2005;12(11):1457–63. https://doi.org/10.1016/j.acra.2005.08.013.
17. Raherison C, Girodet P-O. Epidemiology of COPD. Eur Respir Rev. 2009;18(114):213–21. https://doi.org/10.1183/09059180.00003609.
18. 2020 Gold Reports. Global Initiative for Chronic Obstructive Lung Disease - GOLD. Accessed 28 Jan 2021. https://goldcopd.org/gold-reports/.
19. Morice AH, Celli B, Kesten S, Lystig T, Tashkin D, Decramer M. COPD in young patients: a pre-specified analysis of the four-year trial of tiotropium (UPLIFT). Respir Med. 2010;104(11):1659–67. https://doi.org/10.1016/j.rmed.2010.07.016.
20. Agusti A, Alcazar B, Cosio B, et al. Time for a change: anticipating the diagnosis and treatment of COPD. Eur Respir J 2020;56(1). doi:https://doi.org/10.1183/13993003.02104-2020.
21. Kohansal R, Martinez-Camblor P, Agustí A, Buist AS, Mannino DM, Soriano JB. The natural history of chronic airflow obstruction revisited: an analysis of the Framingham offspring cohort. Am J Respir Crit Care Med. 2009;180(1):3–10. https://doi.org/10.1164/rccm.200901-0047OC.
22. Eisner MD, Anthonisen N, Coultas D, et al. An official American Thoracic Society public policy statement: novel risk factors and the global burden of chronic obstructive pulmonary disease. Am J Respir Crit Care Med. 2010;182(5):693–718. https://doi.org/10.1164/rccm.200811-1757ST.
23. Fuller-Thomson E, Chisholm RS, Brennenstuhl S. COPD in a population-based sample of never-smokers: interactions among sex, gender, and race. Int J Chronic Dis. 2016;2016:5862026. https://doi.org/10.1155/2016/5862026.
24. Blanc PD, Torén K. Occupation in chronic obstructive pulmonary disease and chronic bronchitis: an update. Int J Tuberc Lung Dis. 2007;11(3):251–7.
25. Syamlal G. Chronic obstructive pulmonary disease prevalence among adults who have never smoked, by industry and occupation — United States, 2013–2017. MMWR Morb Mortal Wkly Rep. 2019;68. https://doi.org/10.15585/mmwr.mm6813a2.
26. Thomsen M, Nordestgaard BG, Vestbo J, Lange P. Characteristics and outcomes of chronic obstructive pulmonary disease in never smokers in Denmark: a prospective population study. Lancet Respir Med. 2013;1(7):543–50. https://doi.org/10.1016/S2213-2600(13)70137-1.
27. Overview | Chronic obstructive pulmonary disease in over 16s: diagnosis and management | Guidance | NICE. Accessed 28 Jan 2021. https://www.nice.org.uk/guidance/NG115
28. Vogelmeier CF, Criner GJ, Martinez FJ, et al. Global strategy for the diagnosis, management, and prevention of chronic obstructive lung disease 2017 report. GOLD executive summary. Am J Respir Crit Care Med. 2017;195(5):557–82. https://doi.org/10.1164/rccm.201701-0218PP.
29. Singh D, Agusti A, Anzueto A, et al. Global strategy for the diagnosis, management, and prevention of chronic obstructive lung disease: the GOLD science committee report 2019. Eur Respir J 2019;53(5). https://doi.org/10.1183/13993003.00164-2019.
30. Coxson HO, Dirksen A, Edwards LD, et al. The presence and progression of emphysema in COPD as determined by CT scanning and biomarker expression: a prospective analysis from the ECLIPSE study. Lancet Respir Med. 2013;1(2):129–36. https://doi.org/10.1016/S2213-2600(13)70006-7.
31. Wells JM, Washko GR, Han MK, et al. Pulmonary arterial enlargement and acute exacerbations of COPD. N Engl J Med. 2012;367(10):913–21. https://doi.org/10.1056/NEJMoa1203830.
32. Bodduluri S, Reinhardt JM, Hoffman EA, Newell JD, Bhatt SP. Recent advances in computed tomography imag-

ing in chronic obstructive pulmonary disease. Ann Am Thorac Soc. 2017;15(3):281–9. https://doi.org/10.1513/AnnalsATS.201705-377FR.
33. Lynch DA, Austin JHM, Hogg JC, et al. CT-definable subtypes of chronic obstructive pulmonary disease: a statement of the Fleischner Society. Radiology. 2015;277(1):192–205. https://doi.org/10.1148/radiol.2015141579.
34. Friedlander AL, Lynch D, Dyar LA, Bowler RP. Phenotypes of chronic obstructive pulmonary disease. COPD J Chronic Obstr Pulm Dis. 2007;4(4):355–84. https://doi.org/10.1080/15412550701629663.
35. Remy-Jardin M, Faivre J-B, Kaergel R, et al. Machine learning and deep neural network applications in the thorax: pulmonary embolism, chronic thromboembolic pulmonary hypertension, aorta, and chronic obstructive pulmonary disease. J Thorac Imaging. 2020;35:S40. https://doi.org/10.1097/RTI.0000000000000492.
36. Ogawa E, Nakano Y, Ohara T, et al. Body mass index in male patients with COPD: correlation with low attenuation areas on CT. Thorax. 2009;64(1):20–5. https://doi.org/10.1136/thx.2008.097543.
37. Boschetto P, Quintavalle S, Zeni E, et al. Association between markers of emphysema and more severe chronic obstructive pulmonary disease. Thorax. 2006;61(12):1037–42. https://doi.org/10.1136/thx.2006.058321.
38. Grydeland TB, Dirksen A, Coxson HO, et al. Quantitative computed tomography measures of emphysema and airway wall thickness are related to respiratory symptoms. Am J Respir Crit Care Med. 2010;181(4):353–9. https://doi.org/10.1164/rccm.200907-1008OC.
39. Han MK, Kazerooni EA, Lynch DA, et al. Chronic obstructive pulmonary disease exacerbations in the COPDGene study: associated radiologic phenotypes. Radiology. 2011;261(1):274–82. https://doi.org/10.1148/radiol.11110173.
40. Klooster K, ten Hacken NHT, Hartman JE, Kerstjens HAM, van Rikxoort EM, Slebos D-J. Endobronchial valves for emphysema without interlobar collateral ventilation. https://doi.org/10.1056/NEJMoa1507807.
41. Madani A, De Maertelaer V, Zanen J, Gevenois PA. Pulmonary emphysema: radiation dose and section thickness at multidetector CT quantification--comparison with macroscopic and microscopic morphometry. Radiology. 2007;243(1):250–7. https://doi.org/10.1148/radiol.2431060194.
42. Bankier AA, De Maertelaer V, Keyzer C, Gevenois PA. Pulmonary emphysema: subjective visual grading versus objective quantification with macroscopic morphometry and thin-section CT densitometry. Radiology. 1999;211(3):851–8. https://doi.org/10.1148/radiology.211.3.r99jn05851.
43. Gevenois PA, de Maertelaer V, De Vuyst P, Zanen J, Yernault JC. Comparison of computed density and macroscopic morphometry in pulmonary emphysema. Am J Respir Crit Care Med. 1995;152(2):653–7. https://doi.org/10.1164/ajrccm.152.2.7633722.
44. Castillo-Saldana D, Hague CJ, Coxson HO, Ryerson CJ. Using quantitative computed tomographic imaging to understand chronic obstructive pulmonary disease and fibrotic interstitial lung disease: state of the art and future directions. J Thorac Imaging. 2020;35(4):246–54. https://doi.org/10.1097/RTI.0000000000000440.
45. Mascalchi M, Camiciottoli G, Diciotti S. Lung densitometry: why, how and when. J Thorac Dis. 2017;9(9):3319–45. https://doi.org/10.21037/jtd.2017.08.17.
46. Hoesein FAAM, van Rikxoort E, van Ginneken B, et al. Computed tomography-quantified emphysema distribution is associated with lung function decline. Eur Respir J. 2012;40(4):844–50. https://doi.org/10.1183/09031936.00186311.
47. Regan EA, Lynch DA, Curran-Everett D, et al. Clinical and radiologic disease in smokers with Normal spirometry. JAMA Intern Med. 2015;175(9):1539–49. https://doi.org/10.1001/jamainternmed.2015.2735.
48. Woodruff PG, Barr RG, Bleecker E, et al. Clinical significance of symptoms in smokers with preserved pulmonary function. N Engl J Med. 2016;374(19):1811–21. https://doi.org/10.1056/NEJMoa1505971.
49. Gietema HA, Zanen P, Schilham A, et al. Distribution of emphysema in heavy smokers: impact on pulmonary function. Respir Med. 2010;104(1):76–82. https://doi.org/10.1016/j.rmed.2009.08.004.
50. Koo H-K, Vasilescu DM, Booth S, et al. Small airways disease in mild and moderate chronic obstructive pulmonary disease: a cross-sectional study. Lancet Respir Med. 2018;6(8):591–602. https://doi.org/10.1016/S2213-2600(18)30196-6.
51. Bhatt SP, Washko GR, Hoffman EA, et al. Imaging advances in chronic obstructive pulmonary disease. Insights from the genetic epidemiology of Chronic Obstructive Pulmonary Disease (COPDGene) Study. Am J Respir Crit Care Med. 2018;199(3):286–301. https://doi.org/10.1164/rccm.201807-1351SO.
52. Sharma N, Aggarwal LM. Automated medical image segmentation techniques. J Med Phys Assoc Med Phys India. 2010;35(1):3–14. https://doi.org/10.4103/0971-6203.58777.
53. Refaee T, Wu G, Ibrahim A, et al. The emerging role of radiomics in COPD and lung cancer. Respiration. 2020;99(2):99–107. https://doi.org/10.1159/000505429.
54. Röhrich S, Hofmanninger J, Prayer F, Müller H, Prosch H, Langs G. Prospects and challenges of Radiomics by using nononcologic routine chest CT. Radiol Cardiothorac Imaging. 2020;2(4):e190190. https://doi.org/10.1148/ryct.2020190190.
55. Schroeder JD, McKenzie AS, Zach JA, et al. Relationships between airflow obstruction and quantitative CT measurements of emphysema, air trapping, and airways in subjects with and without Chronic Obstructive Pulmonary Disease. AJR Am J Roentgenol. 2013;201(3):W460–70. https://doi.org/10.2214/AJR.12.10102.
56. Akira M, Toyokawa K, Inoue Y, Arai T. Quantitative CT in chronic obstructive pulmonary disease: inspiratory and expiratory assessment. Am J Roentgenol. 2009;192(1):267–72. https://doi.org/10.2214/AJR.07.3953.
57. Ostridge K, Wilkinson TMA. Present and future utility of computed tomography scanning in the assessment and management of COPD. Eur Respir J. 2016;48(1):216–28. https://doi.org/10.1183/13993003.00041-2016.
58. Haruna A, Muro S, Nakano Y, et al. CT scan findings of emphysema predict mortality in COPD. Chest. 2010;138(3):635–40. https://doi.org/10.1378/chest.09-2836.
59. Johannessen A, Skorge TD, Bottai M, et al. Mortality by level of emphysema and airway wall thickness. Am J Respir Crit Care Med. 2013;187(6):602–8. https://doi.org/10.1164/rccm.201209-1722OC.
60. Jairam PM, Graaf Y van der, Lammers J-WJ, Mali WPTM, Jong PA de. Incidental findings on chest CT imaging are associated with increased COPD exacerbations and mortality. Thorax 2015;70(8):725–731. doi:https://doi.org/10.1136/thoraxjnl-2014-206160.
61. Sørensen L, Shaker SB, de Bruijne M. Quantitative analysis of pulmonary emphysema using local binary patterns. IEEE Trans Med Imaging. 2010;29(2):559–69. https://doi.org/10.1109/TMI.2009.2038575.
62. Sorensen L, Nielsen M, Lo P, Ashraf H, Pedersen JH, Bruijne M de. Texture-based analysis of COPD: a data-driven approach. IEEE Trans Med Imaging 2012;31(1):70–78. doi:https://doi.org/10.1109/TMI.2011.2164931.
63. Sørensen L, Nielsen M, Petersen J, Pedersen JH, Dirksen A, de Bruijne M. Chronic obstructive pulmonary disease quantification using CT texture analysis and densitometry: results from the Danish lung cancer screening trial. Am J Roentgenol. 2020;214(6):1269–79. https://doi.org/10.2214/AJR.19.22300.
64. Ginsburg SB, Lynch DA, Bowler RP, Schroeder JD. Automated texture-based quantification of Centrilobular nodularity and

Centrilobular emphysema in chest CT images. Acad Radiol. 2012;19(10):1241–51. https://doi.org/10.1016/j.acra.2012.04.020.
65. Lafata KJ, Zhou Z, Liu J-G, Hong J, Kelsey CR, Yin F-F. An exploratory radiomics approach to quantifying pulmonary function in CT images. Sci Rep. 2019;9 https://doi.org/10.1038/s41598-019-48023-5.
66. Castaldi PJ, San José Estépar R, Mendoza CS, et al. Distinct quantitative computed tomography emphysema patterns are associated with physiology and function in smokers. Am J Respir Crit Care Med. 2013;188(9):1083–90. https://doi.org/10.1164/rccm.201305-0873OC.
67. Binder P, Batmanghelich NK, Estepar RSJ, Golland P. Unsupervised discovery of emphysema subtypes in a large clinical cohort. Mach Learn Med Imaging MLMI Workshop. 2016;10019:180–7. https://doi.org/10.1007/978-3-319-47157-0_22.
68. Zulueta-Coarasa T, Kurugol S, Ross JC, Washko GG, Estépar RSJ. Emphysema classification based on embedded probabilistic PCA. Conf Proc Annu Int Conf IEEE Eng Med Biol Soc IEEE Eng Med Biol Soc Conf. 2013;2013:3969–72. https://doi.org/10.1109/EMBC.2013.6610414.
69. Peng, L. Lin, H. Hu, et al. Classification of pulmonary emphysema in CT images based on multi-scale deep convolutional neural networks. In: 2018 25th IEEE International Conference on Image Processing (ICIP). 2018. pp. 3119–23. https://doi.org/10.1109/ICIP.2018.8451514
70. Westcott A, Capaldi DPI, McCormack DG, Ward AD, Fenster A, Parraga G. Chronic obstructive pulmonary disease: thoracic CT texture analysis and machine learning to predict pulmonary ventilation. Radiology. 2019;293(3):676–84. https://doi.org/10.1148/radiol.2019190450.
71. Singh G, AL'Aref SJ, Assen MV, et al. Machine learning in cardiac CT: basic concepts and contemporary data. J Cardiovasc Comput Tomogr. 2018;12(3):192–201. https://doi.org/10.1016/j.jcct.2018.04.010.
72. Fischer AM, Varga-Szemes A, van Assen M, et al. Comparison of artificial intelligence-based fully automatic chest CT emphysema quantification to pulmonary function testing. AJR Am J Roentgenol. 2020;214(5):1065–71. https://doi.org/10.2214/AJR.19.21572.
73. Chartrand G, Cheng PM, Vorontsov E, et al. Deep learning: a primer for radiologists. Radiographics. 2017;37(7):2113–31. https://doi.org/10.1148/rg.2017170077.
74. Morris MA, Saboury B, Burkett B, Gao J, Siegel EL. Reinventing radiology: big data and the future of medical imaging. J Thorac Imaging. 2018;33(1):4–16. https://doi.org/10.1097/RTI.0000000000000311.
75. Eltorai AEM, Bratt AK, Guo HH. Thoracic radiologists' versus computer scientists' perspectives on the future of artificial intelligence in radiology. J Thorac Imaging. 2020;35(4):255–9. https://doi.org/10.1097/RTI.0000000000000453.
76. Wang Y, Yu M, Wang M, et al. Application of artificial intelligence-based image optimization for computed tomography angiography of the aorta with low tube voltage and reduced contrast medium volume. J Thorac Imaging. 2019;34(6):393–9. https://doi.org/10.1097/RTI.0000000000000438.
77. González G, Ash SY, Vegas-Sánchez-Ferrero G, et al. Disease staging and prognosis in smokers using deep learning in chest computed tomography. Am J Respir Crit Care Med. 2018;197(2):193–203. https://doi.org/10.1164/rccm.201705-0860OC.
78. Regan EA, Hokanson JE, Murphy JR, et al. Genetic epidemiology of COPD (COPDGene) study design. COPD. 2010;7(1):32–43. https://doi.org/10.3109/15412550903499522.
79. Vestbo J, Anderson W, Coxson HO, et al. Evaluation of COPD longitudinally to identify predictive surrogate end-points (ECLIPSE). Eur Respir J. 2008;31(4):869–73. https://doi.org/10.1183/09031936.00111707.
80. Humphries SM, Notary AM, Centeno JP, et al. Deep learning enables automatic classification of emphysema pattern at CT. Radiology. 2019;294(2):434–44. https://doi.org/10.1148/radiol.2019191022.
81. Tammemagi MC, Schmidt H, Martel S, et al. Participant selection for lung cancer screening by risk modelling (the pan-Canadian early detection of lung cancer [PanCan] study): a single-arm, prospective study. Lancet Oncol. 2017;18(11):1523–31. https://doi.org/10.1016/S1470-2045(17)30597-1.
82. Bibault J-E, Xing L. Screening for chronic obstructive pulmonary disease with artificial intelligence. Lancet Digital Health. 2020;2(5):e216–7. https://doi.org/10.1016/S2589-7500(20)30076-5.
83. Yang D, Xu D, Zhou SK, et al. Automatic Liver Segmentation Using an Adversarial Image-to-Image Network. In: Descoteaux M, Maier-Hein L, Franz A, Jannin P, Collins DL, Duchesne S, editors. Medical image computing and computer assisted intervention – MICCAI 2017. Lecture Notes in Computer Science. Cham: Springer International Publishing; 2017. p. 507–15. https://doi.org/10.1007/978-3-319-66179-7_58.
84. Fischer AM, Varga-Szemes A, Martin SS, et al. Artificial intelligence-based fully automated per lobe segmentation and emphysema-quantification based on chest computed tomography compared with global initiative for chronic obstructive lung disease severity of smokers. J Thorac Imaging. 2020;35:S28. https://doi.org/10.1097/RTI.0000000000000500.
85. Fischer AM, Yacoub B, Savage RH, et al. Machine learning/deep neuronal network: routine application in chest computed tomography and workflow considerations. J Thorac Imaging. 2020;35:S21. https://doi.org/10.1097/RTI.0000000000000498.
86. Smith-Bindman R, Kwan ML, Marlow EC, et al. Trends in use of medical imaging in US health care systems and in Ontario, Canada, 2000-2016. JAMA. 2019;322(9):843–56. https://doi.org/10.1001/jama.2019.11456.
87. Bellolio MF, Heien HC, Sangaralingham LR, et al. Increased computed tomography utilization in the emergency department and its association with hospital admission. West J Emerg Med. 2017;18(5):835–45. https://doi.org/10.5811/westjem.2017.5.34152.
88. Larson DB, Johnson LW, Schnell BM, Salisbury SR, Forman HP. National Trends in CT use in the emergency department: 1995–2007. Radiology. 2011;258(1):164–73. https://doi.org/10.1148/radiol.10100640.
89. Hsueh Y-W, Lin Y-C, Lin C-H, et al. Trends in computed tomography scan uses in Taiwan from 2000 to 2013. J Chin Med Assoc. 2019;82(12):948–56. https://doi.org/10.1097/JCMA.0000000000000199.
90. Rosenkrantz AB, Hughes DR, Duszak R. The U.S. radiologist workforce: an analysis of temporal and geographic variation by using large National Datasets. Radiology. 2015;279(1):175–84. https://doi.org/10.1148/radiol.2015150921.
91. Brady AP. Error and discrepancy in radiology: inevitable or avoidable? Insights Imaging. 2016;8(1):171–82. https://doi.org/10.1007/s13244-016-0534-1.
92. Berlin L. Radiologic errors and malpractice: a blurry distinction. AJR Am J Roentgenol. 2007;189(3):517–22. https://doi.org/10.2214/AJR.07.2209.
93. Borgstede JP, Lewis RS, Bhargavan M, Sunshine JH. RADPEER quality assurance program: a multifacility study of interpretive disagreement rates1 1RADPEER is a quality assurance product of the ACR. For information or to implement RADPEER, contact the ACR's quality and safety department at 1 (800) 227-5463, extension 4384. J Am Coll Radiol. 2004;1(1):59–65. https://doi.org/10.1016/S1546-1440(03)00002-4.
94. Ganeshan D, Duong P-AT, Probyn L, et al. Structured reporting in radiology. Acad Radiol. 2018;25(1):66–73. https://doi.org/10.1016/j.acra.2017.08.005.
95. Nobel W, Marks SC, Kubik S. The anatomical basis for femoral nerve palsy following iliacus hematoma. J Neurosurg. 1980;52(4):533–40. https://doi.org/10.3171/jns.1980.52.4.0533.
96. ESR paper on structured reporting in radiology. Insights Imaging. 2018;9(1):1–7. https://doi.org/10.1007/s13244-017-0588-8.

Artificial Intelligence-Based Evaluation of Patients with Interstitial Lung Disease

41

Mario Silva, Gianluca Milanese, Roberta Eufrasia Ledda, Michele Maddalo, and Nicola Sverzellati

Introduction

Interstitial lung disease (ILD) represents a category of pulmonary conditions that manifest with diffuse involvement of lung parenchyma [1]. It encompasses primary and secondary abnormalities with a wide range of pathological entities into several radiological representations. Radiology is integrated in the multidisciplinary process of diagnosis and follow-up of ILD because it warrants noninvasive, repeatable, panoramic, detailed characterization of lung parenchyma [2]. The finest morphologic standard of radiology in ILD is warranted by volumetric high-resolution computed tomography (HRCT), where the signal (X-ray) shows the most convenient interaction with tissue-air interface.

The macroscopic appearance of ILD on imaging has variable association with its pathological counterpart (radiological patterns < pathological patterns); hence radiological patterns of ILD are recognized and assist in clinical classification, yet with limitations. The use of artificial intelligence (AI) and objective analysis of ILD encounters the need for consistency of reading (and reporting) [3]; furthermore it offers a multilevel complete analysis of the complexity of HRCT data [4] that potentially expands beyond radiology by translational integration of multilevel data (e.g., demographics, physiology, laboratory, etc.). This chapter describes AI approaches to ILD and their development, according to its proposed clinical integration and perspective.

M. Silva, MD, PhD (✉) · G. Milanese, MD, PhD · R. E. Ledda, MD
N. Sverzellati, MD, PhD
Scienze Radiologiche, Department of Medicine and Surgery (DiMeC), University of Parma, Parma, Italy
e-mail: mario.silva@unipr.it; gianluca.milanese@unipr.it; robertaeufrasia.ledda@unipr.it; nicola.sverzellati@unipr.it

M. Maddalo, MSc
Servizio di Fisica Sanitaria, Azienda Ospedaliera-Universitaria di Parma, Parma, Italy
e-mail: mmaddalo@ao.pr.it

Clinical Demand

The most variants of ILDs share clinical, physiological, radiological, and pathological similarities, including varying degrees of fibrosis, inflammation (transient or chronic), and vascular injury. The clinical outcome of ILD is variable among entities: disease regression is expected in a limited proportion of scenarios, whereas "disease control" (stability or delay of progression) is deemed the optimal outcome against disease progression and/or mortality in a substantial number of ILDs. For instance, some smoking- or drug-related lung diseases can revert, whereas the clinical purpose of "disease control" is applied to idiopathic pulmonary fibrosis (IPF) or pulmonary fibrosis associated with connective tissue disease (CTD-ILD). Such outcomes represent the backbone of biomarker development and intercept specific clinical demands of the diverse ILD entities.

The management of patients with ILD relies on multidimensional profiling, which includes several medical domains such as symptoms (e.g., dyspnea, cough), physiology (e.g., forced vital capacity, carbon monoxide diffusion capacity), quality of life, survival, and imaging. Among such domains, imaging outstands for reliability and practicality, notably when using HRCT [5]. This statement was stipulated by the CTD-ILD working group in their Outcome Measures in Rheumatology (OMERACT) filter: imaging with HRCT warrants "truth," "discrimination," and "feasibility" [5]. The high yield of imaging for biomarkers of ILD is warranted for outcome measures for both clinical and research purposes [5]. However, radiologists are well aware of the interobserver variability in imaging interpretation, notably in ILD [3]. Objective analysis of imaging data by AI provides the unique opportunity of standardized interpretation of anatomical data, and it can be adapted to both fine detail and panoramic view of the disease. For this reason, all branches of AI are valued for reducing interobserver variability between "humans" by objective analysis of pulmonary abnormalities, including both their extent and pattern(s). Beyond the need

C. N. De Cecco et al. (eds.), *Artificial Intelligence in Cardiothoracic Imaging*, Contemporary Medical Imaging,
https://doi.org/10.1007/978-3-030-92087-6_41

of consistency of the biomarker, the use of AI can further enrich the information by analyzing the complexity of lung architecture in its volumetric representation. This latter task seems an exclusive field of AI for comprehensive textural analysis. Its development and validation seem beyond human "radiological calibration," potentially endorsed in non-radiological outcomes (e.g., pathology, clinical diagnosis, clinical course, etc.).

In summary, ILD represents a prominent field of AI application with the utmost potential for improvement of clinical practice and support to clinical trials.

Techniques

The definition of AI in ILD includes several mathematical approaches to the imaging data. Since the 1980s, the use of AI in ILD developed across levels of complexity, following the technological evolution driven by quality of image data (e.g., translation from two-dimensional sequential to volumetric three-dimensional acquisition of CT) and computational power [6]. Technical principles are thereafter described in light of their specific application to lung abnormalities in ILD.

Tissue Density

Densitometric techniques represented the first approach to computerized analysis of lung parenchyma. It was first explored in obstructive lung disease and then in restrictive lung disease. It was early developed with two-dimensional method on single-slice or sequential CT imaging of the lung, and thereafter expanded to volumetric analysis. The tissue density technique is still valued in both scientific and clinical fields, especially for obstructive lung disease, whereas its use seems relatively limited for restrictive lung disease.

This simple approach relies on individual pixel/voxel density and its mathematical representation into histogram; hence the reduction of image noise is a mandatory technical requirement. For this purpose, smooth reconstruction algorithm is preferred to minimize noisy voxels related to edge-enhancing kernels. The representation of voxel density can be calculated for selected slice or for the total number of slices that compose the lung volume. The latter method represents the current standard of reference because it grants volumetric comprehensive analysis of the whole lung [7].

Mathematical parameters for analysis of density histogram (a.k.a. first-order statistics) allow for quantitative description of hypo- or hyperdense deviation from "normal" lung parenchyma, hence depicting the reduction or increase of pulmonary tissue against gas component (Table 41.1).

The density histogram of a normal lung is outlined in Fig. 41.1: the "mode" of the histogram is usually represented between −900 and − 850 Hounsfield units (HU) in full inspiration, describing the apex of a tall and narrow bell-shaped component of the histogram. The bell-shaped component continues in a right-sided smear, up to about −200 HU on the density scale.

Variations in the outline of the histogram reflect the overall variation in lung density and include both deformations of the bell-shaped component and of the right-sided smear. Extensive abnormalities with diffuse distribution are reflected by sizeable alteration of the histogram shape. The expected effect of most ILDs on histogram outline could be summarized by reduction of height of the bell-shaped component with concomitant swelling of its right slope, followed by increased height of the right-sided smear (Fig. 41.1: progressive increase of fibrosis severity in yellow and red lines). This visual concept is the semantic translation of the following mathematical parameters: reduction of kurtosis and increase of skewness, respectively [22]. Provided reproducible inspiratory breath-hold and consistent CT protocol, the volumetric density histogram was proposed for objective quantitation of longitudinal change in primary and secondary ILD [23].

Advantage of density histogram is the relatively simple analysis and representation. On the other hand, this simplification becomes the major limit of this technique because of its dimensional deprivation of density distribution: the lung is translated into a "cumulative densitometric view," and HRCT loses its power of "detailed panoramic." For instance, two fairly different types of ILD such as sarcoidosis and usual interstitial pneumonia (UIP) are represented by visual CT patterns with elements of individual distinction (e.g., elementary signs, spatial distribution), yet they might show quite similar density histogram, notably with decreased kurtosis and increased skewness. To overcome the limitation of "cumulative densitometric view" and reconcile with "detailed panoramic," the use of histogram was proposed on small selections of lung parenchyma. This approach aimed to isolate specific quantitative histogram representation of morphological CT patterns such as ground glass, reticulation, and honeycombing [24]. Such technique represented a brilliant intuition, until the development of textural analysis.

Tissue Texture

The elevation of clinical imaging from sequential to thin-slice volumetric acquisition and the frenetic rise of computational power allowed the introduction of three-dimensional analysis of images. The morphological complexity of ILDs took major advantage from this technological boost [25]. After neuroradiology, chest imaging rates second in the

Table 41.1 The main features of density histogram are reported along with extensive definition and their expected application for clinical use

Histogram parameter	Definition	Proposed clinical use
Mean lung attenuation (MLA)/mean lung density (MLD)	Arithmetic mean of attenuation values detected in every voxel Reference values for healthy subjects: 837.5 HU [8]/ -819 HU [9]/ -798 HU [10]	Simple parameter with moderate correlation with visual extent assessment of ILD, where increased MLA values derive from the increased amounts of fibrotic or inflammatory tissue [8, 11, 12] Severity of the disease can be compared by evaluating MLA values: advanced diseases show higher values [13] Overall, MLA is a not-sensitive metric; in ILDs, coexisting abnormalities with different impact on density (e.g., ground-glass opacities and honeycombing) might cause average values underestimating differences in distribution and severity [14]
Median	Median value of the lung attenuation distribution values	Estimate of lung density harboring information on extent and severity of ILD, independently associated with the presence of moderate-to-severe dyspnea [12]
Skewness	Dimensionless quantity measuring the lack of symmetry of the density histogram (how much the distribution histogram is symmetric, with regard to the most frequent value) Values: a perfectly symmetric histogram has a skewness of 0; a long right-tailed histogram has a skewness >0, while a long left-tailed histogram has a skewness <0 [15] Reference values for healthy subjects: 3.5 ± 0.5 [8]	Distribution parameter with moderate correlation with visual extent assessment of ILD [11] ILDs: patients show lower skewness values because of increased amounts of fibrotic or inflammatory tissue [8, 12, 16, 17] Comparison between severity of the disease can be performed by evaluating skewness values, with advanced diseases showing lesser values [13]
Kurtosis	Dimensionless quantity measuring how the distribution is peaked relative to a normal distribution (how much the distribution histogram is peaked) Normal distribution has a kurtosis of zero Reference values for healthy subjects: 18.8 ± 4.5 [8]	Distribution parameter with moderate correlation with visual extent assessment of ILD [11] ILDs: patients show lower kurtosis values (platykurtic: flat and lower curve with a more homogenous distribution of the histogram parameters) because of increased amounts of fibrotic or inflammatory tissue [8, 12, 18] Comparison between diseases' severities can be performed by evaluating kurtosis values, with advanced diseases showing lesser values (kurtosis close to 0 or < 0: moderate/severe fibrosis) [13, 19]
Contrast (CNT)	Describes the bias of a histogram from 0 HU Reference values for normal lung: 743,712 [20]	Lungs with increased density (e.g., with ground-glass attenuation) has lower CNT: a larger number of voxels of high absolute HU are associated with higher CNT values (whereas a histogram with only 0 HU has a CNT = 0) [20], and subjects with diffuse lung diseases show lower CNT values [21]
Variance (VAR)	Describes the variation within the histogram (dispersion)	A histogram concentrating around MLA has lower VAR (with more normal areas), while a histogram with higher tails in the distribution has greater VAR [21]
Entropy (EPY)	Describes the variation within the histogram (dispersion)	Histogram with various lung attenuation values has greater values of EPY [21]
Fibrosis ratio	Ratio between non-fibrotic lung volume (−1024 to 500 HU) and total lung volume (−1024 to 200 HU) Reference values for healthy subjects: 0.99 [8]	Allows to differentiate between fibrotic and non-fibrotic subjects: values lower than 0.99/1.0 could represent the presence of fibrosis [8]

number of publications about development and investigation of informative technology, in the last decade [6].

Texture analysis includes several computational steps; each of these interdependent steps involves progressive complexity of image analysis; therefore, their development demands the utmost robust support to avoid interim deviation. The implementation of quantitative features of texture includes second- or higher-order statistics (beyond descriptors seen in density histogram). Again, textural analysis of ILD is based on density substrate, which is particularly convenient in the context of expected pathological abnormalities of the lung that evolve throughout a naturally extremely hypodense parenchyma.

The development of textural analysis in ILD starts with building libraries of morphological examples represented by discrete region of interest. Each item of the library is classified visually by expert thoracic radiologist(s); this step is variably ranked in the workflow of software development (the rank of this process defines methods in different shades of supervised or unsupervised algorithms) and selected to correspond to a prototypical example of elementary parenchymal abnormalities (e.g., normal lung, ground glass, reticulation, honeycombing). In this phase, visual prototypical abnormalities are preferred to define visual "classes" or "categories" and drive the multiparametric process of construction of a computerized classification model. The

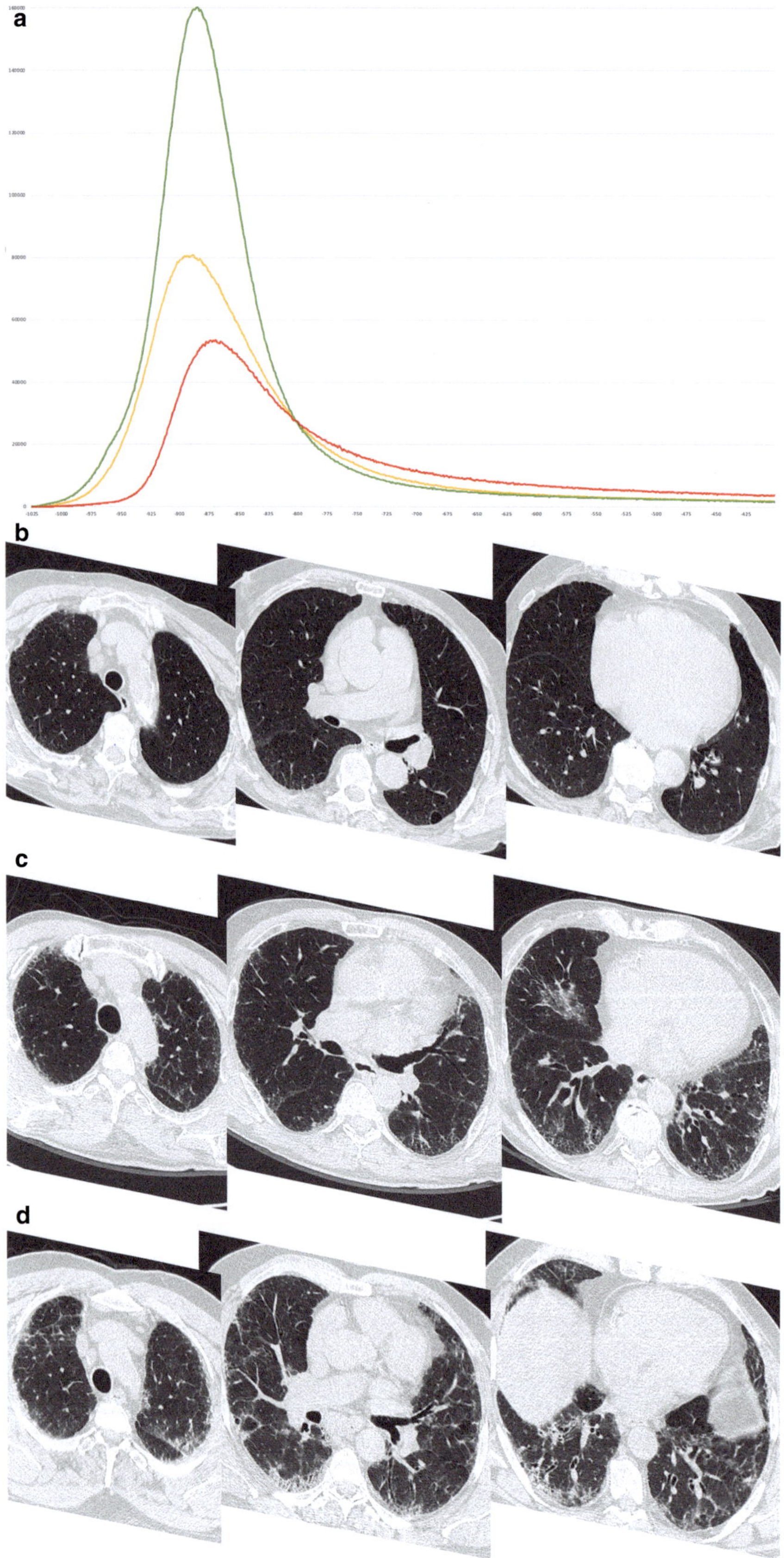

Fig. 41.1 (**a-d**) Histogram of density for three different patients with normal lung (**a** green histogram; **b** three axial CT slices) or ILD with mild (**a** yellow histogram; 1C three axial CT slices) or moderate (**a** red histogram; **d** three axial CT slices) extent of disease. The outline of the histogram progressively decreases in height, from normal lung and progressive increase of ILD severity; this reflects the reduction of air content in the lung. Likewise, the right-sided slope and smear swell up showing progressive increase of tissue matter, which sums up in the high-density proportion of the chart

computational steps into multiparametric analysis of "visual categories" usually result in a larger number of "quantitative categories" that distribute across a continuous range of classification [26]. Therefore, "quantitative categories" augment the size of possible morphological patterns. The full range of "quantitative categories" develops across a continuum of morphological patterns that also identifies *intermediate classifications* that lay in a gray zone in between "visual categories." The *intermediate classifications* can be censored to drive the learning process of the software, with the aim of gaining specificity and robustness in its future application. Therefore, the learning process picks an assortment of "quantitative categories" with enough individual distinction between the reference "visual categories" as these visual categories are state-of-the-art predictors of disease pattern.

Beyond the correspondence with "validated predictors" such as the prototypical "visual categories," the development of textural analysis comes along with further "novel descriptors" of the disease, for instance the quantification of details that are hardly reached by the human sight or maybe subtle abnormalities with specific anatomical distribution. The quantification of vascular texture and perivascular abnormalities emerged in the era of textural analysis of ILD and of other pulmonary diseases [27]. Indeed, the vascular system features a particularly rich network across the lung structure, and this texture is prone to alterations along with ILD development. The tracking and segmentation of lung vessels is relatively easy because their conspicuity and density are substantially higher than the remaining lung components (e.g., airway, airspace, fissures), especially in healthy or minimally injured lung. Noteworthy, pulmonary diseases mostly develop as a combination of abnormalities in all lung components, including airway, airspace, interstitium, and vessels. Therefore, vascular component has a quite robust rationale for characterization of pulmonary involvement in ILD, since its early phase. The advent of computer-based description of vascular structures unveiled a field of investigation that was otherwise quite limited until visual reading. The direct measurement of vascular complexity is currently synthetized into quantification of vascular representation, as a whole or by selected hierarchy or size. Moreover, vessel interface with pulmonary parenchyma offers a further source of information and potential support for understanding of disease behavior and susceptibility to treatment.

Deep Learning: Radiological and Multidimensional Analysis

The use of computer-based analysis for tissue density and tissue texture helps standardization of radiological performance in ILD, but it is quite limited to the description of loss of airspace and type of fundamental pulmonary abnormality. Both approaches were meant for supporting the quantification of disease severity, while neither of them was built with the aim of assisting the diagnosis of ILD [28].

The range of possible diagnoses in ILD is investigated across several domains, including clinical, laboratory, functional, radiologic, and pathologic descriptors. These multidimensional descriptors can be synthetized into a unique final diagnosis or, sometimes, are longitudinally combined into the so-called "working diagnosis". The "working diagnosis" is a clinical demand in ILD, because the hierarchy of presentation of disease components might vary substantially across individual patients, therefore challenging the use of a single labeled ILD throughout the chronic course of disease. For instance, CTD-ILD might result uncomplete in the early phase of investigation, an interim classification was created for these specific ILD scenarios, and it was named interstitial lung disease with autoimmune feature (IPAF); yet, "working diagnosis" is deemed for a much larger use in the universe of ILD. The contribution of radiology is paramount in this challenging clinical setting. Imaging holds potential for driving the clinical scenario when typical radiological patterns are encountered or when the clinical differential includes diseases with frankly different radiological representation. Deep learning was used to classify the macroscopic morphological pattern of disease in radiology [29]. Furthermore, the utmost support from AI is expected from its application across the full range of information discussed by multidisciplinary approach, notably with a method for managing and weighting the relevance of individual clinical domains [30, 31].

Deep learning approaches to ILD are quite heterogeneous; the specific examples will be referred in the following paragraphs about each single disease. As a rule of thumb, deep learning algorithm for ILD can include visual descriptors, quantitative descriptors of tissue density and texture, and further analysis of imaging data derived from complex algorithms of automatic classification. Algorithms of classification can run unsupervised, weakly supervised, or semi-supervised. The method of decisional trees is frequently employed; the complexity of decisional tree is usually directly associated with the amount of data that contribute to the diagnosis and by the degree of overlapping between two or more individual ILDs. Kim et al. compared deep learning by convolutional neural network (CNN) and shallow learning of support vector machine (SVM) for classification of six elementary categories of regional abnormalities: normal lung, ground-glass opacity, consolidation, reticular opacity, emphysema, and honeycombing [32]. They found that CNN outperforms SVM, with 95% and 81% accuracy, respectively. The CNN approach was especially valuable in distinguishing parenchymal abnormalities with pathological ambiguity, for instance normal compared to emphysema or honeycombing compared to reticular opacity. The process of data extraction in CNN was deemed an advantage for interscanner applicability of the classifier, since its unsupervised extraction of features warrants adaptation to different sets of data source. Noteworthy, the more layer in the CNN structure, the higher the accuracy of the classifier, but still balanced gaze should be pursued between complexity of the system and accuracy of the classification. The in-depth discussion of this branch might seem beyond the common understanding of the medical arena; for this reason engineering is deeply involved in medical development of these tools.

Difficulties

Difficulties in imaging of ILD include several factors that are dependent either on patient compliance or on technical factors. First of all, reproducibility of breath depth is a major determinant of quantitation of lung tissue by CT. Spirometric co-registration of image acquisition has been long proposed, yet the complexity of the hardware and its limited availability currently represent major limitations in clinical use. Spirometric co-registration is applied more frequently in pediatric imaging where the compliance of the patient to breath instruction might be minimal. Anyway, the development of the majority of AI algorithms for ILD imaging is based on non-gated imaging, which intrinsically accounts for the longitudinal variability encountered in the application of the software. Spatial warping of volume CT would also be possible to facilitate overlapping of volumetric data, yet this process would not account for regional artifactual variation in lung density and would therefore result in unpredictable classification. The problem of volume consistency is also to be considered in the natural course of ILD with fibrotic behavior, where longitudinal volume reduction occurs as a natural course of the disease. Therefore, this most relevant feature of lung imaging should not be deemed for artificial correction.

Second, the assessment of lung abnormalities is prone to technical variability, either as a result of contemporary different CT protocols (e.g., intra-vendor and inter-vendor, low-dose protocols, etc.) or as an expected longitudinal perspective of technology development (e.g., reconstruction algorithm with iterative or artificial intelligence technology, X-ray beam filtering, etc.). In this field, simple methods by analysis of histogram density seem more robust than complex algorithms for textural analysis [33]. However, some algorithms for textural analysis are expressively designed to minimize such variability, as it will be detailed below [33, 34].

Clinical Perspective of AI in ILD

The technological development of AI analysis for ILD is driven by the clinical need for accuracy in disease characterization and classification, as well as by the growing availability of treatments that reduce the rate of disease progression. Following are the AI application for ILD categories that are currently investigated in research field and are frontline candidates for implementation in the clinical routine.

Idiopathic Pulmonary Fibrosis (IPF)

Several authors investigated the use of AI in the field of idiopathic pulmonary fibrosis (IPF), in the last decades. The rise of AI in characterization of IPF is promoted by emerging therapeutic options, which brought about a paradigm shift in the demand of initial and longitudinal assessment of the disease.

In patients with diagnosis of IPF, the density histogram can help in the stratification of disease course, by longitudinal analysis. The simple histogram approach was reported inferior to expert visual scoring of ILD, at single time-point evaluation on baseline data. On the other hand, the histogram was better suited for characterization of longitudinal changes. Best et al. showed that annual CT could show significant increase of mean lung density, and decrease of kurtosis and skewness, showing worsening of lung fibrosis in IPF patients [35]. Further studies confirmed this observation and showed that the histogram analysis by percentiles could be useful in depicting minor changes in ground-glass or reticular component, respectively by using the 40th or 80th percentile [23]. As mentioned above, the use of histogram deprives the HRCT from the detailed panoramic view (one of the major advantages of HRCT), and therefore its use in single time point shows lower yield compared to the visual rating, because the latter can describe the disease complexity in its regional heterogeneity [36]. The use of histogram for quantification of regional heterogeneity was investigated by selecting individual histograms from small areas in the lung; this approach was shown effective for recognizing areas of normal lung, which was associated with outcome [24].

Textural approaches by either two- or three-dimensional analysis of lung parenchyma were largely applied in the setting of clinical trials, mostly as secondary or surrogate endpoint. As a consequence, their clinical use is foreseen as a natural extension of the experience gained in experimental setting, which indeed provides a robust body of literature to drive practical clinical evaluation. The most known software for this application include the adaptive multiple feature method (AMFM) [37, 38], computer-aided lung informatics for pathology evaluation and rating (CALIPER) [26], data-driven textural analysis (DTA) [34], and quantitative interstitial lung disease (QILD) [19, 39, 40]. It is noteworthy that all the available models perform well for stratification of functional impairment and prognosis; meanwhile they show complementary capability. The use of each algorithm is thereafter discussed.

The *AMFM platform* is based on Bayesian classifier that includes a process of selection for ranking the features on the basis of their power to discriminate between reference examples of tissue [41]. The classification by AMFM was comparable to expert radiologist in rating areas of admixed ground glass and reticulation, at baseline. The classification of ground glass and reticulation was associated with prognostic outcome including functional decline, hospitalization, or survival [38]. Salisbury et al. reported that baseline extent ≥10% of ground glass and reticulation by AMFM yields a twofold risk of disease progression, even after adjustment for gender, age, physiology, and smoking status [38]. Furthermore, the longitudinal quantitation of ground glass and reticulation by AMFM was weakly associated with proportional reduction in forced vital capacity (FVC). One limitation of this software is found in its susceptibility to different acquisition protocols.

The *CALIPER platform* allows for classification of seven elementary patterns as follows: normal lung, ground-glass opacity, reticular density, honeycombing, and three degrees of low attenuation (mild, moderate, severe). The process of digitalization of textural information is based on volumetric reference samples (sized 15 x 15 x 15 mm) selected by human experts. The algorithm analyzes such volume, extracts the features, and operates feature selection to distil the signature with the highest yield in classifying each of the seven elementary patterns. Furthermore, this algorithm can segment the vascular texture for estimating pulmonary vascular volume (PVV) (Fig. 41.2) and an indirect perivascular metric called "vascular related structures" (VRS). The VRS potentially represents fine interstitial abnormalities abutting the vascular surface; therefore, its quantitation might show promise for estimate of early pulmonary changes, likely beyond human sight. The segmentation of vessels represents a new biomarker for lung characterization, and it outstands as unique CT feature without visual correlate. Furthermore, the vascular quantitation maintains clinical intelligibility, which is sometimes quite hard to understand for other new biomarkers based on mathematical lexicon. There is a wealth of literature about CALIPER in IPF; it was validated across several acquisition and reconstruction parameters, including low-dose CT. This software was first tested against physiology on the single time point, showing good correlation

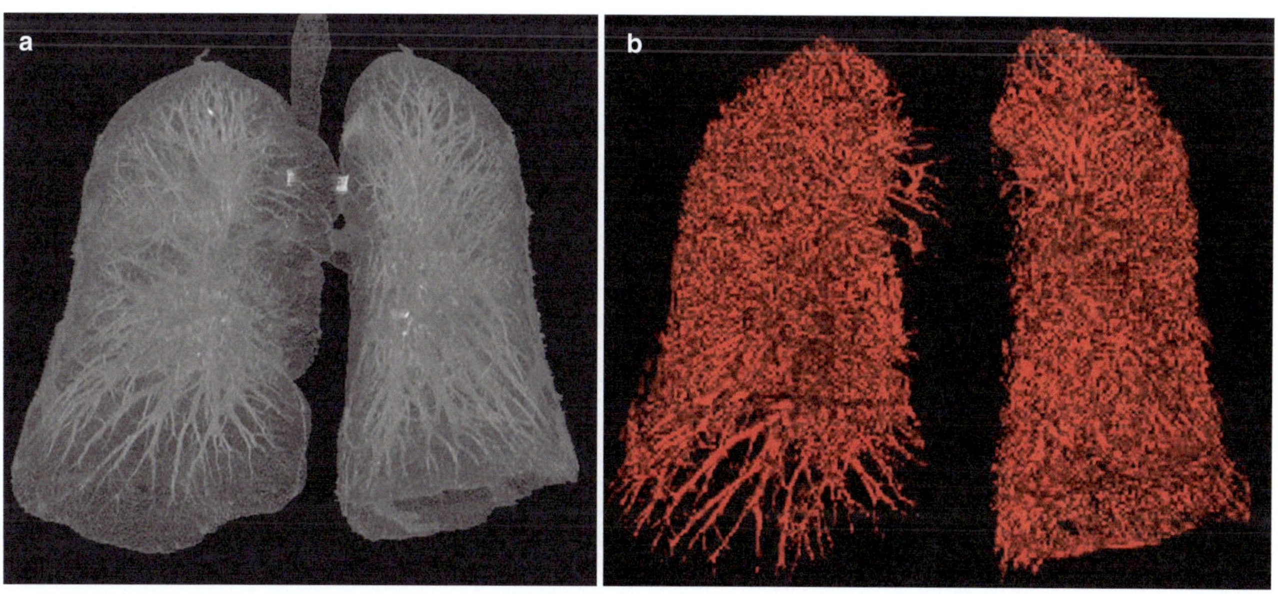

Fig. 41.2 (**a**, **b**) Three-dimensional reconstruction of segmented vessels by CALIPER

between the ILD score and pulmonary function tests. Jacob et al. showed that the extent of ILD by CALIPER could be a valuable surrogate for the "composite physiological index" (CPI), a multifactorial physiology index for the stratification of disease severity and prognosis [42]. On longitudinal characterization of disease, this software correlated with clinical trajectory, including functional decline and survival [43]. Furthermore, Sverzellati et al. showed that HRCT by CALIPER could complement physiology in the longitudinal stratification of long-term disease course, in IPF patients with 2-year clinically stable disease. The authors reported a discrete threshold for practical application in clinical use: an increase of ILD by *20% relative variation of ILD at 1 year* since the baseline was associated with worse outcome. For instance, a baseline ILD extent 15% that grows to 19% after 1 year should be deemed +27% relative variation and therefore is associated with increased risk of disease progression, despite apparent clinical stability. Similarly, *20% relative variation of VRS at 2 years* was also associated with worse outcome strata [44]. The discovery of VRS parameter opened more scenarios for clinical and research practicality; indeed, the use of this metric was proposed for cohort enrichment in clinical trials because it could warrant reduction of the population size and costs [45]. The clinical use of CALIPER is also assisted by a graphic synthesis of the volumetric data into a chart called "glyph." The "glyph" is a rounded chart composed of six wedges, namely, one wedge a lobe (lingual deemed an individual lobe). The size of each wedge varies according to the volume variation of each lobe, helping the topographic reading of tissue damage distribution. The segmented parenchymal abnormalities are schematized by color-coded circles, as a corresponding proportion of volumetric representation in each individual wedge lobe (Fig. 41.3).

The *DTA platform* is based on an unsupervised algorithm for classifying pulmonary abnormalities into a dictionary of elemental low-level pixel patterns from lung CT [46]. The process is based on the unsupervised analysis of innumerable small patches of lung CT, sized 3 x 3 mm. Elementary items of the dictionary are weighted according to their yield for reconstruction of novel image regions; this process grants selection of the most relevant unsupervised features to be used in the classifier. The item selection brings to a consolidated dictionary composed of 512 elements, an apparently huge number of features compared to visual capability and human annotation capacity. The dictionary of unsupervised items is reconciled with clinical meaning by human expert selecting areas of lung CT with typical features of UIP (reticulation, traction bronchiectasis, and honeycomb). Despite that unsupervised data extraction is operated on small samples (3 x 3 mm), the analysis of geometrical complexities is gained by using clinical classifiers of larger size (14 x 14 mm). This process warrants the ability to classify areas of ILD that reflect features of UIP; however, to date, it cannot be assumed that DTA warrants UIP diagnosis because this algorithm is still unexplored out of UIP patients. Because DTA works on planar reference, this software can be applied either to volumetric or sequential HRCT data [46]. Humphreys et al. showed that DTA classifier has moderate correlation with visual scoring of fibrotic lung; noteworthy DTA was associated with mean score from two human experts, despite substantial interobserver variability [46]. The use of DTA for longitudinal evolution of fibrotic lung was associated with functional decline, also showing potential advantage compared to the variability in ILD scoring progression from human experts. Also, DTA score adds information beyond parameters based on the density histogram. Multivariable models for progression-free survival including both DTA and features based on density histogram retained DTA score and discarded histogram variables, thus suggesting that the clinical yield of DTA is high for stratification of prognosis (Humphries SM et al., data submitted). When reading fibrosis score by DTA, the figure of ILD extent seems one order of magnitude higher than visual score (e.g., mean DTA extent 36.6% vs mean visual extent 4.2%) [46]; this mismatch warrants further investigation on the weigh that such a rating system should be interpreted with. The longitudinal assessment of lung fibrosis by DTA was given a reference value for minimally clinically important difference. An increase in ILD extent of 3.4% over a period of

Fig. 41.3 (**a, b**) Synthetized representation of ILD segmentation into glyphs, by CALIPER. Two case scenarios are shown, with disease stability (**a**) or disease progression (**b**), over 2 years. The visual evaluation of glyph allows ready understanding of the three-dimensional evolution of the disease, including involvement of individual lobes (size of wedge) and characterization of each of seven elementary patterns of lung abnormalities (color-coded circles). The use of glyph seems particularly promising for clinical use into structured report.
In case of stable disease (**a**), the glyph shows heterogeneous distribution of disease since baseline (top row) with substantial restrictive involvement of the right lower lobe (RL). The individual lobar involvement is denoted by the size of the wedge; in this case the RL wedge is substantially restricted compared to the 360° degrees of representation of the whole lung volume. The disease severity remains stable at the first (mid-row) and second (bottom row) annual follow-up by HRCT, as it can be noted by the steady representation of color-coded lung abnormalities.
In case of progressive disease (**b**), the glyph shows relatively homogeneous distribution of disease across lung lobes, at baseline (top row). The evolution of diseases shows heterogeneous severity across lobes, which is easily depicted by observing the relative increase in size of the wedge for the right middle lobe (RM) the first (mid-row) and second (bottom row) annual follow-up by HRCT. The glyph graphics show that every lobe but RL were substantially involved with honeycombing (brown circle)

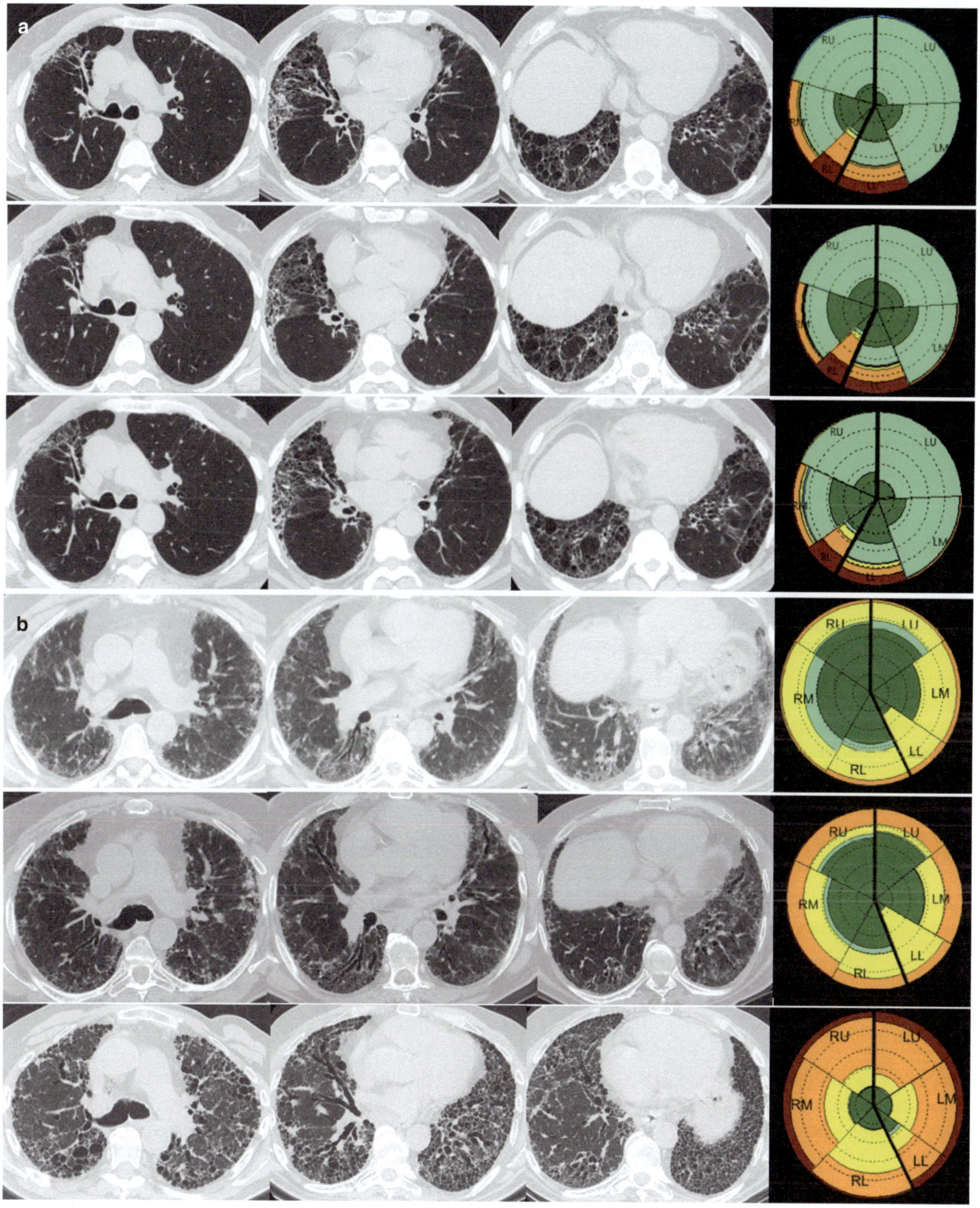
a
b
RU
LU
RM
LM
RL
LL

12.5–15 months was meant clinically relevant when compared to anchor physiology variables at follow-up (e.g., corresponding to 5–10% decrease in FVC relative change compared to baseline) [47]. The prognostic yield of DTA was also confirmed in IPF patients with minimal functional impairment (FVC > 80% at baseline), in whom the increase of 5% fibrosis score by DTA was associated with a hazard ratio of 1.18 for progression-free survival (Humphries SM et al., data submitted). The use of DTA was also extended to subclinical setting in asymptomatic first-degree relatives of patients with familial interstitial pneumonia (FIP), for the detection of interstitial lung abnormalities (ILA) on CT. Salisbury et al. reported that DTA paralleled visual rating of ILA at baseline and showed association with progression to ILD in 5 years [48].

The *QILD platform* is based on a mathematical method called robustness-driven feature selection (RDFS), which was meant for producing a CT texture classifier that is robust across potential variations of CT data [49]. The aim of RDFS is to select a feature subset that is robust to CT technical factors, under the key assumption that robust features produce robust classifiers. The feature computation of QILD is based on extremely small volumetric samples of lung CT (each composed of 9 voxels sized 0.5 x 0.5 x 0.5 mm by data curation) assembled into a library that includes 2008 training volumetric samples with balanced representation of lung fibrosis, ground glass, honeycombing, and normal lung. In this algorithm, each feature is assigned a *robustness index* that is computed directly from a multi-reconstruction dataset: the *robustness index* of a given feature is calculated as the ratio of standard deviation across different protocols divided by the standard deviation within the reference protocol. In other words, the *robustness index* compares the variation due to changing technical factors (inter-protocol) against the intrinsic variation found within a single reference protocol (intra-protocol) [49]. Low values of *robustness index* are preferred in the RDFS for selecting the 50 features of QILD platform. Therefore, the method of QILD shows promise for the utmost performance across independent centers and populations. While QILD is designed to recognize and segment any portion of abnormal lung on CT, it also includes a specific classifier called quantitative lung fibrosis (QLF) that aims to isolate selected fibrotic component. The use of QLF allows specific detection and segmentation of fibrotic reticulation pattern, as per definition from Kim et al. [33]. The accuracy of QILD for detection and quantitation of ILD was as high as 0.96 area under the curve, compared to human expert reference [19]. The short-term repeatability coefficient of QILD was 0.4% for the whole lung and 2% for the most severe lobe within a subject [19]. Kim et al. reported that both QILD and features based on density histogram significantly varied in a 7-month period of follow-up in patients with IPF; nonetheless QLF showed tighter association with functional decay compared with histogram kurtosis and skewness, and overall QILD score [33].

The above methods for trial and clinical use in IPF patients were deemed for disease detection and severity rating, yet none of the above specifically addressed pattern recognition and definition of disease diagnosis. This task was targeted by a deep learning method proposed by Walsh et al. within the radiological scheme of the 2011 American Thoracic Society (ATS)/European Respiratory Society (ERS)/Japanese Respiratory Society (JRS)/Latin American Thoracic Association(ALAT) criteria for a usual interstitial pneumonia pattern and the 2018 Fleischner Society criteria for usual interstitial pneumonia on high-resolution CT [29]. The deep learning method was based on a multicenter database of 1157 cases with CT signs of ILD; the database was preprocessed to create montages of 4 segmented axial high-resolution CT image slices; this process led to final training dataset with 420,096 unique montages, for algorithm training. The deep learning algorithm was supported by a neural network architecture based on CNN and called Inception-ResNet-v2 [29]. The algorithm was trained and retrained several times to allow learning process on this sufficiently large dataset. The use of the algorithm on a test set by 150 CTs of fibrotic lung disease ought to outstand the performance of the deep learning process, which could outperform the classification of 56/91 chest radiologists in adjudicating categories from the 2011 American ATS/ERS/JRS/ALAT criteria for a UIP pattern. The trained deep learning system took 2.31 seconds to analyze 150 cases and output the radiological classification [29]; this operational time might vary according to the computational power of the machine.

ILD Associated with Connective Tissue Disease (CTD-ILD)

Connective tissue diseases (CTD) are associated with systemic disorders, including secondary pulmonary involvement with ILD, which is named CTD-ILD. The pulmonary damage is a major determinant of morbidity and mortality in CTD-ILD. The assessment of CTD-ILD by AI application for CT images began a couple of decades ago. Similarly to IPF, the histogram-based approach was the first method applied to stratification of disease severity and prognostication. Textural analyses were implemented also for this group of secondary ILD; Jacob et al. showed that visual scoring generally identified more extensive ILD and emphysema than CALIPER across several groups of CTD-ILD, including the most representative diseases [50]. In particular, there was opposite proportion of ground glass and reticulation between visual and CALIPER, with the latter scoring more extensive ground-glass component. Furthermore, the parameter PVV showed the highest yield in predicting mortality, after correction for age and gender, suggesting that this parameter might be extremely relevant in the setting of CTD-ILD [50].

ILD associated with systemic sclerosis (SSc-ILD) is the leading cause of death in this CTD; therefore, the assessment of pulmonary damage shows major yield for prognostication. The assessment of pulmonary physiology in SSc-ILD is limited by confounding factors such as myopathy; for this reason the objective measurement of ILD by CT is deemed relevant. The expected radiological pattern in SSc-ILD is called nonspecific interstitial pneumonia (NSIP), which is different from UIP pattern in its distribution (sparing of subpleural lung) and elementary finding (relative abundance of ground glass, rare honeycombing). In 2008, Goh et al. reported a robust method for stratification of prognosis in SSc-ILD; it was based on contingent use of visual ILD extent on CT and physiology [51]. Since this pioneer visual reference method, many authors tried quantitative methods to investigate SSc-ILD with the aim of avoiding interobserver variability. Features based on density histogram were reported in association with lung physiology. Ninaber et al. reported association between the 85th percentile of density histogram and diffusion capacity and FVC (both % predicted) [52]. The method of percentiles was also valuable for testing the response to autologous hematopoietic stem cell transplantation; the 90th percentile of density histogram showed a negative correlation with FVC during an 18-month period of follow-up after transplantation [53]. In SSc-ILD with single lung transplantation, the longitudinal variation of histogram features is significantly different between transplanted and native lung [54]. Quantitative scoring of SSc-ILD by skewness and kurtosis of the density histogram was associated with clinical prediction models of mortality [55]. Furthermore, Saldana et al. showed that the longitudinal change of skewness and kurtosis is associated with functional decline and survival in SSc-ILD (Fig. 41.4), after adjustment for age, sex, pack-years, and change in visual CT [56]. Ufuk et al. showed that the visual method by Goh into limited or extensive disease was better associated with histogram kurtosis in the density range between −1024 HU and − 200 HU, among an assortment of several features based on density histogram [57]. Radiomics application to SSc-ILD showed that multivariable model (combination of neighContrast.LHL and M_correlation.HLL) outperformed visual scoring in predicting the Gender-Age-Physiology (GAP) stage [58]. Textural classifiers in SSc-ILD were capable of differentiating between SSc-ILD patients and controls, with as high as 0.981 area under the curve [59]. Nonetheless, Milanese et al. warned on the substantial variability when applying the machine learning algorithm across different CT protocols, including iterative reconstruction algorithms [59]. The limit of inter-scan variability should be controlled when assessing SSc-ILD texture by the QILD platform. Kim et al. reported that SSc-ILD extent by QLF (e.g., detection and segmentation fibrotic reticulation pattern) was strongly associated with visual scoring and extent >25% yielded 0.96 area under the curve for 25% extent by visual score, in the scleroderma lung study [60]. The full QILD classifier (including also lung fibrosis, ground glass, honeycombing, and normal

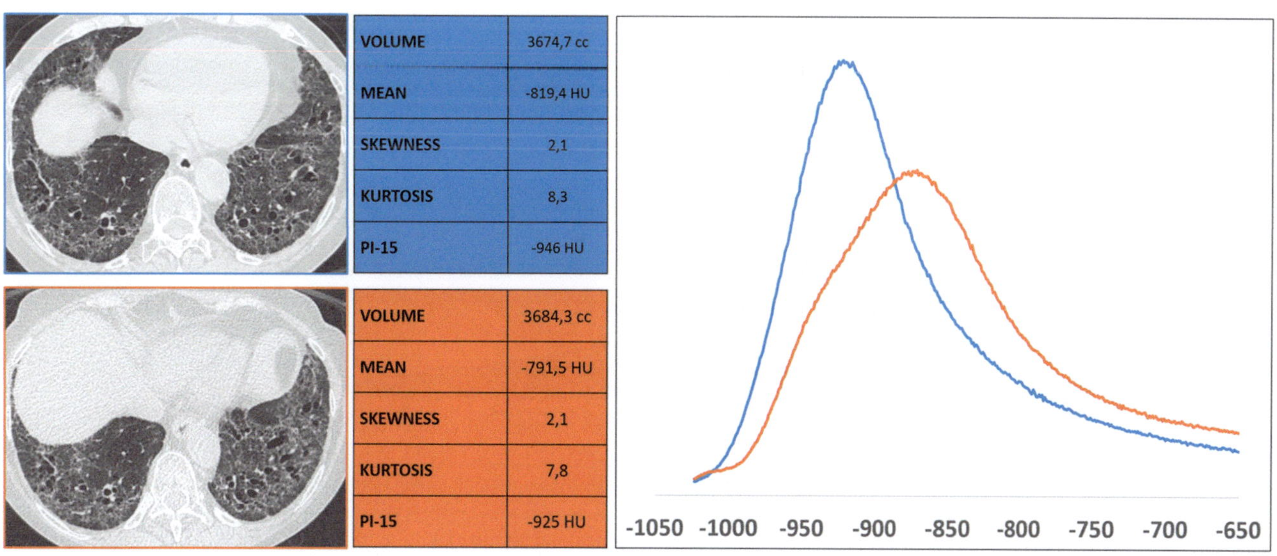

Fig. 41.4 Histogram of density in a patient with progressive SSc-ILD. The outline of the histograms varies from baseline (blue line) to follow-up (orange line), reflecting a substantial variation in tissue-air proportion in the lung. Histogram metrics vary (blue box baseline, orange box follow-up) with increase of mean lung density (from −819 HU to −792), 15th percentile (from −946 HU to −925 HU), and kurtosis (from 8.3 to 7.8). Noteworthy, this example shows a possible pitfall of using the longitudinal evolution of individual parameters of the density histogram: the skewness of the histogram remains stable (2.1) across the time points, which represents a limitation of the global adimensional representation of parenchymal complexities out of their specific geometric distribution

lung) could quantify the change of individual morphological patterns on CT of SSc-ILD patients with or without treatment, notably showing reduction of QILD in patients under treatment, compared to increase of QILD in the placebo group [61]. Conversely, the CALIPER platform could not depict pulmonary improvement after therapy, in a period of 2 years [62].

In patients with rheumatoid arthritis ILD (RA-ILD), Ito et al. compared visual semiquantitative ILD score with a histogram-based feature called fibrosis ratio [63]. The fibrosis ratio by density histogram was calculated as the ratio of the number of voxels with density > − 400 HU divided by the total number of voxels (Fig. 41.5). In a population of RA-ILD patients with a mortality of 24.6% over almost 5 years, the histogram-based fibrosis ratio was associated with poor outcome. Notably, the authors reported that fibrosis score > 20% yielded a ninefold increased risk of mortality [63]. However, the longitudinal use of fibrotic ratio might be limited by unpredictable variations in lung volumetry and components of lung injury, for instance in case of combined pulmonary fibrosis and emphysema [64]. Furthermore, RA-ILD has also a morphological component that cannot be captured by histogram; namely, RA-ILD is most frequently represented by UIP pattern, which is ultimately a negative prognostic factor described by visual assessment and otherwise diluted in the one-dimensional histogram parameters [63].

Conclusion

The application of AI to chest imaging has been rapidly evolving over the last decades, showing the ability to meet research and clinical demands. Several AI approaches have been successfully employed for disease detection and severity rating, offering a solution to the human intra- and interob-

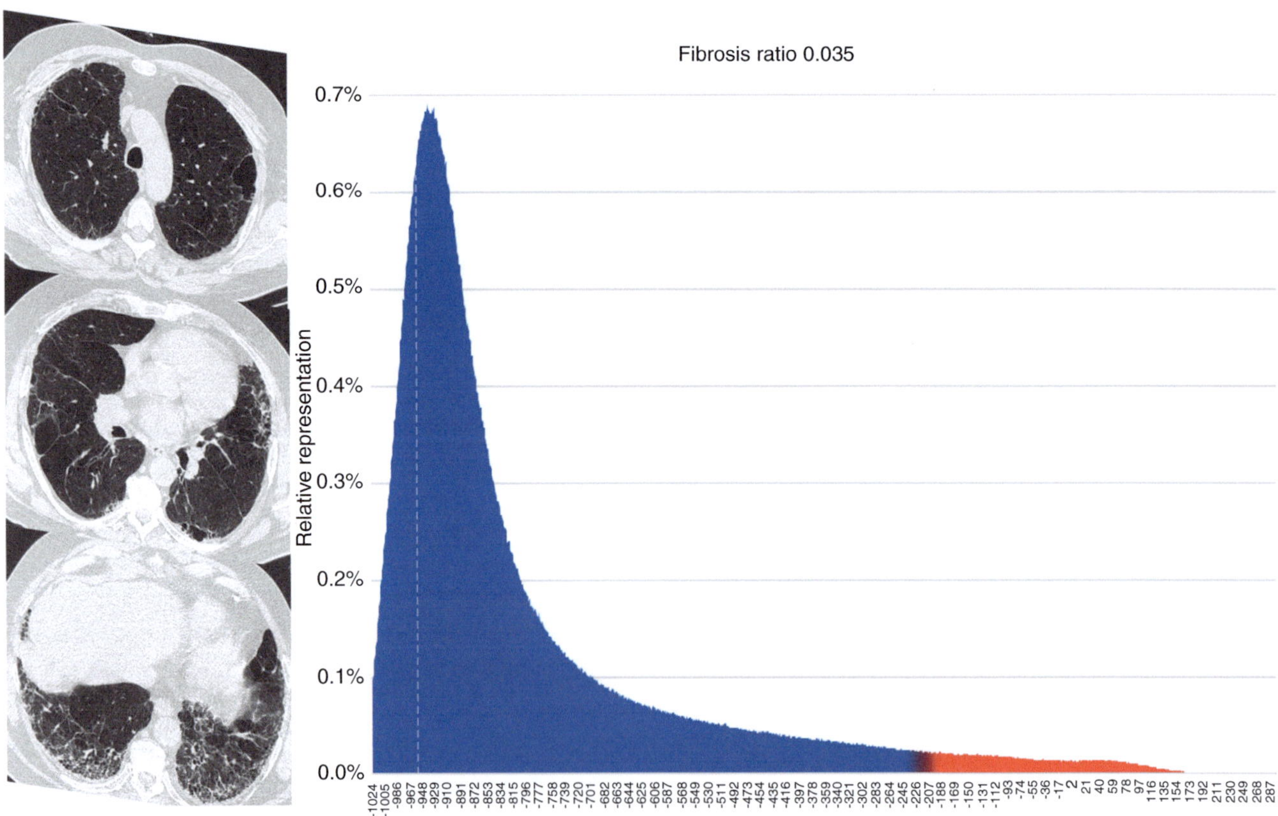

Fig. 41.5 Patient with RA-ILD as depicted by the "UIP-like" pattern on the three axial CT images. The use of "fibrosis ratio" (according to Ito et al., Ref. [63]) is applied by analysis of density histogram: lung voxels above −200 HU (red) are divided by the total amount of lung voxels (blue and red). The fibrosis ration in this patient reports ILD extent 3.5%. Noteworthy, the histogram of density also shows a sizeable proportion of voxels below −950 HU (voxels plotted on the left of the dashed white line define the proportion of emphysematous lung), which quantifies emphysema extent 20.8%. Noteworthy, both fibrosis and emphysema contribute in the impairment of lung diffusion capacity with additive effect on the carbon monoxide diffusion capacity (DLco), which most often reflects the severity of lung impairment, albeit appropriate quality of DLco remains a challenge in clinical practice. Otherwise, fibrosis (restrictive) and emphysema (obstructive) competitively influence respiratory dynamics and lung volume at physiology test, which might result in normal forced vital capacity and forced expiratory volume in the first second despite substantial lung disruption (3.5% fibrosis and 20.8% emphysema). The use of CT for lung impairment definitely provides relevant clinical value in the multidisciplinary management of patients with CTD and complex ILD representation

server variability. Some AI algorithms have been developed with the purpose of evaluating longitudinal changes over time or in response to treatment, with the aim to intercept specific clinical needs of diverse ILD patients, for both IPF and CTD-ILD. The use of AI in ILD is ranking to clinically deploy, notably providing with the potential to parallel the performance of expert chest radiologists and, therefore, to expand the capacity of good diagnostic and prognostic performance. The integration of AI software with radiology and other clinical data is the next level of personalized ILD care, which should be pursued to optimize the benefits of such synergistic multidisciplinary relationship.

References

1. Desai S, Devaraj A, Lynch D, Sverzellati N, Elicker BM. High-resolution CT of the lung. Webb, Müller and Naidich – 6th edition. 2020.
2. Silva M, Milanese G, Seletti V, Ariani A, Sverzellati N. Pulmonary quantitative CT imaging in focal and diffuse disease: current research and clinical applications. Br J Radiol. 2017;91:20170644.
3. Walsh SL, Calandriello L, Sverzellati N, Wells AU, Hansell DM, Consort UIPO. Interobserver agreement for the ATS/ERS/JRS/ALAT criteria for a UIP pattern on CT. Thorax. 2016;71(1):45–51.
4. Chassagnon G, Vakalopoulou M, Paragios N, Revel MP. Artificial intelligence applications for thoracic imaging. Eur J Radiol. 2020;123:108774.
5. Saketkoo LA, Mittoo S, Huscher D, Khanna D, Dellaripa PF, Distler O, et al. Connective tissue disease related interstitial lung diseases and idiopathic pulmonary fibrosis: provisional core sets of domains and instruments for use in clinical trials. Thorax. 2014;69(5):428–36.
6. Soffer S, Ben-Cohen A, Shimon O, Amitai MM, Greenspan H, Klang E. Convolutional neural networks for radiologic images: a Radiologist's guide. Radiology. 2019;290(3):590–606.
7. (QIBA) QIBA. Available from: http://qibawiki.rsna.org/images/a/a8/QIBA_CT_Lung_Density_Profile_090420-clean.pdf.
8. Sverzellati N, Calabro E, Chetta A, Concari G, Larici AR, Mereu M, et al. Visual score and quantitative CT indices in pulmonary fibrosis: relationship with physiologic impairment. Radiol Med. 2007;112(8):1160–72.
9. Beinert T, Behr J, Mehnert F, Kohz P, Seemann M, Rienmuller R, et al. Spirometrically controlled quantitative CT for assessing diffuse parenchymal lung disease. J Comput Assist Tomogr. 1995;19(6):924–31.
10. Rienmuller RK, Behr J, Kalender WA, Schatzl M, Altmann I, Merin M, et al. Standardized quantitative high resolution CT in lung diseases. J Comput Assist Tomogr. 1991;15(5):742–9.
11. Ariani A, Lumetti F, Silva M, Santilli D, Mozzani F, Lucchini G, et al. Systemic sclerosis interstitial lung disease evaluation: comparison between semiquantitative and quantitative computed tomography assessments. J Biol Regul Homeost Agents. 2014;28(3):507–13.
12. Hartley PG, Galvin JR, Hunninghake GW, Merchant JA, Yagla SJ, Speakman SB, et al. High-resolution CT-derived measures of lung density are valid indexes of interstitial lung disease. J Appl Physiol. 1985;76(1):271–7.
13. Best AC, Lynch AM, Bozic CM, Miller D, Grunwald GK, Lynch DA. Quantitative CT indexes in idiopathic pulmonary fibrosis: relationship with physiologic impairment. Radiology. 2003;228(2):407–14.
14. Mascalchi M, Camiciottoli G, Diciotti S. Lung densitometry: why, how and when. J Thorac Dis. 2017;9(9):3319–45.
15. Orlandi I, Camiciottoli G, Diciotti S, Bartolucci M, Cavigli E, Nacci F, et al. Thin-section and low-dose volumetric computed tomographic densitometry of the lung in systemic sclerosis. J Comput Assist Tomogr. 2006;30(5):823–7.
16. Goldin JG. Quantitative CT of the lung. Radiol Clin N Am. 2002;40(1):145–62.
17. Ariani A, Imperatori A, Castiglioni M, Daffre E, Aiello M, Bertorelli G, et al. Quantitative computed tomography detects interstitial lung diseases proven by biopsy. Sarcoidosis, Vasc Diffuse Lung Dis. 2018;35(1):16–20.
18. Nguyen-Kim TDL, Maurer B, Suliman YA, Morsbach F, Distler O, Frauenfelder T. The impact of slice-reduced computed tomography on histogram-based densitometry assessment of lung fibrosis in patients with systemic sclerosis. J Thorac Dis. 2018;10(4):2142–52.
19. Wu X, Kim GH, Salisbury ML, Barber D, Bartholmai BJ, Brown KK, et al. Computed tomographic biomarkers in idiopathic pulmonary fibrosis. The future of quantitative analysis. Am J Respir Crit Care Med. 2019;199(1):12–21.
20. Sumikawa H, Johkoh T, Yamamoto S, Yanagawa M, Inoue A, Honda O, et al. Computed tomography values calculation and volume histogram analysis for various computed tomographic patterns of diffuse lung diseases. J Comput Assist Tomogr. 2009;33(5):731–8.
21. Sumikawa H, Johkoh T, Yamamoto S, Takahei K, Ueguchi T, Ogata Y, et al. Quantitative analysis for computed tomography findings of various diffuse lung diseases using volume histogram analysis. J Comput Assist Tomogr. 2006;30(2):244–9.
22. Lubner MG, Smith AD, Sandrasegaran K, Sahani DV, Pickhardt PJ. CT texture analysis: definitions, applications, biologic correlates, and challenges. Radiographics. 2017;37(5):1483–503.
23. Colombi D, Dinkel J, Weinheimer O, Obermayer B, Buzan T, Nabers D, et al. Visual vs fully automatic histogram-based assessment of idiopathic pulmonary fibrosis (IPF) progression using sequential multidetector computed tomography (MDCT). PLoS One. 2015;10(6):e0130653.
24. Iwasawa T, Asakura A, Sakai F, Kanauchi T, Gotoh T, Ogura T, et al. Assessment of prognosis of patients with idiopathic pulmonary fibrosis by computer-aided analysis of CT images. J Thorac Imaging. 2009;24(3):216–22.
25. Hansell DM, Goldin JG, King TE Jr, Lynch DA, Richeldi L, Wells AU. CT staging and monitoring of fibrotic interstitial lung diseases in clinical practice and treatment trials: a position paper from the Fleischner Society. Lancet Respir Med. 2015;3(6):483–96.
26. Bartholmai BJ, Raghunath S, Karwoski RA, Moua T, Rajagopalan S, Maldonado F, et al. Quantitative computed tomography imaging of interstitial lung diseases. J Thorac Imaging. 2013;28(5):298–307.
27. Sverzellati N, Silva M. The matter of lung: quantification of vascular substance in asthma. Am J Respir Crit Care Med. 2018.
28. Raghu G, Remy-Jardin M, Myers JL, Richeldi L, Ryerson CJ, Lederer DJ, et al. Diagnosis of idiopathic pulmonary fibrosis. An Official ATS/ERS/JRS/ALAT clinical practice guideline. Am J Respir Crit Care Med. 2018;198(5):e44–68.
29. Walsh SLF, Calandriello L, Silva M, Sverzellati N. Deep learning for classifying fibrotic lung disease on high-resolution computed tomography: a case-cohort study The Lancet Respir Med. 2018.
30. Draelos RL, Dov D, Mazurowski MA, Lo JY, Henao R, Rubin GD, et al. Machine-learning-based multiple abnormality prediction with large-scale chest computed tomography volumes. Med Image Anal. 2020;67:101857.
31. Chassagnon G, Vakalopoulou M, Battistella E, Christodoulidis S, Hoang-Thi TN, Dangeard S, et al. AI-driven quantification, staging and outcome prediction of COVID-19 pneumonia. Med Image Anal. 2020;67:101860.
32. Kim GB, Jung KH, Lee Y, Kim HJ, Kim N, Jun S, et al. Comparison of shallow and deep learning methods on classifying the regional pattern of diffuse lung disease. J Digit Imaging. 2018;31(4):415–24.

33. Kim HJ, Brown MS, Chong D, Gjertson DW, Lu P, Kim HJ, et al. Comparison of the quantitative CT imaging biomarkers of idiopathic pulmonary fibrosis at baseline and early change with an interval of 7 months. Acad Radiol. 2015;22(1):70–80.
34. Humphries SM, Yagihashi K, Huckleberry J, Rho BH, Schroeder JD, Strand M, et al. Idiopathic pulmonary fibrosis: data-driven textural analysis of extent of fibrosis at baseline and 15-month follow-up. Radiology 2017:161177.
35. Best AC, Meng J, Lynch AM, Bozic CM, Miller D, Grunwald GK, et al. Idiopathic pulmonary fibrosis: physiologic tests, quantitative CT indexes, and CT visual scores as predictors of mortality. Radiology. 2008;246(3):935–40.
36. Kliment CR, Araki T, Doyle TJ, Gao W, Dupuis J, Latourelle JC, et al. A comparison of visual and quantitative methods to identify interstitial lung abnormalities. BMC Pulm Med. 2015;15:134.
37. Uppaluri R, Hoffman EA, Sonka M, Hunninghake GW, McLennan G. Interstitial lung disease: a quantitative study using the adaptive multiple feature method. Am J Respir Crit Care Med. 1999;159(2):519–25.
38. Salisbury ML, Lynch DA, van Beek EJ, Kazerooni EA, Guo J, Xia M, et al. Idiopathic pulmonary fibrosis: the association between the adaptive multiple features method and fibrosis outcomes. Am J Respir Crit Care Med. 2017;195(7):921–9.
39. Kim GHJ, Weigt SS, Belperio JA, Brown MS, Shi Y, Lai JH, et al. Prediction of idiopathic pulmonary fibrosis progression using early quantitative changes on CT imaging for a short term of clinical 18-24-month follow-ups. Eur Radiol. 2020;30(2):726–34.
40. Walsh SLF, Humphries SM, Wells AU, Brown KK. Imaging research in fibrotic lung disease; applying deep learning to unsolved problems. Lancet Respir Med. 2020;8(11):1144–53.
41. Uppaluri R, Hoffman EA, Sonka M, Hartley PG, Hunninghake GW, McLennan G. Computer recognition of regional lung disease patterns. Am J Respir Crit Care Med. 1999;160(2):648–54.
42. Jacob J, Bartholmai BJ, Rajagopalan S, Kokosi M, Nair A, Karwoski R, et al. Automated quantitative computed tomography versus visual computed tomography scoring in idiopathic pulmonary fibrosis: validation against pulmonary function. J Thorac Imaging. 2016;31(5):304–11.
43. Maldonado F, Moua T, Rajagopalan S, Karwoski RA, Raghunath S, Decker PA, et al. Automated quantification of radiological patterns predicts survival in idiopathic pulmonary fibrosis. Eur Respir J. 2014;43(1):204–12.
44. Sverzellati N, Silva M, Seletti V, Galeone C, Palmucci S, Piciucchi S, et al. Stratification of long-term outcome in stable idiopathic pulmonary fibrosis by combining longitudinal computed tomography and forced vital capacity. Eur Radiol. 2020;30(5):2669–79.
45. Jacob J, Bartholmai BJ, Rajagopalan S, van Moorsel CHM, van Es HW, van Beek FT, et al. Predicting outcomes in idiopathic pulmonary fibrosis using automated computed tomographic analysis. Am J Respir Crit Care Med. 2018;198(6):767–76.
46. Humphries SM, Yagihashi K, Huckleberry J, Rho BH, Schroeder JD, Strand M, et al. Idiopathic pulmonary fibrosis: data-driven textural analysis of extent of fibrosis at baseline and 15-month follow-up. Radiology. 2017;285(1):270–8.
47. Humphries SM, Swigris JJ, Brown KK, Strand M, Gong Q, Sundy JS, et al. Quantitative high-resolution computed tomography fibrosis score: performance characteristics in idiopathic pulmonary fibrosis. Eur Respir J 2018;52(3).
48. Salisbury ML, Hewlett JC, Ding G, Markin CR, Douglas K, Mason W, et al. Development and progression of radiologic abnormalities in individuals at risk for familial interstitial lung disease. Am J Respir Crit Care Med. 2020;201(10):1230–9.
49. Chong DY, Kim HJ, Lo P, Young S, McNitt-Gray MF, Abtin F, et al. Robustness-driven feature selection in classification of fibrotic interstitial lung disease patterns in computed tomography using 3D texture features. IEEE Trans Med Imaging. 2016;35(1):144–57.
50. Jacob J, Bartholmai BJ, Rajagopalan S, Brun AL, Egashira R, Karwoski R, et al. Evaluation of computer-based computer tomography stratification against outcome models in connective tissue disease-related interstitial lung disease: a patient outcome study. BMC Med. 2016;14(1):190.
51. Goh NS, Desai SR, Veeraraghavan S, Hansell DM, Copley SJ, Maher TM, et al. Interstitial lung disease in systemic sclerosis: a simple staging system. Am J Respir Crit Care Med. 2008;177(11):1248–54.
52. Ninaber MK, Stolk J, Smit J, Le Roy EJ, Kroft LJ, Bakker ME, et al. Lung structure and function relation in systemic sclerosis: application of lung densitometry. Eur J Radiol. 2015;84(5):975–9.
53. Wada DT, de Almeida FA, de Moraes DA, Dias JBE, Baddini-Martinez J, Oliveira MC, et al. Automatic quantitative computed tomography evaluation of the lungs in patients with systemic sclerosis treated with autologous stem cell transplantation. J Clin Rheumatol. 2020;26(7S Suppl 2):S158–S64.
54. Hinze AM, Lin CT, Hussien AF, Perin J, Venado A, Golden JA, et al. Longitudinal assessment of interstitial lung disease in single lung transplant recipients with scleroderma. Rheumatology (Oxford). 2020;59(4):790–8.
55. Ariani A, Silva M, Seletti V, Bravi E, Saracco M, Parisi S, et al. Quantitative chest computed tomography is associated with two prediction models of mortality in interstitial lung disease related to systemic sclerosis. Rheumatology (Oxford). 2017.
56. Saldana DC, Hague CJ, Murphy D, Coxson HO, Tschirren J, Peterson S, et al. Association of Computed Tomography Densitometry with disease severity, functional decline, and survival in systemic sclerosis-associated interstitial lung disease. Ann Am Thorac Soc. 2020;17(7):813–20.
57. Ufuk F, Demirci M, Altinisik G. Quantitative computed tomography assessment for systemic sclerosis-related interstitial lung disease: comparison of different methods. Eur Radiol. 2020;30(8):4369–80.
58. Martini K, Baessler B, Bogowicz M, Bluthgen C, Mannil M, Tanadini-Lang S, et al. Applicability of radiomics in interstitial lung disease associated with systemic sclerosis: proof of concept. Eur Radiol. 2020.
59. Milanese G, Mannil M, Martini K, Maurer B, Alkadhi H, Frauenfelder T. Quantitative CT texture analysis for diagnosing systemic sclerosis: effect of iterative reconstructions and radiation doses. Medicine (Baltimore). 2019;98(29):e16423.
60. Kim HG, Tashkin DP, Clements PJ, Li G, Brown MS, Elashoff R, et al. A computer-aided diagnosis system for quantitative scoring of extent of lung fibrosis in scleroderma patients. Clin Exp Rheumatol. 2010;28(5 Suppl 62):S26–35.
61. Kim HJ, Tashkin DP, Gjertson DW, Brown MS, Kleerup E, Chong S, et al. Transitions to different patterns of interstitial lung disease in scleroderma with and without treatment. Ann Rheum Dis. 2016;75(7):1367–71.
62. Baqir M, Makol A, Osborn TG, Bartholmai BJ, Ryu JH. Mycophenolate mofetil for scleroderma-related interstitial lung disease: a real world experience. PLoS One. 2017;12(5):e0177107.
63. Ito Y, Arita M, Kumagai S, Takei R, Noyama M, Tokioka F, et al. Radiological fibrosis score is strongly associated with worse survival in rheumatoid arthritis-related interstitial lung disease. Mod Rheumatol. 2019;29(1):98–104.
64. Cottin V, Cordier JF. Combined pulmonary fibrosis and emphysema in connective tissue disease. Curr Opin Pulm Med. 2012;18(5):418–27.

42 Artificial Intelligence-Based Evaluation of Infectious Disease Imaging: A COVID-19 Perspective

Li Fan, Jun Shi, Nannan Shi, Wenting Tu, Yun Bian, Xiuxiu Zhou, Yu Guan, Yuxin Shi, and Shiyuan Liu

Introduction

Artificial intelligence (AI) has been used in many medical fields, especially in medical imaging. AI was first used in the detection of lung nodules, then differential diagnosis and prognosis prediction, and so on. The application of AI in infectious disease is just rising, considering the outbreak of COVID-19 in early December 2019 [1]. This virus is a novel type of the coronavirus family, which is named 2019 novel coronavirus (2019-nCoV) by the World Health Organization (WHO) on January 7, 2020 [2]. The 2019-nCoV causes acute respiratory system infections and is also called coronavirus disease 19 (COVID-19). The WHO has declared COVID-19 is a public health emergency of international concern, because of rapid spread all over the world. Due to its highly contagious nature, rapid and reliable diagnosis of COVID-19 is very important. It can not only guide the follow-up therapies to improve outcomes but also help to control the disease spread effectively. Today, viral nucleic acid detection using real-time polymerase chain reaction (RT-PCR) is the gold standard for confirming COVID-19 [3]. However, with limitations of being time-consuming and high false-negative rate of RT-PCR, many COVID-19 patients may not be identified and cannot receive appropriate treatment in time. Chest computed tomography (CT), as a routine and highly sensitive imaging tool for pneumonia diagnosis, is relatively easy to perform and can produce fast diagnosis of COVID-19 [4]. Chest CT is one of the key components in the diagnostic workup for patients with suspected infection. In this chapter, we focus on the application of AI in COVID-19.

AI Methods for Infectious Disease

It is well known that X-ray and chest CT are the primary medical imaging techniques for COVID-19 identification (Fig. 42.1, Table 42.1). In addition, lung ultrasound imaging is also applied in clinic for special cases of COVID-19.

Deep learning (DL), as the most popular method of AI in recent years, has contributed to fight against COVID-19 actively, especially in the field of medical imaging. The AI-empowered applications do not aim to replace clinicians but provide decision support and improve efficiency. These applications mainly include the following tasks: dedicated imaging platform, segmentation of lung and infection region, diagnosis and prognosis assessment, and other pioneering basic and clinical researches [5, 6].

It is worth noting that most of the current works are developed based on convolutional neural networks (CNN) and its variants, since CNN is a typical DL method for image processing. In most cases, many labeled training data are generally required to train an accurate and robust CNN model. However, it is difficult to acquire sufficient samples for segmentation of lung and infection regions, detection of lesions, and diagnosis of COVID-19, especially at the early stage of outbreak, because accurate annotation is expensive, labor-intensive, and time-consuming. Therefore, different machine learning methods have been developed to train CNN models with inadequate labeled samples, such as transfer learning [7–9], semi-supervised learning [10–13], active learning [14–16], and so on.

L. Fan, MD (✉) · W. Tu, MM · X. Zhou, MM · Y. Guan, MM
S. Liu, MD
Department of Radiology, Changzheng Hospital, Naval Medical University, Shanghai, China
e-mail: cjr.liushiyuan@vip.163.com

J. Shi, PhD
School of Communication and Information Engineering, Shanghai University, Shanghai, China
e-mail: junshi@shu.edu.cn

N. Shi, MM · Y. Shi, MD
Department of Radiology, Shanghai Public Health Clinical Center, Fudan University, Shanghai, China
e-mail: shinannan@shphc.org.cn; shiyuxin@shphc.org.cn

Y. Bian, MD
Department of Radiology, Changhai hospital, Naval medical University, Shanghai, China

C. N. De Cecco et al. (eds.), *Artificial Intelligence in Cardiothoracic Imaging*, Contemporary Medical Imaging,
https://doi.org/10.1007/978-3-030-92087-6_42

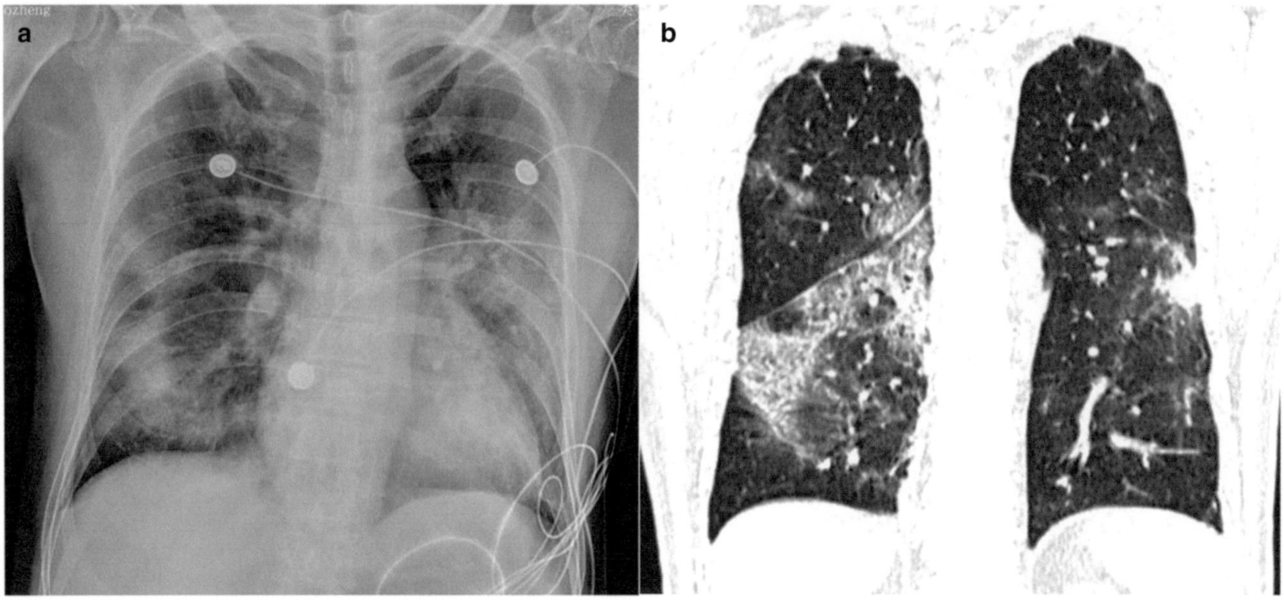

Fig. 42.1 A 61-year-old male was confirmed as COVID-19 after viral nucleic acid detection. (**a**) X-ray image at admission, (**b**) CT image 5 days later, both of which can clearly show typical pneumonia lesions

Radiomics has also been used in COVID-19 for the differential diagnosis. Fang et al. [17] developed a nomogram which performed well in the training set (AUC, 0.959), where out of 56 patients with COVID-19 pneumonia, 49 patients initially showed a negative result by viral nucleic acid detection, and 7 patients were from another hospital. This nomogram performed well in the validation set as well (AUC, 0.955), and it also showed good calibration in both the training and validation samples.

Segmentation of Lung Lesion Based on AI

In general, lung infection segmentation on CT is a necessary initial step for disease analysis. It mainly delineates the regions of interest (ROIs), such as lung, lobes, bronchopulmonary segments, and infected regions or lesions, on the chest X-ray and CT images (Fig. 42.2). There are many CNN-based works reported for segmentation, among which U-Net and its variants, such as UNet++ and V-Net, are the predominant methods used for both X-ray and CT images. The symmetric encoder and decoder structures in U-Net can effectively fuse the high-level and low-level features through the skip-connection operation. Segmentation approaches can be classified into three types: manual, semiautomatic, and fully automatic. The manual segmentation methods are monotonous and time-consuming, and can be affected by inter- and intra-observer variability. Semiautomatic approaches cost less time than manual segmentation methods. Nowadays, fully automatic procedures are raising more and more attention [18]. U-Net, a type of fully convolutional network proposed by Ronneberger [19], has been widely applied for automatic segmentation in COVID-19 applications because of its simple structure and high performance [20–22]. For instance, Li et al. [23] developed a U-Net-based automatic segmentation system to quantify the COVID-19 pneumonia regions on chest CT images. The average dice coefficients between the segmentations of the AI system and those of two experienced radiologists were 0.74 ± 0.28 and 0.76 ± 0.29, respectively. U-Net++, a new and more powerful architecture for medical image segmentation, is equipped with deeply supervised encoder and decoder sub-networks [24]. Chen et al. [25] trained UNet++ to extract infection lesions on CT images using 289 randomly selected CT images. The model successfully extracted infection lesions from 600 images in testing set with an accuracy of 100%. Inf-Net [26], VB-Net, and others were also applied to segment pneumonia lesions. To further improve the performance of segmentation, the attention mechanism is often embedded in the backbone of U-Net to learn the most discriminant part of the features in the network.

Transfer learning is an effective way to mitigate the issue of small size samples, in particularly, the pixel-level annotated images in the segmentation task. It transfers the knowledge of a learned model to another new model to help promote the performance and significantly reduce the requirement for large a number of training data for the task in the target domain. A commonly used method is to transfer the pre-trained segmentation models on chest images for other purposes to the new segmentation task for COVID-19, whose parameters will be fine-tuned with limited samples.

Table 42.1 AI studies of COVID-19 analyzed with sample size, AI algorithm, purpose, and main results

Author	Sample size			AI algorithm	Purpose	Main results	
	Total	Training set	Validation set			Training set	Validation set
Xu Fang [17]	329	239	90	Radiomics	To develop and validate a model for differentiating COVID-19 and other viral pneumonia	AUC: 0.959 Sensitivity: 92.65% Specificity: 93.20% Accuracy: 0.829	AUC: 0.955 Sensitivity: 92.86% Specificity: 97.06% Accuracy: 0.944
Zhang Li [23]	196	–	–	Deep learning; U-Net structure	To develop a fully automated AI system to quantitatively assess the disease severity and disease progression of COVID-19	AUC: 0.97 Sensitivity: 92.41% Specificity: 90.49% Cohen's kappa: 0.8220	–
Jun Chen [25]	164	64	100	Deep learning; UNet++	To construct a system based on deep learning for detecting COVID-19 pneumonia on high-resolution CT	–	Sensitivity: 98% Specificity: 94% Accuracy: 0.96
Shuo Wang [32]	935	709	226	DenseNet121-FPN; COVID-19Net	To propose a fully automatic deep learning system for COVID-19 diagnostic and prognostic analysis	AUC: 0.90 Sensitivity: 78.93% Specificity: 89.93% Accuracy: 81.24%	AUC: 0.87 Sensitivity: 80.39% Specificity: 76.61% Accuracy: 78.32%
Lin Li [33]	3322	2969	353	Deep learning framework COVNet	Using artificial intelligence to detect COVID-19 and community-acquired pneumonia based on pulmonary CT	–	AUC: 0.96 Sensitivity: 90% Specificity: 96%
Shuai Wang [34]	259	–	–	Transfer learning; GoogLeNet Inception v3 CNN	To develop a deep learning algorithm using CT images to screen for coronavirus disease (COVID-19)	–	AUC: 0.93 Sensitivity: 88% Specificity: 87% Accuracy: 89.5%

Semi-supervised learning is another widely used method to alleviate the issue of insufficient labeled data. The semi-supervised learning-based segmentation models only require a small number of pixel-level annotated COVID-19 infection images, and then adopt the unlabeled data to augment the training dataset. For example, they generally can produce the pseudo pixel-level labels from the unlabeled images through the trained network to enlarge the training dataset. Therefore, these algorithms generally achieve superior segmentation performance.

It is known that prior information or the clinical human knowledge is helpful for segmentation task. Therefore, the novel human-in-the-loop strategy has been integrated into the training procedure of a segmentation model. For example, the CNN model can be interactively trained with radiologists to revise the incorrect segmentation [27]; the initial seed point can be given by a radiologist as the clinical knowledge to provide an accurate localization for initializing the segmentation of a region [28].

Quantification, Diagnosis, and Differential Diagnosis of Infectious Disease

CT findings of COVID-19 depend on its disease severity heavily. It has been reported that CT quantitation of pneumonia in the severe and critical type was significantly higher than that of moderate type [29]. The ratio of pneumonia volume to the entire lungs can be used as a quantitative parameter of disease severity evaluation. The quantitative evaluation of pneumonia volume has been defined as an important indicator for management of the severe type patients. Several AI assistant diagnosis systems have already been developed and are being tested in hospitals currently, focusing on the intelligent scanning, diagnosis, and severity evaluation (Figs. 42.3, 42.4, 42.5, and 42.6), in order to minimize the contact transmission, improve the diagnostic accuracy, and guide the treatment.

As a new disease, COVID-19 has many similar manifestations with other types of pneumonia. Therefore, radiologists should accumulate many experiences to achieve a high diagnostic performance. The computer-aided diagnosis

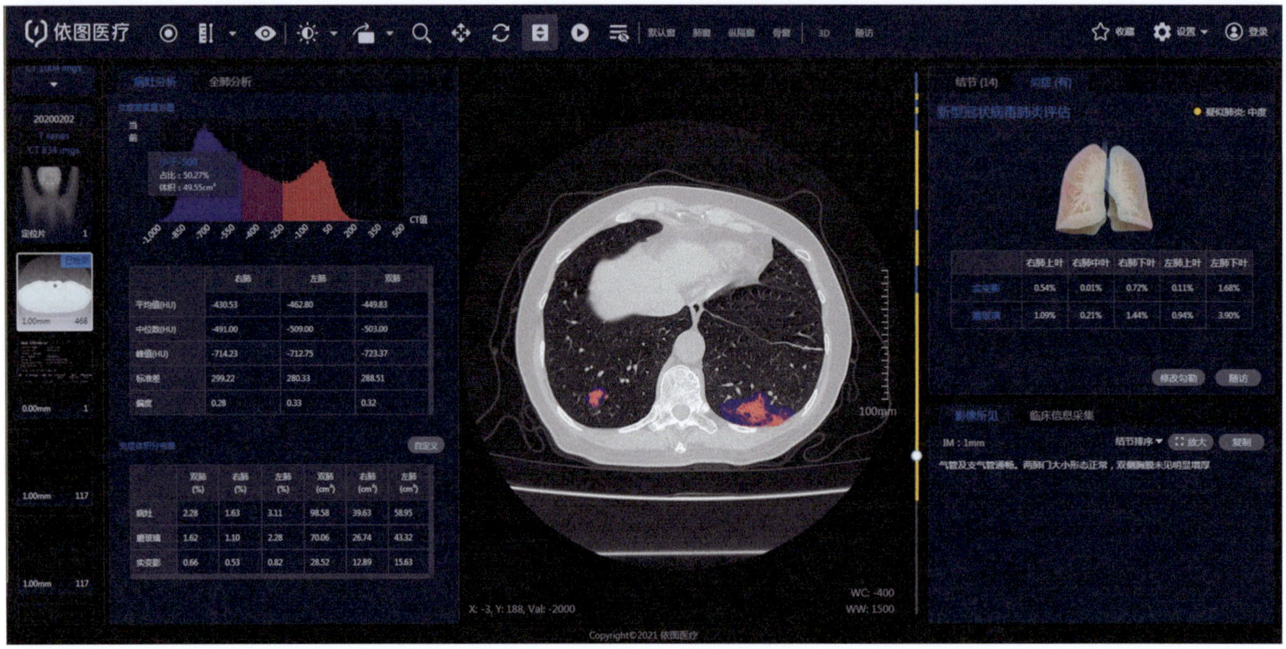

Fig. 42.2 The software of YITU Healthcare based on fully convolutional neural network could segment and identify pneumonia lesions automatically. Blue and red pseudo colors representing ground-glass opacity (GGO) and consolidation components, respectively

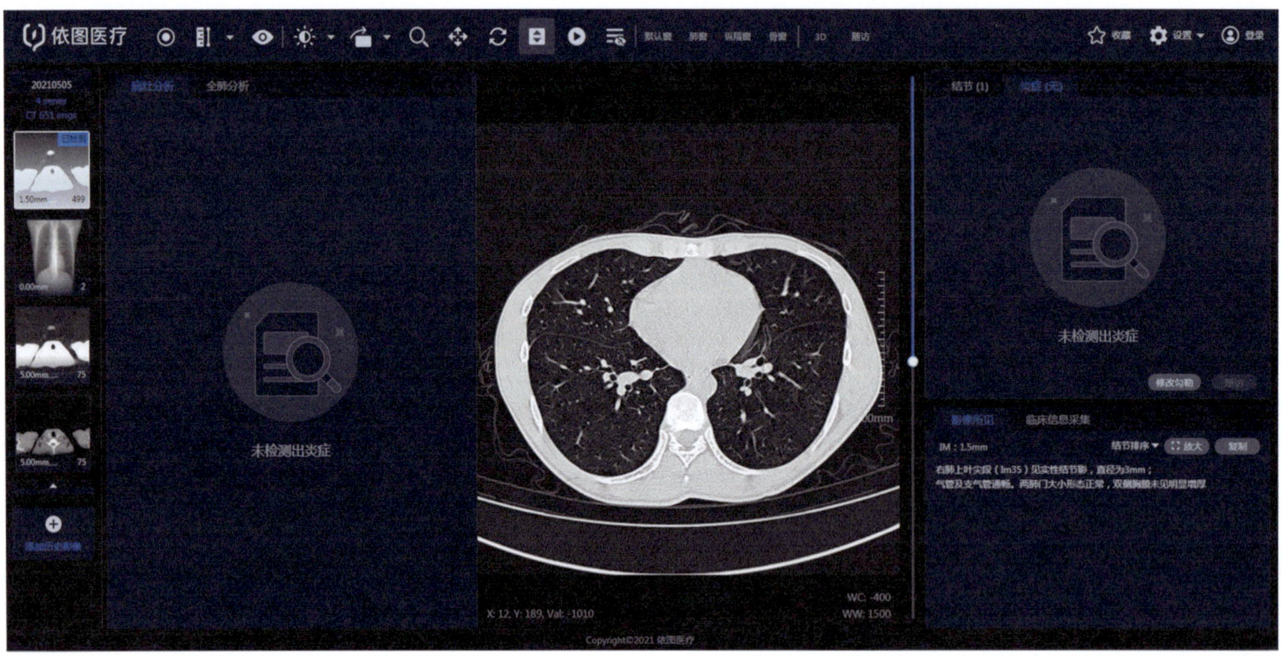

Fig. 42.3 A 24-year-old male was admitted to the hospital with COVID-19 nucleic acid positive and was diagnosed with mild pneumonia clinically. The AI assistant diagnosis system did not detect pneumonia lesions

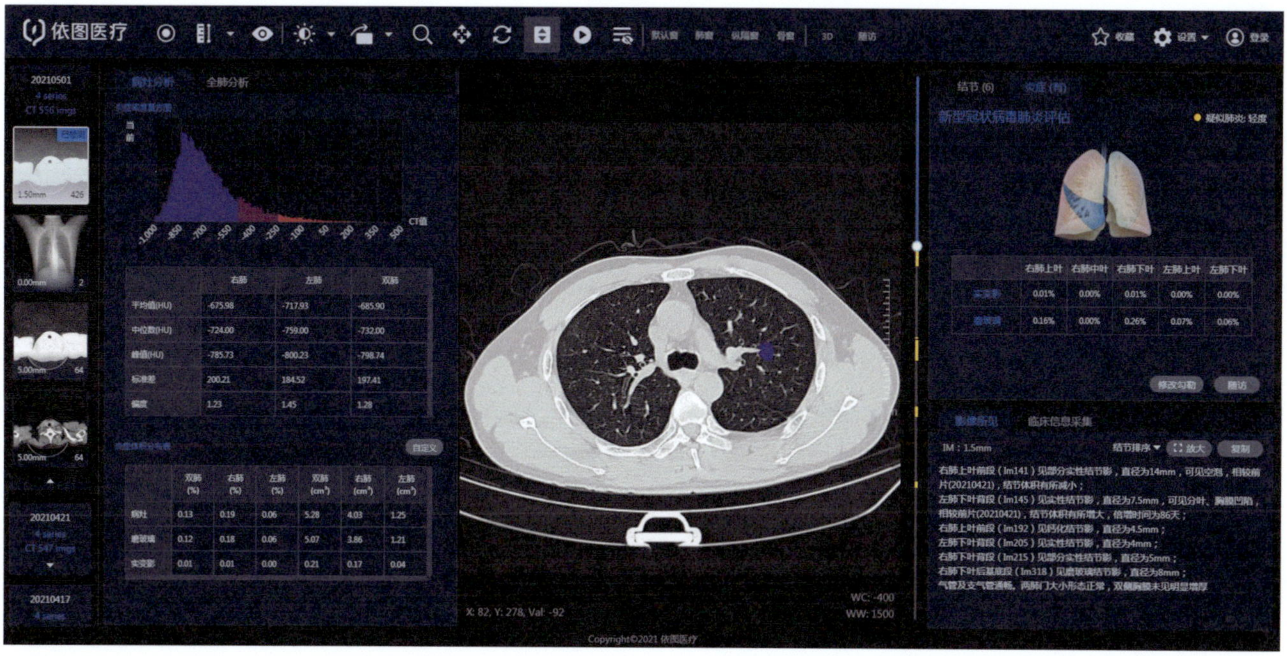

Fig. 42.4 A 45-year-old male was diagnosed with common COVID-19 clinically. The AI assistant diagnosis system detected a small number of pneumonia lesions in the upper lobe of the left lung, and quantified the volume and volume ratio of the ground-glass shadow and the consolidation shadow. According to the above parameters, the software finally diagnosed the patient as mild pneumonia

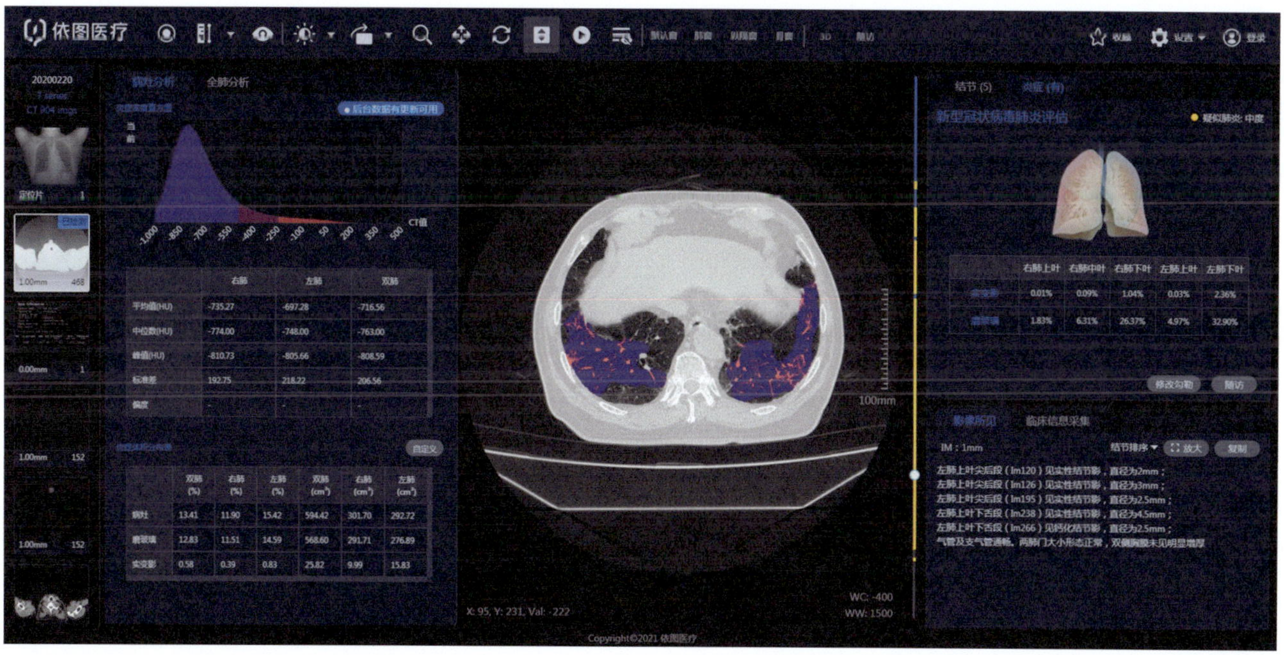

Fig. 42.5 A 70-year-old male was diagnosed with severe type COVID-19 clinically. The AI assistant diagnosis system detected multiple pneumonia lesions in both lungs, and measured the volume ratios of ground-glass shadow and consolidation shadow to the entire lungs as 12.83% and 0.58%, respectively. The software finally diagnosed the patient as moderate pneumonia

(CAD) is highly desired to help improve decision. Much effort has been made to develop various CNN-based models for X-ray- and CT-based CAD for COVID-19. Due to the limited training samples with labels, the strategies of transfer learning are also widely adopted for the diagnosis task of COVID-19, especially the pre-trained model-based approach, which has already trained the CNN models with large-scale training images from other fields. The commonly used pre-trained CNN models for COVID-19 diagnosis include AlexNet, GoogLeNet, VGG-Net, ResNet, DenseNet, etc.

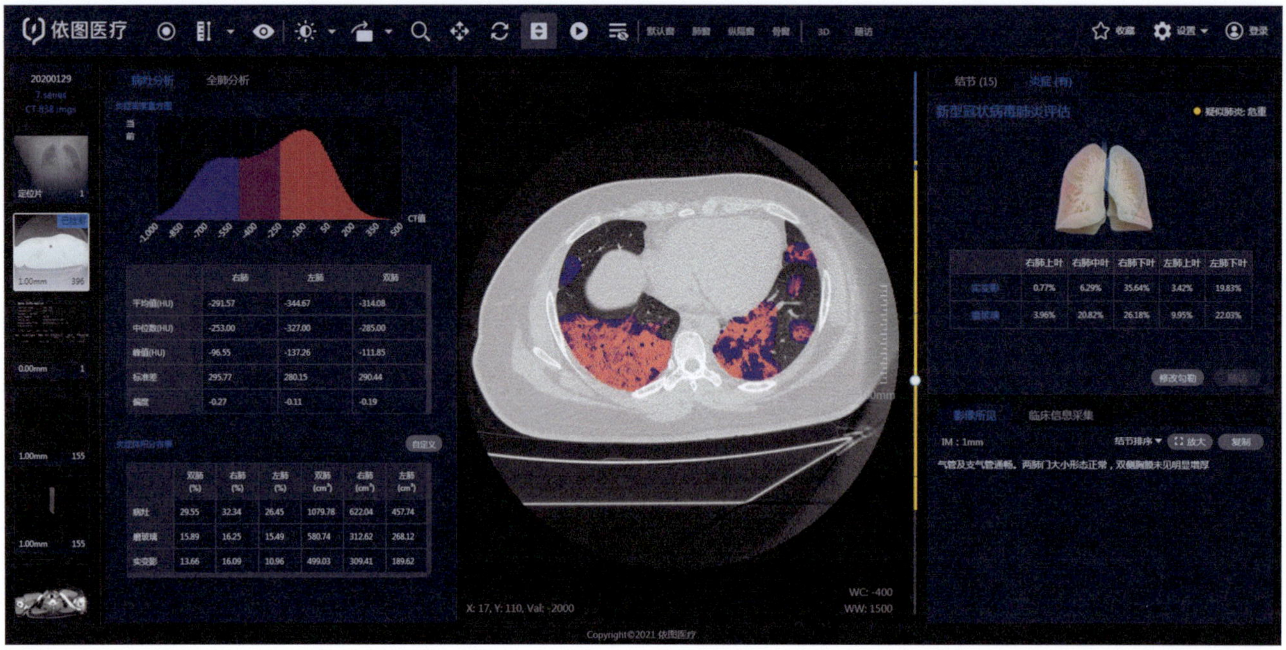

Fig. 42.6 A 25-year-old male was diagnosed with critical type COVID-19 clinically. The AI assistant diagnosis system detected multiple pneumonia lesions in both lungs, and measured the volume ratios of ground-glass shadow and consolidation shadow to the entire lungs as 15.89% and 13.66%, respectively. The software finally diagnosed the patient as critical pneumonia

Compared with the CNN models trained from scratch with a small number of labeled X-ray or CT images, the pre-trained CNN models can achieve superior performance for the diagnosis task of COVID-19 by fine-tuning the model parameters with even limited training samples. Moreover, they can also speed up the convergence procedure. Many improved CNN models have also been proposed based on these pre-trained models for COVID-19 diagnosis. Ni et al. [30] utilized a deep learning model for automatic detection of abnormalities in CT images of COVID-19 patients and compare its quantitative determination performance with radiologists. They found that the deep learning model of CT can also assist radiologists in making quicker diagnosis with superior performance. For these suspected of COVID-19 patients, there is an urgent to segregate the infected patients in time and provide proper treatment. Jin et al. [31] proposed a UNet++ – based segmentation model for pneumonia lesions and a ResNet50 based on 1136 training cases (723 COVID-19 positives, and 413 COVID-19 negatives) from 5 hospitals classification model for differential diagnosis. In the experiment, the sensitivity and specificity of test dataset are 0.974 and 0.922, respectively. Similarly, Wang et al. [32] trained a deep learning model with 1266 patients from 6 cities or provinces. The model achieved good performance in discriminating COVID-19 pneumonia from other pneumonia types. Li et al. [33] developed a deep learning model on chest CT exams, and the model showed good discrimination in COVID-19 (AUC, 0.96) and in community-acquired pneumonia (AUC, 0.95). Wang et al. [34] used a deep learning algorithm to screen CT images for COVID-19 pneumonia. The internal 45 validation achieved a total accuracy of 89.5% with specificity of 0.88 and sensitivity of 0.87. The external testing dataset showed a total accuracy of 79.3% with specificity of 0.83 and sensitivity of 0.67. Gozes et al. [35] used deep learning CT image analysis and achieved classification results for coronavirus vs. non-coronavirus cases per thoracic CT studies of 0.996 AUC (95%CI: 0.989–1.00) on Chinese control and infected patients.

On the other hand, other machine learning methods have also been adopted to develop the customized CNN models for COVID-19 diagnosis to mitigate the problem of small size samples to a certain extent, among which active learning is an effective one. As abovementioned that there are only a limited number of labeled samples together with many unlabeled images, the active learning can effectively cut the cost of annotation by actively selecting the most informative samples to be labeled from the unlabeled data so as to augment the training set and then improve the performance of model. For example, an active learning framework has been proposed to combine the U-Net and hybrid active learning strategy to diagnose COVID-19 with CT scans and patient-level labels, and the sample diversity and predicted loss are simultaneously considered in this work. Some works have integrated both active learning and weakly supervised learning into a framework to further improve the diagnosis performance.

Imaging Outcome and Dynamic Change During Follow-Up

The evolution process of COVID-19 on CT image is not quite clear yet. Pan F et al. [36] reviewed 21 patients recovering from COVID-19 (without severe respiratory distress during the disease course). The mean interval between baseline and follow-up CT scans was 4 ± 1 day, and the mean hospitalization duration was 17 ± 4 days. The majority cases with COVID-19 were controlled with stable and improving conditions after effective personalized treatment. The peak severity was at approximately 10 days, and the improvement happened at approximately 14 days after initial onset of symptoms. The follow-up CT showed that the lesions in lungs were decreased in both number and size. The density of lesions was reduced as well [37]. The CT findings of clinically cured cases showed full recovery or only small amounts of residual stripes. For some cases, the GGO and consolidation in lungs became some thick fibrotic stripes in short term, which need follow-up studies to explore its outcome. Some cases with COVID-19 who failed to receive effective therapy would deteriorate, and the changes would occur rather rapid. The lesions on CT would become more diffusely distributed in a truly short term [38].

AI-based methods can also be applied for the evaluation of change of COVID-19 pneumonia regions over time (Figs. 42.7 and 42.8). Pu et al. [39] developed a computer software to automatically and robustly detect and quantify regions of

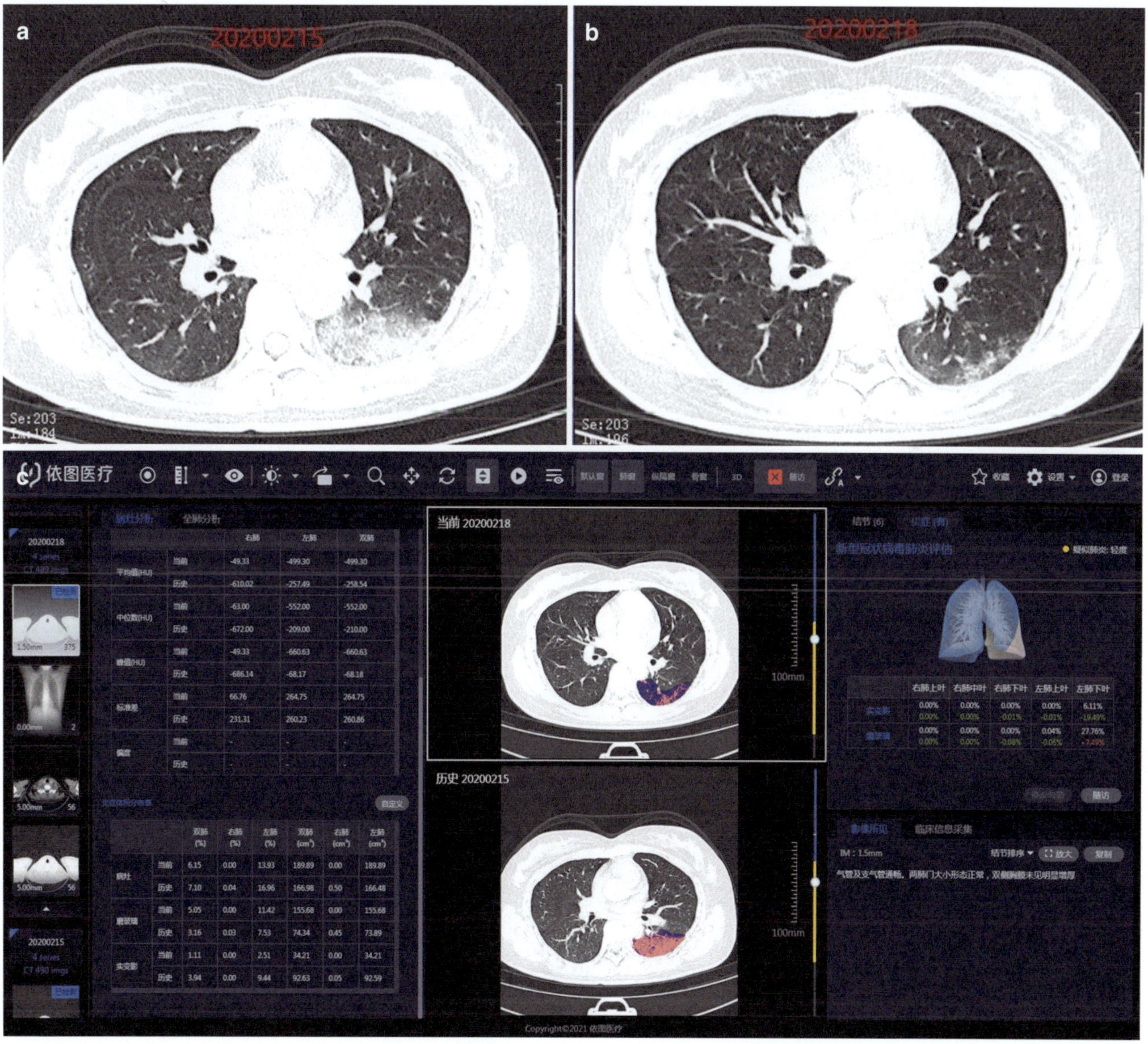

Fig. 42.7 A 40-year-old female COVID-19 patient, (**a**) baseline CT images. (**b**) 3 days later, pneumonia in the left lower lobe was reduced and the density decreased. (**c**) The AI-assisted diagnosis software quantitatively measured the volume and volume ratio of the ground-glass component and the solid component before and after treatment

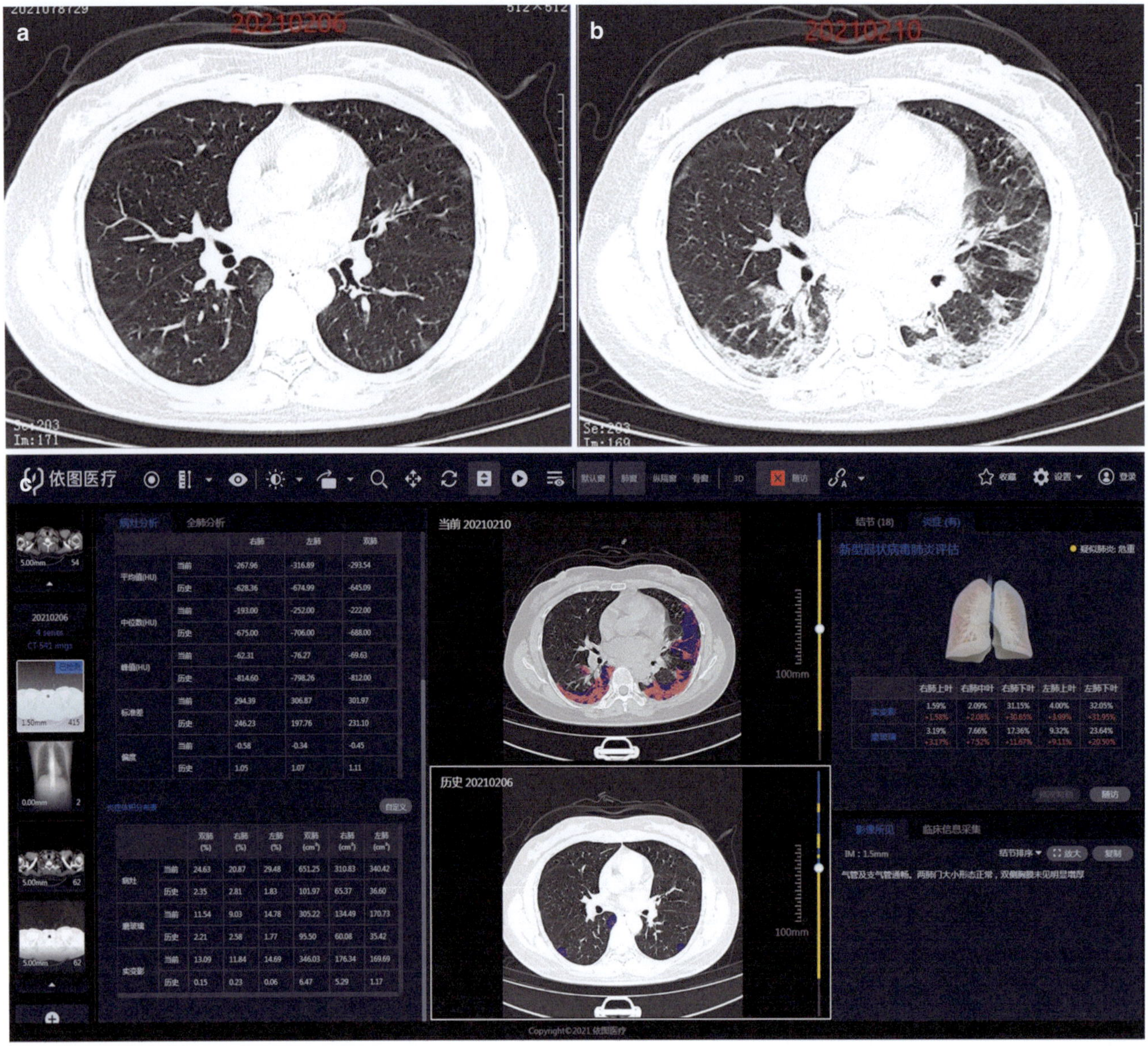

Fig. 42.8 A 48-year-old female patient with COVID-19, (**a**) baseline CT images. (**b**) 4 days later, there is a significant increase in the number and density of pneumonia without effective treatment. (**c**) The AI-assisted diagnosis software quantitatively measured the volume and volume ratio of the ground-glass component and the solid component

pneumonia associated with COVID-19 on CT as well as disease progression. By using AI, it was found that the quantitative volume ratios of COVID-19 lung lesions on CT scans are superior to previous clinical biomarkers including chronic health evaluation II (APACHE-II) score, neutrophil-to-lymphocyte ratio (NLR), and d-dimer levels, and are a novel and promising predictor of COVID-19 progression to severe illness [40]. Huang et al. [41] collect and analyze 126 patients by calculating the CT lung opacification percentage with a deep learning-based tool. They find that this approach could potentially eliminate the subjectivity in the initial assessment and follow-up of pulmonary findings in COVID-19. AI-assisted CT imaging analysis helps to find potential high-risk patients and predicts progression to severe illness. The follow-up strategy would be drawn by these studies focusing on AI to visualize the change of the infection regions of COVID-19 patients. Yuxin Shi's team from Shanghai Public Health Clinical Center attempts to use the AI to visualize the change of the infection regions of COVID-19 patient and provide the follow-up strategy (Fig. 42.9).

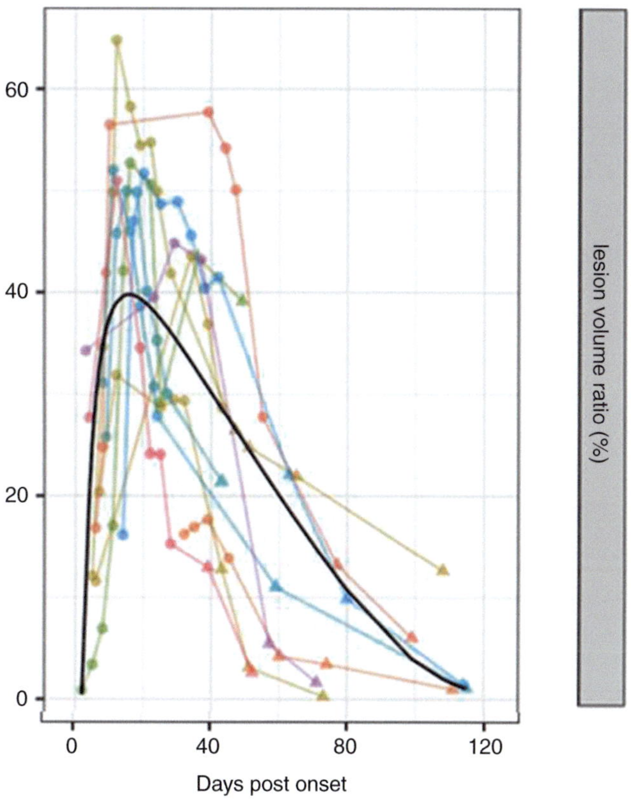

Fig. 42.9 The change of the infection regions of COVID-19 patient. Each curve represents the change trend of the volume ratio of one case, and the black curve simulates the change of the volume ratio of the population of cases

Reducing the Workload of Healthcare Workers

A sudden and vast increase in the numbers of patients during COVID-19 pandemic has brought a very high workload for the doctors. Here, AI is used to reduce the workload of healthcare workers [42]. It not only provides the best training to young doctors regarding this new disease [43] but also helps in diagnosis and treatment at an early stage.

The Role of Chest Imaging in Patient Management During the COVID-19 Pandemic

The role of chest imaging in the management of COVID-19 should be based on the different epidemic stages, countries and regions, hospitals, clinical scenarios, and disease stages, just as recommended in the consensus. In China, in the early outbreak of COVID-19, chest imaging is regarded as one of the criteria of suspected cases, with the huge increase of patients and the lack of RT-PCR test kits, in the fifth version of Chinese protocol [44], pneumonia on CT is regarded as the clinical diagnosis only in Hubei Province, and corresponding isolation and treatment is taken to control the transmission, just as recommended in the clinical scenario 3. This should be considered with much attention by other countries if a huge population is waiting for RT-PCR test, due to the lack of kits, delay awaiting the results, as well as false-negative cases. Chest imaging can be considered as a useful test for relieving quickly difficult situations. With the control of the transmission, in the following sixth and seventh versions of Chinese protocol, the clinical diagnosis based on CT images has been removed. But chest imaging is still regarded as one of the major modalities to evaluate the severity of disease, progression, and outcome. Therefore, the role of chest imaging in the management is dynamic based on the comprehensive situations.

With the development of RT-PCR rapid test, improvement of quality of test kits, and the capacity of hospital for test, RT-PCR as a gold criterion is recommended for the quick screening. Chest imaging is regarded as an adjunct to RT-PCR to evaluate the severity and the progression of pneumonia. In the consensus, chest imaging is stricter to COVID-19 patients, only for the patients with the risk factor for disease progression and with moderate to severe respiratory symptoms. Considering the radiation dose in a short time, controlling the chest imaging is feasible, it is important to only perform it on-demand, and low-dose CT is recommended for the follow-up. Just as the recommendation of chest radiographs for stable intubated patients with COVID-19 is on-demand, not daily routine protocol.

Development of Drugs and Vaccines

AI is used for drug research by analyzing the existing data on COVID-19. It is useful for drug research and development. This technology is used in speeding up drug testing in real time, where standard testing takes plenty of time and hence helps to accelerate this process significantly, which may not be possible by a human. It can help to identify useful drugs for the treatment of COVID-19 patients. It has become a powerful tool for diagnostic test designs and vaccination development.

In summary, not only the abovementioned DL methods but also other advanced machine learning methods, such as multitask learning, semi-supervised, weakly supervised learning, self-supervised learning, and ensemble learning, have also been applied to the tasks of segmentation, detection, and classification of COVID-19. In the future, AI and COVID-19 should be further integrated with clinical information, epidemiology, imaging, prognosis, and other multiple characteristics, in order to achieve comprehensive, intelligent assessment of the disease, early screening and warning, and guidance for clinical accurate diagnosis and treatment. AI-based applications are promising and will enhance the management of infectious patients in clinical practice in the future.

Conclusion

Chest imaging is a routine and highly sensitive method for pneumonia diagnosis. Due to the outbreak of COVID-19, chest imaging-based AI system for diagnosing COVID-19 has flourished. Deep learning and radiomics are the most popular methods used in COVID-19 for the differential diagnosis. Transfer learning and semi-supervised learning can mitigate the issue of small size samples and insufficient labeled data of COVID-19. AI can automatically and accurately segment, identify, and quantitatively analyze pneumonia lesions to assist clinicians in making rapid and accurate diagnosis. In diagnosing the severity of COVID-19 and identifying other pneumonia, AI has also shown good performance. AI-based methods can be applied for the evaluation of change of COVID-19 pneumonia regions over time, in order to better manage COVID-19 patients and suspected cases. AI has also played an irreplaceable role in the development of drugs and vaccines. In summary, AI used to diagnose COVID-19 greatly reduces the pressure on medical staff and saves time and money costs.

References

1. Huang C, Wang Y, Li X, et al. Clinical features of patients infected with 2019 novel coronavirus in Wuhan, China. Lancet. 2020;395(10223):497–506.
2. WHO main website. https://www.who.int. Accessed 5th Feb 2020. https://doi.org/10.1073/pnas.1502972112.
3. Haque N, Bari MS, Ahmed S, et al. Detection of 2019-Novel Coronavirus (2019-nCoV) by rRT-PCR at Mymensingh Medical College, Mymensingh, Bangladesh. Mymensingh Med J. 2020;29(3):589–95.
4. Ai T, Yang Z, Hou H, et al. Correlation of Chest CT and RT-PCR testing for coronavirus disease 2019 (COVID-19) in China: a report of 1014 cases. Radiology. 2020;296(2):E32–40.
5. Shi F, Shi J, Wu Z, et al. Review of artificial intelligence techniques in imaging data acquisition, segmentation and diagnosis for Covid-19. Published in: IEEE Reviews in Biomedical Engineering (Early Access), 16 April 2020. 2020. https://doi.org/10.1109/RBME.2020.2987975.
6. Wynants L, Van Calster B, Collins GS, et al. Prediction models for diagnosis and prognosis of covid-19: systematic review and critical appraisal. BMJ. 2020;369:m1328.
7. Postolopoulos ID, Mpesiana TA, et al. Covid-19: automatic detection from x-ray images utilizing transfer learning with convolutional neural networks. Physical and Engineering Sciences in Medicine. 2020;43:635–40.
8. Jaiswal A, Gianchandani N, Singh D, et al. Classification of the COVID-19 infected patients using DenseNet201 based deep transfer learning. J Biomol Struct Dyn. 2021;39(15):5682–89.
9. Zhu J, Shen B, Abbasi A, et al. Deep transfer learning artificial intelligence accurately stages COVID-19 lung disease severity on portable chest radiographs. PloS one. 2020;15(7):e0236621.
10. Loey M, Manogaran G, Taha MHN, et al. A hybrid deep transfer learning model with machine learning methods for face mask detection in the era of the COVID-19 pandemic. Measurement. 2020;167:108288.
11. Ma J, Nie Z, Wang C, et al. Active contour regularized semi-supervised learning for COVID-19 CT infection segmentation with limited annotations. Phys Med Biol. 2020;65(22):225034.
12. Fan DP, Zhou T, Ji GP, et al. Inf-net: automatic COVID-19 lung infection segmentation from CT images. IEEE Trans Med Imaging. 2020;39(8):2626–37.
13. Luger S, Tapo AA, Homan CM, et al. Towards a crowdsourcing platform for low resource languages–a semi-supervised approach. In Proceedings of the Eighth Conference on Human Computations. In Proceedings of the Eighth Conference on Human Computations. 2020.
14. Santosh KC. AI-driven tools for coronavirus outbreak: need of active learning and cross-population train/test models on multitudinal/multimodal data. J Med Syst. 2020;44(5):1–5.
15. Tan HR, Chng WH, Chonardo C, et al. How chemists achieve active learning online during the COVID-19 pandemic: using the Community of Inquiry (CoI) framework to support remote teaching. J Chem Educ. 2020;97(9):2512–8.
16. Singhal MK. Facilitating virtual medicinal chemistry active learning assignments using advanced zoom features during COVID-19 campus closure. J Chem Educ. 2020;97(9):2711–4.
17. Fang X, Li X, Bian Y, et al. Radiomics nomogram for the prediction of 2019 novel coronavirus pneumonia caused by SARS-CoV-2. Eur Radiol. 2020;30:6888–901.
18. Oulefki A, Agaian S, Trongtirakul T, et al. Automatic COVID-19 lung infected region segmentation and measurement using CT-scans images. Pattern Recognit. 2020;2:107747.
19. Ronneberger O, et al. U-Net: convolutional networks for biomedical image segmentation. in International conference on medical image computing and computer-assisted intervention. 2015. pp. 234–241.
20. Wang X, Deng X, Fu Q, et al. A Weakly-Supervised Framework for COVID-19 Classification and Lesion Localization From Chest CT. IEEE Transactions on Medical Imaging. 2020;39(8):2615–25.
21. Zhang P, et al. CoSinGAN: learning COVID-19 infection segmentation from a single radiological image. Diagnostics (Basel). 2020;10(11):901.
22. Wang M, et al. Deep learning-based triage and analysis of lesion burden for COVID-19: a retrospective study with external validation. Lancet Digital Health. 2020;2(10):e506–15.
23. Li Z, et al. From community-acquired pneumonia to COVID-19: a deep learning-based method for quantitative analysis of COVID-19 on thick-section CT scans. Eur Radiol. 2020;30(12):6828–37.
24. Zhou Z, et al. UNet++: a nested U-Net architecture for medical image segmentation. Deep Learn Med Image Anal Multimodal Learn Clin Decis Support. 2018;11045:3–11.
25. Chen J, et al. Deep learning-based modeel for detecting 2019 novel coronavirus pneumonia on high-resolution computed tomography. Sci Rep. 2020;10(1):19196.
26. Fan DP, et al. Inf-Net: automatic COVID-19 lung infection segmentation from CT images. IEEE Trans Med Imaging. 2020;39(8):2626–37.
27. Shi F, Wei Y, Xia L, et al. Lung volume reduction and infection localization revealed in Big data CT imaging of COVID-19. Int J Infect Dis. 2021;102:316–8.
28. Yue H, Yu Q, Liu C, et al. Machine learning-based CT radiomics method for predicting hospital stay in patients with pneumonia associated with SARS-CoV-2 infection: a multicenter study. Ann Transl Med. 2020;8(14):859.
29. Huang LHR, Yu P, et al. The correlation between clinical characteristics and CT findings in different clinical stage in COVID-

19. Chin J Radiol. 2020;54(00):E003. https://doi.org/10.3760/cma.j.issn.1005-1201.2020.0003. (In Chinese)
30. Ni Q, et al. A deep learning approach to characterize 2019 coronavirus disease (COVID-19) pneumonia in chest CT images. Eur Radiol. 2020;30(12):6517–27.
31. Wang B, et al. AI-assisted CT imaging analysis for COVID-19 screening: building and deploying a medical AI system. Appl Soft Comput. 2020;98:106897.
32. Wang S, et al. A fully automatic deep learning system for COVID-19 diagnostic and prognostic analysis. Eur Respir J. 2020;56(2):2000775.
33. Li L, Qin L, Xu Z et al. Artificial intelligence distinguishes COVID-19 from community acquired pneumonia on chest CT. Radiology. 2020: 200905. https://doi.org/10.1148/radiol.2020200905:200905.
34. Wang S, Kang B, Ma J, et al. A deep learning algorithm using CT images to screen for Corona Virus Disease (COVID-19). Eur Radiol. 2021;31(8):6096–104.
35. Ophir Gozes MF-A, Hayit Greenspan, Patrick D, et al. Eliot Siegel rapid AI development cycle for the Coronavirus (COVID-19) Pandemic: initial results for automated detection & patient monitoring using deep learning CT image analysis.arXiv. 2020;2003.05037.
36. Pan F, Ye T, Sun P, et al. Time course of lung changes on chest CT during recovery from 2019 novel coronavirus (COVID-19) pneumonia. Radiology. 2020. 200370. https://doi.org/10.1148/radiol.2020200370.
37. Duan Y-n, Qin J. Pre- and Posttreatment Chest CT Findings: 2019 Novel Coronavirus (2019-nCoV) Pneumonia. Radiology. 2020. 200323. https://doi.org/10.1148/radiol.2020200323.
38. Jiang N, Zheng C, Fan Y, et al. CT appearance of new coronavirus pneumonia in subclinical period and short-term changes. Chin J Radiol. 2020;54(00):E008. https://doi.org/10.3760/cma.j.issn.1005-1201.2020.0008. (In Chinese)
39. Pu J, Leader J, Bandoset A,et al. Automated quantification of COVID-19 severity and progression using chest CT images. Eur Radiol. 2021;31(1):436–46.
40. Liu F, et al. CT quantification of pneumonia lesions in early days predicts progression to severe illness in a cohort of COVID-19 patients. Theranostics. 2020;10(12):5613–22.
41. Lu H, Han R, Ai T, et al. Serial quantitative chest CT assessment of COVID-19: deep-learning approach. Radiology: cardiothoracic. Imaging. 2020;2(2):e200075.
42. Wan KH, Huang SS, Young A, et al. Precautionary measures needed for ophthalmologists during pandemic of the coronavirus disease 2019 (COVID-19). Acta Ophthalmol. 2020;98:221–2.
43. Gupta R, Ghosh A, Singh AK, et al. Clinical considerations for patients with diabetes in times of COVID-19 epidemic. Diabetes Metab Syndr. 2020;14:211–2.
44. Diagnosis and Treatment Protocols of COVID-19 Infection (Trial Version 5). The National Health Commission of the People's Republic of China [EB/OL]. http://www.nhc.gov.cn/yzygj/s7653p/202002/8334a8326dd94d329df351d7da8aefc2.shtml.

Lung Cancer Screening and Nodule Detection: The Role of Artificial Intelligence

43

Sunyi Zheng, Peter M. A. van Ooijen, and Matthijs Oudkerk

Introduction

Lung cancer accounted for the majority of cancer-related deaths in 2017, more than the combination of the other three leading cancers: colorectal, breast, and prostate cancer [1]. Despite an accelerated decline in the long-term mortality rate, it remains one of the deadliest cancers worldwide. In 2020, it is estimated to cause 135,720 deaths in the United States [1]. The 5-year survival rate for lung cancer at stage IV is only 4% [2]. However, early detection of lung cancer can improve survival rates, as patient treatment plans can be drawn up and implemented at an earlier disease stage [3]. Computed tomography (CT) is an effective method to detect and investigate lung cancer, which generally presents as a pulmonary nodule. CT can also be utilized for the measurement of pulmonary nodule intensity, diameter, or volume, and can provide diagnostic information, based on morphological features, lymph node locations, and distant metastasis, for use in subsequent nodule management. The implementation of lung cancer screening worldwide has led to an ever-increasing workload pressure on radiologists, and the need for accurate nodule detection. To reduce the heavy burden which radiologists face, over the last two decades, artificial intelligence (AI) systems using classic machine learning and advanced deep learning algorithms have been designed [4, 5]. These systems were designed with the aim of achieving a high sensitivity and a low false-positive rate in nodule identification [6]. Systems implemented using classic machine learning techniques more rely on human intervention to define feature extraction algorithms, while systems with advanced deep learning techniques can independently learn the extraction of features. With more data available, the era of deep learning is leading to a renewed interest in leveraging AI systems for accurate and efficient nodule detection, and the integration of them within reporting workstations.

In this chapter, we will focus on the development of AI detection systems for pulmonary nodules, and discuss factors which affect their performance. Moreover, we look at the comparisons in performance between AI and radiologists on pulmonary nodule detection, and explore the role of AI in lung cancer screening programs.

Lung Cancer Screening

With the aim of detecting lung cancer at an early stage, in populations with a high risk of lung cancer, randomized lung cancer screening trials have been established worldwide. In a recently published review regarding lung cancer screening, multiple large-scale screening programs have provided evidence showing lung cancer-related mortality rate is reduced in patients who have undergone CT screening [7]. Variation was however seen in the definitions of clinically relevant nodules (based on size) in the differing CT-based screening trials. One of the major studies included "relevant" nodules based on diameters >4 mm [8], while other studies adopted diameter in addition to volume measurement for nodule managment [9–11]. In this section we briefly review four large-scale lung cancer screening programs. Comparisons of the four lung cancer screening programs including relevant findings are shown in Table 43.1.

S. Zheng, MSc
Department of Radiation Oncology, University Medical Center Groningen/University of Groningen, Groningen, The Netherlands
e-mail: s.zheng@umcg.nl

P. M. A. van Ooijen, MSc, PhD, CPHIMS
Department of Radiation Oncology and Data Science Center in Health, University Medical Center Groningen, Groningen, The Netherlands
e-mail: p.m.a.van.ooijen@umcg.nl

M. Oudkerk, MD, PhD, FNASCI, EBCR (✉)
Faculty of Medical Sciences, University of Groningen, Groningen, The Netherlands

Institute for Diagnostic Accuracy, Groningen, The Netherlands
e-mail: m.oudkerk@rug.nl

C. N. De Cecco et al. (eds.), *Artificial Intelligence in Cardiothoracic Imaging*, Contemporary Medical Imaging,
https://doi.org/10.1007/978-3-030-92087-6_43

Table 43.1 Comparisons of relevant nodules and findings in various lung cancer screening studies

Screening trials	Size of relevant nodules	Relevant findings
NLST	≥4 mm	Diameter-based LDCT reduced lung cancer mortality (hazard ratio [HR] = 0.80, $P < 0.01$)
NELSON	≥4 mm or ≥30 mm^3	Volume-based LDCT reduced lung cancer mortality (HR = 0.76 in men, $P = 0.01$; HR = 0.67 in women)
UKLS	≥3 mm or ≥15 mm^3	LDCT can detect lung cancer (85.7% stage I or II) at an early stage. Mortality results to be published
MILD	≥60 mm^3	Prolonged LDCT screening reduced lung cancer mortality (HR = 0.61, $P < 0.02$)

The National Lung Cancer Screening Trial (NLST) was initiated in 2002, and in total 53,454 participants were enrolled [8]. Half of the participants received LDCT scans and half underwent single-review chest radiography. The study demonstrated that screening using low-dose CT (LDCT) could yield a 20% reduction in lung cancer mortality compared to screening with chest radiography (hazard ratio [HR] = 0.80, P < 0.01). However, more false positives were found due to variation in nodule characterization and reporting manners by radiologists. To solve this issue, Lung Reporting and Data System (Lung-RADS) was released by the American College of Radiology, in order to provide clear definitions of positive findings and effective nodule management for LDCT lung cancer screening. Despite a decrease in sensitivity, a study showed Lung-RADS (2014 version), when considering noncalcified nodules at least 4 mm in any diameter, can result in a lower false-positive rate (with vs. without: 12.8% vs. 26.6%) at baseline when applying it retrospectively on the results of the NLST [12]. In the recent 2019 version of Lung-RADS, taking diameter and volume measurement into consideration, nodules larger than 4 mm or 30 mm^3 (regardless of type) with a risk of malignancy greater than 1% should be reported and recommended for short-term follow-up with additional diagnostic testing or tissue sampling [13].

The Dutch–Belgian randomized controlled lung-cancer screening trial (NELSON) was started in 2003 and recruited 15,789 individuals aged between 50 and 74. Half of the participants underwent volume-based LDCT screening, and the other participants received no screening (control group). Recently published results showed that among men, volume-based screening can substantially reduce the mortality rate of lung cancer, when compared to participants who did not undergo screening (cumulative rate ratio for lung cancer-specific mortality = 0.76, 95% CI: 0.61–0.94, $P < 0.05$ at 10 years) [9]. To support the successful implementation of the NELSON study and other lung cancer screening programs in Europe, the European position statement on lung cancer screening was released [14]. The statement indicated that solid non-calcified nodules larger than or equal to 4 mm or 30 mm^3 and sub-solid nodules greater than 5 mm are clinically relevant in screening programs.

The UK Lung Cancer Screening (UKLS) pilot trial randomized 4055 patients, aged 50–75, into CT screening and no screening groups. The UKLS trial showed that more than 80% of early stage lung cancers could be detected and delivered potentially curative treatment [10]. This study focused on nodules which were larger than 3 mm or 15 mm^3.

The multicenter Italian Lung Detection (MILD) trial recruited 2376 individuals who underwent annual or biennial LDCT. Ten-year results of the MILD trial provided evidence that prolonged LDCT screening led to a 39% mortality reduction in lung cancer (HR = 0.61, 95% CI: 0.39–0.95, $P < 0.02$) [15]. Besides, the lung cancer-specific 10-year mortality was similar in both biennial and annual screening groups. However, LDCT screening occurring every 2 years instead of 1 year could save 44% of follow-up scans for individuals who had a negative baseline examination [11]. A negative case in the MILD trial was classified as a nodule with the volume less than 60 mm^3.

Despite the increased opportunity for early detection of lung cancer through the implementation of lung cancer screening programs, lung cancer may still be missed or detected at a late stage. This is due to the complexity of nodule characterization and their anatomical structures, an increased number of CT slices to be viewed, inconsistent levels of observer reading experience, fatigue, etc. A potential solution to this problem is the use of a well-preforming AI-based system to assist radiologists for nodule detection.

AI-Based Pulmonary Nodule Detection

Machine intelligence, better known as artificial intelligence (AI), is used to describe machines which are designed to mimic and help humans to achieve certain goals. AI has been attempting to support radiologists since the end of the twentieth century. The first AI system for lung nodule detection on chest radiographs was published in 1988. Due to insufficient computational power, poor image quality, and immature detection algorithms, the system yielded a high false-positive rate and its generalizability was unknown [16]. With the developments in computational resources and digital imaging, computers are able to process more difficult tasks, and the introduction of CT imaging brings a clearer view of the three-dimensional bodily structures. Consequently, AI has achieved great success in nodule detection in recent years, especially during the era of deep learning.

Aims of AI

The reasons for implementing an AI nodule detection system for radiologists are as follows:

1. To avoid missing clinically relevant nodules. Nodules have large variations in size, characteristics, and anatomical location, which can easily lead to false-negative outcomes.
2. To reduce the number of false positives that might result in unnecessary follow-up, incorrect clinical staging and treatment, etc.
3. To save the time of radiologists concentrating on diagnosis and subsequent management of nodule characteristics, if the AI system is efficient and can accurately process scans.

Stages of Nodule Detection Systems

An AI nodule detection system can consist of five stages. Firstly, images should be retrieved from the picture archiving and communication system. Then, the image will be preprocessed in appropriate window settings. The next (optional) step is to segment lung parenchyma, so that the system can focus solely on the region of interest and not be disrupted by other organs, clothes, or tables. The most essential two stages come after the segmentation of lung parenchyma, as shown in Fig. 43.1. At the nodule candidate detection stage, AI will try to find as many nodule candidates as possible based on features defined by algorithms. Corresponding nodule coordinates and size can be further calculated to extract features of nodule candidates. In the end, by analyzing extracted features, false-positive candidates will be removed from the final output at the false-positive reduction stage.

Detection Systems Using Classic Machine Learning Algorithms

Machine learning (ML), as a subset of AI, can achieve a good performance on small datasets, but reply on the experience of humans. This might limit the generalizability of the machine learning-based system if it is validated on an external set, or even an internal set. Moreover, due to inadequate computational power, most systems have been established based on small private databases, and their performance varies. In a literature survey regarding the progress of machine learning-based systems on nodule detection, the sensitivity of the systems varied from 70.0% to 90.0%, whereas the false-positive rate ranged from 0.5 to 15 per scan [17].

In one of the fully automated detection systems, multiple thresholds were applied to segment the lung region, and initial nodule candidates were selected using an 18-point algorithm [18]. For nodule candidate characterization, a feature vector was computed based on the mean HU value, standard deviation, volume, radius, sphericity, eccentricity, and circularity. In 43 evaluated CT scans with 171 nodules, the AI system had a sensitivity of 70.0% with 1.5 false positives detected in every scan. A different study dedicated to detecting isolated, juxtapleural, and juxtavascular nodule types using 2D and 3D operations accordingly [19] used 164 nodules detected in 20 patients by 2 radiologists as a reference standard. A sensitivity of 97.4% was achieved for isolated nodules, whereas a sensitivity of 93.0% was achieved for juxtapleural and juxtavascular nodules. Using a novel quantized convergence index filter to enhance round lesions, an automatic system was able to achieve a high sensitivity of 90% on five clinical datasets [20]. Eight rule-based features, such as the output level of quantized convergence index filter, gray-level gradient, and lengths, were applied for false-positive reduction by linear discriminant analysis. Another

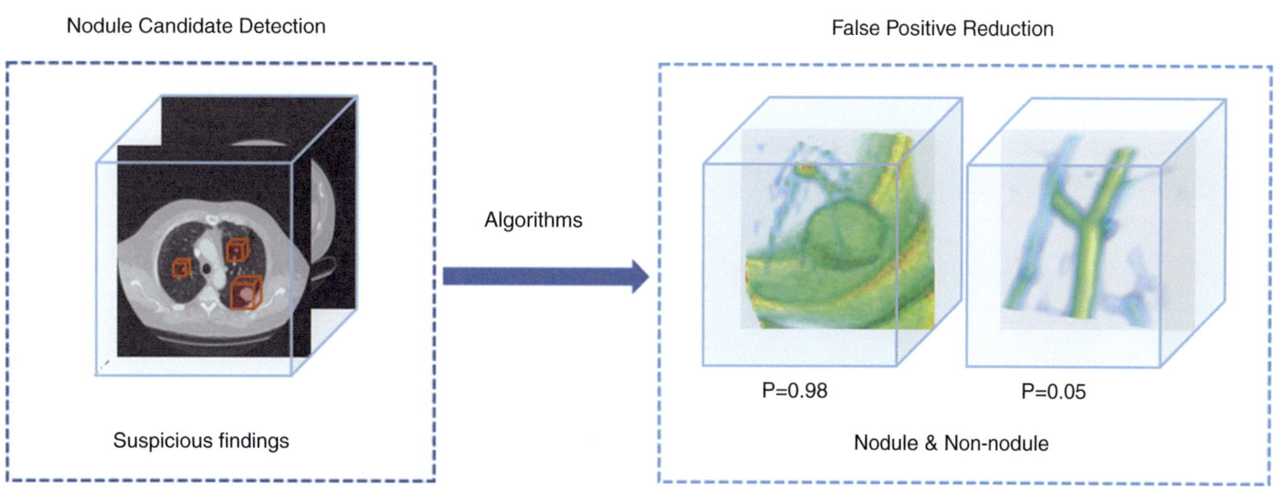

Fig. 43.1 Two main stages in a nodule detection system

interesting study designed an algorithm that included a multi-scale Laplacian of Gaussian filter, prior shape information, and circularity to detect nodule candidates, before applying deep learning techniques for false-positive reduction [21]. One hundred percent of nodules on the 888 CT scans were found, although an average false-positive rate of 50.3 appeared in each scan.

Since many AI systems used different data for development, it is difficult to make a fair comparison. Hence, the public dataset ANODE09 was released, to benchmark the performance of different systems [22]. This dataset included 55 scans collected in the NELSON study. The organizer compared the performance of six AI systems and found the combination of the results can boost the final sensitivity from 20.8% to 72.5% with one false positive per scan [23]. More specially, with the same false-positive rate, the sensitivities of identifying small, large, isolated, vascular, pleural, and peri-fissural nodules were 76.1%, 67.8%, 73.8%, 72.1%, 62.7%, and 82.9%, respectively. More nodules could have been detected if a higher false-positive rate was tolerated. They also studied false-positive findings and found the main causes to be vessel branchings, small lesions such as scar tissue, and apparent protrusions mimicking nodules in areas where high-density body structures are close or in contact with the pleural surface of the lung. As false positives are often small, an extra algorithm might be helpful which discards findings less than 4 mm, in order to further reduce the false-positive rate of the system.

Detection Systems Applying Advanced Deep Learning Algorithms

Deep learning (DL) is a subcategory of machine learning utilizing artificial neural networks to learn presentative features of targets. Compared to ML algorithms, DL is more advanced with automated feature extraction and possibly unlimited accuracy, although a larger training set and more powerful computers are required. A recent systematic review paper showed DL systems can achieve high accuracy from 82.2% to 97.6% [4].

For the purpose of facilitating the development of computer-aided detection systems using DL techniques, large datasets are available, such as the Lung Image Database Consortium and Image Database Resource Initiative (LIDC/IDRI) with 1018 annotated thoracic CT scans collected from 7 participated academic centers, [24] and the National Lung Cancer Screening Trial (NLST) dataset with LDCT scans from 26,254 patients [25]. Furthermore, many competitions have been held for the implementation of DL-based nodule detection systems. For example, the LUng Nodule Analysis 2016 (LUNA16) competition built a benchmark dataset with 888 CT scans which were acquired in thin slices and selected from the LIDC-IDRI database for evaluation [26]. In 2017, a Kaggle's Data Science Bowl (DSB) challenge was organized for lung cancer diagnosis with a subset of the NLST set [27]. Two years later, the Lung Nodule Database (LNDb) competition released 294 annotated CT scans retrospectively collected in Porto for automated nodule management based on the 2017 Fleischner society pulmonary nodule guidelines [28, 29].

In recent years, a large number of researchers have utilized the LUNA16 dataset to build up AI detection systems. In one study, results of five complete AI detection systems and three systems developed only for removal of false positives were combined. The nodule detection rate at the candidate detection stage was increased up to 98.3%, which was higher than that of any single system. At the false-positive reduction stage, probabilities of nodule candidates were simply averaged. As a result, the merged system achieved a sensitivity of 96.9% with one false positive per scan [30]. In another study, a deep learning approach was implemented inspired by the maximum intensity projection (MIP) technique which is one of the useful routine clinical procedures [31]. Their results showed that convolutional neural networks were capable of detecting more small nodules (85.5–88.5%) between 3 and 10 mm on three different MIP slices (5, 10, and 15 mm) than on 1 mm axial slices (79.4%). Examples of various MIP images are shown in Fig. 43.2. After results on various slices were merged, 95.4% of nod-

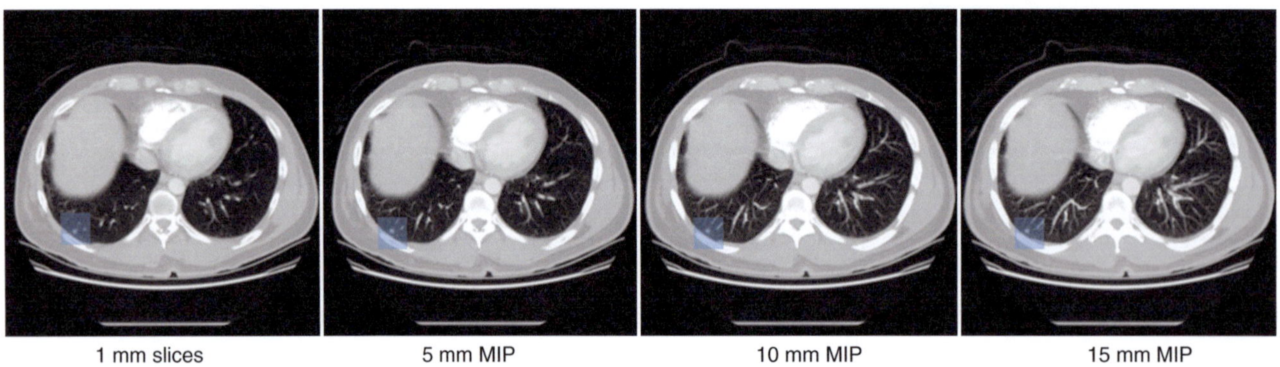

Fig. 43.2 Comparisons between different images generated by maximum intensity projection (MIP) and 1 mm axial slices. Nodules are enhanced and vessels are more continuous in the MIP images

ules (regardless of size) were detected. Moreover, using two kinds of cubic patches for the elimination of false positives resulted in a final sensitivity of 92.7% with one false positive per scan. When the system took 16 MIP slices into consideration, the performance was further improved to 94.4% at a false-positive rate of one [32]. Furthermore, a study proposed a 3D Feature Pyramid Network with 96 × 96 × 96 volumetric patches and an HS2 network to reduce false positives by tracking changes of consecutive slices where the nodule candidate is [33]. Aided by applying spatial features, the system can reach a sensitivity of 90.4% with a very low false-positive rate of one eighth. Additionally, this study implemented a faster region-based convolutional neural network with two regions [34]. To integrate spatial information with the aim of refining results, three continuous slices containing nodule candidates were fed into three classification models, and the final probability was averaged. If the models misclassified any nodules, this data was used again for retraining. The designed system finally found 85.2% of nodules with also one false positive per scan.

In addition, nodules have large variations in morphology, which challenges the ability of the system to reduce the number of irrelevant findings. One method took CT patches in multiple scales for training, and combined the strategy that gradually extracted features in a zoom-in and zoom-out manner [35]. As a consequence, the proposed method yielded a sensitivity of 94.7%. Moreover, based on the ResNet-101 which had high accuracy on natural images, a developed nodule detector found 71.9% of nodules on the subset of the DSB challenge [36].

Some studies have used other databases for system implementation and yielded good performance in nodule identification. For example, a retrospective study collected 9225 chest radiographs with nodules and 34,067 negatives cases, between 2010 and 2015 [37]. Thirteen experienced radiologists labeled these images. The proposed DL system was internally and externally assessed on datasets from three hospitals in South Korea and one in the United States. The area under the receiver of AI (0.92–0.99) was superior to 17 out of 18 physicians who were involved in the evaluation. AI was able to detect 96% of nodules which were >30 mm, 74% of nodules 20–30 mm, 68% of nodules 15–20 mm, 55% of nodules 10–15 mm, and 11% of nodules <10 mm. A different study included 2000 CT scans with 2608 nodules from NLST, LIDC-IDRI, and a private dataset [38]. Challenging negative mining and volumetric patches training were applied to facilitate the performance. When the system was evaluated on 354 validation CT scans, a sensitivity of 93% was achieved for nodules larger than 5 mm. A third study used 12,754 CT scans, of which 11,625 were obtained from 3 hospitals for AI development and 1129 were collected from more than 10 centers for validation [39]. The AI system showed a sensitivity of 74.0% when the false-positive rate is one in terms of different nodules. More specifically, AI had a sensitivity of 71.9%, 88.6%, 61.3%, 85.2%, 86.4%, and 75.3% for solid nodules ≤6 mm, solid nodules >6 mm, sub-solid nodules ≤5 mm, sub-solid nodules >5 mm, calcified nodules, and pleural nodules, respectively. In 2019, the Google AI team proposed an end-to-end system that took the volume of interest for cancer detection [40]. The system was first trained on the LIDC-IDRI dataset and subsequently fine-tuned on 70% of 29,541 NLST cases. Tested on 6729 cases, the cancer detector reached a sensitivity of 97.5% for baseline scans and 94.6% for prior scans when the top 2 detections were hit.

Factors Impacting the Performance of AI

The performance of existing AI systems varies from system to system. Many factors such as CT parameters (slice thickness, slab thickness, scan dose), nodule characteristics (nodule location, nodule size, nodule density), and pulmonary vessel can influence the performance of AI.

Slice Thickness

Due to the difference between vendors and reconstruction algorithms, CT scans have thin and thick slices. Thick-section CT scans have the issue of partial volume effect, which causes the information loss of small objects. Evidence demonstrates sensitivity of the AI detection system is decreased when the same AI was assessed in CT scans with thick slices compared to thin slices. To explore the effect of slice thickness on the performance of a computer-aided detection (CAD) system, Kim et al. evaluated an AI system on multi-detector CT scans in 1 mm and 5 mm groups in 10 patients [41]. In the thin-section group, 126 nodules were detected by 2 radiologists, whereas 114 nodules were found in the thick-section group. The AI system detected 120 out of 126 (95.2%) and 101 out of 114 (88.6%) nodules in two groups separately. The evidence was also supported by Narayanan et al. who assessed a CAD system in 192 CT scans with a slice thickness of 1.25 mm from the LUNA16 dataset [42]. At a down-sampling ratio of 2, 4, and 8, images with a slice thickness of 2.5, 5, and 10 mm were stimulated. The study exemplified the system tested on 1.25 or 2.5 mm slices outperformed the one on 5 or 10 mm slices. The performance of using different slice thickness settings is shown in Fig. 43.3.

Slab Thickness in Maximum Intensity Projections

Maximum intensity projections (MIPs) are one of the clinical procedures used by radiologists to efficiently detect

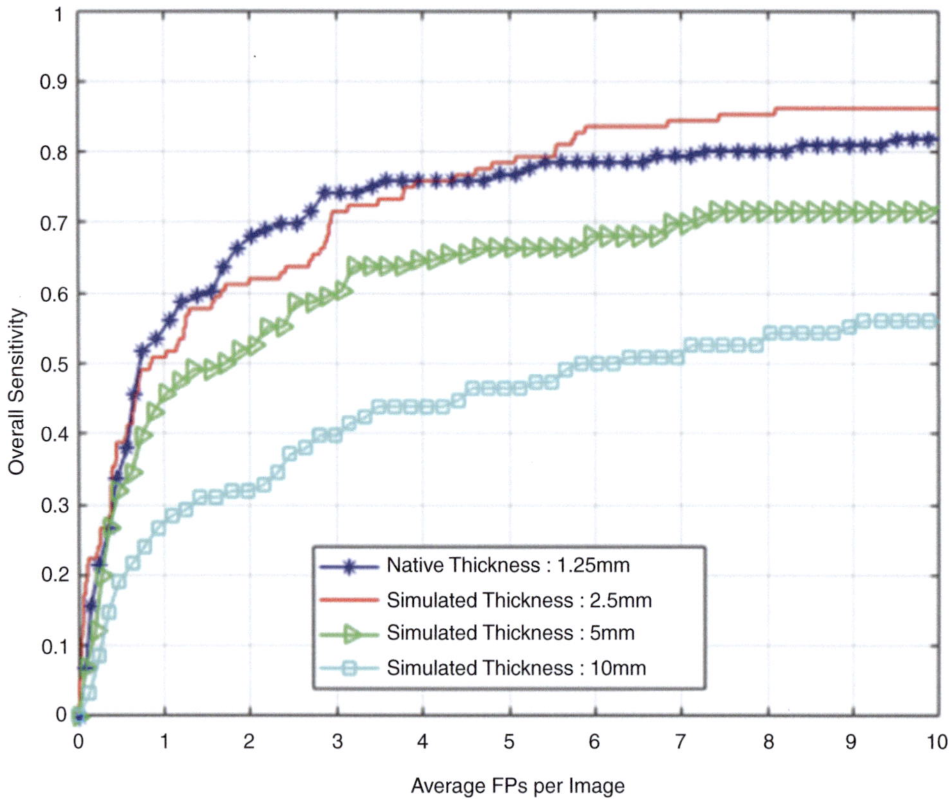

Fig. 43.3 Performance of CAD in different slice thickness settings for nodule detection. (Reprinted with permission of Barath Narayanan. From: Narayananet al. [42])

nodules in vessel-enhanced slices. Human observation using MIPs with a slab thickness of 10 mm showed a higher nodule detection rate than using 5, 15, and 20 mm MIPs [43]. However, the principle of detecting nodules between radiologists and AI is not completely the same. Ten-mm might not be the optimal slab thickness for AI to detect lung lesions. To determine the optimal slab thickness for AI, one study investigated the effect of different slab thicknesses at the nodule candidate detection stage using the large LUNA16 dataset [32]. To avoid partial volume effect, scans with a slice thickness >2.5 mm were excluded. All scans were interpolated to 1 mm slices, and MIPs with a slab thickness from 3 to 50 mm at an interval of 5 mm were generated by the 1 mm slices. The system was developed and validated with one type of MIP each time, and results were acquired by tenfold cross-validation. With increasing slab thickness, the detection rate of the AI system initially gradually increased up to 90% with a slab thickness of 10 mm, and thereafter decreased slowly. Regarding false positives, the number decreased with slab thickness from 1 mm to 25 mm, and remained stable thereafter. When determining the appropriate method for detecting as many nodules as possible at the nodule candidate detection stage, 10 mm was the optimal parameter of MIP for AI.

Radiation Dose

Radiation dose is related to the tube current and voltage, and by lowering one of these values, radiation dose can be reduced. However, in doing so the image quality can be also decreased which may cause more false positives. To attempt to reduce the dose which patients receive from screening, while keeping a high detection rate of lung cancer, studies have been conducted to evaluate the effect of using low-dose CT (LDCT) or ultra-low-dose CT (ULDCT) on the performance of AI detection. It is evident that in spite of an increasing number of false positives, AI can detect a similar number of nodules on CT scans performed at a lower dose. For example, Young et al. collected 481 LDCT scans from the NLST screening and simulated corresponding scans with 50% and 25% of the original dose [44]. On a patient level, the AI system detected 38%, 37%, and 38% of patients who had at least one nodule at the original, 50%, and 25% dose, respectively. Although the sensitivity was comparable, the AI system found 13.5 more false positives per scan with 25% dose, compared to 5 false positives per scan with 50% dose and 3 false positives per scan with routine dose. Therefore, the authors suggested that it might be possible to reduce radiation dose of LDCT by a half in the current NSTL protocol. A different study included scans of 25 patients, and image acquisitions were performed at a dose of 2.2, 1.2, 0.9, and 0.6 mSv by reducing the tube current [45]. When CT scans were reconstructed using the filtered back-projection technique, a similar number of true positives were detected by the AI system at different dose levels, while ten more false positives appeared on the scans at a lower dose compared to routine scans. Furthermore, in a large evaluation study, an AI system was tested on 187 LDCT scans and 942 regular CT scans [39]. There was no significant difference between dose levels for AI when detecting true positives.

Nodule Location

According to anatomical location, nodules can be categorized into pleural, isolated, and juxtavascular types. Some studies have shown that nodule location can affect the performance of AI. In the research of Bae et al., authors found that isolated nodules were easier to detect using the system than juxtavascular and pleural nodules [19]. This was due to isolated nodules having a clear contrast between nodule boundary and lung parenchyma. In addition, these nodules were differentiable on a single slice without the need for comparison between contiguous slices. By contrast, the other two types of nodules, having more complex morphological features, were connected to disturbing vessels or tissues. This trend was also proved by the study of van Ginneken et al. who evaluated an AI system on the ANODE09 dataset [23]. The sensitivities of detection of isolated, juxtavascular, and pleural nodules were 73.8%, 72.1%, and 62.7%, respectively. Another reason for the good accuracy demonstrated when detecting isolated nodules is the high prevalence of these nodules in the training set. This meant that the system had learned more features of isolated nodules, and hence tended to detect them.

Nodule Size

Some AI systems are prone to missing small nodules, since they only show up in a few slices and noise can highly impact the definition of the nodule boundary. In the work of Zheng et al., nodules were stratified according to the Lung-RADS guideline [46]. The majority of missed nodules (15/23) had a diameter between 3 and 6 mm at the nodule candidate detection stage. A similar result was found in the work of Xie et al. [34]. The detection rate was only 44.4% for nodules smaller than 10 mm, whereas it was 86.9% for larger nodules (10–30 mm). Contrarily, van Ginneken et al. found that five out of six of the evaluated AI systems presented lower sensitivities in identifying large nodules at different false-positive rates [23]. A possible explanation from the authors was that small nodules appeared more frequently in the training dataset, which results in a conflict expectation.

Nodule Density

In general, solid nodules are more differentiable than part-solid and non-solid nodules in the lung window settings. A study undertaken by Setio et al. analyzed the density of detected nodules for seven AI nodule detection systems which participated in the LUNA16 challenge [30]. All of the systems showed a similar detection trend; the fewer the solid components in nodules, the greater the sensitivity of the system. In other words, among the three types of nodules, non-solid nodules had the lowest sensitivity. They normally represent areas of ground-glass opacity, which increases the difficulty for AI to differentiate them from almost identical lung parenchyma or focal pneumonia. Another study also investigated the performance of AI on solid and sub-solid nodules [39]. The detection rate of solid nodules was 72.9% (556/763) in LDCT scans, whereas that of sub-solid nodules was only 65.0% (256/394).

Pulmonary Vessels

Pulmonary vessels are one of the main false-positive findings in the results of AI systems. When nodules are close or attached to vessels, it becomes challenging for AI to select these nodules. If vessels are removed from the lung while preserving nodules completely, nodule detection could be much easier for both human readers and AI, with less false-positive results. Inspired by this idea, Gu et al. developed a deep learning-based detection system using the pulmonary vessel suppression technique, and explored the effect of removal of vessels on the performance of AI [47]. The ablation experiment demonstrated that sensitivity improved from 96.9% to 98.6%, with a false-positive rate that dropped from 7.65 to 0.92 per scan after ruling out pulmonary vessels for the same candidate detection and false-positive reduction algorithms. Another recent study showed that the elimination of pulmonary vessels can reduce suspicious regions [48]. Although most nodules (94.0%) can be detected by AI, the false-positive rate, 15.1 per scan, was still high. The reason for this may be that the authors only used 2D slices instead of 3D cubic patches for false-positive elimination; therefore, nodular findings could not be effectively removed.

Role of AI in Nodule Detection

Although AI can achieve promising performance in the detection of different sizes and types of pulmonary nodules, the effect of its performance in the reading of CT scans when compared to or used alongside radiologists should be further studied before applying it in real clinical practice. The performance of AI, such as the percentage of truly detected nodules, the number of false positives, and the order of using aided detection, highly impacts the role that AI plays in clinical settings. For the purpose of exploring the feasibility of applying AI systems in clinical practice, a large number of studies have been conducted to compare their performance with that of radiologists. Despite a few researchers finding that AI failed in improving diagnostic accuracy [49], most results have shown that AI can be a good second or concurrent reader, when results of AI are shown to radiologists subsequently or concurrently. The reading principles of using AI or computer-aided detection (CAD) systems are presented in Fig. 43.4.

In the subsequent model, AI is generally considered as a second reader, and radiologists are only allowed to see the results of computerized detection after finishing their first read. After the initial independent radiologist reads, the computerized findings for the same scans are displayed to radiologists for the purpose of checking whether nodules reported are indeed true nodules. Thus, the consensus panel, including nodules detected by both radiologists and AI, will be included in the reference standard. In the first phase of a comparison study, the authors analyzed the effect of utilizing AI in the subsequent model for nodule detection on thin-section CT scans [50]. When AI was used as a second reader, the final sensitivities were 82%, 97%, and 82% for solid, part-solid, and GGO nodules, respectively. However, the sensitivities were only 57%, 81%, and 69% for corresponding nodules while reading without AI. To assess the effectiveness of AI as a second reader, Awai et al. collected 50 chest CT scans with nodules ranging from 3 mm to 29 mm [51]. Five experienced radiologists and five radiology residents were asked to rate nodule presence with and without using a computer-aided detection system. The observation results showed that there was a significant detection difference between reading alone and using the system afterward, for both experienced and less experienced readers. The study concluded that the use of AI can enhance nodule detection for both reader groups.

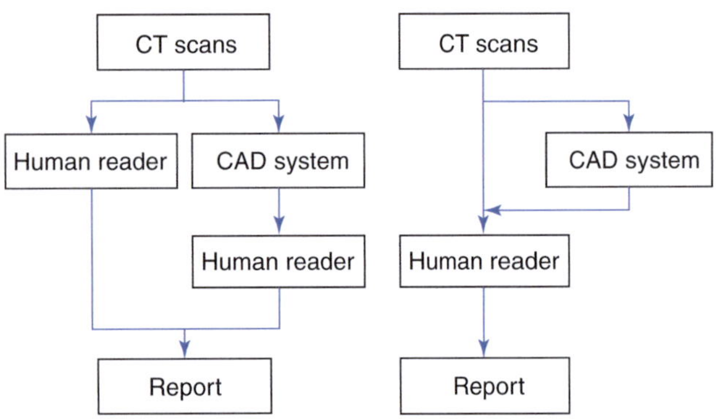

Fig. 43.4 Reading principles with the CAD integrated. The CAD is a second reader in the left workflow, while the CAD is a concurrent reader at the right side

In the concurrent model, radiologists can take image interpretation of AI into account while reading the CT scans. Studies have shown that when AI is used as a concurrent reader, radiologists are capable of detecting more nodules than reading alone. The study of Matsumoto et al. compared the performance of nodule detection on 50 CT scans with and without AI. With the help of the second AI reader, 66.5% of nodules were found by radiologists [52]. In contrast, only 56.5% of nodules were detected in unaided reading. Importantly, radiologists took only approximately 10 seconds longer reading each scan, and the sensitivity of nodule detection was improved.

The concurrent model obviously saves more time than the subsequent model since radiologists do not have to go through slices again without AI-aided detection. This assumption was proved by Matsumoto et al. who compared the performance of AI on 50 CT scans in both models [52]. The results showed that the mean reading time in the concurrent model (132 ± 70 s) was significantly shorter than that of the subsequent model (210 ± 103 s). A similar trend was reported in the study of Beyer et al. where the reading time was 274 seconds vs. 337 seconds on average for the concurrent model vs. the subsequent model [53]. Matsumoto et al. also found no significant difference in the performance of radiologists in these two models. Conversely, Beyer et al., who also reviewed 50 scans, reported the sensitivity when using AI as a second reader was significantly higher than the sensitivity in the case of applying it concurrently [53]. A possible explanation for the varying results is that the AI system of Matsumoto et al. achieved a higher stand-alone sensitivity of 63% with 3.5 false positives per scan, whereas Beyer et al. had a stand-alone sensitivity of 43% with 1.3 false positives per scan. The results of Matsumoto et al. were more conducive to the effectiveness of using AI.

AI detection systems can also detect nodules previously missed in the consensus of radiologists, and could be utilized as an assisting reader. Findings could be referenced by radiologists in lung cancer screening programs, if a higher sensitivity and a lower false-positive rate can be achieved. In the study of Zhao et al., an AI system was evaluated on 400 LDCT scans selected from the NELSON screening study [54]. Five out of one hundred and fifty-one nodules were only detected by double reading, whereas thirty-three true nodules were only identified by AI. Notably, one nodule overlooked by radiologists but found by AI was lung cancer. A second study compared the detection performance of AI and double reading on 346 CT scans retrospectively collected in a lung cancer screening program between March and November 2017 [55]. The ratio of men to women was 221:125, and the average age was 51 years old. The AI system had a higher sensitivity than radiologists, not only for nodules larger than 5 mm (96.5% vs. 88.0%) but also for small nodules (84.3% vs. 77.5%), although the system yielded more false positives for radiologists to check. Seventeen nodules were confirmed as missed by the readers but detected by AI after a third reading by an experienced radiologist. A third comparison study evaluated three AI systems on the large LIDC-IDRI dataset, with 777 nodules accepted by 4 radiologists [56]. The best system reached a sensitivity of 82% with 1108 false-positive findings. After the exclusion of the obvious non-nodules by a researcher, 269 findings were assessed by 4 radiologists. There were 45 marks accepted by 4 radiologists as nodules, of which 70% were not obvious pulmonary nodules. Thirty-seven nodules were larger than 4 mm and required follow-up. These findings indicate AI has the potential to detect subtle nodules previously missed by radiologists. Furthermore, an AI-based system was evaluated on the NLST screening chest radiographs from 5485 participants [57]. The sensitivity and specificity when using AI were 100.0% and 90.9% for malignant nodule detection in digital radiographs. Compared to results of AI, radiologists had a lower sensitivity of 94.1% but a slightly higher specificity of 91.0%. AI also found seven nodules or masses missed by radiologists. The study concluded that the AI system outperformed NLST radiologists in detecting malignant nodules, and might help radiologists to detect lung cancer if used as a second reader.

Despite studies showing that AI can boost radiologist's performance, the feasibility of applying AI systems in daily clinical practice and lung cancer screening has not been sufficiently proven. It is necessary to validate AI systems on screening data from multiple institutes and provide more evidence on the detection of those clinically relevant nodules. In addition, not only technicians but also radiologists should work cooperatively to build up a larger and more widely distributed nodule dataset, which is shared with the community in order to further stimulate the development of nodule detection systems.

Conclusions

Lung cancer accounts for the majority of cancer-related deaths, and the 5-year survival rate is only 4% when detected at stage IV. For the purpose of detecting lung cancer at an early stage, randomized lung cancer screening trials have been established all over the world. The results from some large-scale screening studies, such as NELSON and NLST, show that the mortality rate of patients who undergo CT screening was reduced. These developments give lung cancer patients a greater chance of survival, but as a consequence the reading workload of radiologists is increasing. Artificial intelligence detection systems have been designed with the aim of reducing the pressure on radiologists, so that they can focus more on diagnoses. Despite many factors, such as CT parameters, nodule characteristics, and pulmonary vessels, affecting the sensitivity and false-positive rates of AI, AI can still provide substantial assistance for radiologists in the clinic, both as a second reader and concurrent reader. A few studies have been conducted evaluating AI on lung cancer screening data, and show AI can achieve good performance on nodule detection. In the future, the effect of using AI in lung cancer screening programs should be further studied. AI could be utilized as an assisting reader whose findings can be referenced by radiologists in screening settings, so long as the sensitivity can be continuously improved and the false-positive rate can be minimized.

References

1. Siegel RL, Miller KD, Jemal AJCacjfc. Cancer statistics. 2020. 2020;70(1):7–30.
2. Miller KD, Nogueira L, Mariotto AB, et al. Cancer treatment and survivorship statistics. 2019. 2019;69(5):363–85.
3. Oncology NLSTRTJJoT. Lung cancer incidence and mortality with extended follow-up in the national lung screening trial. 2019;14(10):1732–42.
4. Pehrson LM, Nielsen MB, Ammitzbøl Lauridsen CJD. Automatic pulmonary nodule detection applying deep learning or machine learning algorithms to the LIDC-IDRI database: a systematic review. 2019;9(1):29.
5. Li D, Mikela Vilmun B, Frederik Carlsen J, et al. The Performance of Deep Learning Algorithms on Automatic Pulmonary Nodule Detection and Classification Tested on Different Datasets That Are Not Derived from LIDC-IDRI: A Systematic Review. 2019;9(4):207.
6. Setio AAA, Ciompi F, Litjens G, et al. Pulmonary nodule detection in CT images: false positive reduction using multi-view convolutional networks. 2016;35(5):1160–1169.
7. Oudkerk M, Liu S, Heuvelmans MA, Walter JE, Field JKJNRCO. Lung cancer LDCT screening and mortality reduction—evidence, pitfalls and future perspectives. 2020:1–17.
8. Medicine NLSTRTJNEJo. Reduced lung-cancer mortality with low-dose computed tomographic screening. 2011;365(5):395–409.
9. de Koning HJ, van der Aalst CM, de Jong PA, et al. Reduced lung-cancer mortality with volume CT screening in a randomized trial. 2020;382(6):503–13.
10. Field JK, Duffy S, Baldwin DR, et al. UK Lung Cancer RCT Pilot Screening Trial: baseline findings from the screening arm provide evidence for the potential implementation of lung cancer screening. 2016;71(2):161–70.
11. Pastorino U, Sverzellati N, Sestini S, et al. Ten-year results of the Multicentric Italian Lung Detection trial demonstrate the safety and efficacy of biennial lung cancer screening. 2019;118:142–48.

12. Pinsky PF, Gierada DS, Black W, et al. Performance of Lung-RADS in the National Lung Screening Trial: a retrospective assessment. 2015;162(7):485–91.
13. Lung ct screening reporting & data system (lung-rads). https://www.acr.org/Clinical-Resources/Reporting-and-Data-Systems/Lung-Rads. Accessed 10 Oct 2020.
14. Oudkerk M, Devaraj A, Vliegenthart R, et al. European position statement on lung cancer screening. 2017;18(12):e754-66.
15. Pastorino U, Silva M, Sestini S, et al. Prolonged lung cancer screening reduced 10-year mortality in the MILD trial: new confirmation of lung cancer screening efficacy. 2019;30(7):1162–9.
16. Giger ML, Doi K, MacMahon HJMP. Image feature analysis and computer-aided diagnosis in digital radiography. 3. Automated detection of nodules in peripheral lung fields. 1988;15(2):158–66.
17. Li QJCMI, Graphics. Recent progress in computer-aided diagnosis of lung nodules on thin-section CT. 2007;31(4–5):248–57.
18. Armato III SG, Giger ML, MacMahon HJMp. Automated detection of lung nodules in CT scans: preliminary results. 2001;28(8):1552–61.
19. Bae KT, Kim J-S, Na Y-H, Kim KG, Kim J-HJR. Pulmonary nodules: automated detection on CT images with morphologic matching algorithm—preliminary results. 2005;236(1):286–93.
20. Matsumoto S, Kundel HL, Gee JC, Gefter WB, Hatabu HJMIA. Pulmonary nodule detection in CT images with quantized convergence index filter. 2006;10(3):343–352.
21. Zhang J, Xia Y, Zeng H, Zhang YJN. NODULe: Combining constrained multi-scale LoG filters with densely dilated 3D deep convolutional neural network for pulmonary nodule detection. 2018;317:159–67.
22. The ANODE09 dataset. https://anode09.grand-challenge.org/Home/. Accessed 12 Oct, 2020.
23. Van Ginneken B, Armato III SG, de Hoop B, et al. Comparing and combining algorithms for computer-aided detection of pulmonary nodules in computed tomography scans: the ANODE09 study. 2010;14(6):707–22.
24. Armato III SG, McLennan G, Bidaut L, et al. The lung image database consortium (LIDC) and image database resource initiative (IDRI): a completed reference database of lung nodules on CT scans. 2011;38(2):915–31.
25. The National Lung Screening Trial dataset. https://wiki.cancerimagingarchive.net/display/NLST/National+Lung+Screening+Trial. Accessed 11 Oct 2020.
26. LUNA16 grand challenge. https://luna16.grand-challenge.org/. Accessed 11 Oct 2020.
27. Data Science Bowl 2017. https://www.kaggle.com/c/data-science-bowl-2017. Accessed 11 Oct 2020.
28. Pedrosa J, Aresta G, Ferreira C, et al. Lndb: A lung nodule database on computed tomography. 2019.
29. Fleischner 2017 guideline. https://radiologyassistant.nl/chest/plumonary-nodules/fleischner-2017-guideline. Accessed 11 Oct 2020.
30. Setio AAA, Traverso A, De Bel T, et al. Validation, comparison, and combination of algorithms for automatic detection of pulmonary nodules in computed tomography images: the LUNA16 challenge. 2017;42:1–13.
31. Zheng S, Guo J, Cui X, Veldhuis RN, Oudkerk M, Van Ooijen PM. Automatic pulmonary nodule detection in CT scans using convolutional neural networks based on maximum intensity projection. IEEE Trans Med Imaging. 2019;39(3):797–805.
32. Zheng S, Cui X, Vonder M, et al. Deep learning-based pulmonary nodule detection: effect of slab thickness in maximum intensity projections at the nodule candidate detection stage. Computer Methods Programs in Biomedicine. 2020;196
33. Liu J, Cao L, Akin O, Tian Y. 3DFPN-HS2: 3D feature pyramid network based high sensitivity and specificity pulmonary nodule detection. Paper presented at: International Conference on Medical Image Computing and Computer-Assisted Intervention. 2019.
34. Xie H, Yang D, Sun N, Chen Z, Zhang Y. Automated pulmonary nodule detection in CT images using deep convolutional neural networks [published online ahead of print January 2019]. Pattern Recogn. 2019;85:109–19.
35. Kim B-C, Yoon JS, Choi J-S, Suk H-IJNN. Multi-scale gradual integration CNN for false positive reduction in pulmonary nodule detection. 2019;115:1–10.
36. Kuan K, Ravaut M, Manek G, et al. Deep learning for lung cancer detection: tackling the kaggle data science bowl 2017 challenge. 2017.
37. Nam JG, Park S, Hwang EJ, et al. Development and validation of deep learning–based automatic detection algorithm for malignant pulmonary nodules on chest radiographs. 2019;290(1):218–28.
38. Kaluva KC, Vaidhya K, Chunduru A, Tarai S, Nadimpalli SPP, Vaidya S. An automated workflow for lung nodule follow-up recommendation using deep learning. Paper presented at: International Conference on Image Analysis and Recognition. 2020.
39. Liu K, Li Q, Ma J, et al. Evaluating a fully automated pulmonary nodule detection approach and its impact on radiologist performance. 2019;1(3):e180084.
40. Ardila D, Kiraly AP, Bharadwaj S, et al. End-to-end lung cancer screening with three-dimensional deep learning on low-dose chest computed tomography. 2019;25(6):954–61.
41. Kim J-S, Kim J-H, Cho G, Bae KTJR. Automated detection of pulmonary nodules on CT images: effect of section thickness and reconstruction interval—initial results. 2005;236(1):295–9.
42. Narayanan BN, Hardie RC, Kebede TMJJMI. Performance analysis of a computer-aided detection system for lung nodules in CT at different slice thicknesses. 2018;5(1):014504.
43. Li W, Chu Z, Zhang Y, Li Q, Zheng Y, Lv F. Effect of slab thickness on the detection of pulmonary nodules by use of CT maximum and minimum intensity projection. Am J Roentgenol. 2019;213(3):562–7.
44. Young S, Lo P, Kim G, et al. The effect of radiation dose reduction on computer-aided detection (CAD) performance in a low-dose lung cancer screening population. 2017;44(4):1337–46.
45. Den Harder AM, Willemink MJ, Van Hamersvelt RW, et al. Effect of radiation dose reduction and iterative reconstruction on computer-aided detection of pulmonary nodules: Intra-individual comparison. 2016;85(2):346–51.
46. Zheng S, Cornelissen LJ, Cui X, et al. Deep convolutional neural networks for multi-planar lung nodule detection: improvement in small nodule identification. Med Phys. 2020.
47. Gu X, Xie W, Fang Q, Zhao J, Li QJMp. The effect of pulmonary vessel suppression on computerized detection of nodules in chest CT scans. Med Phys. 2020;47(10):4917–27.
48. Jiang H, Ma H, Qian W, Gao M, Li YJIjob, informatics h. An automatic detection system of lung nodule based on multigroup patch-based deep learning network. 2017;22(4):1227–37.
49. Nietert PJ, Ravenel JG, Taylor KK, Silvestri GAJJoti. Influence of nodule detection software on radiologists' confidence in identifying pulmonary nodules with computed tomography. 2011;26(1):48.
50. Godoy MC, Kim TJ, White CS, et al. Benefit of computer-aided detection analysis for the detection of subsolid and solid lung nodules on thin-and thick-section CT. 2013;200(1):74–83.
51. Awai K, Murao K, Ozawa A, et al. Pulmonary nodules at chest CT: effect of computer-aided diagnosis on radiologists' detection performance. 2004;230(2):347–52.
52. Matsumoto S, Ohno Y, Aoki T, et al. Computer-aided detection of lung nodules on multidetector CT in concurrent-reader and second-reader modes: a comparative study. 2013;82(8):1332–7.
53. Beyer F, Zierott L, Fallenberg E, et al. Comparison of sensitivity and reading time for the use of computer-aided detection (CAD)

of pulmonary nodules at MDCT as concurrent or second reader. 2007;17(11):2941–7.
54. Zhao Y, de Bock GH, Vliegenthart R, et al. Performance of computer-aided detection of pulmonary nodules in low-dose CT: comparison with double reading by nodule volume. 2012;22(10):2076–84.
55. Li L, Liu Z, Huang H, Lin M, Luo DJTc. Evaluating the performance of a deep learning-based computer-aided diagnosis (DL-CAD) system for detecting and characterizing lung nodules: Comparison with the performance of double reading by radiologists. 2019;10(2):183–92.
56. Jacobs C, van Rikxoort EM, Murphy K, Prokop M, Schaefer-Prokop CM, van Ginneken BJEr. Computer-aided detection of pulmonary nodules: a comparative study using the public LIDC/IDRI database. 2016;26(7):2139–47.
57. Yoo H, Kim KH, Singh R, Digumarthy SR, Kalra MKJJNO. Validation of a Deep Learning Algorithm for the Detection of Malignant Pulmonary Nodules in Chest Radiographs. 2020;3(9):e2017135.

44 Lung Cancer Characterization and Prognosis: The Role of Artificial Intelligence

Carolyn Horst, Robert O'Shea, and Vicky Goh

Introduction

Approximately 2.1 million cases of lung cancer are diagnosed worldwide every year, resulting in 1.8 million deaths [1]. Survival outcomes are poor, often because symptoms develop when the disease has already reached a late stage (III/IV) and curative treatment is no longer possible. Imaging, involving multiple modalities and approaches, is key to oncological processes, and lung cancer is no exception. A standard patient pathway from diagnosis to treatment and onward survival may involve screening for or initial identification of the disease via computed tomography (CT) imaging, 18F-fluorodeoxyglucose positron emission tomography (18F-FDG PET) in order to further characterise the lesion detected, CT-guided biopsy in order to gain histological and/or mutation status information and further imaging in aid of treatment and diagnosis, including cone-beam CT (CBCT) and surveillance scans (see Fig. 44.1 for a schematic of the lung cancer patient imaging pathway).

Many studies have been published in the last 10 years investigating the ways in which imaging biomarkers can be applied at each step in the lung cancer journey, from differentiating benign from malignant pulmonary nodules, investigating phenotype and genotype information, determining tumour behaviour including the development of lymph node and distant metastases and predicting response to treatment and overall prognosis. To date, the majority of imaging biomarker identification studies have investigated imaging radiomics, where regions-of-interest (ROI), usually delineated by radiologists, are fed through software that extracts multilevel data types or 'features' from each ROI. Machine learning techniques have been applied at this point, to distinguish between redundant and useful features, due to the considerable amount of data the feature extraction process creates, and to generate helpful statistical outputs. Thus far, in the development of imaging-based biomarkers for lung cancer, there has been limited use of machine learning to identify the classifiers or features themselves, usually due to lack of large volume datasets. This chapter will assess the evidence to date of the application of machine learning in lung cancer.

Staging, Histology and Treatment

Lung cancer is classified based on histological tissue of origin into non-small-cell lung cancer (NSCLC) (approximately 80% of all cases) and small-cell lung cancer. NSCLC is further subdivided into adenocarcinoma, squamous cell carcinoma and large-cell carcinoma, with adenocarcinoma being predominant. Lung cancer staging is completed both radiologically and histologically via the tumour, node, metastases (TNM) staging system, most recently updated in 2017 to the eighth edition [2]. This system considers tumour size and location (e.g. endobronchial or diaphragmatic), nodal involvement and location (single or multiple, local or distant) and location and number of metastases in order to formulate an overall stage of the disease. Disease stage is predictive of prognosis and is considered an important part of the clinical assessment of a patient when treatment decisions are being made.

Further information on lung cancer phenotype is gained from biopsy samples obtained via a needle biopsy (usually guided by CT imaging), bronchoscopy or after surgical

C. Horst, AB, MA, MBBS, PhD (✉)
V. Goh, MA, MBBChir, MD, MRCP, FRCR
Department of Cancer Imaging, School of Biomedical Engineering and Imaging Sciences, King's College London, London, UK

Department of Radiology, Guy's and St Thomas' NHS Foundation Trust, London, UK
e-mail: carolyn.horst@kcl.ac.uk; vicky.goh@kcl.ac.uk

R. O'Shea, MB BCh, BAO, MSc
Department of Cancer Imaging, School of Biomedical Engineering and Imaging Sciences, King's College London, London, UK
e-mail: robert.1.oshea@kcl.ac.uk

C. N. De Cecco et al. (eds.), *Artificial Intelligence in Cardiothoracic Imaging*, Contemporary Medical Imaging,
https://doi.org/10.1007/978-3-030-92087-6_44

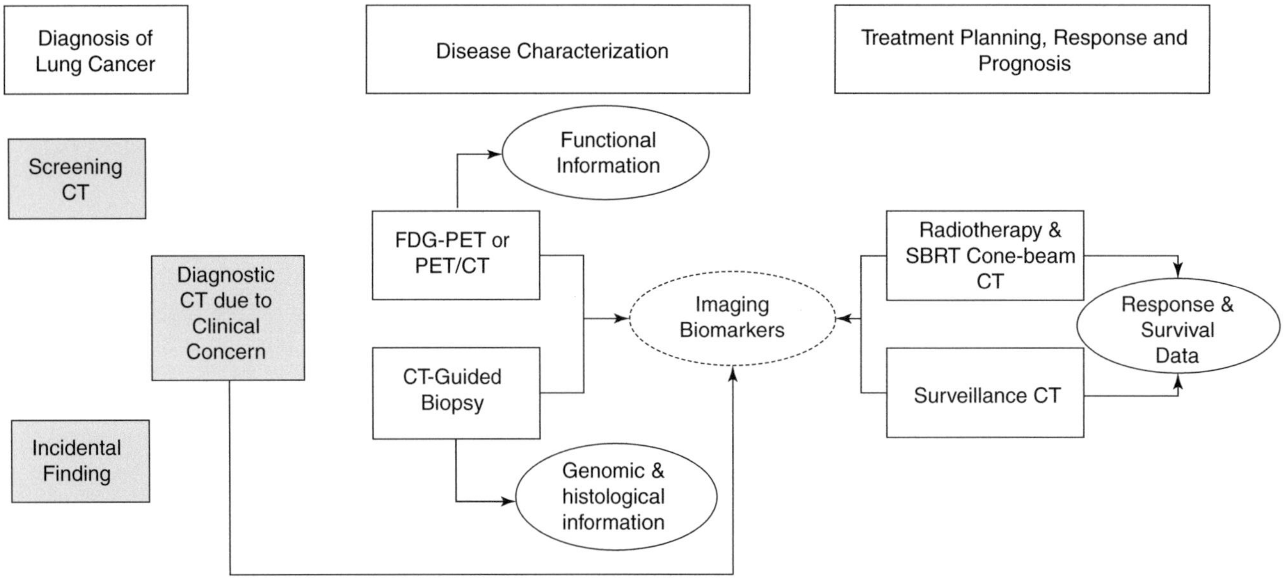

Fig. 44.1 A schematic of imaging in the lung cancer patient pathway. AI applications to the processes outlined in grey boxes are not directly addressed in this chapter. Patients may have many of these imaging studies performed, or only a few, depending on their disease, treatment and prognosis. Categories of data in the circles indicate the information available from each type of imaging. 'Imaging Biomarker' data can potentially be collected from each of the stages of imaging

resection. Histological samples are assessed visually to determine the cell of origin (small cell versus NSCLC and its subtypes) and to assess the structural features of the tissues. Genetic testing allows for detection of any targetable mutations within the tumour. For example, lung cancers with high epidermal growth factor receptor (EGFR) and anaplastic lymphoma kinase (ALK) mutational burdens are likely to benefit from tyrosine kinase inhibitor (TKI) therapies. Similarly, immune checkpoint inhibitors (ICI), including agents that target T-cell membrane protein programmed cell death-1 (PD-1) and its ligand (PD-L1), are more efficacious in tumours where PD-L1 expression is high. Therefore, understanding driver mutations and the underlying tumour composition is integral to targeting therapy appropriately. See Fig. 44.2 for a schematic of the most common targetable pathways in lung cancer.

Lung cancer treatment is split into either surgical resection, radiotherapy or chemotherapeutic treatment. For early-stage disease (I and II) where the patient is fit enough for radical intervention, surgical treatment is carried out with curative intent. For disease stages III and IV, oncological treatment is offered, either via chemotherapeutic agents, including the targeted therapies mentioned above, or radiotherapy, to shrink the tumour and slow its spread. Unfortunately, cure is unlikely in late-stage disease, even with newer pharmacological agents, as drug resistance often develops, and the tumour subsequently grows and seeds to other sites. A treatment option for those patients with early-stage disease but who are unfit for surgery is stereotactic body radiation therapy (SBRT), also known at stereotactic ablative radiotherapy (SABR), where high-dose irradiation of the cancerous lesion is undertaken with curative intent.

Despite the proliferation and improvement of targeted therapeutic agents, the known genotype of driver mutations and less invasive surgical techniques, overall survival from lung cancer is poor compared to other tumour types [3]. There is a need for personalised medicine to improve prognosis: imaging AI may be able to offer insights for staging, genomics, optimal treatment and prognosis, at each step in the lung cancer patient's pathway.

Lung Cancer Characterisation

Phenotyping

Lung cancer phenotypes cover a broad spectrum of histological types and subtypes. AI, in particular radiomics combined with machine learning, is being used to elucidate underlying cell structures and gather data on the phenotype of the entire tumour. Clinically, this is potentially useful where a biopsy is either inconclusive or impossible, but may also be used in addition to an adequate sample, as a biopsy only captures a small portion of the whole tumour, and may therefore only reflect a portion of the tumour cell composition. Gathering whole-tumour phenotypic information via imaging may also enable greater certainty around treatment planning, response to therapies and surgery and overall prog-

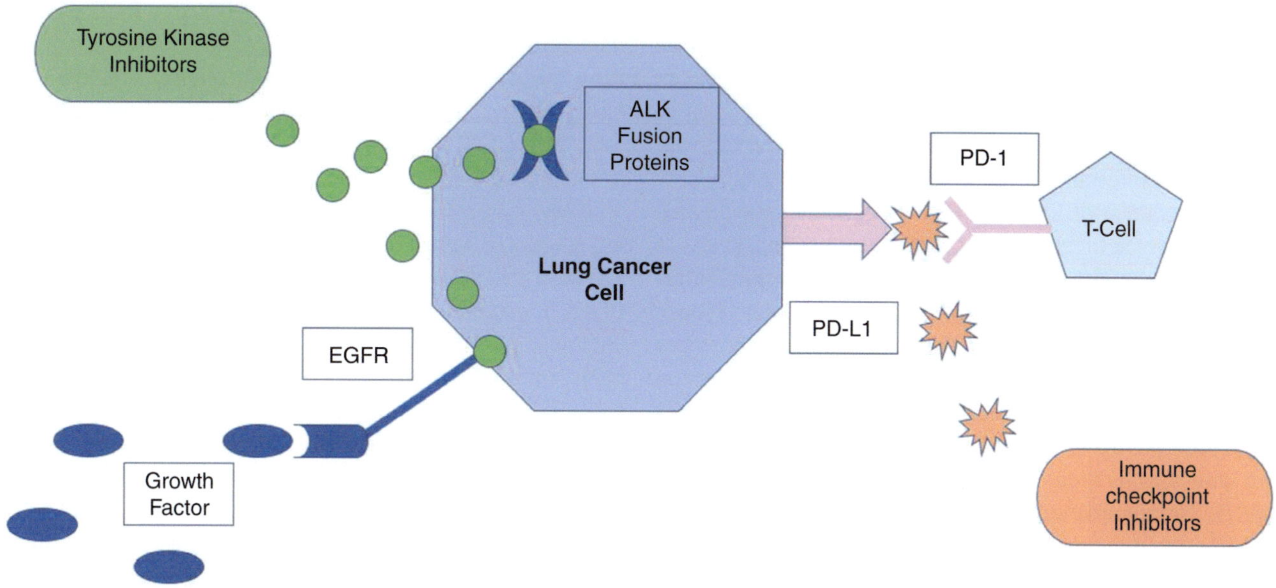

Fig. 44.2 Schematic of the most common targets and targeted therapies in lung cancer. Endothelial growth factor receptor (EFGR) cell membrane protein is stimulated by growth factors to trigger cell division. Tyrosine kinase inhibitors block EGFR initiation of the cell division pathway. Anaplastic lymphoma kinase (ALK) fusion proteins also stimulate cell division, and tyrosine kinase inhibitors can downregulate the signals sent from the mutant proteins to prevent this process. Immune checkpoint inhibitors prevent anomalous signalling of the lung cancer cell to T-cells via PD-L1 to PD-1, allowing the T-cell to recognise it as an abnormal cell for immune destruction

nosis, as lung cancer phenotype is known to correlate with prognosis and be predictive of response and tumour behaviour.

Recent research has attempted to predict the subtypes of NSCLC, distinguishing between adenocarcinoma (ADC), squamous cell carcinoma (SCC), large-cell carcinoma (LCC) and those not otherwise specified (NOS) cancers [4, 5] via CT imaging. Various radiomics and deep learning methods have been used, including first-, second- and higher-order statistical feature extraction, the application of filters for investigating textural and intensity features, and SMOTE algorithms to increase the imaging sample size for the less common subtypes of NSCLC in a cohort. Machine learning methods including support vector machine (SVM) and random forest (RF) have also been applied to 18F-FDG PET/CT datasets, specifically for ADC versus SCC assessment, and compared to each other to determine which individual or composite approaches might achieve the greatest performance [5]. By combining radiomics and machine learning methods, Han et al. achieved an area under the curve (AUC) of 0.90, with a sensitivity of 92% and specificity of 81%, for distinguishing adenocarcinoma from squamous cell carcinoma. These results were not validated on an external dataset, but the early outcomes are promising.

Radiomics and radiomics-plus-machine learning models have also shown the ability to distinguish subtypes of adenocarcinoma. ADC can manifest as adenocarcinoma in situ (AIS), minimally invasive adenocarcinoma (MIS) and invasive adenocarcinoma (IAC), which can be further characterised histologically depending on the presence of certain patterns, for example, micropapillary structures, which carry a poorer prognosis than samples with a lepidic predominant pattern [6]. Identifying these subtypes may allow for better whole-tumour characterisation, and therefore more accurate prognosis. Early research from several groups have demonstrated the potential of different radiomics signatures and quantitative imaging biomarkers at categorising appearances of these subtypes, with AUCs of 0.80–0.89, sensitivities of 82–99% and specificities of 53–80% [7–9].

Nevertheless, these phenotype studies have been heterogeneous in approach, data collection and comparison groups, but the underlying effort to define imaging biomarkers that consistently predict LC subtype will be worthwhile, as long as any model can demonstrate consistency across diverse populations and scanning protocols.

Genotyping and Targeted Therapies

Radiogenomics takes the requirement to demonstrate a correlative link between imaging features and the underlying cancer architecture a step further than histological phenotyping. Early studies by Aerts et al. have demonstrated that quantitative imaging biomarkers may reflect underlying biological processes, specifically distinct molecular pathways and gene-expression patterns taking place within tumours [10–12]. This work has set the stage for the application of radiogenomics to lung cancer, in an effort to derive even more useful information on the behaviour of these tumours.

In the context of lung cancer, radiogenomics models are being employed to link imaging with the mutational status of the cancers. As with phenotyping, valuable genotyping information may be lost by having small or incomplete biopsy samples, which cannot reflect the heterogeneous genotypes of the whole tumour. This information is clinically relevant to treatment for lung cancer, as cancers with certain genotypic characteristics, particularly EGFR and ALK mutations, are known to be more sensitive to tyrosine kinase inhibitors (TKI). Immunotherapies that target PD-1 and its ligand PD-L1 also demonstrate efficacy and are recommended as first-line therapy for metastatic disease, in combination with platinum-based therapies. Tumours often become refractory to these new pharmacological agents, but repeated biopsy to gain more information on genetic mutations is infrequently performed. Radiogenomics may have a future role in assisting the approach to treatment and prognosis.

Mutation Status Classification

Several epidermal growth factor receptor (EGFR) mutations increase sensitivity to tyrosine kinase inhibitor agents such as erlotinib and gefitinib. Multiple groups have demonstrated the ability of CT radiomics features, alone or combined with clinical features such as sex, age and smoking history, to predict EGFR+ versus EGFR- mutational status, with AUCs between 0.75 and 0.83, and accuracies of 75–77% [13–16]. One well-designed study by Rios Velazquez et al. also investigated the ability of their radiomics signature to distinguish between EGFR+ and KRAS+ tumours (AUC 0.86, accuracy 79%) and validated their signature against a separate cohort of patients from different hospital sites [15], which may indicate good replicability of the model in the future.

Several studies have used machine learning with or without radiomics to delve more deeply into imaging phenotypes and underlying genotypes; one group used an end-to-end deep learning model to predict EGFR mutational status, without radiomics input, and achieved an AUC of 0.81 and an accuracy of 74% on an independent validation cohort [17]. Another radiomics signature reported by Li et al. demonstrated an AUC of 0.79 (accuracy 72%) for classifying EGFR+ tumours, and went further to look at the ability to identify specific mutations of the EGFR gene (19Del and L858R), where their model achieved an AUC of 0.71 (accuracy 66%) [16]. At the moment, subcategorising EGFR mutations via imaging biomarkers into specific gene deletions or transfigurations is probably limited; a paper attempting to distinguish between four common EGFR mutations (at exons 18, 19, 20 and 21) achieved AUCs of less than 0.7, even when combined with clinical features [18]. Given the availability of TKI therapy and the importance of establishing EGFR mutational status, further work in this field is anticipated.

Early, single-site data point to 18F-FDG PET/CT providing additional, valuable information about underlying EGFR status. It has previously been demonstrated that 18F-FDG PET/CT parameters such as volume and metabolic activity are lower in EGFR+ tumours compared with EGFR- tumours [19]; initial data demonstrate that 18F-FDG PET/CT radiomics features, particularly tumour heterogeneity and metabolic texture features, when combined with clinical features can achieve an AUC in the validation set of 0.87 (accuracy 81%) [20]. The results of this study have not been reproduced, but, if replicable, may demonstrate the added benefit of metabolic information gained from functional imaging, in the context of driver mutations.

Anaplastic lymphoma kinase (ALK) fusion status, like EGFR, can be used to assess the likelihood of a tumour's response to ALK-TKI therapy. Assessment of the ALK status faces the same challenges as assessing EGFR mutational burden—immunohistochemistry is expensive and relies on adequate biopsy samples for diagnosis, but the potential benefit to patients can be significant. Though very early results, Song et al. have demonstrated considerable success at predicting ALK fusion status using preoperative CT images, clinicopathological information and a deep learning model (AUC in independent validation cohort 0.84, accuracy of 77%) [21].

PD-1 and PD-L1

With the advent and success of immunotherapies aimed at PD-1 and PD-L1, there is mounting interest in being able to use imaging biomarkers to assess the immune status of lung cancers, to identify who will benefit from these therapies, who may be unresponsive, and who may develop resistance in the future. The burden of PD-L1 in a given tumour is generally assessed via immunohistochemistry assays from biopsy samples, and, much like for driver mutations, if the sample is inadequate, the test results may not reflect the true immunological state of the tumour. Using an imaging biomarker to assess the immune status of the whole tumour may be a viable option instead, though, at the time of printing, studies are small and inconclusive [22, 23]. At the moment, research in the PD-1/PD-L1 radiomics sphere is more focused on assessing the prognostic benefit of immunotherapy treatments than attempting to make a link between the expression of PD-L1 and imaging biomarkers. These studies will be discussed in the *Prognosis and Response* section.

In summary, the results discussed above in this section all require robust validation and must demonstrate that they can be replicated in diverse populations, but early data on how radiomics and radiomics-plus-machine learning may be applied to genotyping and phenotyping are promising.

Prognosis and Response

Understanding prognosis enables informed decision-making around the potential benefit of different therapeutic approaches to lung cancer. Prognosis is necessarily tied to treatment response and therefore not independent of prognostic assessments made before treatment is instigated, which highlights the importance of understanding how prognosis may change before and after treatment. Clinically, prognosis is predicted by TNM staging and other clinical factors such as performance status, age and gender. AI methods are being applied to pre-treatment imaging to discover if biomarkers have prognostic benefit, either to glean additional information to TNM staging or clinical factors alone or to predict response to certain treatment types. The discussion about these novel methods for investigating imaging biomarkers is split below according to whether the endpoint of interest is prognosis or treatment response.

Pre-Treatment Imaging and Prognosis

Pre-treatment 18F-FDG PET/CT and CT imaging studies are performed regularly in lung cancer patients and therefore have the potential to provide further data on the tumours' composition, beyond the clinicopathological data and TNM staging that are usually utilised in a prognostic context. Much of the work on pre-treatment imaging biomarkers focuses on understanding two concepts: the first is the tumour microenvironment, often investigated via peritumoural features, where CT imaging features are hypothesised to reflect certain biological processes or states, for example, the immune status or the presence of cancerous cells outside the main tumour burden (see Fig. 44.3 for an illustration of intratumoural versus peritumoural feature extraction and modelling). This is relevant to prognosis because the histologically proven presence of malignant cells outside the tumour has already been shown to correlate with poorer prognosis, as the spread of the cancer has already commenced via the surrounding lymphatics, blood vessels and air spaces [24–26]. The second area of interest is tumour heterogeneity, which is thought to reflect the diversity of phenotypes between malignant cells of the same tumour. Studies examining these factors on pre-treatment CT scans show some success at distinguishing between tumours likely to progress or recur after treatment and those that have a better chance of survival [27–29]. Models were most discriminatory when they incorporated radiomics features (e.g. texture) and clinicopathological variables (e.g. age, sex, smoking history), demonstrating the additive properties of imaging biomarkers in the prediction of disease-free or overall survival.

Despite this promising outlook for using pre-treatment imaging to predict prognosis, many other studies have not demonstrated significantly improved prediction of survival outcomes beyond the clinicopathological factors, such as TNM, or could only improve on these models incrementally but not significantly [30–32]. This variability of results likely reflects both the heterogeneous approach to the data collected and heterogeneity in the data—it is difficult to ensure the replicability of both the positive and negative studies when the models are not regularly validated on independent patient cohorts, where data points are often inconsistent between studies, and where different scanners and protocols are used. Further prospective research is required before any model can be applied as a clinical decision-making aid, either as a supplement to clinicopathological features or as a replacement.

Some studies have shown limited success at demonstrating a correlation between tumour and peritumoural features and the development of distant metastases or nodal disease, the presence of which act as a proxy for survival metrics, as metastatic spread inevitably impacts prognosis. These techniques may enable more nuanced decisions around treatment and surveillance, but this approach will only prove fruitful in the future if their results can be replicated [33–37]. Currently, these approaches are diverse in the clinicopathological data collected, and heterogeneous in the tumour and peritumoural features being investigated, and will require rigorous testing and retesting before clinical implementation is possible. Please see Table 44.1 for details of the studies investigating radiomics features and pre-therapy CT imaging to predict prognosis.

A similar challenge exists for identifying imaging biomarkers in pre-treatment 18F-FDG PET/CT. 18F-FDG PET may provide additional radiomics features reflecting the functional aspects of a tumour, but whether these radiomics features are replicable and therefore useful for prognosis is open for debate. A review by Han et al. could not demonstrate consistent reproducibility of 18F-FDG PET textural features for the prediction of survival, after assessing the results of 17 studies [38]. Newer research is equally inconsistent at demonstrating a prognostic benefit for 18F-FDG PET/CT features, regardless of whether the outcome of interest is survival or other prognostic criteria such as nodal involvement or distant metastases [39–45]. While theoretically promising, considerable obstacles to implementation exist before pre-treatment CT, and 18F-FDG PET/CT imaging can be used clinically for prognosis and subsequent treatment decisions.

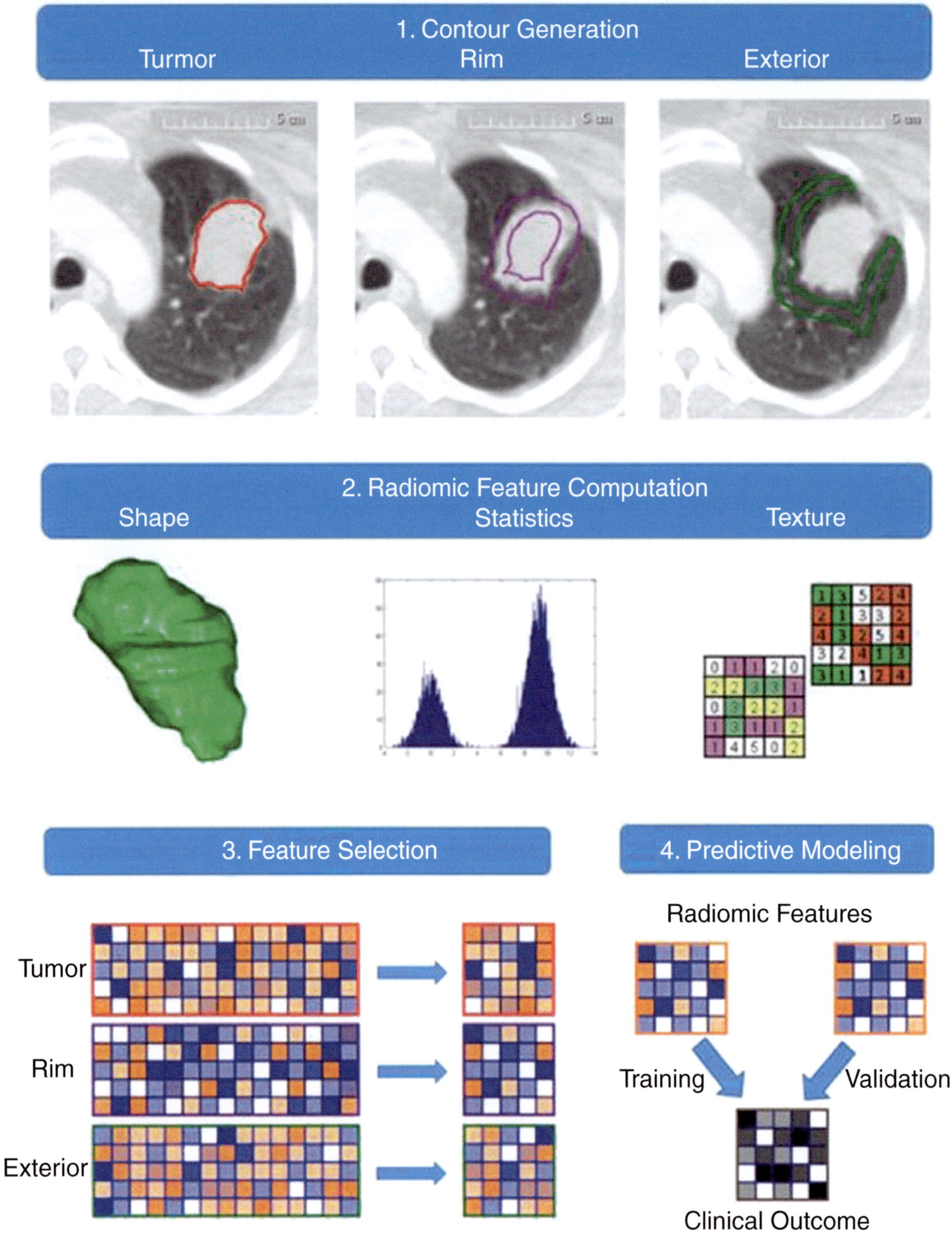

Fig. 44.3 A demonstration of how intratumoural and peritumoural feature extraction is performed. (1) Generation of the rim and exterior contours based on segmented tumour contour. (2) Extraction of the radiomics features from each of the tissue contour region. (3) Dimension reduction of the radiomics features based on feature stability and relevance. (4) Prognostic power of the radiomics features is evaluated through predictive modelling and validation

Table 44.1 Summary of recent studies using AI for lung cancer prognosis

First Author	N	Features	Software	Outcome	Data	Internal validation performance	External validation performance	Outperformed clinical factors model	Comments
Hosny [30]	1194	CNN, Radiomics	TensorFlow, PyRadiomics	2-year survival in non-small-cell lung cancer	Retrospective Multicentre multivendor	NR	AUC = 0.70	Yes	Deep learning outperformed radiomics
Kim [31]	2697	3D CNN	TensorFlow	Disease-free survival post-resection of clinical stage I adenocarcinoma	Retrospective Multicentre multivendor	CI = 0.74	CI =0.71	No	Model saliency maps indicated that the most informative pixels were those of the solid tumour and the peritumoural rim
Huang [32]	282	Radiomics	Custom	Disease-free survival in stage I-II non-small-cell lung cancer	Retrospective Single institution Single vendor	CI = 0.72	NR	Yes	
Dou [33]	200	Radiomics	PyRadiomics	Distant metastasis in stage II–III lung adenocarcinoma	Retrospective Multicentre multivendor	NR	CI = 0.64	Yes	Found peritumour radiomics features to be more informative than intratumoural features
Gu [34]	542	Radiomics	Custom	Metastasis in stage Ia lung adenocarcinoma	Retrospective Single institution Multivendor	AUC = 0.80	N/A	N/A	
Wang [35]	360	Radiomics	PyRadiomics	Preoperative prediction of lymph node metastasis in clinical stage T1 lung adenocarcinoma	Retrospective Single institution Multivendor	AUC = 0.86	N/A	N/A	Clinical parameters improved radiomic model
Yang [36]	467	Radiomics	PyRadiomics	EGFR mutational status in lung adenocarcinoma	Retrospective Single institution Single vendor	AUC = 0.79	N/A	Yes	
Zhong [37]	492	Radiomics	NR	Lymph node metastasis in lung adenocarcinoma	Retrospective Single Centre Single vendor	AUC = 0.97	N/A	Yes	

AUC area under the curve, *CI* concordance index, *CNN* convolutional neural network. *NR* not reported

Pre-treatment lung cancer imaging does not limit itself to the tumour or its immediate peritumoural tissue, and arguably the application of AI to these imaging studies should not be limited to these areas, either. Very early studies are investigating whether other tissues captured on imaging may provide prognostic information, for example, features derived from bone marrow activity on 18F-FDG PET/CT scans, or lymph nodes [46, 47]. Data are preliminary, but these approaches are a salient reminder that potentially important information may be contained in areas other than the most obvious regions of interest.

Treatment Response Prediction and Imaging Biomarkers

The gold standard for assessing treatment response in lung and other cancers is the Response Evaluation Criteria in Solid Tumours (RECIST) framework. RECIST is applied by radiologists and oncologists to post-treatment images to assess tumour size and other characteristics in order to estimate prognosis and treatment response. This method, though standardised, is subjective and open to inter- and intra-observer variation. Therefore, the ability of radiomics to mine quantitative data from pre- and post-therapy images to evaluate therapeutic response is of great interest.

Several reviews have succinctly summarised the current radiomics approaches to predicting treatment response, most recently Chetan et al. [48]. Their robust review of 14 articles on pre-treatment 18F-FDG PET/CT and CT images demonstrated a range of features that may be predictive of treatment response as evaluated by RECIST. They assessed each study with a Radiomics Quality Score (RQS) to indicate the results' replicability and susceptibility to bias. A range of treatment modalities [SBRT, chemoradiation (CRT), radiotherapy (RT), TKI], tumour stages and sample sizes were included in the studies (largest included study n = 127). The median RQS score for the studies was +2.5 (possible range − 8 to +36), demonstrating poor study quality and questionable reproducibility of the results. As the authors noted, the highly heterogeneous nature of the data collected in these 14 articles meant comparison between features was not possible, and the lack of external validation cohorts meant that results were prone to overfitting.

A similar review from Shi et al., though lacking an RQS and therefore less quantitative in its assessment methods, found equally heterogeneous results for pre-treatment imaging and response prediction [49]. In their review, they also summarised studies examining delta radiomics, where changes in radiomics features over time (before, during and after treatment) are investigated to predict response. This approach may be particularly useful in the context of SBRT or radiotherapy, where imaging is performed regularly during treatment for planning purposes and therefore may be able to demonstrate response or progression early, and influence onward management in real time. This review, while comprehensive, indicates that methods of data collection, therapies examined and outcomes measured are currently too diverse to compare, despite individual study results appearing promising.

Since these reviews in 2018, research has continued to focus on the same areas of response prediction, and gains are incremental. Sample sizes are getting larger and increasingly include external validation cohorts [50–54]. Even so, input data (types of images, clinical and genomic data) and endpoints are variable (RECIST, progression-free survival, local control), making assessment and comparison of the underlying radiomics and deep learning tools impossible. For radiomics to play a role in the assessment of treatment response, it will have to show that a given model is consistently reproducible, that it correlates to underlying biological processes, and adds value or supplants the current gold standard (RECIST) for assessing response.

Limitations and Obstacles to AI in Lung Cancer Characterisation and Prognosis

Much of the research cited in this chapter is cutting-edge, aiming to elucidate the ways in which increased processing power and AI may add value to the lung cancer patient's journey. This added value may manifest in several ways; firstly, in increased diagnostic accuracy, by providing enhanced information down to the level of phenotypic and genotypic detail; through improved prognostic capability, by understanding tumour features such as texture heterogeneity and the tumour microenvironment; and through treatment response assessment or real-time adjustments in therapeutic dose or approach through pre-treatment imaging and delta radiomics.

At the moment, however, research cannot be said to be conclusive in any of these endeavours. The limitations to the application of radiomics and other AI processes are similar to those in other areas of medicine: there is a lack of consistency to the way that data is being collected, integrated and reproduced. Many studies are small ($n < 200$), single-site studies using the same imaging protocols and proscribed datasets, meaning generalizability between populations is difficult to demonstrate. Where studies are larger and results externally validated, study endpoints are often heterogeneous, making comparison between radiomics signatures and nomograms difficult.

It has also been shown that different radiomics software packages do not always agree on which features are statistically significant, even when given the same set of images [55]. As many authors point out, better and more standardised data collection and reporting frameworks are required to enable results to be comparable [48].

Furthermore, results must demonstrate an additive benefit to existing clinical assessment criteria, be they biopsy results, TNM staging or RECIST scores. This final challenge—of demonstrating clinical benefit—will need to take into account clinical utility and cost-effectiveness of the proposed models; AUCs alone are not sufficient for clinical implementation decisions however good they may be [56]. In order to depart from radiomics-based AI programmes into true deep learning applications, which may enable identification of biomarkers that we are currently unable to investigate, much larger, curated radiological datasets are required. This will only be possible with coordinated efforts between researchers, clinicians and, in some situations, patients. We are a way away from being able to assemble these datasets at the moment, but efforts are being made to standardise approaches to imaging data collection, and to break down barriers to clinical data collection and processing so that research can progress [57–60].

Conclusion

In conclusion, AI may provide unique and valuable insights into the behaviour of lung cancers by mining imaging data in such a way radiologists cannot do on their own; however, a unified push to enable generalisation of results and greater standardisation of the AI tools being developed is required before clinical implementation will be possible. Once this hurdle is overcome, AI may facilitate improved lung cancer outcomes through greater personalisation of the patient pathway, through nuanced and individualised data collection and analysis, and tailored treatment approaches.

References

1. International Agency for Research on Cancer. All cancer types factsheet. Int Agency Res Cancer Globocan [Internet]. 2018;876:2018–9. Available from: http://gco.iarc.fr/today.
2. Rami-Porta R, Asamura H, Travis WD, Rusch VW. Lung cancer - major changes in the American joint committee on cancer eighth edition cancer staging manual. CA Cancer J Clin. 2017;67(2):138–55.
3. Lung cancer statistics | Cancer Research UK [Internet]. [cited 2018 Nov 19]. Available from: https://www.cancerresearchuk.org/health-professional/cancer-statistics/statistics-by-cancer-type/lung-cancer/survival#heading-Zero.
4. Liu J, Cui J, Liu F, Yuan Y, Guo F, Zhang G. Multi-subtype classification model for non-small cell lung cancer based on radiomics: SLS model. Med Phys. 2019;46(7):3091–100.
5. Han Y, Ma Y, Wu Z, Zhang F, Zheng D, Liu X, et al. Histologic subtype classification of non-small cell lung cancer using PET/CT images. Eur J Nucl Med Mol Imaging. 2020.
6. Hung JJ, Jeng WJ, Chou TY, Hsu WH, Wu KJ, Huang BS, et al. Prognostic value of the new international association for the study of lung cancer/American thoracic society/European respiratory society lung adenocarcinoma classification on death and recurrence in completely resected stage i lung adenocarcinoma. Ann Surg. 2013;258(6):1079–86.
7. Lu L, Wang D, Wang L, Guo P, Li Z, E L, et al. A quantitative imaging biomarker for predicting disease-free-survival-associated histologic subgroups in lung adenocarcinoma (European Radiology). Eur Radiol. 2020;30(7):3614–23. https://doi.org/10.1007/s00330-020-06663-6.
8. Yuan M, Zhang YD, Pu XH, Zhong Y, Li H, Wu JF, et al. Comparison of a radiomic biomarker with volumetric analysis for decoding tumour phenotypes of lung adenocarcinoma with different disease-specific survival. Eur Radiol. 2017;27(11):4857–65.
9. Park S, Lee SM, Noh HN, Hwang HJ, Kim S, Do KH, et al. Differentiation of predominant subtypes of lung adenocarcinoma using a quantitative radiomics approach on CT. Eur Radiol. 2020;30(9):4883–92.
10. Aerts HJWL, Velazquez ER, Leijenaar RTH, Parmar C, Grossmann P, Cavalho S, et al. Decoding tumour phenotype by noninvasive imaging using a quantitative radiomics approach. Nat Commun. 2014;5
11. Grossmann P, Stringfield O, El-Hachem N, Bui MM, Velazquez ER, Parmar C, et al. Defining the biological basis of radiomic phenotypes in lung cancer. elife. 2017;6:1–22.
12. Aerts HJWL, Grossmann P, Tan Y, Oxnard GG, Rizvi N, Schwartz LH, et al. Defining a radiomic response phenotype: a pilot study using targeted therapy in NSCLC. Sci Rep [Internet]. 2016;6(June):1–8. https://doi.org/10.1038/srep33860.
13. Tu W, Sun G, Fan L, Wang Y, Xia Y, Guan Y, et al. Radiomics signature: a potential and incremental predictor for EGFR mutation status in NSCLC patients, comparison with CT morphology. Lung Cancer [Internet]. 2019;132(December 2018):28–35. https://doi.org/10.1016/j.lungcan.2019.03.025.
14. Jia TY, Xiong JF, Li XY, Yu W, Xu ZY, Cai XW, et al. Identifying EGFR mutations in lung adenocarcinoma by noninvasive imaging using radiomics features and random forest modeling. Eur Radiol. 2019;241
15. Rios Velazquez E, Parmar C, Liu Y, Coroller TP, Cruz G, Stringfield O, et al. Somatic mutations drive distinct imaging phenotypes in lung cancer. Cancer Res. 2017;77(14):3922–30.
16. Li S, Luo T, Ding C, Huang Q, Guan Z, Zhang H. Detailed identification of epidermal growth factor receptor mutations in lung adenocarcinoma: combining radiomics with machine learning. Med Phys. 2020;47(8):3458–66.
17. Wang S, Shi J, Ye Z, Dong D, Yu D, Zhou M, et al. Predicting EGFR mutation status in lung adenocarcinoma on computed tomography image using deep learning. Eur Respir J. 2019;53(3)
18. Mei D, Luo Y, Wang Y, Gong J. CT texture analysis of lung adenocarcinoma: can Radiomic features be surrogate biomarkers for EGFR mutation statuses. Cancer Imaging. 2018;18(1):1–9.
19. Kim Y, Paeng JC, Park YS, Cheon GJ, Lee DS, Chung J-K, et al. Relation of EGFR mutation status to metabolic activity in localized lung adenocarcinoma and its influence on the use of FDG PET/CT parameters in prognosis. Am J Roentgenol [Internet]. 2018 Jun 1 [cited 2020 Oct 1];210(6):1346–51. Available from: https://www.ajronline.org/doi/10.2214/AJR.17.18916.
20. Zhang J, Zhao X, Zhao Y, Zhang J, Zhang Z, Wang J, et al. Value of pre-therapy 18F-FDG PET/CT radiomics in predicting EGFR mutation status in patients with non-small cell lung cancer. Eur J Nucl Med Mol Imaging. 2020;47(5):1137–46.
21. Song Z, Liu T, Shi L, Yu Z, Shen Q, Xu M, et al. The deep learning model combining CT image and clinicopathological information for predicting ALK fusion status and response to ALK-TKI therapy in non-small cell lung cancer patients. Eur J Nucl Med Mol Imaging. 2020.

22. Yoon J, Suh YJ, Han K, Cho H, Lee HJ, Hur J, et al. Utility of CT radiomics for prediction of PD-L1 expression in advanced lung adenocarcinomas. Thorac Cancer. 2020;11(4):993–1004.
23. Tang C, Hobbs B, Amer A, Li X, Behrens C, Canales JR, et al. Development of an immune-pathology informed Radiomics model for non-small cell lung cancer. Sci Rep [Internet]. 2018;8(1):1–9. https://doi.org/10.1038/s41598-018-20471-5.
24. Kadota K, Nitadori JI, Sima CS, Ujiie H, Rizk NP, Jones DR, et al. Tumor spread through air spaces is an important pattern of invasion and impacts the frequency and location of recurrences after limited resection for small Stage I lung adenocarcinomas. J Thorac Oncol [Internet]. 2015 May 30 [cited 2020 Oct 7];10(5):806–14. Available from: http://www.jto.org/article/S1556086415323935/fulltext.
25. Shimada Y, Ishii G, Hishida T, Yoshida J, Nishimura M, Nagai K. Extratumoral vascular invasion is a significant prognostic indicator and a predicting factor of distant metastasis in non-small cell lung cancer. J Thorac Oncol [Internet]. 2010 Jul 1 [cited 2020 Oct 7];5(7):970–5. Available from: http://www.jto.org/article/S1556086415305402/fulltext.
26. Saijo T, Ishii G, Ochiai A, Hasebe T, Yoshida J, Nishimura M, et al. Evaluation of extratumoral lymphatic permeation in non-small cell lung cancer as a means of predicting outcome. Lung Cancer [Internet]. 2007 Jan 1 [cited 2020 Oct 7];55(1):61–6. Available from: http://www.lungcancerjournal.info/article/S0169500206005265/fulltext.
27. Khorrami M, Bera K, Leo P, Vaidya P, Patil P, Thawani R, et al. Stable and discriminating radiomic predictor of recurrence in early stage non-small cell lung cancer: multi-site study. Lung Cancer [Internet]. 2020;142(February):90–7. https://doi.org/10.1016/j.lungcan.2020.02.018.
28. Lee G, Park H, Sohn I, Lee S, Song SH, Kim H, et al. Comprehensive computed tomography Radiomics analysis of lung adenocarcinoma for prognostication. Oncologist. 2018;23(7):806–13.
29. Choe J, Lee SM, Do KH, Kim S, Choi S, Lee JG, et al. Outcome prediction in resectable lung adenocarcinoma patients: value of CT radiomics. Eur Radiol. 2020;30(9):4952–63.
30. Hosny A, Parmar C, Coroller TP, Grossmann P, Zeleznik R, Kumar A, et al. Deep learning for lung cancer prognostication: A retrospective multi-cohort radiomics study. PLoS Med. 2018;15(11):1–25.
31. Kim H, Mo Goo J, Hee Lee K, Kim YT, Park CM. Preoperative ct-based deep learning model for predicting disease-free survival in patients with lung adenocarcinomas. Radiology. 2020;296(1):216–24.
32. Huang Y, Liu Z, He L, Chen X, Pan D, Ma Z, et al. Radiomics signature: A potential biomarker for the prediction of disease-free survival in early-stage (I or II) non-small cell lung cancer. Radiology. 2016;281(3):947–57.
33. Dou TH, Coroller TP, van Griethuysen JJM, Mak RH, Aerts HJWL. Peritumoral radiomics features predict distant metastasis in locally advanced NSCLC. PLoS One. 2018;13(11):1–15.
34. Gu Y, She Y, Xie D, Dai C, Ren Y, Fan Z, et al. A texture analysis–based prediction model for lymph node metastasis in stage IA lung adenocarcinoma. Ann Thorac Surg [Internet]. 2018;106(1):214–20. Available from: https://doi.org/10.1016/j.athoracsur.2018.02.026.
35. Wang X, Zhao X, Li Q, Xia W, Peng Z, Zhang R, et al. Can peritumoral radiomics increase the efficiency of the prediction for lymph node metastasis in clinical stage T1 lung adenocarcinoma on CT? Eur Radiol. 2019;29(11):6049–58.
36. Yang X, Dong X, Wang J, Li W, Gu Z, Gao D, et al. Computed tomography-based Radiomics signature: A potential indicator of epidermal growth factor receptor mutation in pulmonary adenocarcinoma appearing as a subsolid nodule. Oncologist. 2019;24(11):1156–64.
37. Zhong Y, Yuan M, Zhang T, Zhang YD, Li H, Yu TF. Radiomics approach to prediction of occult mediastinal lymph node metastasis of lung adenocarcinoma. Am J Roentgenol. 2018;211(1):109–13.
38. Han S, Woo S, Suh CH, Kim YJ, Oh JS, Lee JJ. A systematic review of the prognostic value of texture analysis in 18F-FDG PET in lung cancer. Ann Nucl Med [Internet]. 2018;32(9):602–10. https://doi.org/10.1007/s12149-018-1281-9.
39. Arshad MA, Thornton A, Lu H, Tam H, Wallitt K, Rodgers N, et al. Discovery of pre-therapy 2-deoxy-2- 18 F-fluoro-D-glucose positron emission tomography-based radiomics classifiers of survival outcome in non-small-cell lung cancer patients. Eur J Nucl Med Mol Imaging. 2019;46(2):455–66.
40. Konert T, Everitt S, la Fontaine MD, van de Kamer JB, MacManus MP, Vogel W V., et al. Robust, independent and relevant prognostic 18F-fluorodeoxyglucose positron emission tomography radiomics features in non-small cell lung cancer: Are there any? PLoS One [Internet]. 2020;15(2):1–20. Available from: https://doi.org/10.1371/journal.pone.0228793.
41. Krarup MMK, Nygård L, Vogelius IR, Andersen FL, Cook G, Goh V, et al. Heterogeneity in tumours: validating the use of radiomic features on 18F-FDG PET/CT scans of lung cancer patients as a prognostic tool. Radiother Oncol [Internet]. 2020;144:72–8. https://doi.org/10.1016/j.radonc.2019.10.012.
42. Yang B, Zhong J, Zhong J, Ma L, Li A, Ji H, et al. Development and validation of a Radiomics nomogram based on 18F-Fluorodeoxyglucose positron emission tomography/computed tomography and Clinicopathological factors to predict the survival outcomes of patients with non-small cell lung cancer. Front Oncol. 2020;10(July):1–14.
43. Nie P, Yang G, Wang N, Yan L, Miao W, Duan Y, et al. Additional value of metabolic parameters to PET/CT-based radiomics nomogram in predicting lymphovascular invasion and outcome in lung adenocarcinoma. Eur J Nucl Med Mol Imaging 2020.
44. Tau N, Stundzia A, Yasufuku K, Hussey D, Metser U. Convolutional neural networks in predicting nodal and distant metastatic potential of newly diagnosed non–small cell lung cancer on FDG PET images. Am J Roentgenol [Internet]. 2020 Jul 1 [cited 2020 Oct 7];215(1):192–7. Available from: https://www.ajronline.org/doi/10.2214/AJR.19.22346.
45. Mattonen SA, Davidzon GA, Bakr S, Echegaray S, Leung ANC, Vasanawala M, et al. [18F] FDG positron emission tomography (PET) tumor and penumbra Imaging features predict recurrence in non-small cell lung cancer. Tomogr (Ann Arbor, Mich). 2019;5(1):145–53.
46. Mattonen SA, Davidzon GA, Benson J, Leung ANC, Vasanawala M, Horng G, et al. Bone marrow and tumor radiomics at 18F-FDG PET/CT: impact on outcome prediction in non–small cell lung cancer. Radiology. 2019;293(2):451–9.
47. Carvalho S, Leijenaar RTH, Troost EGC, Van Timmeren JE, Oberije C, Van Elmpt W, et al. 18FDG-PET-Radiomics of metastatic lymph nodes and primary tumour in NSCLC - a prospective externally validated study. PLoS One. 2018;Submitted(1):1–16.
48. Chetan MR, Gleeson F V. Radiomics in predicting treatment response in non-small-cell lung cancer: current status, challenges and future perspectives. Eur Radiol. 2020.
49. Shi L, He Y, Yuan Z, Benedict S, Valicenti R, Qiu J, et al. Radiomics for response and outcome assessment for non-small cell lung cancer. Technol Cancer Res Treat. 2018;17(619):1–14.
50. Song J, Shi J, Dong D, Fang M, Zhong W, Wang K, et al. A new approach to predict progression-free survival in stage IV EGFR-mutant NSCLC patients with EGFR-TKI therapy. Clin Cancer Res. 2018;24(15):3583–92.
51. Sun R, Limkin EJ, Vakalopoulou M, Dercle L, Champiat S, Han SR, et al. A radiomics approach to assess tumour-infiltrating CD8 cells and response to anti-PD-1 or anti-PD-L1 immunotherapy: an imaging biomarker, retrospective multicohort study. Lancet Oncol. 2018;19(9):1180–91.

52. Lou B, Doken S, Zhuang T, Wingerter D, Gidwani M, Mistry N, et al. An image-based deep learning framework for individualizing radiotherapy dose. Lancet Digit Heal. 2019;1(3):1–25.
53. Tunali I, Gray JE, Qi J, Abdalah M, Jeong DK, Guvenis A, et al. Novel clinical and radiomic predictors of rapid disease progression phenotypes among lung cancer patients treated with immunotherapy: an early report. Lung Cancer [Internet]. 2019;129(November 2018):75–9. Available from: https://doi.org/10.1016/j.lungcan.2019.01.010.
54. Mu W, Tunali I, Gray JE, Qi J, Schabath MB, Gillies RJ. Radiomics of 18F-FDG PET/CT images predicts clinical benefit of advanced NSCLC patients to checkpoint blockade immunotherapy. Eur J Nucl Med Mol Imaging. 2020;47(5):1168–82.
55. Fornacon-Wood I, Mistry H, Ackermann CJ, Blackhall F, McPartlin A, Faivre-Finn C, et al. Reliability and prognostic value of radiomic features are highly dependent on choice of feature extraction platform. Eur Radiol. 2020.
56. Halligan S, Altman DG, Mallett S. Disadvantages of using the area under the receiver operating characteristic curve to assess imaging tests: A discussion and proposal for an alternative approach. Eur Radiol. 2015;25(4):932–9.
57. Radiological Society of North America. Quantitative Imaging Biomarkers Alliance [Internet]. [cited 2020 Oct 15]. Available from: https://www.rsna.org/en/research/quantitative-imaging-biomarkers-alliance.
58. Zwanenburg A, Leger S, Vallières M, Löck S. Image biomarker standardisation initiative. Radiology [Internet]. 2016 Dec 21 [cited 2020 Oct 15];295(2):328–38. Available from: http://arxiv.org/abs/1612.07003.
59. Mongan J, Moy L, Kahn CE. Checklist for Artificial Intelligence in Medical Imaging (CLAIM): A Guide for Authors and Reviewers. Radiol Artif Intell [Internet]. 2020 Mar 1 [cited 2020 Oct 15];2(2):e200029. Available from: https://doi.org/10.1148/ryai.2020200029.
60. Lambin P, Leijenaar RTH, Deist TM, Peerlings J, De Jong EEC, Van Timmeren J, et al. Radiomics: The bridge between medical imaging and personalized medicine [Internet]. Vol. 14, Nature Reviews Clinical Oncology. Nature Publishing Group; 2017 [cited 2020 Oct 15]. p. 749–62. Available from: https://www.nature.com/articles/nrclinonc.2017.141

Artificial Intelligence for Opportunistic Chest CT Screening and Prognostication

45

Nikos Sourlos, Peter M. A. van Ooijen, and Rozemarijn Vliegenthart

Introduction

Low-dose chest computed tomography (CT) can help detect cancer in early stages and has been found to significantly improve the survival of long-term smokers [1, 2]. Trials have shown that low-dose CT screening prevented death due to lung cancer in up to 25% of cases [1, 2]. Since the publication of these large-scale trials, there has been increasing interest in implementation of lung cancer screening in healthcare practice. This has resulted in recommendations from major societies particularly in the USA [3], on the criteria for individuals who are recommended to undergo chest CT screening, aimed at early lung cancer detection. In Europe, there is still more hesitation with regard to CT screening implementation, as a number of questions still need answering (ESR/ERS and EUPS statements [4, 5]).

Apart from early detection of lung cancer based on lung nodules, chest CT scans can also help in the early detection of emphysema, as a marker for chronic obstructive pulmonary disease (COPD). Presence of emphysema on CT has been found to be a predictor of mortality [6] and of lung cancer [7] in screening setting. Visual and quantitative evaluation of emphysema may provide complimentary information related to prognosis [8]. Moreover, chest CT can provide useful information on the presence and severity of coronary artery calcium (CAC), which is related to the risk of cardiovascular disease (CVD) [9]. While the standard method for evaluating the CAC score, as quantification of CAC, is an electrocardiographically triggered cardiac CT scan, lung cancer screening studies have shown that a CAC estimate based on low-dose chest CT is also related to risk of CVD events [9].

For COPD and cardiovascular disease screening, results from randomized trials showing benefit of early detection, combined with early treatment, are lacking. The ROBINSCA trial aims to determine the benefit of CAC screening based on non-contrast cardiac CT [10]. For the foreseeable future, it is likely that if chest CT screening is indeed implemented in Europe, it will be aimed at long-term (ex-) smokers, and focused on early detection of lung cancer. This screening population would comprise a huge number of screenees, undergoing potential (bi-)annual CT screening. If eventually CAC screening would be implemented, the population that would qualify for that screening would likely be much larger than for lung cancer screening, as risk factors are much broader than smoking alone and include hypertension, diabetes, and hypercholesterolemia, factors that are highly prevalent in the Western populations.

The challenges associated with CT screening of a large population group are numerous. These include logistics (invitations, administration of baseline and follow-up screenings), capacity of CT systems, standardization of CT protocols, image quality and evaluation protocols, and manpower to evaluate the CT scans [5]. All these issues contribute to screening costs. The screening workload can put a huge burden on radiologists' time to evaluate, register, and check the results of the scans [11]. This will result in fatigue, which in turn will decrease radiologist's performance of detecting nodules and reading speed [12]. In addition, the scans of many of the individuals that will be screened will be without abnormalities, with a negative screening result. The question is whether image reading can be optimized with better selection of scans that need radiologist evaluation.

AI can help to address, among others, the abovementioned issues. It can automatically detect small lung nodules by finding complex patterns or even detect features that would otherwise be missed, reducing the time radiologists need to spend on reading CT scans, and so, reducing the total

N. Sourlos, MSc · R. Vliegenthart, MD, PhD (✉)
Department of Radiology, University of Medical Center Groningen/University of Groningen, Groningen, Netherlands
e-mail: n.sourlos@umcg.nl; r.vliegenthart@umcg.nl

P. M. A. van Ooijen, MSc, PhD, CPHIMS
Department of Radiation Oncology and Data Science Center in Health, University Medical Center Groningen, Groningen, The Netherlands
e-mail: p.m.a.van.ooijen@umcg.nl

C. N. De Cecco et al. (eds.), *Artificial Intelligence in Cardiothoracic Imaging*, Contemporary Medical Imaging,
https://doi.org/10.1007/978-3-030-92087-6_45

cost of screening [13]. Moreover, it can prioritize the workflow by moving screenees with significant findings to the top of the list of scans that the radiologist will assess. In addition, it can save time by automatically quantifying the size of nodules found. Furthermore, AI seems promising in reducing noise in reconstructed images, and so the dose required during the scan can be further reduced and the acquisition time can be decreased [14, 15]. These topics are further explored in the remainder of this chapter.

Another difficulty in clinical practice is to evaluate all relevant biomarkers related to B3 diseases. The National Institutes of Health Biomarkers Definitions Working Group defines a biomarker as "a characteristic that is objectively measured and evaluated as an indicator of normal biological processes, pathogenic processes, or pharmacologic responses to a therapeutic intervention" [16]. A biomarker should provide information about disease risk to a greater extent than the standard risk factors like age, smoking, etc. [17]. A challenge in implementing biomarkers is the fact that different CT systems, scan protocols, reconstructions, and software may yield differences in biomarker results [18]. Thus, standardization, for example, in image quality, is needed. Also, the value of a biomarker in relation to clinical disease and events needs to be determined for different populations in order to understand generalizability. Also, we should take into account the inherent correlation between biomarkers, and perform validation to make certain that the biomarker is reproducible and accurate [17].

Machine learning methods have started to allow automatic extraction of useful features from images like nodule size, diameter, shape, etc., which help to derive new imaging biomarkers, some beyond the visual and (semi-)quantitative analysis by a radiologist. Before the rise of these methods, this task was usually performed manually, by experienced radiologists who used to spend a significant amount of time to find and extract these features. It is worth noticing that a biomarker will be more useful in clinical practice if it is more informative than just the imaging alone [19].

Finally, if biomarkers will be used to predict the outcome of a disease in a screenee, there are some indicators of how well they perform compared to other available biomarkers. These are their discrimination ability and their calibration and reclassification by evaluating statistical models with and without the biomarker [17].

Potential for AI Role in B3 Screening

There are many ways in which AI can help in the workflow of B3 screening (either aimed at lung cancer, emphysema, CVD, or all three). Figure 45.1 shows the different steps where AI may have value in the future.

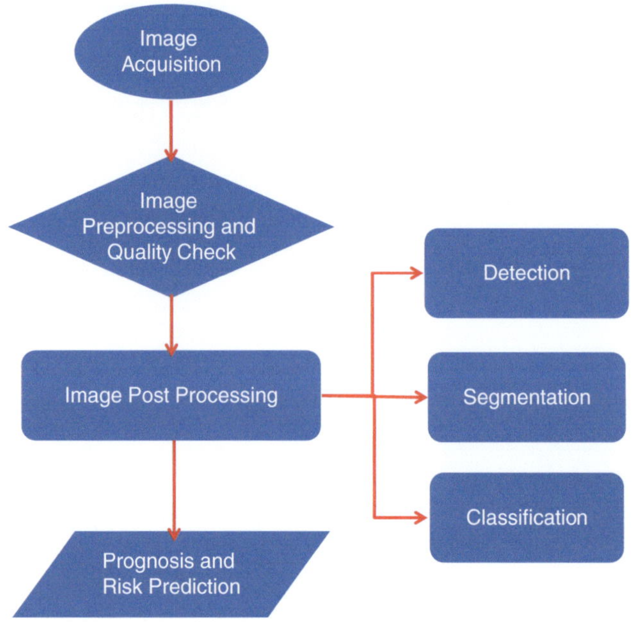

Fig. 45.1 Workflow steps in B3 screening which AI can contribute

Image Acquisition

The first step in the pipeline of low-dose chest CT screening is the image acquisition. Recently a system based on deep learning was developed that uses 3D cameras to find the optimal position in which an individual should be positioned for the CT scan. By doing that, the right amount of dose will be delivered to the right location, and the image quality can also be improved and homogenized, since noise in the output image will be reduced [20].

Image Pre-Processing

The next step in the pipeline is the pre-processing of the acquired CT images into a standard format (normalization, resizing, etc.) and to check if they have an adequate quality to perform diagnosis [21]. In this step noise reduction techniques are applied, in particular iterative reconstruction. AI can also be used instead of classic iterative reconstruction procedures, to improve image quality of low-dose CT scans by reducing noise and improving structural fidelity [22]. Image improvement algorithms which reduce noise and artifacts (Fig. 45.2) are of importance since radiation dose can be reduced, due to the fact that the decreased image quality can be compensated by the noise reduction algorithm. There may even be the possibility in the future to generate contrast-enhanced CT images out of non-enhanced ones [23]. Also, images from different CT scanner vendors can be made more alike in quality, by using vendor-neutral deep learning image reconstruction software [24].

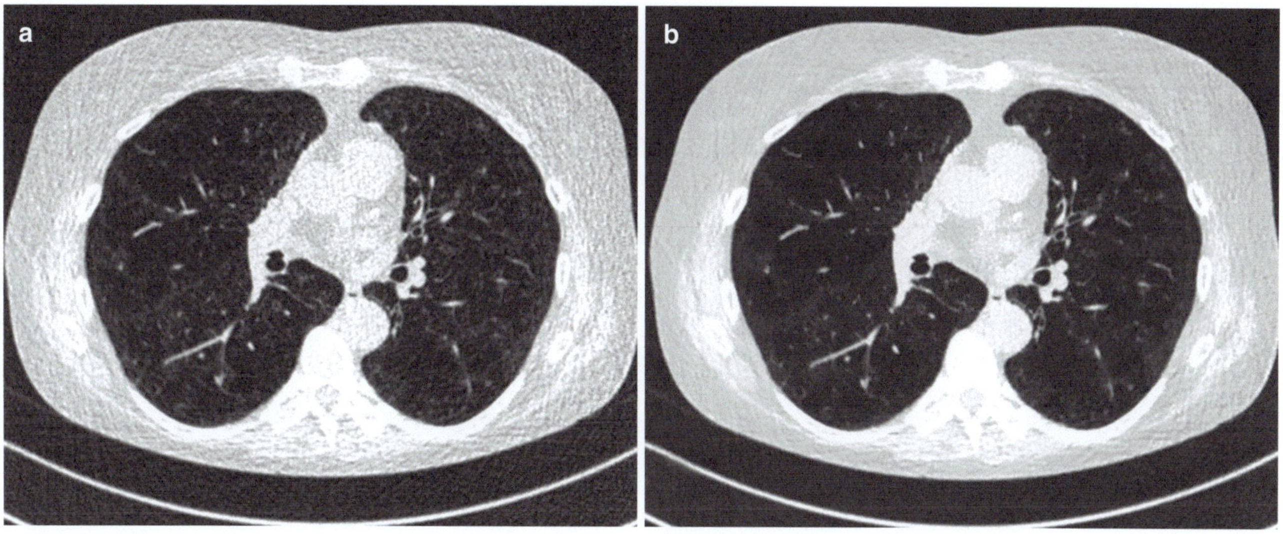

Fig. 45.2 AI for noise reduction. On the left (**a**) the regular chest CT image and on the right (**b**) the improved, reduced-noise version, generated by the AI algorithm [13]

Image Post-Processing

The next step is the post-processing. Here, the preprocessed images are fed to an AI algorithm which either detects the region of interest or segments the lesion or classifies the image according to the goals. After that, the scan result for the particular screenee is determined. Using the results from image post-processing, a risk prediction algorithm is then used to determine the risk of the screenee. The prognosis is estimated, and at the end, it is decided if another routine screening needs to be scheduled or if workup or short-term follow-up is required.

Below, a few specific applications of AI in image post-processing of B3 diseases are presented:

1. Object detection: Object detection algorithms identify specific objects in an image by drawing a bounding box around them. Examples of these algorithms are the R-CNN, the fast R-CNN, the faster R-CNN, and the mask R-CNN [25]. An application of such algorithms could be to find a region of interest in an image (Fig. 45.3). Lung nodules can also be detected using CNNs. An example of lung nodule detection can be seen in Fig. 45.4. Using maximum intensity projection CT images, the number of false positives per scan can be reduced significantly [26]. Except from the higher sensitivity, a recent study has shown that an AI system can have better performance compared to radiologists in the lung nodule detection task [27]. Based on the findings and on risk factors [28], the AI will then decide if additional screening is needed.
2. Segmentation: Segmentation is a per-pixel classification task. A label is given to each pixel as belonging to one of a set of predefined categories, and at the end, a mask is applied to segment the region of the image that contains the pixels of a specific category [30, 31]. An example of a segmentation algorithm is the U-net which can be used to segment coronary artery calcium, a predictor of cardiovascular events [30]. The Dice coefficient can be used to evaluate the results of the segmentation to the ground truth (e.g., manual segmentation) [30]. In Fig. 45.5 a segmentation of the heart is presented.

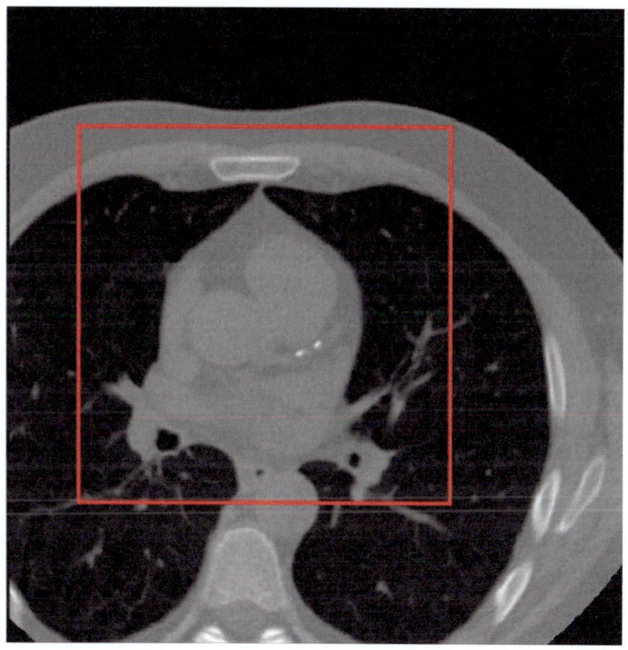

Fig. 45.3 Object detection algorithm outputs a bounding box around the heart [13]

3. Classification: Classification algorithms classify patients to one of a set of predefined categories (e.g., patients with

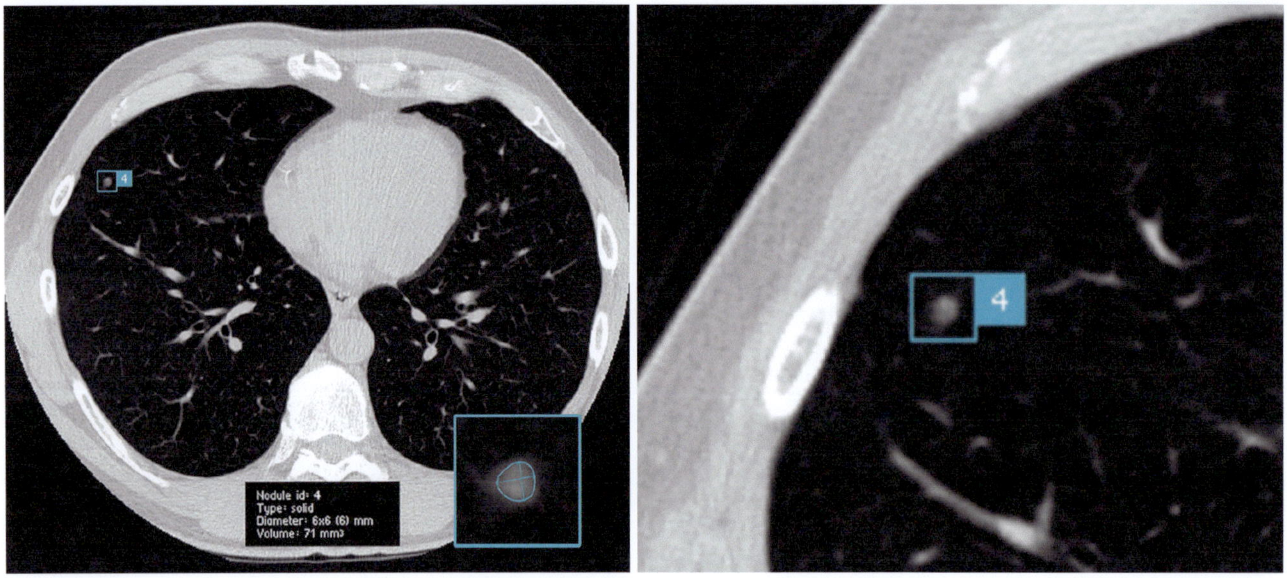

Fig. 45.4 Bounding box around a lung nodule on chest CT, with a magnified view on the right [29]

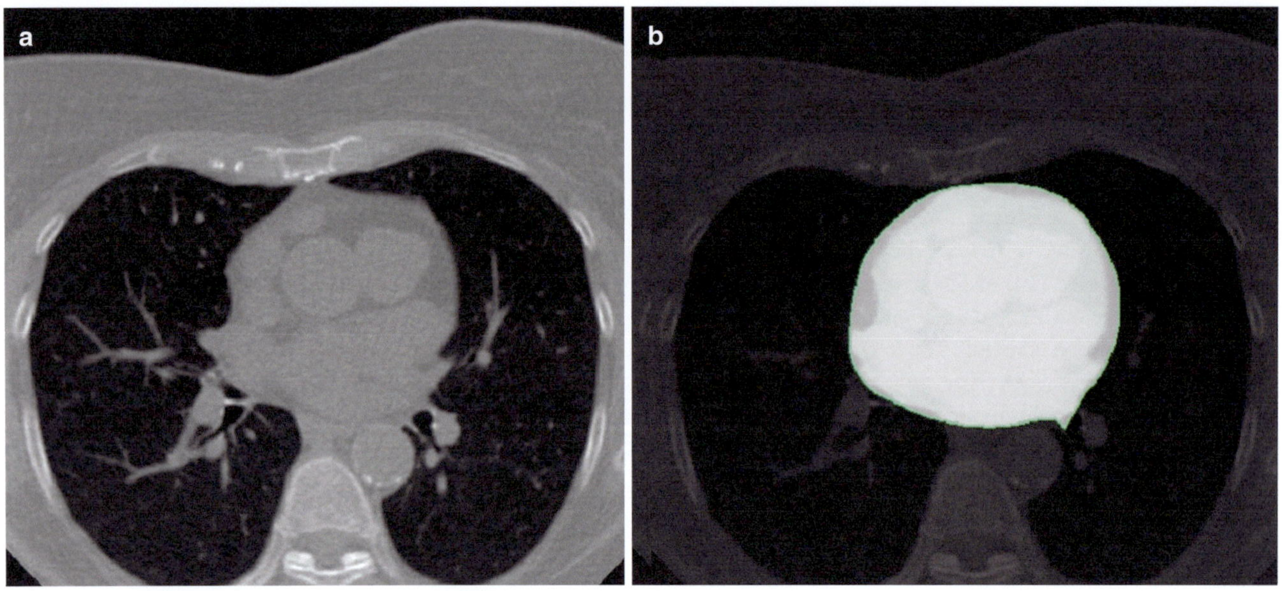

Fig. 45.5 Segmentation of the heart. On the left (**a**) the input image and on the right (**b**) the binary segmented image projected over the original CT image [13]

or without myocardial infarction). A deep neural network (DNN) can be used to directly classify lung nodules in an image as benign or malignant. Nodule features can be extracted from these networks and fed into a machine learning classifier.

Next, another algorithm can be used to further improve the performance of the model [32]. The whole process is demonstrated in Fig. 45.6.

Prognosis and Risk Prediction

Prognosis and risk prediction algorithms based on AI have recently become available. These algorithms output a continuous function with a numerical output indicating, e.g., the cardiovascular disease risk and/or the survival time of patients [33]. Inputs can also be biomarkers instead of images. For assessing the risk of individuals, methods like the Framingham risk score (FRS) and body mass index

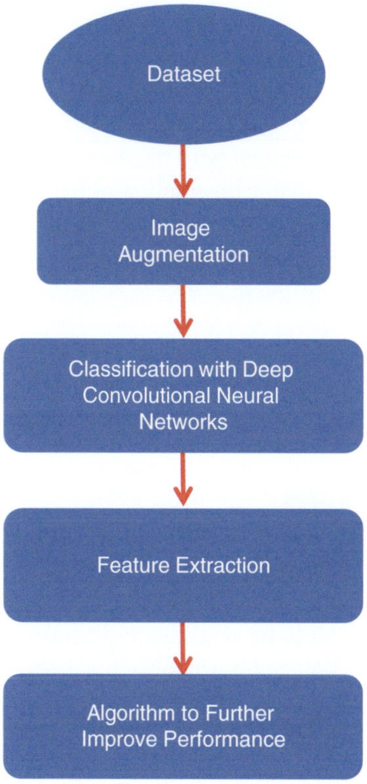

Fig. 45.6 To classify chest CT images with deep learning models, augmentation is often used to increase the examples in the training set; features are extracted after the model is trained. These features are used as input to another algorithm to further improve the performance of the deep learning network

(BMI) for CVD are commonly used. These methods consider a number of biomarkers like cholesterol levels to evaluate the risk score [34, 35]. A recent study showed that automated CT-based biomarkers derived from image processing algorithms are more accurate in predicting cardiovascular events compared to FRS and BMI [36]. Moreover, one other study revealed the potential of using AI methods to uncover new predictive factors in CVD [37]. For lung cancer, the risk can be estimated from an AI algorithm including lung nodule volume [38].

It is worth noting that there are also some cluster analysis algorithms that help us find patterns in data without any prior knowledge about the patterns that exist in the data. An example of these algorithms is hierarchical clustering that is used for heterogenous cardiac diseases; these algorithms could help us understand the mechanisms that cause heart failure [39].

Clinical Implementation

AI has revolutionized the medical field. Nevertheless, there are many challenges to applying AI algorithms in clinical practice. Below the most important ones are presented.

Technical Considerations

The mechanisms that lead most of the AI algorithms to their predictions are not well understood. This is the so-called "black box" problem with AI systems, which means that the processes and calculations that take place may not be easily interpreted by humans. The algorithms lack explainability, and so their predictions cannot be treated without suspicion by the clinicians [40, 41]. For detection objectives, one possible solution to address the lack of explainability is to use Grad-CAM method. In that method the areas in the output image that influenced the output of the algorithm the most are visualized [42]. Furthermore, by having more GPU memory, it is possible to train 3D CNNs which will be able to better detect the regions of interest in images (e.g., nodules) [31].

Population Characteristics

The deep learning training process is highly dependent on the input data and the corresponding labels in that the deep learning network can only learn from examples provided to it. Therefore, imbalance in these input data might influence the decision-making capacity of the deep learning network or make it less generalizable. The influence of imbalance on the deep learning network could, for example, lead to discrimination of certain minority groups in the training data either causing bad performance in certain groups or resulting in misclassification. The decrease in generalizability can lead to decreased performance of a deep learning network when deployed in another environment. For example, one study showed that there is a significant difference in cardiometabolic biomarkers between women and men [43]. It is therefore possible that these differences between biomarkers in women and men will lead to variations in development and complications of CVD and, so, in potential gender-specific early misdiagnosis [44]. If this is the case, we would have bias even if the dataset is balanced in terms of the population of each sex. Another example could be the presence of a specialized doctor for a particular type of rare lung cancer in a hospital. This will lead patients from all around the country to this hospital to be examined by this specialist. Since this is a rare cancer, it is likely that patients who do not live close to the hospital are having this type of cancer, while those who live near that area are not having it. It seems like there is an inverse correlation between distance to the hospital and having the rare cancer, even though these two variables are independent [45]. So, living in a country in which a specialized doctor is only available in one hospital from which data were collected and used to train an AI algorithm could make the algorithm learn wrong patterns. This can only be avoided by adding data from other hospitals and from different countries as well, since in those data it is likely that this correlation does not exist and, so, it would be possible to make the algorithm generalize better.

Dataset Challenges

Acquisition characteristics should be taken into account during dataset creation. If the dataset consists of images from multiple CT systems, it may be the case that they do not have the same characteristics. The resolution, the slice thickness, the reconstruction kernel, etc. may differ between images of different datasets, and so their quality will not be the same [46]. This can severely impact the performance of our AI algorithm since, for example, it may only be able to localize small nodules in high-resolution images.

In addition to that, many medical experts should take part in the annotation procedure of the dataset to ensure that it is done properly [47]. This will inevitably introduce interobserver variability which should be resolved [47]. Lastly, it is essential to preprocess the images that are fed to the model to ensure that they are in the format that the AI algorithm was trained on [39]. Otherwise, wrong results will be obtained.

Application Area

During training of an AI algorithm, the dataset should be representative of the type of data and of the population that the algorithm will see in the future [47]. If, for example, the goal is to detect skin cancer in the general population, the dataset should consist of people of all colors, so that minorities are also included, to prevent selection bias. In addition to that, specific medical requirements should be taken into account. For example, it may be more important to have less false positives even at the cost of increased false negatives and vice versa. It is also very important to notice that an AI algorithm is likely to be trained with more images of patients than of healthy individuals and, so, be biased in favor of diagnosing disease instead of healthiness. In screening, it is not known in advance if someone is healthy or not. It is likely that the individual is healthy since screening is mainly performed on asymptomatic individuals. Therefore, AI software may fail to work in screening because of that class imbalance. It would be better to train AI algorithms with equal amounts of data from each class (here diseases and healthy individuals). One way to test the performance of the algorithm in class imbalance problems is to train it with different splits of images between healthy and diseased. For example, a training set may consist of 40% diseased and 60% healthy individuals or 30% and 70% or any other split. It should be noted that there may be a decrease in accuracy if bias is reduced, considering that having less training data of diseased may not allow the algorithm to achieve the detection performance that would have if the training set consisted of equal amounts of images of diseased and of healthy individuals. Another way to deal with the decreased performance is to use techniques like oversampling of the minority class, in which more copies of the minority class are added in the training set, or undersampling of the majority class, in which some of the data of the majority class are removed, or, similar to upsampling, generate new examples of the minority class [48]. Moreover, data augmentation could be an option for the examples of the minority class.

Legal Challenges

Another limitation that may prevent the use of AI in clinical practice is the massive datasets required to train a model, which are difficult to be acquired, especially when they contain sensitive screenee information. It is important to respect privacy regulations and secure the anonymity of the individuals [47]. Another legal aspect could be the accepted role of AI in a screening setting. AI could play a major role in the cost-effectiveness of large population screening programs if it could safely discriminate between participants who do not have disease and participants who are suspected of having disease with a varying likelihood. The legal issue however would be if an AI system, although capable of doing so with very high accuracy, could be allowed to discard screening participants from further investigation without any human intervention. The question is whether a human expert check would still be required, also for those participants of which the algorithm is 100% sure they do not have any of the diseases screened for. Since most AI nowadays are aimed at a single defined task, it could, for example, be argued that a screening AI that safely rules out lung nodules, COPD, and coronary calcification could miss something a human observer would be able to detect (e.g., thoracic aorta aneurysm). Having AI systems trained and implemented for all possible pathologies that could show up in screening would be very challenging and increase the cost dramatically.

AI Benchmarking

To avoid many of the above problems, validation of software based on a benchmark dataset should be performed. This dataset should be created trying to avoid as many biases as possible. The characteristics of the population data that were collected along with the characteristics of the CT systems used to acquire the data can significantly affect the performance of the AI algorithm. Therefore, standardization/normalization of the data should be performed. Moreover, it should be ensured that the dataset is representative in terms of resolution of images, slice thickness, etc. of the data that will be given as input to the AI algorithm in the clinical practice. Additionally, this dataset should be tailored to a specific area of application (e.g., lung nodule detection) and to a specific target population (e.g., white individuals of ages 30–40). Moreover, harmonization of annotated data from different studies should be performed since each study may have a unique annotation protocol. Furthermore, batch effects and human observer difference may arise because of the different times the annotations were performed and of the different radiologists that contributed in the annotation tasks, respectively. Statistical tests can help check the coherence of these data as well as test their variation. Only if all the above suggestions are followed, the generalization of the algorithm as well as its broad coverage can be tested. At the end, there may still be some inherent biases that cannot be avoided.

Conclusion

Even though AI's potential in assisting medical experts in B3 screening, prediction, diagnosis, and many other tasks is promising, with specific tasks having proven benefit in many studies, a lot of work needs to be done before AI algorithms can be implemented in chest CT screening. It is important to ensure that most of the potential biases are avoided, that the algorithm can be generalized to the scan protocol, and that the dataset it was trained on resembles the target population. AI algorithm validation is an essential step before allowing algorithms to be used in medical practice.

References

1. de Koning HJ, van der Aalst CM, de Jong PA, Scholten ET, Nackaerts K, Heuvelmans MA, Lammers JJ, Weenink C, Yousaf-Khan U, Horeweg N, Van 't Westeinde S, Prokop M, Mali WP, Mohamed Hoesein FAA, Van Ooijen PMA, Aerts JGJV, Den Bakker MA, Thunnissen E, Verschakelen J, Vliegenthart R, Walter JE, Ten Haaf K, Groen HJM, Oudkerk M. Reduced lung-cancer mortality with volume CT screening in a randomized trial. N Engl J Med. 2020;382(6):503–13. https://doi.org/10.1056/NEJMoa1911793. Epub 2020. Jan 29
2. Nelson PS. Targeting the androgen receptor in prostate cancer–a resilient foe. N Engl J Med. 2014;371(11):1067–9. https://doi.org/10.1056/NEJMe1409306. Epub 2014 Sep 3. PMID: 25184629.
3. Dyer O. US task force recommends extending lung cancer screenings to over 50s. BMJ. 2021;11(372):n698. https://doi.org/10.1136/bmj.n698. PMID: 33707175.
4. Kauczor HU, Baird AM, Blum TG, Bonomo L, Bostantzoglou C, Burghuber O, C˘epick'a B, Comanescu a, Couraud S, Devaraj a, Jespersen V, Morozov S, Agmon IN, Peled N, Powell P, Prosch.H, Ravara S, Rawlinson J, Revel MP, Silva M, Snoeckx A, van Ginneken B, van Meerbeeck JP, Vardavas C, von Stackelberg O, Gaga M. European Society of Radiology (ESR) and the European Respiratory Society (ERS). ESR/ERS statement paper on lung cancer screening. Eur Radiol. 2020 Jun;30(6):3277–3294. https://doi.org/10.1007/s00330-020-06727-7.. Epub 2020 Feb 12. PMID: 32052170..
5. Oudkerk M, Devaraj A, Vliegenthart R, Henzler T, Prosch H, Heussel CP, Bastarrika G, Sverzellati N, Mascalchi M, Delorme S, Baldwin DR, Callister ME, Becker N, Heuvelmans MA, Rzyman W, Infante MV, Pastorino U, Pedersen JH, Paci E, Duffy SW, de Koning H, Field JK. European position statement on lung cancer screening. Lancet Oncol. 2017;18:e754–66. https://doi.org/10.1016/S1470-2045(17)30861-6. PMID: 29208441.
6. Haruna A, Muro S, Nakano Y, Ohara T, Hoshino Y, Ogawa E, Hirai T, Niimi A, Nishimura K, Chin K, Mishima M. CT scan findings of emphysema predict mortality in COPD. Chest. 2010;138(3):635–40. https://doi.org/10.1378/chest.09-2836. Epub 2010 Apr 9. PMID: 20382712
7. Li Y, Swensen SJ, Karabekmez LG, Marks RS, Stoddard SM, Jiang R, Worra JB, Zhang F, Midthun DE, de Andrade M, Song Y, Yang. P. Effect of emphysema on lung cancer risk in smokers: a computed tomography-based assessment. Cancer Prev Res (Phila). 2011;4(1):43–50. https://doi.org/10.1158/1940-6207.CAPR-10-0151. Epub 2010 Nov 30. PMID: 21119049; PMCID: PMC3018159.
8. Lynch DA, Moore CM, Wilson C, Nevrekar D, Jennermann T, Humphries SM, Austin JHM, Grenier PA, Kauczor HU, Han MK, Regan EA, Make BJ, Bowler RP, Beaty TH, Curran-Everett D, Hokanson JE, Curtis JL, Silverman EK, Crapo JD; Genetic Epidemiology of COPD (COPDGene) Investigators. CT-based Visual Classification of Emphysema: Association with Mortality is the COPDGene Study. Radiology. 2018 Sep;288(3):859–866. https://doi.org/10.1148/radiol.2018172294. Epub 2018 May 15. PMID: 29762095; PMCID: PMC6122195.
9. Fan L, Fan K. Lung cancer screening CT-based coronary artery calcification in predicting cardiovascular events: a systematic review and meta-analysis. Medicine. 2018;97(20):e10461. https://doi.org/10.1097/MD.0000000000010461.
10. Vonder M, van der Aalst CM, Vliegenthart R, van Ooijen PMA, Kuijpers D, Gratama JW, de Koning HJ, Oudkerk M. Coronary artery calcium imaging in the ROBINSCA trial: rationale, design, and technical background. Acad Radiol. 2018;25(1):118–28. https://doi.org/10.1016/j.acra.2017.07.010. Epub 2017 Aug 23. PMID: 28843465.
11. Pyenson BS, Sander MS, Jiang Y, Kahn H, Mulshine JL. An actuarial analysis shows that offering lung cancer screening as an insurance benefit would save lives at relatively low cost. Health Aff (Millwood) 2012 Apr;31(4):770–779. doi: https://doi.org/10.1377/hlthaff.2011.0814. PMID: 22492894.
12. https://www.radiologybusiness.com/topics/care- optimization/fatigue-radiology-what-its-impact-and-what-can- be-done?nopaging=1, Accessed 25-3-2021.
13. van den Oever LB, Vonder M, van Assen M, van Ooijen PMA, de Bock GH, Xie XQ, Vliegenthart R. Application of artificial intelligence in cardiac CT: from basics to clinical practice. Eur J Radiol 2020 Jul;128:108969. doi: https://doi.org/10.1016/j.ejrad.2020.108969. . Epub 2020 Apr 8. PMID: 32361380.
14. Zhang Z. Euclid Seeram, "the use of artificial intelligence in computed tomography image reconstruction - a literature review". Journal of Medical Imaging and Radiation Sciences. 2020;51(4):671–7, ISSN 1939-8654. https://doi.org/10.1016/j.jmir.2020.09.001.
15. https://knowledge.wharton.upenn.edu/article/saving-robot- radiologists/, Accessed 25-3-2021.
16. Strimbu K, Tavel JA. What are biomarkers? Curr Opin HIV AIDS. 2010;5(6):463–6. https://doi.org/10.1097/COH.0b013e32833ed177.
17. Dhingra R, Vasan RS. Biomarkers in cardiovascular disease: statistical assessment and section on key novel heart failure biomarkers.

Trends in cardiovascular medicine vol. 2017;27(2):123–33. https://doi.org/10.1016/j.tcm.2016.07.005.
18. Erdal BS, Demirer M, Little KJ, Amadi CC, Ibrahim G, O'Donnell TP, Grimmer R, Gupta V, Prevedello LM, White RD. Are quantitative features of lung nodules reproducible at different CT acquisition and reconstruction parameters? PLoS One. 2020;15(10):e0240184. https://doi.org/10.1371/journal.pone.0240184.
19. Kammer MN, Massion PP. Noninvasive biomarkers for lung cancer diagnosis, where do we stand? Journal of Thoracic Disease. 2020;12(6):3317–30. https://doi.org/10.21037/jtd-2019-ndt-10.
20. https://new.siemens.com/global/en/company/stories/research-technologies/artificial-intelligence/artificial-intelligence-imaging-techniques.html, Accessed 25-3-2021.
21. Lee JH, Grant BR, Chung JH, Reiser I, Giger M. Assessment of diagnostic image quality of computed tomography (CT) images of the lung using deep learning. In: Medical Imaging 2018: Physics of Medical Imaging. Vol 10573. Houston, TX: International Society for Optics and Photonics; 2018. p. 105731M.
22. Shan H, Padole A, Homayounieh F, et al. Competitive performance of a modularized deep neural network compared to commercial algorithms for low-dose CT image reconstruction. Nature Machine Intelligence 2019 Jun;1(6):269–276. DOI: https://doi.org/10.1038/s42256-019-0057-9.
23. Santini, Gianmarco Zumbo, Lorena Martini, Nicola Valvano, Gabriele Leo, Andrea Avogliero, Francesco Chiappino, Dante Della Latta, Daniele. (2018). Synthetic contrast enhancement in cardiac CT with Deep Learning.
24. Lim WH, Choi YH, Park JE, Cho YJ, Lee S, Cheon Kim WS, Kim IO, Kim JH. Application of vendor-neutral iterative reconstruction technique to pediatric abdominal computed tomography. Korean J Radiol. 2019;20(9):1358–67. https://doi.org/10.3348/kjr.2018.0715.
25. Zhao Z, Zheng P, Xu S, Wu X. Object detection with deep learning: a review. IEEE Transactions on Neural Networks and Learning Systems. 2019;30:3212–32.
26. Zheng S, Guo J, Cui X, Veldhuis RNJ, Oudkerk M, van Ooijen PMA. Automatic pulmonary nodule detection in CT scans using convolutional neural networks based on maximum intensity projection. IEEE Trans Med Imaging. 2020;39(3):797–805. https://doi.org/10.1109/TMI.2019.2935553. Epub 2019 Aug 15
27. Cui S, Ming S, Lin Y, et al. Development and clinical application of deep learning model for lung nodules screening on CT images. Sci Rep. 2020;10:13657. https://doi.org/10.1038/s41598-020-70629-3.
28. Heuvelmans MA, Vonder M, Rook M, Groen HJM, De Bock GH, Xie X, Ijzerman MJ, Vliegenthart R, Oudkerk M. Screening for early lung cancer, chronic obstructive pulmonary disease, and cardiovascular disease (the Big-3) using low-dose chest computed tomography: current evidence and technical considerations. J Thorac Imaging. 2019;34(3):160–9. https://doi.org/10.1097/RTI.0000000000000379.
29. Winkels M, Cohen TS. Pulmonary nodule detection in CT scans with equivariant CNNs. Med Image Anal. 2019;55:15–26. https://doi.org/10.1016/j.media.2019.03.010. ISSN 1361-8415.
30. van den Oever L, Cornelissen LV, Xia M, Bolhuis C, Vliegenthart J, Veldhuis R, Bock R, Oudkerk G, Van Ooijen M, Peter. Deep learning for automated exclusion of cardiac CT examinations negative for coronary artery calcium. Eur J Radiol. 2020;129:109114. https://doi.org/10.1016/j.ejrad.2020.109114.
31. Zheng S, Cornelissen LJ, Cui X, Jing X, Veldhuis RNJ, Oudkerk M, van Ooijen PMA. Deep convolutional neural networks for multiplanar lung nodule detection: improvement in small nodule identification. Med Phys. 2020; https://doi.org/10.1002/mp.14648. Epub ahead of print.
32. Sathyakumar K, Munoz M, Singh J, Hussain N, Babu BA. Automated lung cancer detection using artificial intelligence (AI) deep convolutional neural networks: a narrative literature review. Cureus. 2020;12(8):e10017. https://doi.org/10.7759/cureus.10017.
33. Liu Y. Application of artificial intelligence in clinical non-small cell lung cancer. Artif Intell Cancer. 2020;1(1):19–30.
34. Lim G. HDL-related biomarkers of cardiovascular risk. Nat Rev Cardiol. 2017;14:382. https://doi.org/10.1038/nrcardio.2017.79.
35. Jahangiry L, Farhangi MA, Rezaei F. Framingham risk score for estimation of 10-years of cardiovascular diseases risk in patients with metabolic syndrome. J Health Popul Nutr. 2017;36:36. https://doi.org/10.1186/s41043-017-0114-0.
36. Pickhardt PJ, Graffy PM, Zea R, Lee SJ, Liu J, Sandfort V, Summers RM. Automated CT biomarkers for opportunistic prediction of future cardiovascular events and mortality in an asymptomatic screening population: a retrospective cohort study. Lancet Digit Health. 2020;2(4):e192-200. https://doi.org/10.1016/S2589-7500(20)30025-X. Epub 2020 Mar 2. PMID: 32864598; PMCID: PMC7454161.
37. Alaa AM, Bolton T, Di Angelantonio E, Rudd JHF, van der Schaar M. Cardiovascular disease risk prediction using automated machine learning: a prospective study of 423,604 UK biobank participants. PLoS One. 2019;14(5):e0213653. https://doi.org/10.1371/journal.pone.0213653.
38. Ardila D, Kiraly AP, Bharadwaj S, et al. End-to-end lung cancer screening with three-dimensional deep learning on low-dose chest computed tomography. Nat Med. 2019;25:954–61. https://doi.org/10.1038/s41591-019-0447-x.
39. Dey D, Slomka PJ, Leeson P, Comaniciu D, Shrestha S, Sengupta PP, Marwick TH. Artificial intelligence in cardiovascular imaging: JACC state-of-the-art review. J Am Coll Cardiol. 2019;73(11):1317–35. https://doi.org/10.1016/j.jacc.2018.12.054. PMID: 30898208; PMCID: PMC6474254.
40. Yan Y, Zhang JW, Zang GY, Pu J. The primary use of artificial intelligence in cardiovascular diseases: what kind of potential role does artificial intelligence play in future medicine? J Geriatr Cardiol. 2019;16(8):585–91. https://doi.org/10.11909/j.issn.1671-5411.2019.08.010. PMID: 31555325; PMCID: PMC6748906.
41. Bjerring JC, Busch J. Artificial intelligence and patient-centered decision-making. Philos Technol. 2020; https://doi.org/10.1007/s13347-019-00391-6.
42. https://medium.com/@mohamedchetoui/grad-cam-gradient-weighted-class-activation-mapping-ffd72742243a, Accessed 25-3- 2021.
43. Lew J, Sanghavi M, Ayers CR, McGuire DK, Omland T, Atzler D, Gore MO, Neeland I, Berry JD, Khera A, Rohatgi A, de Lemos JA. Sex-based differences in Cardiometabolic biomarkers. Circu- lation 2017 135(6):544–555. i: https://doi.org/10.1161/CIRCULATION-AHA.116.023005. PMID: 28153991; PMCID: PMC5302552.
44. Sobhani K, Nieves Castro DK, Fu Q, Gottlieb RA, Van Eyk JE, Noel Bairey Merz C. Sex differences in ischemic heart disease and heart failure biomarkers. Biol Sex Differ. 2018;9(1):43. https://doi.org/10.1186/s13293-018-0201-y.
45. van Amsterdam WAC, Verhoeff JJC, de Jong PA, et al. Eliminating biasing signals in lung cancer images for prognosis predictions with deep learning. NPJ Digit Med. 2019;2:122. https://doi.org/10.1038/s41746-019-0194-x.
46. Pelc NJ. Recent and future directions in CT imaging. Ann Biomed Eng. 2014;42(2):260–8. https://doi.org/10.1007/s10439-014-0974-z.
47. Weikert T, Francone M, Abbara S, Baessler B, Choi BW, Gutberlet M, Hecht EM, Loewe C, Mousseaux E, Natale L, Nikolaou K, Ordovas KG, Peebles C, Prieto C, Salgado R, Velthuis B, Vliegenthart R, Bremerich J, Leiner T. Machine learning in cardiovascular radiology: ESCR position statement on design requirements, quality assessment, current applications, opportunities, and challenges. Eur Radiol. 2020; https://doi.org/10.1007/s00330-020-07417-0. Epub ahead of print. PMID: 33211147.
48. https://towardsdatascience.com/methods-for-dealing-with-imbalanced-data-5b761be45a18, Accessed 25-3-2021.

Artificial Intelligence-Based Detection of Pulmonary Vascular Disease

46

Martine Remy-Jardin and Jacques Remy

Introduction

Artificial intelligence (AI) is a major trigger for the radiological community to reconsider daily practice whose strengths and limitations are known by all practitioners. Nowadays, the radiologists' practice is based on a cognitive integration of complex information combining the semiological analysis of image features in a precise anatomical and physiopathological context. Whereas these methodological approaches are regularly enriched by scientific and technological improvement, one can easily understand that novel computational tools derived from AI are likely to transform radiological practice.

A first step for radiologists is certainly to become familiar with new technological concepts and specific terminology that are accessible in review articles, bridging gaps between physicists and radiologists [1–3]. It is also important to consider the clinical situations that could rapidly benefit from these innovations in order to shape the role of AI-based diagnostics and predictions in clinical practice. The field of acute and chronic diseases of the pulmonary circulation, mostly investigated with CT angiography (CTA), is an important target for specific applications of AI. The purpose of this chapter is to highlight some clinically relevant potential applications of AI aimed at optimizing the CT-based diagnosis of disorders of the pulmonary circulation.

M. Remy-Jardin, MD, PhD (✉) · J. Remy, MD
Department of Thoracic Imaging, Hospital Calmette, University Lille, CHU Lille, Lille, France
e-mail: martine.remy@chru-lille.fr

AI in the Detection of Acute Pulmonary Embolism

Historical Background

The first attempts to use AI in the diagnosis of acute PE used an artificial neural network (ANN) as a CAD tool for predicting PE from ventilation-perfusion lung scans and chest radiographs [4]. The authors used the database of the PIOPED study, namely, the Prospective Investigation of Pulmonary Embolism Diagnosis [5], and compared the performance of the network with that of the physicians involved in this multicentric PE study. They showed that the ANN significantly outperformed the physicians, suggesting that this approach could assist physicians with the diagnosis of PE. The same group also showed that the use of ANN in the diagnosis of PE was a promising way to improve cost-effectiveness in the care of patients with nondiagnostic lung scans [6]. The early neural networks were fed with physicians' classifications of ventilation-perfusion (V-P) lung scintigrams combined with other clinical information. Such networks were used as a source of advice to inexperienced physicians and could provide experts with a second opinion [7]. More recently, completely automated methods for V-P lung scintigram interpretation have been developed with good performance reported with planar scintigraphy [8], while automated detection of match and mismatch defects by means of image-processing techniques has been developed with SPECT imaging [9].

AI Applied to the CTA Diagnosis of Acute PE

Current Needs

Pulmonary embolism is a potentially life-threatening clinical problem, and CT angiography is the standard for diagnosis. Over the past 20 years, there has been an increase in the number of CTA studies indicated for PE evaluation and a

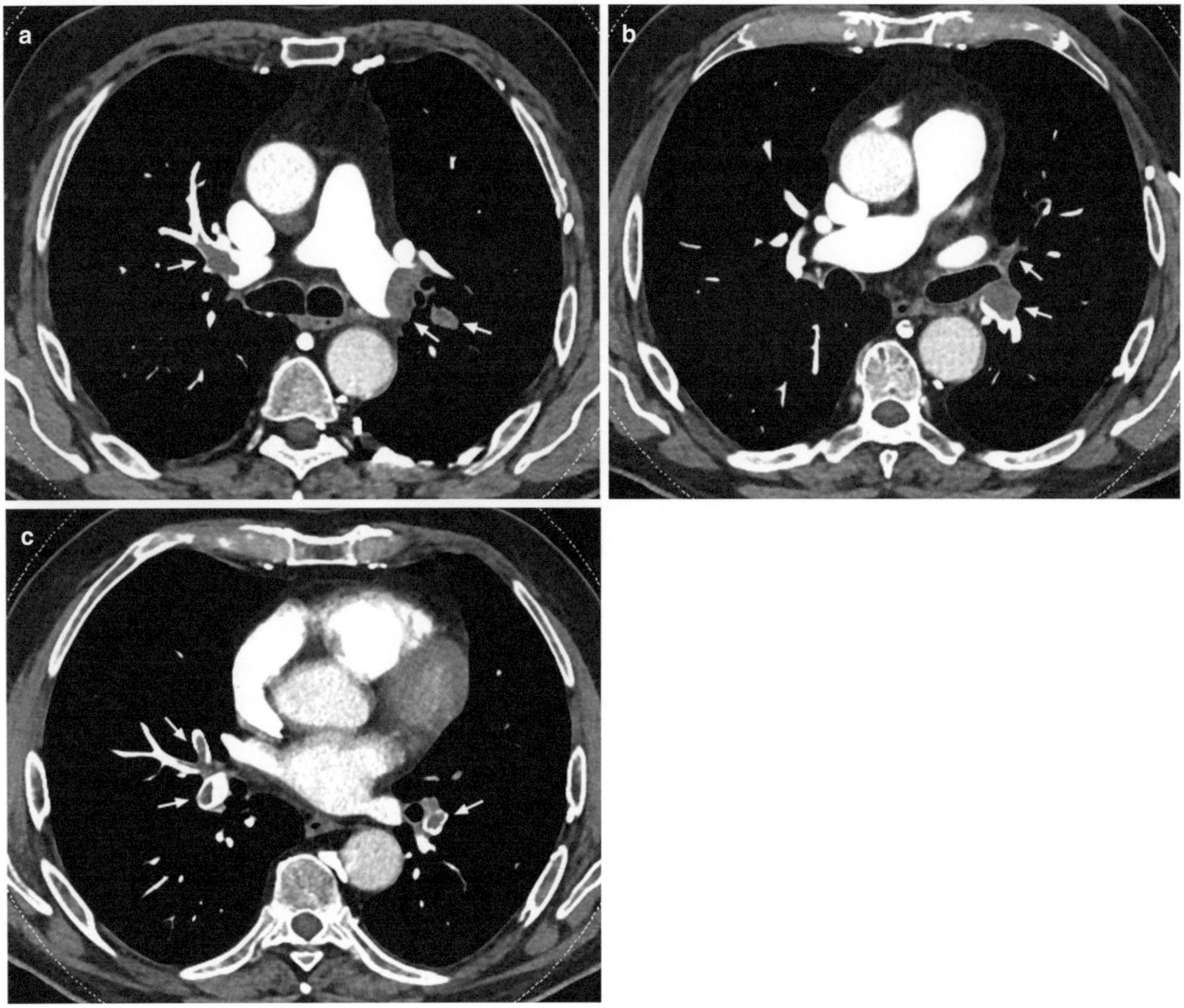

Fig. 46.1 Dual-energy CT angiographic study obtained in a 72-year-old male referred for acute onset of dyspnea (**a** to **c**) illustrates the presence of numerous endoluminal clots in the right and left pulmonary arteries (arrows) indicative of acute pulmonary embolism

decrease in diagnostic yield. Approximately 10% or less of patients who undergo CTA for PE are positive for the disease [10], highlighting the need for improvement in patient selection before CTA. A practical consequence of this rise in CTA indications in the emergency department may be the difficulty in quickly identifying positive CT examinations amidst a large number of unremarkable scans. Regarding image analysis, detection of clots within central pulmonary arteries is an easy task (Fig. 46.1). However, radiologists may encounter interpretive difficulties, especially at the level of peripheral pulmonary arteries, which may lead to false-positive or false-negative results. The current means to overcome this difficulty is to combine the reading of morphologic and perfusion images when the patient is scanned with dual-energy CT (Fig. 46.2). The final step of rapidly communicating critical findings to clinicians is another facet of the current practical difficulties in PE management.

AI-Driven Solutions

AI can be applied to the determination of a PE-risk score to help inform CT imaging decisions. Considering that current PE-risk scores (i.e., Wells or revised Geneva) are underused and thus lead to persistent overuse of CT imaging for PE, Banerjee et al. developed a machine learning model to generate a patient-specific risk score for PE using longitudinal clinical data [11]. This approach arrives at an imaging-specific PE likelihood recommendation that could be used to improve use of PE-CT imaging in referred patients.

The challenge for detection of acute pulmonary embolism (PE) is directly influenced by the location of endovascular

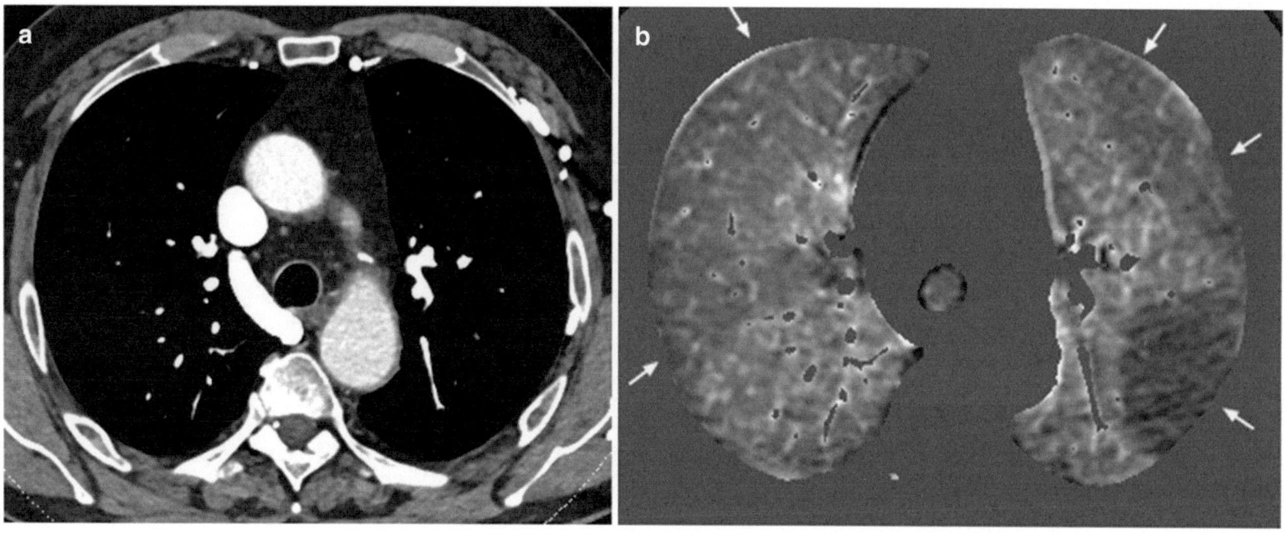

Fig. 46.2 Mediastinal (**a**) and lung perfusion (**b**) images from the same CT examination as that shown in Fig. 46.1, illustrating the difficulty in identifying clots within small-sized pulmonary arteries. Note the number and extent of perfusion defects (arrows on **b**) related to obstruction of peripheral pulmonary arteries by endoluminal clots that are not depictable on the corresponding mediastinal image (**a**)

clots within the pulmonary circulation. When their depiction relies on visual analysis of CT sections, there are obvious differences between the easy depiction of clots within central pulmonary arteries and the time-consuming analysis of segmental and sub-segmental pulmonary arteries to identify small-sized filling defects. Consequently, whereas there is a limited utility in AI for the detection of central PE, this approach could be of major interest for the recognition of peripheral PE, in particular when this diagnosis is not clinically suspected. In a recent study, Weikert et al. evaluated the performance of an AI-powered algorithm for the automatic detection of PE on chest CT angiograms on a large dataset [12]. The PE detection algorithm prototype was based on a deep convolutional neural network comprising a ResNet architecture that was found to have a high degree of diagnostic accuracy for the detection of PE on CT angiograms. Most of the false-positive findings were due to contrast agent-related artifacts, pulmonary veins, and lymph nodes. Owing to a balanced performance in regard to sensitivity (92.7%) and specificity (95.5%), this prototype was considered to fulfill the prerequisite for its usefulness in clinical practice. By complementing traditional ways of worklist prioritization in radiology departments, this approach can speed up the diagnostic and therapeutic workup of patients with PE and help to avoid false-negative calls. Concretely, a notification can be sent to the radiologist in charge via e-mail or a pop-up window whenever the algorithm prototype suspects the presence of PE in a CT angiogram and thereby initiate prompt reading of this case. It should be noted that, in line with previous studies relying on visual reading and automated PE detection with CAD, the detection rate was found to be dependent on the localization of emboli, CT angiograms containing central emboli being more likely to be detected than those with sub-segmental emboli only.

Deep learning can also be considered to calculate the clot burden in order to reduce the physician's workload. Liu et al. have recently reported that clot burden measured with deep learning (i.e., a fully deep learning convolutional neural network called U-Net) correlated with Qanadli and Mastora scores as well as with parameters of right ventricular dysfunction on CTPA [13].

Clear distinction between arteries and veins is a major prerequisite for proper recognition of acute PE. A basic approach to separate the two vascular trees consists in the manual inspection of individual CT slices to trace the vessel back to their origin in search for features that specifically characterize arteries and veins. However, intrinsic issues of CT images, like a large number of slices, scan resolution, and partial volume effect, along with extreme complexity and density of the vessel tree, make this manual separation a long and tedious job, which may be prone to mistakes. For this reason, having a method to semiautomatically segment vascular structures on CT images may be crucial to improve the physician's ability to assess pathological conditions. In a recent study, Jimenez et al. developed a fully automatic algorithm that utilizes a CNN approach to separate arteries and veins in chest CT images [14]. They showed that a 3D CNN can learn specific A/V characteristics from small vessel segments directly extracted from non-contrast CT images without any further operations such as bronchi segmentation and vessel enhancement.

Although somewhat provocative for radiologists, it is also interesting to note that AI can help diagnose acute PE without imaging data. This approach relies on the fact that PE is a disease without specific clinical variables, leading clinicians to collect clinical variables to estimate PE likelihood in agreement with existing guidelines. In a recent study, Rucco et al. used data on 28 diagnostic features of 1427 people considered at risk of pulmonary embolism after a first screening in the emergency room and the outcome for each person of whether or not they developed PE [15]. This data was used to develop a neural hypernetwork, based on a combination of entities that does not use image analysis (i.e., *Q*-analysis with machine learning). This system recognized 94% of those developing PE.

AI Applied to Acute PE Reports

Medical imaging reports contain an abundant amount of diagnostic information that is inaccessible to automated analysis due to free-text narration. Were this unstructured free text be converted into a computer-manageable representation, it could be exploited in a variety of situations requiring automatic information extraction. Convolutional neural networks (CNNs) have been effective in visual object and speech-recognition tasks and may also be an extremely powerful tool for free-text annotation without the drawbacks of traditional natural language processing approaches because they do not require the development of dictionary-based libraries, grammatical feature definitions, concept codes, sentence-level annotation, or the generation of predefined terms [16]. In a recent study, Banerjee et al. evaluated a deep learning approach for classifying free-text radiology reports related to the diagnosis of pulmonary embolism – PE present/absent; PE acute/chronic; and PE central/sub-segmental only [17]. They demonstrated high fidelity compared to state-of-the-art rule-based method and found it generalizable across institutions for the clinically relevant categorization related to the diagnosis of PE. In another study from the same group, the performance of a deep learning convolutional neural network (CNN) model was compared with a traditional natural language processing model in extracting pulmonary embolism (PE) findings from thoracic computed tomography (CT) reports from two institutions [16]. The CNN model demonstrated an accuracy of 99% and an area under the curve value of 0.97 for determining the presence of pulmonary embolism in contrast-enhanced chest CT reports. As underlined by these authors, these techniques may make the valuable diagnostic information in radiology text available at a large scale to be used in models that evaluate imaging utilization, used as part of clinical decision support models, used to predict outcomes, and used as a valuable tool to evaluate ordering provider imaging yield rates. This information can be useful in an array of applications from large-scale retrospective research to focused clinical applications.

In a study conducted at an emergency department, the estimated prevalence of incidentalomas in chest CTA ordered to diagnose PE was 24% (141/589), while the prevalence of PE was only 9% (5/589) [18]. Pham et al. evaluated the combination of natural language processing and machine learning to detect thromboembolic disease diagnosis and incidental clinically relevant findings [19]. Developing a text processing pipeline for identifying incidental findings would help clinicians for epidemiological surveillance.

AI in the Detection of Chronic Thromboembolic Disease

Current Needs

There is a large knowledge gap within the imaging community in the interpretation of CT examinations of patients with chronic thromboembolic disease with or without pulmonary hypertension, mainly related to the erroneous perception of too complex a disease to depict [20]. This needs to be demystified as chronic PE can be easily approached on mediastinal and lung images, based on the identification of the vascular signs of chronic obstruction of pulmonary arteries (i.e., arterial stenosis, web, mural thrombi), the concurrent presence of bronchopulmonary abnormalities (i.e., mosaic perfusion, sequelae of lung infarct, bronchomegaly), and systemic collateral supply (i.e., enlarged systemic bronchial and/or non-bronchial systemic arteries) (Fig. 46.3). This rich semiology is not fully exploited by radiologists and not familiar to clinicians, both situations leading to a persistent reluctance in relying on CTA to diagnose chronic thromboembolic disease (CTED) and/or chronic thromboembolic pulmonary hypertension (CTEPH). It is also important to underline that chronic PE can be depicted in the setting of suspected acute PE [21]. Radiologists should pay attention to features of chronic obstruction superimposed to the presence of fresh clots to avoid delayed diagnosis of irreversible abnormalities in the pulmonary circulation (Fig. 46.4).

Directions for AI-Driven Automated Depiction of Chronic Pulmonary Artery Obstruction

When considering the detection of chronic PE or the assessment of CTEPH, CT interpretation requires a meticulous and time-consuming analysis of arterial branches for proper description of all abovementioned abnormalities. In both situations, an automated approach to the analysis of morphological features and a simplified view of the pulmonary arte-

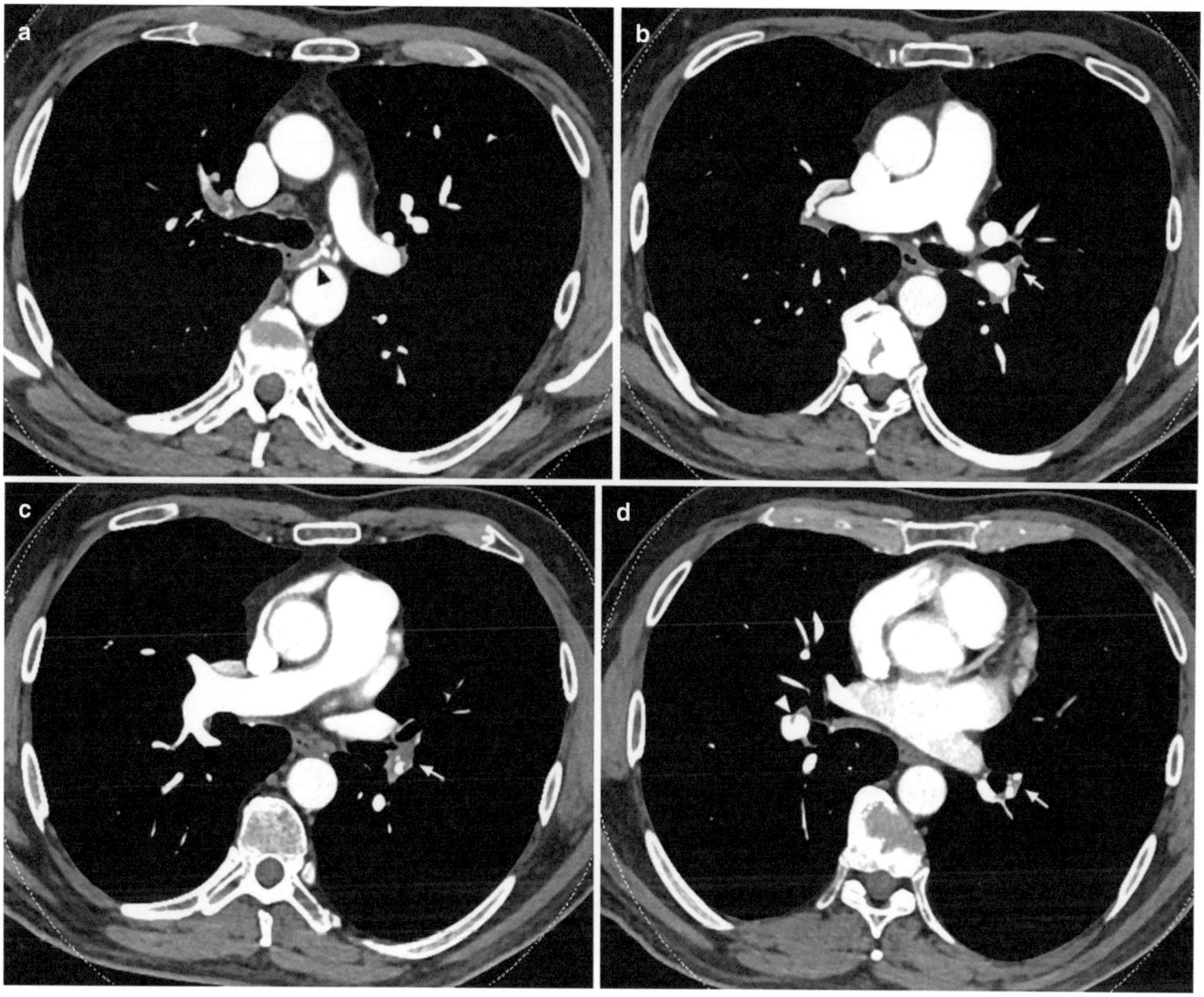

Fig. 46.3 Chest CT angiographic examination obtained in a 45-year-old female suspected of chronic thromboembolic pulmonary hypertension. (**a-d**) illustrates the numerous vascular signs indicative of chronic obstruction of the pulmonary circulation, including endoluminal filling defects, arterial stenosis (arrows), and webs (white arrowhead). Note the additional depiction of bronchial artery dilatation (black arrowhead on **a-d**), indicative of the systemic collateral supply secondary to the chronic obstruction of pulmonary arteries

rial tree could be particularly helpful. The list of CT features suggesting the presence of chronic PE has recently been highlighted [20]. Ende-Verhaar et al. have shown that the presence of three or more of six standardized radiologic parameters (i.e., intravascular webs, pulmonary artery retraction or dilatation, bronchial artery dilatation, right ventricular hypertrophy, and intraventricular septum flattening) was associated with a high specificity for diagnosis of CTEPH [21]. In the pretherapeutic evaluation of CTEPH, the AI approach should include not only the proximal extent of clots in all branches prior to pulmonary thromboendarterectomy but also the precise location of focal stenosis and/or webs when mapping candidate lesions prior to balloon pulmonary angiography. Several AI-driven tools are currently under development.

AI in the Diagnostic Approach of Pulmonary Hypertension

Current Context

Pulmonary hypertension (PH) may be due to parenchymal, cardiac, thromboembolic, and other diseases and is usually evaluated in expert PH centers. The depiction of elevated pulmonary artery pressure, the search for the etiology of PH,

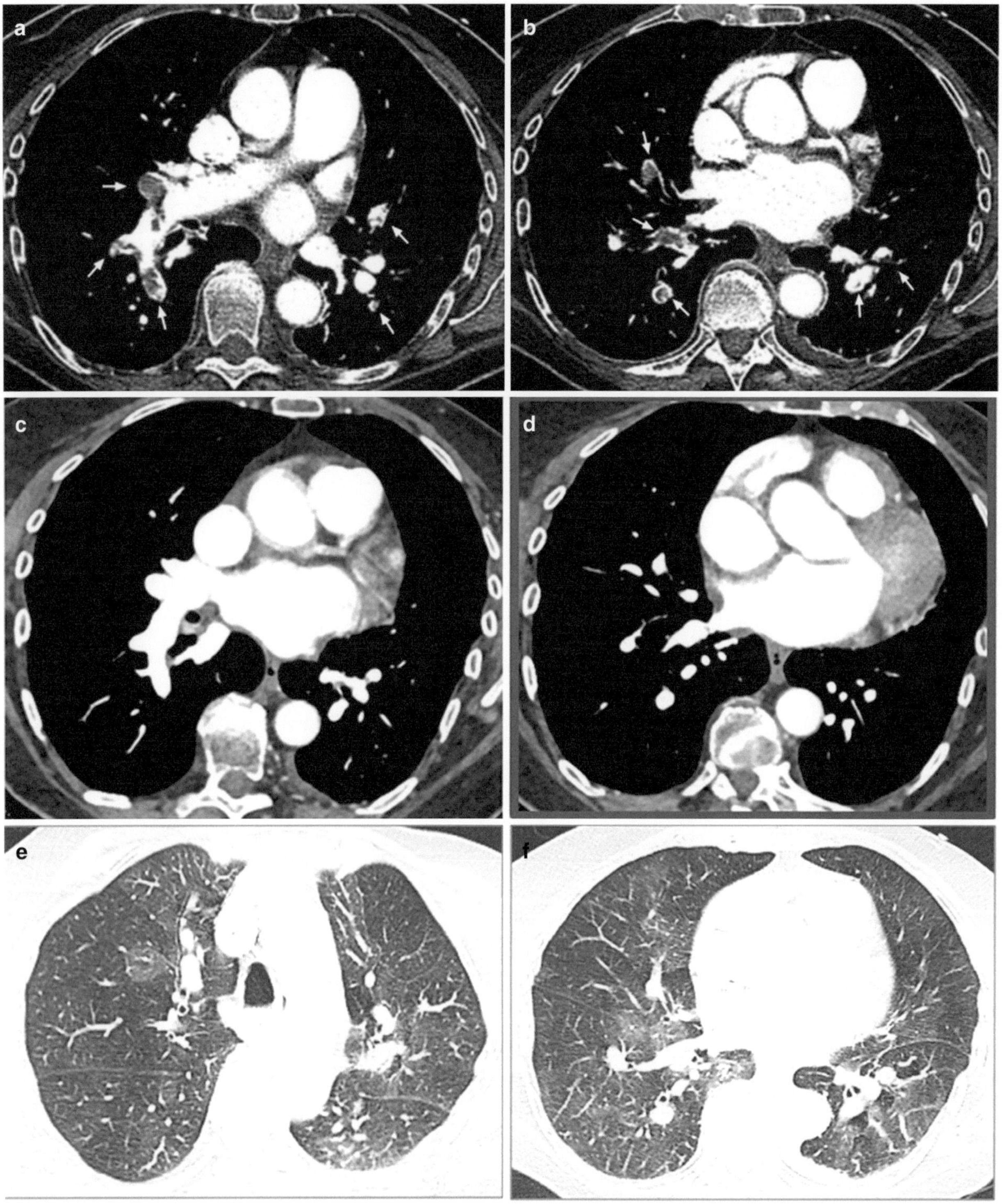

Fig. 46.4 Chest CT angiograms in a 79-year-old female with acute pulmonary embolism superimposed on chronic thromboembolic pulmonary hypertension (CTEPH) illustrating the delayed diagnosis of CTEPH at the time of acute pulmonary embolism. (**a** to **b**): Mediastinal images from a single-energy chest CT angiographic examination obtained at the time of acute pulmonary embolism. This diagnosis is based on the depiction of numerous endoluminal filling defects (arrows) in the context of acute respiratory failure. (**c** to **d**): Mediastinal images from the follow-up dual-energy CT angiogram obtained 6 months after the acute event at the time of patient referral to the expert center for suspicion of chronic thromboembolic pulmonary hypertension (CTEPH). The same anatomical levels as those shown in **a** and **b** showing complete resolution of endoluminal clots
Lung images reconstructed from the initial (**e-f**) and follow-up CT examinations (**g-h**), obtained at similar anatomical levels. Presence of a mosaic perfusion pattern, highly suggestive of CTEPH on both examinations, which was missed at the time of acute PE diagnosis. (**i** to **k**): Lung perfusion images generated from the follow-up dual-energy CT examination showing numerous PE-type defects (arrows), confirming the link between chronic obstruction of the pulmonary circulation and pulmonary hypertension

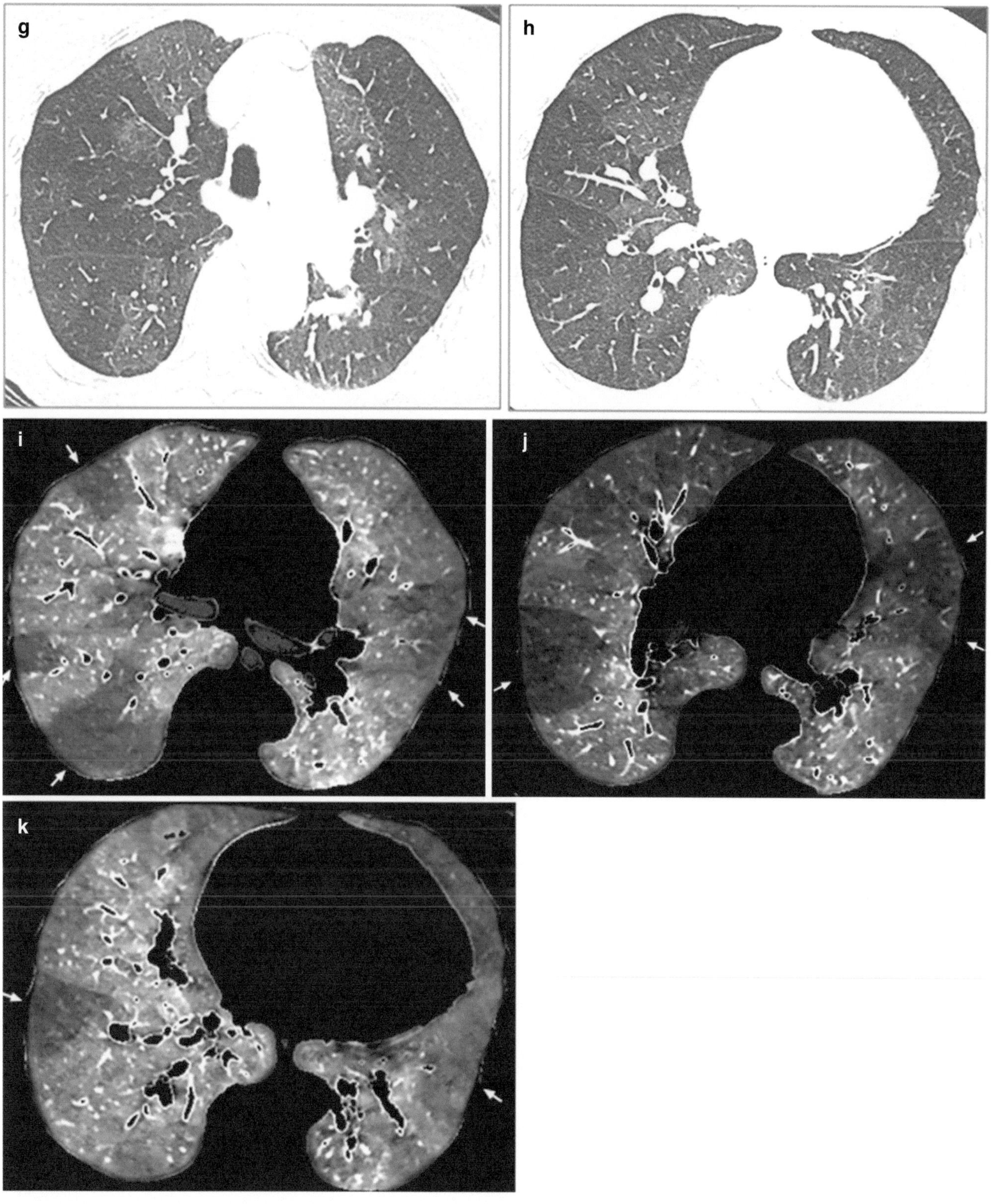

Fig. 46.4 (continued)

and the choice of the optimal therapeutic option necessitate multidisciplinary discussions for proper management. Whereas PH represents an important healthcare burden, the clinical applications of artificial intelligence in this field are very preliminary, but their development would definitely facilitate patient management in several directions. Figures 46.5 and 46.6 illustrate the current limitations of visual assessment of pulmonary circulation on morphologic and perfusion images.

Directions for AI-Driven Solutions

Because of the poor prognosis of PH, it is of great significance to screen patients with PH at an early stage for timely intervention or to assess the value of PAP for following up patients with cardiac or pulmonary disorders. An important field of application could be the early detection of PH, as this diagnosis is often delayed because of the lack of specificity of clinical symptoms. Several facets of this approach have already been investigated. In a recent study, Bergeman et al. investigated the usefulness of machine learning techniques to identify patients with idiopathic pulmonary arterial hypertension (iPAH) [22]. This study found high levels of activity and frequent contacts with healthcare services in the 3 years before a confirmed diagnosis of idiopathic PAH. In addition, patients frequently attended respiratory and cardiology specialties. The combination of high levels of activity and the richness of specialty interactions raises the possibility that patients with iPAH may exhibit characteristic patterns of

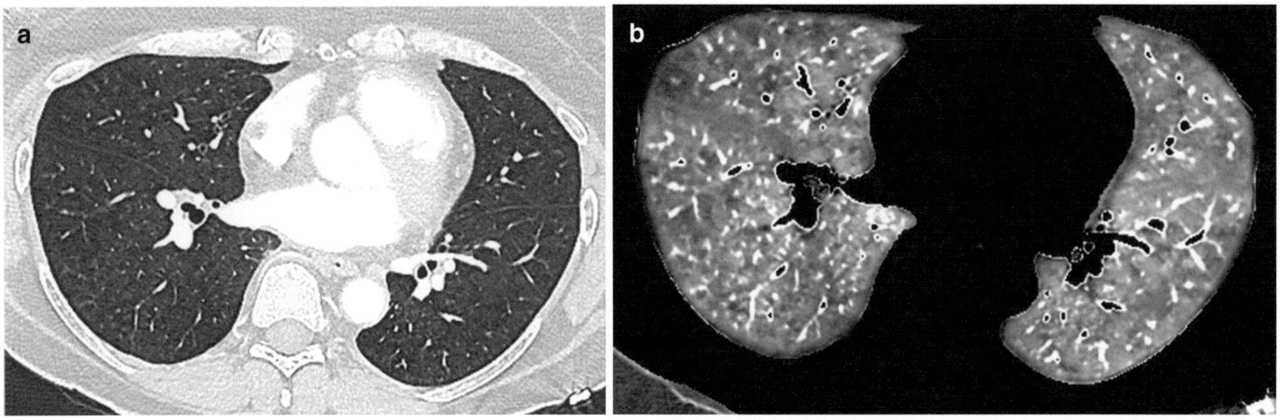

Fig. 46.5 Dual-energy CT angiographic examination obtained in a 65-year-old female referred for pulmonary arterial hypertension. (**a**) Lung image obtained at the level of the lower lobes showing faint parenchymal micronodules, suggestive of plexogenic arteriopathy in this context. (**b**) Corresponding lung perfusion image showing a diffuse pattern of patchy defects in both lungs

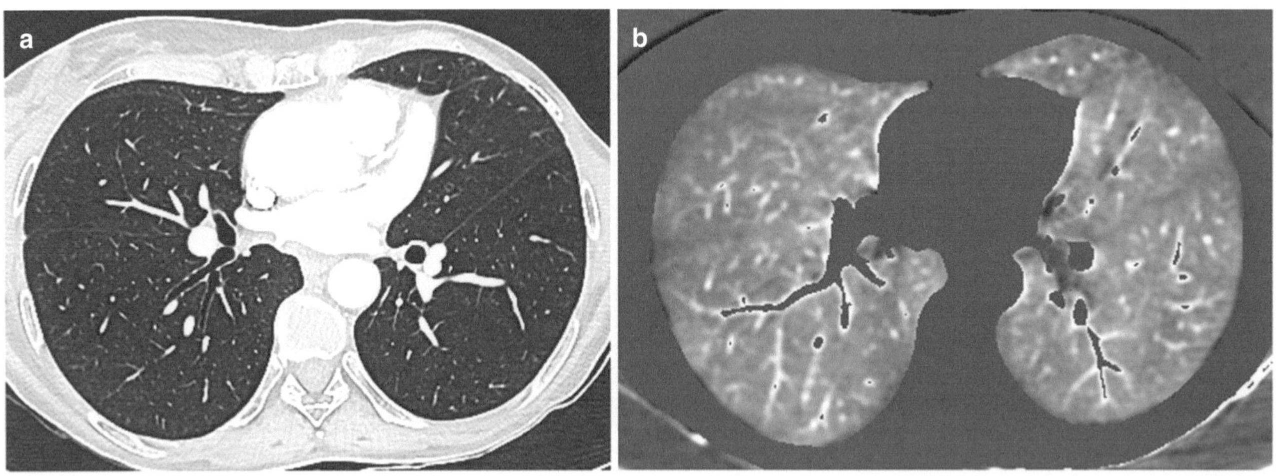

Fig. 46.6 Dual-energy CT angiographic examination obtained in a 59-year-old female referred for pulmonary arterial hypertension. This case illustrates the limitations of visual assessment of lung microcirculation. (**a**) Lung image obtained at the level of the right middle lobe bronchus showing a normal-appearing lung parenchyma. (**b**) Lung perfusion image obtained at the level of the right bronchus intermedius, showing homogeneous enhancement of the lung parenchyma in both lungs. The hypoattenuated areas correspond to the avascular zones of fissures

behavior separate from other cardiorespiratory conditions, providing sufficient data to support the development of a predictive diagnostic algorithm for iPAH. Another application of network science has been proposed to discern pediatric PH subtypes from comorbidity data recorded in longitudinal datasets [23]. These authors aimed to use network statistics to improve clinical definitions and identify clinically relevant patterns of disease in pediatric patients with hope that this would lead to earlier and improved diagnostic specificity. This is the first study in PH using machine learning techniques to improve understanding of a rare disease.

Another field of application could be the prediction of elevated pulmonary artery pressure (PAP). In a retrospective study, Zou et al. used CNNs to predict PH based on frontal chest radiographs [24]. Their study used deep learning algorithms to classify abnormalities suggesting PH in chest radiographs with high accuracy and good generalizability. Kusunose et al. hypothesized that application of AI to the chest X-ray could identify elevated PAP and stratify the risk of heart failure hospitalization with PH [25]. In a preliminary work, they created, trained, validated, and then tested a convolutional neural network to identify elevated PAP (>20 mm Hg). They found that applying AI to the chest X-ray in high-risk groups had limited performance when used alone in identifying elevated PAP.

Current methods to assess PH rely on indirect consequences of raised pulmonary vascular resistance at the level of the right ventricle and proximal pulmonary artery, while morphological assessment of small vascular sections on unenhanced CT can also play a role. Increasing implementation of 4D flow analysis allows for the noninvasive assessment of flow through the pulmonary artery, where the presence of vortices and duration of vortices have been shown to be diagnostic for PH [26]. This application is an active focus in MR development. High diagnostic accuracy has been shown for pulmonary arterial hypertension based on a tensor-based machine learning approach [27]. Combined automated 3D volumetry of the central pulmonary arteries by pulmonary CT angiography and echocardiographic pressure estimate has recently been reported as an interesting approach to predict the presence of pulmonary hypertension [28]. Machine learning by using cardiac MR imaging could also be used as a tool to guide patient management [29].

Whereas alterations of lung microcirculation can be depicted morphologically on HRCT lung images (e.g., in the context of PVOD) or estimated on the basis of perfusion defects on perfusion scintigraphy and dual-energy or MR perfusion images, none of these techniques can provide fine analysis of the most distal compartment of the pulmonary circulation. There is no doubt that machine-learning approaches should open new possibilities in the analysis of distal parts of the pulmonary circulation, thus participating in the confident depiction of diagnostic or prognostic features.

Conclusion

AI in the diagnostic approach of pulmonary vascular diseases opens new horizons in daily practice. It can help optimize the diagnostic resources, thus participating in improved patient management and indirectly in reduction in radiation exposure. It has also the potential of improving daily workflow, assisting radiologists in highlighting positive exams in the emergency department as well as exams with chronic obstruction of pulmonary arteries. Lastly, radiologists are waiting for the exciting step when their visual analysis of images will be combined with patterns only "seen" by AI tools.

References

1. Erickson BJ, Korfiatis P, Akkus Z, Kline TL. Machine learning for medical imaging. Radiographics. 2017;37:505–15.
2. Klang E. Deep learning and medical imaging. J Thorac Dis. 2018;10:1325–8.
3. Retson TA, Besser AH, Sall S, et al. Machine learning and deep neural networks in thoracic and cardiovascular imaging. J Thorac Imaging. 2019;34:192–201.
4. Tourassi GD, Floyd CE, Sostman HD, Coleman RE. Acute pulmonary embolism: cost-effectiveness analysis of the effect of artificial neural networks on patient care. Radiology. 1998;206:81–8.
5. The PIOPED investigators. Value of the ventilation/perfusion in acute pulmonary embolism. JAMA. 1990;263:2753–9.
6. Tourassi GD, Floyd CE, Coleman RE. Acute pulmonary embolism: cost-effectiveness analysis of the effect of artificial neural networks on patient care. Radiology. 1998;206:81–8.
7. Scott JA. Artificial neural networks and image interpretation: a ghost in the machine. Semin Ultrasound CT MRI. 2004;25:396–403.
8. Holst H, Aström K, Järund A, et al. Automated interpretation of ventilation-perfusion lung scintigrams for the diagnosis of pulmonary embolism using artificial neural networks. Eur J Nucl Med. 2000;27:400–6.
9. Reinartz P, Kaiser HJ, Wildberger JE, et al. SPECT imaging in the diagnosis of pulmonary embolism: automated detection of matched and mismatch defects by means of image processing techniques. J Nucl Med. 2006;47:968–73.
10. Mountain D, Keijzers G, Chu K, et al. RESPECT-ED (rates of pulmonary emboli (PE) and sub-segmental PE with modern computed tomographic pulmonary angiograms in emergency departments): a multi-center observational study finds significant yield variation, uncorrelated with use or small PE rates. PLoS One. 2017;12(8):e0184219. https://doi.org/10.1371/journal.pone.0184219.
11. Banerjeel SM, Yang J, et al. Development and performance of the pulmonary embolism result forecast model (PERFORM) for computed tomography clinical decision support. JAMA Netw Open. 2019;2:e198719. https://doi.org/10.1001/jamanetworkopen.2019.8719.
12. Weikert T, Winkel DJ, Bremercih J, et al. Automated detection of pulmonary embolism in CT pulmonary angiograms using an AI-powered algorithm. Eur Radiol. 2020;30:6545–53.
13. Liu W, Liu M, Guo X et al. Evaluation of acute pulmonary embolism and clot burden on CTPA with deep learning. Eur Radiol. 2020. https://doi.org/10.1007/s00330-020-06699-8.
14. Jimenez-Carretero D, Bermejo-Pelaez D, Waksko GR, et al. Pulmonary artery-vein classification in CT images using deep learning. IEEE Trans Med Imaging. 2018;37:2428–40.

15. Rucco M, Sousa-Rodrigues D, Merelli E, et al. Neural hypernetwork approach for pulmonary embolism diagnosis. BMC Res Notes. 2015;6:617.
16. Chen MC, Ball RL, Yang L, et al. Deep learning to classify radiology free-text reports. Radiology. 2018;286:845–52.
17. Banerjee I, Chen MC, Lungren MP, Rubin DL. Radiology report annotation using intelligent word embeddings: applied to multi-institutional chest CT cohort. J Biomed Inform. 2018;77:11–20.
18. Hall WB, Truitt SG, Scheunemann LP, et al. The prevalence of clinically relevant incidental findings on chest computed tomographic angiograms ordered to diagnose pulmonary embolism. Arch Intern Med. 2009;169:1961–5.
19. Pham AD, Neveol A, Lavergne T, et al. Natural language processing of radiology reports for the detection of thromboembolic diseases and clinically relevant incidental findings. BMC Bioinformatics. 2014;15:266.
20. Remy-Jardin M, Ryerson CJ, Schiebler M, et al. Imaging of pulmonary hypertension in adults: a position paper from the Fleischner society. Radiology. 2021;00:1–19.
21. Ende-Verhaar YM, Meijboom LJ, Kroft LJM, et al. Usefulness of standard computed tomography pulmonary angiography performed for acute pulmonary embolism for identification of chronic thromboembolic pulmonary hypertension: results of the InShape III study. J Heart Lung Transplant. 2019;38(7):731–8. https://doi.org/10.1016/j.healun.2019.03.003. Epub 2019 Mar 15. PMID: 30962147.
22. Bergemann R, Allsopp J, Jenner H, et al. High levels of healthcare utilization prior to diagnosis in idiopathic pulmonary arterial hypertension support the feasibility of an early diagnosis algorithm: the SPHInX project. Pulm Circ. 2018;8(4):1–9. https://doi.org/10.1177/2045894018798613.
23. Ong MS, Mullen MP, Austin ED, et al. Learning a comorbidity-driven taxonomy of pediatric pulmonary hypertension. Circ Res. 2017;121:341–53.
24. Zou XL, Ren Y, Feng DY, et al. A promising approach for screening pulmonary hypertension based on frontal chest radiographs using deep learning: a retrospective study. PLoS One. 2020;15(7):e0236378.
25. Kusunose K, Hirata Y, Tsuji T, et al. Deep learning to predict elevated pulmonary artery pressure in patients with suspected pulmonary hypertension using standard chest X ray. Nature Research. 2020;10:19311.
26. Reiter G, Reiter U, Kovacs G, et al. Blood flow vortices along the main pulmonary artery measured with MR imaging for the diagnosis of pulmonary hypertension. Radiology. 2015;275(1):71–9. https://doi.org/10.1148/radiol.14140849.
27. Swift A, Lu H, Uthoff J, et al. A machine learning cardiac magnetic resonance approach to extract disease features and automate pulmonary arterial hypertension diagnosis Eur Heart J Cardiovasc Imaging. 2020. [Epub ahead of print]; https://doi.org/10.1093/ehjci/jeaa001.
28. Melzig C, Wörz S, Egenlauf B, et al. Combined automated 3D volumetry by pulmonary CT angiography and echocardiography for detection of pulmonary hypertension. Eur Radiol. 2019;29(11):6059–68. https://doi.org/10.1007/s00330-019-06188-7.
29. Dawes TJW, de Marvao A, Shi W, et al. Machine learning of three-dimensional right ventricular motion enables outcome prediction in pulmonary hypertension: a cardiac MR imaging study. Radiology. 2017;283(2):381–90. https://doi.org/10.1148/radiol.2016161315.

Artificial Intelligence-Based Evaluation of the Aorta

47

Domenico Mastrodicasa, Marina Codari, Valery L. Turner, Virginia Hinostroza, Kathrin Bäumler, Martin J. Willemink, and Dominik Fleischmann

Introduction

Aortic dissection and aortic aneurysms are the most common aortic diseases and are associated with high morbidity and mortality [1]. Imaging and accurate measurements of aortic size play a key role in the diagnosis, treatment planning, and surveillance of patients with aortic diseases. Manual measurements of aortic diameters are time-consuming, and reproducibility is suboptimal [2, 3]. Machine learning (ML)-based image processing workflows have recently gained traction due to their potential to automatically extract imaging features with similar or higher accuracy and reproducibility compared to manual annotations or rule-based approaches [4]. Furthermore, deep learning (DL) algorithms can identify patterns in large clinical and imaging datasets that cannot be recognized by human observers. The availability of such tools could improve the risk stratification and treatment planning of patients with aortic diseases [5, 6]. This chapter summarizes recent promising artificial intelligence (AI) applications in the evaluation of the aorta, with a focus on aortic dissection and abdominal aortic aneurysm (AAA).

D. Mastrodicasa, MD (✉)
Department of Radiology, Stanford University School of Medicine, Center for Academic Medicine, Palo Alto, CA, USA
e-mail: mastro@stanford.edu

M. Codari, MSc, PhD · V. L. Turner, MD · V. Hinostroza, MSc
K. Bäumler, PhD
Department of Radiology, School of Medicine, Stanford University, Stanford, CA, USA

M. J. Willemink, MD, PhD
Segmed, Inc, Menlo Park, CA, USA

Department of Radiology, Stanford University School of Medicine, Stanford, CA, USA

D. Fleischmann, MD
Department of Radiology, School of Medicine, Stanford University, Stanford, CA, USA

Cardiovascular Institute, Stanford University, Stanford, CA, USA

Aortic Landmark Detection

The localization of anatomical landmarks is a prerequisite for several medical image analysis tasks, including initializing image registration and segmentation. The detection of aortic landmarks is becoming increasingly relevant for an accurate planning of endovascular and surgical procedures, as well as for patients' surveillance. One of the first attempts to localize aortic landmarks using ML techniques was proposed by Zheng et al. [7]. The authors used a hierarchical approach to localize 8 aortic valve landmarks (2 coronary ostia, 3 hinges, and 3 commissures) on 278 contrast-enhanced C-arm computed tomography (CT) scans performed in transcatheter aortic valve implantation (TAVI) candidates. First, the landmark location was roughly estimated using marginal space learning. Then, landmark detection was refined using a probabilistic boosting tree classifier. A mean (±standard deviation [SD]) detection error of 2.09 ± 1.18 mm, 2.07 ± 1.53 mm, and 2.17 ± 1.31 mm was reported for aortic hinges, commissures, and coronary ostia, respectively [7]. The proposed method showed a fast processing time of approximately 1 sec per CT scan, and was robust with respect to variation of field of view, scan timing, contrast agent, and valve regurgitation. Later, Al et al. proposed a two-step approach to automatically estimate aortic valve landmarks in TAVI patients using colonial walk [8]. In this study, the first step involved the detection of a single landmark identifying a 3D region of interest; in the second step, eight colonial walkers estimated the location of the same landmark detected by Zheng et al. [7]. The model was trained using 40 CT angiography (CTA) scans of non-TAVI patients and was tested on 31 pre-TAVI patients. Reported mean (±SD) detection errors in TAVI patients were 2.81 ± 1.85 mm, 2.77 ± 1.82 mm, and 2.54 ± 1.60 mm for aortic hinges, commissures, and coronary ostia, respectively. The proposed approach showed high computational efficiency, requiring only 12 msec to detect all landmarks [8].

C. N. De Cecco et al. (eds.), *Artificial Intelligence in Cardiothoracic Imaging*, Contemporary Medical Imaging,
https://doi.org/10.1007/978-3-030-92087-6_47

Ghesu et al. proposed deep reinforcement learning (DRL) as an alternative technique to perform landmark detection. The authors developed several artificial agents navigating the CT image volume toward the target landmark locations using a multi-resolution approach. The proposed method was used to identify eight anatomical landmarks, including three vessel bifurcations on the aortic arch. The authors reported a mean (±SD) localization error of 3.71 ± 2.01 mm, 3.89 ± 1.95 mm, and 3.09 ± 1.50 mm for the origin of the brachiocephalic artery, of the left common carotid artery, and of the left subclavian artery, respectively, and median runtime of just 33 msec [9]. The same approach was then integrated by Rueckel et al. into the commercial software AI-Rad Companion Chest CT (Siemens Healthineers, Erlangen, Germany) (Fig. 47.1), which was applied to estimate the size of 9 aortic landmarks (Fig. 47.2) in 36 CT scans from 18 patients with ectasia of the ascending aorta [10]. This technique was then combined with other DL algorithms to estimate aortic diameters at target landmark location. Results showed a mean reporting time reduction of 63%, including the 33.6% of cases needing a manual correction, and a mean reduction of interobserver variability, defined as the average deviation from the three reader's common mean, of 42.5% [10]. A partial policy-based DRL approach was also proposed by Al et al. to localize eight aortic valve landmarks in CTA studies. This approach divided the original search problem into several simpler problems involving multiple sub-agents. The model was trained and evaluated using a fourfold cross-validation strategy on 71 CTA scans of non-TAVI and pre-TAVI patients. In non-TAVI patients, reported mean (±SD) detection errors were 1.96 ± 0.98 mm, 1.95 ± 0.93 mm, and 1.91 ± 0.95 mm for aortic hinges, commissures, and coronary ostia, respectively, while in pre-TAVI scans, the corresponding detection errors were 2.08 ± 1.24 mm, 2.02 ± 1.15 mm, and 1.94 ± 1.01 mm [11]. Finally, Codari et al. trained five DRL agents to detect the aortic annulus location in CTA scans of patients with aortic dissection implementing the method proposed by Alansary et al. (Fig. 47.3) [12]. The agents were trained on 75 CTA scans and validated on 24 CTA scans. Reported results showed a median localization error (and interquartile range [IQR]) of 2.98 (2.15–3.51) mm in validation data [2].

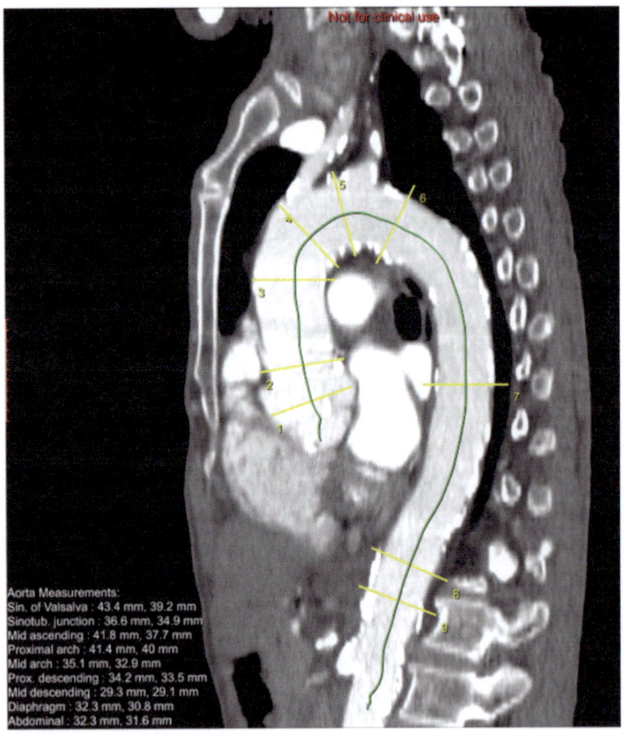

Fig. 47.1 CT angiography of the thoracic aorta, sagittal view (AI-Rad Companion Chest CT, Siemens Healthineers). The landmarks are detected automatically based on deep reinforcement learning and are placed at nine anatomical landmark positions, according to the ESC/AHA guidelines

More recently, DL approaches based on convolutional neural networks (CNNs) have been proposed to detect aortic landmarks. Astudillo et al. semiautomatically detected five aortic valve landmarks in pre-TAVI CTA scans. After the manual identification of the subvolume containing the aortic root, three CNNs were used to segment and derive three landmark masks [13]. The masks were averaged and normalized to obtain landmark probability maps, which was then post-processed by combining hierarchical clustering and map thresholding techniques to identify final landmark locations. The proposed model was trained with 344 CT scans and validated on 100 CT scans, which were also used to estimate interobserver variability. Reported median and interquartile range (IQR) annotation errors were 1.6 (1.2–2.3) mm for the left-coronary cusp; 1.5 (0.9–2.1) mm for the non-coronary cusp; 1.6 (1.3–2.2) mm for the right coronary cusp; and 1.3 (0.9–1.9) mm and 1.4 (0.9–2.0) mm for the left and right coronary ostia, respectively. The proposed method showed lower or comparable annotation error when compared to interobserver variability. According to the authors, the high performance and low processing time (below 1 sec) highlight the potential of DL for TAVI planning [13].

Noothout et al. developed a global-to-local landmark detection strategy using fully convolutional CNNs [14]. A CNN first simultaneously estimated the global location of all landmarks. The final location of each landmark was then finalized using dedicated CNNs. They exploited the computational efficiency of a patch-based classification while mitigating its lack of precision by regressing the displacement vectors pointing to the target landmarks for each patch. Final landmark locations were identified as the weighted average of displacement vectors. The authors used this method to estimate eight aortic valve commissures, hinge, and coronary ostia landmarks in cardiac CTA scans. The method was trained using 412 CTA scans, validated on 60 CTA scans, and tested on 200 CTA scans. A subset of 100 scans was randomly selected among to estimate intra- and interob-

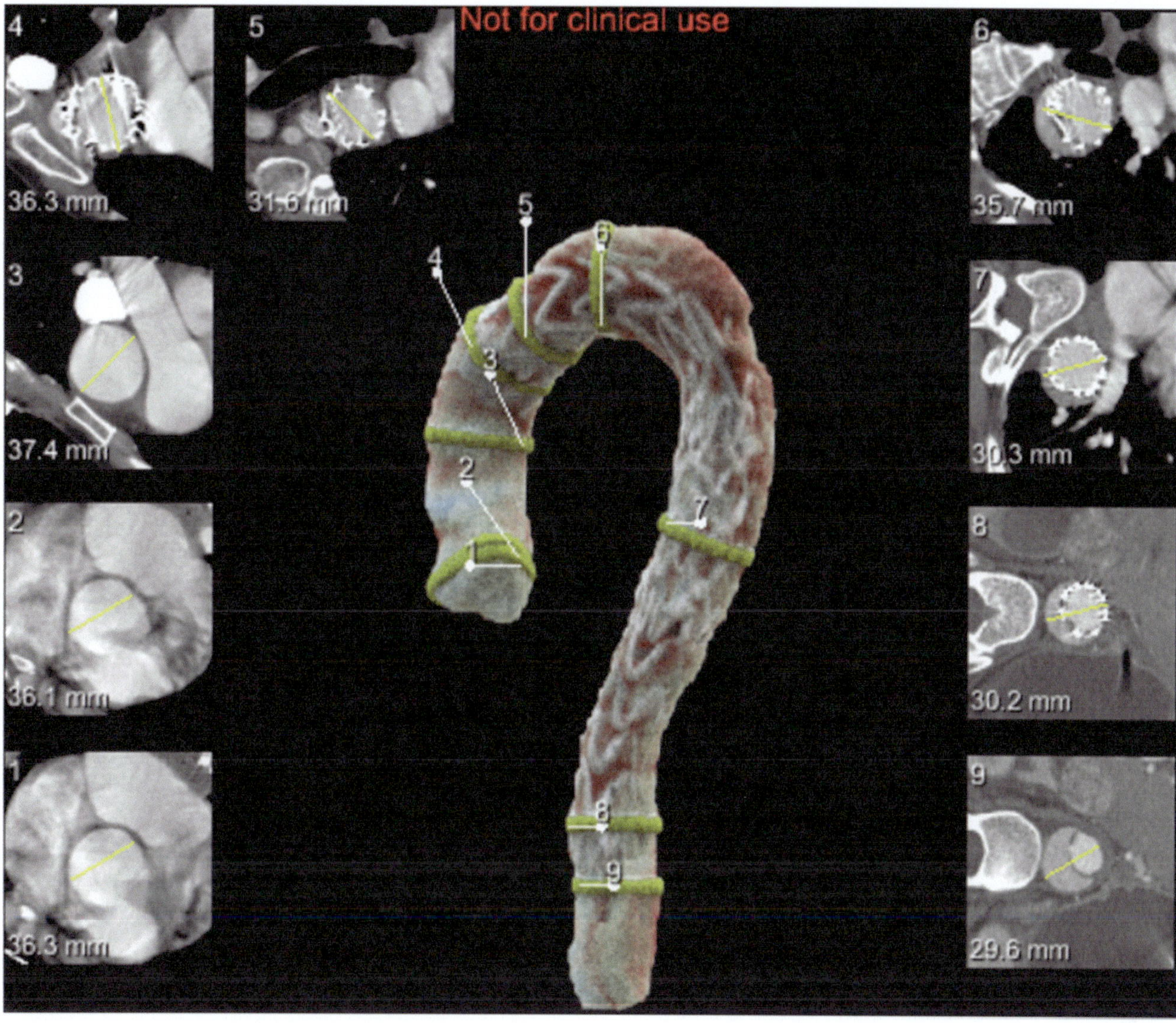

Fig. 47.2 Postoperative CT angiography of the aorta after endovascular stent placement, 3D rendering and cross-sectional views (1–9) (AI-Rad Companion Chest CT, Siemens Healthineers). The cross-sectional images are perpendicular to the aortic centerline. The aortic landmarks are as follows: aortic root, aortic arch center, brachiocephalic artery bifurcation, left common carotid artery, left subclavian artery, and celiac trunk

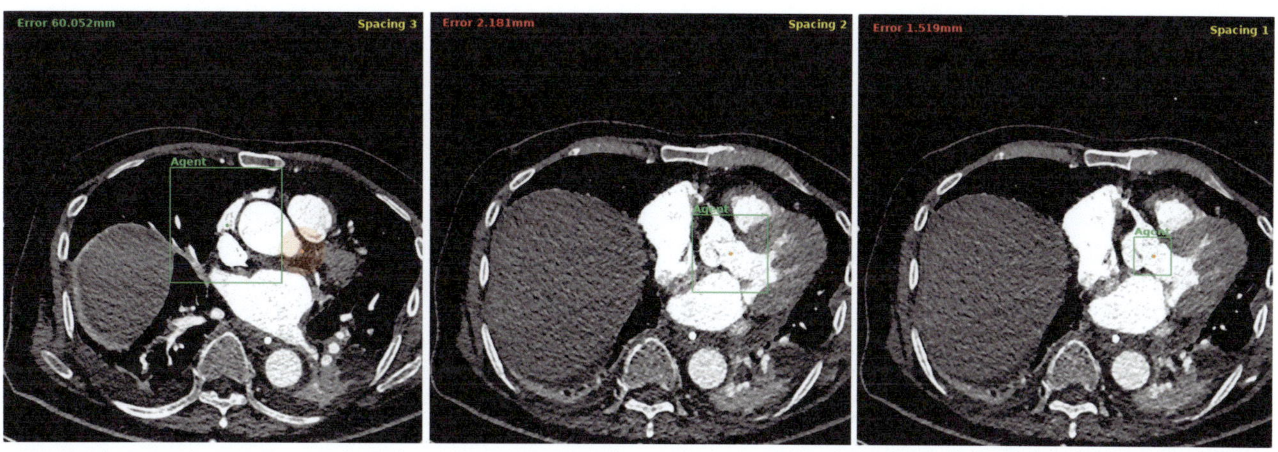

Fig. 47.3 Example of hierarchical resolution steps performed to localize the aortic annulus landmark using the deep reinforcement learning agent proposed by Codari et al. (2020)

server variability. The simultaneous estimation of multiple landmarks resulted in the most accurate landmark detection, with an overall mean (±SD) error of 1.87 ± 1.67 mm. The average processing time per scan was 0.06 ± 0.05 seconds, and for six landmarks automatic detection errors were lower than intra-observer variability. Due to its fast annotation time and high accuracy, this method may be suitable for large clinical studies as well as real-time annotations [14]. While DLR approaches result in the optimal search path from an initial location toward a single landmark of interest at a time, CNN can be used for both single and multi-landmark localizations without the need of navigating the entire volume and without prior segmentation steps. For this reason, CNN could be considered a more efficient approach.

Aortic Segmentation

Aortic segmentation is a critical step that enables the evaluation of a wide range of aortic morphologic features, including lumen size. These features are routinely used to diagnose diseases and guide treatment decisions. However, manual annotation is time-consuming and hard to implement in the current clinical workflow. Therefore, segmentation methods based on ML algorithms have been recently introduced to automate segmentations and standardize both diagnosis and risk assessment. In most of these studies, an expert-based manual annotation is used as the ground truth.

Unenhanced and Contrast-Enhanced CT

One of the first methods to automatically segment the aorta using a DL approach was proposed by Noothout et al. The authors used a dilated convolutional neural network (CNN) to segment the aorta into ascending aorta, aortic arch, and descending thoracic aorta [15]. The study was conducted on 24 low-dose, unenhanced chest CT scans from the National Lung Screening Trial [16]. The dilated CNN was applied to axial, coronal, and sagittal CT images to classify voxels into one of the three aortic segments or background; then, the results of each image plane were averaged to provide the final segmentation. The CNN was able to accurately segment the thoracic aorta with an average overall Dice similarity score (DSC) of 0.87 ± 0.03. Interestingly, the best performance was reported for the descending thoracic aorta, while results were the least accurate in the ascending aorta. The cardiac pulsation, the low soft-tissue contrast caused by lack of intravascular iodinated contrast, and the potentially higher image noise deriving from the low radiation dose protocol posed specific challenges to the investigation and could explain the discrepancy between performance on ascending and descending aorta.

A similar segmentation approach was recently proposed by Fantazzini et al. [17]. However, in this investigation, the authors used 80 contrast-enhanced CTA scans of the aorta. A DL approach was used to locate and segment the lumen of the thoracoabdominal aorta as well as the branch vessels of the aortic arch and of the abdominal aorta. A three-step workflow was used, starting with a coarse localization of the aorta performed by a CNN on down-sampled images. Next, three CNNs independently segmented the aorta in the axial, sagittal, and coronal planes. The final segmentation was obtained by integrating these segmentations. The multi-view aggregation provided better results than those obtained with single-view segmentations.

Aortic Dissection

Recently, DL approaches have been proposed to segment the aorta in patients with aortic dissection. Image segmentation is challenging in aortic dissection, which is characterized by two flow channels, the true (TL) and the false lumen (FL), which can be asymmetric in size and contrast opacification. Cao et al. used a cascade of fully CNN to process CTA scans of 276 patients with type B aortic dissection (TBAD) [18]. The authors developed three CNN models to segment the whole aorta, TL, and FL at the same time. The authors reported DSC of 0.93 ± 0.01, 0.93 ± 0.01, and 0.91 ± 0.02 for the whole aorta, TL, and FL, respectively, demonstrating the feasibility of fully automatic TL and FL segmentation. Similarly, Hahn et al. proposed a stepwise CNN-based approach to generate multiplanar reformations (MPRs) of the aorta and segment TL and FL on MPRs orthogonal to the aortic axis [3]. The study was conducted on 153 CTA scans of 45 patients with uncomplicated TBAD (Fig. 47.4). Patients were followed up to a median of 4 years, and the manual segmentation of four experienced radiologists was used as the reference standard. The authors reported an average DSC ranging from 0.873 to 0.900 for both validation and test sets. Despite the presence of FL thrombosis in the dataset, this model performed well and proved its potential to be used in follow-up assessments.

In another study, the segmentation was focused exclusively on the TL. Cheng et al. used a CNN with a customized U-Net architecture to segment the TL on 2D axial images [19]. The author included only 20 CTA scans; half of them were positive for aortic dissection. The algorithm correctly detected nine patients with and eight without aortic dissection, with a sensitivity and specificity of 90% and 80%, respectively, and overall accuracy of 85%.

The investigations described so far focused on the segmentation of static images on CT datasets. Bai et al. proposed an image sequence segmentation algorithm combining a fully convolutional network with a recurrent neural network [20]. This combination allowed to incorporate spatial and temporal information into the segmen-

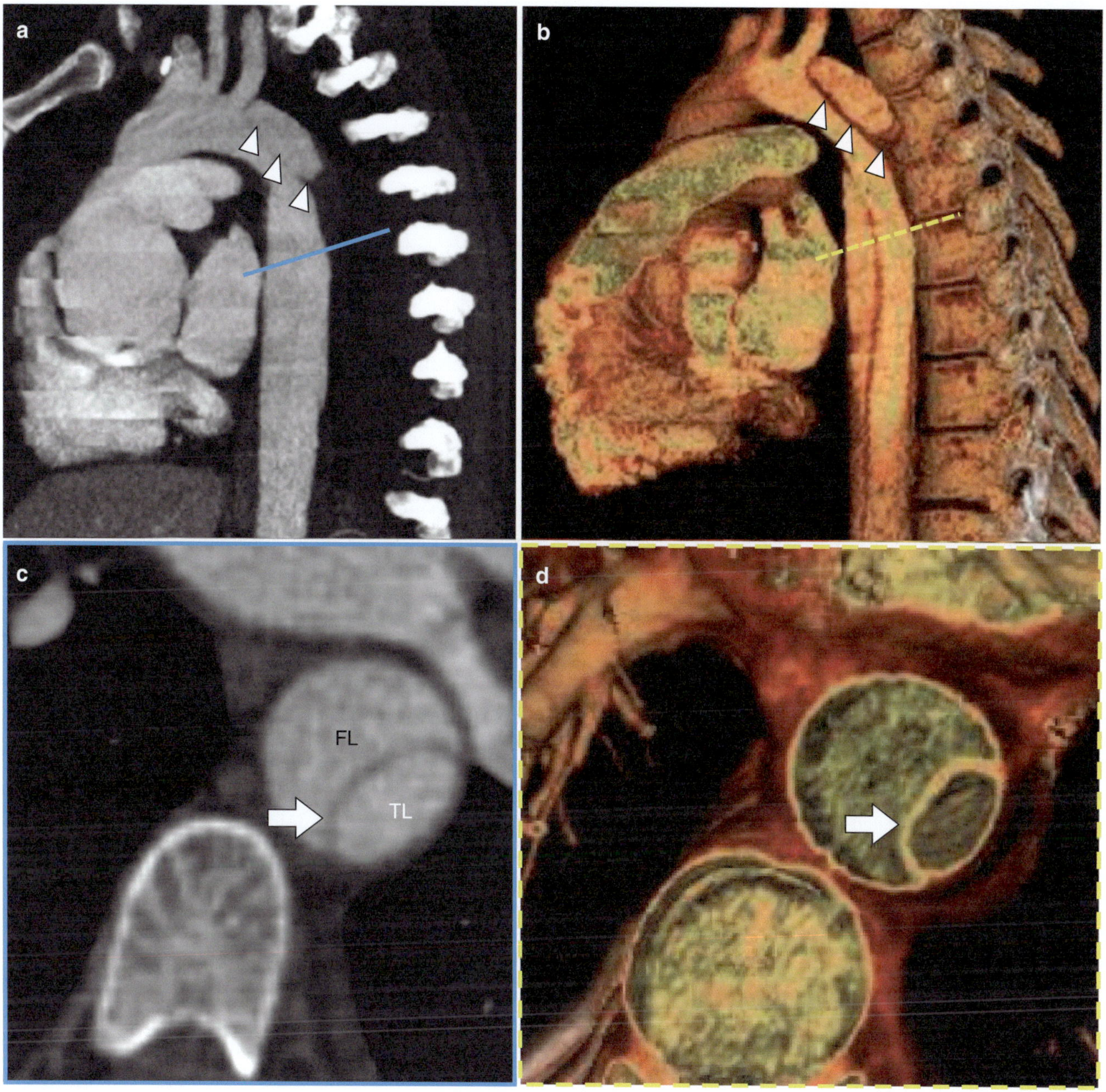

Fig. 47.4 Sagittal MIP view (**a**) and axial image (**c**) of a CT angiography obtained in a 67-year-old man with a type **b** aortic dissection. The dissection flap (white arrowheads in **a** and **b**) is visible distal to the left subclavian artery. The dissection flap is much better seen on three-dimensional volume-rendered slabs (**b** and **d**). (*FL* false lumen, *TL* true lumen)

tation task. The study was performed using a large dataset of aortic magnetic resonance (MR) image sequences of 500 patients from the UK Biobank. The authors reported an average DSC of 0.960 and 0.953 for the ascending and descending aorta, respectively. More importantly, the authors addressed the challenge of training the network based on temporally sparse annotations, and the results outperformed state-of-the-art baseline methods both for segmentation accuracy and for temporal smoothness.

Abdominal Aortic Aneurysm

Several methods have been proposed for AAA segmentation. de Bruijne et al. proposed a semiautomatic technique to segment the AAA sac on CTA scans based on shape model fitting in sequential slices [21]. In this method, the contour obtained manually in the first 2D axial image is used as a reference for determining the contour of the aneurysm sac in the subsequent image. This method was inspired by the active shape model (ASM) segmentation scheme which is a model-based method combining the statistical knowledge of object shape and variations with local appearance models near the object contours. The study was conducted on 1175 axial slices obtained from 23 CTA scans: 2 pre-operative scans and 21 scans acquired after endovascular stenting, either directly after the procedure or during a 1–12-month follow-up. An expert-guided manual segmentation was used as the gold standard for AAA sac's contours. The method proposed by the authors showed accurate segmentation, with a manual intervention required only in one of the six slices. This work highlighted the potential to reduce the time requirements of expert segmentation by a factor of 6.

In a previous study, Subasic et al. proposed another semi-automatic approach for AAA segmentation based on CTA images [22]. This time, the approach was based on a 3D deformable model implemented using the level-set algorithm, which is specifically fit to model complex structures such as AAA. The segmentation process was based on two separate steps for the inner and outer aortic wall on a total of 11 CTA datasets. After a 3D segmentation of the AAA, the authors extracted a 3D model of the aortic wall with relative errors close to those obtained by human experts.

Later, Zhuge et al. proposed an automatic AAA segmentation system using a 3D level-set method [23]. This hybrid framework for segmentation combined global region analysis, local feature analysis, and a level-set boundary evolution method. The authors tested the proposed algorithm on 20 CTA datasets and compared the results with expert manual tracing. The average segmentation time per patient was 7.4 ± 3.8 min as opposed to the 20–30 min of the manual method, and the volume overlap was 95.3% ± 1.4%. Notably, this model required no user manual intervention other than identifying the most proximal and distal slices containing the aneurysm.

Aortic Thrombus Segmentation

The aortic enlargement occurring in AAA favors the formation of a thrombus. Although the role of thrombus volume on aneurysm rupture is still debated, the accurate measurements of its maximal diameter are still relevant to assess patients' prognosis. However, accurate segmentation of the thrombus is a difficult task due to the similar densities of the thrombus and surrounding structures. Maiora et al. proposed an active learning image segmentation system for a quick AAA volume segmentation [24]. In this study, the random forest classifier iteratively returned the pixels with uncertain classification outcome to the human reader. The training was based on the iterative interaction with the human operators until the desired segmentation performance was reached. This approach resulted in reduced time for volume segmentation while progressively minimizing the human intervention.

Establishing an accurate patient-specific segmentation of the thrombus is also useful for pre-operative AAA planning and postoperative assessment. Lalys et al. proposed a near-automatic 3D deformable model-based approach for thrombus segmentation [25]. The study included 145 patients with AAA who underwent a CTA scan. Both pre-operative and postoperative scans were included in the study. The approach proposed by the authors was designed to be generic and required minimal manual interaction to guarantee a fast and versatile method for thrombus segmentation. Compared to manual delineations, the algorithm showed accurate results, with DSC of 0.86 and 0.87 for pre- and postoperative CTA scans, respectively.

Although generic and fast, the approach described by Lalys et al. still required some manual input. Lopez-Linares et al. proposed a fully automatic approach for thrombus segmentation based on CNN [4]. The proposed method first used a CNN to detect the thrombus from CTA datasets of 13 patients, followed by another CNN for thrombus segmentation. A DSC of 0.82 was obtained for postoperative thrombus segmentation. The quality of the 3D automatic segmentation was validated against the expert-based manually delimited volume as the ground truth.

If left untreated, AAA continues to expand until rupture. However, the accurate estimation of the risk of rupture in AAA is currently limited. Joldes et al. proposed a method to analyze AAA and predict the risk of rupture in 48 patients [26]. The model was able to extract information from different imaging modalities such as CT and MRI, and it was tailored to simulate several modeling scenarios, including the presence of thrombus. This method involves several image processing steps, including image segmentation, geometry creation, meshing, finite element analysis, and rupture potential index computation. Eventually, a 3D color-contoured model of the AAA was generated. Except for the initial image segmentation, this model did not require any further user intervention; therefore, it showed the potential to reduce the analysis time and avoid the need for technical knowledge.

Some of the AAA components, like thrombus and calcifications, are visualized differently based on the imaging modality employed. For instance, MR is known for the high soft-tissue discrimination; therefore, it is ideal for the visualization of the intraluminal thrombus. On the other hand, CT is better suited for the visualization of wall calcifications. A more comprehensive evaluation of the AAA would require a combination of both imaging modalities. Wang et al. developed network fusion methods for the image segmentation of 21 patients with AAA in both MR and CT scans [27]. CT images were segmented into five classes, including aortic wall, lumen, thrombus, calcifications, and background. MR images had a similar segmentation, but the calcifications were excluded. An expert-acquired segmentation was used as the ground truth. Their approach resulted in a shorter training time to handle non-registered CT and MR images. Further, the network fusion allowed a fused representation of AAA in both CT and MR images to be learned. These results showed the potential to achieve multimodality image registration and analysis.

Lareyre et al. attempted to advance AAA image analysis further by making it fully automatic [28]. The authors proposed a pipeline to detect the aortic lumen and to characterize AAA components without manual input. This multi-institutional and multivendor study was conducted on CTA datasets of 40 patients with AAA. The software allowed the automatic detection of key elements of AAA, including the presence of intraluminal thrombus and wall calcifications. The authors reported a DICE score of 0.93 for the segmentation of the aortic lumen and 0.88 for the thrombus, while the computational time ranged from 5 sec to 1 min per patient. Moreover, there was an excellent correlation between the manual and the automatic segmentation methods, for both aortic lumen ($r = 0.99$) and thrombus ($r = 0.90$). The precision and robustness of the proposed method could characterize a high number of AAAs in a short time. In clinical practice, this has the potential to translate into a more reproducible endograft sizing.

Over time, segmentation methods have evolved toward more sophisticated and fully automated approaches. Nonetheless, some parts of the pipeline, such as the expert annotation or the initial AAA segmentation, are still manual. Additionally, the datasets available to develop and train these algorithms are still limited; larger multi-institutional datasets are required to test if these methods would translate their value on a much larger scale.

Image Classification to Detect Aortic Dissection

Recently, a few studies investigated automatic methods to detect the presence of aortic dissection on contrast-enhanced CT datasets. Harris et al. proposed a CNN model to process 2D axial slices and detect aortic dissection or aortic rupture [29]. The study was conducted in the context of a teleradiology practice where exam prioritization could increase the chances of patient survival due to the high volume of studies performed. The proposed method aimed to classify more than 30,000 CTA scans of the chest prospectively for 4 weeks and to prioritize cases positive for aortic dissection or aortic rupture. The authors reported that CT scans labeled as positive from the algorithm had a significantly reduced delay time ($P < 0.0001$). The study prioritization resulted in a time difference of more than 6 min in reporting time. Hata et al. proposed a DL-based algorithm to detect aortic dissection in 170 patients [30]. In this study, only unenhanced CT scans were used, and real-time exam prioritization was not feasible due to the retrospective design of the study. The algorithm showed an area under the curve of 0.94 for detecting aortic dissection, with accuracy, sensitivity, and specificity comparable to those of the radiologists.

These investigations represent only the first attempts to detect aortic dissection on CT studies automatically. Although promising, these methods have still substantial limitations. For instance, aortic dissections with a limited cranio-caudal extension may be missed, and further characterization in acute or chronic, or type A vs type B, is still not possible. Moreover, other aortic findings, such as the presence of an aortic aneurysm, could trigger false positives. Future study should address these limitations before clinical implementation is considered.

Prediction in Aortic Dissection and AAA

Outcome Prediction in Patients with Aortic Dissection

Another area of great interest for ML methods is the prediction of outcomes in patients with aortic diseases. The random forest classification has a high accuracy in disease risk prediction and diagnosis. Wojnarski et al. investigated the risk of developing type A aortic dissection (TAAD) in a large cohort of 1181 patients with bicuspid aortic valve [5]. These patients tend to develop aortic complications more frequently than the general population; however, the timing of prophylactic ascending aortic replacement lacks consensus. Therefore, the authors used random forest classification to determine risk factors for aortic dissection, including initial CT data and clinical variables. The authors reported that the risk of developing TAAD at the time of initial imaging was highly dependent on the diameter of the ascending aorta with a threshold of 5.3 cm, followed by the aortic diameter at the sinuses of Valsalva with a threshold of 5.0 cm.

The random forest classifier was also used by Wu et al. to establish the risk prediction for in-hospital rupture of TAAD patients [31]. Aortic rupture is a catastrophic event and requires appropriate emergency surgical triage. The investigation included 1133 patients diagnosed with TAAD based on CTA scans. All CT scans were assessed by two experts who were blinded to the study purpose. The presence of a periaortic hematoma was the strongest predictor of in-hospital aortic rupture, followed by 15 more clinical variables, including a high blood pressure (>160 mmHg) at admission.

Short-term and long-term postoperative mortalities were investigated in two separate studies focused on patients who underwent surgical treatment of TAAD. In the first study, Macrina et al. tested a large series of clinical and surgical risk factors to predict mortality at 30 days after surgery [32]. The potential predictors were divided into four categories as follows: demographic characteristics, pre-operative, intraoperative, and immediate postoperative variables. The authors reported that the presence of pre-operative shock, the duration of the extracorporeal circulation, the presence of postoperative chronic renal failure, the year of surgery, the intubation before surgery, the need for immediate dialysis in continuous after surgery, the amount of postoperative bleeding in the first 24 hours, and the presence of pre-operative neurological symptoms were selected as prognostic variables. The same group of authors later assessed the long-term postoperative mortality over a maximum follow-up time of 7 years [33]. The authors reported 84 deaths (36%), of which 81 (95%) were linked to a cardiac origin. Further, the presence of Marfan habitus, the duration of circulatory arrest, the choice of a surgical procedure involving the ascending aorta and the hemiarch, and the sudden onset of postoperative chronic renal failure were risk factors indicating a worse prognosis.

Prediction of AAA Growth and Rupture

AI algorithms have also been tested to predict growth and prognosis of AAA patients. A study from Lee et al. aimed to predict the AAA growth in individual patients at 12 and 24 months from the baseline using a set of benchmark learning techniques [34]. AAA growth size measured by the anteroposterior diameter on ultrasound was prospectively recorded at 12 months for 94 patients, while 79 of those patients were further followed up at 24 months. A 2 mm error margin was allowed in the algorithm to account for the widely accepted technical variability between anteroposterior diameter ultrasound measurements in AAAs. The algorithm accurately predicted individual AAA diameters in 85% of patients at 12 months, and 71% at 24 months. If confirmed in larger studies, these results could lead to a more personalized stratification of surveillance intervals for AAA patients.

Large AAAs are more prone to rupture than small ones; however, small AAA may rupture as well. Kelinestreurer et al. proposed an AAA monitoring program based on eight biomechanical factors to provide a more accurate prediction for individual patients with small AAA [35]. Their approach was tested on a cohort of three patients and correctly classified the patient's status in the following categories: low risk, observation, elective repair, and imminent rupture. The prediction of AAA rupture based on this method provides more accurate results than the maximum AAA diameter alone.

Prediction of Postoperative Outcomes

AAA is associated with high-mortality rates; however, the natural history and progression are influenced by a large number of clinical and imaging factors. In this context, the use of AI-based predictive mortality scores in AAA repair candidates or patients with ruptured AAA represents a novel and thriving field. Hadjianastassiou et al. investigated the ability to predict in-hospital mortality in a group of 1751 postoperative AAA patients [6]. The authors compared the performance of multiple regression modeling and an artificial neural network (ANN) with the trainee clinicians' prognosis estimates. Both elective and emergency procedures were included. Multiple regression modeling predicted in-hospital mortality more accurately than both clinicians' estimates and ANN modeling. However, since the prediction was compared to the estimation of trainee clinicians, these models may be more suitable as tools to assist intensive care unit trainee clinicians rather than support experienced physicians who might be more accurate in their clinical judgment.

Wise et al. used a similar approach but focused on patients with ruptured AAA [36]. In this investigation, the authors proposed an ANN to assess the likelihood of in-hospital mortality of 125 patients based on pre-operative factors. Age at rupture, cardiac arrest, loss of consciousness, and shock were included in a four-variable ANN. Compared to a multiple logistic regression model and to the established Glasgow Aneurysm Score, the four-variable ANN predicts in-hospital mortality with greater discriminant ability. This ANN model could provide accurate prognostic guidance in patients with ruptured AAA and might help determine appropriate candidates for surgery.

The prediction of in-hospital mortality was further investigated by Monsalve-Torra et al. who tested different ML algorithms and developed a clinical decision support system based on 310 patients undergoing open repair of AAA [37]. The authors used two ANNs, namely, multilayer perceptron and radial basis function networks, and a Bayes-based method. After a feature selection process to reduce the computational complexity, the Bayes-based network resulted in the best algorithm with an accuracy of 96.1%, and a sensitivity and a specificity of 86.8% and 96.8%, respectively. The availability of a good prediction tool could improve the surgery results by achieving a better planning of care.

Turton et al. aimed to identify key predictors to estimate mortality at 30 days in 102 patients after surgery for ruptured AAA [38]. The authors used these predictors to construct a neural network and validated their prognostic importance for each case. The authors reported a 30-day mortality rate of 53%. A neural network including pre-operative cardiac arrest, the occurrence of an intraperitoneal bleed, pre-operative thrombocytopenia, and compromised blood pressure on arrival predicted individual survival correctly in 82.5% of individual cases, with sensitivity and specificity of 86.4% and 79.3%, respectively.

ANNs have also been used to predict endograft complications and long-term mortality after endovascular repair (EVAR) of AAAs. Karthikesalingam et al. aimed to use ANN analysis to develop and externally validate a predictive tool for determining the risk of endograft complications and mortality after EVAR in 761 patients [39]. Pre-operative aneurysm morphology was quantified, and endograft complications were recorded on routine surveillance CT scans up to 5 years after surgery. ANN was used to predict whether patients would be at low or high risk of endograft complications (aortic/limb) or mortality. ANN models predicted endograft complications and mortality with excellent discrimination between a low-risk and high-risk group. In the external validation, the 5-year rates of freedom from aortic complications, limb complications, and mortality were 95.9% vs 67.9%; 99.3% vs 92.0%; and 87.9% vs 79.3%, respectively ($p < 0.001$). Stratifying the risk of long-term outcomes after EVAR using advanced ML techniques might positively impact both patient selection and surveillance after EVAR. However, further validation of the model and feasibility study are required before clinical use of these tools.

Feature selection (FS) is a ML technique used to automatically identify relevant attributes from data to increase the accuracy of a predictive model. Attallah et al. proposed a new hybrid FS method presenting a solution to high-level censoring on two EVAR datasets of 457 and 286 patients collected from 2 different centers [40]. They used a multiple classifier system as a wrapper method and merged it with iterated feature ranking filter method to select features. The results showed that the proposed technique outperformed individual classifiers and variable selection methods based on a Cox model and was more accurate in predicting the risk of re-intervention after EVAR.

Subsequently, Attallah et al. used a different novel feature selection technique and uncensoring approach to deal with the same EVAR datasets of 457 and 286 patients from 2 distinct centers [41]. Their aim was to use a wrapper FS method with ANN to select a reduced subset of features to predict the risk of EVAR re-intervention after 5 years of the procedure. The proposed approach for feature selection resulted in a predictive model outperforming other predictive methods, like Cox's regression model, in predicting long-term risk of aortic complications after EVAR. This approach could save physicians' time and effort to collect unnecessary variables and increase the accuracy of risk prediction models.

Long-term imaging surveillance after EVAR is necessary to identify potential complications such as endoleaks. García et al. aimed to evaluate the capability of texture features obtained from the aneurysmatic thrombus CT images to discriminate favorable from unfavorable evolution caused by endoleaks in 70 patients who underwent EVAR [42]. Texture parameters were obtained by applying three different techniques on extracted regions of interest: gray-level co-occurrence matrix (GLCM), gray-level run length matrix (GLRLM), and gray-level difference method (GLDM). The texture feature set obtained by each method was separately fed to an artificial neural network classifier, a backpropagation neural network, to discriminate the AAAs with unfavorable evolution. The criteria for unfavorable evolution cases were based on the detection of contrast medium within the aneurysm sac or on a regular increase in aneurysm diameter. Anteroposterior aneurysm diameter measurements were obtained from axial CT images orthogonal to the aortic axis, and only diameter changes ≥2 mm were considered significant. For favorable cases, the criteria were based on the absence of contrast and on a stable reduction of aneurysm diameter during the entire follow-up. GLCM, GLRLM, and GLDM features presented a good discrimination ability to differentiate between favorable or unfavorable evolutions. Therefore, texture analysis could be useful as complementary information to classify abdominal aneurysm evolution after EVAR.

Pre-operative planning of EVAR is critical to prevent and anticipate postoperative complications. Perrin et al. aimed to develop a finite element methodology to simulate the deployment of marketed bifurcated stent grafts in patient-specific aneurysm models to predict biomechanically induced complications of the procedure [43]. The simulation process was applied on three clinical cases using pre-operative CT scans to generate patient-specific vessel models. The numerical results were compared to the actual deployed geometry of the stent grafts after surgery that was extracted from postoperative scans. The numerical results showed good agreement with actual postoperative CT scans. These tools may be of use to improve pre-operative planning of EVAR and anticipate post-EVAR complications.

Conclusion

Over the past few years, a growing number of ML/DL algorithms have been proposed to process imaging and clinical data of patients with aortic diseases. Most of these algorithms have been focusing on the segmentation of the aorta as well as on the assessment of patients with aortic dissection or AAA. While these methods look certainly promising, there are several obstacles to their implementation in daily clinical practice. For instance, only a small number of imaging studies are currently used to develop ML/DL algorithms, and expert-based annotated datasets are rare. Furthermore, most ML/DL algorithms focus on developing single components of image analysis rather than fully addressing real clinical issues. The US Food and Drug Administration (FDA) and the European Medicines Agency (EMA) pose further challenges for their stringent regulatory requirements on medical algorithms.

Nonetheless, these obstacles are also opportunities for the scientific community. High-performance computing technologies are increasingly accessible in parallel with curated large-scale and publicly available databases. Such databases include imaging and clinical data and may overcome some of the limitations listed above by addressing the need for validation on a more extensive training dataset. Novel ML/DL algorithms developed based on these premises may allow a more tailored approach and assist the clinicians in automatically achieving a more accurate, timely, and comprehensive evaluation of patients with aortic disease.

References

1. Nienaber CA, Clough RE, Sakalihasan N, Suzuki T, Gibbs R, Mussa F, Jenkins MP, Thompson MM, Evangelista A, Yeh JS, Cheshire N, Rosendahl U, Pepper J. Aortic dissection. Nat Rev Dis Primers. 2016;2:16053. https://doi.org/10.1038/nrdp.2016.53.
2. Codari M, Pepe A, Mistelbauer G, Mastrodicasa D, Walters S, Willemink MJ, Fleischmann D. Deep reinforcement learning for localization of the aortic annulus in patients with aortic dissection. In: Thoracic image analysis. Cham: Springer International Publishing; 2020. p. 94–105.
3. Hahn LD, Mistelbauer G, Higashigaito K, Koci M, Willemink MJ, Sailer AM, Fischbein M, Fleischmann D. CT-based true- and false-lumen segmentation in type B aortic dissection using machine learning. Radiol Cardiothora Imaging. 2020;2(3):e190179. https://doi.org/10.1148/ryct.2020190179.
4. Lopez-Linares K, Aranjuelo N, Kabongo L, Maclair G, Lete N, Ceresa M, Garcia-Familiar A, Macia I, Gonzalez Ballester MA. Fully automatic detection and segmentation of abdominal aortic thrombus in post-operative CTA images using deep convolutional neural networks. Med Image Anal. 2018;46:202–14. https://doi.org/10.1016/j.media.2018.03.010.
5. Wojnarski CM, Svensson LG, Roselli EE, Idrees JJ, Lowry AM, Ehrlinger J, Pettersson GB, Gillinov AM, Johnston DR, Soltesz EG, Navia JL, Hammer DF, Griffin B, Thamilarasan M, Kalahasti V, Sabik JF 3rd, Blackstone EH, Lytle BW. Aortic dissection in patients with bicuspid aortic valve-associated aneurysms. Ann Thorac Surg. 2015;100(5):1666–73. https://doi.org/10.1016/j.athoracsur.2015.04.126; discussion 1673-1664.
6. Hadjianastassiou VG, Franco L, Jerez JM, Evangelou IE, Goldhill DR, Tekkis PP, Hands LJ. Informed prognosis [corrected] after abdominal aortic aneurysm repair using predictive modeling techniques [corrected]. J Vasc Surg. 2006;43(3):467–73. https://doi.org/10.1016/j.jvs.2005.11.022.
7. Zheng Y, John M, Liao R, Nottling A, Boese J, Kempfert J, Walther T, Brockmann G, Comaniciu D. Automatic aorta segmentation and valve landmark detection in C-arm CT for transcatheter aortic valve implantation. IEEE Trans Med Imaging. 2012;31(12):2307–21. https://doi.org/10.1109/TMI.2012.2216541.
8. Al WA, Jung HY, Yun ID, Jang Y, Park HB, Chang HJ. Automatic aortic valve landmark localization in coronary CT angiography using colonial walk. PLoS One. 2018;13(7):e0200317. https://doi.org/10.1371/journal.pone.0200317.
9. Ghesu FC, Georgescu B, Zheng Y, Grbic S, Maier A, Hornegger J, Comaniciu D. Multi-scale deep reinforcement learning for real-time 3D-landmark detection in CT scans. IEEE Trans Pattern Anal Mach Intell. 2019;41(1):176–89. https://doi.org/10.1109/TPAMI.2017.2782687.
10. Rueckel J, Reidler P, Fink N, Sperl J, Geyer T, Fabritius MP, Ricke J, Ingrisch M, Sabel BO. Artificial intelligence assistance improves reporting efficiency of thoracic aortic aneurysm CT follow-up. Eur J Radiol. 2021;134:109424. https://doi.org/10.1016/j.ejrad.2020.109424.
11. Abdullah Al W, Yun ID. Partial policy-based reinforcement learning for anatomical landmark localization in 3D medical images. IEEE Trans Med Imaging. 2020;39(4):1245–55. https://doi.org/10.1109/TMI.2019.2946345.
12. Alansary A, Oktay O, Li Y, Folgoc LL, Hou B, Vaillant G, Kamnitsas K, Vlontzos A, Glocker B, Kainz B, Rueckert D. Evaluating reinforcement learning agents for anatomical landmark detection. Med Image Anal. 2019;53:156–64. https://doi.org/10.1016/j.media.2019.02.007.
13. Astudillo P, Mortier P, Bosmans J, De Backer O, de Jaegere P, Iannaccone F, De Beule M, Dambre J. Automatic detection of the aortic annular plane and coronary ostia from multidetector computed tomography. J Interv Cardiol. 2020;2020:9843275. https://doi.org/10.1155/2020/9843275.
14. Noothout JMH, De Vos BD, Wolterink JM, Postma EM, Smeets PAM, Takx RAP, Leiner T, Viergever MA, Isgum I. Deep learning-based regression and classification for automatic landmark localization in medical images. IEEE Trans Med Imaging. 2020;39(12):4011–22. https://doi.org/10.1109/TMI.2020.3009002.
15. Noothout JM, De Vos BD, Wolterink JM, Išgum I. Automatic segmentation of thoracic aorta segments in low-dose chest CT. In: Medical Imaging 2018: Image Processing. International Society for Optics and Photonics; 2018. p. 105741S.
16. Aberle DR, Berg CD, Black WC, Church TR, Fagerstrom RM, Galen B, Gareen IF, Gatsonis C, Goldin J, Gohagan JK, Hillman B, Jaffe C, Kramer BS, Lynch D, Marcus PM, Schnall M, Sullivan DC, Sullivan D, Zylak CJ, National Lung Screening Trial Research T. The National Lung Screening Trial: overview and study design. Radiology. 2011;258(1):243–53. https://doi.org/10.1148/radiol.10091808.
17. Fantazzini A, Esposito M, Finotello A, Auricchio F, Pane B, Basso C, Spinella G, Conti M. 3D automatic segmentation of aortic computed tomography angiography combining multi-view 2D convolutional neural networks. Cardiovasc Eng Technol. 2020;11(5):576–86. https://doi.org/10.1007/s13239-020-00481-z.
18. Cao L, Shi R, Ge Y, Xing L, Zuo P, Jia Y, Liu J, He Y, Wang X, Luan S, Chai X, Guo W. Fully automatic segmentation of type B aortic dissection from CTA images enabled by deep learning. Eur J Radiol. 2019;121:108713. https://doi.org/10.1016/j.ejrad.2019.108713.
19. Cheng J, Tian S, Yu L, Ma X, Xing Y. A deep learning algorithm using contrast-enhanced computed tomography (CT) images for segmentation and rapid automatic detection of aortic dissection. Biomed Signal Processing Cont. 2020;62:102145. https://doi.org/10.1016/j.bspc.2020.102145.
20. Bai W, Suzuki H, Qin C, Tarroni G, Oktay O, Matthews PM, Rueckert D. Recurrent neural networks for aortic image sequence segmentation with sparse annotations. In: Medical image computing and computer assisted intervention – miccai 2018. Cham: Springer International Publishing; 2018. p. 586–94.
21. de Bruijne M, van Ginneken B, Viergever MA, Niessen WJ. Interactive segmentation of abdominal aortic aneurysms in CTA images. Med Image Anal. 2004;8(2):127–38. https://doi.org/10.1016/j.media.2004.01.001.
22. Subasic M, Loncaric S, Sorantin E. 3-D image analysis of abdominal aortic aneurysm. Stud Health Technol Inform. 2000;77:1195–200.

23. Zhuge F, Rubin GD, Sun S, Napel S. An abdominal aortic aneurysm segmentation method: level set with region and statistical information. Med Phys. 2006;33(5):1440–53. https://doi.org/10.1118/1.2193247.
24. Maiora J, Papakostas GA, Kaburlasos VG, Grana M. A proposal of texture features for interactive CTA segmentation by active learning. Stud Health Technol Inform. 2014;207:311–20.
25. Lalys F, Yan V, Kaladji A, Lucas A, Esneault S. Generic thrombus segmentation from pre- and post-operative CTA. Int J Comput Assist Radiol Surg. 2017;12(9):1501–10. https://doi.org/10.1007/s11548-017-1591-8.
26. Joldes GR, Miller K, Wittek A, Forsythe RO, Newby DE, Doyle BJ. BioPARR: a software system for estimating the rupture potential index for abdominal aortic aneurysms. Sci Rep. 2017;7(1):4641. https://doi.org/10.1038/s41598-017-04699-1.
27. Wang D, Zhang R, Zhu J, Teng Z, Huang Y, Spiga F, Hong-Fei Du M, Gillard JH, Lu Q, Lio P. Neural network fusion: a novel CT-MR aortic aneurysm image segmentation method. Proc SPIE Int Soc Opt Eng. 2018;10574 https://doi.org/10.1117/12.2293371.
28. Lareyre F, Adam C, Carrier M, Dommerc C, Mialhe C, Raffort J. A fully automated pipeline for mining abdominal aortic aneurysm using image segmentation. Sci Rep. 2019;9(1):13750. https://doi.org/10.1038/s41598-019-50251-8.
29. Harris RJ, Kim S, Lohr J, Towey S, Velichkovich Z, Kabachenko T, Driscoll I, Baker B. Classification of aortic dissection and rupture on post-contrast CT images using a convolutional neural network. J Digit Imaging. 2019;32(6):939–46. https://doi.org/10.1007/s10278-019-00281-5.
30. Hata A, Yanagawa M, Yamagata K, Suzuki Y, Kido S, Kawata A, Doi S, Yoshida Y, Miyata T, Tsubamoto M, Kikuchi N, Tomiyama N. Deep learning algorithm for detection of aortic dissection on non-contrast-enhanced CT. Eur Radiol. 2021;31(2):1151–9. https://doi.org/10.1007/s00330-020-07213-w.
31. Wu J, Qiu J, Xie E, Jiang W, Zhao R, Qiu J, Zafar MA, Huang Y, Yu C. Predicting in-hospital rupture of type a aortic dissection using random. Forest J Thorac Dis. 2019;11(11):4634–46. https://doi.org/10.21037/jtd.2019.10.82.
32. Macrina F, Puddu PE, Sciangula A, Trigilia F, Totaro M, Miraldi F, Toscano F, Cassese M, Toscano M. Artificial neural networks versus multiple logistic regression to predict 30-day mortality after operations for type a ascending aortic dissection. Open Cardiovasc Med J. 2009;3:81–95. https://doi.org/10.2174/1874192400903010081.
33. Macrina F, Puddu PE, Sciangula A, Totaro M, Trigilia F, Cassese M, Toscano M. Long-term mortality prediction after operations for type a ascending aortic dissection. J Cardiothorac Surg. 2010;5:42. https://doi.org/10.1186/1749-8090-5-42.
34. Lee R, Jarchi D, Perera R, Jones A, Cassimjee I, Handa A, Clifton DA, Oxford Abdominal Aortic Aneurysm Study A, Oxford Regional Vascular S. Applied machine learning for the prediction of growth of abdominal aortic aneurysm in humans. EJVES Short Rep. 2018;39:24–8. https://doi.org/10.1016/j.ejvssr.2018.03.004.
35. Kleinstreuer C, Li Z. Analysis and computer program for rupture-risk prediction of abdominal aortic aneurysms. Biomed Eng Online. 2006;5:19. https://doi.org/10.1186/1475-925X-5-19.
36. Wise ES, Hocking KM, Brophy CM. Prediction of in-hospital mortality after ruptured abdominal aortic aneurysm repair using an artificial neural network. J Vasc Surg. 2015;62(1):8–15. https://doi.org/10.1016/j.jvs.2015.02.038.
37. Monsalve-Torra A, Ruiz-Fernandez D, Marin-Alonso O, Soriano-Paya A, Camacho-Mackenzie J, Carreno-Jaimes M. Using machine learning methods for predicting inhospital mortality in patients undergoing open repair of abdominal aortic aneurysm. J Biomed Inform. 2016;62:195–201. https://doi.org/10.1016/j.jbi.2016.07.007.
38. Turton EP, Scott DJ, Delbridge M, Snowden S, Kester RC. Ruptured abdominal aortic aneurysm: a novel method of outcome prediction using neural network technology. Eur J Vasc Endovasc Surg. 2000;19(2):184–9. https://doi.org/10.1053/ejvs.1999.0974.
39. Karthikesalingam A, Attallah O, Ma X, Bahia SS, Thompson L, Vidal-Diez A, Choke EC, Bown MJ, Sayers RD, Thompson MM, Holt PJ. An artificial neural network stratifies the risks of Reintervention and mortality after endovascular aneurysm repair; a retrospective observational study. PLoS One. 2015;10(7):e0129024. https://doi.org/10.1371/journal.pone.0129024.
40. Attallah O, Karthikesalingam A, Holt PJ, Thompson MM, Sayers R, Bown MJ, Choke EC, Ma X. Using multiple classifiers for predicting the risk of endovascular aortic aneurysm repair re-intervention through hybrid feature selection. Proc Inst Mech Eng H. 2017;231(11):1048–63. https://doi.org/10.1177/0954411917731592.
41. Attallah O, Karthikesalingam A, Holt PJE, Thompson MM, Sayers R, Bown MJ, Choke EC, Ma X. Feature selection through validation and un-censoring of endovascular repair survival data for predicting the risk of re-intervention. BMC Med Inform Decis Mak. 2017;17(1):115. https://doi.org/10.1186/s12911-017-0508-3.
42. Garcia G, Maiora J, Tapia A, De Blas M. Evaluation of texture for classification of abdominal aortic aneurysm after endovascular repair. J Digit Imaging. 2012;25(3):369–76. https://doi.org/10.1007/s10278-011-9417-7.
43. Perrin D, Badel P, Orgeas L, Geindreau C, Dumenil A, Albertini JN, Avril S. Patient-specific numerical simulation of stent-graft deployment: validation on three clinical cases. J Biomech. 2015;48(10):1868–75. https://doi.org/10.1016/j.jbiomech.2015.04.031.

Artificial Intelligence- and Radiomics-Based Evaluation of Carotid Artery Disease

48

Michele Porcu, Riccardo Cau, Jasjit S. Suri, and Luca Saba

Introduction

Carotid artery disease (CAD) is commonly encountered in clinical practice, in particular carotid atherosclerosis (CAS). The prompt recognition and characterization of CAD is fundamental for the correct management of these patients, in particular to limit complications such as ischemic stroke due to the rupture of an atherosclerotic plaque (AP) [1].

In the last decades, several epidemiological, molecular, and imaging studies allowed the scientific community to better understand the pathological mechanisms underlying CAD, impacting daily clinical practice. For example, although the degree of stenosis remains the main imaging parameter for choosing the more appropriate treatment of carotid artery stenosis due to the presence of AP [2, 3], in the last years researchers focused their attention on the study of the AP composition, introducing the concept of *vulnerable plaque* (i.e., a plaque at high risk of rupture) [4–7].

Following the recent introduction of artificial intelligence (AI) algorithms, researchers are now able to perform not only a qualitative but also a quantitative analysis of imaging data [8–10]. By using dedicated software, several quantitative features of the images can be extracted, and this process is called *texture analysis* (TA). The data derived from TA can be exploited alone or combined with other "-omics" data (e.g., genomics or metabolomics data) by means of AI algorithms creating advanced models for computer-aided diagnosis (CADx). The final goal is to assess the risk of rupture of carotid atherosclerotic plaque (CAP), stratify the risk of stroke, or monitor the response to therapy. Up to date, these algorithms have still not been introduced in clinical practice, but the knowledge created by and understanding of these technologies play a pivotal role in facilitating their clinical implementation and utilization by radiologists.

In the next sections, we will discuss the state of the art of carotid artery imaging, focusing in particular on CAS. Subsequently, we will show the main AI applications for CAP analysis.

M. Porcu, MD · R. Cau, MD · L. Saba, MD (✉)
Department of Radiology, Azienda Ospedaliero Universitaria di Cagliari, Cagliari, Italy

J. S. Suri, PhD, MBA, FIEEE, FAIMBE, FAIUM
Stroke Monitoring and Diagnostic Division, AtheroPoint™, Roseville, CA, USA

Carotid Artery Imaging in Clinical Practice

From the Degree of Stenosis to the Plaque Characterization

As stated in the introduction, the evaluation of CAS has moved from the evaluation of carotid artery obstruction only to the study of the CAP composition. The latest guidelines for the treatment of CAS published by the American Heart Association (AHA) in 2014 [11] and by the European Society of Cardiology (ESC) in 2017 [12] still indicate the degree of stenosis measured according to the method of the North American Symptomatic Carotid Endarterectomy Trial (NASCET) [13] or by the European Carotid Surgery Trial (ECST) [14], as the only imaging biomarker to be taken into account for the therapeutic management of the patient. However, several steps forward have been made for the identification of other risk factors for CAP rupture and onset of subsequent pathological conditions, such as transient ischemic attack (TIA) and stroke. In fact, thanks to the ability of the new advanced imaging techniques, it is possible to look *beyond the lumen* for identifying the vulnerable plaque.

The importance of assessing the carotid artery wall for CAD evaluation is not a recent discovery. In 1986 *Pignoli* et al. [15] were the first authors demonstrating that the intima-media thickness (IMT) measured by ultrasound (US) closely reflects the histological results. Further studies revealed that increased common carotid artery intima-media thickness (CCA-IMT) is associated with the risk of stroke and myocardial infarction [16]. A CCA-IMT value >1 mm is

C. N. De Cecco et al. (eds.), *Artificial Intelligence in Cardiothoracic Imaging*, Contemporary Medical Imaging,
https://doi.org/10.1007/978-3-030-92087-6_48

commonly considered as abnormal [17]. In 2018, the Vessel Wall Imaging Study Group of the American Society of Neuroradiology published a white paper with recommendations and guidelines for carotid artery wall imaging [4] that tried to summarize years of research studies focused on the analysis of the single components of CAP and on their role in plaque instability. In particular, three concepts have been underlined in this paper [4]: (a) the degree of stenosis is a weak indicator of the extension of CAP [4, 18]; (b) several plaque features identifiable by imaging techniques are associated with the development of ischemic symptoms; and (c) these plaque features increase the risk of stroke regardless the degree of stenosis [4, 19, 20].

Degree of Carotid Stenosis and Imaging Biomarkers of Vulnerable Plaque

According to the American Heart Association (AHA) and European Society of Cardiology (ESC) guidelines, the degree of stenosis still represents the only imaging biomarker considered in the management of patients with carotid artery stenosis secondary to AP [11, 12]. In particular, according to the ESC guidelines [12], carotid endarterectomy (CEA) and medical treatment are recommended for patients with recent symptoms of stroke/TIA and carotid stenosis between 70 and 99% (level of evidence: IA). However, as mentioned above, this paradigm is changing, and in the last decades, several histopathological and imaging studies analyzed and identified several features of AP vulnerability (Table 48.1) that should be considered in addition to the degree of stenosis for the therapeutic management of the patient [5].

The first feature to be considered is the CAP thickness, defined as the maximum thickness of the plaque [5]. According to the Mannheim consensus, a CAP is defined when the IMT is greater than 1.5 mm [21]. CAP thickness has been demonstrated to be more strongly associated with cerebral ischemic symptoms than the degree of stenosis [5, 22]. The second feature is CAP volume, which has been demonstrated to be directly and independently associated with plaque vulnerability and stroke [23].

Table 48.1 List of the main plaque vulnerability biomarkers [4, 5]

List of the main biomarkers of plaque vulnerability	
Plaque features	*Note*
Plaque thickness	Definition of plaque: IMT >1.5 mm
Plaque volume	–
Fibrous cap status (thickness and surface morphology)	1. Smooth 2. Irregular 3. Ulcerated
Plaque inflammation	–
Plaque neovascularization	–
Lipid-rich necrotic core	–
Intraplaque hemorrhage	–

IMT intima-media thickness

Two aspects of the CAP surface, the fibrous cap thickness and the surface morphology, are other important features to be considered in the evaluation of plaque stability [4, 5]. The fibrous cap is a layer of connective tissue that covers the core of the plaque and separates it from the arterial lumen. A thin or ruptured cap is an important characteristic of plaque vulnerability [5, 24, 25]. The surface of the CAP can be classified as (a) smooth; (b) irregular (with the surface thickening fluctuating between 0.3 mm and 0.9 mm); and (c) ulcerated (when there are cavities that measures at least 1 mm in thickness) [5, 26]. The presence of an irregular surface is considered a marker of plaque vulnerability [5, 26], whereas the presence of ulceration could represent a clue of previous plaque rupture, and its predictive value remains uncertain [5, 27].

The plaque inflammation and the consequent intraplaque neovascularization due to the angiogenesis phenomenon represent another marker of vulnerability, which is also referred to as plaque activity [5, 28]. From a pathological point of view, neoangiogenesis is characterized by the production of irregular microvessels inside of the AP core, and the inflammation is characterized by the presence of inflammatory cells (especially macrophages and lymphocytes) that accumulates mainly in the shoulder or in the fibrous cap [5, 29, 30].

The final result of continuous accumulation of cholesterol inside the CAP core and of plaque inflammation is the volumetric gain and necrosis of the core [5, 29, 30]; this lipid-rich necrotic core (LRNC) consists of debris of apoptotic cells, cholesterol crystals, and calcium deposits, and itself stimulate the inflammatory response in a self-feeding process that leads to the increase of plaque volume and plaque instability [29, 31]. It has been demonstrated that the presence of LRNC is predictive of an increased risk of stroke [5, 25] and that carotid plaques with a maximum percentage of LRNC (%LRNC = LRNC core area/wall area) greater than 40% are more likely to develop rupture of the fibrous cap during 3-year follow-up when compared to those plaque whose %LRNC is lesser than 40% [5, 32].

The rupture of the microvessels inside of the AP can lead to intraplaque hemorrhage (IPH), which contributes to LRNC enlargement and plaque progression [5, 30, 33], and it is considered the most important imaging parameter associated with the onset of stroke symptoms [5, 30, 34].

Finally, a recent research by *Saba* et al. [35] suggested that perivascular fat inflammation could represent another risk factor associated with plaque instability.

What Imaging?

Carotid artery stenosis degree can be evaluated well by ultrasound (US), computed tomography (CT), and magnetic resonance imaging (MRI) [4, 5, 11, 12].

Regarding the analysis of the CAP composition, there is not a single method of choice for carotid artery wall analysis, due to the fact that not all the components of the CAP can be visualized in the same way.

US is considered the standard imaging tool for first-line assessment of carotid artery wall disease, due to its safety and wide availability [4, 36], and has shown to be very efficient for identifying "high-risk" plaque in patients with atherosclerosis [4, 37]. For example, US is able not only to assess the degree of stenosis but also to assess the CCA-IMT [15–17] and carotid artery stiffness [38], to identify LRNC and calcifications [29]. By evaluating the elasticity of the wall through the use of the elastography [39], a three-dimensional US (3D-US) technique is able to assess CAP volume with good reproducibility [40, 41]. The use of contrast-enhanced US (CEUS) technique is also able to evaluate neovascularization and inflammation [4]. However, US suffers of its intrinsic operator-dependent limitation, and several additional limitations for the assessment of the intraplaque hemorrhage (IPH) and of the fibrous cap status [4, 30]. Intravascular US (IVUS) can be used for CAP analysis due to its excellent spatial resolution, in particular for the evaluation of the fibrous cap status, but it is an invasive technique and the benefit-risk assessment of this procedure need to be assessed [4].

Despite the usage of ionizing radiations, CT is considered a reliable and fast technique for analysis of CAP components due to its great spatial resolution. The use of iodinated contrast medium through the CT angiography (CTA) technique allows improvement of the contrast resolution, allowing analysis of the degree of carotid stenosis, the luminal surface of the plaque, the plaque volume the LRNC, and the degree of intraplaque vascularization (although these last two conditions can be indistinguishable from each other) [4, 5, 29, 30].

MRI is an optimal technique for carotid artery imaging due to its intrinsic multiparametricity and intrinsic high-contrast resolution [4, 5]. In particular, the use of high-field scanners (1.5/3 Tesla) and dedicated neck coils improves the signal-to-noise ratio, making the analysis of plaque components possible [4]. A study protocol including T1-weighted images (T1-WI), T2-weighted images (T2-WI), proton density-weighted images (PD-WI), and time of flight (TOF) can deliver important information about the luminal surface of the plaque (with a sensitivity similar to CT [36]), the plaque volume, LRNC, and fibrous cap status, and it is considered the best technique for IPH detection [4]. Further, the use of contrast medium can offer important information about the neovascularization [4, 42], and the use of new contrast mediums known as ultrasmall superparamagnetic iron oxide (USPIO), which consists of molecules bound with iron particles, can also evaluate plaque inflammation via uptake by inflammatory cells localized inside the CAP [4, 43].

A summary table of the pros and cons of all the imaging modalities and of their appropriateness for the analysis of plaque features is provided in Table 48.2.

Carotid Artery Imaging: The Role of Artificial Intelligence

The development of AI algorithms able to identify the degree of stenosis and plaque features of vulnerability has dramatically increased in the last years, thanks to the improved computational power of modern hardware, and to novel software solutions [9, 10].

In particular, TA and machine learning (ML) have been used in carotid artery imaging for the creation of models able

Table 48.2 Imaging techniques for identification of plaque vulnerability biomarkers [4, 5, 76]

Imaging techniques for identification of biomarkers of plaque vulnerability			
Imaging modality	*Pros*	*Cons*	*Evaluable biomarkers*
US	Safe Economic Wide availability	Operator-dependent	Plaque thickness. Plaque volume (especially with 3D-US) Neovascularization (especially with CEUS) Fibrous cap status (especially with IVUS)
CTA	Fast High reproducibility Operator-independent	Use of ionizing radiations Use of contrast medium (mandatory)	Plaque thickness Plaque volume Fibrous cap status
MRI	Safe High reproducibility Operator-independent	Contraindications in case of metallic implants/ claustrophobia Use of contrast medium (optional) Time-consuming	Plaque volume Intraplaque hemorrhage Fibrous cap status (it requires contrast medium administration)

US ultrasound, *CEUS* contrast-enhanced ultrasound, *IVUS* intravascular ultrasound, *3D-US* three-dimensional ultrasound, *CTA* computed tomography angiography, *MRI* magnetic resonance imaging to identify vulnerable plaques and to stratify the stroke risk [10, 44]. Representative training datasets are necessary for the development of these models [44], and preprocessing of the images for noise and/or artifacts removal is often required, in particular for models based on US imaging [44]. The first step is represented by the identification and segmentation of the target region of interest (ROI) or volume of interest (VOI), which can be performed manually or (semi-) automatically [10]. The ROI/VOI then undergoes TA analysis, which allows to extrapolate up to a thousands of descriptive features by the mathematical analysis of the distribution and differences in grayscale values of the pixel of an image; shape-based features, first-order statistics (homogeneity, entropy, etc.) (Fig. 48.1), and higher-order statistics can be extracted from the selected ROI/VOI. All these data are then used in the data mining process [10, 44, 45]. The models are then created by exploring the mutual relationships between radiomic features and a selected outcome variable. This process is realized by using one or more combined machine learning techniques (e.g., supervised learning, unsupervised learning, and reinforcement learning) [10, 44]. Finally, the model is validated using a validation dataset, and the performance can be measured in terms of discrimination and calibration. Discrimination is defined as the ability of the model to classify cases that match an outcome from those who do not match it; it is typically measured in terms of sensitivity and specificity by using the receiver operating characteristic (ROC). Calibration is defined as the agreement between model predictions and observed outcomes; it is typically reported by using calibration plots [10, 44, 46].

In the next subsections, we will discuss the main results obtained in this field in the last years, focusing in particular on the TA for identification of vulnerable plaques, and on CAD models developed for stroke risk stratification.

Artificial Intelligence in Ultrasound

As previously mentioned, US is the most safe and fast imaging technique for the analysis of CAD, and it is therefore not surprising that the scientific community made great efforts in applying AI technologies to this imaging modality [47]. We will focus our attention on the IMT calculation, due to its recognized association with the risk of stroke and myocardial infarction [16], and on the analysis of the IMC and CAP.

Evaluation of Intima-Media Thickness

One of the first AI applications in carotid artery US has been focused on the semiautomatic and automatic calculation, and characterization of the CCA-IMT [16] (Fig. 48.2). Manual IMT evaluation suffers from high inter- and intra-observer variability [48], and therefore the development of semiautomatic and automatic methods could help improve measurement accuracy and reliability. One of the first attempts was performed in 1994 by *Selzer RH* et al. [49, 50]; they developed an automated algorithm for edge detection based on the identification of the maximum intensity gradient point, perpendicular to the direction of the vessel boundary, manually segmented by the operator. Since then, several complex algorithms for fully automatic IMT identification have been developed; for example, the model developed by *Wang K* et al. [51] based on Otsu's method (an algorithm able to perform automatic image thresholding) and an adaptive wind-

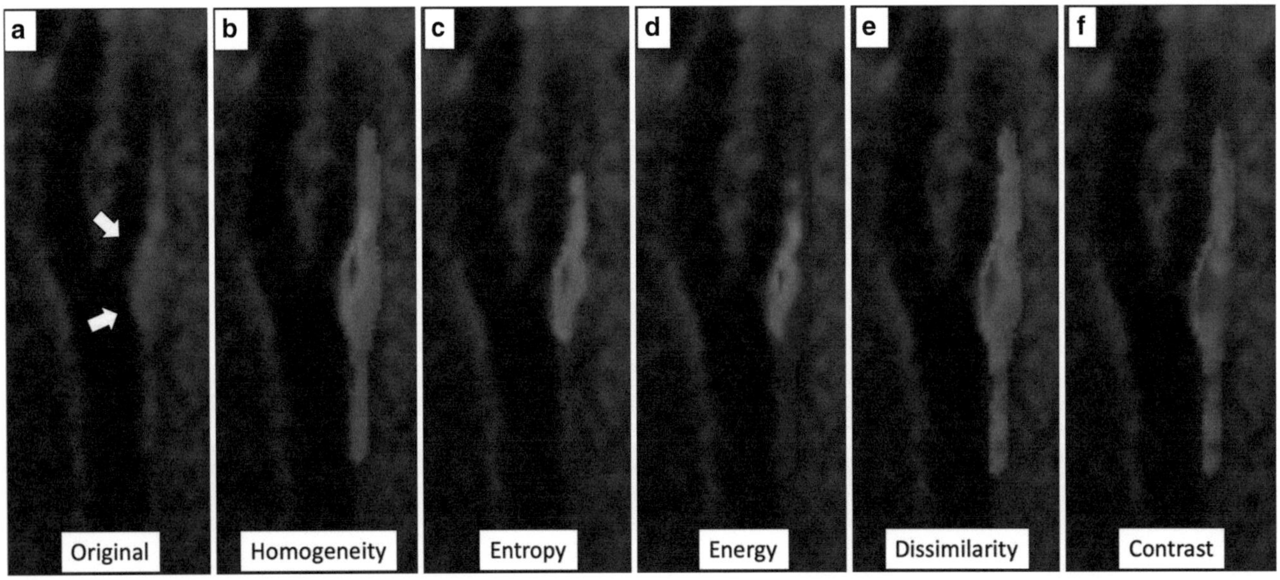

Fig. 48.1 Example of texture analysis (TA) on an MRI examination of a 52-year-old male patient with left side carotid stenosis. The sequence analyzed was a non-contrast fat-sat T1-WI. (**a**) The plaque (white arrows) is evident at the bifurcation of the common carotid artery. (**b**) Homogeneity; (**c**) entropy; (**d**) energy; (**e**) dissimilarity; (**f**) contrast

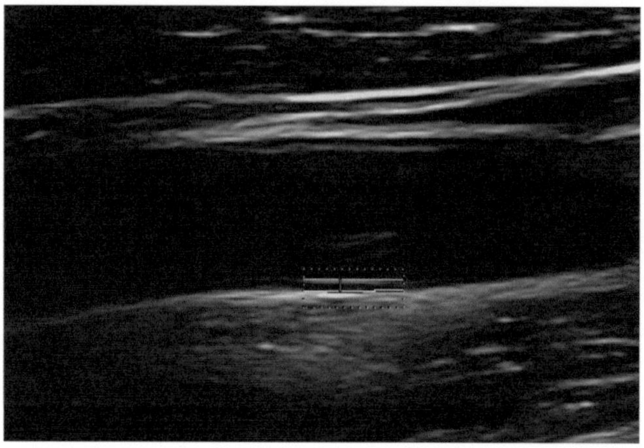

Fig. 48.2 Example of automated intima-media thickness (IMT) detection of the far wall of a common carotid artery in an ultrasound image of a 40-year-old male patient with a medical history of dyslipidemia

driven optimization technique (an iterative heuristic global optimization method), or the model by *Savaş S* et al. [52], utilizing a deep learning algorithm with multiple hidden layers. It is noteworthy to underline that some models are able to automatically detect IMT with very small measurement errors when compared to manual measurement, like the one created by *Menchón-Lara RM* et al. [53] that is able to automatically measure IMT with a measurement error of only 5.79 ± 34.42 μm. The evolution of AI technologies allows to obtain automatic accurate measures of not only the IMT but also of the total plaque area. In particular, the system created by *Biswas M* et al. [54], consisting of two stages of independent deep learning models, was able to measure the plaque area with an error of 2.79 ± 2.37 mm^2 when compared to manual tracing.

Evaluation of Intima-Media Complex and Carotid Artery Plaque

During the last decades, many other techniques have been developed for the analysis of not only the IMT but more for the more general analysis of the intima-media complex (IMC), i.e., the composition and organization of the carotid artery wall components (intima, media, and adventitia) [47, 55], using TA [10]. For example, in 2002 *Lal BK* et al. [56] were among the firsts that demonstrated a correlation between grayscale intensity ranges of the components of the plaque analyzed by US and histological findings by using TA. The authors extrapolated the grayscale intensity ranges of blood, calcium, fibromuscular tissue, and lipids from the US images of the carotid arteries of 10 healthy subjects, and then they performed a pixel distribution analysis (PDA) of the US images of 20 carotid artery plaques for assessing the amount of these same components within the plaques. The comparison between the PDA-derived predictions for blood, lipids, fibromuscular tissue, and calcium, and the histological estimates has been shown to be significantly correlated (p-value <0.02 for every single component).

One of the first goals achieved by TA was to demonstrate the possibility to discriminate between vulnerable and stable CAPs. An interesting example is represented by the study of *Kakkos SK* et al. [57], which showed how TA can be helpful in identifying CAP associated with a neurological event, demonstrating independent direct association between different texture features and amaurosis fugax, TIA, and stroke; in particular the area under the curve (AUC) of the regression-derived predicted probability resulted to be 0.92 for amaurosis fugax, 0.82 for TIA, and 0.85 for stroke (p-value <0.001). Subsequently, in 2016, *Doonan RJ* et al. [58] reported that some US imaging TA features (in particular echolucency and homogeneity) are associated with histologic features of plaque instability; the authors performed a digital image analysis software for extracting echodensity and textural features from carotid arteries of 160 patients; then, they performed a principal component analysis (PCA) for reducing imaging variables, and they used logistic regression models to determine whether PCA variables and individual imaging features were able to predict histologic features of plaque instability. It has also been demonstrated by *Madycki G* et al. [59] that TA can be helpful in predicting complications related to surgical procedures, showing that the use of TA applied to the CAP is able to predict the degree of microembolization during endarterectomy. Interestingly, TA features of plaque instability have been found not only on conventional US images but also on derived US techniques such as elastography; for example, in 2017 *Huang C* et al. [60] applied TA to carotid elastography for discriminating stable from unstable plaques by using MR as an "in vivo" reference; more specifically, the researchers found that the contrast and 99th percentile of the absolute strain rate were the best-performing features for plaque classification, with an AUC = 0.81. Lastly, it has been demonstrated that TA technique can be helpful also in monitoring the evolution of CAD: for example, in 2014 *van Engelen A* et al. [61] reported that changes in texture and total plaque volume observed by US monitoring are predictive of vascular events; in particular, in multivariate Cox regression, changes in plaque texture and total plaque volume showed to be both significant predictors, with mean hazard ratio of 1.4 and 1.5 per 100 mm^3, respectively (p-value <0.001). Another example is the research conducted by *Awad J* et al. [62] that showed that it is possible to quantitatively evaluate the effects of statin therapy by using the TA on three-dimensional US images.

The implementation of machine learning (ML) techniques [63] to the TA results allowed the creation of models that can be used for different purposes [10, 46]. The research conducted in 2003 by *Christodoulou CI* et al. [64] was among the first ones developing a CADx model for identifying asymptomatic patients with carotid stenosis at risk of stroke. The authors retrospectively analyzed 230 US plaque images, classified as asymptomatic and symptomatic (plaques that determined ipsilateral hemispheric symptoms). For every image, different texture feature sets were extracted, and the data were analyzed by a modular neural network that consisted of self-organizing map (SOM) classifiers for the classification task [64]. The average diagnostic yield was 73.1% by combining the results of the SOM classifiers [64]. The subsequent studies developed by adopting the same scheme model (TA + AI modeling) took advantage of the improved computational abilities, and of the hardware and software evolution, creating more complex models able to obtain better diagnostic accuracy. In 2011, *Acharya RU* et al. [65] created a CADx able to analyze CAP, and to classify them into symptomatic or asymptomatic by analyzing the textural features. The system consisted of three modules: (a) preprocessing; (b) feature extraction (standard deviation, entropy, symmetry, and run percentage); and (c) classification, performed by using AdaBoost and support vector machine (SVM) for automated decision-making. The system showed a classification accuracy of 82.4%, with a sensitivity of 82.9% and a specificity of 82.1% [65]. Further, the authors purposed an integrated index called symptomatic/asymptomatic carotid index (SACI) to discriminate symptomatic from asymptomatic patients using just one index or number [65]. A more recent model by *Saba L* et al. [66] adopted a polling-based PCA strategy in the ML framework for selection of dominant radiomic features, and the system showed an accuracy of 98.55% for far-wall plaques and 98.83% for near-wall plaques.

It is reasonable to forecast that in the future, US will continue to be one of the main research fields for AI applied to the study of carotid arteries due to its intrinsic qualities (safety, availability, and low cost).

Artificial Intelligence in Computed Tomography

The importance of CT and MR imaging for the identification and characterization of CAP features, together with the operator independency and the good reproducibility, makes these techniques a perfect target for the development of accurate AI-based CADx systems, aimed at vulnerable plaque identification and CVD/stroke risk stratification.

One of the first examples of AI applications to carotid CT is the research by *Vukadinovic D* et al. [67], published in 2010, which created a semiautomated segmentation model for the segmentation of the outer vessel wall, which is able to automatically detect the calcium components and the outer vessel wall utilizing a GentleBoost framework. Recently, it has been possible to develop also fully automated systems for carotid segmentation and analysis of the extracranial carotid arteries from CT angiography (CTA). For example, the model by *Caetano Dos Santos FL* et al. [68] showed a success rate of 83% for detection of the carotid arteries, with a specificity, sensitivity, and accuracy of 25%, 83%, and 71%, respectively.

Although the application of TA and machine learning on carotid CTA has still not been extensively investigated, it has revealed to be important for the study of CAD (Fig. 48.3).

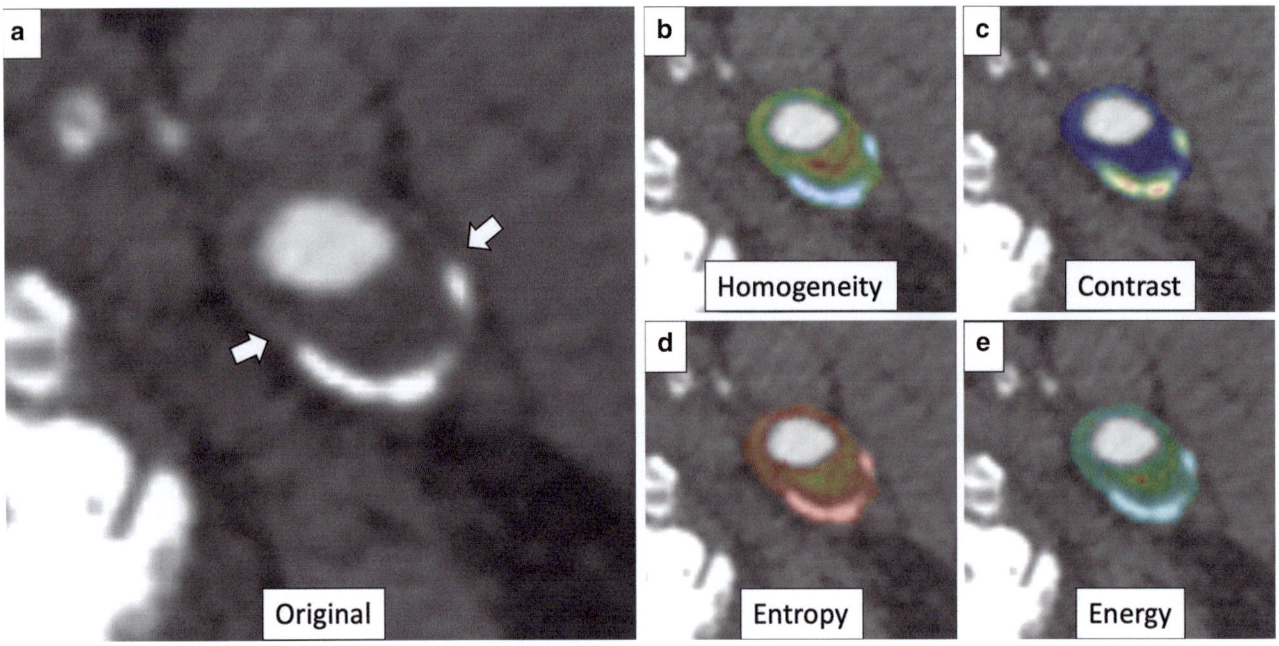

Fig. 48.3 Example of texture analysis (TA) on a CTA examination of a 78-year-old male patient with left side carotid stenosis. (**a**) The plaque (white arrows) is evident at the origin of the internal carotid artery. (**b**) Homogeneity; (**c**) contrast; (**d**) entropy; (**e**) energy

For example, the study by *Thornhill RE* et al. [69] showed that ML classifiers using five radiomic discriminative features were able to discriminate between free-floating intraluminal thrombi and carotid plaque with a sensitivity and a specificity of 87.5% and 71.4%, respectively, and an AUC = 0.85 at ROC analysis. The use of radiomic features can be helpful also in creating CADx models for discriminating symptomatic or asymptomatic plaque as reported by *Acharya UR* et al. [70], who created a model using local binary pattern features and wavelet energy features extracted from a CTA dataset of 20 consecutive patients. These features were used to train and test several supervised learning algorithm-based classifiers. The support vector machine (SVM) classifier, a supervised learning model with associated learning algorithms, presented the highest accuracy (88%) with sensitivity and specificity of 90.2% and 86.5%, respectively.

Artificial Intelligence in Magnetic Resonance Imaging

As previously mentioned, MRI is an optimal technique for carotid artery imaging because of its intrinsic multiparametricity and high-contrast resolution [4, 5]. These properties are fundamental for developing automated systems for carotid artery detection and boundary identification, for example, the model developed by *Cheng DC* et al. [71]; this model consisted of two phases: (1) the position detection of the carotid artery, which works by exploiting the intensity, area size, and shape as features for discriminating carotid artery from the other structures of the neck, and (2) the accurate boundary identification of the carotid artery, based on the use of directional gradient, Hough transform, and circle model-guided dynamic programming. In a more recent study published in 2020, *Samber DD* et al. [72] analyzed 4422 axial T2-WI images of 189 subjects with clinically evident atherosclerosis disease by using CNN algorithms, one for the segmentation of the vessel lumen and the other for the segmentation of the vessel wall. The comparison of the overall quantitative assessment between CNN segmentations and manual segmentations was determined by calculating the DICE metric [73]. The average DICE coefficient was 0.96 for the lumen and 0.87 for the vessel wall [72].

MRI multiparametricity and high-contrast resolution revealed to be of great advantage for the identification of plaque vulnerability features, such as IPH and fibrous cap thickness. In 2004, *Adame IM* et al. [74] were able to develop a model to automatically detect outer boundaries and plaque components in carotid MR short-axis black-blood images by using a combined model-based segmentation and fuzzy clustering for the detection of the vessel wall, lumen, and lipid core, with an excellent correspondence between automatic and manual measurement of lumen and outer wall, and acceptable results for fibrous cap thickness measurement. This model is of particular interest because the study of plaque vulnerability features (in particular IPH) is the future target of prospective research trials conducted for improving the clinical management of patients with CAS [75].

Advanced Computed Modeling and "Model of Risk" (MOR) Approaches

Besides radiomics analysis and the development of models able to discriminate between vulnerable and stable plaques, it is noteworthy to underline that in the last years, several researches developed sophisticated models for stratifying the risk of stroke that do not include CAP imaging vulnerability biomarkers.

Two very recent examples are represented by the risk model proposed by *Yin J* et al. *in 2020* [76] and by *Burke JF* et al. [77] in 2019. The first model [76] was created by using the data of the China National Stroke Screening and Prevention Project (CNSSPP) [78]; the subjects of the study were randomly divided into a testing and a validation dataset. The model included 19 risk factors. A predictive scoring system (from 0 to 10) was generated, applying a cutoff value of 6.5 for identifying high-risk patients. The model showed good performance, with an AUC of 0.738 for training dataset and 0.737 for validation dataset. *Burke* et al. [77] developed a model for identifying high-risk patient that would benefit from CEA. In this case, the authors developed a model based on data from the Asymptomatic Carotid Atherosclerosis Study (ACAS) [79] and validated by using the data from the Atherosclerosis Risk in Communities (ARIC) study [80]. The model was developed on ACAS data by exploiting three baseline risk factors (body mass index, creatinine, and degree of contralateral stenosis); model discrimination was calculated with Harrell's c-statistic (c-statistic = 0.59), and the model stratified the risk between the lowest and highest risk quintiles (5.1%–12.5%). The model was then validated on the data of the ARIC study, finding similar predictiveness (c-statistic = 0.58). CEA resulted superior to medical treatment across the spectrum of baseline risk, with wide variation of the magnitude of the treatment effect between the lowest and the highest risk quintiles (3.2%–10.7%). Even if the model was developed by exploiting only three baseline risk factors, the results demonstrated the potential to influence clinical decision-making in patients with asymptomatic CAD.

Future Perspectives

According to the studies discussed above, it is clear that radiomics and AI will become an integral part of the radiologist's daily practice. Following future technological advancements, it will be possible to create even more refined and complex algorithms for stratifying the risk of CAP rupture and stroke, and for predicting and monitoring the response to treatment. In particular, the integration of radiomics data from different imaging techniques, clinical data, and other "-omics" data, together with the use of ML techniques, will definitely improve the performances of these models [10].

Some of these models have already been developed, although they have still not been introduced into clinical practice. For example, *Jamthikar A* et al. [81, 82] created a low-cost ML-based CVD/stroke assessment system by exploiting 47 risk factors, 34 image-based and 13 conventional (i.e., demographic data and blood biomarkers). This system, based on the analysis of 395 images from US scans of carotid arteries in 202 Japanese patients, showed good performances in stratifying cardiovascular/stroke risk, using carotid artery stenosis as an event-equivalence gold standard, with AUC = 0.80 (p-value <0.0001). In 2020, the same group [83] developed a similar multiclass ML algorithm for CVD/stroke risk assessment. This model was developed and tested on 500 patients who underwent both carotid US and coronary angiography. For every patient, a multiclass coronary angiographic score [84] was calculated and used as CVD endpoint to develop and evaluate the performances of the model. The model showed better outcome results when compared to conventional cardiovascular risk calculators such as Framingham risk score [85] and the Systematic Coronary Risk Evaluation [86].

Conclusion

Initial AI and radiomics results applied to carotid artery diseases are promising, and in the next years, we will assist to a very fast technical evolution that, together with the advancements in the comprehension and identification of plaque features of vulnerability, will revolutionize the diagnostic approach to the patient in the view of personalized medicine.

References

1. Ooi YC, Gonzalez NR. Management of extracranial carotid artery disease. Cardiol Clin. 2015;33(1):1–35. https://doi.org/10.1016/j.ccl.2014.09.001.
2. Eckstein HH. European society for vascular surgery guidelines on the management of atherosclerotic carotid and vertebral artery disease. Eur J Vasc Endovasc Surg. 2018;55(1):1–2. https://doi.org/10.1016/j.ejvs.2017.06.026.
3. Abbott AL, Paraskevas KI, Kakkos SK, et al. Systematic review of guidelines for the management of asymptomatic and symptomatic carotid stenosis. Stroke. 2015;46(11):3288–301. https://doi.org/10.1161/STROKEAHA.115.003390.
4. Saba L, Yuan C, Hatsukami TS, et al. Carotid artery wall imaging: perspective and guidelines from the asnr vessel wall imaging study group and expert consensus recommendations of the american society of neuroradiology. AJNR Am J Neuroradiol. 2018;39(2):E9–E31. https://doi.org/10.3174/ajnr.A5488.
5. Saba L, Saam T, Jäger HR, et al. Imaging biomarkers of vulnerable carotid plaques for stroke risk prediction and their potential clinical implications. Lancet Neurol. 2019;18(6):559–72. https://doi.org/10.1016/S1474-4422(19)30035-3.
6. Naghavi M, Libby P, Falk E, et al. From vulnerable plaque to vulnerable patient: a call for new definitions and risk assessment strategies: Part I. Circulation. 2003;108(14):1664–72. https://doi.org/10.1161/01.CIR.0000087480.94275.97.
7. Naghavi M, Libby P, Falk E, et al. From vulnerable plaque to vulnerable patient: a call for new definitions and risk assessment strategies: Part II. Circulation. 2003;108(15):1772–8. https://doi.org/10.1161/01.CIR.0000087481.55887.C9.
8. Gillies RJ, Kinahan PE, Hricak H. Radiomics: images are more than pictures, they are data. Radiology. 2016;278(2):563–77. https://doi.org/10.1148/radiol.2015151169.
9. Saba L, Biswas M, Kuppili V, et al. The present and future of deep learning in radiology. Eur J Radiol. 2019;114:14–24. https://doi.org/10.1016/j.ejrad.2019.02.038.
10. Porcu M, Solinas C, Mannelli L, et al. Radiomics and "radi-...omics" in cancer immunotherapy: a guide for clinicians [published online ahead of print, 2020 Aug 7]. Crit Rev. Oncol Hematol. 2020;154:103068. https://doi.org/10.1016/j.critrevonc.2020.103068.
11. Kernan WN, Ovbiagele B, Black HR, et al. Guidelines for the prevention of stroke in patients with stroke and transient ischemic attack: a guideline for healthcare professionals from the American Heart Association/American Stroke Association [published correction appears in Stroke. 2015 Feb;46(2):e54]. Stroke. 2014;45(7):2160–236. https://doi.org/10.1161/STR.0000000000000024.
12. Aboyans V, Ricco JB, Bartelink MEL, et al. 2017 ESC Guidelines on the Diagnosis and Treatment of Peripheral Arterial Diseases, in collaboration with the European Society for Vascular Surgery (ESVS): Document covering atherosclerotic disease of extracranial carotid and vertebral, mesenteric, renal, upper and lower extremity arteries Endorsed by: the European Stroke Organization (ESO)The Task Force for the Diagnosis and Treatment of Peripheral Arterial Diseases of the European Society of Cardiology (ESC) and of the European Society for Vascular Surgery (ESVS). Eur Heart J. 2018;39(9):763–816. https://doi.org/10.1093/eurheartj/ehx095.
13. Barnett HJ, Taylor DW, Eliasziw M, et al. Benefit of carotid endarterectomy in patients with symptomatic moderate or severe stenosis. North American Symptomatic Carotid Endarterectomy Trial Collaborators. N Engl J Med. 1998;339(20):1415–25. https://doi.org/10.1056/NEJM199811123392002.
14. Randomised trial of endarterectomy for recently symptomatic carotid stenosis: final results of the MRC European Carotid Surgery Trial (ECST). Lancet. 1998;351(9113):1379–87.
15. Pignoli P, Tremoli E, Poli A, Oreste P, Paoletti R. Intimal plus medial thickness of the arterial wall: a direct measurement with ultrasound imaging. Circulation. 1986;74(6):1399–406. https://doi.org/10.1161/01.cir.74.6.1399.
16. Pignoli P, Tremoli E, Poli A, Oreste P, Paoletti R. Intimal plus medial thickness of the arterial wall: a direct measurement with ultrasound imaging. Circulation. 1986;74(6):1399–406. https://doi.org/10.1161/01.cir.74.6.1399.
17. Boulos NM, Gardin JM, Malik S, Postley J, Wong ND. Carotid plaque characterization, stenosis, and intima-media thick-

ness according to age and gender in a large registry Cohort. Am J Cardiol. 2016;117(7):1185–91. https://doi.org/10.1016/j.amjcard.2015.12.062.
18. Mono ML, Karameshev A, Slotboom J, et al. Plaque characteristics of asymptomatic carotid stenosis and risk of stroke. Cerebrovasc Dis. 2012;34(5–6):343–50. https://doi.org/10.1159/000343227.
19. Saba L, Anzidei M, Marincola BC, et al. Imaging of the carotid artery vulnerable plaque. Cardiovasc Intervent Radiol. 2014;37(3):572–85. https://doi.org/10.1007/s00270-013-0711-2.
20. Saba L, Tamponi E, Raz E, et al. Correlation between fissured fibrous cap and contrast enhancement: preliminary results with the use of CTA and histologic validation. AJNR Am J Neuroradiol. 2014;35(4):754–9. https://doi.org/10.3174/ajnr.A3759.
21. Touboul PJ, Hennerici MG, Meairs S, et al. Mannheim carotid intima-media thickness and plaque consensus (2004–2006-2011). An update on behalf of the advisory board of the third, fourth and fifth watching the risk symposia, at the 13th, 15th and 20th European Stroke Conferences, Mannheim, Germany, 2004, Brussels, Belgium, 2006, and Hamburg, Germany, 2011. Cerebrovasc Dis. 2012;34(4):290–6. https://doi.org/10.1159/000343145.
22. Zhao X, Hippe DS, Li R, et al. Prevalence and characteristics of carotid artery high-risk atherosclerotic plaques in Chinese patients with cerebrovascular symptoms: a Chinese atherosclerosis risk evaluation II Study. J Am Heart Assoc. 2017;6(8):e005831. Published 2017 Aug 14. https://doi.org/10.1161/JAHA.117.005831.
23. Yoneyama T, Sun J, Hippe DS, et al. In vivo semi-automatic segmentation of multicontrast cardiovascular magnetic resonance for prospective cohort studies on plaque tissue composition: initial experience. Int J Cardiovasc Imaging. 2016;32(1):73–81. https://doi.org/10.1007/s10554-015-0704-0.
24. van Dijk AC, Truijman MT, Hussain B, et al. Intraplaque hemorrhage and the plaque surface in carotid atherosclerosis: the plaque at RISK Study (PARISK). AJNR Am J Neuroradiol. 2015;36(11):2127–33. https://doi.org/10.3174/ajnr.A4414.
25. Gupta A, Baradaran H, Schweitzer AD, et al. Carotid plaque MRI and stroke risk: a systematic review and meta-analysis. Stroke. 2013;44(11):3071–7. https://doi.org/10.1161/STROKEAHA.113.002551.
26. Barnett HJ, Taylor DW, Eliasziw M, et al. Benefit of carotid endarterectomy in patients with symptomatic moderate or severe stenosis. North American Symptomatic Carotid Endarterectomy Trial Collaborators. N Engl J Med. 1998;339(20):1415–25. https://doi.org/10.1056/NEJM199811123392002.
27. van Gils MJ, Homburg PJ, Rozie S, de Weert TT, Dippel DW, van der Lugt A. Evolution of atherosclerotic carotid plaque morphology: do ulcerated plaques heal? A serial multidetector CT angiography study. Cerebrovasc Dis. 2011;31(3):263–70. https://doi.org/10.1159/000322152.
28. Truijman MT, Kwee RM, van Hoof RH, et al. Combined 18F-FDG PET-CT and DCE-MRI to assess inflammation and microvascularization in atherosclerotic plaques. Stroke. 2013;44(12):3568–70. https://doi.org/10.1161/STROKEAHA.113.003140.
29. Porcu M, Mannelli L, Melis M, et al. Carotid plaque imaging profiling in subjects with risk factors (diabetes and hypertension). Cardiovasc Diagn Ther. 2020;10(4):1005–18. https://doi.org/10.21037/cdt.2020.01.13.
30. Porcu M, Anzidei M, Suri JS, et al. Carotid artery imaging: The study of intra-plaque vascularization and hemorrhage in the era of the "vulnerable" plaque. J Neuroradiol. 2020;47(6):464–72. https://doi.org/10.1016/j.neurad.2019.03.009.
31. Xu D, Hippe DS, Underhill HR, et al. Prediction of high-risk plaque development and plaque progression with the carotid atherosclerosis score. JACC Cardiovasc Imaging. 2014;7(4):366–73. https://doi.org/10.1016/j.jcmg.2013.09.022.
32. Sun J, Balu N, Hippe DS, et al. Subclinical carotid atherosclerosis: short-term natural history of lipid-rich necrotic core--a multicenter study with MR imaging. Radiology. 2013;268(1):61–8. https://doi.org/10.1148/radiol.13121702.
33. Saam T, Hetterich H, Hoffmann V, et al. Meta-analysis and systematic review of the predictive value of carotid plaque hemorrhage on cerebrovascular events by magnetic resonance imaging. J Am Coll Cardiol. 2013;62(12):1081–91. https://doi.org/10.1016/j.jacc.2013.06.015.
34. Saba L, Zucca S, Gupta A, et al. Perivascular fat density and contrast plaque enhancement: does a correlation exist? AJNR Am J Neuroradiol. 2020;41(8):1460–5. https://doi.org/10.3174/ajnr.A6710.
35. Saba L, Montisci R, Sanfilippo R, Mallarini G. Multidetector row CT of the brain and carotid artery: a correlative analysis. Clin Radiol. 2009;64(8):767–78. https://doi.org/10.1016/j.crad.2009.03.009.
36. Bluth EI. Value of US in selecting patients for carotid angioplasty and stent placement. Radiology. 2005;237(1):374–5. https://doi.org/10.1148/radiol.2371050432.
37. Teixeira R, Vieira MJ, Gonçalves A, Cardim N, Gonçalves L. Ultrasonographic vascular mechanics to assess arterial stiffness: a review. Eur Heart J Cardiovasc Imaging. 2016;17(3):233–46. https://doi.org/10.1093/ehjci/jev287.
38. Mahmood B, Ewertsen C, Carlsen J, Nielsen MB. Ultrasound vascular elastography as a tool for assessing atherosclerotic plaques - a systematic literature review. Ultrasound Int Open. 2016;2(4):E106–12. https://doi.org/10.1055/s-0042-115,564.
39. Makris GC, Lavida A, Griffin M, Geroulakos G, Nicolaides AN. Three-dimensional ultrasound imaging for the evaluation of carotid atherosclerosis. Atherosclerosis. 2011;219(2):377–83. https://doi.org/10.1016/j.atherosclerosis.2011.05.006.
40. Chiu B, Shamdasani V, Entrekin R, Yuan C, Kerwin WS. Characterization of carotid plaques on 3-dimensional ultrasound imaging by registration with multicontrast magnetic resonance imaging. J Ultrasound Med. 2012;31(10):1567–80. https://doi.org/10.7863/jum.2012.31.10.1567.
41. Etesami M, Hoi Y, Steinman DA, et al. Comparison of carotid plaque ulcer detection using contrast-enhanced and time-of-flight MRA techniques. AJNR Am J Neuroradiol. 2013;34(1):177–84. https://doi.org/10.3174/ajnr.A3132.
42. Wasserman BA, Smith WI, Trout HH, third, Cannon RO third, Balaban RS, Arai AE. Carotid artery atherosclerosis: in vivo morphologic characterization with gadolinium-enhanced double-oblique MR imaging initial results. Radiology. 2002;223(2):566–73. https://doi.org/10.1148/radiol.2232010659.
43. Chan JMS, Monaco C, Wylezinska-Arridge M, et al. Imaging vulnerable plaques by targeting inflammation in atherosclerosis using fluorescent-labeled dual-ligand microparticles of iron oxide and magnetic resonance imaging. J Vasc Surg. 2018;67(5):1571–1583.e3. https://doi.org/10.1016/j.jvs.2017.04.046.
44. Sharma AM, Gupta A, Kumar PK, et al. A review on carotid ultrasound atherosclerotic tissue characterization and stroke risk stratification in machine learning framework. Curr Atheroscler Rep. 2015;17(9):55. https://doi.org/10.1007/s11883-015-0529-2.
45. Varghese BA, Cen SY, Hwang DH, Duddalwar VA. Texture analysis of imaging: what radiologists need to know. AJR Am J Roentgenol. 2019;212(3):520–8. https://doi.org/10.2214/AJR.18.20624. Epub 2019 Jan 15
46. Lambin P, Rios-Velazquez E, Leijenaar R, et al. Radiomics: extracting more information from medical images using advanced feature analysis. Eur J Cancer. 2012;48(4):441–6. https://doi.org/10.1016/j.ejca.2011.11.036.
47. Huang Q, Zhang F, Li X. Machine learning in ultrasound computer-aided diagnostic systems: a survey. Biomed Res Int. 2018;2018:5137904. https://doi.org/10.1155/2018/5137904. Published 2018 Mar 4.
48. Saxena A, Ng EYK, Lim ST. Imaging modalities to diagnose carotid artery stenosis: progress and prospect. Biomed Eng Online.

2019;18(1):66. https://doi.org/10.1186/s12938-019-0685-7. Published 2019 May 28.
49. Schmidt C, Wendelhag I. How can the variability in ultrasound measurement of intima-media thickness be reduced? Studies of interobserver variability in carotid and femoral arteries. Clin Physiol. 1999;19(1):45–55. https://doi.org/10.1046/j.1365-2281.1999.00145.x.
50. Selzer RH, Hodis HN, Kwong-Fu H, et al. Evaluation of computerized edge tracking for quantifying intima-media thickness of the common carotid artery from B-mode ultrasound images. Atherosclerosis. 1994;111(1):1–11. https://doi.org/10.1016/0021-9150(94)90186-4.
51. Wang K, Pu Y, Zhang Y, Wang P. Fully automatic measurement of intima-media thickness in ultrasound images of the common carotid artery based on improved otsu's method and adaptive wind driven optimization. Ultrason Imaging. 2020;42(6):245–60. https://doi.org/10.1177/0161734620956897.
52. Wang K, Pu Y, Zhang Y, Wang P. Fully automatic measurement of intima-media thickness in ultrasound images of the common carotid artery based on improved otsu's method and adaptive wind driven optimization. Ultrason Imaging. 2020;42(6):245–60. https://doi.org/10.1177/0161734620956897.
53. Menchón-Lara RM, Sancho-Gómez JL, Bueno-Crespo A. Early-stage atherosclerosis detection using deep learning over carotid ultrasound images. Appl. Soft Comput. 2016;49:616–28.
54. Biswas M, Saba L, Chakrabartty S, et al. Two-stage artificial intelligence model for jointly measurement of atherosclerotic wall thickness and plaque burden in carotid ultrasound: A screening tool for cardiovascular/stroke risk assessment. Comput Biol Med. 2020;123:103847. https://doi.org/10.1016/j.compbiomed.2020.103847.
55. Loizou CP. A review of ultrasound common carotid artery image and video segmentation techniques. Med Biol Eng Comput. 2014;52(12):1073–93. https://doi.org/10.1007/s11517-014-1203-5.
56. Lal BK, Hobson RW. Pappas PJ, et al. Pixel distribution analysis of B-mode ultrasound scan images predicts histologic features of atherosclerotic carotid plaques [published correction appears in J Vasc Surg. 2003 Sep;38(3):497; Chakhtura Ellie Y [corrected to Chakhtoura Elie Y]]. J Vasc Surg. 2002;35(6):1210–7. https://doi.org/10.1067/mva.2002.122888.
57. Kakkos SK, Nicolaides AN, Kyriacou E, et al. Computerized texture analysis of carotid plaque ultrasonic images can identify unstable plaques associated with ipsilateral neurological symptoms. Angiology. 2011;62(4):317–28. https://doi.org/10.1177/0003319710384397.
58. Doonan RJ, Gorgui J, Veinot JP, et al. Plaque echodensity and textural features are associated with histologic carotid plaque instability. J Vasc Surg. 2016;64(3):671–677.e8. https://doi.org/10.1016/j.jvs.2016.03.423.
59. Madycki G, Staszkiewicz W, Gabrusiewicz A. Carotid plaque texture analysis can predict the incidence of silent brain infarcts among patients undergoing carotid endarterectomy. Eur J Vasc Endovasc Surg. 2006;31(4):373–80. https://doi.org/10.1016/j.ejvs.2005.10.010.
60. Huang C, He Q, Huang M, et al. Non-invasive identification of vulnerable atherosclerotic plaques using texture analysis in ultrasound carotid elastography: an in vivo feasibility study validated by magnetic resonance imaging. Ultrasound Med Biol. 2017;43(4):817–30. https://doi.org/10.1016/j.ultrasmedbio.2016.12.003.
61. van Engelen A, Wannarong T, Parraga G, et al. Three-dimensional carotid ultrasound plaque texture predicts vascular events. Stroke. 2014;45(9):2695–701. https://doi.org/10.1161/STROKEAHA.114.005752.
62. Awad J, Krasinski A, Parraga G, Fenster A. Texture analysis of carotid artery atherosclerosis from three-dimensional ultrasound images. Med Phys. 2010;37(4):1382–91. https://doi.org/10.1118/1.3301592.
63. Saba L, Biswas M, Kuppili V, et al. The present and future of deep learning in radiology. Eur J Radiol. 2019;114:14–24. https://doi.org/10.1016/j.ejrad.2019.02.038.
64. Christodoulou CI, Pattichis CS, Pantziaris M, et al. Texture-based classification of atherosclerotic carotid plaques. IEEE Transactions on Medical Imaging. 2003;22(7):902–12. https://doi.org/10.1109/TMI.2003.815066.
65. Acharya RU, Faust O, Alvin AP, et al. Symptomatic vs. asymptomatic plaque classification in carotid ultrasound. J Med Syst. 2012;36(3):1861–71. https://doi.org/10.1007/s10916-010-9645-2.
66. Saba L, Jain PK, Suri HS, et al. Plaque tissue morphology-based stroke risk stratification using carotid ultrasound: a polling-based PCA learning paradigm. J Med Syst. 2017;41(6):98. https://doi.org/10.1007/s10916-017-0745-0.
67. Vukadinovic D, van Walsum T, Manniesing R, et al. Segmentation of the outer vessel wall of the common carotid artery in CTA. IEEE Trans Med Imaging. 2010;29(1):65–76. https://doi.org/10.1109/TMI.2009.2025702.
68. Caetano Dos Santos FL, Kolasa M, Terada M, Salenius J, Eskola H, Paci M. VASIM: an automated tool for the quantification of carotid atherosclerosis by computed tomography angiography. Int J Cardiovasc Imaging. 2019;35(6):1149–59. https://doi.org/10.1007/s10554-019-01549-1.
69. Thornhill RE, Lum C, Jaberi A, et al. Can shape analysis differentiate free-floating internal carotid artery thrombus from atherosclerotic plaque in patients evaluated with CTA for stroke or transient ischemic attack? Acad Radiol. 2014;21(3):345–54. https://doi.org/10.1016/j.acra.2013.11.011.
70. Acharya UR, Sree SV, Mookiah MR, et al. Computed tomography carotid wall plaque characterization using a combination of discrete wavelet transform and texture features: A pilot study. Proc Inst Mech Eng H. 2013;227(6):643–54. https://doi.org/10.1177/0954411913480622.
71. Cheng DC, Billich C, Liu SH, et al. Automatic detection of the carotid artery boundary on cross-sectional MR image sequences using a circle model guided dynamic programming. Biomed Eng Online. 2011;10:26. https://doi.org/10.1186/1475-925X-10-26; Published 2011 Apr 11.
72. Samber DD, Ramachandran S, Sahota A, et al. Segmentation of carotid arterial walls using neural networks. World J Radiol. 2020;12(1):1–9. https://doi.org/10.4329/wjr.v12.i1.1.
73. Dice LR. Measures of the amount of ecologic association between species. Ecology. 1945;26:297–302.
74. Adame IM, van der Geest RJ, Wasserman BA, Mohamed MA, Reiber JH, Lelieveldt BP. Automatic segmentation and plaque characterization in atherosclerotic carotid artery MR images. MAGMA. 2004;16(5):227–34. https://doi.org/10.1007/s10334-003-0030-8.
75. Saba L, Moody AR, Saam T, et al. Vessel wall-imaging biomarkers of carotid plaque vulnerability in stroke prevention trials: a viewpoint from the carotid imaging consensus group. JACC Cardiovasc Imaging. 2020;13(11):2445–56. https://doi.org/10.1016/j.jcmg.2020.07.046.
76. Yin J, Yu C, Liu H, et al. A model to predict unstable carotid plaques in population with high risk of stroke. BMC Cardiovasc Disord. 2020;20(1):164. https://doi.org/10.1186/s12872-020-01450-z; Published 2020 Apr 7.
77. Burke JF, Morgenstern LB, Hayward RA. Can risk modelling improve treatment decisions in asymptomatic carotid stenosis?. BMC Neurol. 2019;19(1):295. Published 2019 Nov 22. https://doi.org/10.1186/s12883-019-1528-7.
78. Wang X, Li W, Song F, et al. Carotid atherosclerosis detected by ultrasonography: a national cross-sectional study. J Am Heart Assoc. 2018;7(8):e008701. https://doi.org/10.1161/JAHA.118.008701; Published 2018 Apr 5.

79. Endarterectomy for asymptomatic carotid artery stenosis. Executive committee for the asymptomatic carotid atherosclerosis Study. JAMA. 1995;273(18):1421–8.
80. The Atherosclerosis Risk in Communities (ARIC) Study: design and objectives. The ARIC investigators. Am J Epidemiol. 1989;129(4):687–702.
81. Jamthikar A, Gupta D, Khanna NN, et al. A low-cost machine learning-based cardiovascular/stroke risk assessment system: integration of conventional factors with image phenotypes. Cardiovasc Diagn Ther. 2019;9(5):420–30. https://doi.org/10.21037/cdt.2019.09.03.
82. Jamthikar A, Gupta D, Khanna NN, Saba L, Laird JR, Suri JS. Cardiovascular/stroke risk prevention: A new machine learning framework integrating carotid ultrasound image-based phenotypes and its harmonics with conventional risk factors. Indian Heart J. 2020;72(4):258–64. https://doi.org/10.1016/j.ihj.2020.06.004.
83. Jamthikar AD, Gupta D, Mantella LE, et al. Multiclass machine learning vs. conventional calculators for stroke/CVD risk assessment using carotid plaque predictors with coronary angiography scores as gold standard: a 500 participants study [published online ahead of print, 2020 Nov 12]. Int J Cardiovasc Imaging. 2020; https://doi.org/10.1007/s10554-020-02099-7; https://doi.org/10.1007/s10554-020-02099-7.
84. Johri AM, Chitty DW, Matangi M, et al. Can carotid bulb plaque assessment rule out significant coronary artery disease? A comparison of plaque quantification by two- and three-dimensional ultrasound. J Am Soc Echocardiogr. 2013;26(1):86–95. https://doi.org/10.1016/j.echo.2012.09.005.
85. D'Agostino RB Sr, Vasan RS, Pencina MJ, et al. General cardiovascular risk profile for use in primary care: the Framingham Heart Study. Circulation. 2008;117(6):743–53. https://doi.org/10.1161/CIRCULATIONAHA.107.699579.
86. Conroy RM, Pyörälä K, Fitzgerald AP, et al. Estimation of ten-year risk of fatal cardiovascular disease in Europe: the SCORE project. Eur Heart J. 2003;24(11):987–1003. https://doi.org/10.1016/s0195-668x(03)00114-3.

Part V

Artificial Intelligence: General Considerations

Artificial Intelligence in Medicine: Laws, Regulations, and Privacy

49

Enzo Maria Le Fevre and Giselle Heleg

Data: The Basic Asset for AI

Many times, when we think of artificial intelligence (herein after AI), we imagine a world full of robots and machines; however, the truth is that AI has been with us for a long time and even appears in a much more common way than we imagine. Computers learn to detect non-decipherable patterns using biostatistics through the processing of massive data sets (big data) by using mathematical models called *algorithms*. The particularity of this *cutting-edge* technology is given by data which is considered the basic asset for AI. While digitalization has considerably increased the collection capacity of data and the volume of digital devices able to do so is spreading dramatically, the massive application of AI systems has exponentially increased automated treatment capabilities and processing speed of data. This combination of innovation produces a series of unprecedented risks and opportunities due to the form and massive amount of data that can be collected [20]. Governments and international organizations have started launching specific data and AI governance strategies [19] in order to address some of the challenges that are exposed in this chapter.

In order for an AI solution to be successful, a vast amount of data is required so as to optimize the performance of the algorithms. In other words, when the AI system is trained with structured and quality data, it is in a position to provide a more accurate and precise answer. Therefore, if hospitals and research institutions combined all their bases to achieve a sufficiently large and diverse data set, the benefits will multiply.

Although AI has made health data simultaneously more valuable, abusing these data is now much easier causing rejection toward the centralization of large amount of confidential medical information in the hands of technology companies or governments. However, an adequate safeguard of the right to privacy might end up with these barriers and use data for statistical and scientific purposes. This will allow the system to be trained with a diverse set of data, being able to be implemented anywhere in the world, increasing its generality [21].

Health Data: Risks and Opportunities

Today, data plays a fundamental role in practically all aspects of AI development, and its transformative power is creeping into many industries, promising a truly life-changing impact in medicine. In order to maximize its benefits and mitigate its risks, it is essential to create a shared understanding regarding the importance of digital health solutions and highlight the need of creating an interoperable digital health ecosystem so as to assure seamless and secure exchange of health data between users, healthcare providers, health systems managers, and health data services.

Since AI systems are not applied on patients themselves but on their digital or digitized data, countries with infrastructures that support digitized and interoperable health databases will, therefore, be best positioned to take advantage of AI's potential to transform health care. At this point, it is essential to encourage patient's consent for data sharing so as to protect their privacy, provide secure digital systems, and avoid inappropriate use of sensitive personal data. Such sharing is vital as it can contribute to the enhancement of quality of processes, the outcomes of health services, and the continuity of care for patients and may also lead to the building of an interoperable knowledge base.

However, data sharing stresses the need for a strong legal and regulatory base to protect privacy, confidentiality, integ-

E. M. Le Fevre, PhD (✉) · G. Heleg, LLB
Laboratory on Innovation and Artificial Intelligence (IALAB), Faculty of Law, University of Buenos Aires, Buenos Aires, Argentina
e-mail: enzo@enzolefevre.eu; giselleheleg@ialab.com.ar

C. N. De Cecco et al. (eds.), *Artificial Intelligence in Cardiothoracic Imaging*, Contemporary Medical Imaging, https://doi.org/10.1007/978-3-030-92087-6_49

rity, and availability of data while at the same time requires an effective communication of data security strategies so as to preserve transparency [29]. In this regard, one of the main risks associated to health data refers to whether it has been treated in a manner that is respectful of human rights and democratic values. The decision to adopt such an approach stems from the understanding of many international bodies and entities that AI actors must respect the rule of law, human rights, and democratic values throughout the entire life cycle. Specifically, the Organization for Economic Cooperation and Development [22], the European Commission [14], the Council of Europe [7], and the Inter-American Development Bank [2] speak on this matter.

Last, but not least, the data used to train the AI algorithms might be biased. Cultural differences might make some patients less likely to report certain symptoms that may be used by the software as input factors; language challenges may limit the information offered or cause wrong information to be entered. Economic and accessibility factors may imply certain tests or treatments were not possible for some patients. Therefore, AI-enabled healthcare products should be rigorously tested to understand their performance across populations with medical and demographic differences [25].

Health Data Protection

The increased visibility and availability of information has emphasized the need for an adequate protection of health data. Patient's personal data must be protected, and sufficient safeguards should be provided so as to avoid risks that may result from unauthorized access to personal information on sensitive health topics, such as sexual and reproductive health issues, among others.

There are two fundamental principles in data processing. On the one hand, we find the principle of confidentiality which implies that if the owner has given the personal consent only for the data to be subjected to a specific treatment, the owner of the data must be guaranteed and ensured that such data will not be transferred to another subject without a proper consent. In other words, only authorized people or entities can access the information [5]. The right of consent is one of the key points in all types of data processing and presents enormous difficulties in terms of artificial intelligence [10]. In this line, databases and public and private registries that wish to process data of human or legal persons, as a general rule, must first require their consent for the treatment. Exceptions must be provided by law and must be interpreted restrictively. The right to informational self-determination, linked to privacy, determines that the owners of data – especially sensitive data – are not required to provide them, unless there is an informed consent [6].

On the other hand, confidentiality is part of security. Those responsible for the treatment must adopt a set of preventive and reactive measures that allow safeguarding and protecting the information. This principle is increasingly gaining prominence in the digital world since the European Union considers that security of information and sensitive data of citizens has become a matter of highest priority. Its loss or improper treatment can incur fines of up to 20 million euros or 4% of the annual turnover [26]. Security includes the following:

- Availability, since it is necessary to guarantee access to information when required. This includes preventing system crashes that might allow illegitimate access.
- Integrity, since correct information must be provided without unauthorized modifications or errors.
- Authentication, which includes the need to verify and guarantee that the origin of data is correct.

Besides, there are a series of guidelines, embodied in international documents, that should be followed so as to guarantee data protection.

- *Relying on legislation.*

Given the nature of the personal data at stake – health data – relying on legislation would contribute to legal certainty, since (a) the treatment of health-related data would be prescribed in detail and the purpose of treatment would be specified; (b) it would be clearly determined who is responsible and who can access them; (c) the possibility of processing data for different purposes would be excluded, and (d) specific guarantees would be provided [13].

When drafting legislation, decision-makers need to try to do it as inclusive as possible. Through legislation, the right to data protection may be limited so as to safeguard national security, public safety, public health, rights and freedoms of third parties, as well as matters of public interest.

In addition, legislation allows those in charge of processing personal data to know the limits within which they can operate [11].

- *Determine who is responsible for the processing of personal data.*

Determining who decides the means and purposes of data processing is crucial to establish who is responsible for complying with the rules and who should provide information to the user about its rights and personal data processing [13]. This point is essential for users to know who they can enforce their rights against.

- *Respect the explicit and specific purpose of the processing of personal data.*

The personal data necessary to achieve the objectives pursued by the AI system must be processed for explicit and specific purposes [18], in order to prevent data from being used for hidden purposes that violate the users' rights.

- *Provide information.*

The owners of systems, applications, and solutions that collect and process personal data should encourage transparency and provide information to the user in a clear, accessible, and easily understandable way on all aspects entailed. The information should be based on data processing activities and their characteristics, including the retention period of data collected and the purposes of the processing.

- *Guarantee the possibility of reporting those who fail to comply with the measures.*

It is necessary that those who developed applications and those responsible for the treatment guarantee to anyone who considers that their privacy or their data is being affected the possibility of making a complaint.

Control over Health Data

AI represents a major challenge as this cutting-edge technology is continuously changing and its black box nature reaches conclusions that are so mathematically complex, they cannot always be understood by humans [2]. This black box challenge does not only mean that the user doesn't understand how the system works, but the problem goes much further as the system might provide unusual and unpredictable answers even for experts. Sometimes this may occur because developers did not recognize training data included information or because clinically relevant information was not included in digital health data [8]. Besides, these types of mistakes can only be found when the software is tested with new data and, consequently, when an AI system lacks of an explanation on how it works; careful and extensive testing is the only way to discover its flaws and weaknesses. Regarding regulation, the General Data Protection Regulation (GDPR) includes an "explainability requirement" that applies to AI at some level but does not precisely clarifies its extent [17]. This means that AI solutions should be able to explain people how a certain decision was made. For all these reasons, traditional regulatory regimes for medical products may not be sufficiently risk-averse or timely. Governments should provide clarity on applicable laws and regulations and consider new methods of regulations that take these challenges into account [25].

In addition, when using AI systems to make predictions, developers should comply with the principle of transparency, i.e., users should be given information about how certain an algorithm's prediction is or what factors were the most important for reaching a decision. By doing this, users might have an insight into when a particular recommendation should not be trusted [24].

Different sort of patient's consent might be required depending on the data that will be collected. At this point, it is extremely important to ensure human control in each of the stages of the system's life cycle, so as to make sure that the software continues to work as expected in the changing environment. Besides, countries should consider liability for the performance of the system, as well as the sort of consent that should be required to access the data.

Health Data Privacy

Over the years and with the rise of AI, privacy has reached a turning point. By accepting the terms and conditions of a website or mobile application, users, almost without noticing it, share personal data that is stored in large databases. This data can be mined for an infinite number of uses, purchasing recommendations or other services as well as marketing opportunities. Even though these functionalities might provide a helpful service, the potential risks carried are not trivial. Sharing personal data does not only allow tracking and monitoring people but also enables the creation of digital profiles and can even predict behaviors.

Although privacy can be difficult to safeguard, there are binding documents such as the GDPR and other recommendations from international organizations that enshrine a series of principles which should be followed so as to protect privacy when processing data:

- Transparency: refers to the standards that must be met regarding the information directed to the data holder. Specifically, it must be concise, easily accessible, and easily understood.
- Purpose: implies that the data must be collected for an explicit and legitimate purpose. The data collected and subjected to treatment must be limited exclusively to those that are necessary to achieve the intended purpose, without being able to extend to other personal data [1].
- Minimization: requires that the data is used in an adequate way, relevant and limited to what is necessary [4].
- Accuracy: the user must have the real possibility of requesting its rectification.
- Suppression: data must be deleted upon consumer request.
- Need for collection: data collection must be carried out under conditions of necessity, proportionality in a democratic society and under the control of governments [23].

- Safety: technological solutions must include the most advanced information security mechanisms [9–11, 13, 15]; this is also valid for all the infrastructure involved in the process, such as data centers or communication networks.

Accessing personal sensitive data of patients such as medical records is strictly protected. However, in the past years, data sharing between hospitals and AI companies has increased and has generated controversy, highlighting some ethical concerns. Who owns and controls the patient's data that is used to develop an AI solution? How can patients' right to privacy be protected? **If a patient's data is used to train an AI program, what legal rights does he have? In this regard, the Health Insurance Portability and Accountability Act (HIPAA) only protects individually identifiable health information** [28]. **This means that there are no** restrictions on the use or disclosure of anonymous health information, i.e., health information that does not identify or provide a reasonable basis for identifying an individual. By saying this, once the personal health data has been anonymized, the patient has no further legal recourse to limit its use.

Privacy issues might be solved if people believe in the importance of sharing their health data. In other words, patients should understand the great impact that these data can have on the development and strengthening of health systems. However, this necessarily requires countries to ensure an adequate legal and ethical framework that assures patients' safety, data security, appropriate use and ownership of health data, privacy data recoverability, as well as protection of intellectual property rights.

From EU to the USA: Data Circulation after the End of the Privacy Shield

On 12 July 2016, the adequacy decision on the EU-US Privacy Shield was adopted. This framework aimed to protect the fundamental rights of European people whose personal data was being transferred to the USA for commercial purposes and allowed free transfer of data to certified companies in the USA. To reach this aim, strong data protection obligations were imposed to companies that received personal data from Europe. Besides, safeguards on access to data were established as well as means to guarantee effective protection and redress for individuals. Afterward, on December 2016, the EU-US Data Protection Umbrella Agreement was concluded which contained a comprehensive set of data protection rules that apply to all transatlantic exchanges between criminal law enforcement authorities. By doing this, Europeans' levels of protections were enforced [12].

However, this data transfer framework ended in July. The Schrems II decision has invalidated the EU-US Privacy Shield immediately and has also hinted at greater scrutiny for alternate data transfer mechanisms like standard contractual clauses and binding corporate rules, leaving many companies uncertain over how to conduct business involving transatlantic data transfers. The Court of Justice of the European Union concluded that the EU-US framework failed to ensure the protections imposed by the GDPR as it did not provide adequate safeguards to prevent European data from being provided to US government or law enforcement agencies [27]. Schrems II decision prevents companies from transferring personal information to countries with more flexible data protection rules as they must ensure to comply with European privacy standards. This ruling affects big tech companies like Facebook and Google, and the data subject to the transfer rules can include communications such as emails and social media posts, financial records, business files, human resource materials about employees, marketing databases, and customer records.

As a consequence, companies now have to carry out a reevaluation and revision of agreement terms related to data transfer across large numbers of agreements. By doing this, companies are enabled to fully assess their rights and responsibilities and better understand corresponding privacy compliance risk. Furthermore, reviewing agreements can help them determine whether they should enhance their data transfer strategy with supplemental measures such as including data encryption or other security commitments, breach notification, and termination rights.

Actually, in the American continent there are three countries that obtained the declaration of adequacy of the European authorities for international transfer: Canada, Argentina, and Uruguay. Schrems court decision has not affected the adequacy resolutions which remain in force and with full effect. Therefore, for the moment data transfers from the member states of the European Union to these three jurisdictions are legitimized under the decisions taken by the European authorities in a timely manner. As most of the countries have not yet obtained an adequacy decision, the following mechanisms established in articles 46 and 49 of the GDPR must be used so as to validate the transfers:

- A legally binding and enforceable instrument between public authorities or bodies.
- Binding corporate rules.
- The standard data protection clauses adopted by the European Commission.
- The standard data protection clauses adopted by a supervisory authority and approved by the European Commission.
- An approved code of conduct, or an approved certification mechanism.

Now, the controller in the European Union must check in each case and, if necessary, in collaboration with the recipient of the transfer, whether the law of the third country of destination guarantees adequate protection in light of the regulations of the European Union. Where appropriate, additional guarantees to those offered by said clauses must be provided. If the controller cannot adopt sufficient additional measures to guarantee that protection, the control authority is obliged to suspend or end the transfer of personal data to the country in question. In particular, this happens when the law of the destination country imposes obligations on the recipient of a transfer of personal data that are contrary to the aforementioned clauses.

Finally, Schrems II decision reinforces the powers of the supervisory authorities regarding the possibility of suspending or prohibiting, where appropriate, a transfer of personal data to a third country based on the standard contractual data protection clauses.

Security and Resilience in eHealth Infrastructures and Services

The development and deployment of AI tools should be carried out within a socio-technical framework which includes technologies, human skills, organizational structures, and regulations, where individual interests and the social good are preserved and enhanced. The eHealth field is no exception; to provide regulatory support for the creation of such a framework, ethical and legal principles are needed that include autonomy, harm prevention, and equity.

Besides, the success of these sets of technologies highly depends on ensuring an appropriate design for the context in which they are applied. On the one hand, this includes structural issues in the settings where these technologies are used, the health needs which are addressed, the available infrastructure, and the ease of use of the technology [30]. On the other hand, a more universal data infrastructure will make developing and scaling software more efficient. In this sense the new European Data Strategy [9–11, 15] launched in early 2020 provides new and important guidelines. At the same time, countries must examine how they protect the privacy of citizen's health data. This includes both data that has traditionally been considered health data and new types of data such as personal activity trackers or geolocation data.

Medical devices, which were traditionally standalone systems, are becoming network-integrated within hospital IT systems and are no longer immune to traditional cyberattacks. At the same time, new technologies are implemented faster than security systems can be created or updated to protect them. For this reason, security is now a primary concern as healthcare systems are becoming vulnerable to security incidents. These issues range from malware that compromises systems integrity and patient's privacy to distributed denial of service attacks, what hinders patient care. In the health field, these attacks pose unique challenges as they can have ramifications beyond financial loss and violation of privacy.

In order to avoid the breach of healthcare data, the Health Insurance Portability and Accountability Act of 1996 [3] implemented physical and technical safeguards to ensure sensitive information is protected from cybercriminals. Physical safeguards include workstation use and security, device and media controls, and facility access controls. Technical safeguards include a unique user identification number, emergency access procedure, automatic logoff, encryption, and decryption. However, these safeguards are continuously being breached by cybercriminals. For these reasons, it is crucial for nations to realize how vital their national eHealth systems are and take all necessary measures to protect them. On the one hand, this requires adequate infrastructure for data protection. On the other hand, constant software updates are essential so as to keep up with recent advances and security holes that cybercriminals have exposed. Besides, healthcare providers must be aware of cybersecurity trends and threats as they emerge, including ransomware threats.

The European Union Agency for Cybersecurity (ENISA) has made a series of recommendations [16] regarding security in eHealth which are targeted to member states and operators of critical eHealth infrastructures. Among them, states are advised to conduct an asset identification and a risk assessment to classify their critical eHealth infrastructures and services and develop a national catalogue. In addition, they should introduce clear cyber security guidelines, exchange knowledge and lessons learned, perform an impact/cost-benefit analysis of healthcare cyber security incidents, and use this as leverage for increasing investment on eHealth systems and secure infrastructure. States should also develop incident response mechanisms to bring together healthcare organizations and national cyber security competent centers. Lastly, they should raise awareness among citizens and healthcare organizations about the importance of providing cyber security training to personnel and users.

Moreover, ENISA's report showed that the most important cyber security challenges in eHealth infrastructures and systems are the following.

Systems Availability

It is the basic feature for achieving continuity of electronic healthcare and implies continuous accessibility of critical health information by authorized professionals in order to ensure the best healthcare services. Generally, the more digitized the health sector in a country, the more the health services are affected by interruptions in eHealth infrastructures.

Consequently, network and information system availability are considered to be very critical.

Lack of Interoperability
eHealth infrastructures include many diverse systems and applications interconnected at various scales, i.e., a medical device collecting clinical data can be linked in the same network a computer uses to access the Internet. On the one hand, a core issue for an effective and secure use of health services is to ensure a high level of interoperability and guarantee that information is transmitted safely through individual information systems, health service institutions, healthcare providers, and patients. On the other hand, the recipient's system should be able to use the information received in order to proceed in various actions. The lack of interoperability may also affect the security updates in an eHealth services network. The results of the report outlined that 25% of the survey respondents claimed that there is no interoperability framework in place at their organization.

Access Control and Authentication
One of the greatest vulnerabilities in data security is sharing data between third parties and insiders. Consequently, access control and authentication are key security features in eHealth infrastructures. At the same time, the need to retain a user-friendly system is of great importance since it helps avoiding errors introduced by the user. Besides, providers of health data must be sure that parties who consume data enforce, in turn, access constraints conformant to the purposes under which that data was provided.

Data Integrity
It is key to ensure quality and integrity of the data that is stored and exchanged as mistakes in personal or clinical data may affect a person's medical treatment, insurance, or employability. These errors are often related to incorrect entry by staff.

Network security
Network security becomes critical when the security of other critical assets relies on the security of the network. One of the main vulnerabilities of an eHealth network is the inadequate firewall, and external attackers are considered to be one of the major threats.

Security Expertise and Awareness
Security practices by personnel are considered a source of potential problems and appear to be a significant challenge, as in some countries the human factor is considered the most important cause of security incidents. Thus, it is of high importance to ensure that the security architecture and all the respective procedures and measures that must be followed are well designed, understood, and applied by all relevant stakeholders in an organization.

Data Loss
Digitalization of information and eHealth services imply that a significant amount of vital, personal, and confidential data is stored in digital format. Therefore, protection of data from loss is very important. Common causes of data loss are unauthorized access to clinical patient data by IT providers and by healthcare organizations and the backup policy.

Standardization, Compliance, and Trust
One of the main concerns in attaining security in eHealth infrastructures is the proper use and persistence to create, maintain, and enforce an interoperability framework so that integrated systems contribute to cost reduction in eHealth.

Cross-Border Incidents
The challenges that should be tackled in order to facilitate transferability of data in cross-border healthcare are mainly related to building a common interoperability and access control and authentication framework.

Health Data Management for AI

Despite the cybersecurity challenges in eHealth, AI has the potential to expand access to care, improve health outcomes, create more efficient work processes, and lower costs. To do this, proper data management is essential. In this line interoperability of health data is essential, and possible existing biases must be carefully examined prior to the implementation of AI as the system behavior might diverge depending on the region and the population and its recommendations may influence final decisions differently.

On the one hand, for effective data management, it is necessary that users are trained in both knowledge and possible limitations of the software. On the other hand, continuous training of the people who work with the system is necessary. Education on data and AI and how to assess the system is essential for deploying safety AI tools.

Surveillance is also key for an effective management of data. This includes analyzing the supply chain so as to optimize supply chain movement and the potential to mine health records and social media to look for adverse reaction signals.

Besides, having a digital data infrastructure is also critical. For efficient use of the system, data must be structured, standardized, and accessible to innovators. At the same time, privacy concerns around digitalizing and consolidating health information should be seriously considered, and data should be protected from cyberattacks. Special attention should be given to ensure that all patients have complete and unbiased health records. In the meantime, countries should support research so as to understand how health data may be biased, so this information can be used when designing, testing, and evaluating AI products [25].

Health data might change substantially depending on where and when, on whom and by whom, and for what purpose it was collected. Structured and unstructured data can be completely different depending on national or regional standards, insurance requirements, local workflow norms, and other factors. This means that data can be so heterogeneous, and consequently, some changes to an AI system might have to be made depending on how data is defined, formatted, and stored.

Finally, when managing data, it is key to always have in mind people's fundamental rights together with the aforementioned principles that must be followed when collecting, processing, and transferring personal data.

Conclusion

In conclusion, the use of cutting-edge technologies in the field of health implies many monumental challenges. However, the benefits of these set of technologies are much greater. We should continue rethinking how we use and manage data to redefine healthcare without losing sight of the principles of confidentiality, security, privacy, transparency and fairness, and the protection of people's fundamental rights. In order to achieve these aims, having a digital data infrastructure is crucial as well as taking all the necessary measures to prevent cybersecurity attacks. A proper harmonization of regulatory framework on data and on the way interoperability of data needs to work is needed at international level. AI cannot be seen as an end in itself but as a means that should serve to increase people's well-being. For this, AI has to have a human-centered approach, which allows generating the trust of people, in relation to the results that the system produces. AI must be developed so that people are its center, which implies that systems must be subject to the following principles: (i) algorithmic transparency; (ii) algorithmic traceability or explicability; (iii) maximum algorithmic access, and (iv) algorithmic non-discrimination. Making predictions or even more simple data automated elaboration with improperly designed tools can, in fact, lead to erroneous and, in many cases, ethically incorrect decisions.

References

1. Amnesty International. COVID-19: surveillance and threat to your rights, official page available at: https://www.amnesty.org/es/latest/news/2020/04/covid-19-surveillance-threat-to-your-rights/. 2020.
2. Cabrol M, González N, Pombo C et al. Roberto Sánchez a., ethical and responsible adoption of artificial intelligence in Latin America and the Caribbean, Fair Lac BID, p. 14. 2020. https://publications.iadb.org/publications/spanish/document/fAIr_LAC_Adopci%C3%B3n_%C3%A9tica_y_responsable_de_la_inteligencia_artificial_en_Am%C3%A9rica_Latina_y_el_Caribe_es.pdf. Accessed on 17 Jan 2021.
3. CDC. Health Insurance Portability and Accountability Act of 1996 https://www.cdc.gov/phlp/publications/topic/hipaa.html. 2015. Accessed 17 Jan 2021; European Union Agency for Network and Information Security. Security and Resilience in eHealth. https://www.enisa.europa.eu/publications/security-and-resilience-in-ehealth-infrastructures-and-services. Accessed 17 Jan 2021
4. Corvalán J. Perfiles digitales humanos. La Ley, Buenos Aires: Thomson Reuters; 2020.
5. Corvalán J. Perfiles digitales humanos. La Ley: Buenos Aires; 2020. p. 105.
6. Corvalán JG. Perfiles digitales humanos. La Ley: Buenos Aires. p. 114.
7. Council of Europe. European Ethics Charter on the use of artificial intelligence in justice systems and their environment. 2018. https://campusialab.com.ar/wp-content/uploads/2020/07/Carta-e%CC%81tica-europea-sobre-el-uso-de-la-IA-en-los-sistemas-judiciales-.pdf. Accessed on 17 Jan 2021.
8. Esteva A, Kuprel R, et al. Dermatologist-level classification of skin cancer with deep neuronal networks. Nature. 2017;542:115–8. https://www.nature.com/articles/nature21056 Accessed on 17 Jan 2021.
9. European Commission. Communication from the Commission to the European Parliament, the Council, the European Social and Economic Committee and the Committee of the region, A European strategy for Data. 2020. https://eur-lex.europa.eu/legal-content/EN/TXT/?qid=1593073685620&uri=CELEX%3A52020DC0066. Accessed 17 Jan 2021.
10. European Commission. Communication from the Commission. Guidance on apps supporting the fight against COVID19 pandemic in relation to data protection. 2020. https://op.europa.eu/es/publication-detail/-/publication/f8f4dc8b-80a4-11ea-bf12-01aa75ed71a1/language-en. Accessed on 17 Jan 2021.
11. European Commission. European data protection board. Statement on the processing of personal data in the context of the COVID19 outbreak. 2020. https://edpb.europa.eu/system/files/2021-03/edpb_statement art 23gdpr_20200602_en.pdf. Accessed 17 Jan 2021.
12. European Commission. EU-US Privacy Shield. 2016. https://ec.europa.eu/info/law/law-topic/data-protection/international-dimension-data-protection/eu-us-data-transfers_en#law-enforcement-cooperation-eu-us-umbrella-agreement. Accessed 17 Jan 2021.
13. European Commission. Communication from the Commission. Guidance on mobile applications to support the fight against the covid-19 pandemic with regard to data protection. 2020. https://eur-lex.europa.eu/legal-content/ES/TXT/PDF/?uri=CELEX:52020XC0417(08)&from=EN. Accessed 17 Jan 2021.
14. Indipendent high-level expert group on artificial intelligence. Ethics guidelines for trustworthy AI. 2019. https://ec.europa.eu/newsroom/dae/document.cfm?doc_id=60419. Accessed 17 Jan 2021.
15. European Commission. White Paper on artificial intelligence, Brussels. 2020. https://ec.europa.eu/digital-single-market/en/news/white-paper-artificial-intelligence-public-consultation-towards-european-approach-excellence. Accessed 17 Jan 2021.
16. European Union Agency for Network and Information Security. Security and Resilience in eHealth. 2015. https://www.enisa.europa.eu/publications/security-and-resilience-in-ehealth-infrastructures-and-services. Accessed 17 Jan 2021.
17. Forbes. Can You Sue An Algorithm For Malpractice? 2019. https://www.forbes.com/sites/insights-intelai/2019/02/11/can-you-sue-an-

algorithm-for-malpractice/?sh=688aa8c07013. Accessed 17 Jan 2021.
18. Jellinek. Statement on the processing of personal data in the context of the COVID19 outbreak. 2020. https://edpb.europa.eu/our-work-tools/our-documents/outros/statement-processing-personal-data-context-covid-19-outbreak_en. Accessed 17 Jan 2021.
19. Le Fevre E, Ubaldi B, et al. State of the art in the use of emerging technologies in the public sector. OECD working papers on public governance No. 31. Paris: OECD Publishing; 2019. https://doi.org/10.1787/932780bc-en. Accessed 17 Jan 2021.
20. Lugo R, Maldonado G, Murata C. Artificial intelligence to assist clinical diagnosis in medicine. Rev Alerg Mex. 2014:110–20. https://www.redalyc.org/articulo.oa?id=4867/486755034010. Accessed 16 Oct 2020.
21. Miller D, Brown E. Artificial intelligence in medical practice: the question to the answer? Am J Med. 2017:129–33. https://doi.org/10.1016/j.amjmed.2017.10.035. PMID: 29126825.
22. OECD. Artificial intelligence in society; 2019. pp 87–96. https://read.oecd.org/10.1787/eedfee77-en?format=pdf. Accessed 17 Jan 2021.
23. Pereira D. COVID and data privacy. 2020. https://blog.everis.com/es/blog/tecnolog%C3%ADa/covid-19-y-privacidad-de-datos. Accessed 17 Jan 2021.
24. Rudin C. Stop explaining black box machine learning models for high stakes decisions and use interpretable models instead. Nature. 2019;1:206–15. https://www.nature.com/articles/s42256-019-0048-x. Accessed 17 Jan 2021.
25. Silcox C. Artificial Intelligence in Health Care, Inter-American Development Bank. 2020. https://publications.iadb.org/publications/english/document/Artificial-Intelligence-in-Health-Care-Promises-and-Challenges.pdf. Accessed 17 Jan 2021
26. Tecon. Simplifying technologies: Information security. 2018. https://www.tecon.es/la-seguridad-de-la-informacion/. Accessed on 17 Jan 2021.
27. The New York Times. E.U. court strikes down trans-Atlantic data transfer pact. 2020. https://www.nytimes.com/2020/07/16/business/eu-data-transfer-pact-rejected.html?auth=link-dismiss-google1tap. Accessed on 17 Jan 2021.
28. United States Department of Health & Human Services. Summary of the HIPAA Privacy Rule. 1996. https://www.hhs.gov/sites/default/files/privacysummary.pdf. Accessed 17 Jan 2021.
29. World Health Organization. Global strategy on digital health 2020–2025. 2020. https://www.who.int/docs/default-source/documents/gs4dhdaa2a9f352b0445bafbc79ca799dce4d.pdf?sfvrsn=f112ede5_68. Accessed 17 Jan 2021.
30. World Health Organization. WHO releases the first guideline on digital health intervention. 2019. https://www.who.int/news/item/17-04-2019-who-releases-first-guideline-on-digital-health-interventions. Accessed 17 Jan 2021.

Health Economics, Economic Evaluation and Artificial Intelligence Technology

50

Ijeoma Uchegbu, Yael Rodriguez-Guadarrama, Tiago Rua, Muralikrishnan R. Kartha, Musa Abdulkareem, and Steffen E. Petersen

Introduction

Kenneth Arrow's 1963 seminal paper launched modern health economics by identifying the particular economic problem within healthcare as uncertainty [1]. Since then, health economics has quickly gained popularity in healthcare decision-making [2] with recent applications in guiding health technology development at early stages [3–5]. This chapter introduces health economics and its economic evaluation framework. It outlines the current challenges of the economic evaluation of medical technology (MedTech) and artificial intelligence (AI). Also, it discusses the use of the value proposition as a means to address some of these challenges. The goal of this chapter is to inform the reader of the essential components required for the proper economic evaluation of AI in cardiothoracic imaging.

What Is Health Economics?

Economics is the study of scarce goods and how they are allocated in a particular economy (or market). Therefore, health economics is the study of the allocation of scarce goods within the healthcare market [6]. The healthcare market has unique characteristics which makes the application of economic theory challenging [1]. Firstly, patients (the "consumers") demand health and not healthcare. Therefore, the demand for healthcare is derived, and the presence of significant uncertainty primarily influences it. On the supply side, healthcare is provided by the health system, which, in several countries, has zero cost at the point of care. Such health systems face the dilemma of maximising a particular societal objective (e.g. health outcomes) subject to available (and limited) resources. Committing resources to one disease area or subgroup means it cannot be utilised in another. This concept

I. Uchegbu, MPharmS, MSc · M. Abdulkareem, MSc, PhD
National Institute for Health Research (NIHR) Barts Biomedical Research Centre, William Harvey Research Institute, Queen Mary University of London, London, UK

Barts Heart Centre, St Bartholomew's Hospital, Barts Health National Health Service (NHS) Trust, London, UK
e-mail: i.uchegbu@qmul.ac.uk; m.abdulkareem@qmul.ac.uk

Y. Rodriguez-Guadarrama, BEng, MSc
Wellcome EPSRC Centre for Medical Engineering, School of Biomedical Engineering and Imaging Sciences, King's College London, London, UK

King's Technology Evaluation Centre, School of Biomedical Engineering and Imaging Sciences, King's College London, London, UK

Department of Primary Care and Population Health, Faculty of Population Health Sciences, University College London, London, UK
e-mail: yael.rodriguez@maplehealthgroup.com

T. Rua, MSc, PhD
Covid-19 Vaccination Programme, Guy's and St Thomas' NHS Foundation Trust, London, UK

King's Health Economics, Kings College London, London, UK
e-mail: tiago.duarte@gstt.nhs.uk

M. R. Kartha, MHM, MSc, PhD
King's Technology Evaluation Centre, School of Biomedical Engineering and Imaging Sciences, King's College London, London, UK

King's Health Economics, Kings College London, London, UK
e-mail: muralikrishnan.radhakrishnan_kartha@kcl.ac.uk

S. E. Petersen, Msc, MPH, MD, DPhil (✉)
National Institute for Health Research (NIHR) Barts Biomedical Research Centre, William Harvey Research Institute, Queen Mary University of London, London, UK

Barts Heart Centre, St Bartholomew's Hospital, Barts Health National Health Service (NHS) Trust, London, UK

The Alan Turing Institute, London, UK
e-mail: s.e.petersen@qmul.ac.uk

C. N. De Cecco et al. (eds.), *Artificial Intelligence in Cardiothoracic Imaging*, Contemporary Medical Imaging,
https://doi.org/10.1007/978-3-030-92087-6_50

is known as the opportunity cost, the value of which is unknown in the absence of market prices. However, decisions need to be made about resource allocation, which requires some assessment of the value for money of committed resources [6].

One of the analytical tools available in health economics is economic evaluation. Economic evaluation allows the assessment of value for money through the comparative analysis of the costs and consequences of alternative courses of action [7]. Different types of economic evaluation exist (e.g. cost-effectiveness analysis) depending on how consequences are valued and measured. The increasing financial pressure of funding health systems has led to economic evaluation being widely adopted by agencies around the world as a pragmatic vehicle to inform decisions, particularly to assess the value for money of pharmaceutical technologies. However, the methodological framework developed for the evaluation of pharmaceutics is not well suited to address issues about the evaluation of medical technology (MedTech) and digital health technologies (DHTs). As a result, the economic tools that can be used to provide economic evidence for MedTech and AI-enabled MedTech (MedTech-AI) remain an open area for research.

In the remainder of this chapter, we present an overview of the principles behind an economic evaluation and how these methods inform decision-making. Also, these concepts have been linked to the challenges arising when AI-enabled technologies are evaluated and to the potential avenues to address them by succinctly quantifying their potential value. We will present a case study throughout the chapter to exemplify aspects of the economic evaluation process relevant to the challenges related to the economic evaluation for MedTech and MedTech-AI. The chapter ends with a summary of the requirements for an economic evaluation of MedTech-AI.

Economic Evaluation

General Overview

> *"All models are wrong, but some are useful"*
> *George E. P. Box [8]*

Technological advancements often imply an improvement in output and, hence, health outcomes within the healthcare context. Additional costs are also assumed. In a hypothetical case of a health system with an unlimited budget, the decision would be to choose the most effective alternative. In reality, decision-makers face the difficult task of healthcare allocation under constrained budgets. As a result, decisions are not only based on clinical (or operational) value but also the economic costs [7]. Decision-makers have resorted to the use of economic theory and the concept of allocative efficiency to inform efficient use of healthcare budgets.

As illustrated in Fig. 50.1 (adapted from Drummond et al., 2015) [7], cost and consequences are the conceptual pillars of the components of an economic evaluation.

The provision of healthcare requires the commitment of resources such as health technology and health professionals. Costs are dependent on the care pathways under investi-

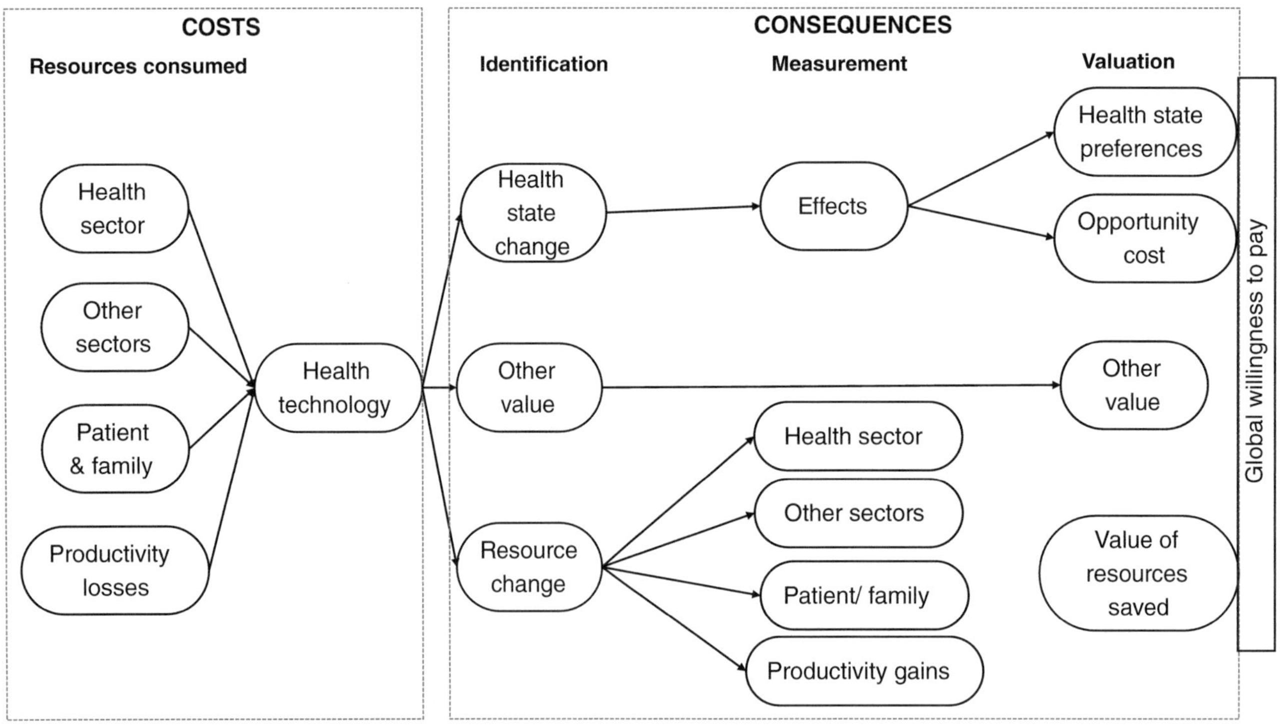

Fig. 50.1 Components of costs and consequences in economic evaluation

gation and the events that may occur as individuals move through these pathways. The identification of resource use depends on the perspective of the evaluation. For example, the perspective of the hospital will concentrate on the healthcare resource use within the acute clinical pathway a patient is cared for. The National Health Service (NHS, i.e. the United Kingdom's publicly funded healthcare systems) perspective would consider costs outside the acute hospital environment to include primary and social care over a time horizon that is appropriate for the disease being evaluated. Sometimes the costs that patients or their families may incur (i.e. additional out-of-pocket expenses such as transportation costs or lost income due to sick days) are essential for the decision-maker. In each case, resource use should be appropriately identified and correctly valued [9].

Similarly, the resulting consequences of adopting health technology must be correctly identified, measured and valued. Consequences of health technologies might have a direct impact on the health state of the target population, create efficiency gains by reducing costs or create value in other areas. Box 50.1 illustrates downstream consequences due to an application of AI to cardiovascular magnetic resonance imaging (CMR) pathways [10].

Box 50.1 Downstream Consequences of AI-Adapted Cardiovascular Magnetic Resonance

Cardiovascular Magnetic Resonance (CMR) Image Quality Control based on AI Image Segmentation Algorithms

Several AI-based quality control tools proposed by researchers rely on image segmentation algorithms to automate the process of identifying problems resulting from the acquisition or image reconstruction process. These AI-based automated quality control tools are capable of using the level of artefacts in a CMR image to categorise the image as having, for example, 'good' 'bad' or 'excellent' qualities. The downstream consequence of improved image quality through the rejection of poor-quality images can lead to improved image analysis and the avoidance of healthcare events such as repeated outpatient appointments and repeated image acquisition. In the economic evaluation of this pathway, probabilities will inform the likelihood of inadequate image quality for the imaging technologies, the likelihood of observing mistakes within the imaging report due to this failure and the likelihood of prescribing the wrong treatment if an inadequate image was used to inform clinical decision-making. Treatment choice will define health outcomes. The value of treatments are often obtained from systematic reviews of the literature and, where required, a synthesis of published data using tools like meta-analysis.

The health economics literature has primarily focused on measures of health state changes. This type of consequences might include gains or losses in mortality and morbidity or intermediate outcomes (e.g. avoidance of adverse effects or improvement in the number of correct diagnoses). The gold standard for the measurement of health state changes is randomised controlled trials (RCTs). It is possible to conduct an economic evaluation within an RCT by simultaneously collecting data on the resource use. Alternatively, health economists use decision analysis to overcome RCT design issues and when multiple sources of evidence are relevant and available to inform a decision of a problem. Decision-analytic models is a simple tool that integrates the available data in a logical and consistent manner. The analysis draws on the probability of events occurring within a clinical pathway to estimate the expected costs and outcomes. These data are derived from clinical research, ideally RCTs. The most frequent model types used are decision trees and Markov chain models [11]. Their use is illustrated in the case study at the end of this chapter.

Types of Economic Evaluation

The economic evaluation framework consists of analytical techniques that utilise the current evidence base for the decision problem being addressed and which differ according to the measurement and valuation of costs and outcomes (consequences). Partial and full economic evaluations exist. An example of partial evaluations, which assess only costs [12], is presented in Box 50.2.

Box 50.2 Considerations When Evaluating Diagnostic Strategies

Diagnostic strategies for coronary artery disease

A cost analysis of two imaging strategies to detect significant coronary artery stenosis in individuals suspected of coronary artery disease (CAD) was carried out by Moschetti and colleagues. The focus of the cost analysis was the diagnostic workup of people with indications for CMR tests within the European CMR Registry. The test strategies were CMR as the gatekeeper for coronary angiography or coronary angiography for all patients. Resource use was quantified according to CMR test output: a positive result led to coronary angiography, a negative result led to no additional tests, and an inconclusive result led to various other tests (stress echocardiography, cardiac CT or SPECT). Cost of each test was based on the setting they were carried out in (i.e., inpatient or outpatient) for each country included in the cost analysis. From the perspective of a department that seeks to reduce the cost of a diagnostic pathway, this analysis is sufficient. For the healthcare system, concerned with planning care for a population, the cost of consequences further downstream is also important. The impact of diagnosis and subsequent treatment and management have not been accounted for in this cost analysis. By focusing on the diagnostic pathway, Moschetti et al (2016) have not included the cost of adverse events and treatment. They have not evaluated the health outcomes that could lead to changes in healthcare resource use during the lifetime of the population. A longer time horizon would account for the reduction in adverse events caused by the unnecessary application of an invasive test, coronary angiography, as well as the health outcomes due to treatments informed by the intervention.

The choice of evaluation method depends on the goal of the analysis. There are five economic evaluations which consider both costs and effects: cost-consequence analysis, cost-effectiveness analysis, cost-utility analysis and cost-benefit analysis. The measurement of costs and consequences by analytical method is presented in Table 50.1.

Table 50.1 Types of economic evaluation according to the measurement of costs and consequences

Type of economic evaluation	Costs	Effects
Cost-consequence analysis	Monetary units	List of multiple outcomes
Cost-minimisation analysis	Monetary units	None – Assumed or demonstrated equal effectiveness to comparators
Cost-effectiveness analysis	Monetary units	Natural (single) unit of effect, e.g. reduction in blood pressure, life years gained
Cost-utility analysis	Monetary units	Life years adjusted for quality of life according to multiple outcomes
Cost-benefit analysis	Monetary units	Monetary units

Cost-consequence analysis (CCA) is a systematic description, measurement and presentation of disaggregated costs and outcomes in their natural units (e.g. blood pressure) [9]. CCA supports clinical decision-makers who use components of the analysis output that best suits the context of their decision problem. This method is increasingly used in the evaluation of MedTech to support decision-making due to variability in infrastructure. One limitation of this type of analysis is that it requires implicit judgements on how to value each component [9]. Cost-minimisation analysis (CMA) is based on an underlying assumption that the two competing alternatives generate the same level of effect; therefore, the analysis focuses on the quantification of costs with the least costly considered best value for money. However, the uncertainty around the estimates of costs and consequences means this assumption is unlikely to hold in all contexts. The preference is for a cost-effectiveness analysis (CEA) so that uncertainty in both costs and effects is addressed. CEA involves the assessment of a single (often clinical) natural unit such as blood pressure to identify the least costly strategy for achieving the objective of the evaluation, e.g. reduction in blood pressure. Cost-benefit analysis (CBA) involves the measurement of outcomes with a common monetary measure [7].

A particular type of CEA referred as cost-utility analysis (CUA) allows the assessment of multiple outcomes by capturing both length and quality of life with the composite measure known as quality-adjusted life years (QALYs). The use of QALYs enables comparison of interventions across the health system. In the calculation of QALYs, the length of time an individual finds themselves in a particular health state is adjusted for the quality of life they obtain in that particular health state. Health states are valued by the population using generic preference-based measures such as EuroQol-5D (EQ-5D) [13]. Valuation of health states and details of the methodology for their estimation are not the focus of this chapter, but a vast critical mass exists in the literature for further details [7].

How Economic Evaluation Informs Decisions

Many countries globally require the economic evaluation of interventions to inform decision-making of their uptake by the healthcare system. However, the context of decision-making differs between countries and depends on how the healthcare system is financed and organised. Systems with single payers such as the UK, Australia and Canada have more readily adopted economic evaluations to centralise health policy [7]. Several agencies and organisations worldwide conduct health technology assessment to determine decisions on adoption and reimbursement of health technology. For instance, in the UK, these agencies include the National Institute for Health and Care Excellence (NICE) in England, the Scottish Medicines Consortium (SMC) and the All Wales Medicines Strategy Group (AWMSG).

Full economic evaluations such as CEA enable the calculation of the incremental costs and outcomes of new health technologies, usually in comparison to current practice. This comparison allows four different outcomes, as illustrated in the cost-effectiveness plane shown in Fig. 50.2.

Straightforward decisions occur in two situations: (i) adopt "dominant" new technology when it is cheaper and more effective than usual care (South-East quadrant, SE) and (ii) reject the new "dominated" technology when the new technology is more expensive and less effective than usual care (North-West quadrant, NW). In the South-West (SW) and North-East (NE) quadrants, a decision rule is needed as decisions are value judgements on what clinical effectiveness we buy or lose for an increase or decrease in the unit of cost, respectively. Exceptional circumstances lead to the adoption of less expensive and less effective interventions, as observed in the SW quadrant. Therefore, economic evaluation tends to focus on the problem of paying more for more effect in the NE quadrant. A favourable decision is made if the extra benefits outweigh the additional costs incurred by the new technology. Hence, the technology is adopted if the ratio between difference in costs and outcomes, the incremental cost-effectiveness ratio (ICER), lies below a cut-off value (the decision rule). This cut-off is the cost-effectiveness threshold (the dotted line in the cost-effectiveness plane; see Fig. 50.2). The UK's NICE, for example, makes decisions utilising a cost-effectiveness threshold ranging between £20,000 and £30,000 per additional QALY gained for the adoption of pharmaceutical products.

Decision rules are the engine that operationalises the cost-effectiveness framework. What the cost-effectiveness threshold should reflect has been subject to extensive discussion. Some authors argue that the cost-effectiveness thresh-

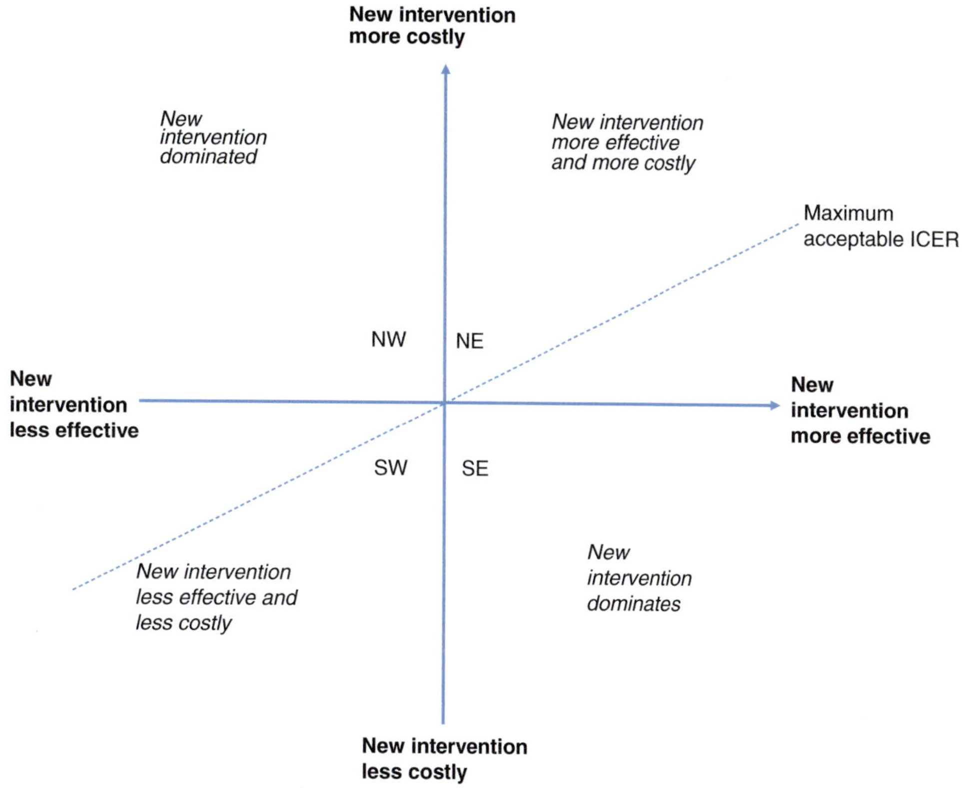

Fig. 50.2 Cost-effectiveness plane

old ought to represent the opportunity cost of the health displaced by the extra costs attributed to the new technology [14]. To this end, the opportunity cost could be interpreted as the rate at which growth in the healthcare expenditure is converted into gains in health outcomes.

Challenges of Economic Evaluation of Artificial Intelligence

One Fit for All Economic Evaluation Framework?

In an ideal world, decision-makers could assess the costs and outcomes of all interventions and rank them by their net benefit. The decision then would consist of implementing as many of the most effective interventions and technology as possible up to the exhaustion of a defined budget constraint [15, 16]. Considerations are hampering this approach. Firstly, it requires information availability of the costs and benefits of all existing and new initiatives within the healthcare portfolio. Secondly, such an approach implies that the measurement of the impact of all interventions is in a single standard outcome metric. This is the most prominent and most crucial limitation as not all healthcare interventions have a direct link to clinical outcomes or health-related quality of life measures, the preferred measurement of impact. While this link between pharmaceutical products and their impact at different outcomes often exists as a consequence of well-designed trials, it is harder to establish such a connection in the case of MedTech [17].

Furthermore, decision-making in a healthcare context is fraught with uncertainty. Three types of uncertainty exist in an economic evaluation: variability, heterogeneity and methodology. Variability describes how the outcomes of individuals vary, while heterogeneity describes the known differences between individuals. Uncertainty in methodology refers to the values used to inform parameters and the model structure or framework [11].

Characteristics of MedTech

The evidence base for the effectiveness of MedTech is limited [18–20]. This is partly due to the less demanding requirements to enter the healthcare market compared to pharmaceutical technologies [21] but also due to difficulty assessing the value of MedTech. For example, the application of a diagnostic tool does not necessarily lead to changes in health outcomes, as this is due to treatment. Figure 50.3 illustrates the evidence required to prove an impact on health outcomes which are attributable to the diagnostic output.

Unlike pharmaceutical interventions, the value of MedTech stems from the ability to reduce uncertainty downstream within a clinical pathway. However, benefits outside the clinical pathway may be realised due to efficien-

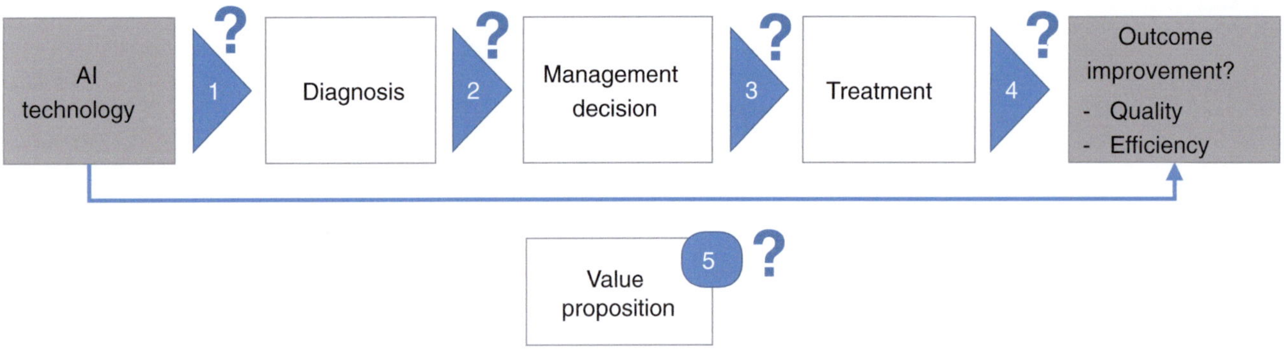

Fig. 50.3 Uncertainty in the assessment of value in the use of a diagnostic tool

cies. The only economic evaluation method to incorporate benefits outside the clinical pathways being evaluated is the disaggregated reporting of CCA.

The MedTechHTA project [22] summarised challenges in MedTech economic evaluation by setting out major features of devices which do not easily lend themselves to the standard analysis methods. These include how the user interacts with the device to generate learning curve effects, the incremental nature of innovation and broader organisational impact. Learning curves complicate the assumptions around the use of MedTech output to inform clinical decisions and, as a result, complicate the assessment of the impact on clinical decision-making and health outcomes. The incremental nature of innovation is infrequently evaluated in clinical trials, and so the added value is harder to decipher while the organisational impact suggests the need for a more flexible costing approach that incorporates costs outside of the pathway MedTech is applied to.

Challenges in AI-Enabled MedTech

Challenges are more pronounced when MedTech AI is concerned. For example, the learning curve is not only present between the user and the device but also the device and the data it trains on – the impact of the latter less easily managed if the learning is unsupervised. The incremental nature of innovation can be company- or data-driven, and broader organisational implications may need to consider the infrastructure requirements necessary to enable such innovative technology to be utilised within a clinical environment. We could regard AI as a health system transformation lever rather than individual technological devices. This change in perspective impacts on technical, clinical, human and cognitive (patient and clinician), professional and organisational, economic, legal and ethical [23] aspects. While some proposed methods exist to evaluate health system changes [24], there still are significant challenges to generalisability as this type of interventions is often context-dependent. So, data trained on for an AI solution may not be relevant for its use in all contexts.

Guidance for the Economic Evaluation of AI-Enabled MedTech

Several publications highlight the underlying differences between MedTech and pharmaceutical products and the evident need for adequate economic evaluation frameworks to correctly measure value in the former [17, 19, 25]. Nonetheless, the literature of methods to overcome such issues is scarce [23]. A study that assesses the status quo of HTA guidelines across Europe found that only four countries have issued official guidance on the recommended analysis to appraise medical devices [26]. Furthermore, the Expert Panel on Effective Ways of Investing in Health, set up by the European Commission, was requested to provide opinion on how to evaluate the overall impact of digital health technology, where AI was included, upon the health system. The Expert Panel's recommendations similarly pointed to the need for adapting the existing evaluative framework to capture the real impact of these technologies [27].

One of the few countries that have generated a reference case for MedTech is the UK. In 2009, the UK's NICE, which produces guidance and other resources to inform health policy, created the Medical Technologies Evaluation Programme (MTEP). This programme was the result of a technical consultation seeking to improve adoption of MedTech in the UK's National Health Service (NHS) [18]. Unlike other NICE methods guide, the MTEP does not state a particular study design as the preferred source of evidence [28]. NICE encourages the use of CCA as the primary analytical

Table 50.2 Economic evidence standards for digital health technologies, NICE Evidence Standards Framework

Economic analysis level	Risk to the payer	Analytical approach
Basic	Low	Budget impact analysis
Low financial commitment	Medium	Cost-consequence and budget impact analysis
High financial commitment	High	Cost-utility/cost-consequence and budget impact analysis

approach to enable the disaggregated reporting of economic and clinical benefits. This recommendation is more flexible than recommendations for technologies that have an impact on health outcomes.

More recently, NICE developed a framework of effectiveness and economic evidence standards within a tier-based system as part of the pilot programme for evaluating digital health technology (DHT) within the UK's NHS. Evidence tier 1 corresponds to DHTs that provide system services such as the referral and scheduling of appointments. Evidence tier 2 comprises DHT that is used to inform, monitor and communicate. Lastly, tiers 3a and 3b are formed by DHTs that are used to provide preventative, behavioural change and self-manage interventions and to treat, actively monitor, diagnose or to calculate, respectively. The framework for economic standards was set as an aid to promote a consistent and systematic guideline to properly quantify the economic impact of DHTs. The framework revolves around three core concepts: (1) economic information, (2) value proposition and (3) appropriate economic analysis.

Along with the correct identification of the information, a value proposition assessment should be carried out to identify the most relevant type of economic analysis feasible. The standards framework indicates that the level of economic analysis should match the financial commitment for the NHS linked to the risk that it poses to the payer (see Table 50.2) [29].

Value Proposition Framework

The use of value propositions by those who inform health policy suggests an interest in clarifying what value should be expected of new DHT. Recent publications have sought to illustrate the potential uses and opportunities of AI and ML techniques throughout radiology pathways. A myriad of ways in which ML techniques can transform clinical environments have been identified [30, 31]. Much of the potential value is the automation of tasks within radiology pathways to release clinician time for other duties and reduce the time taken to complete tasks. Box 50.3 summarises some areas of potential value for cardiothoracic pathways according to Moore et al. (2020) [30].

Box 50.3 Identifying Value According to Impact

Potential value of AI within a cardiothoracic context

Within cardiothoracic imaging pathways, Moore et al. (2020) listed the value of several potential AI applications that impact patient care. For example, the application of ML to improve scanner utilisation reduces waiting times through better time allocation for different procedures and patients with characteristics that require more attention. This reduces revenue loss due to missed appointments. In the optimisation of image acquisition, quality can be preserved with ML whilst reducing the radiation dose. Additionally, the positioning of patients – patient centring – has been improved by AI, leading to a lower amount of radiation. Automated quality assessment removes the need for a technologist to review images before the clinical review by the radiologist, thereby reducing the need for reattendance for rescanning for low-quality images. Moore et al. (2020) also highlighted the role of ML in diagnosis through detection, quantification, characterisation, and follow-up of findings. The ability to prioritise abnormal scans reduces the time to diagnosis for patients at high risk.

These applications improve processes that inform the diagnosis, treatment, and management of patients, and increase the likelihood of positive outcomes. These process (intermediate) outcomes are challenging to assess in health economic evaluations due to the difficulty in attributing health outcome to these applications.

Value has been described as the health outcomes achieved per monetary unit spent [32]. To enable the identification of value within CMR imaging pathways, researchers in the USA used data from Medicare reimbursement to identify five categories of clinical impact due to CMR data: (i) results in a new diagnosis, (ii) avoids the need for an invasive procedure, (iii) avoids the need for further "layered" testing, (iv) results in a minor change in clinical management or (v) no difference in clinical outcome [33].

Figure 50.4 illustrates five domains of value to consider in AI-enabled technologies applied to imaging which has been adapted from a report by PricewaterhouseCoopers about the value of AI in healthcare [34]. These domains go further than the five categories of clinical impact above as it enables the demonstration of value within different elements of healthcare. The first four domains reflect the continuum of care across the NHS, ranging from the prevention of disease and health promotion up to the ongoing treatment of known clinical conditions. The fifth domain reflects the transformational capabilities of AI in the context of research and innovation.

The above domains of value enable the development of a value proposition for technology to support the identification of appropriate methods for economic analysis as the areas of clinical impact, and hence data requirements, are explicit.

In marketing, a value proposition is defined as an innovation, service or feature that makes a company or product attractive to the customer [35]. Some argue the value proposition must move beyond the articulation of solely the business, economic and clinical values. Ethical, professional and cultural values should also be taken into account along with the usability and acceptance of new technology [36]. This

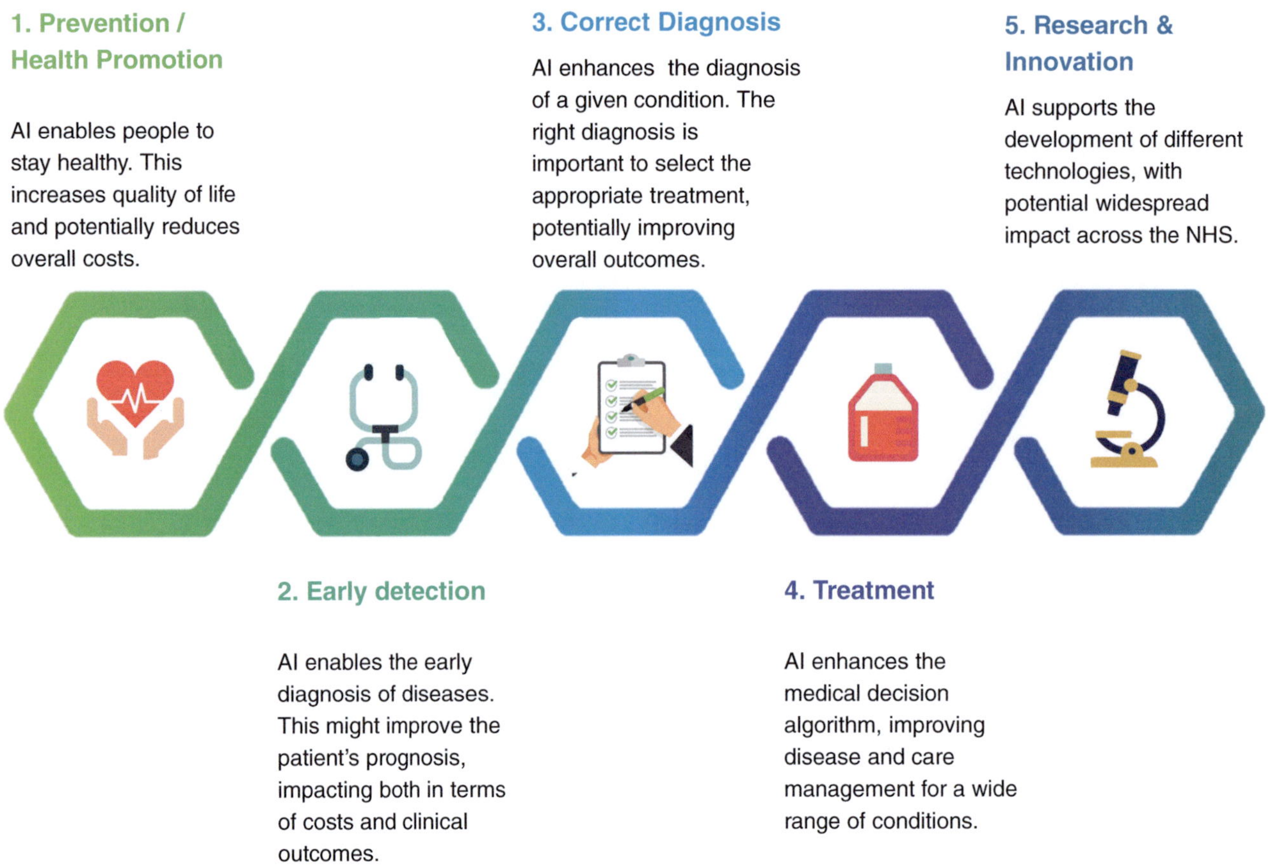

Fig. 50.4 Five domains of value where AI is transforming healthcare

view mirrors the challenges in the evaluation of medical devices summarised by various researchers [25, 37]. These challenges include, but are not limited to, data quality issues, the learning curve of healthcare professionals, the ability to measure long-term outcomes and the broader impact these technologies have on the organisation [37]. It is clear that without the use of a transparent framework, we may not fully realise the benefits of new technologies.

Table 50.3 sets out examples of AI/ML applications to CMR imaging and the real-world benefit if the proposed AI/ML applications come to fruition. The aim is to illustrate the first step of creating the value proposition – assigning value to the healthcare impact.

Table 50.3 illustrates the variety of ways MedTech can bring value within a real-world context. It highlights the need to systematically identify areas of impact and the value that can be achieved. Frameworks such as presented in Fig. 50.4 and utilised in Table 50.3 ensure the development of a value proposition that considers a more global assessment of value. With this information, health economists can better model and address evidence requirements for economic evaluation, thereby generating evidence of the true cost-effectiveness of MedTech such as MedTech-AI within cardiothoracic imaging pathways.

Economic Evaluation of Artificial Intelligence-Enabled MedTech

Published Literature

Economic evidence of AI-enabled MedTech remains limited within the published literature. Wolff et al. (2020) conducted a systematic review aiming at identifying literature assessing AI technologies deployed in the healthcare industry and reported that only six papers fulfilled the inclusion criteria, mainly, a detailed description of the technology under scrutiny and transparent reporting of economic outcomes. The research also analysed the quality of the six papers based on the description of the analysis performed, hypothesis formulation, cost perspective, whether or not comparators were included, calculation of the net present value of the technology and verification of the base case. Whereas all studies describe the analysis performed and state the perspective

Table 50.3 Real-world benefit of AI application to CMR imaging

Dimension of value	Proposed AI/ML application to CMR	Proposed real-world benefit, i.e. value propositions of AI/ML application
Prevention/ health promotion	• ML techniques to improve subgrouping a heterogeneous patient population	• Improved stratification to appropriate preventative treatment • Slowing down of disease progression • Improved prognosis
Correct diagnosis	Referral and scheduling	
	• AI-based decision support tools for the selection of appropriate imaging modality [31, 38] • Suggest appropriate cardiac imaging test [31] • Estimate pre-test likelihood [31]	• Reduces need for unnecessary downstream diagnostic testing • Reduces the need for repeat testing • Reduces exposure to contrast and radiation • Reduces time to test
	Image acquisition	
	• AI-optimised image reconstruction [31, 38]	• Uses less ionising radiation • Increases image quality • Reduces the number of inconclusive results
	Image analysis	
	• Automatic image segmentation and quantification [31] • Flag incidental findings [31]	• Reduces inter-operator variability in decision-making • Increases the chance of appropriate clinical decision-making.
	Image reporting	
	• AI-supported description of findings [31] • Likelihood of differential diagnoses [31] • Reporting diagnostic and prognostic information [31]	• Reduces incorrect diagnoses • Reduces inappropriate healthcare use due to incorrect diagnosis • Reduces adverse events due to inappropriate treatment • Increases likelihood of treatment being appropriate
Treatment and treatment management	• Development and update of clinical decision support systems using all available information including cost-effectiveness data	• Improved stratification to appropriate treatment • Improves management • Reduces frequency of acute events
Research and innovation	• Combining diagnostic and clinical data to the following: Predict prognosis Inform clinical guidance Identify unmet needs for new innovation	• Addresses unmet need within clinical pathways • Increases innovation in health care • Improves health outcomes in the general population

adopted, none of the studies carried out a full economic evaluation; in fact, all the six cases only conducted cost analyses of AI-enabled MedTech products. The researchers also highlight that none of the studies included the development and operational costs for the implementation of AI technologies.

Other examples which were not reported in the literature review of Wolff et al. (2020) arrived at a similar conclusion. A targeted literature review identified eight additional studies containing economic evidence of AI-enabled technologies. Of these, only one study reports the use of a full cost-effectiveness analysis [39]. For the study reported, the authors assessed an AI-enabled platform to monitor treatment of tuberculosis versus directly observed therapy from a healthcare perspective in the USA. While details of the type of analytical approach (cost-utility analysis through decision modelling) and results of the base case and scenario analyses are provided, other information, such as a description of the intervention and the comparator, are limited as the study is a conference abstract. The remaining studies only reported the assessment of cost [40–45]. Some studies conducted model-based minimisation analysis [40–42, 45, 46]. Still, only one study quantified the difference in healthcare resource utilisation after the implementation of an AI-based app to classify and manage patients according to risk [44]. The majority of the cost-minimisation studies assess AI technologies as a first-line diagnostic to guide subsequent management. In all cases, the use of AI leads to a cost reduction. Nonetheless, the type of evidence utilised to inform the analyses came from either observational data or feasibility studies.

NICE evaluated three technologies as part of a brand-new pilot programme for evaluating digital health technology. Of these, only one included an AI component. The technology consisted of a remote cardiac monitoring service to detect cardiac arrhythmias. The recordings are analysed by an algorithm that produces a technical report with recommendation on the diagnosis. The technology submission included a cost-consequence model in the absence of data capturing clinical outcomes. While NICE acknowledged the technology might be cost-saving, the final recommendation considers entities that choose to use it should collect more data to resolve uncertainty around long-term costs and consequences [47].

Case Study Summary

The case study below summarises the information required to plan the economic evaluation of AI in cardiac pathways (Table 50.4). The rationale for model selection is also included.

Table 50.4 Information required to plan the economic evaluation of AI in cardiac pathways

Context and unmet need	Risk prediction tools are essential for the prevention of cardiovascular diseases (CVD). Several risk prediction tools exist, and each has its limitations, and different algorithms may only be suitable for a given population [48]
Decision problem	*Is an AI-based CVD risk calculator more cost-effective than its equivalent classical statistics-based CVD risk calculator for the prediction of CVD events in a healthy population?*
PICO	Population: Healthy population over the age of 40 Intervention: The CVD risk calculator developed using non-adaptive machine learning (ML) algorithms (ML-CVD) Comparator: Statistics-based CVD risk calculator (S-CVD) Outcomes: CVD events including MI, stroke and stroke death (note: Both calculators use the same factors (input variables) to compute CVD risk)
Value	Areas of value: Prevention/health promotion Reduction in the incidence and prevalence of CVD and CVD-related events in the population Reduction in healthcare resource use Early detection Reduction in disease severity, therefore a change in health state and an increase in quality of life Increased survival and quality of life Reduction in healthcare resource use Correct diagnosis Increase in accuracy of CVD risk prediction Increase in appropriate treatment Reduction in inappropriate treatment Reduction in healthcare resource use Treatment Increased survival and quality of life Research and innovation Treatment data informs adaptation of algorithm
Evaluation methods	The value domains show multiple areas of impact. Cost-utility analysis will capture the multiple areas of impact by assessing change in survival and quality of life according to events following testing and in the health states to be evaluated

Table 50.4 (continued)

<table>
<tr>
<td>Model</td>
<td>
The clinical efficacy study that informs this case study has a short time horizon, and so a decision-analytic model is required to combine data from different sources to extrapolate to the lifetime of the population
First the population must be stratified according to test results. The decision tree in the below figure stratifies individuals according to test output and quantifies the costs and outcomes of each diagnostic strategy

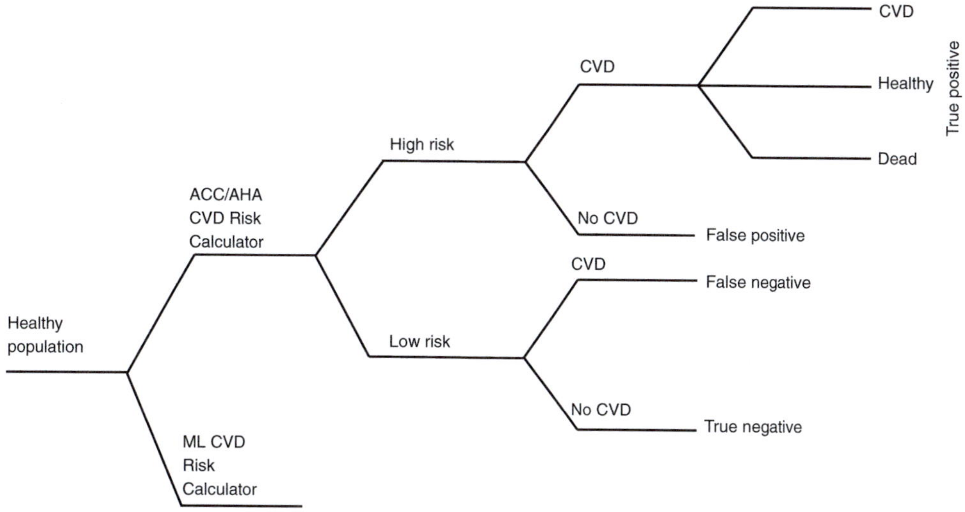

Illustration of decision tree for CVD stratification

In the interest of space, the outcome branches (CVD, healthy and dead) are presented for only one of the four test accuracies (true positive) and stratification for only one of the two interventions
The decision tree incorporates the areas of value identified in the prevention, correct diagnosis and treatment value domains. Individuals are stratified according to test results. Health outcomes and cost of care are dependent on the accuracy of the test output. Rules (based on literature or expert opinion) can be made to allocate health outcomes and healthcare resource use according to test accuracy. For example, in this case study, quality of life is worst for those who have a CVD diagnosis during their lifetime (true positive and false negative), and a reduction in quality of life is required for patients who are treated inappropriately (false positive)
A limitation of the decision is its inability to assess long-term impact without the tree becoming unwieldly. To assess long-term impact on cost and consequences of recursive events, a Markov chain model can be used to quantify costs and consequences. In the below Figure, an individual remains in the "healthy" state for each cycle of the model (e.g. 1 year) until they have their first CVD event or die from CVD- or non-CVD-related causes

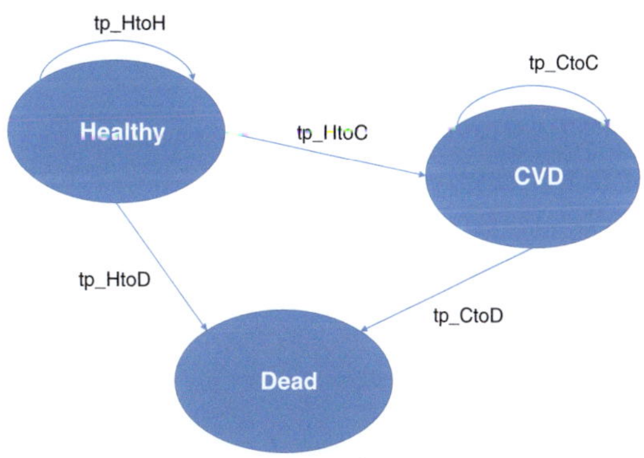

Illustration of an analytical model for decision-making

State transmission probabilities inform the probability of remaining in the same health state or moving to a different health state in each cycle, for example, transmission probability from healthy to CVD (tp_HtoC)
Each health state is associated with specific healthcare resource use and quality of life enabling the costs and consequences of the treatment decisions stratified by the decision tree to be calculated
Evidence requirements for this evaluation include diagnostic accuracy studies to link clinical decision-making to diagnostic output for both technologies and clinical effectiveness studies
– Preferably, randomised controlled trial to reduce bias – To link the clinical decision to health outcomes, i.e. risk of CVD in the presence/absence of preventative treatment
The cost-effectiveness of new technology can now be assessed.
</td>
</tr>
</table>

Summary

In summary, the goal of health economics is to support the allocation of scarce resources within a healthcare environment. Economic evaluations are a set of analytical tools which differ according to the outcomes being assessed and allow the assessment of alternative courses of action under budget constraints. Outcomes can be natural units such as blood pressure or life years saved but can also be quality of life measurements which inform resource allocation across a health system. MedTech evaluation, particularly when married with AI software, is challenging due to difficulty linking output with health outcomes. This difficulty is due to general characteristics of MedTech and the many applications of AI within health and care systems. Health policy organisations such as the UK's NICE have addressed this problem by recommending cost-consequence analysis as the preferred economic evaluation method. To support the identification of evidence to inform this disaggregated economic method, NICE also recommends the use of value proposition to determine the health economic analysis most suitable for the evaluation problem. In this chapter, we have presented value domains within a value proposition framework, which identify types of clinical value. This has supported the identification of appropriate economic evaluation methods in a case study showing that the value proposition of an intervention can play a role in setting research priorities in the area of MedTech and AI, support the design of future trials of MedTech-AI and enable better health economic evaluation of MedTech-AI.

References

1. Arrow KJ. Uncertainty and the welfare economics of medical care. Uncertainty in economics. Elsevier; 1978. p. 345–75.
2. Culyer AJ, Newhouse J. Handbook of Health Economics. Elsevier; 2000.
3. Vallejo-Torres L, Steuten LM, Buxton MJ, Girling AJ, Lilford RJ, Young T. Integrating health economics modeling in the product development cycle of medical devices: a Bayesian approach. Int J Technol Assess Health Care. 2008;24(4):459–64.
4. Ijzerman MJ, Steuten LM. Early assessment of medical technologies to inform product development and market access: a review of methods and applications. Appl Health Econ Health Policy. 2011;9(5):331–47.
5. Hartz S, John J. Contribution of economic evaluation to decision making in early phases of product development: a methodological and empirical review. Int J Technol Assess Health Care. 2008;24(4):465–72.
6. Folland S, Goodman AC, Stano M. In: Abingdon O, editor. The economics of health and health care. 7th ed. New York, NY: Routledge; 2016.
7. Drummond MF, Sculpher MJ, Claxton K, Stoddart GL, Torrance GW. Methods for the economic evaluation of health care programmes. Oxford University Press; 2015.
8. George EPB. Science and statistics. J Am Stat Assoc. 1976;71(356):791–9.
9. Gray A, Clarke PM, Wolstenholme JL, Wordsworth S. In: Gray A, Briggs A, editors. Applied methods of cost-effectiveness analysis in healthcare. Oxford University Press; 2010.
10. Robinson R, Valindria VV, Bai W, Oktay O, Kainz B, Suzuki H, et al. Automated quality control in image segmentation: application to the UK biobank cardiovascular magnetic resonance imaging study. J Cardiovasc Magn Reson. 2019;21(1):18.
11. Briggs A, Claxton K, Sculpher M. Decision modelling for health economic evaluation. Oxford University Press; 2006.
12. Moschetti WE, Konopka JF, Rubash HE, Genuario JW. Can robot-assisted Unicompartmental knee arthroplasty be cost-effective? A Markov decision analysis. J Arthroplast. 2016;31(4):759–65.
13. Brazier J, Ratcliffe J, Saloman J, Tsuchiya A. Measuring and valuing health benefits for economic evaluation. Oxford University Press; 2016. p. 2016–2.
14. Ochalek J, Lomas J, Claxton K. Estimating health opportunity costs in low-income and middle-income countries: a novel approach and evidence from cross-country data. BMJ Glob Health. 2018;3(6):e000964.
15. Stinnett AA, Paltiel AD. Mathematical programming for the efficient allocation of health care resources. J Health Econ. 1996;15(5):641–53.
16. Epstein DM, Chalabi Z, Claxton K, Sculpher M. Efficiency, equity, and budgetary policies: informing decisions using mathematical programming. Med Decis Mak. 2007;27(2):128–37.
17. Drummond M, Griffin A, Tarricone R. Economic evaluation for devices and drugs--same or different? Value Health. 2009;12(4):402–4.
18. Campbell B, Dobson L, Higgins J, Dillon B, Marlow M, Pomfrett C. A new health technology assessment system for devices: the first five years. Int J Technol Assess Health Care. 2017;33(1):19–24.
19. Campbell B, Campbell M, Dobson L, Higgins J, Dillon B, Marlow M, et al. Assessing the value of innovative medical devices and diagnostics: the importance of clear and relevant claims of benefit. Int J Technol Assess Health Care. 2018;34(4):419–24.
20. Keltie K, Bousfield DR, Cole H, Sims AJ. Medical technologies evaluation Programme: a review of NICE progression decisions, 2010–2013. Health Policy Technol. 2016;5(3):243–50.
21. Rothery C, Claxton K, Palmer S, Epstein D, Tarricone R, Sculpher M. Characterising uncertainty in the assessment of medical devices and determining future research needs. Health Econ. 2017;26(Suppl 1):109–23.
22. Tarricone R, Torbica A, Drummond M. Group ftMP. Key recommendations from the MedtecHTA project. Health Econ. 2017;26(S1):145–52.
23. Alami H, Lehoux P, Auclair Y, de Guise M, Gagnon MP, Shaw J, et al. Artificial intelligence and health technology assessment: anticipating a New level of complexity. J Med Internet Res. 2020;22(7):e17707.
24. Meacock R. Methods for the economic evaluation of changes to the organisation and delivery of health services: principal challenges and recommendations. Health Econ Policy Law. 2019;14(1):119–34.
25. Tarricone R, Torbica A, Drummond M. Challenges in the assessment of medical devices: the MedtecHTA project. Health Econ. 2017;26(Suppl 1):5–12.
26. Blüher M, Saunders SJ, Mittard V, Torrejon Torres R, Davis JA, Saunders R. Critical Review of European Health-Economic Guidelines for the Health Technology Assessment of Medical Devices. Front Med. 2019;6(278)
27. De Maeseneer J. European expert panel on effective ways of investing in health: opinion on primary care. Primary health care research &amp. Development. 2015;16(2):109–10.
28. Green W, Hutton J. Health technology assessments in England: an analysis of the NICE medical technologies evaluation Programme. Eur J Health Econ. 2014;15(5):449–52.

29. National Institute for Health and Care Excellence (NICE). Evidence standards framework for digital health technologies. Available from: https://www.nice.org.uk/about/what-we-do/our-programmes/evidence-standards-framework-for-digital-health-technologies.
30. Moore W, Ko J, Gozansky E. Artificial intelligence pertaining to cardiothoracic imaging and patient care: beyond image interpretation. J Thorac Imaging. 2020;35(3):137–42.
31. Petersen SE, Abdulkareem M, Leiner T. Artificial intelligence will transform cardiac imaging—opportunities and challenges. Front Cardiovascul Med. 2019;6(133).
32. Porter ME. What is value in health care? N Engl J Med. 2010;363(26):2477–81.
33. Hegde VA, Biederman RW, Mikolich JR. Cardiovascular magnetic resonance imaging-incremental value in a series of 361 patients demonstrating cost savings and clinical benefits: an outcome-based study. Clin Med Insights Cardiol. 2017;11:1179546817710026.
34. PricewaterhouseCoopers. No longer science fiction, AI and robotics are transforming healthcare. Available from: https://www.pwc.com/gx/en/industries/healthcare/publications/ai-robotics-new-health/transforming-healthcare.html.
35. Lexico.com. Value proposition 2020 [cited 2020 15/10/2020]. Available from: https://www.lexico.com/definition/value_proposition.
36. Buttigieg SC, Jv H. The conceptualization of value in the value proposition of New health technologies comment on "providing value to New health technology: the early contribution of entrepreneurs, investors, and regulatory agencies". Int J Health Policy Manag. 2018;7(2):186–8.
37. Craig JA, Carr L, Hutton J, Glanville J, Iglesias CP, Sims AJ. A review of the economic tools for assessing new medical devices. Appl Health Econ Health Policy. 2015;13(1):15–27.
38. Siegersma KR, Leiner T, Chew DP, Appelman Y, Hofstra L, Verjans JW. Artificial intelligence in cardiovascular imaging: state of the art and implications for the imaging cardiologist. Neth Heart J. 2019;27(9):403–13.
39. Salcedo J, Rosales M, Nuno D, Suen SC, Chang AH. PIN23 Cost-effectiveness evaluation of artificial intelligence monitoring of active tuberculosis treatment in los angeles county, california: a pilot study. Value Health. 2019;22(Supplement 2):S198.
40. Teferra RA, Grant BJB, Mindel JW, Siddiqi TA, Iftikhar IH, Ajaz F, et al. Cost minimization using an artificial neural network sleep apnea prediction tool for sleep studies. Ann Am Thorac Soc. 2014;11(7):1064–74.
41. Mori Y, Kudo S, Misawa M, Saito Y, Ikematsu H, Hotta K, et al. Optical biopsy of diminutive colorectal polyps with real-time use of "artificial intelligence"-assisted endoscopy. United European Gastroenterol J. 2018;6(8 Supplement):A188–A9.
42. Philipsen RH, Sánchez CI, Maduskar P, Melendez J, Peters-Bax L, Peter JG, et al. Automated chest-radiography as a triage for Xpert testing in resource-constrained settings: a prospective study of diagnostic accuracy and costs. Sci Rep. 2015;5:12215.
43. Xie Y, Nguyen QD, Hamzah H, Lim G, Bellemo V, Gunasekeran DV, et al. Artificial intelligence for teleophthalmology-based diabetic retinopathy screening in a national programme: an economic analysis modelling study. The Lancet Digital Health. 2020;2(5):e240–e9.
44. Enriquez A, Dhond MJ, Gill Y, Dhond M, Mancherje C, Breneisen J, et al. Cost savings to medicare by implementing kencor artificial intelligence software: a pilot study of 30 patients. J Investig Med. 2019;67(4):801–2.
45. Zhang C, Paolozza A, Tseng P-H, Reynolds JN, Munoz DP, Itti L. Detection of children/youth with fetal alcohol spectrum disorder through eye movement, psychometric, and neuroimaging data. Front Neurol. 2019;10(80).
46. Xie G, Chen T, Li Y, Chen T, Li X, Liu Z. Artificial intelligence in nephrology: how can artificial intelligence augment Nephrologists' intelligence? Kidney Dis (Basel). 2020;6(1):1–6.
47. [NICE]. NIfHaCE. Zio Service for detecting cardiac arrhythmias (2017). Available from: https://www.nice.org.uk/advice/mib101.
48. Rossello X, Dorresteijn JA, Janssen A, Lambrinou E, Scherrenberg M, Bonnefoy-Cudraz E, et al. Risk prediction tools in cardiovascular disease prevention: a report from the ESC prevention of CVD Programme led by the European Association of Preventive Cardiology (EAPC) in collaboration with the acute cardiovascular care association (ACCA) and the Association of Cardiovascular Nursing and Allied Professions (ACNAP). Eur Heart J Acute Cardiovasc Care. 2019;0(0):2048872619858285.

Commercialization and Intellectual Property of Artificial Intelligence Applications in Cardiovascular Imaging

51

Jaap de Bruin, Nynke Breimer, and Holger Veenhuis

Introduction

Artificial intelligence (AI), and in particular deep learning, is expected to touch every aspect of healthcare in the future, whether improving diagnostics, finding new or more personalized therapeutics, or helping to manage population health [1, 2]. Commercial AI-based applications are entering the clinic, in particular in clinical domains that are traditionally heavily (digital) data driven, such as radiology and cardiology. Between 2015 and 2020, 129 AI/ML-based medical devices were approved in the United States for radiology compared to 40 (non-AI/ML) cardiovascular devices [3]. This uptake and potential of commercial AI propositions is driven by urgent needs in health systems globally, e.g., increased demands on staff such as workload increases in radiology, and unsustainably rising costs [2, 4]. Across the care continuum (Fig. 51.1), opportunities to implement AI propositions are expected to emerge that could help address some of these needs. This potential has not gone unnoticed to the medical industry and venture capital: the number of venture deals in health AI increased fourfold over the past 5 years, and venture funding increased tenfold over the same period [5], a trend that appears not to be at the end of its growth. These developments provide ample opportunities for academia, healthcare providers (HCPs), and industry to collaborate and innovate.

In this chapter, we aim to explore the success factors for commercial AI applications, expand on its development, highlight the role of intellectual property rights in this field, and, lastly, identify what market dynamics we may expect in this industry – in particular the impact on the AI company-healthcare provider relation. We focus on the relevant aspects for cardiovascular imaging but provide a more generic viewpoint where relevant.

Success Factors for Commercial AI Applications in *Cardiovascular* Imaging

As healthcare systems around the globe increasingly align with value-based principles, new applications and commercial propositions are expected to follow the core value principles of driving efficiency (i.e., affordability, capacity), efficacy (i.e., improved outcomes), patient experience, or access to care when it comes to improving *healthcare operations*. Peripheral to healthcare operations, *strengthened research and innovation* and *improvements in population health* are areas of opportunity [6]; refer also to Fig. 51.1 and the examples provided in Box 51.1.

Box 51.1 Examples

AI Improving Healthcare Operations

Echocardiography remains the predominant imaging modality for the timely and cost-effective evaluation of cardiac anatomy and function. However, the acquisition and interpretation of echocardiography remains highly dependent on operator experience [7] and is a repetitive task. AI could improve standardization and quality of care and reduce operational costs, e.g., by providing standardized suggestions for annotations, segmentations, or views. Several AI companies

J. de Bruin, MSc (✉)
Utrecht Health Seed Fund, Utrecht, the Netherlands

Utrecht Holdings, Utrecht University, Utrecht, the Netherlands
e-mail: j.debruin@uu.nl

N. Breimer, LLM, MBA
Global Product Manager Radiology AI & Amplifier Marketplace, Sectra, Linköping, Sweden/Almere, the Netherlands

H. Veenhuis, Dipl.-Phys., Dr. rer. nat.
Eisenführ Speiser, Bremen, Germany

Bremen University, Bremen, Germany
e-mail: hveenhuis@eisenfuhr.com

C. N. De Cecco et al. (eds.), *Artificial Intelligence in Cardiothoracic Imaging*, Contemporary Medical Imaging,
https://doi.org/10.1007/978-3-030-92087-6_51

have been or are developing solutions that (partly) automate the interpretation and annotation of echocardiography, such as Ultromics (EchoGo), Caption Health (Caption AI), and DiA Imaging Analysis (LVivo). Modality vendors like Philips and GE Healthcare (Vivid™ Ultra Edition) are also developing native AI software for their modalities.

AI Strengthening Research and Innovation

Genetic factors are a major risk factor for cardiovascular disease. Heart failure with preserved ejection fraction (HFpEF) is a highly prevalent condition which represents a high cost to the healthcare system. One of the challenges with developing effective therapies for HFpEF has been the substantial phenotypic and pathophysiological heterogeneity in the disease process that may not be well suited for the conventional "one size fits all" approach in therapy. AI technology is particularly well suited to find patterns in complex data and to find distinct phenotypic subgroups [8]. This approach could support and accelerate the development of new therapies, e.g., by identifying new drug targets [9].

AI Improving in Population Health Management

The electrocardiogram (ECG) provides a cost-effective and scalable opportunity to improve population health management [7]. Consumers increasingly have access to wearable ECG devices which unlock an opportunity for screening for underdiagnosed conditions, enabling earlier diagnosis or identifying risks from a certain lifestyle. Examples of wearable developers are KardiaBand (AliveCor), Eko DUO, Apple (Apple Watch), Happitech (AF Detection), and Qardio (QardioCore) [10, 11]. A challenge that remains to be addressed is how to manage and store the large sets of data and incorporate the output in meaningful clinical decision-making and patient pathways, including taking into consideration the impact of false-positive and false-negative results and the potential increase of diagnoses without actionable therapeutic solutions.

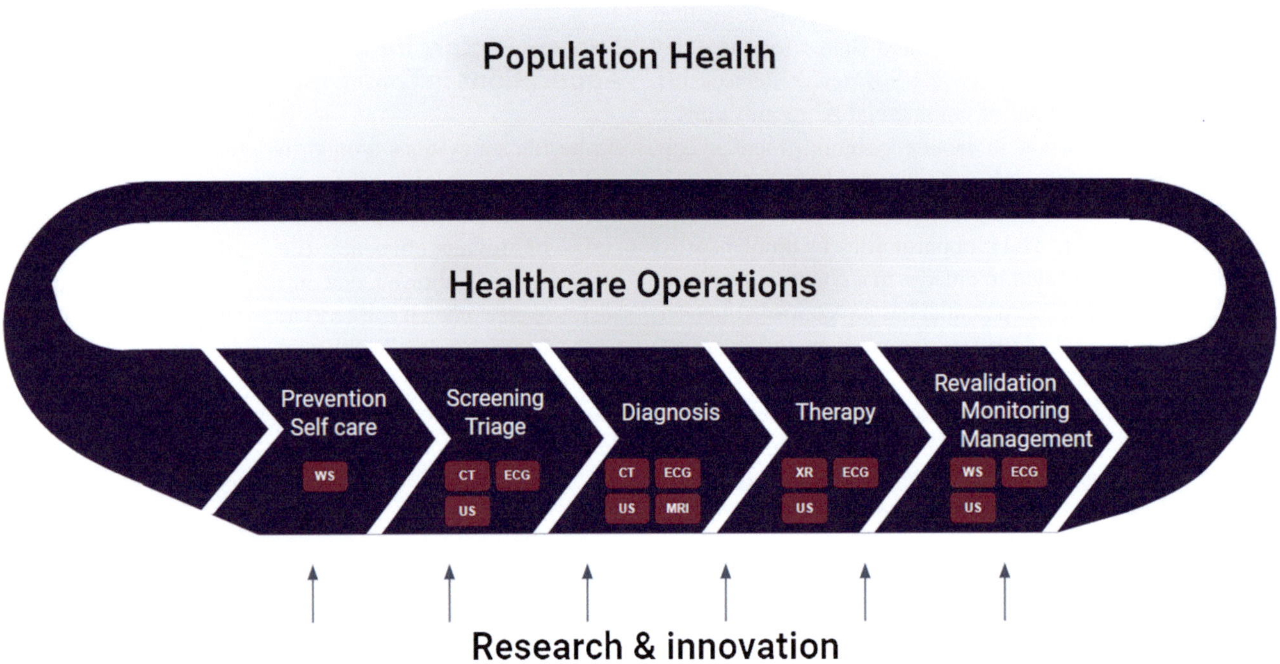

Fig. 51.1 Areas of opportunity for AI in cardiovascular health. Key cardiovascular imaging/sensing modalities are highlighted. WS wearable sensors, CT computed tomography, ECG electrocardiography, US ultrasound/echography, MRI magnetic resonance imaging, XR (interventional/diagnostic) X-ray

Many success factors can be distinguished for scalable, widely adopted commercial AI applications. Propositions that are best positioned to get scalable, fast, and wide adoption are expected to fulfil the following three key criteria.

1. *Proven alignment with value based principles*

The proposition provides *clear*, *proven*, and *direct* benefit(s) from a value-based perspective. Concretely, the proposition should provide an improvement in the following areas: (clinical) outcomes; cost or capacity improvement; patient experience; or access to care. Specifically for AI propositions, it is important to start and define the right use case and determine whether AI is the solution to the identified problem. Second, validation and thereby applicability (or scalability) to various HCPs' patient populations in specific regions is a key prerequisite for scaling: the data on which the application is trained, tested, and validated should be predictive of the performance in a certain patient population. Some have therefore argued that regional clustering of applications related to the accessibility of data may be a likely – or even desirable – result [12]. It should be noted however that the relation between development dataset and performance in a certain population is not always straightforward, e.g., a recent external evaluation of three commercial AI algorithms for screening mammograms on Swedish women population concluded that the algorithm trained on data from an Asian population outperformed the other two, including one that was trained on a Swedish population [13]. Third, evidence regarding the economical impact may be required to convince administrators to invest and adopt a solution, especially if it requires significant change management.

2. *Balanced incentives for payer, beneficiary and user*

The proposition of the AI application has clear and balanced incentives for payer, beneficiary, and user. Users, such as physicians, nursing staff, and care support staff should be incentivized to use and apply the AI application. Payers, such as administrators, policy makers, and/or insurers, will need to get a proper return on investment. A payer-beneficiary relationship is strongest when objectives are aligned and the proposition directly leads to (proof of) improved patient care. An additional complexity is the mix of personas that are part of the purchasing cycle like clinical, administration, and IT. Adoption of AI is still in its early stage; therefore it is important to understand what drives the purchasing decision, since that is the key to move toward the mature and mass adoption stage in this industry. For example, although quality is a high priority for the radiology department, quality improvement alone may not be sufficient to drive software adoption in mature healthcare economies unless direct cost or time savings can also be attributed to the software [14].

3. *Gradual embedding & proper fit in healthcare ecosystem*

The proposition should have a clear fit with and – preferably iterative or gradual – embedding in (a) *existing care structures* and (b) *HCP's technical ecosystems*, to lower the actual and perceived investment required. Potential benefits from AI-supported workflows typically entail new routing and flow of data and patients and therefore require new ways of working and changes in HCP staff routines. Propositions that keep these changes and investments relatively gradual are expected to face lower barriers for adoption.

The second component of fit in the ecosystem, i.e., the technical/infrastructure ecosystem, is equally not to be underestimated. Typically, hospital institutions rely on two main IT solutions: enterprise image management (EIM) and the electronic medical record (EMR). HCPs globally trend toward consolidation and reducing the variety of IT systems and reducing the number of vendor relations accordingly. In cardiology, with the variety of modalities and data, there seems to be more fragmentation compared to radiology; however also here these trends are observed. AI applications often need to fit in and seamlessly integrate in the established systems for availability and easier transfer of results [15] and improved clinical effect [16]. Interoperability between systems in this domain has been driven largely by standardization such as DICOM and IHE. With the entrance of AI, new standards for integration need to be developed [17].

Development of AI Applications in Cardiovascular Imaging

Several phases can be distinguished in the evolution from an AI algorithm to an adopted, established change in the clinic. Some publications have mapped out the different phases of AI application development [2, 18, 19]. Though the terminology differs, the core concepts of development are largely similar. Figure 51.2 provides an overview that will be used throughout this chapter as a general framework.

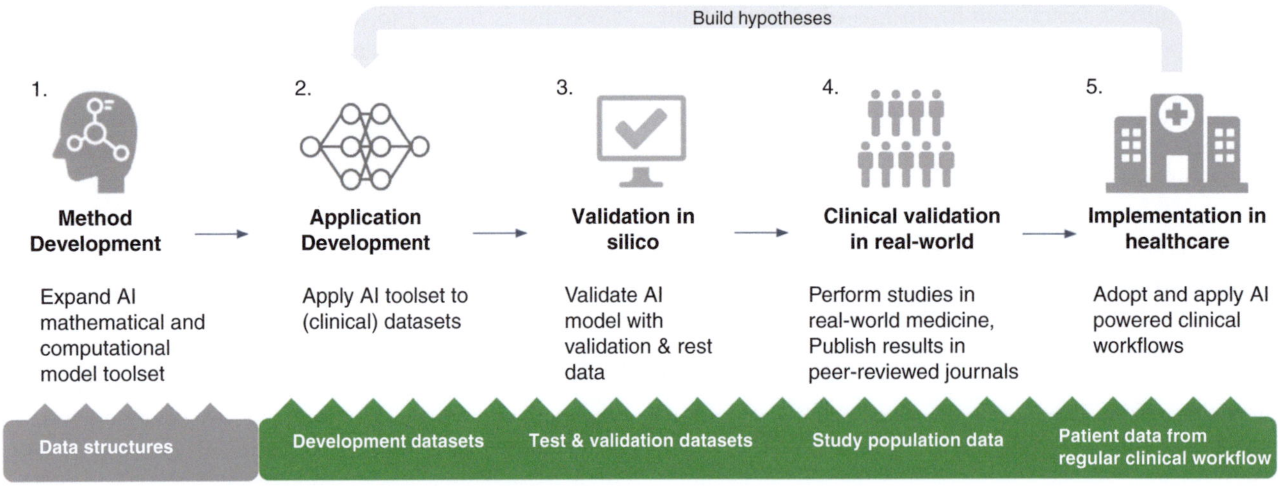

Fig. 51.2 From AI algorithm to changing medical practice – development phases and relevant datasets [19]

Data plays a key role throughout the process, whether that be development and validation datasets to develop an application in the first place, to study population data and finally patient data from the regular clinical workflow.

Method Development

"Method development" refers to the development of the fundamental AI toolset, e.g., mathematical approaches. Method development will not be further discussed here, as this is in the realm of the fundamental mathematical sciences, although hypotheses and challenges in this scientific field are obviously fed by real-world challenges and barriers in other phases of development. Data plays a role in this phase, but only from a proof-of-technical-principle perspective.

Application Development and Validation in Silico

Application development encompasses the proper definition or hypothesis of a proposition, the definition for the right input data and collection of that data (i.e., *development dataset*), and the application of AI tools to the development dataset.

Defining a meaningful use case that ensures benefits for users and payers, creates return on investment for investors and AI companies, and attracts buyers when commercialization takes place is critical and laborious. Successful use case definition depends on the ability to involve multiple stakeholders that understand the cardiology and/or radiology care continuum and the interaction between AI vendors and HCPs. In practice, the multi-stakeholder impact on the targeted care paths should be considered. A common pitfall is that use case development is heavily influenced by what type of data is accessible for the AI application developer. This pitfall can be avoided by starting with "the end in mind," i.e., to assess the implementability and impact in the implementation in healthcare stage as input to the application development [19].

The next stage can be dubbed "validation in silico" [2, 19], i.e., the validation of the AI model in test and validation datasets. Larson and others speak of "feasibility" (performance on a small test on ideal conditions) and "capability" (performance in a controlled environment simulating real-world conditions) as the stages of validation [18].

Clinical Validation in the Real World

Several publications have argued for the proper validation of AI algorithms in the "real world," i.e., recommend prospective studies [2, 18, 19]. Larson dubs this "effectiveness (efficacy)" and identifies two levels of performance:

1. Real-world performance: performance in the clinical environment relative to capability
2. Local validation: performance at a given site relative to capability and established real-world performance

Access to representative is essential datasets for reference and testing that evolve over the lifecycle of the product each time new information is available. For AI companies this can be a major hurdle [17]. The recommendation for prospective studies in the effectiveness phase will impact the time to market and cost of an AI application. In the pharmaceutical industry, this is standard practice, balanced by a significant monetary upside potential. The state of commercialization of current AI applications is in its infancy and hasn't shown this upside (yet) [14]. A longer go-to market cycle, although justified for promoting quality and safety, will typically require a more robust business case in terms of higher profitability. A consequence may be that the current AI applications are "too narrow" in their impact (in terms of efficiency and quality) and it may require the technology to evolve. The lack of highly cited clinical studies that investigate the integration of AI in clinical medicine underscores this point [20]. Nevertheless, prospective studies will most likely be a requirement before major guideline changes are implemented. An example is HeartFlow's FFRCT product, where NICE (United Kingdom) stated that the use of FFRCT may avoid the need for invasive coronary angiography and revascularization, which was concluded after prospective studies like PLATFORM were performed [21, 22].

Alternatively, local validation on a retrospective dataset could be performed to adjust for a patient population with differing disease prevalence, demographic factors, and comorbidities. Academia, AI companies, and developers may develop technical solutions to make this process easy and low cost. Local validation approaches will introduce new challenges, such as the question how guidelines may be altered based on locally proven implementations, rather than a more universal, multicenter level of proof.

Implementation in Healthcare

The last stage, i.e., "implementation in healthcare," is about adoption of AI-powered workflows in the clinic.

Technically, the AI product is to be monitored for its "durability" [18], i.e., performance over time, including quality of the output, monitoring and algorithm "learning," and improvement. Regarding durability, AI companies have the obligation to support their products across its life cycle including adherence to newer types of scanners and extension of geographies and patient populations. This can be a daunting and difficult task to achieve for individual startup AI companies. Monitoring clinical performance (i.e., performance on a local patient population) may be the most challenging task in this context. The Food and Drug Administration (FDA, United States) will work with stakeholders on creating clarity around real-world performance monitoring for AI applications. The FDA's aim is to develop a framework that can be used for seamless gathering and validation of relevant real-world performance parameters and metrics [23].

Clinical adoption is often the most time-consuming and complex task in the commercialization of AI applications, not the least as in most cases AI-powered workflows require a change of way of working of multiple stakeholders or even across organizations. Referrals (from peers and key opinion leaders) are key to make AI solutions mainstream to a wider community. Successful digital transformation requires many elements, such as setting the right (digital) strategy, adapting organizational (infra-)structure, attracting the right capabilities and talent, initiating cultural changes, and adopting an aptitude for testing and learning [24–26].

For the adoption of AI applications, three unique implementation aspects are highlighted. First, the performance of an AI application may be different due to, e.g., a locally different patient or scanner mix compared to the original training and validation data. The reader of the output could encounter built-in bias. Furthermore, there is the risk of "automation bias," meaning that humans start to rely entirely on the output of the application instead of applying their own critical judgment. It is important that end-users gain an understanding of the basic principles, potentials, and limits of AI [27]. Development of this capability is required for a successful transformation process. Second, building trust in the application is key to maximize the impact and usage. AI is a new technology, and for some users it creates a "black box" feeling when reading the outcomes, and especially when an application generates unexplainable outputs (even though accurate), trust might be difficult to gain. Both general AI skills training and specific training on the performance and functionalities of the application are required. Third, AI technology is in its infancy, which has an impact on budget allocation and implementation experience in HCP institutes. Many projects today start as pilot projects driven by enthusiasts or early adopters, and budget allocation and scalability requirements are often considered as an afterthought, reducing the odds for or delay HCP adoption significantly. A dedicated roadmap and strategy for HCPs to implement AI transformation are therefore warranted [25].

Classification and Regulatory Aspects

AI-based cardiovascular imaging software applications are subject to several legislations and regulations, primarily depending on the geography where the application is to be used or sold and the classification in that particular geography. A comprehensive overview of regulations and laws governing these applications is beyond the scope of this chapter. Instead, we aim to pinpoint some of the key aspects that are relevant for health AI applications specifically and refer to other sources for further reading.

Currently, medical, AI-based (commercial) software applications are largely bound to the same scrutiny as non-AI-based healthcare products, i.e., legislation, regulations, and standards [28–30]. Four aspects specific for AI-based applications warrant highlighting in the context of this chapter from a regulatory perspective.

First, healthcare institutions that participate in data collection, labeling, and/or AI algorithm development will be under more scrutiny in the near future, as the boundaries between medical device developer and data supplier become increasingly gray and legislators are putting intensified demands on institutions that are creating their own devices. This is most distinct in the EU, where MDR introduces new legislation regarding "home-brew" medical devices which in practice applies the same legal framework on healthcare institutions as commercial companies with the exception of receiving a CE mark.

Second, AI inherently involves the acquisition, storing, and processing of data; in a way, a deep neural network is a reflection of the data it is trained on. The European Union has been leading in protective legislation with the introduction of the General Data Protection Regulation (GDPR), and other legislative regions are studying how to approach this topic.

Third, ownership of data and the approval to store or process datamay in some cases be diffuse. Requirements for opt-in and opt-out patient consent or mandatory population consent differ per region or even institution. There are geographical variations in who owns the data, e.g., within the United States, there are state-to-state variations in declarations of the ownership of the medical record data ranging from the hospital/physician owning the data to the patient owning the information and gaps that are not addressed at all from a legal perspective [7].

Fourth, regulatory bodies and legislative organizations are currently studying how to approach and adapt regulatory standards to the emerging phenomenon of *continuous learning* devices, i.e., devices that are continuously evolving [31].

The Role of Intellectual Property

Most medical technologies are characterized by high development costs, and AI applications form no exception. Companies and investors therefore seek ways to create and exploit barriers for competitors to their technologies, target applications, and target markets to increase the likelihood of a return on investment. The depth and need for such barriers typically depend on (a) the required *investment depth and horizon*, (b) the *size of the business opportunity*, and (c) the relative *strength of other barriers* to entry to protect the target proposition.

Generally, there are different options for protecting inventions, particularly AI inventions, to create these barriers. In the intellectual property domain, three types of rights are identified to be potentially relevant: copyrights, design rights, and patent rights. With respect to the first, AI inventions like other software-related inventions are protected by copyrights in most jurisdictions. Although a copyright can provide an effective barrier against one-to-one copying of a respective software (e.g., the exact source code), it does not protect the underlying idea and can hence relatively easily be circumvented. With respect to design rights, the design of a

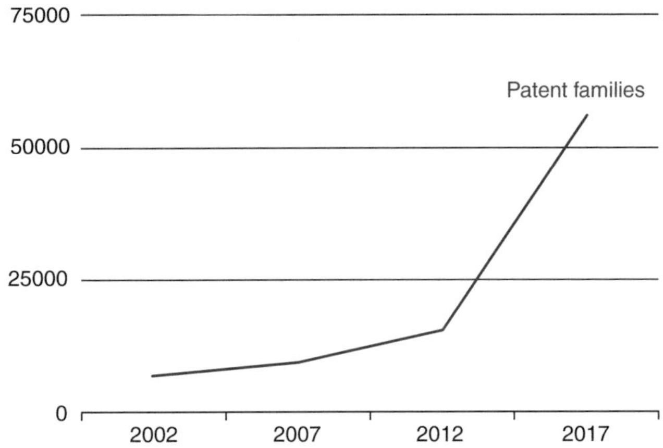

Fig. 51.3 Number of AI patent families over time based on information from the World Intellectual Patent Organization (WIPO) [32]

graphical user interface used by an AI can be protected. However, this does not protect the actual AI invention and therefore is a fairly limited means to create a barrier against competition. Finally, patent rights are well applicable and generally a strong tool for invention protection in the AI domain.

In recent years the number of patents in the field of AI therefore has massively increased. The number of filings of AI-related patent families grew by an average of 28% between 2012 and 2017, as illustrated in Fig. 51.3.

Although AI inventions are well protectable by patents, several challenges have to be met, besides the requirement of being new (*novelty*). To be patentable, the AI invention must be a *technical* invention, i.e., it must have technical features. Moreover, the technical features must be *inventive*, and in several economically important markets the AI invention should *not relate to a medical method.*

In the following sections, it will be explained how these challenges can be met in Europe, the United States, China, and Japan. The general framework will be explained based on the European patent system, and in subsequent sections, the patent systems of the United States, China, and Japan are brought to the fore by pointing to similarities and differences to the European patent system.

European Patent System

Technicity

In the European patent system, software as such is not patentable [33]. Since AI inventions are software inventions, AI inventions as such are hence not patentable. In this context, the term "as such" refers to nontechnical software and therefore nontechnical AI inventions. Conversely, this means that an AI invention can be patented if the AI invention is technical, i.e., has technical character.

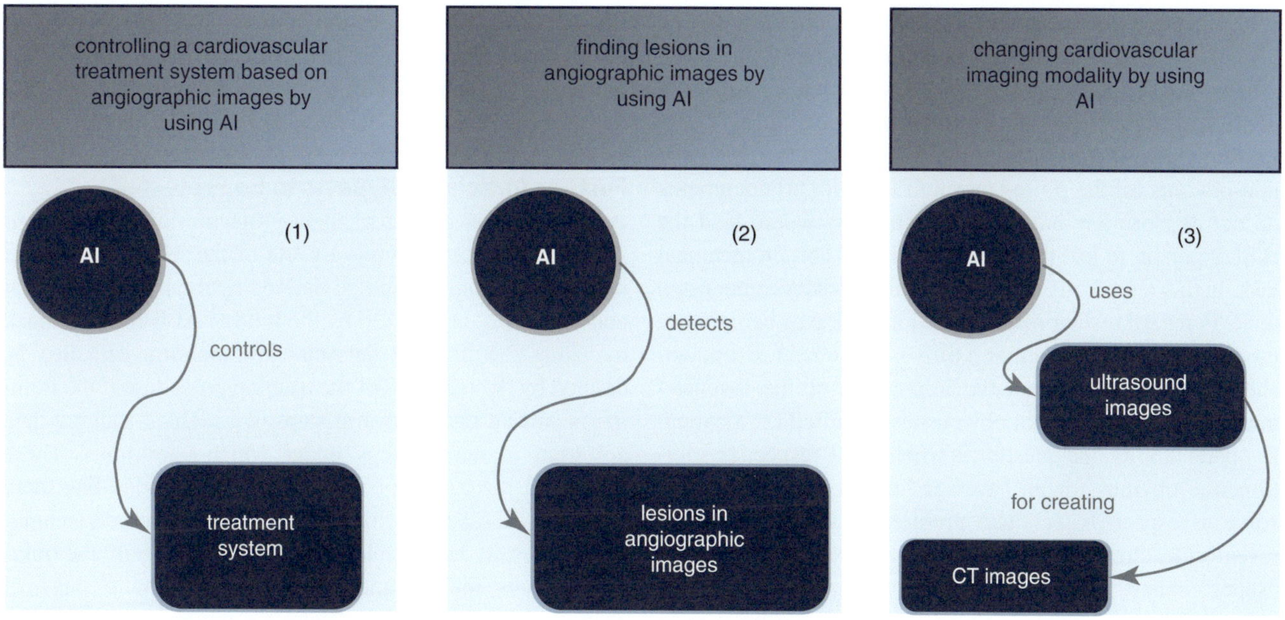

Fig. 51.4 Examples for technicity in AI inventions

An AI invention has technical character if it contributes to producing a technical effect that serves a technical purpose. This technical character can be caused, for instance, by applying the AI to a field of technology and/or by having adapted the AI to a specific technical implementation. The examples below are provided to further clarify.

An AI invention can have technical character due to an application to a field of technology, if the AI controls a specific technical system or process. For example, a cardiovascular imaging system can be controlled using AI, or a system for treating a cardiovascular disease or for assisting a physician in treating a cardiovascular disease can be controlled using AI based on a cardiovascular image (example 1 in Fig. 51.4).

An AI invention can also have technical character if the AI is used for improving the quality of cardiovascular images like in an AI-based denoising procedure; for detecting lesions in cardiovascular images (example 2 in Fig. 51.4); for determining physiological parameters like blood flow values from cardiovascular images; or for image reconstruction. For instance, an AI can be developed to reconstruct a cardiovascular magnetic resonance (MR) or computed tomography (CT) image based on acquired MR or CT raw data, respectively. Technical character could also be lent by using AI for changing a medical imaging modality, for instance, using AI for reconstructing a cardiovascular image having MR or CT characteristics based on ultrasound images (example 3 in Fig. 51.4).

An AI invention can also have technical character due to its specific technical implementation, if, for instance, the AI has a certain structure which is especially suitable for carrying out a technical task and/or for being used on a certain computer having certain characteristics. For example, if a neural network is used as AI, the layer structure of the neural network can be configured such that the respective technical task like finding a lesion in a cardiovascular image can be carried out very efficiently, i.e., for instance, with a very low amount of misclassifications, particularly if the neural network is used in a specific computer structure.

Inventiveness

A second major requirement for patentability is that the technical elements of the AI invention must be *inventive*. Inventiveness means that the invention should not be obvious to a person skilled in the art, given the existing published prior art [34]. It is of crucial importance that the developing company, university, or institute (in the following referred to as "developing entity") does not publish the AI invention before having filed a patent application. If the developing entity publishes the AI invention before filing a corresponding patent application, the developing entity creates prior art so that the AI invention is not even novel and can no longer be patented.[1]

An invention will not be considered inventive if it only replaces a human or known computational expert solving a certain technical problem by an AI expert (i.e., by an expert using AI). In order to be non-obvious, it requires more than

[1]This also refers to China. However, in the United States and Japan, "grace periods" exist, which define that within 12 months before filing a patent application, an applicant's own disclosure is not novelty destroying.

solely using a generally known AI. For example, it can be inventive to use an AI having a certain structure if it is non-obvious for the skilled person to use this certain structure for the technical problem that the invention is directed at.

Applying a certain AI to a certain technical task could be non-obvious for the skilled person if the prior art documents do not disclose any indication which really would lead the skilled person to use the certain AI for the certain technical task. In this regard it is noted that an inventor/developer often tends to regard his/her respective AI invention as being obvious, because for the inventor it truly is obvious. A distinction should be made between the impression of the inventor/developer and the level of obviousness required for a patent. For patentability, the question is whether the respective solution was obvious for an "average" expert, who intends to solve a respective technical problem, wherein the actual inventor/developer is not an "average" expert but often a "super" expert. Moreover, the inventive step must not be assessed by ex post facto analysis. For a person, who already knows the AI invention, it may seem to be obvious, but without knowing the AI invention it would more likely be regarded as being non-obvious and hence inventive.

Medical Methods

In the European patent system, medical methods are generally excluded from patentability [35]. However, this exclusion from patentability does not include systems, apparatuses, and computer programs. The general exclusion of medical methods can therefore be addressed by directing the patent to the apparatus/system comprising the AI and the software/hardware in which the AI has been implemented. Since what will actually be sold by the developing entity is not the AI method, but the AI apparatus/system and/or AI software/hardware, not being allowed to patent the AI medical method is in practice not a huge disadvantage.

Moreover, not any "medical" method is a medical method in accordance with patent law, i.e., not any medical method is excluded from patentability. A few examples are provided to illustrate this. For instance, a diagnostic AI method must be practiced on the human or animal body to be excluded from patentability, wherein, for instance, an AI method directed to finding lesions in a cardiovascular image is not practiced on the human or animal body but on the cardiovascular image. In addition, to be excluded from patentability because of being a diagnostic method, also the last step of a diagnostic method, i.e., assigning an outcome of previous method steps to a particular clinical picture, must be part of a respective claim to be patented [36]. Thus, diagnostic AI methods can be patented, if the last step of such a method, i.e., for instance, assigning the outcome to being a lesion or not, is omitted. Also a surgical AI method like controlling a surgical procedure by using AI based on, for instance, a cardiovascular image can be patentable, if a respective method claim does not comprise an invasive step representing a substantial physical intervention on the body which requires professional medical expertise to be carried out and which entails a substantial health risk even when carried out with the required professional care and expertise [37].

Further AI-Related Aspects to Be Protected

A different viewpoint for patent protection of AI inventions is to focus on the training aspects of the AI algorithm. For instance, the training can be defined by the training datasets and optionally in addition by the kind of AI which is trained by using the training datasets. The training can also be defined by the structure of the training procedure if the training is carried out in several steps, e.g., which training data are used in which steps under which conditions. These aspects of the training can be patented, provided that there are technical features which are inventive. However, technicity is generally less problematic, because typically the training datasets include measured data, data with physical characteristics, or simulated data, wherein the simulated data are the result of a simulation of a measurement. As to the inventive step, the training of the AI with the respective training dataset and the respective kind of AI must not be obvious for the skilled person, given the published prior art, in order to be inventive, as explained in Sect. Inventiveness.

Often, AI is included in a feedback system, i.e., while the AI is in use, it is further trained based on results which are obtained by its normal intended use. For instance, if the AI has been trained and is used already for finding lesions in cardiovascular images, the results of finding the lesions in the medical images can be used for further training the AI. For such training, a quality measure can be used, wherein the quality measure indicates the quality of the respective result of finding the lesions in the cardiovascular images. This quality measure can be automatically determined based on further information from, for instance, physical measurements, databases, user input, etc. Such a feedback system can be patented in addition to the AI itself. For example, different functions of the feedback system can be distributed over different components at different locations, wherein this distribution might be patentable, the used specific quality measure can be patentable, etc. Obviously, such a feedback system must satisfy the criteria of technicity and inventiveness.

The training aspects as discussed in this section will generally not collide with the exclusion of medical methods, as they are inherently not directed at a medical aspect of the AI invention.

Patent System of the United States

With respect to the requirement of *technicity*, the US Patent and Trademark Office of the (USPTO) used to be, in comparison to the European Patent Office, less restrictive. This changed with the US Supreme Court decision on Alice Corporation Pty. Ltd. v. CLS Bank International in 2014, which led to a shift toward the European practice and hence to stricter technicity requirements [38]. In particular, the USPTO carries out a test for assessing subject matter eligibility, wherein it is asked whether a claim is "directed to a judicial exception," such as a law of nature, a natural phenomenon, or an abstract idea, and wherein an abstract idea is defined as being either a mathematical concept, a method of organizing human activity, or a mental process. The claim is patent eligible if it is found not to be directed to a judicial exception, wherein, in accordance with the guidelines on subject matter eligibility of the USPTO, a claim is judged not to be directed to a judicial exception if, for instance, the claim recites a practical application of that judicial exception. The AI invention is hence patentable if it is not an abstract idea like a pure mathematical concept but instead, for instance, refers to a practical application. If therefore the AI invention is not just an abstract idea and has technical character as described above with respect to the European patent system, it is generally also patent eligible in the United States.

With respect to *inventiveness*, similar rules apply in the US system compared to the European system. The most important distinction in the context of health AI is that the US system does not exclude patentability for medical methods. Therefore, a technical AI invention, which is inventive, is patentable in the United States, even if it refers to a medical method.

Patent System of China

In China, the technicity requirements are similar to the European requirements. An AI invention must comprise technical features, i.e., it must comprise features solving a technical problem. Moreover, also in China the technical features of the AI invention must be inventive, and medical methods are excluded from patentability, but, for instance, corresponding medical systems and apparatus are patentable.

In China, AI inventions are therefore patentable under conditions similar to the conditions of the European patent system as described in Sect. Inventiveness.

Patent System of Japan

According to Japanese Patent Law, the term "invention" means the "highly advanced creation of technical ideas utilizing the laws of nature" [39]. Hence, also in Japan, the AI invention must comprise *technical features*, wherein the AI invention must also be *inventive*. Moreover, also in Japan medical methods are excluded from patentability, but, for instance, corresponding medical systems and apparatus are patentable.

In Japan, AI inventions are therefore patentable under conditions similar to the conditions of the European patent system as described in Sect. Inventiveness.

Industry Dynamics and AI Company-HCP Relation

Barriers to Market Entry

When it comes to the scaling of medical technologies, healthcare markets generally favor incumbents over newcomers, due to its heavy regulations, its deep investments in clinical and economical evidence, and its long horizons to return on investment (ROI). Indeed, in life sciences and medical devices, the go-to innovation model has been to develop a technology through venturing and seek for an early "exit" (acquisition) – in many cases pre-market. Investors, startups, and corporates alike aim to set up or exploit barriers to entry in their target markets, to protect against market entry, or to increase market share. Most of the levers at AI companies' disposal to protect a certain niche market or technology may not differ from any medical company. Data obviously plays a more important role though, and there is a different strength in each of these protection mechanisms for AI-based products vs generic medical technologies. In the previous section, the use of intellectual property rights as a market barrier were introduced. Here, a broader perspective on the key areas of barriers to entry for AI based applications is given. The following areas are identified.

- *Intellectual Property Rights, in Particular Patents*

  This is extensively discussed in Sect. The Role of Intellectual Property. Trade secrecy (concretely, keeping source code confidential) is used often as a complementary strategy.
- *Access to (High-Quality, Labeled) Datasets, from Diverse Patient Backgrounds and Geographies*

  This is discussed in more detail in Sect. Development of AI Applications in Cardiovascular Imaging. For example, AI development for echocardiography requires large amounts of data with a wide range of characteristics from a variety of ultrasound machines. Furthermore, echocardiography AI research has largely relied on human interpretation as the ground truth despite the inherent human variability in interpretation and measurement [7].
- *Access to Know-How and Data Science Talent*

  Successful development of AI applications is a multidisciplinary team effort; therefore it relies heavily on access to know-how [15]. This applies across the whole development cycle from method development to implementation in healthcare.

- *Clinical Evidence and Regulatory Approval*

  This is discussed in more detail in Sect. Development of AI Applications in Cardiovascular Imaging.

- *Reimbursement and Business Models*

  Business models for clinical AI applications have as of yet not converged. The subscription model seems to be the preferred model for commercializing AI applications, which is fairly new to the medical technology industry [40]. Though early adopters have different funding streams, mainstream adoption will require either reimbursement or a significant effective cost reduction directly for the payer-HCP. Recently, the Centers for Medicare & Medicaid Services (CMS) in the United States approved the first reimbursement in AI medical imaging for the stroke platform (Viz LVO) of Viz.ai. This reimbursement approval is a breakthrough for AI vendors who struggle to get payment for their subscription models. The approval however also brings concerns to the viability of the business model for AI companies and ROI for venture capitalists. Reimbursements are determined by estimates of volume per subscription, and reimbursements may come down as volumes increase in the system [40]. This is sensible on a healthcare system level, but it will be a challenge for AI companies to maintain price levels that provide healthy returns on investment.

- *Access to (Data) Platforms, Standardization, and Network Effects*

  Incumbents have existing customer networks and relationships ("channels"), including existing integrations to EIM and/or EMR systems, which will be key to adoption. The healthcare AI market is currently fragmented, with a high variety of vendors. Although the expectation is that consolidation will take place at some point, there is also an acknowledgment that development of AI applications will require a lot of subject matter expertise and it may be difficult for small- and mid-size companies to build up that expertise for a high number of use cases. Expected is that health institutions will look for "one-stop shops" to purchase and adopt AI applications, since the process of vetting, contracting, and deploying each individual vendor is time-consuming and not feasible for most individual institutions [41]. A variety of vendors like imaging modality vendors (Philips, Siemens, GE Healthcare), EIM vendors (Sectra, AGFA, Fujifilm), visualization vendors (TeraRecon), and workflow (Nuance Healthcare) have announced a marketplace type of offering to provide a one-stop shop. Additionally, standalone marketplaces like Blackford Analysis, IBM Watson Health, Arterys Marketplace, and Incepto have entered the industry. The concern might be that application integration in the existing IT ecosystem of the hospital is not as deep as would be required [14]. Platforms that have a close link or are provided by EIM providers might therefore be best positioned to address this integration concern. These platforms provide an opportunity for AI ventures in terms of access and speed of implementation but may develop into a threat for their ability to command their terms, conditions, and price/margins.

These barriers have an impact on the way AI-based application markets will shape and on the AI company-healthcare provider relationship.

AI Company-Healthcare Provider Relation

Various barriers that were discussed in the previous section require AI companies' access to, or deep interaction with, HCPs and academia. More than traditional medical device development, this creates a larger (inter)dependency between company and healthcare provider(s). This is relevant in the various phases of AI application development. In Table 51.1, an overview is given of the key interdependencies of AI companies and HCPs in the different development phases of AI applications.

As a consequence of these interdependencies, AI companies and HCPs face questions regarding the value that is exchanged and how institutions and actors are incentivized. Several incentives to collaborate are used throughout the industry, such as (but not limited to) royalty payments; lump sum payments; discounts or access to AI products; and research project sponsorships. These incentivizations are as of yet in its early stages, and a plethora of models and valuations are currently seen in AI company-HCP collaborations [27]. Over time, as this field matures and these collabora-

Table 51.1 What AI companies need from academia and HCPs

Development phase	AI company needs from HCP/academia
1. Method development	Academics in engineering and mathematical sciences to develop new AI methods
2. Application development	Know-how to develop the right hypotheses/proposition designs (use cases) Large, high-quality, labeled datasets (technical and clinical expertise, how to extract, and selection of datasets)
3. Validation in silico	Large, high-quality, labeled datasets Ground truth design and execution
4. Clinical validation in real-world medicine	Clinical trials and evidence; economic proof points
5. Implementation in healthcare	Continuous feedback on model performance – including data to improve Investments in infrastructure and change management Early adopter mentality "wanting to try and fail fast"

tions become more commonplace, these models and the valuations are expected to consolidate and converge.

Discussion

AI applications are attracting tremendous interest from clinical-scientific, policy, and industry actors, but commercialization of AI applications is still in its infancy. Cardiology and radiology are fertile breeding grounds for successful and profitable AI development, mostly because these fields are data driven and well-organized. Mainstream adoption is still expected to take its time. The needs in healthcare systems are pressing, however, and developments (clinical, technical, markets, policy) are moving at a fast pace.

Moving forward, defining value and attribution of that value in the development and adoption process of AI applications is important to ensure realistic monetization and definition of the right business models. AI companies, encouraged by their investors, try to appropriate most of the value in the chain. Platform and EIM providers that support adoption and realization of impact in clinical practice, necessary for commercialization, will define their value in this process. How each player will get a return on investment remains to be seen.

A multitude of developments in regulation and registration of medical data is ongoing and will heavily affect the ability to commercialize AI applications in the cardiovascular space. Legislators are facing questions regarding the freedom to opt out or in. HCPs are wrestling with implementation and supplier standardization challenges. The medical research community should strive for the compilation of multicenter datasets that are currently scarce in the field of cardiovascular imaging [15], though several attempts are being made to address this gap. To accelerate the advancement of AI application development, publicly available datasets could form an attractive strategy. In the United States and the United Kingdom, there are ongoing discussions to establish a national database platform that will be mandatory for HCPs. For example, in the United Kingdom, a national COVID-19 chest imaging database is established to support the advancement of diagnosis and treatment of COVID. The NHS AI Lab leverages the project to explore a wider national platform [42].

The ease and speed of mainstream adoption will be dependent on HCPs and national health agencies' and guidelines committees' ability to develop their workforces and adapt their ways of working [43]. Collaboration creates accountability on the medical professionals for both AI development and adoption. Understanding technical and ethical aspects of AI should be part of the medical training, so that clinicians can work in partnership with engineers and clinical physicists to train and improve algorithms [17]. The need for different roles and responsibilities and the way how to work with AI-powered care paths will likely be a topic of study and experimentation in the years to come.

Finally, there is potentially a big role to play for AI in population health management, e.g., in early screening or preventative care. However, many healthcare systems today aren't focused nor incentivized to capture the full value of this opportunity, and commercial activity in this space seems to be lagging the activity in healthcare operations. Patient/consumer ownership most likely will not be enough to capture this, and governments need to consider institutionalizing preventative care. The COVID pandemic might be a catalyst for this process.

References

1. Topol EJ. Deep medicine: how artificial intelligence can make healthcare human again; 2019.
2. Topol EJ. High-performance medicine: the convergence of human and artificial intelligence. Nat Med. 2019;25:44–56. https://doi.org/10.1038/s41591-018-0300-7.
3. Muehlematter UJ, Daniore P, Vokinger KN. Approval of artificial intelligence and machine learning-based medical devices in the USA and Europe (2015–20): a comparative analysis. The Lancet Digital Health, ISSN: 2589-7500. 2021. https://doi.org/10.1016/s2589-7500(20)30292-2.
4. Bruls RJ, Kwee RM. Workload for radiologists during on-call hours: dramatic increase in the past 15 years. {journal}. {year}.
5. CB Insights. https://www.cbinsights.com/research/report/ai-trends-healthcare/.
6. EIT Health/McKinsey. Transforming healthcare with AI: the impact on the workforce and organisations; 2020.
7. Lopez-Jimenez F, Attia Z, Arruda-Olson AM, Carter R, Chareonthaitawee P, Jouni H, Kapa S, Lerman A, Luong C, Medina-Inojosa JR, Noseworthy PA, Pellikka PA, Redfield MM, Roger VL, Sandhu GS, Senecal C, Friedman PA. Artificial intelligence in cardiology: present and future. Mayo Clin Proc. 2020;95(5):1015–39. https://doi.org/10.1016/j.mayocp.2020.01.038. PMID: 32370835.
8. Segar MW, Patel KV, Ayers C, Basit M, Tang WW, Willett D, Berry J, Grodin JL, Pandey A. Phenomapping of patients with heart failure with preserved ejection fraction using machine learning-based unsupervised cluster analysis. Eur J Heart Fail. 2020;22:148–58. https://doi.org/10.1002/ejhf.1621.
9. Schneider P, Walters WP, Plowright AT, et al. Rethinking drug design in the artificial intelligence era. Nat Rev Drug Discov. 2020;19:353–64. https://doi-org.proxy.library.uu.nl/10.1038/s41573-019-0050-3.
10. Ladejobi AO, Cruz J, Attia ZI, et al. Digital health innovation in cardiology. Cardiovasc Digit Health J. 2020;1(1):6–8. https://doi.org/10.1016/j.cvdhj.2020.07.003.
11. Mincholé A, Rodriguez B. Artificial intelligence for the electrocardiogram. Nat Med. 2019;25:22–3. https://doi.org/10.1038/s41591-018-0306-1.
12. Global perspectives on clinical AI. AIMI Happy Hour; Episode 7. https://www.youtube.com/watch?v=I9aW0gIlmtI.
13. Salim M, Wåhlin E, Dembrower K, et al. External evaluation of 3 commercial artificial intelligence algorithms for indepen-

dent assessment of screening mammograms. JAMA Oncol. 2020;6(10):1581–8. https://doi.org/10.1001/jamaoncol.2020.3321.
14. Tadavarthi Y, Vey B, Krupinski E, et al. The state of radiology AI: considerations for purchase decisions and current market offerings. Radiol. Artif Intell. 2020;2(6):e200004. https://pubs.rsna.org/doi/10.1148/ryai.2020200004
15. Weikert T, Francone M, Abbara S, et al. Machine learning in cardiovascular radiology: ESCR position statement on design requirements, quality assessment, current applications, opportunities, and challenges. Eur Radiol. 2020. https://doi.org/10.1007/s00330-020-07417-0.
16. O'Neill TJ, Xi Y, Stehel E, Browning T, Ng YS, Baker C, Peshock RM. active reprioritization of the reading worklist using artificial intelligence has a beneficial effect on the turnaround time for interpretation of head CT with intracranial hemorrhage. Radiol Artif Intell. 2021;3:2. https://doi.org/10.1148/ryai.2020200024.
17. Kotter E, Ranschaert E. Challenges and solutions for introducing artificial intelligence (AI) in daily clinical workflow. Eur Radiol. 2021;31:5–7. https://doi.org/10.1007/s00330-020-07148-2.
18. Larson DB, Harvey H, Rubin DL, et al. Regulatory frameworks for development and evaluation of artificial intelligence–based diagnostic imaging algorithms: summary and recommendations. JACR October 20, 2020. https://doi.org/10.1016/j.jacr.2020.09.060.
19. Tjong FVY. From AI algorithm to clinical practice. 2020. Publication in preparation.
20. Sreedharan S, Mian M, Robertson R, Yang N. The top 100 most cited articles in medical artificial intelligence: a bibliometric analysis. J Med Artif Intell. [Online] 3:0; 2019.
21. HeartFlow FFRCT for estimating fractional flow reserve from coronary CT angiography. National Institute for Health and Care Excellence, Medical technologies guidance [MTG32]. 13 February 2017.
22. The PLATFORM Study: prospective LongitudinAl Trial of FFRct: Outcome and Resource IMpacts) (PLATFORM). https://clinicaltrials.gov/ct2/show/NCT01943903.
23. U.S. Food & Drug Administration (FDA). Artificial Intelligence/Machine Learning (AI/ML) - Based Software as a Medical Device (SaMD) action plan. January 2021. https://www.fda.gov/media/145022/download.
24. Burkacky O, et al. A blueprint for successful digital transformations for automotive suppliers. August 2018. McKinsey. https://www.mckinsey.com/business-functions/mckinsey-digital/our-insights/a-blueprint-for-successful-digital-transformations-for-automotive-suppliers.
25. Shuaib H. During sectra webinar "Implementing AI in clinical radiology", July 2020. https://medical.sectra.com/solutionarea/ai-medical-imaging/.
26. Omoumi P. et al. To buy or not to buy—evaluating commercial AI solutions in radiology (the ECLAIR guidelines). Eur Radiol. 2021. https://doi.org/10.1007/s00330-020-07684-x.
27. Recht MP, Dewey M, Dreyer K, et al. Integrating artificial intelligence into the clinical practice of radiology: challenges and recommendations. Eur Radiol. 2020;30:3576–84. https://doi.org/10.1007/s00330-020-06672-5.
28. Regulation (EU) 2017/745 of the European Parliament and of the Council of 5 April 2017 on medical devices, amending Directive 2001/83/EC, Regulation (EC) No 178/2002 and Regulation (EC) No 1223/2009 and repealing Council Directives 90/385/EEC and 93/42/EEC (Text with EEA relevance.) OJ L 117, 5.5.2017, p. 1–175 (BG, ES, CS, DA, DE, ET, EL, EN, FR, GA, HR, IT, LV, LT, HU, MT, NL, PL, PT, RO, SK, SL, FI, SV) ELI. http://data.europa.eu/eli/reg/2017/745/oj.
29. 21 C.F.R. § 800 - § 1299. https://www.fda.gov/medical-devices.
30. International Medical Device Regulators Forum. IMDRF Management Committee. IMDRF Strategic Plan 2021–2025. September 2020. IMDRF/MC/N39FINAL:2020 (Edition 2).
31. http://www.imdrf.org/workitems/wi-aimd.asp.
32. WIPO. WIPO Technology Trends 2019: Artificial Intelligence. Geneva: World Intellectual Property Organization. 2019. ISBN: 978-92-805-3007-0.
33. Article 52(1)(c) and (3) of the European Patent Convention.
34. Article 56 of the European Patent Convention.
35. Article 53(c) of the European Patent Convention.
36. decision G 01/04 of the Boards of Appeal of the European Patent Office.
37. decision G 01/07 of the Boards of Appeal of the European Patent Office.
38. Alice Corp. v. CLS Bank Int'l, 573 U.S. 208 (2014).
39. Article 2(1) of the Japanese Patent Act.
40. Oakden-Rayner L. It's complicated. A deep dive into the Viz/Medicare AI reimbursement model. 2020. https://lukeoakden-rayner.wordpress.com/2020/09/24/its-complicated-a-deep-dive-into-the-viz-medicare-ai-reimbursement-model/.
41. Leiner T, Bennink E, Mol CP, Kuijf HJ, Veldhuis WB, Bringing AI. To the clinic: blueprint for a vendor neutral AI deployment infrastructure. Publication submitted.
42. https://www.nhsx.nhs.uk/ai-lab/ai-lab-programmes/ai-in-imaging/.
43. Topol E. Preparing the healthcare workforce to deliver the digital future. NHS. 2019. https://topol.hee.nhs.uk/.

Ethical Considerations of Artificial Intelligence Applications in Healthcare

52

Judy Wawira Gichoya, Carolyn Meltzer, Janice Newsome, Ramon Correa, Hari Trivedi, Imon Banerjee, Melissa Davis, and Leo Anthony Celi

Introduction

Traditionally, ethical evaluations and guidelines for advances in medicine have been directed by Institutional Review Boards (IRBs) who provide a structure to evaluate research and clinical trials to ensure patient safety. The recent advances in artificial intelligence (AI) and its expanding adoption in medicine demand new approaches to ethical consideration. This is because the intersection between AI and medicine is increasingly occurring outside academic hospitals that serve as the scope for most IRBs. For example, smart devices are becoming cheaper and more ubiquitous, and many patients now have smart devices that monitor their health. Moreover, small privately held companies and large companies like Apple and Google are rapidly developing AI-driven health applications, including ECG recordings using the Apple Watch [1], consolidating multiple medical records via Apple Health, and the development of a new electronic medical record (EMR) system aggregating data from other digital sources like social media.

The COVID-19 pandemic highlighted the effects of systemic racism on health, as manifested by the disproportionate burden of COVID-19 disease among traditionally marginalized populations, namely, Black and Hispanic groups [2]. This and other disparities should serve as catalysts to rethink how we build AI systems. In an attempt to overcome the barriers of access disruption from COVID-19, there has been rapid adoption of digital technologies including telemedicine and remote patient monitoring [3, 4]. These changes provide an opportunity to rethink what ethical oversight may be needed beyond the traditional IRB structure. Technologies such as AI to track and assess participant engagement for virtual meetings [5] could hypothetically be used to track scores of provider-patient engagement mined to improve hospital Press Ganey scores [6].

Several radiology societies in North America and Europe worked on a statement of Ethics of AI in Radiology with public feedback on the consensus statement [7]. It was clear during the statement writing that there was a need to come up with a framework that would provide practical and actionable points for AI practitioners to adopt. Therefore, the statement was themed around three topics: ethics of data, ethics of algorithms and trained models, and ethics of practice. In this chapter, we describe examples of ethical challenges and opportunities, with a caveat that the rate of change in AI techniques and tools is too fast to comprehensively provide an up-to-date view of the ethical landscape.

Racial Bias in Healthcare Algorithms

One of the most notable works in this space is by Obermeyer, who evaluated a commercial risk prediction tool applied to

J. W. Gichoya, MD, MS (✉) · H. Trivedi, MD
Department of Radiology, Emory University, Atlanta, GA, USA

Department of Biomedical Informatics, Emory University, Atlanta, GA, USA
e-mail: judywawira@emory.edu; hari.trivedi@emory.edu

C. Meltzer, MD · J. Newsome, MD · M. Davis, MD
Department of Radiology & Imaging Sciences, Emory University, Atlanta, GA, USA
e-mail: cmeltze@emory.edu; janice.newsome@emoryhealthcare.org; melissa.a.davis@emory.edu

R. Correa, PhD Student
Department of Biomedical Informatics, Emory School of Medicine, Atlanta, GA, USA
e-mail: ramon.luis.correa@emory.edu

I. Banerjee, PhD
Department of Biomedical Informatics & Department of Radiology & Imaging Sciences, Emory School of Medicine, Atlanta, GA, USA
e-mail: imon.banerjee@emory.edu

L. A. Celi, MD, MS
Institute for Medical Engineering and Science, Massachusetts Institute of Technology, Cambridge, MA, USA

Division of Pulmonary, Critical Care and Sleep Medicine, Beth Israel Deaconess Medical Center, Boston, MA, USA

Department of Biostatistics, Harvard T.H. Chan School of Public Health, Boston, MA, USA

C. N. De Cecco et al. (eds.), *Artificial Intelligence in Cardiothoracic Imaging*, Contemporary Medical Imaging,
https://doi.org/10.1007/978-3-030-92087-6_52

200 million people in the United States [8]. This algorithm was created to improve care for patients with complex needs by enrolling them into high-risk management care programs where they can receive additional resources and care coordination. The algorithm was developed with past data to predict future healthcare needs and was trained using healthcare cost as the proxy for the need for more comprehensive care. It was designed specifically to *exclude* race as a feature to avoid bias — but cost was clearly not a race-neutral measure of healthcare need. It was later found that Black patients were sicker per healthcare dollar spent, meaning that their costs were only lower due to lack of access. These authors created an index variable that combined health prediction with cost prediction, without changing the data or the model, and were able to increase the percentage of Black patient receiving additional help from 17.7% to 46.5% [8].

Prediction algorithms and systems are frequently used in medicine, including the Model for End-Stage Liver Disease (MELD), Child Pugh score, Pulmonary Embolism Severity Index (PESI), Sequential Organ Failure Assessment (SOFA) score, and many others. For example, the American Heart Association Get with the Guidelines-Heart Failure Risk Score [9] predicts the risk of death in patients admitted to the hospital. Clinicians are advised to use this risk score to guide decisions about referral to cardiology and allocation of healthcare resources. It assigns three additional points to any patient identified as "non-Black," thereby categorizing all Black patients as being at lower risk. Since being Black is equated with lower risk, following the guidelines could direct care away from Black patients. Black patients incur approximately $1800 USD less in medical costs per year compared to White patients with the same number of chronic conditions and are less likely to be identified as high risk for complex care in the future [8]. The challenge is that development of such an algorithm would likely still pass ethical review in most IRBs today. This example demonstrates the challenge of problem formulation, which determines the choice of the label on which the algorithm is trained [8].

We recently analyzed racial bias when using ICU scoring systems (OASIS, SOFA, and APACHE IV) across the MIMIC III and MIMIC IV ICU dataset from Beth Israel and the e-ICU dataset [10]. We found no bias in the discrimination of these scores across races. When a patient had a high score, they were very sick, with uniform prediction on illness severity across races. However, the standardized mortality ratio for patients had significant differences across racial groups – with overprediction of mortality for Blacks and Hispanics, compared to Whites and Asians. As states and hospitals developed guidelines for ventilator usage during the COVID-19 pandemic, these scoring systems were adopted to triage ICU bed and ventilator assignments [11]. Since these scores have been shown to overpredict mortality, care could have been diverted away from patients who were higher risk and toward patients who were likely to survive. Calibration of prediction systems occurs at the time of development; adjusting AI algorithms during ongoing use remains a challenge yet is critical to build systems that have low rates of bias.

Bias in healthcare algorithms can arise due to the data used to build the algorithms. Some notable examples in recent publications include the glomerular filtration rate (GFR) [12] and disparities on pulse oximetry measurements [13]. These data are not currently captured by AI but are fed into AI systems, for example, when predicting risk of intubation for patients or using AI to guide ventilator settings. Equations that estimate the GFR from serum creatinine are race-adjusted [14]. Explanations to justify this race adjustment include the notion that Black people release more creatinine into their blood at baseline, in part because they are reportedly more muscular. Race adjustments that yield higher estimates of kidney function in Black patients might delay their referral for specialist care or transplantation and lead to worse outcomes, while Black people already have higher rates of end-stage kidney disease and death due to kidney failure than the overall population. Similar disparities are observed when pulse oximetry (SPO2) values are compared with arterial blood gas O2 levels collected within 10 minutes of each other [13]. In two large cohorts, Black patients had nearly three times the frequency of occult hypoxemia (i.e., an arterial oxygen saturation of <88% despite an oxygen saturation of 92–96% on pulse oximetry) that was not detected by pulse oximetry when compared to White patients. Generalized population cutoffs (e.g., discharge of patients with COVID-19 to home versus admission based on pulse oximetry) can be amplified when AI systems are developed and not adjusted to account for subpopulation differences [15]. At a reading of 88 or 89% for pulse oximetry, Medicare will reimburse for home oxygen [16]; hence amplification of such discrepancies using AI can cause harm to larger groups of patients.

While the above examples focus on individual data components used for AI development and on problem formulation, it is worthwhile to remember that these data are routinely collected in the process of care which is heavily influenced by long-standing social, cultural, and institutional biases [17–19]. In an ideal world, only individual patient health and disease factors would determine — and guide prediction of — clinical outcomes. Unless the underlying inequities in our communities are addressed, algorithms will perpetuate, if not magnify, existing health disparities.

Operationalizing Fairness in Medical AI Algorithms

While the number of studies showing bias in healthcare algorithms has increased, there is a paucity of solutions and strategies to fix these biases. A few studies have reviewed the impact of removing race from the algorithms as well as in data capture [20]. As of this moment, more work is required to evaluate the impact of de-racing datasets. The availability of curated datasets is critical to understand how current algorithms work. A review of datasets being used for machine learning found that AI systems are developed largely on data from 3 states – California, Massachusetts, and New York – and 34 states were not represented in geographically identifiable cohorts [21]. Labeling data are expensive, and alternatives that have been used include using medical students as labelers and Amazon Mechanical Turk workers who have no background in medicine [22]. The cost of making datasets available is expensive, as each image is reviewed by a person to ensure anonymization. Despite several anonymization strategies, new studies show that medical data cannot be fully deidentified [23]. This ethical conundrum will shape medical AI for decades, either by penalizing data sharing which will in turn limit AI testing and validation or by developing new frameworks that preserve the social good gained from the availability of diverse datasets.

Evaluation of bias in medical AI remains largely technocentric, whereby statistical metrics are created for developers to evaluate if their model is biased. Examples of these metrics include true-positive rate (TPR), false-negative rate (FNR), false discovery rate (FDR), and false omission rate (FOR), among others [24]. These metrics require the selection of a reference group – say White patients with pneumothorax – and then comparisons are made in reference to this group. In a fair system, the ratio would be 1. If the ratio is less than - 0.8, the group is negatively affected by the algorithm, while ratio values >1.2 are seen in groups that are positively favored by the algorithm. Laleh et al. analyzed bias in the MIMIC chest X-ray (CXR) dataset and showed that in patients younger than 20 years, Black and/or low-income patients under Medicaid insurance have the largest underdiagnosis rate [25]. These patterns persist (with different magnitude) when we repeat the same experiments in the CheXpert dataset and the Emory CXR dataset, which has an almost equal distribution of Black and White patients. Sustained bias which is not attributable to the dataset size or proportion of disease exemplifies the challenge of operationalizing fairness, with the need to develop new metrics for evaluating and fixing bias in AI algorithms.

Given concerns for intellectual property of commercial algorithms, it is difficult to evaluate model failures. This is further complicated by the black box nature of underlying techniques that use millions of parameters and finetuning. For computer vision tasks in radiology, saliency maps are largely nonspecific and provide little information to explain a model performance [26]. Several studies are currently evaluating algorithmic failure when data distribution shifts out of distribution (OOD), as may occur after a pandemic stabilizes [27]. These techniques are well established for tabular data but are difficult for computer vision tasks like radiology images. OOD in radiology images requires detection of interclass and intraclass classes (i.e., distinguish between a dog picture and CXR, and distinguish between pneumonia and pneumothorax labels on a CXR, respectively). Moreover, publishing and sharing failure is not encouraged, and reporting in IRB approved studies as well as peer-reviewed articles misses this critical component.

There is a need to develop strategies that factor in human-machine interaction. Technocentric approaches do not fully reflect the reality of medical practice. For example, multiple studies have reviewed the burden of the EMR on physicians causing burnout [28]. This is further limited by the narrow nature of AI, which is built to perform a single task. AI is deployed into the healthcare enterprise as a clinical decision support tool, as a second reader (e.g., in the United Kingdom for mammograms), and rarely as a replacement for radiologists (although some venture-funded radiology groups are trying to implement this model). Incentives and penalties can drive AI use, as seen in the case of computer-aided diagnosis (CAD) for breast cancer where the performance of radiologists is better than CAD, yet the use of digital mammograms plus CAD continues to grow due to the additional reimbursement per study [29]. Viz.ai recently approved reimbursement for a workflow for large vessel occlusion that bypasses the radiologist to notify the neurointerventionalist and other members of stroke care [30]. We need to adopt sociotechnical approaches of evaluating AI that support social transparency in how humans work with AI if we are going to make the augmented radiologist better in performance [31]. Focusing on the human allows us to explore the tensions that arise between fairness versus explainability, fairness versus accuracy/performance, fairness versus generalizability, and fairness versus trust.

As algorithms are deployed from one site to another, their performance can drop and fail to generalize to new populations [32]. This is an area that is widely debated, with proponents who argue that algorithms should be allowed to overfit on specific populations without a plan to use algorithms on new populations [33]. This would require for us to move away from a business model where medical AI algorithms are sold and bought. Instead, the business model would be around assisting healthcare organizations to build, deploy, continuously evaluate, and re-calibrate algorithms. Generalizability is a transient concept in healthcare. Medical algorithms, like the findings of clinical trials, have an expiration date.

AI as a Solution to Healthcare Bias

The limitations of available ground truth for AI training have spurred new research using new forms of labeling. For example, Obermeyer used a deep learning approach to measure the severity of osteoarthritis by using knee X-rays to predict patients' experienced pain, which in turn reduced unexplained racial disparities in pain [34]. Their algorithmic prediction score accounted for 43% (or 4.7x) of disparities more than the radiologist score, suggesting that much of underserved patients' pain stems from factors within the knee that are not reflected in standard radiographic measures of severity. This ability of algorithms to see where radiologists are unable to see holds promise for better performance of the augmented radiologist and also a positive impact on population health [35].

Similar results are observed in breast cancer risk prediction AI studies. Classical prediction models have been shown to perform lower among Hispanic and Black Americans [36]. The MIRAI system combines imaging and clinical risk factors to predict 5-year breast cancer risk and outperforms traditional models. Despite better performance, subgroup analysis shows that the risk prediction is poor for Black women with dense breasts and exemplifies the double disadvantage that can occur among minorities. If we limit reporting of statistical performance on whole groups of data without mandatory subgroup analysis, the AI systems we build and deploy will continue to perpetuate bias.

The Future of Ethical AI in Healthcare

The ethical landscape of AI in healthcare is continuously evolving. The work to be done requires interdisciplinary teams and new forms of governance, because the laws cannot keep up with the rate of progress of AI techniques. For example, the transformer language models that power the Internet today require large amounts of computation only available to limited companies and governments [37]. These systems are not available for evaluation to many researchers, and internal organizational ethics teams have been disbanded in companies like Google [38]. Lots of healthcare institutions are adopting a cloud strategy where these same algorithms will be applied to patient data. It may be that power for AI ethics is shifted away from patients and regulators to companies with large computation power, yet we lack the framework to maintain protections in such an environment.

A review of the FDA and published guidelines did not locate any requirements for failure analysis or fairness evaluation [39]. For example, the CONSORT-AI Extension guideline discusses fairness but does not include it in the checklist points [40]. There is no mention of fairness in the SPIRIT-AI Extension [41], STARD-AI [42], or TRIPOD-ML [43] guidelines. The FDA encourages post-market surveillance, yet the approval of these algorithms is such that it requires minimal change without undergoing the approval process again. Even more concerning is the proposal by the FDA to not regulate medical AI [44] and the subtle deployments occurring from existing EMR vendors of algorithms that cannot be audited and are not FDA approved because they are considered decision support tools. Governance structures will be critical to help clinicians and patients reap the promise of AI [45].

Conclusion

The ethical needs of explosive AI technologies are rapidly evolving with no clear regulatory guidelines. Therefore, work to evaluate bias and fairness of medical algorithms requires interdisciplinary work with data science experts, clinicians, algorithm developers, and AI implementers. This interdisciplinary approach informed by various forms of governance will be critical to ensure that patients can benefit from the promise of AI. Ethical review boards for projects that use AI will need to improve to support failure reporting, as well as adapt to encourage data sharing to maintain the social good of having inclusive and diverse datasets.

Acknowledgments We thank Alicia Lillich from the NIH Library service for assisting with manuscript editing.

References

1. Healthcare - Apple Watch - Apple [Internet]. [cited 2021 May 5]. Available from: https://www.apple.com/healthcare/apple-watch/.
2. Wiley Z, Kubes JN, Cobb J, Jacob JT, Franks N, Plantinga L, et al. Age, comorbid conditions, and racial disparities in COVID-19 outcomes. J Racial Ethn Health Disparities. 2021 Jan 7.
3. Golinelli D, Boetto E, Carullo G, Nuzzolese AG, Landini MP, Fantini MP. Adoption of digital Technologies in Health Care during the COVID-19 pandemic: systematic review of early scientific literature. J Med Internet Res. 2020;22(11):e22280.
4. Mosnaim GS, Stempel H, Van Sickle D, Stempel DA. The adoption and implementation of digital health Care in the Post-COVID-19 era. J Allergy Clin Immunol Pract. 2020;8(8):2484–6.
5. AI Can Run Your Work Meetings Now | WIRED [Internet]. [cited 2021 May 6]. Available from: https://www.wired.com/story/ai-can-run-work-meetings-now-headroom-clockwise/.
6. Hospital CAHPS (HCAHPS) | CMS [Internet]. [cited 2021 May 28]. Available from: https://www.cms.gov/Research-Statistics-Data-and-Systems/Research/CAHPS/HCAHPS1.
7. Geis JR, Brady AP, Wu CC, Spencer J, Ranschaert E, Jaremko JL, et al. Ethics of artificial intelligence in radiology: summary of the joint european and north american multisociety statement. Radiology. 2019;293(2):436–40.
8. Obermeyer Z, Powers B, Vogeli C, Mullainathan S. Dissecting racial bias in an algorithm used to manage the health of populations. Science. 2019;366(6464):447–53.

9. Smaha LA. American Heart association. The American Heart Association get with the guidelines program. Am Heart J. 2004;148(5 Suppl):S46–8.
10. Sarkar R, Martin C, Mattie H, Gichoya JW, Stone DJ, Celi LA. Performance of intensive care unit severity scoring systems across different ethnicities in the USA: a retrospective observational study. Lancet Digit Health. 2021;3(4):e241–9.
11. AI used to predict Covid-19 patients' decline before proven to work - STAT [Internet]. [cited 2021 May 6]. Available from: https://www.statnews.com/2020/04/24/coronavirus-hospitals-use-ai-to-predict-patient-decline-before-knowing-it-works/.
12. Diao JA, Inker LA, Levey AS, Tighiouart H, Powe NR, Manrai AK. In search of a better equation - performance and equity in estimates of kidney function. N Engl J Med. 2021;384(5):396–9.
13. Sjoding MW, Dickson RP, Iwashyna TJ, Gay SE, Valley TS. Racial bias in pulse oximetry measurement. N Engl J Med. 2020;383(25):2477–8.
14. Levey AS, Stevens LA, Schmid CH, Zhang YL, Castro AF, Feldman HI, et al. A new equation to estimate glomerular filtration rate. Ann Intern Med. 2009;150(9):604–12.
15. Shah S, Majmudar K, Stein A, Gupta N, Suppes S, Karamanis M, et al. Novel use of home pulse oximetry monitoring in COVID-19 patients discharged from the emergency department identifies need for hospitalization. Acad Emerg Med. 2020;27(8):681–92.
16. National Coverage Determination (NCD) for Home Use of Oxygen (240.2) [Internet]. [cited 2021 May 6]. Available from: https://www.cms.gov/medicare-coverage-database/details/ncd-details.aspx?NCDId=169.
17. Brahmania M, Wiskar K, Walley KR, Celi LA, Rush B. Lower household income is associated with an increased risk of hospital readmission in patients with decompensated cirrhosis. J Gastroenterol Hepatol. 2021;36(4):1088–94.
18. Rush B, Danziger J, Walley KR, Kumar A, Celi LA. Treatment in disproportionately minority hospitals is associated with increased risk of mortality in sepsis: a national analysis. Crit Care Med. 2020;48(7):962–7.
19. Danziger J, Armengol Á, de la Hoz M, Li W, Komorowski M, Deliberato RO, Rush BNM, et al. Temporal trends in critical care outcomes in U.S. minority-serving hospitals. Am J Respir Crit Care Med. 2020;201(6):681–7.
20. Ioannidis JPA, Powe NR, Yancy C. Recalibrating the use of race in medical research. JAMA. 2021;325(7):623–4.
21. Kaushal A, Altman R, Langlotz C. Geographic distribution of US cohorts used to train deep learning algorithms. JAMA. 2020;324(12):1212–3.
22. Preliminary experience with Amazon's Mechanical Turk for annotating medical named entities | Proceedings of the NAACL HLT 2010 Workshop on Creating Speech and Language Data with Amazon's Mechanical Turk [Internet]. [cited 2021 May 6]. Available from: https://doi.org/10.5555/1866696.1866724.
23. Rocher L, Hendrickx JM, de Montjoye Y-A. Estimating the success of re-identifications in incomplete datasets using generative models. Nat Commun. 2019;10(1):3069.
24. Bellamy RKE, Dey K, Hind M, Hoffman SC, Houde S, Kannan K, et al. AI fairness 360: an extensible toolkit for detecting, understanding, and mitigating unwanted algorithmic bias. arXiv. 2018 Oct 3.
25. Seyyed-Kalantari L, Liu G, McDermott M, Ghassemi M. CheXclusion: Fairness gaps in deep chest X-ray classifiers. arXiv. 2020 Feb 14.
26. Arun N, Gaw N, Singh P, Chang K, Aggarwal M, Chen B, et al. Assessing the (un)trustworthiness of saliency maps for localizing abnormalities in medical imaging. medRxiv. 2020 Jul 30.
27. Zimmerer D, Petersen J, Köhler G, Jäger P, Full P, Roß T, et al. Medical out-of-distribution analysis challenge. Zenodo. 2020.
28. Melnick ER, Dyrbye LN, Sinsky CA, Trockel M, West CP, Nedelec L, et al. The association between perceived electronic health record usability and professional burnout among US physicians. Mayo Clin Proc. 2020;95(3):476–87.
29. Lehman CD, Wellman RD, Buist DSM, Kerlikowske K, Tosteson ANA, Miglioretti DL, et al. Diagnostic accuracy of digital screening mammography with and without computer-aided detection. JAMA Intern Med. 2015;175(11):1828–37.
30. Viz.ai Granted Medicare New Technology Add-on Payment [Internet]. [cited 2021 May 6]. Available from: https://www.prnewswire.com/news-releases/vizai-granted-medicare-new-technology-add-on-payment-301123603.html.
31. Ehsan U, Gichoya JW, Riedl M. Reflective human-centered explainable AI: social transparency, trust, and value tensions in radiology. Unpublished 2020.
32. Nestor B, McDermott MBA, Boag W, Berner G, Naumann T, Hughes MC, et al. Feature Robustness in Non-stationary Health Records: Caveats to Deployable Model Performance in Common Clin Machi Learning Tasks. arXiv. 2019 Aug 2.
33. Futoma J, Simons M, Panch T, Doshi-Velez F, Celi LA. The myth of generalisability in clinical research and machine learning in health care. Lancet Digit Health. 2020;2(9):e489–92.
34. Pierson E, Cutler DM, Leskovec J, Mullainathan S, Obermeyer Z. An algorithmic approach to reducing unexplained pain disparities in underserved populations. Nat Med. 27(1):136–40.
35. Gichoya JW, Celi LA. Beyond the AJR: "an algorithmic approach to reducing unexplained pain disparities in underserved populations". AJR Am J Roentgenol. 2021 Apr 28.
36. Barlow WE, White E, Ballard-Barbash R, Vacek PM, Titus-Ernstoff L, Carney PA, et al. Prospective breast cancer risk prediction model for women undergoing screening mammography. J Natl Cancer Inst. 2006;98(17):1204–14.
37. OpenAI's GPT-3 Language Model: A Technical Overview [Internet]. [cited 2021 May 6]. Available from: https://lambdalabs.com/blog/demystifying-gpt-3/.
38. Google fires second AI ethics researcher following internal investigation - The Verge [Internet]. [cited 2021 May 6]. Available from: https://www.theverge.com/2021/2/19/22292011/google-second-ethical-ai-researcher-fired.
39. Wawira Gichoya J, McCoy LG, Celi LA, Ghassemi M. Equity in essence: a call for operationalising fairness in machine learning for healthcare. BMJ health care. Inform. 2021;28(1)
40. Liu X, Rivera SC, Moher D, Calvert MJ, Denniston AK. SPIRIT-AI and CONSORT-AI working group. Reporting guidelines for clinical trial reports for interventions involving artificial intelligence: the CONSORT-AI extension. BMJ. 2020;9(370):m3164.
41. Rivera SC, Liu X, Chan A-W, Denniston AK, Calvert MJ. SPIRIT-AI and CONSORT-AI working group. Guidelines for clinical trial protocols for interventions involving artificial intelligence: the SPIRIT-AI extension. BMJ. 2020;9(370):m3210.
42. Sounderajah V, Ashrafian H, Aggarwal R, De Fauw J, Denniston AK, Greaves F, et al. Developing specific reporting guidelines for diagnostic accuracy studies assessing AI interventions: the STARD-AI steering group. Nat Med. 2020 Jun 8.
43. Collins GS, Reitsma JB, Altman DG, Moons KGM. Transparent reporting of a multivariable prediction model for individual prognosis or diagnosis (TRIPOD): the TRIPOD statement. Ann Intern Med. 2015;162(1):55–63.
44. Artificial Intelligence/Machine Learning (AI/ML)-Based Software as a Medical Device (SaMD) Action Plan [Internet]. [cited 2021 May 5]. Available from: https://www.fda.gov/medical-devices/software-medical-device-samd/artificial-intelligence-and-machine-learning-software-medical-device.
45. Aiming for truth, fairness, and equity in your company's use of AI | Federal Trade Commission [Internet]. [cited 2021 Apr 25]. Available from: https://www.ftc.gov/news-events/blogs/business-blog/2021/04/aiming-truth-fairness-equity-your-companys-use-ai.

How to Write and Review an Artificial Intelligence Paper

53

Thomas Weikert and Tim Leiner

Introduction

Artificial intelligence (AI) has become one of the main drivers of innovation in healthcare as in other industries. This is especially relevant in the field of cardiovascular imaging where great workload is caused by time-consuming, but essential preprocessing steps like vessel centerline definition in CT angiography and segmentation of heart chambers at multiple timepoints in cardiac MRI. As AI image segmentation is advancing, these algorithms offer great opportunities for cardiovascular imagers. But researchers sitting in front of a blank sheet of paper with the intention to write a scientific article as well as readers of these articles demand guidance to write and review.

This situation is not unprecedented. Over the years, the scientific community has agreed on common quality standards for studies of different kinds. Well-known examples are statements such as the *Standards for Reporting of Diagnostic Accuracy Studies* (STARD) [4], *Standard Protocol Items: Recommendations for Interventional Trials* (SPIRIT) [5], and *Transparent Reporting of a Multivariable Prediction Model for Individual Prognosis or Diagnosis* (TRIPOD) [6]. These frameworks come with checklists that provide excellent guidance for both writing and reviewing scientific papers. Althoughbeit many checklist elements are generally valid and therefore transferable to studies with application of AI in cardiovascular radiology, AI studies have their own methodological peculiarities that mandate a specific approach. The discussion on this topic is still ongoing in the scientific community [3], and a first AI-specific framework, the *Checklist for Artificial Intelligence in Medical Imaging* (CLAIM) [8], has been published recently. This is important because AI studies should be held to the same quality standards as any other diagnostic or prognostic study. While there are some parallels between CLAIM and the ideas put forward in this chapter, the following deliberations are discussed in more detail and put a focus on transparency, e.g., by explicitly demanding information on existing approaches to the same task (AI and non-AI) and disclosure of where, when, and under which conditions the source code is made available.

This chapter discusses 12 considerations that should be part of an AI paper. We hope it helps both authors and readers, and also those not yet familiar with the application of AI in radiology, to report the right information and to ask the right questions. Furthermore, 25 items are derived from these considerations and presented as a readily applicable checklist (Box 53.1). This chapter mostly refers to machine learning (ML), a subset of AI approaches.

Key Considerations

An important preliminary consideration before starting to write or read a study on AI is in which journal the research article is or is planned to be published. Whereas it is reasonable to expect a high level of technical detail in publications with a focus on information technology and engineering, it is appropriate to refer to the supplement or previous publications for full technical details in a journal with a clinical focus.

Clear Definition of the Problem and Study Background

A clear description of the clinical problem and the background of the study must be provided. Studies dealing with a specific condition (e.g., pulmonary embolism) should pre-

T. Weikert, MD (✉)
Department of Radiology, University Hospital Basel, University of Basel, Basel, Switzerland
e-mail: thomas.weikert@usb.ch

T. Leiner, MD, PhD
Department of Radiology, Mayo Clinic, Rochester, MN, USA
e-mail: leiner.tim@mayo.edu

C. N. De Cecco et al. (eds.), *Artificial Intelligence in Cardiothoracic Imaging*, Contemporary Medical Imaging,
https://doi.org/10.1007/978-3-030-92087-6_53

Box 53.1 Checklist of items to include when reporting AI research in radiology

Section	#	Item	Relates to consideration(s)
Title			
	1	Identification as a study using AI to solve a task related to radiology, mentioning the specific AI-approach applied	1, 3
Abstract			
	2	Specification of study objective and disease studied (if any)	1, 5
	3	Information on data origin (single-center? Multi-center? Public database?)	6
	4	Specification of the AI approach used	3
	5	Key performance measure(s)/result(s) with indication of statistical precision (such as 95% confidence intervals)	7
Introduction			
	6	If diagnostic algorithm: Stage of algorithm in the clinical diagnostic pathway, preferably according to international guidelines	1
	7	Rationale for using the specific AI approach	2
	8	Information on existing approaches to the problem (AI and non-AI)	2
Methods			
	9	Details on sample size determination (sample size determination method applied? Rationale behind sample size used?)	4
	10	Detailed information on inclusion and exclusion criteria used for identification of eligible patients/examinations/data	5
	11	Procedure used for splitting data into training, validation, and testing dataset (criteria? Split ratio? Rationale?)	5
	12	Details on how independence of the testing dataset was ensured	5
	13	Method of ground truth determination (how exactly? By whom, including information on professional experience). Was a data quality check workflow in place?	6
	14	Quantification of interrater variability regarding ground truth	6
	15	Information on data preprocessing (data augmentation? Cropping? Re-sizing?)	3
	16	Detailed information on the AI/ML model used, including software libraries and hyperparameters (grade of detail depending on journal's scope)	3
	17	Details on external validation (was it performed? If so, which data was used? Who evaluated the data?)	5, 10
Results			
	18	Basic demographic and clinical characteristics of patients, also listed individually for training, validation, and testing dataset(s)	10
	19	Confusion matrices for index test results (test being evaluated) vs. ground truth	7
	20	Indication of precision for diagnostic measures (such as 95% confidence intervals)	7
	21	Assessment of the algorithm's logic (e.g., saliency maps, structured visual review of results, etc.)	8
Discussion			
	22	Discussion of representativeness of the study dataset for the algorithm's target population and of potential biases	9, 10
	23	Discussion of (potential) implementation of the algorithm in clinical workflows	9
	24	Discussion of (potential) impact of the algorithm results on patient management and outcomes	11
Other information			
	25	Code availability: Where, when, under which conditions. If code is not available, specification of reasons	12

cisely define the disease in focus, preferably using standard terminology like the *International Classification of Diseases* (ICD), for reasons of comparability. If applicable, the exact stage of disease analyzed should be mentioned (e.g., "*central* pulmonary embolism" or "heart failure *NYHA [New York Heart Association] classes III and IV*"). Precision is crucial, as an AI algorithm trained and evaluated for advanced stages of disease might very well miss diagnostically highly relevant early stages and vice versa. In the case of diagnostic algorithms, their exact position in the diagnostic pathway should be stated, preferably referencing international diagnostic guidelines.

If the article is focussed on a more general topic like improving image quality or optimized patient scheduling in a radiology department, the setting in which the analysis takes place should be specified, including details on the investigation site. This is especially important in the field of AI, as algorithms are sensitive to regional bias. Concretely, an algorithm for the detection of pathologic changes on chest X-rays trained in regions with a high prevalence of tuberculosis will be confronted with many examples showing signs of patchy consolidations during training. If this algorithm is later applied in a region with a near-zero prevalence of this disease, false-positive predictions of tuberculosis are a likely consequence.

Discussion of the Rationale behind Using Artificial Intelligence

From an engineer's perspective, a problem has many solutions. It is important to keep in mind that AI is just one of them. It's a powerful technique that rightfully has gained a lot of attention over recent years due to its enormous potential. This is especially true for radiology with its digital data and a central role of visual recognition tasks: many AI algorithms originate from the field of image classification and detection of everyday objects. On the other hand, AI has also become hype. Therefore, reasons for using AI to solve the given problem and a hypothesis on how this may improve upon other non-AI approaches should be formulated.

Consideration of other approaches is especially critical in the healthcare sector, where high-quality data for training and evaluation is scarce. Conventional statistical approaches for predictive modeling and simple Hounsfield units (HU) thresholding for segmentation of findings such as coronary artery calcifications (CACs) on CT are just two examples. In many cases, a combination of AI and non-AI techniques is a powerful approach, for example, using AI to detect heart contours on CT, subsequently defining the area immediately surrounding the heart (e.g., as 1 cm rim around the heart contour), and identifying CACs using a density threshold of >130 HU.

To summarize, when deploying AI in radiology, which is a great option for many tasks, it is important to outline the reasons for doing so. Furthermore, existing approaches previously applied to the same problem, if any, and how they fall short should be mentioned.

Choice of ML Model and Technical Details

Just as the reasoning for using AI should be clear, the choice of the specific approach should be motivated. AI is an umbrella term encompassing a wide variety of techniques that enable computers to perform tasks commonly associated with human intelligence. This is true for the cutting-edge, highly complex, and computationally intensive deep convolutional neural network (DCNN) but also for non-deep learning algorithms based on random forest (RF) and even for simple, non-machine learning approaches. It is obvious that many problems can be solved by more than one AI approach and the author or reader of an article should be aware of the pros and cons of each to identify an appropriate option. It is also legitimate to test multiple approaches if the process is structured and documented in the article.

Even in research articles published in journals with a strict clinical focus, a minimum of technical details is required and must be part of the methods section. The ML algorithms commonly used in the field of radiology are practically never designed from scratch but compiled from building blocks found in online software libraries such as *scikit-learn* [10], *TensorFlow* [1], and *PyTorch* [9]. Therefore, referencing the sources of these building blocks, including the names and versions of packages used, is crucial.

In ML, researchers modify so-called hyperparameters of models, that is, parameters set before the learning phase begins. Two examples are the *learning rate* in DCNNs and the *number of branches* of decision trees in RF models. As *hyperparameters* are important adjusting mechanisms influencing a model's performance, they should be reported, at least in the supplement. The endeavor of designing an algorithm from scratch is usually reported in journals with a focus on information technology and requires in-depth information in order to allow computer scientists to fully comprehend the architecture and possibly propose own improvements. Lately the practice of providing full public access to the code is considered essential to facilitate the peer-review process (see consideration No. 12).

Another important technical consideration to be addressed is if and how *data augmentation* was used. The term denotes techniques that increase the amount of data by adding slightly modified copies of existing data. In radiology, this can be realized by rotating radiographs by a randomly defined angle or adding copies of images with artificially reduced signal-to-noise ratio to the dataset. The obvious effect is an amplification of data without the need to acquire more source data.

This is especially relevant in the context of data scarcity and/or expensive data acquisition, both common challenges of AI projects in radiology.

As a welcome side effect, *data augmentation* can contribute to mitigate the problem of *overfitting*. It occurs when models absorb the subtleties of the training data in too much detail. This results in perfect performance on the training data itself but an inability to generalize to new, unseen data. As data augmentation provides the algorithm with other perspectives on data, it can help to reduce overfitting – but only given that the new, simulated data represents real world data. For example, adding copies of artificially created, slightly rotated radiographs used to develop a model for detection of distal radius fractures can help in the setting of limited source data, as the alignment of the forearm shows slight variations between acquisitions in the real world, too. Furthermore, all preprocessing steps such as cropping of images have to be described.

Concluding, characteristics of the algorithm must be provided, with the level of technical detail in the methods section depending on the journal's scope. Even in the case of journals with a clinical focus, one should provide basic information in the methods section and detailed information either in the supplement or by referring to a technical paper on the same algorithm.

Sample Size Motivation

Power analysis aims at determining the sample size needed to detect a statistical effect. To do so, the estimated effect size and the desired degree of confidence need to be defined. While sample size determination methods are an integral part of many scientific guidelines, most ML studies have not explicitly considered sample size and are often based on convenience samples. In a recent review of articles applying ML to medical imaging, only 4 of 167 (2.4%) had explicitly discussed sample size determination methodologies [2]. In fact, it is challenging to estimate the amount of data required to reach a desired model performance due to the plethora of parameters involved. Therefore, computer scientists often act up to the principle "the more data, the better."

However, there are indicators which help to arrive at an appropriate estimate: first is task complexity. Problems easy to solve for a human usually don't require much data (e.g., classifying pixels as black or white in a sample containing only black and white pixels = high signal-to-noise-ratio [SNR]). On the other hand, detecting subtle changes like small tumors seen in only a few voxels of a whole-body CT scan (= low SNR) usually needs a lot of data. Second is model complexity. A DCNN with multiple layers and features requires larger sample sizes than a linear regression model with just a few input parameters. Third is envisaged model performance. Usually, more samples will help to improve an algorithm. But one should also keep in mind that sample procurement can be very costly and result improvement becomes marginal after a certain point so that it doesn't stand up a cost-benefit analysis. Depending on the ultimate purpose of the algorithm and using domain expertise, a "good enough" performance can be defined in advance. Fourth is quality of data. The better the quality of included samples, the fewer samples are required to reach a given performance. Fifth is previous literature, or more specifically sample sizes used in similar projects. AI has become a frequently deployed approach in radiology, too. There is plenty of information on other projects with various goals using various techniques that can serve as a reference.

While there are no easy answers on this and sample sizes in ML continue to be based mostly on experience or data availability, the mentioned reference points can provide some guidance.

Specification of Training, Validation, and Testing Datasets

Machine learning algorithm development demands data for training, validation, and testing. Investigators should precisely specify how the data was split into these categories. As for sample size determination, there are no general standards regarding the exact ratio. Common splits are as follows [training-validation-testing]: 80%–10%–10% and 60%–20%–20%, the first preferred in situations with little data available. As for all studies, detailed inclusion and exclusion criteria have to be provided.

The function of the validation dataset is to allow for an evaluation of model fit while still trying different hyperparameters. For example, a researcher could evaluate the influence of different learning rates on a model's performance. To exploit as much data as possible for training, cross-validation is a valuable option: the samples reserved for training and validation are combined, and different subsets of this dataset are used to train a model – with the complementary data used for validation. This process is repeated. Cross-validation is especially beneficial when samples are a scarce resource. Because there are plenty of cross-validation techniques, a researcher needs to provide detailed information on which technique was used.

The testing dataset needs to be strictly separate from other datasets because its purpose is to obtain a realistic estimate of the final models' performance and generalizability. This test is performed after training, when the models' hyperparameters and parameters are fixed. Strict separation of the testing dataset is also a requirement for regulatory approval of ML-based computer-assisted detection devices from the

US Food and Drug Administration [7]. How full independence of the testing dataset was ensured must be part of the methods section.

As a last remark, there is quite some confusion about the terms *validation dataset* and *external validation* of a model. While the first is part of the datasets used during algorithm development as described previously, the latter one is used to prove generalizability of an approach on external data, ideally performed by independent researchers. This step is crucial prior to an algorithm's distribution due to the fact that acquisition parameters differ considerably between radiology departments and hardware vendors, (we refer to consideration No. 10).

Ground Truth

A key consideration in ML studies is selection and quality of the reference standard or ground truth. As supervised ML algorithms solely learn relationships in the data they are trained with, quality of ground truth is a limiting factor to an algorithm's performance and therefore of utmost importance. It is good practice to devote some thought and discussion at the very beginning of an AI project to define rules for compiling the ground truth, based on domain expertise, and to make sure everybody involved has fully understood these rules. Therefore, communication between all persons involved is important. In the methods section, researchers should precisely specify how and by whom ground truth data was labeled, including the level of experience of each observer. Experience is specified in years, usually counted from achievement of specialization. Radiology residents' experience can be provided as postgraduate year (PGY), with PGY-3 describing a third-year resident.

Interobserver variability is a known phenomenon in radiology that has to be accounted for. This includes a description of how disagreements were resolved (e.g., by demanding that observers reach a consensus or by adjudicating any differences by a separate observer) and preferentially a quantification of the degree of variability. Exemplified on an AI project aiming at automated cardiac segmentation, a random sample of 25 left ventricles could be annotated by three coauthors and measures of agreement calculated such as the Dice similarity coefficient (see consideration No. 7). Furthermore, details on software used to define the standard of reference such as DICOM viewers need to be provided (software, version, packages used).

If existing labels were used (e.g., from radiology reports or electronic health records), there should be a structured quality check confirming the labels' validity. Concretely, if a research project relies on radiology reports to identify high-grade coronary stenoses, at least a subset of these cases must be thoroughly and visually approved by a competent observer. This is also true when using public datasets that have shown to be of varying quality.

In general, it is advised to implement some kind of audit workflow ensuring that the standard of reference is double-checked and, if needed, corrected. Describing this workflow in the methods section enhances the quality of a research paper. When in doubt, given the importance of ground truth in ML, more rather than less information should be provided. Furthermore, it is good practice to reflect on the chosen methods and weaknesses in the discussion section.

Reporting of Results

In radiology, AI algorithms are mostly applied to classify cases (e.g., separating healthy from sick individuals), detect findings (e.g., tumors in a CT scan), and segment areas of interest (e.g., left ventricles in cardiac MRI).

Regarding classification tasks, confusion matrices with numbers of true-positive, true-negative, false-positive, and false-negative classifications should be provided at a prespecified classifier threshold, analogous to conventional diagnostic studies. Many relevant performance measures are calculated based on this information. Two terms used in ML literature sometimes deviate from standard terminology: sensitivity is named "recall" and positive predictive value (PPV) "precision." An author can opt for both terminologies but should stay consistent throughout the manuscript.

The F1 score is a compound measure of sensitivity and PPV. It exhibits high values only if an algorithm is both sensitive and a positive prediction has a high probability of being correct. The measure cannot be tricked by tweaking an algorithm toward sensitivity only and its use is therefore recommended. Another standard metric is the area under the curve (AUC) of a receiver characteristic curve (ROC). A ROC plots sensitivity (Y-axis) of a parameter against 1-specificity (X-axis) at multiple threshold settings and therefore represents the inherent tradeoff between sensitivity and specificity. Technically, AUC ranges between 0 (all predictions are wrong) to 1 (all predictions are correct). Practically, due to the fact that an algorithm with wrong predictions only is a perfect classifier when inverting its results, an AUC of 0.5 is synonymous to a useless classifier. Similarly, in a binary classification problem (e.g., is a patient healthy or sick?), a coin flip will result in a sensitivity of 50% – it is important to keep this in mind when interpreting results.

Regarding segmentation tasks, intersection over union (IoU) is an important concept. It is defined by $A \cap B$ / $A \cup B$ – that is, by dividing the total number of pixels/voxels common between the algorithm's prediction and the ground truth through all pixels/voxels in both masks, counted separately. Other important metrics include the Dice coefficient (a measure of how well the AI generated contours overlap with the standard of reference contours, similar to IoU), the mean contour distance (the mean distance between two segmentation contours), and the Hausdorff distance (the maximum distance between the two segmentation contours).

Irrespective of the metric used, confidence intervals should be reported as early as in the abstract. This allows readers to assess the statement's accuracy. If a researcher wants to narrow the interval, she or he can add a larger number of samples to the testing dataset. For tasks with an established alternative approach, a comparison should be provided, ideally with the older method applied to the test dataset of the current study. Alternatively, the performance of a new approach can be demonstrated by applying it to a public dataset or participating in a public competition. At least, performance measures of the old approach as reported in previous papers should be mentioned and comparability discussed.

Are the Results Explainable?

AI is often associated with the term "black box." The comparison is drawn because of model complexity, which results in a user experience "input-black box processing-output." This is especially true for state-of-the-art DL algorithms. However, the "black box" allegory is not correct, as the operational mechanisms underlying any algorithm are known and in fact engineered. Most importantly, this should not deter researchers and readers to ask themselves whether the results are explainable.

To do so in the context of deep learning, the concept of *saliency maps* can be used to highlight regions in an image that are mostly involved in the "decision-making" of the algorithm, which means those having most influence on the output. This visual feedback on a model's predictions is important to understand whether networks learn patterns representing pathophysiological features or biologically unknown, potentially irrelevant features. This consideration is particularly pertinent when important treatment decisions are contingent upon the results generated by the algorithm.

In radiology, the most important assessment of explainability of results is a thorough visual review of the output by a domain expert. Thereby, it is also possible to identify reasons for failure of an algorithm and come up with counterstrategies. For example, if the majority of false-positive findings of an algorithm for quantification of coronary calcification in CT scans is caused by aortic calcifications, a combination with an algorithm segmenting the aorta improves performance significantly. Therefore, a sub-analysis investigating reasons for false-positive and false-negative findings strengthens a research article.

Can and Will the Results be Applied in a Clinical Setting?

Machine learning studies designed to solve a specific clinical problem should explicitly consider whether the results can be applied in a real-world clinical setting. This includes two important aspects.

First, the representativity of the dataset used during algorithm development and testing for the clinical setting in which it will be applied should be discussed. Any sources of bias, in particular class imbalance and spectrum bias, meaning variety in performance due to a different case-mix, should be identified and discussed. This underlines the need for a detailed description of the dataset (see consideration No. 5). It is also important to discuss potential consequences of regional differences regarding imaging protocols, radiology hardware, and clinical guidelines. Considering these factors enables a more precise indication of patient populations in which the algorithm can be clinically used.

Second, investigators should provide information on prerequisites of algorithm deployment at the point of care, including issues like availability of the algorithm (e.g., on-premise or via cloud solutions), how fast results are available (e.g., in real time or with delay), and how results are visualized in order to check the model's predictions. As during development of consumer electronics, it's a good idea to identify the user and consider the exact setting in which an algorithm is applied. Additionally, one should reflect on user interaction: if users are deterred by long waiting times, too many false alerts, or the need to log in to yet another piece of software, they will ignore the algorithm, irrespective of its great performance. In general, integration of algorithm results in software used during clinical standard workflows is a promising idea. Furthermore, a good, self-explanatory user interface and output visualization help to gain acceptance.

It is increasingly recognized that algorithm development is just the first and commonly easier part of making AI in radiology work. Therefore, these considerations aiming at clinical implementation should at least be part of the discussion section. It is of course legitimate to limit them to a few remarks in feasibility studies focused on diagnostic performance.

Is the Performance Generalizable?

In the field of radiology, ML model development and testing are mostly performed on convenience samples of locally available data. Although many of these reports have demonstrated encouraging results, it's important to additionally investigate the approaches' external generalizability, preferably on datasets from other independent institutes and investigators in multiple regions.

External validation is important to investigate the robustness of a model to, e.g., differences in image acquisition and reconstruction methods between different vendors and institutes, differences in referral patterns, and variation in the prevalence of the condition of interest. Researchers need to provide full details on the data used for external validation such as the type of hospital, the hardware used for image acquisition, patient demographics, and disease severity.

Conversely, we also believe it is advisable to thoroughly validate externally developed algorithms prior to local clinical use, especially if the algorithms` results are used for automated analysis with results directly transferred to the clinical decision-making processes. Another option is to explicitly develop a local solution to a specific problem, not aiming at further distribution and therefore generalizability. However, this limits the significance of the approach to the scientific community. Even if external validation is not performed, the reasons for this should be provided.

Is there any Evidence that the Model Has an Effect on Patient Management and Outcomes?

Although one of the first steps in ML algorithm development is investigation of diagnostic accuracy, investigators and readers should ask themselves whether there is any evidence or prospect of an effect on patient outcomes. This is especially important for algorithms used for treatment recommendations and detection of critical findings.

It takes the considerations on application in a clinical setting (consideration No. 9) one step further: even if an algorithm exhibits high diagnostic performance and is well embedded in radiology workflows, this doesn't mean it has an effect on patient outcomes. Possible causes preventing real-world impact include delayed communication of results by the radiologist, insufficient clinical workflows, and work overload of referring physicians. Therefore, a holistic perspective on how the algorithm eventually contributes to better patient management is important.

Ideally, the impact on patient management and outcome should be investigated in prospective clinical trials, including evaluation periods without and with the algorithm in use. A close collaboration between all stakeholders and an in-depth understanding of how radiology reports and communicated findings influence clinical care workflows is important to make a difference for the patients. Even research articles focusing on pure diagnostic performance can provide a short reflection on how the algorithm can have an impact.

Is the Code Available?

Transparency regarding an ML model's design and function is a key element for acceptance. Making the computer code available to other investigators is a major step toward this goal and is increasingly becoming a condition for obtaining funding as well as acceptance of studies in high-quality, peer-reviewed journals. It's a good idea in many respects: it allows other researchers to investigate replicability, use them for their own purposes, or build improved versions based on the code provided. Furthermore, uploading software code to platforms with version control function enables documentation of a model's evolution over a long period of time. *GitHub* (github.com) is an example of an online repository enabling researchers to share software code. It includes basic quality checks and has a version control function.

In a scientific paper, investigators should clearly state whether the source code of their algorithm will be made available. If so, they need to indicate where, when, and under which conditions. If not, they need to provide specific reasons.

Checklist

The items of the checklist provided in Box 53.1 are derived from the considerations of the previous section. The purpose of the checklist is to serve as an easy-to-use tool for both authors and reviewers. To this end, it is structured according to the standard sections of a research article.

References

1. Abadi M, Agarwal A, Barham P, Brevdo E, Chen Z, Citro C, Corrado GS, Davis A, Dean J, Devin M, Ghemawat S, Goodfellow I, Harp A, Irving G, Isard M, Jia Y, Jozefowicz R, Kaiser L, Kudlur M, Zheng X. TensorFlow: large-scale machine learning on heterogeneous distributed systems. 2016.
2. Balki I, Amirabadi A, Levman J, Martel AL, Emersic Z, Meden B, Garcia-Pedrero A, Ramirez SC, Kong D, Moody AR, Tyrrell PN. Sample-size determination methodologies for machine learning in medical imaging research: a systematic review. Canadian Associat Radiolog J. 2019;70(4):344–53). Canadian Medical Association. https://doi.org/10.1016/j.carj.2019.06.002.
3. Bluemke DA, Moy L, Bredella MA, Ertl-Wagner BB, Fowler KJ, Goh VJ, Halpern EF, Hess CP, Schiebler ML, Weiss CR. Assessing radiology research on artificial intelligence: a brief guide for authors, reviewers, and readers—from the *radiology* editorial board. Radiology. 2020;294(3):487–9. https://doi.org/10.1148/radiol.2019192515.
4. Bossuyt PM, Reitsma JB, Bruns DE, Gatsonis CA, Glasziou PP, Irwig L, Lijmer JG, Moher D, Rennie D, de Vet HCW, Kressel HY, Rifai N, Golub RM, Altman DG, Hooft L, Korevaar DA, Cohen JF, STARD Group. STARD 2015: an updated list of essential items for

reporting diagnostic accuracy studies. Radiology. 2015;277(3):826–32. https://doi.org/10.1148/radiol.2015151516.

5. Chan A-W, Tetzlaff JM, Altman DG, Laupacis A, Gøtzsche PC, Krleža-Jerić K, Hróbjartsson A, Mann H, Dickersin K, Berlin JA, Doré CJ, Parulekar WR, Summerskill WSM, Groves T, Schulz KF, Sox HC, Rockhold FW, Rennie D, Moher D. SPIRIT 2013 statement: defining standard protocol items for clinical trials. Ann Intern Med. 2013;158(3):200–7. https://doi.org/10.7326/0003-4819-158-3-201302050-00583.
6. Collins GS, Reitsma JB, Altman DG, Moons KGM. Transparent reporting of a multivariable prediction model for individual prognosis or diagnosis (TRIPOD): the TRIPOD statement. BMJ. 2015;350(jan07 4):g7594. https://doi.org/10.1136/bmj.g7594.
7. FDA. Proposed regulatory framework for modifications to Artificial Intelligence/Machine Learning (AI/ML)-Based Software as a Medical Device (SaMD) - Discussion Paper and Request for Feedback. 2019.
8. Mongan J, Moy L, Kahn JEJ. Checklist for artificial intelligence in medical imaging (CLAIM): a guide for authors and reviewers. Radiology: Artificial Intelligence. 2020:2. https://doi.org/10.1148/ryai.2020200029.
9. Paszke A, Gross S, Massa F, Lerer A, Bradbury J, Chanan G, Killeen T, Lin Z, Gimelshein N, Antiga L, Desmaison A, Köpf A, Yang E, DeVito Z, Raison M, Tejani A, Chilamkurthy S, Steiner B, Fang L, et al. PyTorch: an imperative style. High-Performance Deep Learning Library. 2019; http://arxiv.org/abs/1912.01703.
10. Pedregosa F, Varoquaux G, Gramfort A, Michel V, Thirion B, Grisel O, Blondel M, Prettenhofer P, Weiss R, Dubourg V, Vanderplas J, Passos A, Cournapeau D, Brucher M, Perrot M, Duchesnay É. Scikit-learn: machine learning in python. J Mach Learn Res. 2011;12(Oct):2825–30.

54 Cybersecurity in the Era of Artificial Intelligence

Anton S. Becker

Definitions

Artificial Intelligence

The term artificial intelligence (AI) has different meanings for different people. To purists, it may mean the ability of a computer program to solve a variety of tasks in different domains at a human or near-human level. To researchers writing grant proposals, it may mean anything remotely to do with computers. In the current book, slightly different, nuanced definitions may be needed for individual chapters. In the present chapter, we synonymously refer to AI and machine learning for all advanced methods where computational algorithms are employed to analyze data and make inferences for either attack or defense. A special subclass described in more detail below are powerful generative models (GMs), such as generative adversarial networks (GANs).

Generative Models

GMs describe a class of models that contrast with discriminative models. In short, a generative model can create new data instances, whereas a discriminative model can distinguish between different kinds of data instances. For example, a discriminative deep learning model can distinguish mammographic images with cancer from ones with benign or no lesions [1], whereas a GAN may generate new mammographies of breasts with and without cancer. Certain variations of GANs have slightly different properties, for example, a specialized GAN may modify a single pixel to swap image classes [2]. While this attack would unlikely fool a human observer, a CycleGAN [3] can modify images from one class to the other by inserting or removing high-level features, e.g., insert or remove cancerous lesions from mammographies [4]. In theory, given unlimited resources, GMs will sample from the real distribution, meaning they will produce completely realistic fake examples indistinguishable from real ones [5].

Cybersecurity

Like AI, cybersecurity may mean different things in different contexts. For example:

- For individuals, cybersecurity means that their personal data (photos, e-mails, chat logs, etc.) are protected from unauthorized access and their devices are free from malware.
- For patients, cybersecurity means their health-related information is only accessible by people who provide healthcare services to them.
- For hospitals, cybersecurity may include secure locations of their servers, redundant systems to ensure data integrity and/or accessibility in case of power or hardware failure, employing encryption methods to secure traffic, and educating their users about protecting their passwords and accounts.
- For governments, cybersecurity may range from creating laws, policies, and procedures related to data and cybercrimes to establishing an extensive infrastructure to perform surveillance on citizens in order to ensure Internet communication conforms to certain ideological standards.

There are, of course, no clean boundaries and certain aspects intermix throughout these layers. But it helps to remember that the expectations vary, when different people hear the word cybersecurity.

Taxonomically, cybersecurity is a subset of information security. Information security encompasses all forms of data (e.g., storing a paper patient file in a locked cabinet), whereas cybersecurity explicitly refers to digital data. Again, on this

A. S. Becker, MD, PhD (✉)
Memorial Sloan Kettering Cancer Center, New York, NY, USA
e-mail: beckera1@mskcc.org

C. N. De Cecco et al. (eds.), *Artificial Intelligence in Cardiothoracic Imaging*, Contemporary Medical Imaging,
https://doi.org/10.1007/978-3-030-92087-6_54

day and age, the lines are fuzzy (think of computer passwords and PINs written down on a personal notepad), and many use these terms interchangeably.

For this chapter, we will define cybersecurity by its purpose: The aim of cybersecurity is to ensure confidentiality, integrity, and availability of digital data and the underlying systems. Attempts to tamper with any of those aspects represent different kinds of cyberattacks, for example, stealing electronic health records, modifying image data, or ransomware attacks.

Cryptography

Cryptography is the practice and study of techniques for secure data communication and storage. It is an important tool in cybersecurity, involving sophisticated mathematical algorithms crafted around computational hardness assumptions, i.e., it is theoretically possible to break any of these codes, but the time needed to do so *given current technological limits* makes this practically impossible (e.g., time needed may be ten times the current life span of the universe). Note the highlight: new breakthroughs in technologies like AI or quantum computing may render current codes breakable and require development of new algorithms.

Of note, the classical corporate IT security system is modeled after a fortress, i.e., firewalls control the network activities and block most communication to the outside, but the internal IT network is considered "safe" and traffic is usually unencrypted [6]. Whenever encryption is employed, it increases computational load and decreases data throughput, so there is a tradeoff between speed and encryption level.

Arms Race

A fundamental principle underlying the field of cybersecurity is that the field is constantly changing. As new technologies become available, it usually does not take long until they are "repurposed" (abused) for cyberattacks. Afterward, cybersecurity professionals develop and deploy protective and countermeasures. For example, before the Internet, it was extremely difficult for an attacker to gain access to a corporate network, usually requiring some level of physical access to one of the workstations or servers. With the advent of the Internet, cybersecurity firms had to develop strong hardware and software firewalls that protect these private networks from the open Internet. The increase in bandwidth and advent of mobile working has required controlled "puncturing" of those firewalls, for example, with VPN (virtual private network) protocols. AI will inevitably spur the next wave of the arms race, but the phenomenon is not only familiar but an inherent property of cybersecurity.

Cybersecurity in Healthcare

While in the government and various industry sectors cybersecurity has kept up with the rapid technological development to slow the prevalence and effect of cyberattacks, healthcare has chronically lagged behind [7]. In the United Kingdom, many national healthcare system organizations spend as little as 1–2% of their annual budget on IT, compared with 4–10% in other sectors [8]. Due to dependency on legacy systems, many institutions still run outdated software like Microsoft Windows XP or Internet Explorer, which pose a large security risk in itself.

Common Types of Cyberattacks

In the next section, we will list various types of existing cyberattacks. The first paragraph of each subheading is a short explanation; in the second paragraph, we explore how AI may be used in each case, offensively and/or defensively.

Interception/Data Theft

Interception occurs when attackers capture data in-transit between computers. The aim of interception is often data theft, one of the most common attacks. In healthcare, data theft could involve obtaining protected sensitive health information and using it for criminal activity (e.g., blackmailing patients). Moreover, many large academic hospitals run clinical trials, which can make or break regulatory approval of a drug or device. Knowledge of the success or failure in advance is worth a lot of money in the stock market.

AI could be used to intercept and manipulate data of patients to, e.g., hide real diagnoses or add spurious fake diagnoses. Since most diagnoses are multimodal, i.e., made on the combination of clinical presentation, examination, laboratory parameters, imaging, histopathology, etc., it would be insufficient to only manipulate one modality. For example, inserting a cancer into a CT image would only work if the subsequent histopathology images of the biopsy cores are also manipulated to contain cancerous patterns. A mischievous AI would need to be modeled with a complex multidimensional internal representation of diseases and several separate outputs, like a piano player where each finger presses a different key and doesn't "know" what the other finger is pressing, yet the player orchestrates their actions to elicit a symphony from a series of well-orchestrated keypresses (Fig. 54.1).

One of the most effective methods against interception and data theft is sufficient encryption. Another method is the

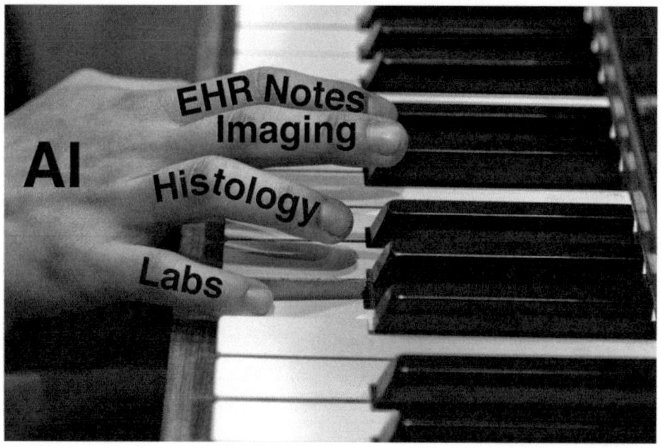

Fig. 54.1 Piano player model of an AI agent manipulating various components of patient data to create a realistic false diagnosis. Own work, (Modified after https://commons.wikimedia.org/wiki/File:Hand_of_Music.jpg by Robert Couse-Baker, released under the Creative Commons Attribution 2.0 Generic license)

creation of fake bait systems, so-called honeypots. A honeypot appears to be a legitimate part of the computer network but is actually an isolated and monitored system used to catch attackers and block them. Although the main aim is often to catch the attacker and block them, one could additionally just play the waiting game and waste their time and resources. For example, a GAN could generate DICOM images of fake patients on-the-fly, thus giving the attacker the impression they hit the hospitals' PACS, when they are in actuality only downloading the hallucinations of an artificial neural network.

Malware/Ransomware

Malware (short for malicious software) is an all-encompassing term for software that intentionally inflicts damage on users, who are typically unaware that they are running it.

Malware can include computer viruses, worms, Trojans, spyware, cryptocurrency miners, or adware. One particular species of malware has unfortunately repeatedly made headlines rampaging across hospital networks: ransomware. Ransomware encrypts the content of a hard drive and displays a message to the user, requesting a ransom payment for decryption of the data. Some variants of ransomware steal the victim's data instead of encrypting it and threaten to either publish it online or delete it. The ransomware WannaCry, which initially spread in 2017, inflicts at least hundreds of millions of dollars in damages. While some ransomware attacks such as WannaCry spread relatively untargeted via worms or Trojans, some attacks are highly targeted and involve knowledge about which data is most valuable to the victim (e.g., patient data in the case of hospitals) and how much a person or institution is able to pay.

Through AI it may become possible for attackers to perform more "targeted" attacks on a widespread level. The ransomware may communicate with a central server and learn which data is most important to different users and which targets are able to pay large sums of money.

Conversely, AI may be used to detect suspicious encryption activity or even before that detect anomalous network activity and prevent ransomware from entering the network.

Botnets and Zombies

Botnets are a collection of compromised computers (called "zombies") that belong to unsuspecting third parties but can be controlled remotely by the owner of the botnet to perform (illicit) tasks without the knowledge of said third parties. Criminals who successfully infect several hundred thousand computers with a botnet malware can use those combined resources, for example, to send millions of network requests to a single website and overload their server (known as a DDoS or denial-of-service attack).

Botnets could also be used by hackers to get access to large computational resources. By hijacking the infected computer's computational power, they could train illegal AIs via distributed learning [9].

Impersonation, Phishing, and Social Engineering

One of the greatest dangers that the Internet and e-mail communication have created is the ease with which attackers can impersonate innocent third parties. Creating a website that closely resembles the login page of an organization's webmail service is very easy, as is sending e-mails from a fake address (known as "spoofing"). The process of obtaining secret passwords in this way is called "phishing," an artificial respelling of the word "fishing" after the pattern of "phreaking," itself a respelling of "freaking" describing an older technique or culture to experiment with phones/telecommunication devices. Social engineering, in a broader context, describes the process of manipulating individuals to divulge sensitive information or facilitate cyberattacks without their knowledge. For example, an IT hotline could be reached with a simple phone call, and the attacker could impersonate their victim to get their username and password.

Attacks like these will get more sophisticated and harder to detect with AI: for example, it is already possible to generate arbitrary realistic video sequences or voice prompts, a technique popularly known as "deepfakes." Although the algorithms for voice generation currently need several hours of high-quality audio data for training, as demonstrated by a group of researchers generating voice prompts from the popular podcast host Joe Rogan [10], it is only a question of time until this will be possible with a short speech excerpt.

Also in this regard, an arms race will ensue between detection of deepfakes and generation of realistic data.

How to Protect your Institution

A comprehensive list of protective measures or concepts is beyond the scope of this short chapter. However, we list a few generalizable principles below that may hopefully be useful to the interested reader.

Clinical, business, and technology leaders within an organization must collaborate. The very first step of a proactive cybersecurity plan is understanding what security risks exist inside a hospital/department. This step cannot be done by cybersecurity experts alone but needs understanding of the various core processes and responsibilities within a department.

A chain is only as strong as the weakest link. Think of the infamous yellow post-it notes on the monitor with the password, rendering a whole sophisticated IT security system nearly useless.

Greatest security risks are inside. Most institutions these days have recognized that training their staff to recognize malicious e-mails and links and avoid phishing attacks, etc., is a cornerstone for institutional cybersecurity.

Backup and recovery plan. Have a solid and tested backup and recovery plan in place.

Require locking of all devices with a long PIN/password. Don't allow reuse of passwords. Currently standard in most institutions, this is also a wise approach for personal devices.

The rapid advance in technology and increase in complexity have caused many healthcare institutions to adopt a reactive leadership style instead of a proactive one, coined the "muddling through" approach by Abraham et al. [11]. This reactive approach is insufficient when it comes to cybersecurity in healthcare. When a security breach compromises systems in healthcare, it does not "shut down IT"; it shuts down patient care. Hence, even though the AI-mediated attacks explored above are hypothetical at this point, further research is necessary so that countermeasures can be developed before AI cyberattacks become a problem.

Conclusion

Cyberattacks involve a heterogenous arsenal of methods to obtain data of access to computer systems. Cyberterrorists will sooner or later include AI algorithms in their arsenal, enabling sophisticated and difficult-to-detect attacks on healthcare systems. Healthcare organizations can prevent attacks by strong collaboration of technology, business, and clinical leaders and a proactive leadership approach to this problem.

References

1. Becker AS, Marcon M, Ghafoor S, Wurnig MC, Frauenfelder T, Boss A. Deep learning in mammography: diagnostic accuracy of a multipurpose image analysis software in the detection of breast cancer. Invest Radiol. 2017;52(7):434–40.
2. Su J, Vargas DV, Sakurai K. One pixel attack for fooling deep neural networks. IEEE Trans Evol Computat. 2019;23(5):828–41.
3. Zhu J-Y, Park T, Isola P, Efros AA. Unpaired Image-to-Image Translation Using Cycle-Consistent Adversarial Networks. In: 2017 IEEE International Conference on Computer Vision (ICCV). IEEE; 2017. p. 2242–51.
4. Becker AS, Jendele L, Skopek O, Berger N, Ghafoor S, Marcon M, et al. Injecting and removing suspicious features in breast imaging with CycleGAN: A pilot study of automated adversarial attacks using neural networks on small images. Eur J Radiol. 2019;120:108649.
5. Goodfellow I, Pouget-Abadie J, Mirza M, Xu B, Warde-Farley D, Ozair S, et al. Generative Adversarial Nets. Advances in Neural Information Processing Systems. 2014.
6. Becker AS, Gugelmann D. AI-cyberterrorism in radiology: Threat or red herring? [Internet]. 2019 [cited 2020 Nov 21]. Available from: https://www.auntminnie.com/index.aspx?sec=sup&sub=aic&pag=dis&ItemID=127678.
7. Kruse CS, Frederick B, Jacobson T, Monticone DK. Cybersecurity in healthcare: A systematic review of modern threats and trends. Technol Health Care. 2017;25(1):1–10.
8. Martin G, Martin P, Hankin C, Darzi A, Kinross J. Cybersecurity and healthcare: how safe are we? BMJ. 2017;358:j3179.
9. Dean J, Corrado G, Monga R, Chen K, Devin M, Mao M, et al. Large scale distributed deep networks. Advances in Neural Information Processing Systems. 2012.
10. Kadhim H, Mama R, Palermo J. RealTalk (Pt. II): How We Recreated Joe Rogan's Voice Using AI | Dessa News | Medium [Internet]. 2019 [cited 2020 Nov 21]. Available from: https://medium.com/dessa-news/realtalk-how-it-works-94c1afda62f0.
11. Abraham C, Chatterjee D, Sims RR. Muddling through cybersecurity: Insights from the U.S. healthcare industry. Bus Horiz. 2019;62(4):539–48.

How Artificial Intelligence will Reshape the Field of Cardiothoracic Imaging: A Global Perspective

55

Carlo N. De Cecco, Jie Zhang, Marly van Assen, Jack Wessell, Tim Leiner, and Bin Lu

Introduction

The use of artificial intelligence (AI) is growing exponentially worldwide. AI has the potential to be a global game changer as a foundational technology that can increase productivity, solve global dilemmas, and increase process quality. The recent years have seen a massive growth in AI applications in a wide variety of industries, including self-driving cars, search engines, and personal assistants.

A 2019 report from the Center for Data Innovation compares China, the European Union (EU), and the USA in terms of their relative standing in the AI economy [1]. They used six metric categories to make this assessment: talent, research, development, adoption, data, and hardware. They concluded based on all metrics that the USA still leads the AI race with China coming in second, while the European Union lags further behind. They also note that this order could change in coming years as China appears to be making more rapid progress than either the USA or EU [1]. All three major players dominate the AI field in one or more of the metrics. One reason that explains the current US dominance is the AI startup ecosystem, having received the most private equity and venture capital funding. China comes in a close second in receiving startup funding, having both higher venture capital and private equity funding than the USA in 2017. In addition, it leads in the development of both traditional semiconductors and computer chips that power AI systems. Also, China has more access to large quantities of data, a major component for AI development. The EU is leading the race when it comes to recruitment of AI talent, which is also reflected in the production of research. However, the EU lags behind in commercial AI adoption and funding [1].

Considering the growth of the global AI industry, it comes as no surprise that the field of medicine also has shown an increased interest in AI. Multiple reports show a steep increase in the expected investments into AI technology in the healthcare sector. KPMG reports that healthcare-related AI investments have reached almost \$1.3 billion in 2017, encompassing 103 deals [2]. Investments in this field are estimated to approach \$36 billion by 2025, which would be a 50% increase from 2018 [3, 4]. When it comes to medical research, a study shows that a total of 27,451 papers were published between 1977 and 2018, of which 84.6% were dated between 2008 and 2018 [5]. Most of these papers have a single country of authorship origin (67.5%). In this list, the top five countries of authorship origin were the USA and Canada, Europe (Italy and Germany), and China. Surprisingly, while the USA and China score very high in the number of publications, the EU scores very low on the number of collaborating institutes.

AI can be used to assist the healthcare industry in a variety of ways. Many countries worldwide deal with understaffed and overburdened healthcare systems [6–10]. According to a WHO report, 44% of WHO member states report to have less than 1 physician per 1000 inhabitants. According to the same report, China has 1.8 doctors per 1000 inhabitants, compared to 2.5 in the USA and 3.4 in Australia. In addition, healthcare costs have been rising in most countries. AI applications can be used to optimize the healthcare system by automizing processes such as patient

C. N. De Cecco, MD, PhD (✉) · M. van Assen, MSc, PhD
Division of Cardiothoracic Imaging, Department of Radiology and Imaging Sciences, Emory University, Atlanta, GA, USA
e-mail: carlo.dececco@emory.edu; marly.van.assen@emory.edu

J. Zhang, PhD (✉) · B. Lu, MD
Department of Radiology, Fuwai Hospital, State Key Laboratory of Cardiovascular Disease, National Centre for Cardiovascular Diseases, Chinese Academy of Medical Sciences and Peking Union Medical College, Beijing, China

J. Wessell, BS
College of Arts and Sciences, Emory University, Atlanta, GA, USA
e-mail: jack.wessell@emory.edu

T. Leiner, MD, PhD
Department of Radiology, Mayo Clinic, Rochester, MN, USA
e-mail: leiner.tim@mayo.edu

C. N. De Cecco et al. (eds.), *Artificial Intelligence in Cardiothoracic Imaging*, Contemporary Medical Imaging,
https://doi.org/10.1007/978-3-030-92087-6_55

scheduling, data analysis, and patient diagnosis and can also be used to increase the quality of healthcare by providing applications that can increase the accuracy of the diagnostic and prognostic workflow. These factors combined can help make the system more efficient and reduce cost while maintaining or even increasing the quality of care.

AI has successfully penetrated almost every industry in varying degrees depending on the nation. However, although AI in medicine is a growing field, the clinical adaptation is still lagging in other industries. Due to the complexity of the field of medicine, differences between nations, and the consequences medicine has on human lives, individuals, corporations, and countries are struggling with the regulatory, legal, and ethical issues of AI implementation. For AI to be a game changer in medicine, these issues need to be dealt with on a local and global level. For widespread adaptation and implementation of AI technology to occur, it might be necessary to share data or AI algorithms across not only institutions but also nations. This will require a global effort to standardize the anonymization and de-identification of data while also introducing standards for the data itself. Efforts should be made to ensure patient confidentially and privacy in this process. For example, the International Medical Device Regulators Forum (IMDRF) is one of the largest organizations working toward international standardization. The IMDRF is a voluntary group of medical device regulators working toward harmonizing international medical device regulation (http://www.imdrf.org/) with members from Australia, Brazil, Canada, China, Europe, Japan, Russia, Singapore, South Korea, and the USA.

In addition to the IMDRF, the Chinese, European, and American regulatory systems are trying to build a framework for medical AI that hopefully will guide safe implementation of AI-based applications into clinical practice.

China

In recent years, the volume of medical AI publications in China has increased exponentially, reaching almost 20% of all global AI publications [11]. With AI programs, "radiomic" information from images which is not discernible to humans can be extracted for research, potentially increasing the diagnostic and prognostic value of the doctor [12]. Therefore, AI research has produced breakthroughs in the medical industry, as cardiothoracic imaging is especially suitable for AI research due its massive imaging datasets and definitive clinical added value. Recently, AI research in cardiothoracic imaging has played a leading role in AI medical applications in China. However, apart from several typical applications, such as recognition of coronary stenosis, pulmonary nodules, and breast tumor, no other mature applications have been achieved in China. The chief reason behind is that the standards and infrastructure need to be established. In addition, most current AI research in imaging focuses on a single narrow task, which is insufficient for achieving a more comprehensive goal or one specific task that needs extensive expertise. Moreover, the opaque mechanism of AI causes doctors to be reluctant to adopt such products, which hinders AI application. Overall, there is still a long way to go until AI in cardiothoracic imaging is accepted and implemented into clinical practice. Using with these challenges and limitations, here we put some insights into the future tendency of cardiothoracic imaging development with AI in China.

Standardized Data System

A unique research infrastructure boasting large centralized cardiothoracic imaging datasets along with rapid implementation across commercial industries has already helped China become very productive in AI research in a short time period [13]. However, these large imaging datasets originate from a variety of technologies built by several companies with different acquisition and reconstruction parameters, limiting the training and testing of the developed AI models; usually, these models work optimally on medical image dataset from one or several specific medical centers that they have been trained with, limiting models' generalizability. In 2017, the National Center for Quality Control of Cardiovascular Diseases was established to strengthen the quality management of cardiovascular diseases in China. The National Center for Cardiovascular Disease and the Fuwai Hospital have undertaken this task, in which quality control of cardiovascular imaging has been implemented by the radiology department of the Fuwai Hospital. In 2018, the China Food and Drug Testing Institute completed the construction of a pulmonary nodule-imaging database, which has been the foundation of several AI medical products for pulmonary nodule analysis. Currently, there is no standardized cardiothoracic imaging database for AI research and applications. Therefore, it is imperative to strictly control the quality of imaging data and establish a national unified standardized imaging database. It is foreseeable that more quality control platforms and cardiothoracic imaging databases will follow to comprehensively improve the level of cardiothoracic medical care, which consequently facilitates AI research in cardiothoracic imaging.

Platform for Labeling, Communication, and Sharing

Though unsupervised learning methods do not need labeled examples, supervised methods, which require doctors to label the data manually, are the main solution to many current problems. Weak-supervised methods which will reduce the need of annotated examples may be the future of AI, as the vice president of Microsoft Research (Asia) has mentioned. This indicates that labeling data is essential. Presently, manual labeling is the main method of producing datasets, which is labor-consuming and depends on the professional level of the participants for accuracy. Under a standardized operation, four experienced radiologists are involved in labeling the same imaging dataset independently in order to improve the credibility of labels, which further increases the workload and introduces the possibility of debate. Moreover, most of the current labeling work is implemented on third-party software, such as ITK-Snap and Labelimage, which is not conducive for communication. In 2011, seven academic centers and eight medical imaging companies in America collaborated on a commonly used database called Lung Image Database Consortium-Image Database Resource Initiative, which would be used for lung nodule annotation. In 2017, a Chinese startup PereDoc took the lead in establishing the diagnostic gold standard by annotating a database of pulmonary nodules on 3D CT medical images. More professional data labeling tools and databases in cardiothoracic imaging as a platform for researchers to learn, communicate, and share are in exploration by AI enterprises in China. On the premise of convenient management and protection of patient privacy, databases with recognized labeling will be established for AI researchers to study.

Improving the Depth and Breadth of AI Applications

Nowadays most AI research focuses on one narrow task, and it is capable of accomplishing neither a complete job nor specific subdivided work. The detection of pulmonary nodules for early lung cancer diagnosis is probably one of the most notable examples of AI applications in cardiothoracic radiology [14, 15]. Clinically, the doctor's job is to identify all lesions which are nodules or embolus. However, current AI products obtain good results in nodules, while other pulmonary lesions or diseases are rarely involved. In addition, the main challenge for the doctor is to identify early lung cancer while lung nodules lack specific imaging features for diagnosis. The lack of depth or breadth of AI models places doctors into awkward situations to adopt such products in clinic use. In order to enhance the added value of AI technology in cardiothoracic imaging, researchers are working toward increasing both the scope and specificity of AI models. On the one hand, domestic AI researchers are constantly expanding the variety of diseases for which AI is an effective tool, such as COVID-19 [16] and aortic dissection [17]. On the other hand, AI research will work toward specific subdivided disease classification or specific conditions, such as lung nodule segment from heterogeneous CT images [18].

Interpretability of Learning Results

Currently, deep learning-based AI approaches generally lack interpretability of the patient's clinical context, limiting their capability to perform subjective associations like a human [19]. For instance, with enough training data, an appropriate AI model is capable of diagnosing cardiomyopathy according to many imaging features, but it could not give a reasonable explanation about what effective features it has learned to make such a judgment, which is like the diagnosis made by a doctor. Since the learning and prediction process is non-transparent and lacks interaction with doctors, it is challenging for an evidence-based medical system to trust uninterpretable results from an experience-based black box. As deep learning models achieve state-of-the-art performance in a variety of cardiothoracic imaging fields, a growing desire to make the models more interpretable is following. Therefore, the interpretability of the results is an important research direction in China. It is also expected that the exploration of black box models for interpretability will facilitate better performance of AI algorithms.

Applications of AI in Clinical Cardiothoracic Imaging

Due to a lack of multicenter standardized imaging data in China and poor universality of deep learning results from a single center or a small number of centers, it is challenging to popularize AI research achievement comprehensively. In 2019, China Medical Device Technology Evaluation Center released *The Key Points of Deep Learning Aided Decision-Making Medical Device Software Evaluation*, which indicates that the evaluation standards of AI medical devices have been officially established, and the policy bottleneck of AI industrial development in healthcare has been broken. So far, seven AI medical devices or systems have been approved with Level 3 certification in China. Among them, three of them are related to cardiothoracic imaging (DeepVessel to calculate fractional flow reserve based on CT images for myocardial ischemic diagnosis, Shenzhen Keya Technology Co. LTD; auxiliary triage software for coronary stenosis detection, Shukun (Beijing) Network Technology Co., LTD; CT imaging assisted detection software for pulmonary nodules detection, Beijing Infervision Technology Co., LTD). In addition, more than 60 AI medical devices have been in the "Green Channel" for medical device approval, half of which are coronary artery-related products. It is expected that more

AI-assisted diagnosis and treatment products will be approved in China, and lots of the products will be no longer confined to development stage or only for clinical research. With the endeavor of AI commercial industries, it is an inevitable trend to actively promote the implementation of AI products in clinical cardiothoracic imaging applications.

European Union

As in other parts of the world, AI for medicine is gaining popularity in Europe. There are several initiatives that aim to streamline the development and implementation of medical AI applications across the continent. The difference between Europe compared to China and the USA is that, although there are centralized organizations for medical device development/certification, the countries forming Europe all have different cultures and languages that need to be considered. This results in challenges regarding data sharing, user interface development, and ethical and financial frameworks. So far, the European Commission has been working hard to set out a generalized European approach for AI, although the implementation of this approach in healthcare will have a whole new set of challenges. It will require a careful balancing of advancements in health and AI technologies, patient privacy, and unintended consequences.

Data Privacy and Cybersecurity

One of the main challenges for the success of AI is ensuring patient privacy and cybersecurity. AI development is highly reliant on large amounts of representative data. The recent scandal of Cambridge Analytica/Facebook that came to light in 2018 over the misuse of data, predominantly for political advertising, sparked a still ongoing debate about the balance between the costs and benefits of large-scale data collection. This discussion is especially important and impactful when it comes to sensitive data such as medical information.

In recent years, the European regulatory systems have decided to update the legislation regarding data privacy and cybersecurity. The General Data Protection Regulation (GDPR) came into work in May 2016 but became fully effective in May 2018, allowing 2 years for EU member states to implement the new regulations [20–22]. The GDPR states that all data processing and use should be opt in and that consumer consent for data use should be clear. The GDPR is more suitable to regulate AI-related data use compared to previous regulations because of the extended territorial scope and rights for subjects; it includes enhanced notification requirements stating that personal data breaches must be reported to the supervising authority within 72 hrs and includes regulations on compensation for material or non-material damage and additional liability for data controllers and processors.

The GDPR will affect AI development and clinical use of AI algorithms. For example, informed consent is required before any collection of personal data. Although informed consent is a well-integrated practice in healthcare when compared to an area such as social media, making informed consent on data collection mandatory will affect medical AI development. In addition, the new regulation allows patients to maintain control over their collected data. Also, the GDPR allows patients to track their data, know which parts are collected, and request the removal of their data. This goes back to the balance between the privacy of a single patient and the benefit they experience versus the benefit that data collection can give to a larger population. The increased data governance by patients also required more effort to be made on educating patient on the purpose of the data collection. Since the implementation of the GRPD in 2018, we see that many hospitals have made the electronic health records available to patients.

With the GDPR being a new regulation, we have seen that companies and healthcare systems need to make significant changes and innovation to meet the new regulatory standards. This might slow down the initial development and implementation process of AI in healthcare. However, by creating a solid regulatory foundation, the patients' trust in AI might grow, which will have a long-term positive effect on AI adaptation [20–22].

In addition to the GPDR, in 2018 the EU adopted the Cybersecurity Directive [23]. This directive aims to regulate requirements that EU member states need to take to prevent cyberattacks. Like the GDPR this also included timely notification of incidents to the authorities. One of the major components of the Cybersecurity Directive affecting AI is Article 22: "Automated individual decision making, including profiling." This requires member states to provide EU citizens with an explanation on algorithmic decisions, including AI-based ones. This article is expected to limit the types of models that can be used in healthcare regarding AI or at least will require effort from AI developers to open the black box of advanced AI algorithms. We already see an increased use of heat-maps in radiology application, aiming to give insight in the decision-making process of deep neural network algorithms [21, 23, 24].

Regulations and Clinical Approval

In February 2020, the European Commission released a white paper on AI, including statements on the use of AI for medical purposes [25, 26]. In the paper, the committee states that the EU needs to "act as one and define its own way, based on European values, to promote the development and deployment of AI." The application of AI for medical purposes is considered an important field of development of AI [24].

The Commission recognizes the value-laden nature of AI regulation and that Europeans have distinct views about privacy, transparency, fairness, etc. They state that current EU regulations already provide a high level of protection through medical device laws and data protection laws; however, they additionally propose to add specific regulations including requirements for training data, record-keeping of used datasets, transparency, robustness and accuracy, as well as human oversight.

Even though many regulations are already in place for medical devices and should cover AI, the European parliament established a special committee on Artificial Intelligence in a Digital Age (AIDA) [27]. The AIDA's main purpose is filling current regulatory gaps to develop a European framework on artificial intelligence (AIDA, 2021). Following its public hearing, AIDA has recently published a Working Paper on AI and Health. They focus on the harmonization of governing rules among the EU member states, creating an ethical framework from the very first stages of AI development to the last, and the adequate protection and safeguards for consumers. Based on this the European Commission proposed a regulation standardizing the rules placed on the use of AI in 2021 [27, 28]. These regulations, if accepted, aim to clear any doubts concerning the implementation of rules, the risks, and the safe use of self-learning medical devices. These regulations would apply to developers of AI applications and devices in addition to the medical device regulations already in place [21, 22, 24].

United States of America

AI can significantly benefit healthcare in the USA as shown in a recent document released by the consulting company Accenture. Their analysis shows that key clinical AI applications can potentially create $150 billion in annual savings for the US healthcare economy by 2026 [29]. In 2018, healthcare spending averaged $11,172 per person in the USA, accounting for 17.7% of GDP. That cost plays an important role in the US healthcare system and is reflected in both the increasing cost of healthcare and the growing number of patients that delay medical treatments. According to a Gallup report, a staggering 25% of Americans say they or a family member put off treatment for a serious medical condition in the past year because of the cost [30]. By delaying care, additional stress is placed on the use of emergency departments, further increasing healthcare cost. According to the American Hospital Association, patient visits to emergency departments in community hospitals increased 19% between 2001 and 2016, further increasing costs. In addition to the financial burden, the workload burden on physicians is also increasing. A study conducted in 2016 by Sinski et al. found that physicians spent only 27% of their clinical days in direct contact with their patients. Much of their time, 49.2%, is spent on electronic hospital records and deskwork. While in the examination room with patients, physicians spent on average 52.9% of their time on electronic records and administrative work. Administrative AI applications could assist in reducing this time and increase the time physicians spend on their patients.

Data Privacy and Cybersecurity

The Health Insurance Portability and Accountability Act (HIPAA) regulated patient privacy and data safety in the USA. HIPAA created rules requiring, among other things, the formulation of policies and the setup of training systems for those who have access to healthcare data of coveted institutes [22]. However, HIPAA only applies to covered institutes, such as hospitals, insurance companies, and pharmacies. Several commercial parties have already started mining personal data, which can be sold and used for AI purposes. Since these industry businesses are not healthcare-related, HIPAA privacy rules do not apply, and thus they are able to sell their data to third parties such as marketers, employers, lenders, and health insurers without violating patient privacy regulations such as HIPAA. Additionally, AI can predict the risk of future medical events [31, 32]. Although the Americans with Disabilities Act prohibits discrimination based on previous and current health issues, it does not prohibit discrimination based on future medical problems. This gap in regulations could severely impact the healthcare system.

In the USA, cybersecurity regarding healthcare applications is dealt with by the Food and Drug Administration (FDA). Currently the FDA requires manufacturers and developers to report only a limited number of risks that their devices present and actions taken to minimize the risk of data safety issues. However, the black box nature of most advanced AI algorithms, especially the neural networks used in radiology, causes a lack of transparency in the working process of AI. Considering the current amount of data collected combined with the increasing number of applications submitted and approved by the FDA for clinical use, regulatory actions regarding cybersecurity are expected to expand.

Regulations and Clinical Approval

A 2020 paper analyzing FDA-approved AI applications showed that only 29 (45%) mentioned any AI/ML-related expressions in the official FDA announcement. The majority

(85.9%) of AI applications were approved by the FDA with a 510(k) clearance, while eight (12.5%) received de novo pathway clearance and only one (1.6%) received premarket approval (PMA) clearance. A 510(k) clearance for an algorithm is granted when it has been shown to be at least as safe and effective as another similar, legally marketed algorithm. Premarket approval is more extensive and is for those applications that can have a large impact on human health, and as such, their evaluation undergoes more thorough scientific and regulatory processes to determine their safety and effectiveness [33]. The two main medical specialties with approved AI-based applications are radiology and cardiology, with 21 (72.4%) and 4 (13.8%) FDA-approved medical devices and algorithms, respectively. Radiology has shown the most progress with AI implementation, especially with the Arterys Inc. algorithms, which are connected to the workflow Picture Archiving and Communication Systems from vendors such as Siemens Healthineers AG (Germany) and GE Healthcare (USA). Of the approved publications listed by the FDA, the majority focus on simple detection of disease or classification of disease severity. Currently, there are no prognostic software examples on the list. However, in research literature we see examples from the field of radiology that use imaging and clinical information to assess cardiovascular risk [34, 35].

Public Datasets

Data is an essential part of AI development and implementation, and the long-term success of AI in radiology will depend on data availability, quality, and thorough clinical validation of AI applications [36]. For AI applications to penetrate the medical field and truly benefit patient care, it is essential to promote data sharing to optimize algorithm validation and clinical implementation. Existing data-sharing efforts include biobanks and international consortia for medical imaging databases, such the UK Biobank (http://www.ukbiobank.ac.uk/) and the Kaggle Data Science Bowl (https://www.kaggle. com/datasets). In addition, we see that many societies are building open-source databases, such as the NIH and the RSNA. These efforts were propelled forward by the COVID-19 pandemic where it was essential to share data to collect information about this fast-spreading disease. In the USA, the National Science and Technology Council Committee on Technology recommended that open data standards for AI should be a key priority for federal agencies [37]. These collaborative data-sharing projects will require significant human effort and regulatory frameworks to allow data sharing not only between institutes but also between different countries. In 2019, Kim et al. evaluated the validation of AI algorithms reported in AI research papers covering all medical fields, including radiology, dermatology, and pathology. They reported that only 6% of all studies used external validation to assess the performance of the AI application. Since then, several guidelines have been published to improve the validation process of medical AI applications [38, 39]. Recently, we have seen an increase in publications that externally validate industry-developed AI algorithms [40, 41]. This will be of great help for the implementation of AI in clinical workflows and will assess the true aid that AI can offer to a radiologist.

Future Perspectives

Artificial intelligence has the potential to automate tasks and assist with patient's treatment planning, diagnosis, and prognosis, possibly making healthcare more efficient. Although AI offers many possibilities to assist in the field of radiology, as with many other fields, it also raises some practical, legal, and ethical challenges. For the medical field, these concerns are mostly related to privacy, discrimination, ethics, and the physician-patient relationship.

One of the main determining points of success of digitalizing healthcare using AI is the creation of an infrastructure supporting AI. AI uses data collected from different sources for different purposes depending on the application, and this data can be stored in a wide range of formats and systems. Healthcare data has been shown to be more heterogeneous than data produced within other fields [37, 42]. The healthcare community has experience with providing a standardized common format for this data. The Digital Imaging and Communications in Medicine (DICOM) standards and the Picture Archiving and Communication System (PACS) revolutionized medical imaging by providing a common standard and format for data management. This standardization should be performed as early as possible in the process, so that all developed platforms and applications can be used using this common format. In a whitepaper by the Canadian Association of Radiologists, Tang et al. [43] stated that in an AI-assisted radiology workflow, algorithms for various purposes could each be a product of individual specialized vendors. The use of a common standard would in these cases be necessary to allow integration between these different algorithms and to allow algorithms to run on different systems.

For AI to be successful in clinical practice, regulations must allow optimal use of an AI model while also considering healthcare coverage, medical licensing, and liability. National and international organizations are working on creating legislation that will ensure safe and effective implementation of AI in many fields, including healthcare. Special focus is being put on patient's privacy, data safety, and cybersecurity.

Data protection is essential for healthcare in general, and it becomes more important with the increased risks that digital care offers. A standardized approach to evaluate the risks of platforms enhances the use and trust in these systems. Regulations should be in place to minimize the risk to patient's privacy and security.

Finally, the development of appropriate funding mechanisms is important for the creation of a sustainable approach to AI research. The development of financial incentives to implement a far-reaching use of AI in the medical practice is beneficial for both patients and providers. The optimal performance of AI applications is reliant on both the underlying infrastructure as discussed above and the ongoing maintenance not only in increasing the amount of patient data but also in terms of updating software algorithms and ensuring hardware operability [37]. This maintenance also needs to be supported by a funding mechanism. Currently it is unclear how AI applications will be paid for clinically. The funding of AI applications is important to regulate because it can potentially be abused to profit off of certain drugs, tests, or devices without clinical users being aware of this manipulation [44].

Education should be the basis of any AI implementation approach both for healthcare personnel and patients. For AI to be successfully used in practice, all stakeholders, hospitals, patients, IT services, physicians, and government, need to be actively involved in the AI implementation process. This will require a certain amount of education for all parties involved. Mutual understanding and collaboration between all parties is imperative because the medical system is based on physicians' ability to make well-informed decisions and convey their reasoning to colleagues and patients [45]. It therefore remains extremely important to provide a functional understanding of the algorithms used in a clinical context. It is also crucial to educate all AI stakeholders in healthcare to have a basic understanding of the different fields involved in order to adapt to the regulations and the implementation of AI into the complex healthcare framework.

Summary

In conclusion, the road ahead for a successful AI implementation in healthcare, and specifically cardiothoracic imaging, relies not only on technical development but also in creating a sustainable regulatory, legal, and ethical framework capable of dealing with the issues that can arise from the clinical implementation of this new technology. China, the EU, and the USA are working on creating the ideal framework for AI to be implemented into our daily lives. However, many of the regulations and guidelines are still in the early stages, and the long-term impacts are still unknown. Thus, a continuous effort in developing a dynamic operative, legal, and ethical framework is necessary for the successful implementation of AI in medicine.

References

1. Castro D, McLaughlin Mi, Chivot E. Who is winning the AI race? Vol. 120, Center for data innovation. 2017.
2. Lavender J. Investment in AI for healthcare soars Healthcare has become a major proving ground for AI capabilities. [Internet]. 2018 [cited 2020 Aug 13]. Available from: https://home.kpmg/xx/en/home/insights/2018/11/investment-in-ai-for-healthcare-soars.html#:~:text=Since 2015%2C VC investment in, at least match 2017's totals.&text=The use of AI and,is not a new endeavor.
3. Bresnick J. Artificial intelligence in healthcare spending to hit $36B. Health IT Analytics. [Internet]. 2018 [cited 2020 Aug 13]. Available from: https://healthitanalytics.com/news/artificial-intelligence-in-healthcare-spending-to-hit-36b
4. Mayo RC, Chang Sen LQ, Leung JWT. Financing artificial intelligence in medical imaging: show me the money. J Am Coll Radiol [Internet]. 2020;17(1):175–7. Available from: https://doi.org/10.1016/j.jacr.2019.07.004.
5. Tran B, Vu G, Ha G, Vuong Q-H, Ho M-T, Vuong T-T, et al. Global evolution of research in artificial intelligence in health and medicine: a bibliometric study. J Clin Med. 2019;8(3):360.
6. Jin Y, Zhu W, Yuan B, Meng Q. Impact of health workforce availability on health care seeking behavior of patients with diabetes mellitus in China. Int J Equity Health. 2017;16(1):1–10.
7. Litewka SG, Heitman E. Latin American healthcare systems in times of pandemic. Dev World Bioeth. 2020;20(2):69–73.
8. Shepherd A. Crisis in Venezuela. BMJ [Internet]. 2019;364(March):l1277. Available from: https://doi.org/10.1136/bmj.l1277
9. Latin America (17 countries): expenditure on health of central government, 2018 (Percentages of GDP). Caribbean, Social Investment Portal in Latin America and. 2018.
10. WHO, The World Bank. Tracking Universal Health Coverage: 2017. Global monitoring report. World Health Organisation. 2017:88.
11. West E, Mutasa S, Zhu Z, Ha R. Global trend in artificial intelligence-based publications in radiology from 2000 to 2018. Am J Roentgenol. 2019.
12. Thrall JH, Li X, Li Q, Cruz C, Do S, Dreyer K, et al. Artificial intelligence and machine learning in radiology: opportunities, challenges, pitfalls, and criteria for success. J Am Coll Radiol [internet]. 2018;15(3):504–8. Available from: https://doi.org/10.1016/j.jacr.2017.12.026.
13. P D. China is quickly becoming an AI superpower. SingularityHub website [Internet]. 2018;acccessed June 24,2019. Available from: singularityhub.com/2018/08/29/china-ai-superpower/#sm.0000853f1o4hydamwwh2n368j9yt7.
14. Auffermann WF, Gozansky EK, Tridandapani S. Artificial intelligence in cardiothoracic radiology. Am J Roentgenol. 2019;212(5):997–1001.
15. Liu K, Li Q, Ma J, Zhou Z, Sun M, Deng Y, et al. Evaluating a fully automated pulmonary nodule detection approach and its impact on radiologist performance. Radiol Artif Intell. 2019;1(3):e180084.
16. Jin C, Chen W, Cao Y, Xu Z, Tan Z, Zhang X, et al. Development and evaluation of an artificial intelligence system for COVID-19 diagnosis. Nat Commun. 2020.
17. Yu Y, Gao Y, Wei J, Liao F, Xiao Q, Zhang J, et al. A three-dimensional deep convolutional neural network for automatic segmentation and diameter measurement of type B aortic dissection. Korean J Radiol. 2021.
18. Wang S, Zhou M, Liu Z, Liu Z, Gu D, Zang Y, et al. Central focused convolutional neural networks: developing a data-driven model for lung nodule segmentation. Med Image Anal. 2017.
19. Martín Noguerol T, Paulano-Godino F, Martín-Valdivia MT, Menias CO, Luna A. Strengths, Weaknesses, Opportunities, and

Threats Analysis of Artificial Intelligence and Machine Learning Applications in Radiology. J Am Coll Radiol. 2019.
20. European Parliament and of the Council. Regulation (EU) 2016/679 of 27 April 2016 on the protection of natural persons with regard to the processing of personal data and on the free movement of such data, and repealing Directive 95/46/EC (General Data Protection Regulation). Off J Eur Union [Internet]. 2016;OJ L 119/1:1–88. Available from: http://data.europa.eu/eli/reg/2016/679/oj.
21. Schneeberger D, Stöger K, Holzinger A. The European legal framework for medical AI. In: Holzinger A, Kieseberg P, Tjoa AM, Weippl E, editors. Machine learning and knowledge extraction. Cham: Springer International Publishing; 2020. p. 209–26.
22. Pesapane F, Volonté C, Codari M, Sardanelli F. Artificial intelligence as a medical device in radiology: ethical and regulatory issues in Europe and the United States. Insights Imaging. 2018;9(5):745–53.
23. Commission E. Cybersecurity strategy of the European Union: an open, safe and secure cyberspace. Jt Commun TO Eur Parliam Counc Eur Econ Soc Comm Comm Reg. 2020.
24. Cohen IG, Evgeniou T, Gerke S, Minssen T. The European artificial intelligence strategy: implications and challenges for digital health. Lancet Digit Heal [Internet]. 2020;2(7):e376–9. https://doi.org/10.1016/S2589-7500(20)30112-6.
25. European-Commission. White Paper on Artificial Intelligence. 2020.
26. van Assen M, Lee SJ, De Cecco CN. Artificial intelligence from a to Z: from neural network to legal framework. Eur J Radiol. 2020;
27. Special Committee on Artificial Intelligence in a Digital Age. AIDA Working Paper on Artificial Intelligence and Health. 2021;(December 2020). Available from: WWW.EUROPARL.EUROPA.EU
28. European-Commission. Regulation of the european parliament and of the council laying down harmonised rules on artificial intelligence (artificial intelligence act) and amending certain union legislative acts. 2021;0106. Available from: WWW.EUROPARL.EUROPA.EU
29. Accenture. Artificial Intelligence: Healthcare's New Nervous System. Accent Rep [Internet]. 2017;1–8. Available from: https://www.accenture.com/us-en/insight-artificial-intelligence-future-growth.
30. Saad L. More Americans delaying medical treatment due to cost. Gallup. 2019;
31. Davis DA, Chawla N V., Blumm N, Barabási AL, Christakis N. Predicting individual disease risk based on medical history. Int Conf Inf Knowl Manag Proc. 2008;769–78.
32. Axelrod RC, Vogel D. Predictive modeling in health plans. Dis Manag Heal Outcomes. 2003;11(12):779–87.
33. Benjamens S, Dhunnoo P, Meskó B. The state of artificial intelligence-based FDA-approved medical devices and algorithms: an online database. NPJ Digit Med [Internet]. 2020;3(1):1–8. Available from: https://doi.org/10.1038/s41746-020-00324-0
34. van Rosendael AR, Maliakal G, Kolli KK, Beecy A, Al'Aref SJ, Dwivedi A, et al. Maximization of the usage of coronary CTA derived plaque information using a machine learning based algorithm to improve risk stratification; insights from the CONFIRM registry. J Cardiovasc Comput Tomogr. 2018;
35. Motwani M, Dey D, Berman DS, Germano G, Achenbach S, Al-Mallah MH, et al. Machine learning for prediction of all-cause mortality in patients with suspected coronary artery disease: a 5-year multicentre prospective registry analysis. Eur Heart J. 2017;
36. Kim DW, Jang HY, Kim KW, Shin Y, Park SH. Design characteristics of studies reporting the performance of artificial intelligence algorithms for diagnostic analysis of medical images: results from recently published papers. Korean J Radiol. 2019;20(3):405–10.
37. He J, Baxter SL, Xu J, Xu J, Zhou X, Zhang K. The practical implementation of artificial intelligence technologies in medicine. Nat Med [Internet]. 2019;25(January). Available from: https://doi.org/10.1038/s41591-018-0307-0.
38. Park SH, Han K. Methodologic guide for evaluating clinical performance and effect of artificial intelligence technology for medical diagnosis and prediction. Radiology. 2018;286(3):800–9.
39. England JR, Cheng PM. Artificial intelligence for medical image analysis: a guide for authors and reviewers. Am J Roentgenol. 2019;
40. Martin SS, van Assen M, Rapaka S, Hudson HT, Fischer AM, Varga-Szemes A, et al. Evaluation of a deep learning–based automated CT coronary artery calcium scoring algorithm. JACC Cardiovasc Imaging. 2019;13(2 Pt 1): https://doi.org/10.1016/j.jcmg.2019.09.015.
41. Fischer AM, Varga-Szemes A, van Assen M, Griffith LP, Sahbaee P, Sperl JI, et al. Comparison of artificial intelligence–based fully automatic chest CT emphysema quantification to pulmonary function testing. Am J Roentgenol. 2020:1–7.
42. Kruse CS, Goswamy R, Raval Y, Marawi S. Challenges and opportunities of big data in health care: a systematic review. JMIR Med Informatics. 2016.
43. Tang A, Tam R, Cadrin-Chênevert A, Guest W, Chong J, Barfett J, et al. Canadian Association of Radiologists White Paper on Artificial Intelligence in Radiology. Canadian Associat Radiolog J. 2018.
44. Char DS, Shah NH, Magnus D. Implementing machine learning in health care — addressing ethical challenges. N Engl J Med. 2018;
45. van Assen M, Cornelissen LJ. Artificial intelligence: from scientific curiosity to clinical precocity? JACC Cardiovasc Imaging. 2020;13(5):1172–4.

Index

C. N. De Cecco et al. (eds.), *Artificial Intelligence in Cardiothoracic Imaging*, Contemporary Medical Imaging,
https://doi.org/10.1007/978-3-030-92087-6

B

U

V

W

X

Z

MIX
Papier aus verantwortungsvollen Quellen
Paper from responsible sources
FSC® C105338

If you have any concerns about our products,
you can contact us on
ProductSafety@springernature.com

In case Publisher is established outside the EU,
the EU authorized representative is:
Springer Nature Customer Service Center GmbH
Europaplatz 3, 69115 Heidelberg, Germany

Printed by Libri Plureos GmbH
in Hamburg, Germany